DALE M. SCHULZ

VOLUME TWO

Ackerman's
SURGICAL PATHOLOGY

VOLUME TWO

Ackerman's
SURGICAL
PATHOLOGY

JUAN ROSAI, M.D.

Professor of Laboratory Medicine and Pathology and
Director of Anatomic Pathology,
University of Minnesota Medical School,
Minneapolis, Minnesota

SIXTH EDITION

with 1608 figures

The C. V. Mosby Company

ST. LOUIS • TORONTO • LONDON   1981

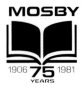

MOSBY

1906 **75** 1981
YEARS

A TRADITION OF PUBLISHING EXCELLENCE

SIXTH EDITION (two volumes)

Copyright © 1981 by The C. V. Mosby Company

Previous editions copyrighted 1953, 1959, 1964, 1968, 1974

Printed in the United States of America

The C. V. Mosby Company
11830 Westline Industrial Drive
St. Louis, Missouri 63141

Library of Congress Cataloging in Publication Data

Ackerman, Lauren Vedder, 1905-
    Ackerman's Surgical pathology.

    Bibliography: p.
    Includes index.
    1. Pathology, Surgical.   I.   Rosai, Juan, 1940-
II.   Title   III.   Title: Surgical pathology.
[DNLM: 1.   Pathology, Surgical.   W0142 A182s]
RD57.Az   1980   617'.07   80-16948
ISBN 0-8016-0045-6

GW/CB/B   9   8   7   6   5   4   3   01/D/091

To the memory
of my father
EZIO ROSAI (1908-1977)

Preface

TO SIXTH EDITION

Twenty-nine years have passed since the first edition of this book was written by Dr. Lauren V. Ackerman. During this time, two major events have taken place in surgical pathology that have influenced the content of this work through its several editions and particularly the present one. The first relates to the remarkable growth and diversification that the field of surgical pathology has undergone during these years; this has been highly beneficial to the specialty in particular and to medicine in general and is discussed in some detail in Chapter 1. The second event can hardly be described as beneficial. I am referring, of course, to Dr. Ackerman's decision not to co-author this edition, although he has thoroughly reviewed the entire manuscript and has contributed numerous references and photographs.

Knowledge and experience aside, there are intellectual works that bear the indelible mark of their creators. This book belongs to that privileged category, and it would have been futile for me to attempt to match that ineffable quality. My aim has been a more modest one: to incorporate the new findings, new thoughts, and new questions that innumerable workers in this vast field have originated in recent years while preserving, as much as I could, the philosophy and flavor that have made this book unique. The general structure and practical emphasis have been maintained. The chapter on "Ultrastructure and surgical pathology" has been deleted because the largely normal ultrastructural features that were described therein are now adequately and more extensively covered in specialized books dealing with the subject. Instead, the specific ultrastructural features of various lesions have been incorporated in the respective discussions. At the time the chapter was written by Walter C. Bauer, M.D., and Malcolm H. McGavran, M.D., it constituted a novel and extremely useful addition. It has been replaced in this edition by one on "Gross techniques in surgical pathology." It is

hoped that this new chapter, along with the Appendix, in which some general guidelines for the handling of the most common and important surgical specimens received in the laboratory are presented, will prove especially useful for pathologists in training and for achieving some degree of standardization in the evaluation of the material.

As with the text, the references have undergone thorough revision, with the deletion of those no longer pertinent and the addition of hundreds of new ones. Further, approximately 380 new figures, some additions and some substitutions, have been included. From the standpoint of physical aspects, because of the ever-increasing size of this book it was deemed desirable to publish this edition in two volumes to facilitate its use.

At this point, it is only fair to note that the attempt of continuity that this edition represents is not simply mine alone. It is rather the work of a large team, in which no participants are less important than others. First of all, several of the chapters and sections have been written or revised, in their entirety or in part, by or with other authors: "Gross techniques in surgical pathology," Hector A. Rodriguez Martinez, M.D.; "Mandible and maxilla," Robert A. Vickers, D.D.S., M.S.D.; "Liver," Hatton W. Sumner, M.D.; "Kidney, renal pelvis, and ureter," Richard K. Sibley, M.D.; "Bone marrow," Richard D. Brunning, M.D.: "Eyes and ocular adnexa," Morton E. Smith, M.D. Further, indebtedness to the following contributors to previous editions, substantial portions of whose material remain in the present text, is gratefully acknowledged: Harvey R. Butcher, Jr., M.D., "Vessels" and also Dr. Ackerman's collaborator on the second, third, and fourth editions of the book; Frederick T. Kraus, M.D., "Female reproductive system"; Michael Kyriakos, M.D., "Cytology"; Malcolm H. McGavran, M.D., "Skin" ("Dermatoses"; "Tumors"); David E. Smith, M.D., "Central nervous system''; and Lorenz E. Zimmerman, M.D., and Eleanor V. Paul, B.S., M.S., ''Eyes and ocular adnexa.''

For many of the chapters that I have revised myself, I have relied heavily on the following members of our Department of Laboratory Medicine and Pathology who are much more knowledgeable than I in their respective fields and who have freely given me their advice, criticisms, and material: Barbara A. Burke, M.D. (pediatric pathology and placenta); Glauco Frizzera, M.D. (lymph nodes); Kazimiera J. Gajl-Peczalska, M.D. (cytology and immunopathology); Richard K. Sibley, M.D. (electron microscopy); and, last but certainly not least, Louis P. Dehner, M.D. (pediatric surgical pathology, gynecologic pathology, and nearly everything else). In addition, C. Elliott Foucar, M.D., and Kiyoshi Mukai, M.D., have also generously contributed valuable material.

Being a clinically oriented specialty, surgical pathology can flourish only if associated with clinical departments with a busy practice and, more importantly, a strong academic orientation. I have been very fortunate in having had such an association during all my years as a surgical pathologist, first in the Regional Hospital of Mar del Plata in Argentina, then at Barnes Hospital in St. Louis, Missouri, and presently at the University of Minnesota Hospitals. Particular recognition is due Dr. John S. Najarian and his staff of the Department of Surgery of the University of Minnesota Medical School for giving me the opportunity to interact with the most academically oriented surgery department I have ever encountered. Within our own Department, my gratitude goes to the Chairman, Dr. Ellis S. Benson, for having provided the Division of Surgical Pathology with generous and uninterrupted scientific, moral, and economic support; to my dearest friend and associate, Dr. Louis ''Pepper'' Dehner, for having helped me immeasurably with the book and in the running of the Division; to Joanne J. Samuelson and her staff in the Laboratories of Diagnostic Cytology and Histology for the invariably high quality of their work; to Josephine Walaszek and her wonderful secretarial staff; and especially to Jill Dinneen, who has typed the entire revision, searched references, coded photographs, and collaborated in many other aspects of the preparation of this book with skill, speed, and grace despite the burden that this imposed on an already heavy schedule.

The bulk of the photographic material represents the work of Cramer Lewis, an artist operating under the guise of Chief Medical Photographer at Washington University School of Medicine, St. Louis, Missouri. The original drawings for the Appendix were made by Mary Albury of the Department of Medical Biographics at the University of Minnesota.

The lessons that I have received in pathology, medicine, and life from Dr. Eduardo F. Lascano and Dr. Lauren V. Ackerman can never be fully retributed. All I can offer them is my deepest gratitude. I could not have worked under two better men.

Finally, and at a more personal level, I need to apologize to my wife Hilda and my sons Alberto, Carlos, and Johnny. Much of the work on this edition took place during evenings and weekends, on hours stolen from them. My wife's understanding and relentless support have only increased my feeling of guilt. I promise them that this will not happen again — not until the next edition, anyway!

Juan Rosai

Minneapolis, Minn.

Preface
TO FIRST EDITION

This book can be only an introduction to the vast field of surgical pathology: the pathology of the living. It does not pretend to replace in any way the textbooks of general pathology, its purpose being merely to supplement them, assuming that the reader has a background in or access to those texts. The contents are not as complete as they might be because emphasis has been placed on the common rather than the rare lesions and are, to a great extent, based on the author's personal experiences.

This book has been written for the medical student as well as for those physicians who are daily intimately concerned with surgical pathology. This must of necessity include not only the surgeon and the pathologist, but also those physicians in other fields who are affected by its decisions, such as the radiologist and the internist. Gross pathology has been stressed throughout with an attempt to correlate the gross findings with the clinical observations. The many illustrations have been selected as typical of the various surgical conditions, although in a few instances the author has been unable to resist showing some of the more interesting rare lesions he has encountered. Concluding each chapter there is a bibliography listing those references which are not only relatively recent and readily available, but also those which will lead the reader to a more detailed knowledge of the subject.

Dr. Zola K. Cooper, Assistant Professor of Pathology and Surgical Pathology, has written one of the sections on Skin, and Dr. David E. Smith, Assistant Professor of Pathology and Surgical Pathology, has written the chapter on Central Nervous System. Both of these members of the Department are particularly well qualified for their respective roles because of their background and present responsibilities in these fields. Their efforts on my behalf are most gratefully acknowledged.

Many members of the Surgical Staff at Barnes Hospital have given much help both knowingly and unwittingly. I am particularly grateful to Dr. Charles L. Eckert, Associate Professor of Surgery, for letting me bother him rather constantly with my questions and for giving freely of his experience. Dr. Richard Johnson, who succeeded me as Pathologist at the Ellis Fischel State Cancer Hospital, agreeably made available all the material there, and Dr. Franz Leidler, Pathologist at the Veterans Hospital, has been most cooperative.

Thanks must be given to Dr. H. R. McCarroll, Assistant Professor of Orthopedics, for constructively criticizing the chapter on Bone and Joint, and to Dr. C. A. Waldron for helping me with the chapters related to the Oral Cavity. Among other faculty friends and colleagues who were especially helpful, I would like to mention Dr. Carl E. Lischer, Dr. Eugene M. Bricker, Dr. Heinz Haffner, Dr. Thomas H. Burford, Dr. Carl A. Moyer, Dr. Evarts A. Graham, Dr. Robert Elman, Dr. Edward H. Reinhard, Dr. J. Albert Key, Dr. Glover H. Copher, Dr. Margaret G. Smith, and Dr. Robert A. Moore.

Mr. Cramer K. Lewis, of our Department of Illustration, has been very patient with my demands, and his efforts and skill have been invaluable. Miss Marion Murphy, in charge of our Medical Library, and her associates gave untiringly of their time.

Because of recent advances in anesthesia, antibiotics, and pre- and postoperative care, modern surgery permits the radical excision of portions or all of various organs. There is a need today for contemplative surgeons, men with a rich background in the fundamental sciences, whether chemistry, physiology, or pathology. The modern surgeon should not ask himself, "Can I get away with this operation?" but rather, "What does the future hold for this patient?" It is hoped that this book may contribute in some small fashion toward the acquisition of this attitude.

Lauren V. Ackerman

St. Louis, Mo.

Contents

VOLUME TWO

Ackerman's
SURGICAL PATHOLOGY

19 Breast

Introduction

The breast is the most important organ from the standpoint of surgical pathology because of the frequency of both benign and malignant lesions. Breast cancer is the most common malignant tumor of women. Since 1947, in the United States it has replaced the uterus as the leading cause of death from cancer. Whether a lesion is benign or malignant is usually the problem faced by both the pathologist and the surgeon. This decision may be quite difficult but must be resolved before therapy is instituted.

Method of pathologic examination

The examination of a mastectomy specimen should be thorough. Much information may be gained by meticulous study. A method for the standardized management of breast specimens has been recommended recently by the Pathology Working Group of the Breast Task Force; adherence to the guidelines presented will result in a thorough examination of the specimen and will facilitate comparisons between different institutions.[9] Serial whole-organ slicing techniques also are used in several laboratories,[1] but one can hardly recommend them for the average surgical pathology laboratory.

A *radical mastectomy specimen* does include adequate skin, all breast parenchyma, the underlying and surrounding fat, the pectoralis major and minor muscles, and the axillary contents in continuity and en bloc. A specimen from a *modified radical mastectomy* (extended simple mastectomy; total mastectomy) consists of all the mammary tissue, including the axillary tail, together with the nipple, the surrounding skin, and a variable amount of lymph node–bearing fat from the lower axilla; in the usual specimen, the axillary portion represents about two-thirds of the entire axillary content. A *simple mastectomy* specimen contains all or almost all the mammary tissue and also includes the nipple and a variable amount of surrounding skin. A *subcutaneous mastectomy* specimen includes most of the mammary tissue, without overlying skin or nipple and often without the axillary tail. A *tylectomy* (lumpectomy; excisional biopsy) specimen consists of a piece of mammary tissue that includes the totality of the mass and a variable amount of surrounding breast tissue. A *supra-radical mastectomy specimen* (rarely seen these days) contains all the components of a radical

1087

mastectomy specimen, plus a resected segment of chest wall, usually the sternal ends of the second, third, fourth, and fifth ribs, an adjacent segment of sternum, and the subpleural connective tissue that contains the internal mammary vessels and nodes; a segment of pleura also may be present.

During the performance of a radical mastectomy, the surgeon should tag the high point of the axillary contents as he removes it from about the medial end of the axillary vein. This allows the pathologist to orient the specimen. Evidence of edema and ulceration of the skin should be noted. If a mass is felt, its borders should be measured. At least three sections should be taken from the tumor with an attempt to include underlying muscle, fascia, and overlying skin if they appear involved. All breast quadrants are sampled, particularly the most prominent parenchymal areas, for such sections may show unexpected extension of the tumor, multiple foci of origin, or various proliferative and possible precancerous lesions.

The next step is a thorough search of the axillary contents for nodes, with a single section taken from each node. An average of at least twenty-five axillary nodes can thus be examined. The axillary contents from radical mastectomy specimens are divided arbitrarily into high, mid, and low areas according to their relation to the pectoralis minor muscle. The nodes from a modified radical mastectomy are arbitrarily divided into a high and a low group (see Appendix). By studying the fresh material in a strong light, one can see and feel the small gray nodes even 0.2 cm in diameter against the glistening yellow fat. Small nodes missed by superficial study may contain carcinoma.

The final step in the examination of the specimen is to place sections of the main tumor, the three other quadrants, the nipple, and the lymph nodes from the high, mid, and low areas of the axilla into separate cassettes. While this procedure is time consuming to both pathologist and technician, the information gained is worthwhile, particularly from the standpoint of prognosis.

An alternative method for studying the parenchymal changes consists in serially slicing the whole organ and submitting each slice for whole-mount examination.[1] This procedure has been extremely worthwhile for the determination of incidence of multicentricity but can hardly be recommended for routine use.

It is also the responsibility of the pathologist to see that representative fresh tumor tissue is quickly frozen and submitted in this state to a laboratory for the performance of hormone-receptor assays.[2]

Two time-consuming and costly techniques, which can be used singly or combined, have been proposed over the years as means to increase the detection of positive nodes. One consists of carrying out the dissection after having cleared the axilla by dissolving the fat in an organic solvent. The other consists of sectioning each node serially for the detection of microscopic metastases. We doubt whether the extra time and expense necessary to carry out these studies are justified by the information gained. There is no question that one can find more nodes after clearing of the specimen. Monroe[8] found an average of 30.4 nodes per specimen and as many as 65 in a single case! It also appears obvious that serial sectioning of apparently negative nodes will show that some (as many as 22, or 24%[4,10,13]) actually contain metastatic deposits, but the important and somewhat surprising finding has been that the survival rate for the patients with occult metastases has been the same as that for patients in whom no metastases were detected with these techniques.[4,10]

The widespread use of mammography has resulted in the discovery of extremely small carcinomas (1-2 mm in diameter). The proper handling of these lesions requires a close cooperation between radiologist, surgeon, and pathologist.[5,11,14] Once the radiologist identifies the abnormal area on mammography, he should provide the surgeon with a "map" showing the relative position of the suspicious area within the breast. Once the appropriate area is excised, the cephalad and lateral margins should be marked by sutures and a roentgenogram should be taken of the specimen. If no lesion is seen, the surgeon should obtain additional tissue. If the abnormal area is present in the specimen, this can be accurately located by slicing the specimen, identifying the slices with a lead number, taking another roentgenogram, and selecting for frozen sections the slice (and the specific area within the slice) containing the abnormal area. The whole procedure takes no more than fifteen minutes and is well worth the small delay. Otherwise, small carcinomas can be entirely missed.[6,12] Roentgenograms can even be taken of the paraffin blocks to document the fact that

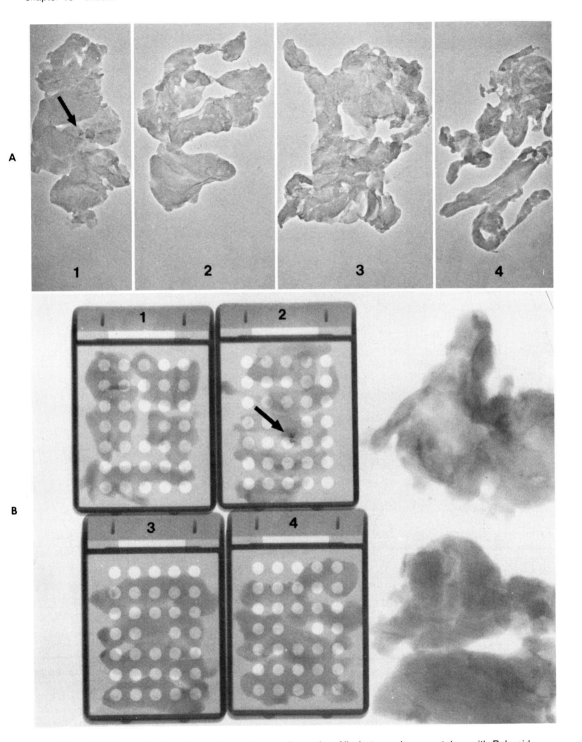

Fig. 1028 Demonstration of use of specimen radiography. All photographs were taken with Polaroid camera and film. Mammographically detected breast lesion was excised. **A,** Specimen was sliced in four portions and roentgenogram taken. Pattern of calcification identical to that seen in original mammography was detected in slice 1. **B,** Portion corresponding to this area of calcification was further divided in four fragments, and all four were embedded in paraffin. Roentgenogram of cassettes shows that suspicious area is in cassette 2. Remainder of slide (two fragments at right) shows no calcification.

the area seen in the mammogram has been embedded (Fig. 1028). Every attempt should be made to identify in the microscopic slide the area regarded by the radiologist as "suspicious" of carcinoma. However, if this is satisfactorily accomplished and the pathologist still fails to find cancer, neither he nor the radiologist should be overly surprised. Only 20% of the lesions labeled "suspicious" mammographically are malignant, and the large major-

ity of these are carcinomas in situ. McDivitt[7] estimated that the chances for the pathologist of finding an invasive carcinoma in a biopsy from a nonpalpable lesion that was interpreted "suspicious" by mammography is less than 2%.

Wolfe[15] has divided breasts into four groups on the basis of the mammographic appearance which he believes correlates with the risk for development of cancer. This correlation might

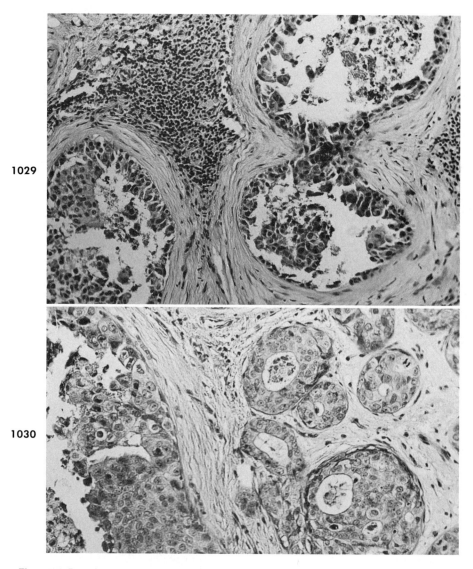

1029

1030

Fig. 1029 Ductal carcinoma of breast diagnosed by frozen section. Patient was young woman with single nodule clinically thought to be benign. (×165; WU neg. 49-4436.)
Fig. 1030 Radical mastectomy demonstrated carcinoma in other quadrants and in one axillary lymph node. Tumor in this section is from quadrant remote from primary tumor shown in Fig. 1029. (×195; WU neg. 49-4437.)

well exist, but it is perplexing that, if this is the case, there seems to be no correlation between these four patterns and the types of histologic alterations.[3]

Cytology

On occasion, an unexpected intraductal cancer may be diagnosed by the examination of nipple secretions. However, the number of times that this is possible is so small that there is little justification for the routine use of this technique.

In some institutions, it is common practice to diagnose breast lesions by cytology from material obtained with aspiration biopsy.[16,24] There is no question that in experienced hands the technique is reliable.[16,18-21,25,26] In a series of 1,745 carcinomas, 88% were correctly identified as such cytologically.[27] A positive cytologic diagnosis will be confirmed in nearly every case, but a relatively high proportion of cytologically negative or inconclusive cases will be subsequently shown to be cancer.[17,22] A negative cytologic diagnosis may give a false sense of security and delay the recognition of the cancer. We agree with McDivitt[23] that this procedure cannot be recommended as a routine technique for most practicing pathologists, and we also agree with Kline et al.[20] that it should be used to complement, and not compete with, routine histologic biopsy.

Frozen section

Mastectomy for presumed cancer should never be done without a histologic diagnosis. Needle biopsy is permissible in order to avoid the necessity of frozen section in those instances in which the mass in the breast is large and the operability of the lesion has been determined. In these cases, the needle biopsy is usually diagnostic.[28]

In most instances, the surgeon requests a frozen section at the time of operation. If the lesion is small (2.5 cm or less), it is entirely excised. If it is larger, then careful incisional biopsy is the best procedure. Incisional biopsy is preferable for large lesions because it disturbs the tumor bed the least. Frozen section diagnosis is accurate. In 679 consecutive frozen sections, done at Barnes Hospital, there were no false positives and three (0.4%) false negatives. The diagnosis was deferred for the permanent sections in six (0.9%) instances. The use of the cryostat has reduced substantially the need to delay diagnosis.

There is no evidence that waiting for the results of the permanent sections (twenty-four hours) causes harm. The greatest difficulty is encountered with papillary and sclerosing lesions (Figs. 1029 and 1030). Both the surgeon and the pathologist should take great precaution to avoid an erroneous diagnosis of cancer that will result in an unnecessary radical mastectomy.

Inflammatory lesions
Tuberculosis

Tuberculosis of the breast is rare and is invariably secondary to bloodstream dissemination or invasion from an adjacent tuberculous process. Grossly, in advanced tuberculosis of the breast, there are suppurating multiple sinuses and areas of necrosis and caseation. This lesion may be mistaken clinically for advanced breast cancer. The regional nodes are quite often involved in caseating forms of tuberculosis.

Abscess

With the advent of chemotherapy, suppurative mastitis during lactation is no longer frequent. Grossly, in the breast parenchyma near the abscess, chronic inflammation with duct stasis and obliteration of lobular pattern is usually present. Microscopically, all signs of inflammation are present. Plasma cells usually are abundant. A localized abscess may simulate cancer.[32]

Plasma cell mastitis

Plasma cell mastitis is a vanishingly rare lesion.[29] It has been described most often in patients between 35 and 40 years of age.[30] It probably does not represent an entity but rather a pattern of reaction to the ductal changes of fibrocystic disease or to fat necrosis. A history of trauma is sometimes present. Clinically, the edema, firmness, and tenderness frequently suggest a diagnosis of carcinoma. The regional lymph nodes also may be enlarged by inflammatory infiltration. Rarely, the disease is bilateral. It may be associated with underlying cancer.[31] Grossly, extensive edema, duct stasis, and interstitial induration are present. Areas of fat necrosis also may be evident. Microscopically, there is duct stasis, focal fat necrosis, and an intense inflammatory infiltrate composed predominantly of plasma cells. Local excision is all that is needed, provided the possibility of an underlying carcinoma has been ruled out.

Fat necrosis

Fat necrosis of the breast usually occurs in obese patients with pendulous breasts. The lesion was described well by Lee and Adair in a number of articles dating from 1920.[37,38] Adair and Munzer[33] reported its incidence to be 2.76% of the patients with primary operable carcinoma.

Fat necrosis is nonbacterial. It is caused by slow aseptic saponification of nodular fat by blood and tissue lipase.[36] In most instances, it is probably a secondary event following the rupture of a dilated duct or cyst in an area of fibrocystic disease, perhaps precipitated by minor trauma. Severe trauma in a previously normal breast is the causative agent in most other instances. Such a history was given by thirty-eight of 110 patients reported by Adair and Munzer.[33] An increased incidence of mammary fat necrosis has been noted after surgical excision of breast nodules. Rarely, fat necrosis of the subcutaneous tissue overlying the breast is a local manifestation of Weber-Christian disease.[34]

Grossly, the lesion may be in the subcutaneous tissue or in the breast. When it is located within the breast, it measures 1-8 cm in diameter, is firm but not stony hard, is rather sharply defined, and at times occurs as multiple masses. The gross appearance is sufficiently character-istic to distinguish it from carcinoma. Early fat necrosis is confined to several well-defined fat lobules. Later, the lesion may become cystic. The cysts may be small or large. They contain yellow granular material and pools of fat. The firmer areas may be opaque, yellowish brown, and greasy. There is considerable surrounding fibrous induration. Calcareous masses eventually may develop in the cystic areas.

Microscopically, there are fat-filled cystic spaces surrounded by foreign body giant cells, collections of fat-filled macrophages, and interstitial infiltration by plasma cells. Duct stasis is often present, a finding probably related to the pathogenesis of some of these lesions.[35] Interstitial tissues may also show an increased number of plasma cells. The prominent proliferation of the connective tissue around the lesion may cause it to be confused with a malignant neoplasm.

The firm lesions of fat necrosis closely mimic carcinoma. Over one-half of the lesions are attached to the overlying skin. The nipple seldom is retracted, and deep attachment is rare (Fig. 1031). Breast pain and axillary lymph node enlargement are usually absent. The close clinical resemblance of this lesion to carcinoma was emphasized by Hadfield.[36] In a review of forty-five cases, he found that twelve patients

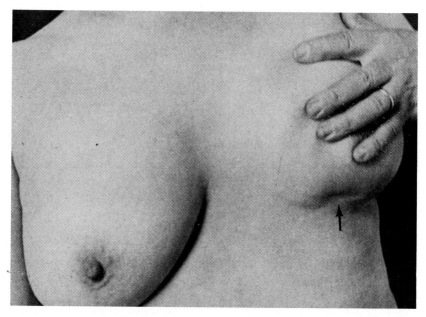

Fig. 1031 Retraction of skin in patient with fat necrosis (arrow). (WU neg. 50-2035; from Lee B J, Adair F: Traumatic fat necrosis of the female breast and its differentiation from carcinoma. Ann Surg **80:** 670-691, 1924.)

had a radical mastectomy for supposed cancer. Of twelve consecutive cases of fat necrosis at Barnes Hospital seen before 1948, five were thought to be carcinoma and two of the patients had a radical mastectomy.

Mammary duct ectasia

Haagensen[39] gave the name of *mammary duct ectasia* to a lesion previously described under designations such as varicocele tumor, comedomastitis, periductal mastitis, stale milk mastitis, chemical mastitis, granulomatous mastitis, and mastitis obliterans.[40] In this process, there are dilatation of the ducts, fibrous thickening of the walls, and ductal accumulation of fatty detritus (Fig. 1032). When this material escapes form the ducts, it causes inflammation. Ductal thickening and shortening may be associated with retraction of the skin and nipple, resulting in a clinical diagnosis of carcinoma.

We have been impressed by the similarity among mammary abscess, plasma cell mastitis, fat necrosis, and mammary duct ectasia. We believe that in most instances they represent different stages of the same process, which is different from fibrocystic disease. Many of the cases are seen in premenopausal parous women and probably represent a localized response to different components of stagnant colostrum.

Duct stasis is the common denominator in all of them. If the material escapes from the ducts, fat necrosis and inflammation may result. The inflammatory component often contains a larger number of plasma cells.

Fibrocystic disease

Fibrocystic disease of the breast is an extremely important lesion because of its frequency, its alleged relationship with carcinoma, and the fact that, when florid, may be confused by the pathologist with carcinoma. It is also known as mammary dysplasia (a term to be avoided), cystic disease, cystic mastopathy, cystic hyperplasia, Reclus' disease, and Schimmelbusch's disease. It is most frequently seen between the ages of 25 and 45 years. Hormones obviously play a role in its development, but the exact pathogenesis remains obscure.[49] Its real incidence is difficult to estimate because the diagnosis depends a great deal upon the liberality of the individual pathologist.[47,54] The process is most often bilateral, but one breast may be much more diseased than the other and appear clinically to be the only one involved.

There is a great degree of variability in the gross and microscopic appearance depending on which manifestation of the disease predominates. The basic morphologic changes are

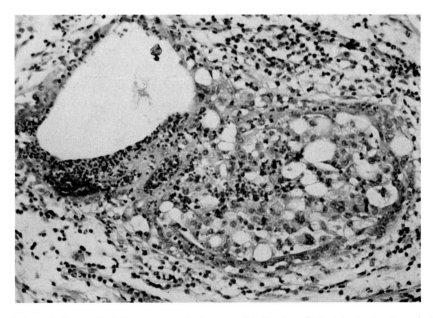

Fig. 1032 Duct stasis with fat necrosis and plasma cell infiltration. Patient had retraction of nipple and indefinite mass. There was no carcinoma. (×225; WU neg. 51-4212.)

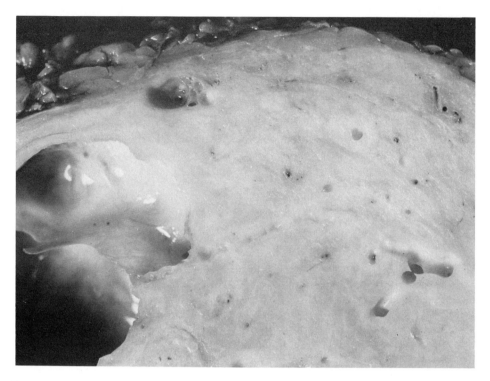

Fig. 1033 Fibrocystic disease demonstrating large smooth-walled cyst, multiple small cysts, and increased stromal tissue. (WU neg. 52-3540.)

as follows:

1 *Dilatation of ducts*. In advanced cases, this may lead to the formation of microscopic or grossly visible cysts containing a cloudy yellow or clear fluid. Some of these cysts have a bluish cast when seen from the outside (blue dome cysts of Bloodgood). Often, numerous small thin-walled cysts are seen in the breast parenchyma surrounding a larger cyst (Fig. 1033). Microscopically, the epithelial lining of most cysts, especially the larger ones, is flattened or altogether absent, the cyst having only a thick fibrous wall. It is not infrequent for these cysts to rupture and elicit an inflammatory response in the stroma, with abundant foamy macrophages and cholesterol clefts.

2 *Apocrine metaplasia*. This is a very common change. It is most often seen in dilated ducts, but it may appear in normal-sized ducts as well. The appearance is identical, at least in hematoxylin-easin sections, to the lining of apocrine sweat glands. The individual cells are large and contain medium-sized nuclei and abundant bright pink cytoplasm; the apical portion shows secretory snouts. A certain degree of nuclear enlargement, papillary infolding, and even cribriform pattern may exist in these

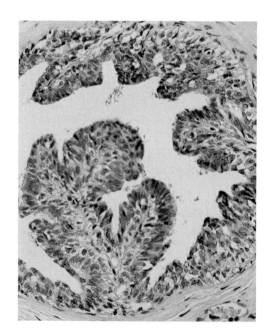

Fig. 1034 Intraductal papillomatosis. This lesion is an expression of fibrocystic disease. (×240; WU neg. 51-931.)

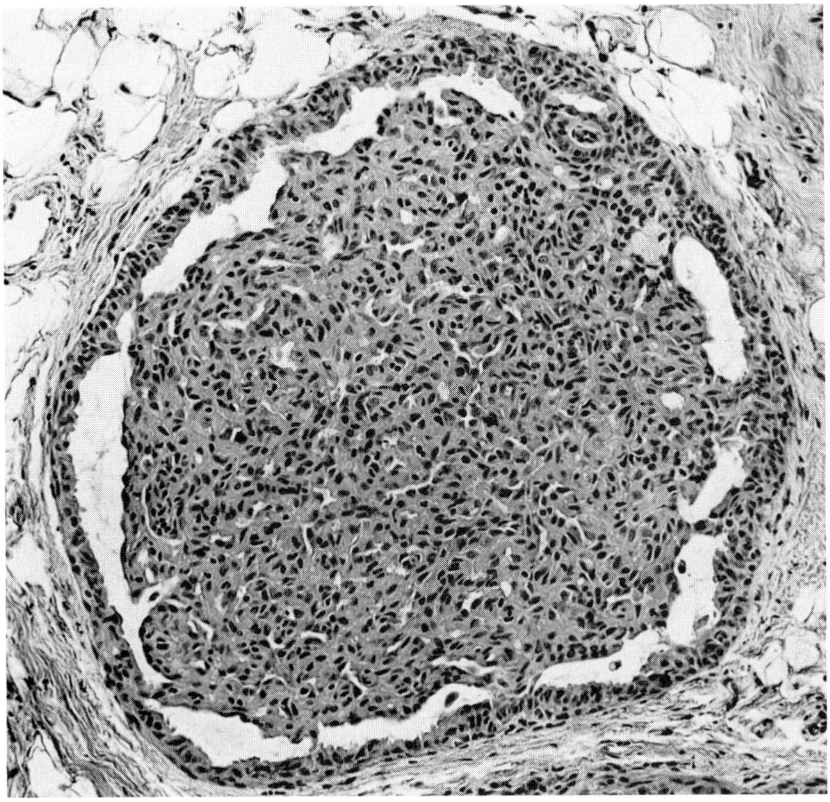

Fig. 1035 Photomicrograph demonstrating marked epithelial hyperplasia within dilated duct. There is no evidence of necrosis, and individual cells are well supported by their stroma. Lesion is completely benign. Prominent cleft has formed between solid intraluminal proliferation and outer epithelial row. In our experience, this is usually indicative of benign condition. (×160; WU neg. 72-9814.)

areas of apocrine metaplasia. Although exceptions exist and apocrine carcinomas have been described, the presence of apocrine metaplasia in a difficult breast lesion strongly favors that the process is benign.

3 *Fibrosis of the stroma.* This change is nearly always present, but its extent varies tremendously. It is probably a secondary event to the rupture of the cysts. In some cases it dominates the gross and microscopic picture, almost to the exclusion of the cystic changes. Such cases are referred to as *fibrous mastopathy* and are regarded by some as distinct from fibrocystic disease,[55] but whether such a pathologic entity exists remains doubtful. The fibrous tissue can become hyalinized. Calcification is a common finding in this condition, but, in contrast to the calcification accompanying carcinoma, it tends to have a coarse, highly irregular pattern.

4 *Chronic inflammation.* This is also an almost invariable finding in this condition. It is not related to infection, and in many cases it is the result of rupture of ducts with release of secretion in the stroma. Lymphocytes, plasma cells, and foamy histiocytes are the predominant cells. When plasma cells predominate, the term "plasma cell mastitis" has been used, but this seems unnecessary.

5 *Duct hyperplasia.* This is the most important and troublesome component of fibrocystic disease, and the one that is considered to be the most significant regarding the possible relationship between this condition and carcinoma. It may involve large, medium-sized, or terminal ducts (Fig. 1034). English pathologists prefer the term *epitheliosis* for this morphologic change.[41a] The proliferation may be solid, be accompanied by the formation of peripheral slits (Fig. 1035), or acquire a papillary configuration. When the latter feature predominates, the condition is referred to nipple adenoma, intraductal papilloma, or papillomatosis, depending on the location. These changes are

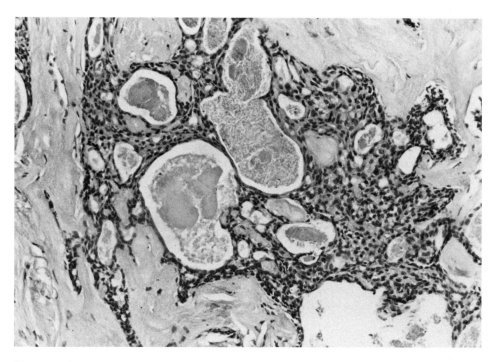

Fig. 1036 Complicated pattern resulting from ductal epithelial proliferation and stromal fibrosis in fibrocystic disease.

discussed separately. Sometimes the continued proliferation of glands and stroma results in a picture reminiscent of fibroadenoma but lacking the circumscription of the latter; this change is sometimes referred to as *fibroadenomatosis* or *fibroadenomatoid hyperplasia*. Proliferation within the terminal ducts, which become bulbous and end blindly, has been designated "blunt-duct adenosis" by Foote and Stewart.[47] Both the secretory epithelial cell and the basal myoepithelial cell participate in the proliferation. In some instances, the latter predominates, resulting in a multilayered duct of cuboidal clear cells lined on the luminal side by a single layer of flattened or cuboidal, more darkly staining cells. Sometimes the myoepithelioid cells acquire a very elongated spindle shape, and this is referred to as *myoid* differentiation or metaplasia. In most cases, even those showing exuberant hyperplasia, cell atypia is minimal. The nuclei are large, but usually vesicular and normochromatic, with some variability in size and shape and scanty mitoses. Cases maintaining this overall architecture but exhibiting some degree of nuclear atypicality are designated "atypical duct hyperplasia." They still lack cribriform pattern and necrosis; if any of the latter features are present, the possibility

of intraductal carcinoma becomes a likely one.

Disturbing microscopic patterns arise when the duct proliferation is accompanied by extensive fibrosis, resulting in a degree of distortion such as to simulate invasion (Fig. 1036). Extreme examples of this phenomenon include sclerosing adenosis and "sclerosing papillary proliferation."[44] The latter condition is easily confused with tubular carcinoma. Actually, some investigators maintain that there is little difference between the two.[46] We believe that such a difference exists and use as the main criterion for identification of the "sclerosing papillary proliferation" the one set forth in the article by Fenoglio and Lattes[44]: the small distorted glands surrounded by cicatricial stroma and pseudoinvasive appearance should be in the center of a scar that is totally surrounded by radiating ducts showing benign papillary proliferation. Prominent elastosis can accompany this lesion.[61]

There are even more disturbing patterns that this highly proliferative type of fibrocystic disease can exhibit but that per se are not indicative of malignancy. One is the presence of proliferating glands in perineurial spaces (Fig. 1037). These are not lymphatic vessels but rather represent planes of decreased tissue resis-

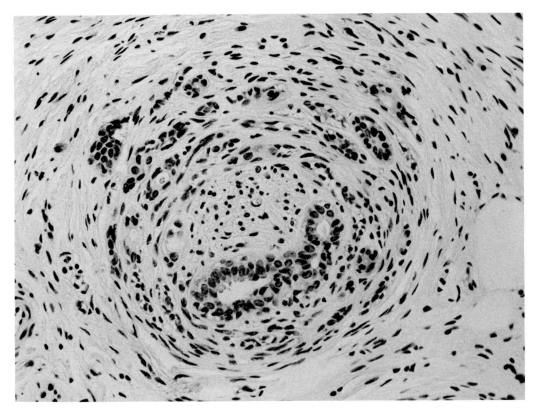

Fig. 1037 Perineurial involvement in patient with fibrocystic disease. Nests of well-differentiated glands are present. This is not evidence of malignancy. (×335; AFIP 55-22047.)

tance.[59] The other is the presence of infiltration of the wall of blood vessels by the proliferating glands; Eusebi and Azzopardi[43] detected this change in 10% of their cases of sclerosing adenosis and/or "severe epitheliosis" after staining the sections with Weigert's method for elastic tissue.

6 Lobular (acinar) abnormalities. In most examples of fibrocystic disease, the lobules are atrophic and distorted by the fibrous proliferation. In others, they participate in the proliferation and may even dominate the microscopic picture. Such cases are referred as lobular hyperplasia. When extreme, they constitute the lesion known as lobular carcinoma in situ, which is discussed on p. 1120. It is well to point out here that nearly all cases of lobular proliferations of the breast, even those fulfilling the generally accepted criteria for carcinoma in situ, arise within the context of fibrocystic disease and probably represent another expression of it.

. . .

Much has been written and argued about a possible relationship between fibrocystic disease and carcinoma. Let us examine the facts.

1 It is common for breasts excised for carcinoma to also exhibit changes of fibrocystic disease. The incidence varies from 20%-40%,[54] but it does not seem to be higher than that observed at autopsy among women who had no recorded breast symptoms.[57] What seems to be of importance, however, is that the fibrocystic disease in the breasts of patients with carcinoma has a greater tendency to show florid duct proliferation and atypia than in those of the control population.[48] Sometimes, all transitional stages can be traced between the carcinoma and the areas of benign proliferation within adjacent tissue, some of the ducts having a borderline appearance in which the decision as to whether or not a carcinoma is present becomes a very subjective interpretation.

2 Some patients with breast carcinoma give

a history of having had a breast biopsy in the past. When such slides are reviewed, it is found, more often than not, than they show florid and even atypical proliferative changes rather than the usual pattern of fibrocystic disease.[51,58]

3 Careful follow-up studies of large series of patients with fibrocystic disease suggest that this population is at a somewhat higher risk of developing carcinoma. In three of the most reliable series,[50,50a,52] this risk was estimated to be from two to four times greater than for the general population (Table 49). It has been further suggested that in those patients with fibrocystic disease associated with atypical duct hyperplasia, the risk may be greater than for the whole group.[41]

4 Chromosomal studies from cases of fibrocystic disease with marked intraductal and/or lobular epithelial hyperplasia have shown aneuploidy and structurally aberrant chromosomes in most cases; these were qualitatively similar to those seen in cells from obvious invasive breast cancers.[45]

What should be the therapeutic approach to fibrocystic disease in the light of these findings?

It seems to us that there is convincing evidence of an increased risk of carcinoma but that this risk is relatively small and that it does not justify the performance of a mastectomy in the ordinary case. Furthermore, it has been shown that if a patient with a microscopic diagnosis of fibrocystic disease in one breast were to develop cancer, the chances are about equal that it will be in the contralateral breast[47]; therefore, the only rational form of prophylactic treatment would be a bilateral mastectomy. This seems hardly justified. Local excision with careful follow-up is the logical alternative, as well as a relatively safe one. However, in our opinion, cases that justify a more aggressive approach do exist. Factors such as extensive, recurrent, and highly atypical duct proliferation, strong family history of breast carcinoma, and cancerophobia may well justify the performance of a simple mastectomy in the individual case.

Further studies of this problem are needed, specifically in trying to determine which morphologic features of fibrocystic disease are more closely associated with the development of carcinoma. A prospective multiinstitutional evaluation of this problem is now in progress in the United States. The special considerations that arise when the changes of fibrocystic diseases are accompanied by so-called lobular carcinoma in situ are discussed in the corresponding section.

Sclerosing adenosis

Sclerosing adenosis is merely a rather uncommon, highly proliferative form of fibrocystic disease. It is found about once in every 100 benign breast lesions. In a large series reported by Urban and Adair,[62] the average age of the patient was 31 years (20-50 years). The process usually occurs in the upper outer quadrant (which is also the most common site of carcinoma of the breast), has a disclike configuration, and cuts with increased resistance.

The most important identifying feature is the architecture of the lesion seen at very low magnification. A distorted central area of lobules and ducts is seen completely surrounded by an extremely cellular glandular proliferation *that retains a lobular pattern*. There is no cytologic atypia and no necrosis. If the characteristic configuration of sclerosing adenosis is recognized, then the cellularity of the lesion, the distortion of the epithelial component by proliferating connective tissue, and the presence of an occasional mitotic figure will not

Table 49 Relationship of gross cystic disease in 1,693 patients to the subsequent development of carcinoma of the breast, 1930-1968*

Age	Person years	Observed breast carcinomas	Expected breast carcinomas
25-29	88.50		.004
30-34	586.75		.098
35-39	1552.50	2	.594
40-44	2999.50	8	2.138
45-49	3946.50	12	4.185
50-54	3377.00	23	3.963
55-59	2125.00	14	2.977
60-64	1107.25	5	1.835
65-69	492.25	7	.987
70 +	207.00	1	.569
Total	16482.25	72	17.35
	Observed incidence	72	
	Expected incidence	17.35	

The observed incidence is four times the expected incidence.

Note: 23 carcinomas were found concomitantly with cysts and are excluded.

*From Haagensen CD: Diseases of the breast, ed. 2. Philadelphia, 1971, W. B. Saunders Co.

result in a mistaken diagnosis of carcinoma (Fig. 1038).

Adenoma of nipple

Adenoma of the nipple (papillomatosis of the nipple ducts) is a form of fibrocystic disease with distinct clinical and pathologic findings. Taylor and Robertson[60] have reported twenty-nine cases (twenty-six women and three men).

The majority occurred in the fourth and fifth decades. The nipple may become eroded.[53] For this reason, it has been mistaken clinically for Paget's disease. The most common complaint is that of serous or bloody discharge from the nipple. It is practically always unilateral.

Microscopically, the lesion shows marked proliferative changes and distortion of ductal

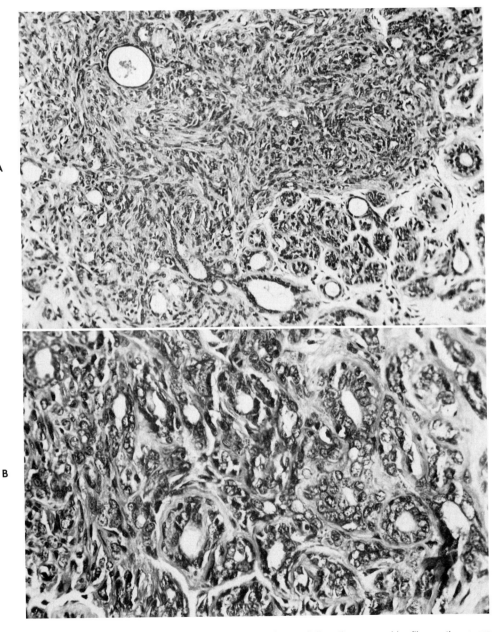

Fig. 1038 A, Sclerosing adenosis. Note distortion and poor delineation caused by fibrous tissue proliferation. **B,** Same lesion illustrated in **A** showing absence of necrosis, uniformity of cells, and lack of mitotic activity. (**A,** ×200; WU neg. 49-4500; **B,** ×400; WU neg. 49-4501.)

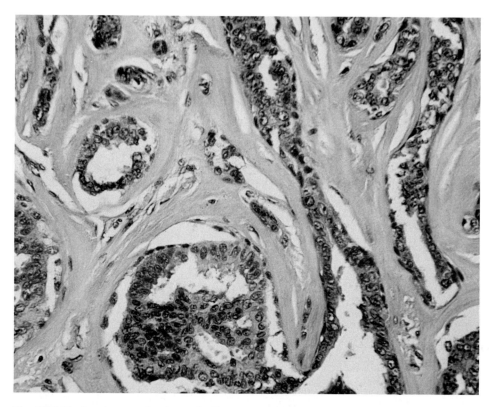

Fig. 1039 Nipple adenoma showing well-differentiated glands growing in dense stroma. This distortion by stroma is one reason why this lesion often is incorrectly called carcinoma. Note double layering, which helps to indicate that lesion is benign. (×275; WU neg. 66-7569.)

elements by dense stroma that may be mistaken for invasive cancer (Fig. 1039).

Presence of a two-cell layer in most ducts, uniformity of the cells, and lack of atypia and necrosis identify the lesion as benign, despite the occasional presence of mitoses and the presence of solid nests of cells. In the series reported by Taylor and Robertson,[60] ten of the patients had been erroneously treated by mastectomy. Local excision is curative.[56]

A note of warning to the pathologist is in order. Just because an intraductal papillary lesion is located in or close to the nipple, it does not necessarily mean that it is a nipple adenoma and therefore benign. Intraductal papillary carcinomas also occur in this location.[42] The criteria for differentiation are analogous to those employed for papillary lesions elsewhere in the breast.

Benign tumors
Fibroadenoma

Fibroadenomas of the breast are frequent in women 20-35 years of age. These tumors in-

crease in size during pregnancy and tend to regress as the age of the patient increases. Grossly, they are usually single but in 20% of the cases they are multiple in the same breast or in both breasts. In the younger age group, a type of fibroadenoma sometimes designated as giant, fetal, or juvenile may weigh as much as 1,000 gm (Figs. 1040 and 1041). It is important not to confuse this tumor with cystosarcoma phyllodes. The usual fibroadenoma, however, is a sharply demarcated, firm tumor, usually no more than 3 cm in diameter. In time, it may calcify or ossify and become extremely hard (Fig. 1042). Rarely, in the younger woman a fibroadenoma may undergo partial or complete mucoid degeneration. Exceptionally, part or all of a fibroadenoma undergoes infarction, presumably as a result of vascular insufficiency. The cut surface of a typical fibroadenoma is grayish white with a whorllike pattern in which poorly defined nodules project slightly above the cut surface (Fig. 1043). Slitlike spaces are often present. The absence of necrosis is valuable diagnostically. The type of breast cancer

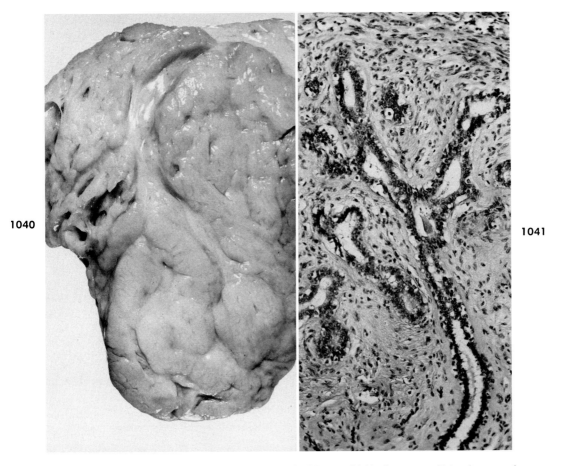

Fig. 1040 Large lobulated fibroadenoma occurring in 37-year-old black woman. Note absence of necrosis. (WU neg. 51-5002.)

Fig. 1041 Fibroadenoma with cellular stroma and elongated branching glands. (×150; WU neg. 49-5941.)

that is occasionally mistaken for fibroadenoma is the medullary type. It is softer and more opaque and frequently contains minute areas of necrosis.

Microscopically, the pattern of the fibroadenoma varies greatly because of different amounts of the epithelial and connective tissue components. Fibroadenomas are labeled *intracanalicular* when the growth of connective tissue is so rapid that it invaginates the ducts into slitlike spaces (Fig. 1044) and *pericanalicular* when the regular round configuration of the glands is maintained. Often, both types of growth are seen in the same lesion. The distinction has no practical connotations.

The well-defined ducts of a fibroadenoma are composed of cuboidal or cylindrical cells with round uniform nuclei. Apocrine metaplasia may be present, but squamous metaplasia

is distinctly uncommon. Foci reminiscent of sclerosing adenosis can be found in the midst of a fibroadenoma. The stroma is made of loose connective tissue rich in acid mucopolysaccharides, although in ancient lesions it may undergo hyaline, calcific, or osseous metaplasia. The cellularity varies a great deal from case to case. Elastic tissue is invariably absent. Exceptionally, mature adipose tissue is seen intermingled with the fibrous stroma.[79] Ultrastructurally, the most interesting feature of these tumors is the constant presence of multilayered basal lamina around the epithelial and endothelial cells.[65]

Malignant transformation of a fibroadenoma is exceptional (0.1%)[64,69] and for practical purposes can be disregarded in the management of this lesion. Florid epithelial hyperplasia in fibroadenomas is not rare and is usually devoid

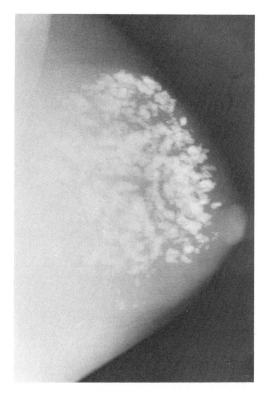

Fig. 1042 Heavy, coarse calcification in large breast fibroadenoma as seen in mammogram.

of clinical significance. However, unquestionable cases in which part of the epithelial component is malignant have been reported. Most of them have been of the *in situ* lobular variety.[68] In some cases the malignant tumor was entirely within the confines of the fibroadenoma and in others involved the surrounding breast as well. The latter may simply represent invasion of the fibroadenoma by a cancer originating elsewhere in the breast. McDivitt et al.[76] collected twenty-six cases of cancers arising in fibroadenomas. Of the sixteen lobular tumors, nine were limited to the fibroadenoma (seven being in situ and two infiltrative) and seven were also present in the surrounding breast (six in situ and one infiltrative). Of the ten ductal carcinomas, eight were present only in the fibroadenomas (six in situ and two infiltrative) and two (both infiltrative) also involved the neighboring gland. The prognosis of the tumors limited to the fibroadenoma was excellent. If the lesion is of the "lobular carcinoma in situ" variant and appears to be limited to the fibroadenoma, there is no indication that a reoperation is necessary if adequate follow-up can be assured.

Eusebi and Azzopardi[66a] have made the startling observation that some of the lobular proliferations seen in fibroadenomas have endocrine features, as shown by their argyrophilia and presence of dense-core granules.

Sarcomatous transformation of the stroma of a fibroadenoma is an even rarer phenomenon.[66] We have seen only one possible case in which a well-circumscribed small nodule had in some areas the appearance of an osteosarcoma, whereas in others it was composed of hyaline stroma enclosing slitlike glandular spaces, a configuration strongly reminiscent of an ancient fibroadenoma.

Adenomas

Adenomas of the breast (exclusive of those having a sweat gland appearance) can be divided into two major types: tubular adenoma and lactating adenoma.[72] *Tubular adenoma* presents in young adults as a solitary, well-circumscribed, tan-yellow, firm mass. Microscopically, a close packing of uniform small tubules lined by a single layer of epithelial cells and an attenuated layer of myoepithelial cells is seen; the stroma is characteristically sparse (Fig. 1045). Sometimes this pattern is seen combined with that of a fibroadenoma, suggesting that the two processes are closely related.

Lactating adenoma presents as a solitary or multiple, freely movable breast mass during pregnancy or puerperium. The lesion is actually a localized focus of hyperplasia in the lactating breast. Grossly, the lesion is well-circumscribed and lobulated. The cut surface is gray or tan, in contrast to the white color of fibroadenoma. Necrotic changes are frequent.[74] Microscopically, proliferated glands are seen lined by actively secreting cuboidal cells (Fig. 1046). This lesion should be distinguished from proliferative and secretory changes brought upon by pregnancy on a preexisting fibroadenoma.

Benign papillary lesions

Papillary proliferations within the breast ducts are extremely important because of their frequency and the difficulty that pathologists often experience in separating the benign from the malignant forms. This is well shown by the fact that they constitute over three-fourths of the breast lesions submitted in consultations by pathologists. Several morphologic types of benign proliferations of the ductal epithelium

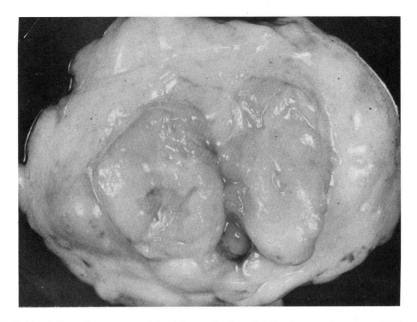

Fig. 1043 Usual fibroadenoma, grayish white, projecting slightly above cut surface. (WU neg. 48-4541.)

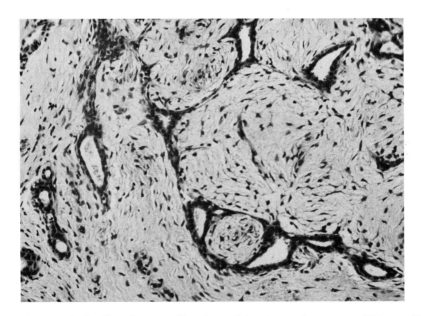

Fig. 1044 Intracanalicular fibroadenoma with rather cellular stroma. (Low power; WU neg. 47-102.)

can be recognized. These include intraductal papilloma, multiple papillomas, diffuse papillomatosis, terminal duct hyperplasia, and atypical duct hyperplasia.[78] The basic pattern of proliferation is similar in all these conditions, the differences being related to the number of lesions, size of duct involved, degree of proliferation, and presence of cell atypia. Nipple adenoma is a special type of duct papillomatosis and has been discussed separately.

Intraductal papillomas are often small but may become 4-5 cm in diameter (Fig. 1047).

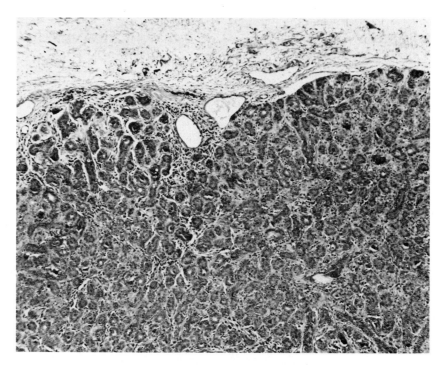

Fig. 1045 Tubular adenoma of breast. Small uniform ducts are present with only minimal intervening stroma. (From Hertel BF, Zaloudek C, Kempson RL: Breast adenomas. Cancer **37:**2891-2905, 1976.)

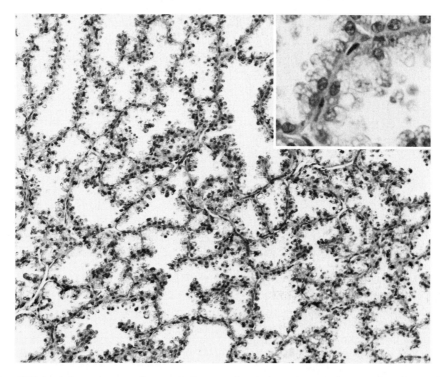

Fig. 1046 Lactating adenoma. Lumen is large and cytoplasm is actively secreting. **Inset** shows abundant secretory cytoplasm in greater detail. (Courtesy Dr. B. F. Hertel, Woodruff, Wis.)

They usually are quite soft and fragile, being supported only by filamentous fibrous tissue trabeculae. Areas of hemorrhage are common. The larger ones appear to lie inside a cystic dilatation of the duct. The multiplicity and the danger of malignant change of these lesions

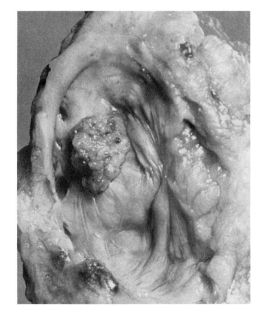

Fig. 1047 Soft, rather large intraductal papilloma. (WU neg. 47-3569.)

have been markedly exaggerated.[75] Haagensen et al.[71] reported recurrences in only three of 108 instances. These recurrences may have represented new lesions, but, in any event, the disease did not progress.

Microscopically, frozen section diagnosis of the intraductal papilloma often is difficult because of the extreme cellularity of the lesion (Fig. 1048). The papillary projections may be trapped in the wall of the cyst, suggesting invasion and malignancy. Infarction and squamous metaplasia may be confusing.

The difficulty in diagnosis increases with the size and complexity of the papilloma. Kraus and Neubecker[73] summarized the various criteria by which an intraductal papilloma can be distinguished from a papillary cancer (Table 50). Presence of two types of cells in papillomas and cribriform pattern and cytologic atypia in carcinomas have been the main distinguishing features in our experience (Fig. 1048). Azzopardi[62a] has described in great detail and with exceptional clarity the fine points in the differential diagnosis between benign and malignant intraductal lesions. Careful reading of his book is a must for all surgical pathologists. He pointed out that benign lesions are characterized by the following features:

1 Extreme rarity of necrosis
2 Rarity of frank evidence of hemorrhage
3 Frequent presence of foamy cells

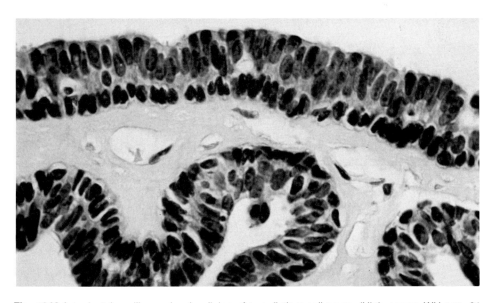

Fig. 1048 Intraductal papilloma showing lining of two distinct cell types. (High power; WU neg. 61-6991.)

4 "Streaming" growth pattern; i.e., the fact that the cells and their nuclei have a parallel orientation of their long axes

5 Indistinct cytoplasmic borders so that the nuclei seem to lie in a syncytial mass

6 Nuclei *rarely* rounded, except when cut transversely

7 Nucleoli small, generally single, and very inconspicuous

8 Irregular nuclear spacing with slight overlap

9 Scant mitotic activity

10 "Tufts" and "mounds" projecting into the lumen

11 Spindle cell bridging, without trabeculae formation

12 Cytoplasmic blebbing

13 Apocrine metaplasia

14 Frequent calcification, but extreme rarity of calcific spherules or psammoma bodies

Juvenile papillomatosis (Swiss cheese disease) of the breast is a special form of papil-lomatosis usually seen in young individuals (average age, 19 years) but occurring in a wide age range (10-44 years). Clinically, the localized, multinodular masses simulate the appearance of a fibroadenoma. Microscopically, there is florid papillomatosis (sometimes with severe atypia), cysts with or without apocrine metaplasia, duct stasis, and sclerosing adenosis. In a series of thirty-seven cases reported by Rosen et al.,[79a] two patients had an independent breast carcinoma; none of the other patients have developed breast cancer after an average follow-up of eight years. Kiaer et al.,[72a] with a smaller experience, showed a more ominous outcome: two of their three patients with this condition developed breast carcinoma many years later.

If a major duct contains a papilloma, local excision is adequate therapy. Long-term follow-up without the development of further difficulty emphasizes the wisdom of conservative treatment[77,81] (Table 51). Simple mastectomy is not indicated.

Gynecomastia

Gynecomastia may result from innumerable causes.[80,83] In a report of 160 cases, Wheeler et al.[82] emphasized that enlargement of the male breast before 25 years of age is usually related to hormonal pubertal changes, but after 25 years of age it is often a manifestation of a serious underlying disease. In a series of 351 cases reported by Bannayan and Hajdu,[63] fifty were classified as juvenile, 103 as idiopathic, and thirty-eight as drug-induced (digitalis, reserpine, Dilantin, etc.). The remaining were secondary to a large variety of causes. The disease was unilateral (the left breast being involved more often than the right) in 244 patients and bilateral in 107. Gynecomastia was centrally located in 311 patients and eccentrically located in the remaining. The authors noted that pubertal and hormone-induced gyne-

Table 50 Differential diagnosis between intraductal papilloma and papillary carcinoma*

Papilloma	Papillary carcinoma
Two types of epithelial cells	Single type of epithelial cell
Nuclei normochromatic	Nuclei hyperchromatic
Aprocrine metaplasia present	Apocrine metaplasia absent
Complex glandular pattern	Cribriform pattern
Prominent connective tissue stroma	Delicate or absent connective tissue stroma
Periductal fibrosis with epithelial entrapment	Epithelial invasion of stroma
Intraductal hyperplasia in adjacent ducts	Intraductal carcinoma in adjacent ducts
Sclerosing adenosis sometimes present in adjacent breast tissue	Sclerosing adenosis generally absent in adjacent breast tissue

*From Kraus FT, Neubecker RD: The differential diagnosis of papillary tumors of the breast. Cancer **15**:444-455, 1962.

Table 51 Follow-up of seventy-six patients with intraductal papilloma treated by local excision (Presbyterian Hospital, New York, N. Y., 1916-1941)*

Site in breast	Total patients treated by local excision	Recurrence of papilloma		Developed carcinoma	% follow-up
		Under 5 yr	After 5 yr		
Central	56	2	0	0	94.6
Peripheral	20	0	1	0	95.0
All sites	76	2	1	0	94.7

*Compiled from Haagensen CD, Stout AP, Phillips JS: The papillary neoplasms of the breast. Ann. Surg. **133**:18-36, 1951.

comastias tend to be bilateral, whereas idiopathic and nonhormonal drug-induced gynecomastias are usually unilateral.

Gynecomastia is characterized by considerable epithelial intraductal hyperplasia and stromal edema (Fig. 1049). This swollen stroma around ducts produces a characteristic "halo" effect. It is mainly composed of acid mucopolysaccharides (particularly hyaluronic acid) and remarkably similar to that found in fibroadenoma of the female breast.[67] The wall of the ducts lacks elastic tissue.

In rare cases, the intraductal epithelial hyperplasia is so extreme as to simulate carcinoma. The microscopic changes are related to the duration of the gynecomastia. Cases of short duration tend to have a prominent hyperplastic epithelial component and stromal edema, whereas in those of long duration stromal fibrosis is prominent. Formation of lobules was observed in twenty-one of the 351 patients reviewed by Bannayan and Hajdu.[63]

Granular cell tumor

Granular cell tumor (a better designation than the misleading granular cell myoblastoma) is a rare but important lesion because no other benign lesion so closely mimics grossly mammary carcinoma. On section, it is firm, homogeneous, and usually white or grayish yellow. As a rule, it is not attached to the overlying skin. Occasionally, it is fixed to the underlying fascia. It may be as large as 10 cm in diameter.

Microscopically, the tumor cells are uniform and large, with vesicular nuclei, abundant granular cytoplasm, and well-defined cytoplasmic outlines. Mitotic figures usually are absent. Necrosis may occur at times. Sudanophilic material seldom is present in the tumor cells. The cytoplasmic granules are PAS positive, contain abundant acid phosphatase and other hydrolytic enzymes, and have an heterogeneous appearance under the electron microscope (Fig. 1050). They represent markedly increased, bizarre lysosomes. Only microscopic examination will distinguish granular cell tumor from carcinoma.[70]

Malignant tumors
Carcinoma

The overwhelming number of malignant tumors of breast parenchyma are carcinomas (95% or more). These tumors can be roughly divided into two major categories: those arising from the major ducts and those originating from the smaller ducts and lobules or acini (the

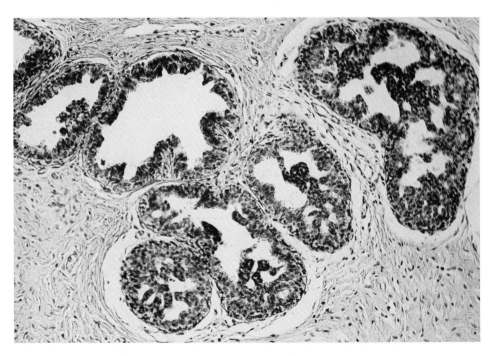

Fig. 1049 Prominent intraductal hyperplasia and stromal edema in gynecomastia. (×145; WU neg. 56-4822.)

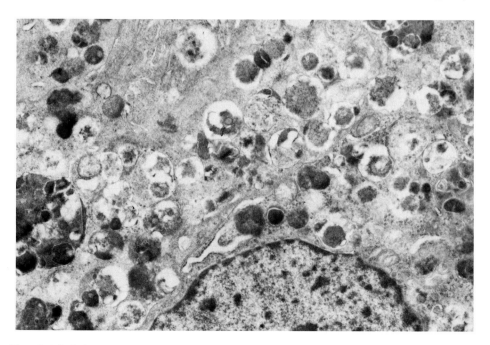

Fig. 1050 Cells from granular cell tumor containing numerous osmiophilic cytoplasmic granules. Some contain myelin figures. Myofilaments are not present. Part of nucleus may be seen at bottom. (Approximately ×12,000.)

so-called terminal secretory unit). Their gross and microscopic features are influenced by their growth within the ducts and lobules, the amount of connective tissue and mucin which they form, their cellular type, and their degree of invasiveness, if any. Extraneous adjectives that have no significance are often applied to breast carcinomas: scirrhous means hard, encephaloid means soft, and carcinoma simplex means a simple carcinoma. These titles are of no prognostic value and should be discarded. Many classifications of breast carcinomas have been proposed, but none has yet gained widespread acceptance. Descriptions of the better recognized variants of breast cancer follow. Comparisons between the light and electron microscopic features of these types have been carried out.[84,86]

Multicentricity (as defined by presence of carcinoma in a breast quadrant other than the one containing the dominant mass) was detected by Fisher et al.[85] in 121 (13.4%) of 904 cases of infiltrating carcinoma; one-third of the smaller foci were invasive and the rest were in situ. Multicentricity was more common in the lobular than in the ductal cancers.

The incidence of bilaterality in breast duct carcinoma is about five times that of the general population and is even higher if there is a family history of breast carcinoma. In lobular carcinoma, incidences of bilaterality have varied from 25%-50% in different series, but most of these lesions represent the controversial "lobular carcinoma in situ" to be discussed later. It is doubtful whether a biopsy of the opposite breast should be taken routinely in patients with breast cancer; it seems more logical to limit this practice only to those patients in whom an abnormality is suspected on clinical or mammographic grounds or to those with types of cancer for which the incidence of bilaterality is particularly high.[87]

There is growing evidence for a pathogenetic link between viruses and human breast cancer. A most interesting application to histopathology of the studies that are being carried out in this field has been the identification in human breast cancer of a mammary tumor virus–related protein.[87a,87b] Close to 50% of the invasive breast cancers are positive, whereas benign breast lesions and cancers from other organs are consistently negative. The level of antigen is higher in the most aggressive histologic types. This technique is already being used for determining the breast origin of metastatic lesions.[87a]

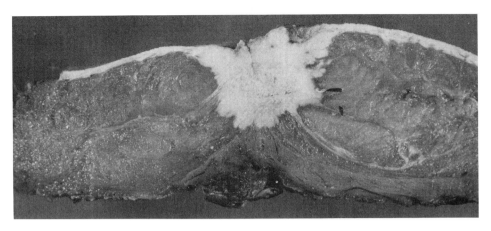

Fig. 1051 Carcinoma of breast with retraction of nipple. There are fine grayish white streaks of tumor ramifying into fat. (Courtesy Dr. R. Johnson, Columbia, Mo.)

Invasive ductal carcinoma

Invasive ductal carcinoma makes up about 75% of all breast cancers. Grossly, it is a poorly defined mass, the hardness of which depends upon the amount of connective tissue present. The tumor cuts with a resistant gritty sensation (unripe pear), is usually yellowish gray, and has fibrous trabeculae radiating through the bright yellow fat of the breast parenchyma (Fig. 1051). It is not rare for these fibrous strands to connect with other nodules of carcinoma at some distance from the primary tumor. The characteristic "chalky streaks" frequently seen in the cut surface do not represent foci of tumor necrosis, as generally believed, but rather bulky masses of elastic tissue surrounding large mammary ducts[92] (Fig. 1052). This change, known as "elastosis," occurs in about 90% of invasive ductal and lobular carcinomas.[88] It is much less common in the other types of breast cancer. It affects the walls of the ducts as well as the vessels (mainly veins). Intraductal cancer is rarely associated with this change, and therefore its presence should stimulate the search for invasion. However, it should be remembered that this alteration also can be seen in benign conditions, particularly the so-called sclerosing papillary proliferation.[89,94] Predominantly cellular tumors are much softer and often contain larger areas of necrosis. The tumor may invade the underlying fascia or muscle.

Microscopically, the tumor cells vary in size and shape and may or may not form glandular spaces. The individual cells of a cellular tumor have prominent nucleoli and many mitotic figures. Areas of necrosis occur in about 60% of the cases.[90] It may be difficult to identify tumor cells if the connective tissue is greatly increased. They may occur in groups of only five or six cells containing very little cytoplasm and surrounded by hyalinized connective tissue.

Multiple foci of origin are common, especially in younger women. They have been clearly demonstrated by whole organ preparations examined by roentgenography and light microscopy.[91,93]

Intraductal carcinoma with or without invasion

The intraductal carcinoma is a relatively infrequent form of breast cancer that grows predominantly within ducts. In most instances, it presents as a palpable mass. In one series, 28% were more than 5 cm in diameter and another 33% were 2-5 cm.[99] Westbrook and Gallager[102] showed that slightly over a half of intraductal carcinomas are centrally located, whereas this was true for only 16% of the infiltrating cancers. The incidence of multicentricity and bilaterality are high: 33% and 10%, respectively, in one particular series.[95a]

Grossly, the tumor contains thick-walled ducts with normal breast parenchyma between them. When the ducts are compressed, wormlike masses of necrotic tumor sometimes extrude from them—thus the name comedocarcinoma given to this variety. If the tumor is contained within the duct lumina and the duct walls are not too greatly thickened, tumor may not be recognized grossly.

Microscopically, the tumor cells resemble

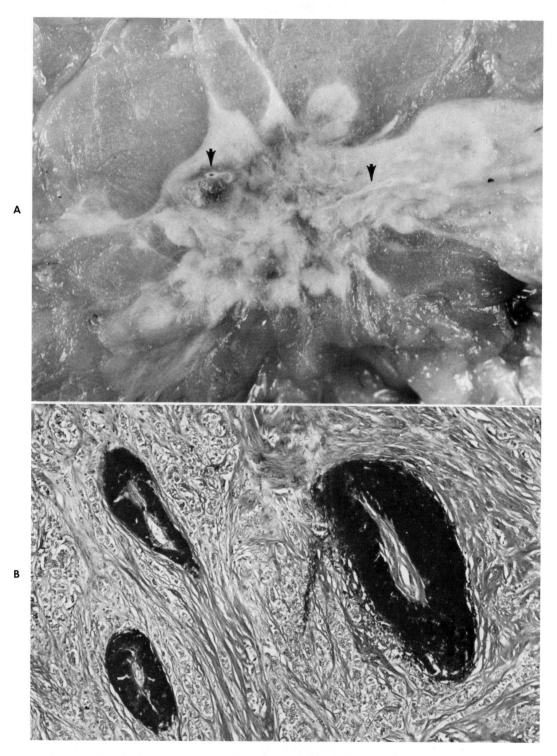

Fig. 1052 A, Gross appearance of typical invasive ductal carcinoma. "Chalky streaks" can be seen throughout tumor. Central space can be identified in some of them (arrows). **B,** Elastic tissue stain of lesion illustrated in **A** showing that "chalky streaks" correspond to grossly thickened elastic layer in wall of nonneoplastic ducts crossing tumor. (**A,** WU neg. 72-10775; **B,** Verhoeff–van Gieson; ×90; WU neg. 72-6052.)

those of the usual breast carcinoma. In this instance, however, the cells are confined to the ducts and are apparently noninvasive. Individual tumor cells have nuclei of variable size and shape with numerous mitotic figures. There is very little supporting connective tissue, and areas of central necrosis in the ducts are common (Figs. 1053 and 1054). Calcium salts frequently are deposited in these necrotic areas and can be identified by mammography. Carcinomas with a papillary or cribriform pattern of growth represent distinct varieties of intraductal carcinomas and are discussed separately.

Intraductal carcinomas may be accompanied by areas of stromal invasion. Silverberg and Chitale[101] found no correlation between tumor size and the degree of infiltration present but demonstrated a good correlation between the incidence of axillary metastases and the degree of infiltration.

Some ductal carcinomas, both in situ and invasive, are formed by cells with abundant acidophilic cytoplasm resembling apocrine epithelium. There is no need to separate these "apocrine carcinomas" from the rest, since there are no differences in their natural history.[97,98]

If a breast biopsy shows tumor confined to the ducts and there is no definite mass palpable in the breast, invasion outside of the ducts in other levels may still be present elsewhere, with the resulting possibility of low axillary lymph node metastases. This was true in seven (18%) of thirty-eight cases evaluated by Carter and Smith.[96] Even if the entire specimen shows only carcinoma in situ, this does not entirely preclude the possibility of metastases in axillary lymph nodes.[99a] Therefore, removal of these nodes (at least for staging purposes) should be carried out. Even if no infiltration is found after a meticulous pathologic study, the likelihood of progression to invasive car-

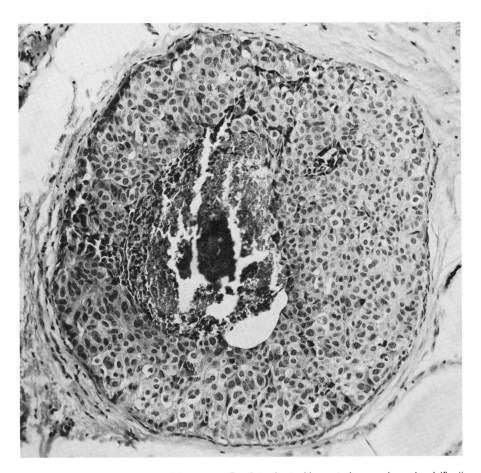

Fig. 1053 Intraductal carcinoma of breast confined to duct with central necrosis and calcification. This is so-called "comedo" type. (×180; WU neg. 50-687.)

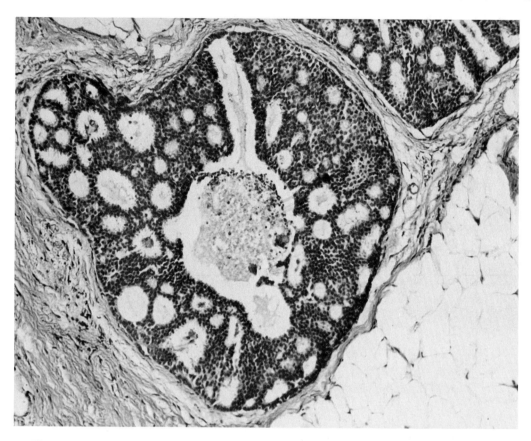

Fig. 1054 Intraductal carcinoma. There is cribriform pattern and central necrosis. Compare with Fig. 1035. (×160; WU neg. 72-9813.)

cinoma is sufficiently high to justify the performance of a mastectomy.[95,99b,100]

Medullary carcinoma

Medullary carcinoma of the breast has a distinctive gross and microscopic pattern.[104] Patients often are under 50 years of age. The tumor is very well circumscribed and may be mistaken clinically and grossly for fibroadenoma. It may become large, usually has a homogeneously gray color, and contains small focal areas of necrosis.

Microscopically, the cells of medullary carcinoma are large and pleomorphic, with large nuclei, prominent nucleoli, and numerous mitotic figures. The pattern of growth has been described as syncytial, a graphic even if inaccurate term. Glandular differentiation and intraductal growth are minimal or absent. Foci of squamous metaplasia, spindle cell metaplasia, or bizarre giant cells may be present.[106] The borders are always well circumscribed. An important part of the picture is a prominent lymphoid infiltrate (Fig. 1055), which may represent a reaction of the host tissues to the neoplasm. If unduly prominent, it can be mistaken microscopically for malignant lymphoma.

Of a series of twenty-three cases of medullary carcinoma seen at Barnes Hospital, thirteen had axillary lymph node metastases. However, in nine of the thirteen cases, only one node was involved, always in the low group. The prognosis of this tumor type is better than for the ordinary invasive ductal carcinoma.[103,105] In the series of Ridolfi at al.,[106] the ten-year survival was 84% as opposed to 63%. The prognosis was particularly good for tumors that were smaller than 3 cm, and remained better than that for ductal carcinoma even when nodal metastases were present.

The term "atypical medullary carcinoma" has been used for tumors that depart somewhat from the foregoing definition,[106] but the delin-

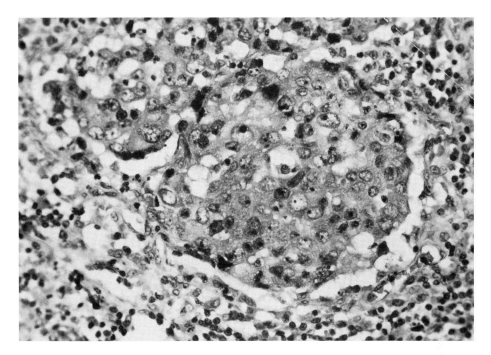

Fig. 1055 Medullary carcinoma with considerable lymphoid stroma. Note large size and lack of glandular differentiation of tumor cells. (×400; WU neg. 50-1419.)

eation of the criteria for its recognition remain somewhat nebulous. We have seen too often the term medullary carcinoma misused for highly cellular breast carcinomas that behaved in a very aggressive fashion and caution the reader to use this term only when all the pathologic criteria for this diagnosis are present.

Paget's disease

Paget's disease of the breast is a name given to the crusted lesion of the nipple caused by cancer.[110] It is merely a peripheral manifestation of an underlying carcinoma of the breast (Fig. 1056). A malignant intraductal component is always present, with or without associated stromal invasion. In this regard, the presence of Paget's disease is only a secondary, albeit dramatic feature of the tumor. The management and prognosis depend largely on the intraductal versus invasive nature of the underlying carcinoma rather than on the presence or appearance of the intraepithelial component.

Grossly, these weeping, eczematoid lesions appear to start on the nipple but later involve the areola and surrounding epidermis. They rarely extend more than a few centimeters. If a definite mass can be palpated beneath the diseased nipple, the underlying tumor will almost always be invasive. This was true in 106 of the 113 cases reviewed by Ashikari et al.[107] On the other hand, absence of a palpable mass is most often than not an indication that the carcinoma is purely intraductal. In the same series, this was found to be the case in sixty-three of ninety-six patients.

Microscopically, these tumors have the general characteristics of the usual ductal carcinoma. Invariably, if enough sections are studied, a connection between the carcinoma within the duct and carcinoma in the overlying nipple can be demonstrated. The large tumor cells lying within the epithelium are identical to the tumor cells lying within the ducts (Fig. 1057). However, because of their close spatial relationship with melanocytes, the malignant cells may acquire intracytoplasmic melanin granules; this phenomenon can also occur in carcinomas located in the large ducts. The clear appearance of the cytoplasm, occasional presence of melanin, and diffuse permeation of the malpighian layer can lead to confusion with malignant melanoma and Bowen's disease. We suppose that both of these conditions could occur in the nipple; in fact, examples of them have been reported. We can only say that, in our experience, whenever this differential diagnosis

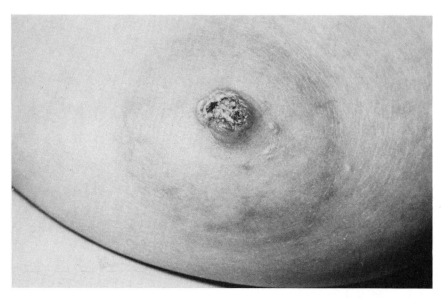

Fig. 1056 Early Paget's disease of nipple. There was underlying carcinoma. (WU neg. 48-1456.)

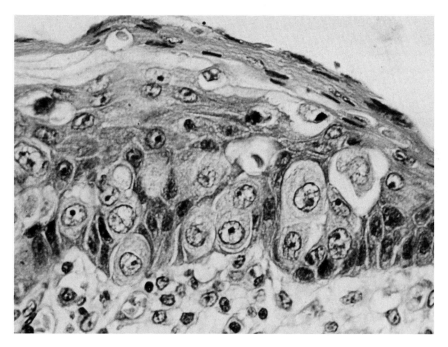

Fig. 1057 Large Paget cells involving epidermis. (×450.)

was considered for a lesion of the *nipple*, the definitive diagnosis invariably turned out to be Paget's disease.

The heated controversies held in the past regarding the histogenesis of Paget's disease of the breast have largely subsided. Careful histo-

chemical and electron microscopic studies have demonstrated that the intraepidermal Paget's cells are of mammary duct origin and not keratinocytes or melanocytes.[109] Another supportive piece of evidence has been provided by the immunocytochemical demonstration in Paget's

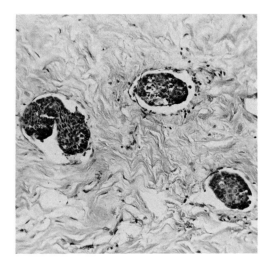

Fig. 1058 Widespread invasion of dermal lymphatics in inflammatory carcinoma. (×140; WU neg. 49-5372.)

cells of casein, a milk protein.[108] The minor controversial point still unsettled is whether the intraepidermal carcinoma cells originate in deeper structures and gradually work their way upward or whether they represent a simultaneous malignant transformation of the intraepidermal portion of the mammary ducts.[111]

Inflammatory carcinoma

The term inflammatory carcinoma was originally used in a clinical sense for a type of breast cancer in which the entire breast was reddened and warm, with widespread edema of the skin, thus simulating the appearance of mastitis. Pathologic studies in some of these cases revealed the lesion to be an undifferentiated carcinoma with widespread carcinomatosis of the dermal lymphatic vessels (Fig. 1058). This led to the belief that an "inflammatory" clinical appearance always corresponded pathologically to dermal lymphatic permeation and vice versa. This assumption is not always correct. Patients may have inflammatory carcinoma clinically in the absence of dermal invasion; conversely, widespread permeation of dermal lymphatics can be seen in the absence of the clinical features of inflammatory carcinoma (so-called "occult" inflammatory carcinoma[114]). From a prognostic standpoint, the presence of dermal lymphatic permeation on microscopic examination is a sign of ominous prognosis, whether the clinical appearance is that of an inflammatory carcinoma or not.[112,114] The clinical recognition of this entity by an

experienced observer is also reliable and associated with a poor prognosis, but ideally it should be accompanied by a skin biopsy showing dermal lymphatic involvement before the tumor is deemed inoperable.[113] It would probably be better to discard the term inflammatory carcinoma altogether.[112]

Papillary carcinoma with or without invasion

Papillary carcinomas make up only a small percentage of breast carcinomas. They can present as a well-circumscribed mass or ramify within ducts to involve an entire breast segment. Several morphologic patterns have been described.[116] The criteria for the diagnosis must be strict, because most papillary breast lesions are benign. The most important differential features are listed in Table 50. Paradoxically, there is more uniformity in cell size and shape in papillary carcinoma than in benign papillary lesions. An extremely elongated nuclear shape, running perpendicular to the duct lumen, favors carcinoma[115] (Figs. 1059 and 1060). Other features favoring cancer are loss of nuclear polarity, lack of a two-cell pattern, and presence of a cribriform pattern of growth without intervening stroma. Azzopardi[114a] emphasized the importance of the *trabecular bars* for the diagnosis of carcinoma. These are defined as rigid rows of cells with their long axes arranged more or less perpendicular to the long axis of the row. He also pointed out that carcinoma does not usually have the "syncytial" character of benign duct hyperplasia and that sharp cell edges are very suggestive of malignancy. Pallor or slight granularity of the cytoplasm should also be cause of concern. The nuclei of carcinoma tend to be round, evenly spaced, and hyperchromatic, the nucleoli being more prominent and mitotic activity more pronounced than in benign conditions. Differentiation into two cell types is characteristically absent.

The invasive component of an intraductal papillary carcinoma also may be papillary or have the features of an ordinary ductal carcinoma; the prognosis is substantially better for the former, which has been found to occur with a significantly high frequency among non-Caucasians and postmenopausal women.[114b]

Frequently, these tumors are inadequately excised. Recurrence may not appear for many years (five or more are not rare). Such recurrence may be local or be accompanied by lymph

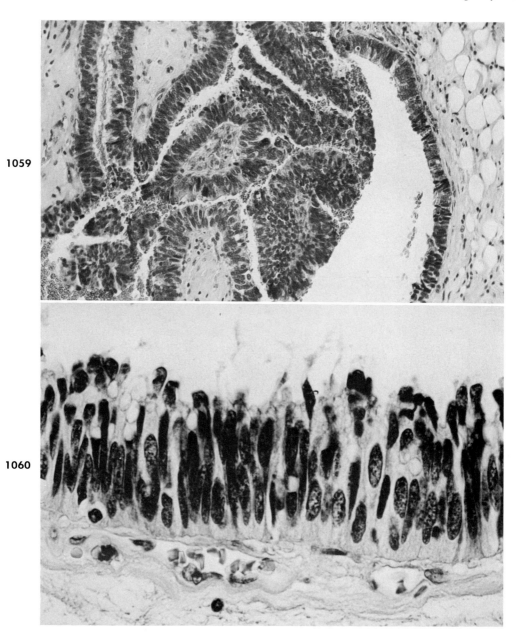

Fig. 1059 Papillary carcinoma without invasion. Note layering of lining cells with loss of nuclear polarity. (×180; WU neg. 52-5317.)

Fig. 1060 Papillary carcinoma demonstrating extreme layering of cells with loss of nuclear polarity. (×775; WU neg. 55-2816.)

node metastases.[115] This is the tumor that has often been diagnosed as benign intraductal papilloma undergoing malignant change. In truth, however, it was malignant from the start.

Mucinous carcinoma

If multiple sections of the breast are stained for mucin, small amounts nearly always will be found within the cytoplasm of the ductal epithelial cells. The diagnosis of mucinous carcinoma of the breast is justified only when the changes due to mucin are dominant. These tumors are well circumscribed, are palpably crepitant, and consist grossly of a currant jelly-like mass often held together by delicate connective tissue septa (Fig. 1061). Hemorrhage

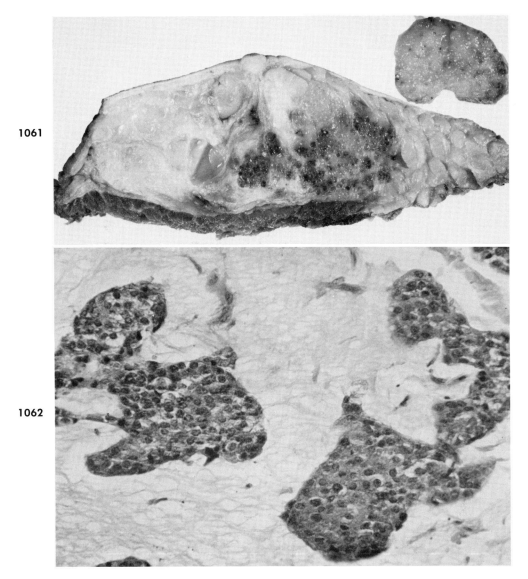

Fig. 1061 Pure mucinous carcinoma of breast in 55-year-old woman. Note typical gelatinous appearance. Tumor measured 7 cm in greatest diameter and was associated with axillary metastases (right upper corner). (WU neg. 66-7609.)

Fig. 1062 Typical appearance of mucinous carcinoma. Note well-differentiated character of cells floating in sea of mucin. (×310; WU neg. 62-9046.)

within the mass is frequent. Microscopically, tumor cells, often few in number, are seen floating in a sea of mucin (Fig. 1062). The individual cells usually form well-defined acini.

The patient with a tumor with these gross and microscopic characteristics has a good prognosis.[117] However, recurrences or metastases can appear many years after the original therapy. In a series of sixty-four cases studied by Rosen and Wang,[117a] nearly 50% of deaths

due to pure colloid tumors occurred twelve years or more after diagnosis. The pure form of mucinous carcinoma occurs most often in older women as a solitary circumscribed lesion which rarely, if ever, metastasizes when the tumor is less than 5 cm in maximal dimension. In such selected instances, this lesion may be treated by wide local excision or by simple mastectomy. Conversely, if areas of mucinous carcinoma alternate with others of ordinary

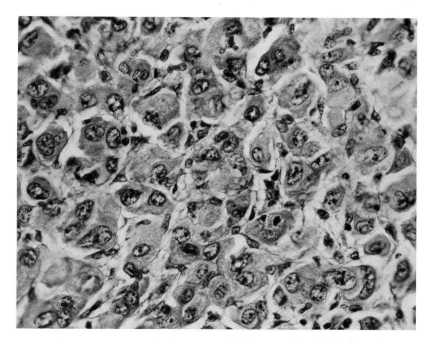

Fig. 1063 Extremely undifferentiated carcinoma of breast that contains large amounts of cytoplasmic mucin. (×400; WU neg. 50-959.)

infiltrating ductal carcinoma, the incidence of metastases and ultimate prognosis are dependent on the latter. Mucinous carcinoma as just described should be clearly separated from the tumor consisting primarily of cells with large amounts of intracellular mucin (the rare signet-ring type). The prognosis of this variety is extremely poor if not hopeless[118] (Fig. 1063.)

The startling observation recently has been made that a substantial number of mucinous carcinomas of the breast contain argyrophilic cells, as well as neurosecretory granules, by electron microscopic examination.[116a,116b] Obviously, this raises the possibility of at least some examples of mucinous carcinomas being related to the carcinoid tumors of the breast described elsewhere in this chapter.

Epidermoid carcinoma

Epidermoid carcinoma is a tumor of elderly women and carries a similar prognosis to that of the ordinary ductal adenocarcinoma.[119] Tumors of epidermal origin and those in which the squamous component is a portion of an otherwise typical cystosarcoma phyllodes should be excluded. The gross appearance of epidermoid carcinoma differs little from the usual breast carcinomas. Sometimes a large central cyst filled with keratin can be identified. Microscopically, most cases seem to represent instances of squamous metaplasia in ductal adenocarcinoma.[121] The squamous foci are often seen lining the wall of cystic formations. Intercellular bridges usually can be identified. The stroma can be quite prominent and cellular.

In some instances, a well-differentiated squamous component is seen associated with a prominent spindle cell sarcomatoid component.[120] This in all likelihood represents a type of spindle cell carcinoma analogous to that seen in the oral cavity and upper respiratory tract rather than a variant of cystosarcoma phyllodes or true carcinosarcoma. Axillary node metastases are usually absent.

Adenoid cystic carcinoma

The adenoid cystic type of carcinoma is an exceedingly rare variant of breast cancer. Microscopically, it resembles the homonymous tumor of salivary gland origin. The similarity is maintained at the electron microscopic level.[125] Perineurial infiltration is prominent.

Lymph node metastases practically never occur. Nayer[126] reported a patient with this type

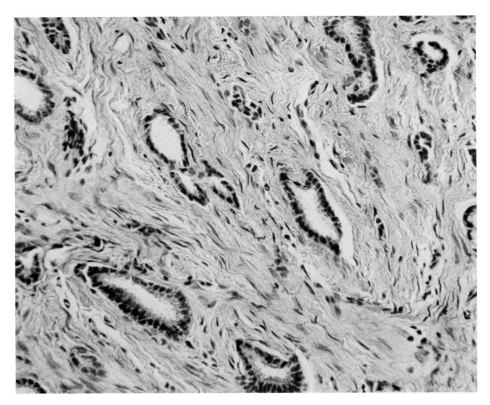

Fig. 1064 Well-differentiated (tubular) carcinoma of breast. (WU neg. 59-7303.)

of carcinoma who had no lymph node metastases at the time of radical mastectomy but who died thirteen years later of pulmonary metastases. We have had seven patients, none of whom had axillary metastases. One patient developed pulmonary metastases six years after mastectomy.[123] Of the twenty-one patients reported by Cavanzo and Taylor,[122] none had evidence of axillary metastases and none died of the tumor. Two patients had local recurrence after simple excision but remained well after mastectomy. It is important not to confuse adenoid cystic carcinoma with intraductal carcinoma with a prominent cribriform pattern. Special stains and electron microscopic examination may be necessary to make this differential diagnosis.[124]

Well-differentiated (tubular) carcinoma

A microscopically deceptive neoplasm, well-differentiated (tubular) carcinoma is often confused with sclerosing adenosis. Grossly, it suggests carcinoma by virtue of its poorly circumscribed margins and hard consistency, but microscopically it simulates a benign condition because of the well-differentiated nature of the glands and the absence of necrosis, mitoses, and cytologic atypia. The striking ductal differentiation of this malignant neoplasm is also maintained at the electron microscopic level.[128] The clues to the diagnosis are the haphazard arrangement of the glands in the stroma, the resulting complete lack of lobular configuration, and the frequent occurrence of typical intraductal carcinoma in large ducts situated within the lesion (Fig. 1064). Morphologic differences with sclerosing adenosis are also detectable at the electron microscopic level: prominent myoepithelial cells and basal lamina reduplication are conspicuous features of sclerosing adenosis but appear to be absent in tubular carcinoma.[129,131] The lack of basement membrane in tubular carcinomas as opposed to its presence in sclerosing adenosis can be appreciated by light microscopic examination of a PAS preparation.[128a]

A high incidence of multicentricity (56%), history of bilateral breast cancer (38%), and family history of breast cancer (40%) were found by Lagios et al.[129a] in a series of seventeen tubular carcinomas.

Metastases to axillary lymph nodes were documented in ten of thirty-three cases reviewed by Taylor and Norris.[130] The involved nodes were usually few and situated low in the axilla. Only one patient was known to have died as a result of the mammary tumor. Sometimes a pattern of tubular carcinoma is seen in association with an ordinary invasive ductal carcinoma[129b,129c]; the prognosis of these combined tumors is worse than that of pure tubular carcinoma but better than for invasive ductal carcinomas without a tubular component.[127] For a possible relationship between tubular and lobular carcinoma, see following discussion.

Lobular carcinoma

Lobular carcinoma arises in lobules and terminal ducts and comprises 6%-14% of all breast cancers.[146] Three stages of evolution are recognized: lobular carcinoma *in situ,* lobular carcinoma *in situ* with infiltration, and infiltrative lobular carcinoma without an identifiable *in situ* component.[147,157] The *in situ* form tends to oc-

cur in younger women. It has no gross distinguishing features and is usually found incidentally in breasts removed for other reasons. The disease, which is often multicentric and bilateral, concentrates within 5 cm of the nipple from the skin surface in the outer and inner upper quadrants.[151,152] Residual foci of tumor are found regularly in breasts removed following a diagnosis of lobular carcinoma in situ made on a biopsy specimen.

Microscopically, the lobules are greatly enlarged and filled with closely packed cells having few mitotic figures and practically no necrosis (Fig. 1065). The cells are quite uniform. Their nuclei are round and normochromatic, with minimal atypical features. Minor morphologic variations exist, depending on the nuclear size and chromatin content, amount and staining reactions of the cytoplasm, number of mitotic figures, presence or absence of necrosis, pattern of growth, and shape of the lobules, but they do not seem to carry any prognostic connotations.[133,148] Examination of the neighboring terminal ducts often reveals proliferation of similar cells, in some cases forming a continu-

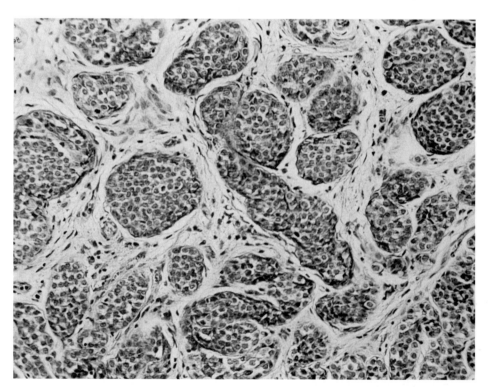

Fig. 1065 Lobular carcinoma in situ of breast. Note lobular pattern, small cells, and lack of necrosis. (×200; WU neg. 52-3452.)

ous row beneath the secretory epithelium and in others resulting in a solid intraluminal growth.[156] (Fig. 1066). Fechner[142] found these ductular changes in thirty-four of forty-five breasts with lobular carcinoma and remarked that their presence should stimulate a careful search for more diagnostic areas. The finding carries no prognostic implication of its own.[136] The diagnosis of lobular carcinoma *in situ* (or whatever equivalent term one might like to use) should be made only in those cases in which the cellular proliferation has resulted in the formation of large solid nests, whereas the designation of lobular hyperplasia can be given to those lesions having normal-sized lobules and ducts and preserving a central lumen (Fig. 1067). Lobular carcinoma in situ should be distinguished from ductal carcinoma with secondary invasion of the lobules. The latter event, which occurs in about 20% of ductal cancers, is identified by the presence of necrosis, cellular pleomorphism, obviously atypical nuclear configuration, formation of small

lumina, and the presence of typical changes of ductal carcinoma in the surrounding large ducts.[132,141]

The infiltrative component of lobular carcinoma is characterized by a haphazard cell growth without tendency to gland formation. In most cases, the cells are arranged in "Indian files" in a dense fibrous stroma, quite often in a concentric manner around lobules involved by *in situ* tumor (Fig. 1068). Periductal and perivenous elastosis can be identified in virtually every case.[139] Variants with a trabecular or a loose alveolar pattern also are recognized.[151a] Another pattern of infiltration is characterized by confluent nests of cells, which can be seen in association with single filing or by itself.[144] Occasionally, small tubular formations[145] or foci of intraductal carcinoma[152a] are seen in what is an otherwise typical invasive lobular carcinoma. This is explained by postulating the fact that lobular carcinoma is not a cancer of just the lobules but rather of the "terminal secretory unit" of the mam-

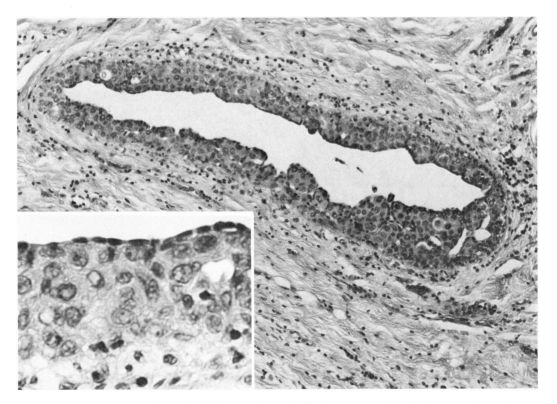

Fig. 1066 Involvement of duct by lobular carcinoma in situ. In presence of such change, a thorough search for typical areas of lobular involvement should be undertaken. **Inset,** High-power examination shows proliferating cells sandwiched between flattened layer of superficial secretory cells and ill-defined basal layer of probable myoepithelial nature. (×150; **inset,** ×500.)

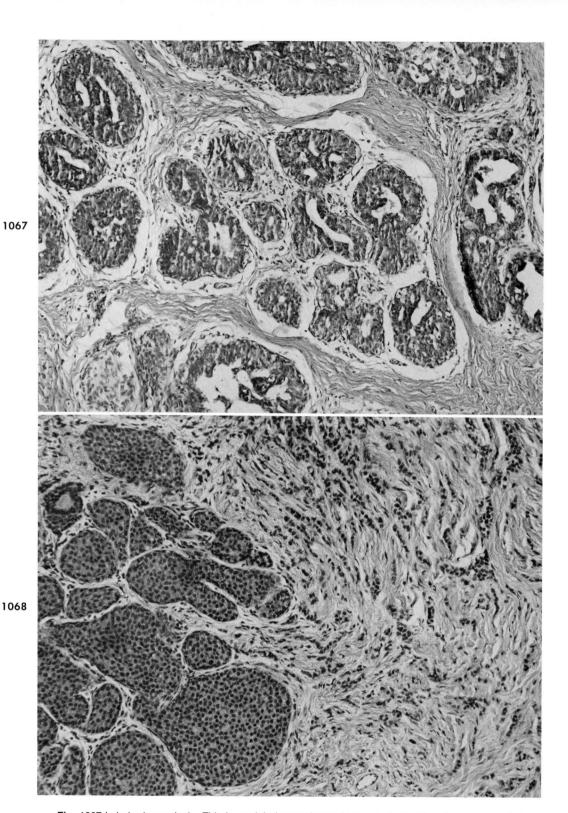

Fig. 1067 Lobular hyperplasia. This is not lobular carcinoma in situ. Individual lobules are not solidly filled with cells, and lesion is confined to lobules (×145; WU neg. 72-9812.)

Fig. 1068 Lobular carcinoma in situ with areas of invasive small cell cancer. In situ areas demonstrate complete packing of individual lobules by uniform cells. These same cells have invaded surrounding tissue and have typical pattern of small cell cancer. (×150: WU neg. 73-60.)

mary gland, which is composed of the lobules and the terminal ducts. As a matter of fact, it has been postulated on the basis of immunocytochemical and ultrastructural features that tubular carcinoma is a well-differentiated (secretory) variant of invasive lobular carcinoma.[139a] It also has been suggested that most of the cases of signet-ring carcinoma of the breast represent yet another morphologic variety of invasive lobular carcinoma.[154] As a matter of fact, small amounts of intracellular mucin production can be found in most invasive lobular carcinomas and in a good number of lobular carcinomas in situ.[138,155a] However, signet-ring cells also can be found in association with invasive ductal carcinoma.[149a] It is imperative that the highly aggressive signet-ring cell carcinoma of the breast be sharply distinguished from the relatively indolent mucinous carcinoma; in the latter, the mucin deposition is almost entirely extracellular.

When lobular carcinoma metastasizes to the axillary nodes, it may grow in a fashion that closely stimulates a malignant lymphoma of the histiocytic type. In such cases, staining of the sections for mucin or ultrastructural demonstration of intracytoplasmic lumina may provide the correct diagnosis.[137] Once the pathologist has learned to recognize the architectural features of invasive lobular carcinoma by careful examination of lesions associated with an *in situ* component, he will be able to suggest a diagnosis of lobular carcinoma even in the absence of the noninvasive element.[143] It is probable that most of the tumors designated as "small cell" cancers represent infiltrative lobular carcinomas (Fig. 1069). About 5% of invasive breast cancer cannot be classified into a ductal or lobular category.[151a]

Mammography can detect approximately one-half of the cases of lobular carcinoma in situ. The positive mammograph shows finely stippled calcification, different from that seen in ductal carcinoma. Microscopically, the calcification may not be in the cancer itself but in the surrounding normal lobules.[149,150] The cell of origin of lobular carcinoma is still disputed. It is quite clear that the tumor arises from a cell normally situated beneath the layer of secretory epithelium, the two candidates being the myoepithelial cells and the undifferentiated ("reserve") epithelial cells.[155] The fact that the cells of lobular carcinoma often contain mucin and the milk protein casein, that they fail to stain for actin, and that a high propor

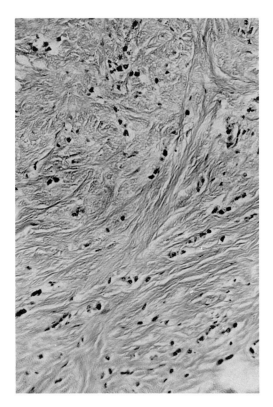

Fig. 1069 Carcinoma of breast (small cell type) with extreme production of fibrous tissue. Individual tumor cells are arranged in "Indian file." This probably represents invasive lobular carcinoma. (×200; WU neg. 49-5467.)

tion of cases contain estrogen receptors argue strongly in favor of epithelial rather than myoepithelial differentiation.[140]

There is little question that invasive lobular carcinoma with or without an *in situ* component is an aggressive form of breast cancer and that it should be treated as such. The big controversy concerns the nature, significance, and proper therapy of the lesion generally designated as carcinoma *in situ*. The concept espoused by the originators of the term and presently supported by a group of investigators, many of whom work or have been trained at Memorial Hospital for Cancer and Allied Diseases in New York City where the entity was first described, is that lobular carcinoma *in situ* is a bona fide carcinoma, that if left alone will progress to invasive carcinoma in a high proportion of cases, and that a mastectomy is indicated in patients in whom this condition is diagnosed unless some contraindications exist.[153]

Many pathologists have been reluctant to accept these concepts and recommendations, and it would seem that evaluation of several recent series amply justifies this reluctance. These series are based on retrospective diagnoses of carcinoma *in situ* in breast biopsies from patients in whom no additional surgery was carried out and long-term follow-up is available. In the series of Wheeler et al.[158] there were twenty-five women with lobular carcinoma *in situ* on biopsy who did not undergo mastectomy; only one women (4%) in a complete follow-up averaging 17.5 years developed ipsilateral invasive carcinoma. Of thirty-two women with a contralateral breast at risk, three (9.7%) developed invasive carcinoma. Andersen[134] had studied forty-seven similar patients: ten subsequently developed twelve invasive carcinomas (eight ipsilateral and four contralateral). Haagensen et al.[148] studied 211 patients with a mean follow-up of fourteen years; an invasive carcinoma developed in 9.08% of the ipsilateral breasts and in *exactly* the same percentage of the contralateral breasts. None of the patients who has had regular follow-up after the *in situ* lobular lesion was detected has died of the disease. Rosen et al.[153] from Memorial Hospital for Cancer and Allied Diseases, have analyzed ninety-nine patients with an average follow-up of twenty-four years; nineteen (19.2%) of them developed invasive carcinoma of the ipsilateral breast and sixteen (16.2%) of the contralateral breast.

What all these figures seem to indicate is (1) that lobular carcinoma in situ, when treated by biopsy only, will lead to invasive carcinoma in only one-tenth to one-fifth of the patients; (2) that if invasive carcinoma does develop, it is just as likely to arise in the contralateral breast than in the breast than had the biopsy; (3) that if a patient with a biopsy diagnosis of lobular carcinoma in situ is examined periodically, the chances of her dying as a result of breast cancer are minimal.

Thus, lobular carcinoma in situ emerges as a condition that is associated with an increased risk of development of breast carcinoma, but the rationale for regarding it as *carcinoma* is open to serious question. In that regard, it is more akin to atypical ductal hyperplasia than it is to intraductal carcinoma. The latter has all the cytologic criteria of malignancy and, if untreated, will lead to invasive carcinoma in the *majority* of the patients. We have already seen that lobular carcinoma in situ does not

fullfill these criteria. Therefore, the very use of the word carcinoma for it has been questioned, because it leaves the surgeon with no options. Alternative terms such as lobular neoplasia,[148] atypical lobular hyperplasia, or lobular dysplasia might be preferable, because they convey the message without forcing the surgeon's hand.

Most investigators agree that careful lifelong follow-up appears to be a safe and rational option for this lesion.[135,148] The performance of a simple mastectomy can be considered in the presence of a strong family history of cancer, extensive fibrocystic disease, or cancerophobia of if a prolonged follow-up evaluation cannot be assured.

Other types of carcinoma

A type of breast carcinoma in which the tumor cells contain abundant cytoplasmic fat has been described as *lipid-rich carcinoma*,[166] but it is doubtful whether it constitutes a specific entity. The metastases to lymph nodes or orbit can closely simulate the appearance of histiocytic lymphoma.[162] Some amount of cytoplasmic fat can be found in most cases of ordinary breast carcinoma[160]; it is apparently a secretory product and not a sign of degeneration; when present in large amounts, it is associated with aggressive behavior.

Patchefsky et al.[165] identified two cases of primary breast cancer having a pattern indistinguishable from that of low-grade *mucoepidermoid carcinoma* of the salivary gland type.

The name of *metaplastic carcinoma* is given to a poorly differentiated type of breast carcinoma in which the predominant component of the neoplasm acquires a sarcomatoid appearance. This may resemble fibrosarcoma, malignant fibrous histiocytoma, chondrosarcoma, or osteosarcoma or a combination of these neoplasms.[164,167] Sometimes the carcinoma is admixed with a prominent component of osteoclast-like giant cells.[158a] Cystosarcoma phyllodes does not belong into this category, but the already mentioned variant of epidermoid carcinoma with spindle cell stroma can be regarded as a distinct type of metaplastic carcinoma.

The latest member to the microscopic family of breast cancers is the *carcinoid tumor*. Cubilla and Woodruff[159] reported no fewer than eight patients with this disease, one of them having two primary tumors in the same breast and another having bilateral disease. None of the patients had the carcinoid syndrome or other endocrine symptoms, but other investigators have subsequently described cases associated with nonepinephrine and ACTH secretion.[163] Microscopically, the tumors were composed of small cells arranged in solid nests separated by fibrous tissue. An intraductal component was identified in three cases, and mucin production was detected in two. Argyrophilic granules were demonstrated in each case, but the argentaffin reaction was negative; electron microscopy showed dense-core granules of neurosecretory type in the three cases in which it was performed. The behavior was rather aggressive.

The differential diagnosis has to be made principally with lobular carcinoma and with carcinoid tumor metastatic to the breast.[161] The histogenesis of this tumor is arguable. Perhaps it arises from neuroendocrine cells normally located in breast ducts and lobules, as Cubilla and Woodruff[159] suggest. Another possibility is that it originates from primitive basal ductal cells with the capacity to partially differentiate into so-called neuroendocrine structures. As such, carcinoid tumor could be regarded as simply another morphologic variant of breast carcinoma. This is the interpretation we prefer.

The possible relationship between carcinoid tumor and mucinous carcinoma has already been discussed.

Classification and grading

It is important to divide breast carcinomas into different types in order to be able to make some predictions regarding the presence and extent of lymph node metastases and thereby the prognosis and treatment. The value of the latter practice in estimating prognosis has been demonstrated repeatedly.[168] Certain features, such as "pushing" peripheral margins, lymphocytic infiltration, and good microscopic differentiation correlate with a good prognosis regardless of tumor type[170-172] (Fig. 1070). By applying these general criteria to the most common forms of classification by tumor type, we have divided breast cancer into four well-defined categories:

Type I

This type includes all *in situ* neoplasms, whether arising from ductal or lobular epithelium. The members of this group are (1) intraductal carcinoma (with or without Paget's disease), (2) intraductal papillary carcinoma, and (3) lobular carcinoma in situ. Numerous blocks should be obtained in all tumors of the Type I group in order to rule out the presence of invasion. If no invasion can be demonstrated, the incidence of metastases is extremely low and the prognosis after mastectomy is excellent. Actually, mastectomy is not necessarily indicated in the third member of this group.

Type II

This group is composed of four microscopically unrelated neoplasms, having in common invasive features, well-delineated margins, and excellent

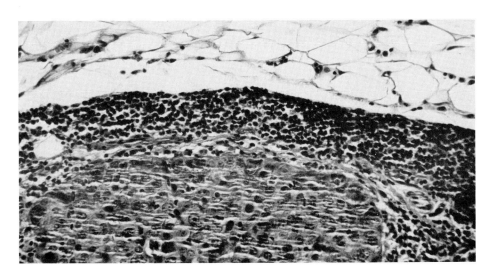

Fig. 1070 Circumscribed, pushing border of medullary carcinoma of breast. There is also mantle of lymphocytes present. (×250; WU neg. 62-9048.)

prognosis after surgical therapy. Metastases to the axillary nodes are either absent or, when present, usually limited to the low group. The four tumors, in decreasing order of curability, are (1) pure mucinous carcinoma, (2) well-differentiated (tubular) carcinoma, (3) invasive papillary carcinoma, and (4) medullary carcinoma.

Type III

This group, which is the most numerous, includes (1) the ordinary invasive ductal carcinoma, (2) intraductal carcinoma with invasion (with or without Paget's disease), and (3) invasive lobular carcinoma. Actually, all carcinomas not definitely classified as

Type I, II, or IV constitute Type III. The prognosis of invasive ductal carcinoma and invasive lobular carcinoma is very similar but apparently is slightly better in the latter. When invasive ductal carcinoma is seen associated with any of the Type II tumors, the prognosis is improved somewhat as a result and becomes better than that of invasive lobular carcinoma.[169]

Type IV

This group is composed of the undifferentiated carcinomas composed of cells without ductal or lobular arrangement, including the rare signet-ring type of carcinoma. Tumors indisputably invading blood

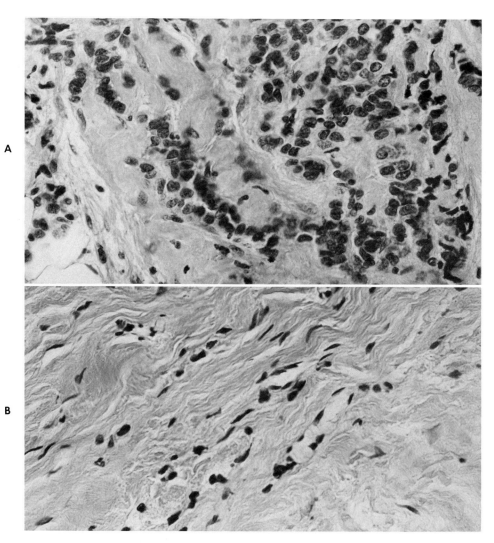

Fig. 1071 A, Undifferentiated carcinoma of breast before treatment with testosterone. **B,** Same tumor shown in **A** after treatment with testosterone demonstrating prominent regression. Note naked nuclei and increased fibrosis. (**A** and **B,** ×400; **A,** WU neg. 50-2970; **B,** WU neg. 50-2971; slides contributed by Dr. R. Johnson, Columbia, Mo.)

vessels, regardless of type, also belong to this category.

Effects of irradiation

There is no doubt that radiation therapy can sterilize breast carcinoma. The tumor either completely disappears or is replaced by fibrosis.

Tumors prominently affected by irradiation contain giant cells with atypical nuclei, naked nuclei, and abnormal mitotic figures. The viability of these tumor cells is difficult to assess. In spite of large amounts of axillary irradiation, tumors often are unaffected in some of the regional lymph nodes. Occasionally, tumor appears to have been sterilized in one portion of a lymph node yet unaffected in another area of the same node. Because of these findings, we have been unable to assess objectively the value of irradiation to involved axillary lymph nodes.[173,175] Undoubtedly, irradiation can wall off carcinoma for variable periods by partially sterilizing the tumor and by creating fibrosis. Such a palliative effect is well justified. Guttman[174] showed that it is possible to achieve a five-year survival rate of approximately 50% by means of roentgentherapy of mammary carcinomas that have been shown to be locally inoperable by biopsy.

Effects of steroid hormones

Estrogens, androgens, and steroids have been tried in different dosages for variable periods to relieve extensive inoperable carcinoma of the breast.[178] Testosterone may cause regression of bone metastases in all age groups. Of course, regression of either the primary tumor or its metastases is only temporary.

Microscopically, the changes produced by any steroid hormone are comparable. There may be prominent collagen hyalinization, increase in the amount of collagen, increase in the prominence of the elastic tissue, necrosis, and even complete disappearance of tumor cells. The changes in tumor cells often are scattered. One group of cells may disappear completely, another may disappear partially, and still another may be morphologically unaffected. The microscopic pattern of affected tumors does not show why there was a response to therapy. Cytoplasmic vacuolation, nuclear aberrations, and cell wall ruptures are present. These changes are roughly analogous to those caused by irradiation.

Rarely, prominent regressive changes, including complete disappearance of tumor cells,

have been demonstrated in both the primary lesion and in the axillary lymph nodes[177] (Fig. 1071). These morphologic changes also are seen infrequently after adrenalectomy for carcinoma of the breast. They are most likely to occur when adrenalectomy has been performed for inflammatory carcinoma of the breast.[176] It is impossible to predict by histologic examination which cancer of the breast will respond to hormonal or endocrine ablative therapy.

Cystosarcoma phyllodes

Cystosarcoma phyllodes is an unsatisfactory name for this uncommon neoplasm of the breast because the majority of the cases are benign.[195] Azzopardi[178b] made the sensible proposal of renaming it *phyllodes tumor* and to qualify it according to the pathologist's assessment of the microscopic appearance and likely behavior. It occurs in the same age group as breast carcinoma. In the series of ninety-four cases reported by Norris and Taylor,[193] the median age at the time of diagnosis was 45 years. Only three patients were younger than 20 years of age, in striking contrast with the age distribution of patients with ordinary fibroadenoma. Although cystosarcoma phyllodes is well known for its propensity to reach giant proportions, it is well to remember that more than one-half of these tumors measure less than 5 cm in diameter.[189] It follows, then, that the diagnosis of cystosarcoma phyllodes can neither be made nor ruled out by size alone.[206,207] A lesion with the microscopic appearance of fibroadenoma should still be diagnosed as such even if it reaches 5 cm or more in diameter (a rare event, predominantly seen in young black females).

Grossly, the typical cystosarcoma presents a teardrop appearance to the breast. The nipple may be flattened, but the overlying skin is almost never attached. On the other hand, attachment of the tumor to the underlying fascia is not infrequent. Cystosarcomas are usually well circumscribed, gray-white, and firm (Fig. 1072). Areas of necrosis, cystic degeneration, and hemorrhage are seen in the larger tumors. Cleftlike spaces may be present. Infection may develop secondary to ulceration. We have seen several cases in which the entire neoplasm had undergone massive hemorrhage infarct.

The microscopic main points for the diagnosis of cystosarcoma are the prominent stromal cellularity and the presence of benign ductal elements as an integral component of the

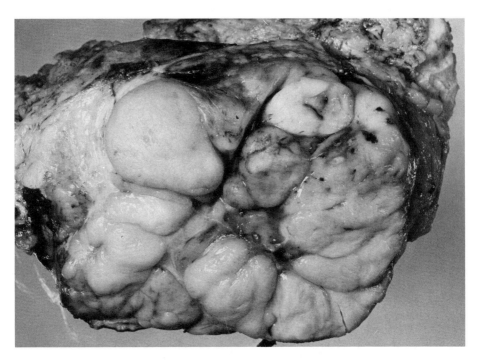

Fig. 1072 Large cystosarcoma phyllodes of breast showing pseudoencapsulation and nodularity. (WU neg. 52-3814.)

neoplasm.[195] Although the distinction between benign and malignant cystosarcoma can be very difficult to make in a given case, sufficient information is now available on the natural history of this neoplasm as to allow a statement to be made about the likelihood of metastases and proper management on the basis of the pathologic features. Tumors with the configuration of fibroadenomas having a cellular stroma without atypical features concentrated in the periductal areas generally lack the capacity to metastasize but have a marked incidence of local recurrence. If an enucleation has been done under the clinical impression of fibro-adenoma, the patient can be safely followed for the possibility of recurrence. If the latter develops, or if this type of cystosarcoma is recognized at the time of initial surgery, local excision with a wide margin of normal tissue is the treatment of choice. Recurrent cysto-sarcoma, which is the consequence of inadequate excision,[188] may still be cured by wide local excision even if resection of the chest wall is required.

On the other hand, obvious sarcomatous tumors with marked nuclear atypia, large number of mitoses, and loss of the relationship between glands and stroma are potentially metastasizing neoplasms and should be treated accordingly (Fig. 1073). An important diagnostic criterion of malignancy is overgrowth of the glands by the sarcomatous stroma, so that low-power views of the tumor show only stroma without epithelial elements.[184] Simple mastectomy is sufficient in most instances, but if there is any question of invasion of the fascia, it should be removed together with the underlying muscle. Metastases of cystosarcoma to axillary nodes are exceptional. They are documented only once in the ninety-four cases reported by Norris and Taylor.[193] Therefore, there is hardly any justification for routine axillary dissection. The incidence of distant metastases has varied from 3% to 12% in the different series. The most common sites are lung and bone, but the central nervous system also can be affected.[200] The metastases are of stromal elements only, although entrapping of normal structures in the lung may simulate a dual composition. For those cystosarcomas that do not fall easily into one of these two extreme categories, the decision has to be made on the basis of size, pushing versus peripheral margins, cellular atypia, and mitotic count.[193,199]

In the benign neoplasms, the stromal component has almost always a fibrous appearance,

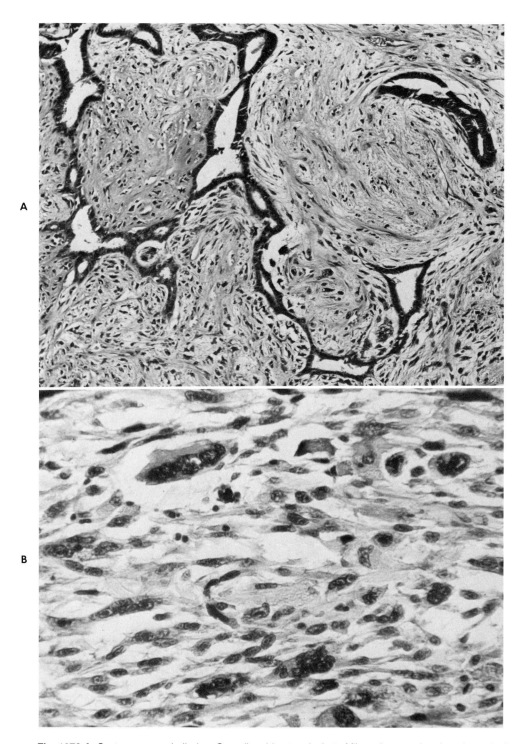

Fig. 1073 A, Cystosarcoma phyllodes. Overall architecture is that of fibroadenoma, but there is marked stromal cellularity. **B,** Another area of tumor shown in **A.** Stroma is highly atypical and grows independently from epithelial components, two signs indicative of malignancy. (**A,** ×130; WU neg. 73-3408; **B,** ×300; WU neg. 73-3407.)

with occasional admixture of mature adipose foci. In the malignant variant, the stroma may have the appearance of fibrosarcoma, liposarcoma, chondrosarcoma, osteosarcoma, malignant fibrous histiocytoma, and rhabdomyosarcoma.[179] The epithelial element is practically always benign, although it may appear quite hyperplastic. Norris and Taylor[193] identified a carcinomatous element in only two of their ninety-four cases. We are unaware of any case of cystosarcoma phyllodes in which the epithelial component of the tumor led to purely carcinomatous metastases.

Other stromal tumors and tumorlike conditions

Stromal sarcomas of the breast are usually large and firm and often circumscribed. Grossly, the tumors appear grayish white and homogeneous. Necrosis may be present. Microscopically, most of them have the features of fibrosarcoma; focal osseous metaplasia can occur. These lesions may be distinguished clinically from carcinomas by their large size and by their failure to become attached to the skin. Microscopically, they are distinguished from cystosarcoma phyllodes by the lack of an epithelial component. Infiltrative margins and severe atypia indicate a greater tendency for local recurrence and distant metastases.[194]

Both *fibromatosis* and *nodular fasciitis* can involve the breast as primary lesions. Their natural history is analogous to that expected when occurring in the usual soft tissue location. Thus, fibromatosis of the breast is infiltrative, aggressive, and prone to local recurrence.[178a,202]

There exists a spectrum of benign breast tumors formed by different proportions and types of stromal elements and glands. Included in this spectrum are the previously discussed fibroadenoma, the fibroadenoma containing adipose tissue, the adenoma with cartilage (analogous to the pleomorphic adenoma of salivary glands), and the rare lesion composed of a mixture of fat, cartilage, and bone but lacking an epithelial component.[186]

There have been reports of primary *liposarcoma*,[191] *leiomyoma* of the nipple,[192] *leiomyosarcoma*,[197] *rhabdomyosarcoma, malignant pleomorphic fibrous histiocytoma (fibroxanthosarcoma), chondrosarcoma*,[180] and *osteosarcoma*.[185] The latter two should be distinguished from benign tumors with osseous or cartilaginous metaplasia, from cystosarcomas

phyllodes in which the cartilage or bone is part of the neoplastic stroma, from carcinomas with osseous or cartilaginous metaplasia,[203] and from a rare benign lesion characterized by an accumulation of multinucleated mammary stromal giant cells.[200a]

Hemangiosarcoma is a distinctive breast neoplasm with an ominous prognosis. Grossly, the tumor is soft, spongy, and hemorrhagic. Microscopically, the diagnostic areas are characterized by anastomosing vascular channels lined by atypical endothelial cells. The appearance may vary in the same tumor from that of a highly undifferentiated solid neoplasm to one indistinguishable from a hemangioma. Metastases occur early through the bloodstream.[182,204] The diagnosis of *hemangioma* of the breast should be made with great caution, both because of its extreme rarity and the fact that a well-differentiated angiosarcoma can closely simulate its pattern. Most hemangiomas described in the breast have a perilobular distribution and a microscopic size such as to escape gross detection by the prosector.[201]

Over 200 cases of *lymphangiosarcoma* of the upper extremity following radical mastectomy have been reported. This sarcoma usually follows long-standing edema but may occur after mastectomy without edema.[205] The tumor appears at an average of ten years after radical mastectomy. In most patients, lymphedema had appeared within one year after mastectomy.

Clinically, the early lesions appear as bluish or purple papules in an edematous skin. They are often multiple and accompanied by deeper independent foci, the latter accounting for the failure of local excision to control the disease. The region most affected at first is the arm, followed by the forearm and elbow. Microscopically, dilated lymphatic channels lined by atypical cells alternate with solid tumor masses. The microscopic diagnosis of this lesion may be difficult in its early phases, for only a small nodule of innocuous-appearing collections of vessels lined by a single layer of endothelium may exist. We agree with Sternby et al.[205] that if such apparent benign vascular proliferation occurs in areas of chronic lymphedema, it has to be regarded and treated as a lymphangiosarcoma.

The prognosis is poor. Approximately 50% of the patients die within two years of the onset, with recurrence in the chest wall and pulmonary metastases. Of the eleven patients known to have survived for more than five years, nine had been treated by radical surgery (wide excision, forequarter amputation, or shoulder disarticulation).[209]

Malignant lymphoma and related lesions

Malignant lymphoma can present as a primary mammary neoplasm or involve the breast as part of a generalized process.[181] Grossly, it is soft and grayish-white. It grows rapidly and is not accompanied by skin retraction or nipple discharge. For some peculiar reason, the right breast is involved more commonly than the left. Multiple nodules are sometimes encountered. The involvement is bilateral in one of every four patients. In a series of sixteen cases of primary lymphoma of the breast,[208] nine were classified as histiocytic, five as poorly differentiated lymphocytic, and two as well-differentiated lymphocytic neoplasms. The prognosis

was poor. Only two patients had a documented long-term survival; in both, the tumor was of lymphocytic type. In a more recent series, the outcome was better, probably because of an improved chemotherapeutic approach: the five-year survival rate for the thirteen patients with follow-up was 49%.[190]

We have never seen Hodgkin's disease presenting as a primary breast tumor, although we have seen several cases of breast involvement in Stage IV disease.

Pseudolymphoma, a reactive process better designated as lymphoid hyperplasia, can present as a distinct mass in the breast.[196] It appears grossly as a firm, solid nodule and microscopically as a lymphoid infiltrate often containing germinal centers and accompanied by vascular proliferation. Some of the cases seem to represent an exuberant local reaction to injury.[188a] As to be expected from a reactive

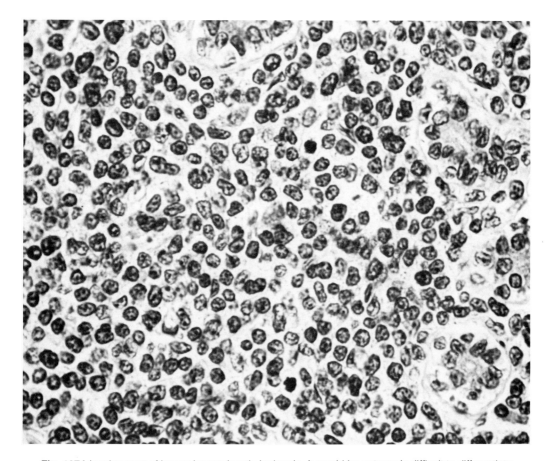

Fig. 1074 Involvement of breast by myelocytic leukemia. It would be extremely difficult to differentiate this lesion from histiocytic lymphoma on hematoxylin-eosin sections. Von Leder stain for chloroacetate esterase was positive. (×720; WU neg. 68-7080.)

lesion, both B and T cells are present, the former exhibiting polyclonal features.[181a]

Acute and chronic *myelocytic leukemia* can present as a localized mass in the breast and be microscopically confused with histiocytic lymphoma[198] (Fig. 1074). The most important clue to the diagnosis of "granulocytic sarcoma" in hematoxylin-eosin sections is the presence of eosinophilic myelocytes or metamyelocytes, identified as cells with a round or slightly indented nucleus and bright eosinophilic cytoplasmic granules. We have found the von Leder stain very useful in the confirmation of this diagnosis. This is a chloroacetate esterase reaction that can be easily performed in formalin-fixed, paraffin-embedded material and that stains the specific lysosomal granules of the cells belonging to the granulocytic series a bright red color.[187]

Exceptionally, a mass of *myeloid metaplasia* can form in the breast in patients with idiopathic myelofibrosis.[180a]

Other lesions

Skin lesions such as *basal cell carcinoma*,[210] *epidermoid carcinoma*, *keratinous cysts*, and *sweat gland tumors* may arise in the skin of the breast and should not be considered as primary breast neoplasms.

Since the breast is a modified sweat gland, it is not surprising that, occasionally, benign tumors having the appearance of sweat gland neoplasms arise from it. These include *clear cell hydradenoma* (eccrine acrospiroma)[213] and the already mentioned *pleomorphic adenoma* (benign mixed tumor).[222]

Metastatic carcinomas rarely affect the breast except in widely disseminated tumors. They typically appear as superficial, well-defined multinodular masses. In the series reported by Hajdu and Urban,[214] there were fourteen malignant melanomas and six lung carcinomas.

Fungous disease (coccidioidomycosis, actinomycosis) may occur and form multiple sinus tracts. We have seen several instances of *foreign body reaction* to polyvinyl plastic (Ivalon). This spongy plastic material was used for mammoplasty. It becomes impregnated with granulation and fibrous tissue. Instead of enhancing beauty, the plastic contracts, hardens, becomes fixed, and may even result in the formation of sinus tracts.[215] A similar foreign body reaction has been described following silicone injections.[223]

Breast infarct can complicate a large variety of conditions, including intraductal papilloma, sclerosing adenosis, fibroadenoma, cystosarcoma phyllodes, hyperplastic lobules during pregnancy,[218,220] syphilis, and Wegener's granulomatosis.[211,221] It also has been reported in association with anticoagulant therapy,[219] postpartum abscess and gangrene, thrombophlebitis migrans disseminata, and mitral stenosis with heart failure.[221]

The eponym *Mondor's disease* is given to a peculiar thrombophlebitis involving breast and the contiguous thoracicoabdominal wall.[212] The condition, which may simulate a malignant neoplasm, often has a sudden onset and appears as a firm slightly nodular cord beneath the skin. Ecchymosis may or may not be present. Microscopically, the process is one of phlebitis with thrombosis.[217] With time, the thrombus recanalizes completely. The condition is self-limited and practically never recurs. It may be related to mechanical injury. In eight of the fifteen cases reported by Herrmann,[216] the disease appeared a few months following a radical mastectomy.

Hormone therapy and breast

Painful engorgement of the breasts occurs not infrequently during the first cycles of contraceptive therapy. This is usually a mild and transient symptom. Pathologically, the only definite mammary change that can be ascribed to the "contraceptive pill" on the basis of the presently available evidence is the development of true acini resembling lactating breast.[227] Hyperplastic epithelial changes in fibroadenomas have been described,[229] but whether they are indeed the result of the therapy is not yet established. Fechner[224] found no differences in the incidence, gross appearance, and microscopic configuration of fifty-four fibroadenomas removed in patients who were receiving oral contraceptives and fifty-four control cases, except for the occasional formation of acini in the former. He obtained similar results when comparing twenty-five cases of fibrocystic disease in patients receiving progestogens with twenty-five control cases.[225]

It has been stated that there is decreased frequency of fibrocystic disease among long-term oral contraceptive users[232]; however, LiVolsi et al.[231] have shown that this does not necessarily apply to the type of fibrocystic disease associated with marked epithelial hyperplasia and atypia.

Nothing definite can be said at the present time about a possible relationship between contraceptive agents and breast carcinoma. Naturally, several cases of breast cancers occurring in patients on progestogen therapy have already been reported. With an estimated 8,500,000 women taking these drugs in the United States, this is hardly surprising. Pathologically, these cancers do not seem to differ from those seen in control cases.[226,227] Obviously, only a carefully designed epidemiologic study will answer the question whether oral contraceptive therapy results in an increased risk of mammary carcinoma and whether it exerts any influence on an existing neoplasm. So far, no convincing evidence has been put forward for either alternative with the possible exception of a slight increase in long-term users who have had previous surgery for benign breast disease.[228]

The situation is somewhat similar regarding a possible relationship between exogenous estrogens and breast cancer. A study of a large group of women who had received conjugated estrogens for menopausal symptoms showed no statistical increase in the overall incidence of breast cancer.[230] However, this same study showed that those women who had had a previous biopsy diagnosis of fibrocystic disease either before or after receiving estrogen therapy had a twofold to ninefold increase in the incidence of breast carcinoma. Another study has shown that breast cancers in menopausal women taking estrogens show no distinctive microscopic features as compared with a control group.[228]

Breast diseases in children and adolescents

Infant breast tissue may undergo *focal intraductal hyperplasia* associated with stromal alterations.[237] This may result in the formation of a unilateral mass beneath the nipple. Also, at the time of puberty, the physiologic development may be initially unilateral, simulating a breast neoplasm. Should such nodules be removed by mistake, no development of the breast will occur.

Fibroadenomas are exceptional before the age of puberty but are the most common pathologic condition seen between puberty and 20 years of age.[233,236] So-called *virginal hypertrophy* may result in massive unilateral or bilateral enlargement. Microscopically, it is characterized by a combined proliferation of

ducts and stroma with little, if any, lobular participation. Farrow and Ashikari[233] encountered thirteen *intraductal papillomas* in patients between the ages of 15 and 19 years.

Most reported cases of *breast carcinoma* in children fall into one of two well-defined categories. Some are infiltrative ductal tumors with a microscopic appearance quite similar to that seen in carcinoma of adults, except that there is a greater proportion of well-differentiated neoplasms (Fig. 1075, *A*). There is also a tendency of the tumor cells to have a clear cytoplasm with evidence of secretory activity[234] (Fig. 1075, *B*). It should be pointed out, though, that breast carcinomas with a secretory pattern also can be observed in adults. Because of this, the term *secretory carcinoma* is to be preferred over that of juvenile carcinoma.[237a] The prognosis in this tumor type is excellent. In the series of seven cases reported by McDivitt and Stewart,[234] there was not a single instance of metastatic spread, and the five-year survival rate was 100%, despite the fact that three of the patients were treated only by local excision. In the series of Tavassoli and Norris,[237a] four of the nineteen patients had nodal metastases, and one patient died with disseminated tumor.

The other type of malignancy that has been described in this age group is a highly undifferentiated solid neoplasm formed by medium-sized round cells without ductular or acinar formation. Many of these cases have been reported or diagnosed as small cell undifferentiated carcinomas. After having personally reviewed some examples, we have the impression that at least some of them actually represent embryonal or alveolar rhabdomyosarcomas or other types of soft tissue sarcomas of the chest wall. The prognosis is extremely poor. Extensive lymphatic and blood-borne metastases develop early in the course of the disease.[235]

Tumors of male breast

In the United States, only 1% of all breast cancer occurs in males, but in Egypt and certain other tropical regions, the incidence rises to nearly 10%.[239] There is no documented association between clinically apparent pubertal gynecomastia and cancer. There are some reports of mammary carcinoma appearing in breasts with estrogen-induced gynecomastia in patients treated for prostatic carcinoma. Although a few unquestionable cases are on record,[244] it is likely that many of these represent

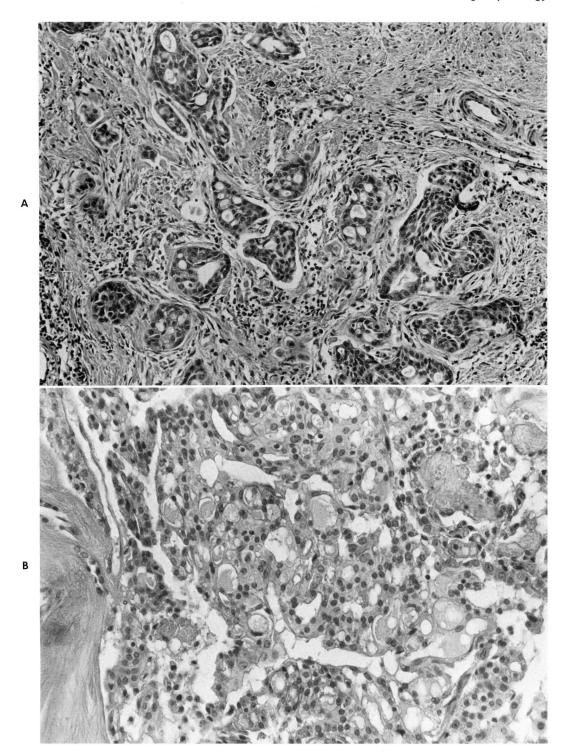

Fig. 1075 A, Breast carcinoma in 10-year-old girl. Small glands composed of atypical cells infiltrate mammary stroma. Total mastectomy was performed. Patient is alive and well six years later. **B,** Secretory carcinoma of breast. Note well-differentiated nature of neoplastic cells and large amount of intracellular and extracellular secretory material. This tumor occurred in 16-year-old girl, and regional lymph nodes were negative. (**A,** ×150; WU neg. 72-9816; courtesy Dr. W. S. Medart, Savannah, Ga.; **B,** slide courtesy Dr. L. Beauchesne and Dr. C. Beauchesne, Sherbrooke, Canada.)

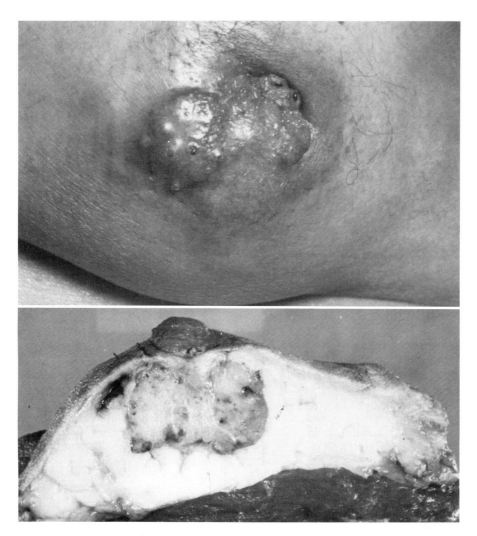

Fig. 1076 Right breast of 65-year-old man showing marked nipple deformity and ulceration with nodularity of areolar skin secondary to infiltrating duct carcinoma. (Courtesy Dr. J. C. Ashhurst, Tuskegee, Ala.)

instead metastatic foci from the prostatic cancer.[238] An increased incidence of breast cancer is seen in patients with Klinefelter's disease.[242]

Clinically, most tumors present in elderly individuals as breast nodules, with or without associated nipple abnormalities. Nipple discharge in an adult male, especially if bloody, should arouse a strong suspicion of carcinoma.[247] Grossly and microscopically, cancers of the male breast are remarkably similar to those seen in females (Fig. 1076). All of the microscopic types identified in female breast have been encountered in males; the least common variety is invasive lobular carcinoma, only a few suggestive cases having been ob-

served.[240] We are unaware of any report on pure lobular carcinoma in situ of the male breast. Skin involvement by fixation and Paget's disease are much more common in males. Microscopic gynecomastia is present in 40% of the cases.[240a] The incidence of axillary metastasis is the same in men as in women, but the prognosis is slightly worse in the former, especially in Stages II and III.[243,245] A correlation between microscopic grade and prognosis exists, following a pattern similar to that in cancer of the female breast.[248] In a series of ninety-seven cases of male breast cancer reported by Heller et al.,[240a] the ten-year survival for the whole group of patients with invasive carcinoma was 40% (79% for those with negative axillary nodes and 11% for those with positive nodes). No differences were found in the incidence of axillary node involvement or stage of the disease when compared with breast cancer in females.

Several cases of nipple adenoma (florid nipple papillomatosis) have been observed, one of them following estrogen therapy for prostatic carcinoma.[249] We have never seen fibrocystic disease, fibroadenoma, or cystosarcoma phyllodes occurring in a male breast, but a case of mammary duct ectasia has been reported.[246] A leiomyosarcoma arising from the nipple also has been observed.[241]

Clinicopathologic correlation

It is imperative that the clinician be skilled in accurate palpation of the breast and axilla when examining a patient with a lump in the breast. We have demonstrated that the benign or malignant nature of a dominant mass can be diagnosed correctly by fourth-year medical students in 55% of instances (5% better than tossing a coin). The experienced clinician can diagnose only 70% correctly. Therefore, a policy of look and see must replace that of wait and see. Once lumps are exposed and sectioned, the surgeon proficient in surgical pathology can grossly identify their benign or malignant nature in over 85% of the patients.

The widespread use of mammography has radically changed the diagnostic approach to breast cancer. Extremely small tumors (1-2 mm) can be detected with this technique, which relies primarily on the presence of calcification. The incidence of calcification in preoperative mammograms in cases of breast cancer was 48.5% in the series of Millis et al.,[277c] whereas the corresponding figure for benign breast disease was 20%. Thus, it should be obvious that a negative mammogram provides no assurance about the absence of breast cancer in a screened patient. Also, some concern has been expressed about the potential carcinogenesis of this diagnostic method in view of the fact that breast cancer has been reported in individuals following exposure of the breast to radiation, whether it be for the treatment of acne or gynecomastia or after repeated fluoroscopic examination, and in individuals exposed to radiation from the atomic bomb.[283c] It should be emphasized, though, that in most of the instances the doses of radiation received were substantially higher to those resulting from mammography or xeroradiography with modern techniques.

The fallacy of attempting to determine the presence of absence of axillary node metastases by palpation is illustrated by the following findings:

Clinically negative and microscopically negative — 84 cases
Clinically negative and microscopically positive — 71 cases
} Examiner correct in 54%

Clinically positive and microscopically positive — 124 cases
Clinically positive and microscopically negative — 22 cases
} Examiner correct in 85%

The error in saying that an axilla is negative when an involved node is present approaches 50%. Conversely, the error is only about 15% when the axilla is thought to contain disease because of the presence of enlarged nodes. The overall error in axillary papation is 30%.

When the axillary lymph nodes contain metastatic cancer in the presence of a clinically and roentgenographically normal breast, the management becomes a difficult problem. The differential diagnosis is usually between breast carcinoma and amelanotic malignant melanoma. Dopa or tyrosinase reaction, immunoperoxidase stain for mammary tumor virus–related protein,[277b,284a] and electron microscopic examination can be helpful in this regard.[268,280,281] If a metastatic tumor in an axillary node is compatible with breast carcinoma and the possibility of melanoma has been reasonably ruled out, removal of the homolateral breast is justified even in the absence of positive findings. A primary malignant tumor, which can be extremely small, will be found in most of the cases.[267] This was true in twenty-three of thirty-four cases reviewed by Ashikari et al.[251] Two-thirds of these tumors were less than 2 cm in diameter. Interestingly, the survival rates were the same whether or not a primary tumor was found in the breast.

The examining physician must be well aware of certain ominous clinical findings of breast carcinoma. The clinical signs indicating inoperability have been listed by Haagensen and

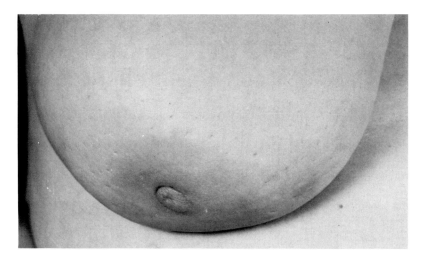

Fig. 1077 Breast in which there was rather prominent edema surrounding nipple. This is an ominous finding. (WU neg. 50-3770.)

Stout.[270] Extensive edema of the breast usually means that tumor has permeated and blocked cutaneous lymphatics and is a sign of an advanced stage of the disease (Fig. 1077).

The pathologic parameters of the usual (Type 3) invasive breast carcinoma that correlate better with survival rates are, in decreasing order of influence, presence and extent of axillary node metastases, size of the primary tumor, stromal reaction, site of the primary tumor, and histologic grade of malignancy.[250,271b] The extent of axillary lymph node involvement can best be estimated by dividing the axillary content into a low, medium, and high group as previously described. In the series of Berg and Robbins,[253] the twenty-year survival rates with negative nodes and with positive nodes at levels I, II and III were 60%, 38%, 30%, and 12%, respectively. Correlations also have been drawn between survival and absolute number of nodes involved (fewer than four versus four or more,[264,284] bulk of the metastatic deposits,[272] and extranodal spread of tumor.[265,277] It has been suggested that the pattern of lymph node response influences survival[286]; even if this were indeed the case, this would still be a poorer prognostic indicator than any of the parameters previously mentioned.[264]

Tumor size correlates well with the incidence of node metastases and with survival rates (Table 52), although exceptions are so many as to make this parameter of little value in the individual case.[263] Because of this, the concept of ''minimal breast carcinoma,'' which includes both in situ carcinomas and invasive carcinomas not larger than 0.5 cm, may be more misleading than useful. Saigo and Rosen[283a] studied 111 patients with invasive breast cancer 1 cm or less in diameter associated with negative nodes who were treated with a minimum of a modified radical mastectomy and followed for at least ten years: 75% were alive with no evidence of disease, 4% were alive with recurrent cancer, 6% had died of disease, and 15% had died of other causes.

The least favorable primary site is the axillary tail; this is followed by the upper outer quadrant, lower inner quadrant, upper inner quadrant, and center.

Histologic grades rely both on the degree of nuclear atypia and extent of tubular formation.[254] There is some suggestion that combining the two provides a better prognostic determination than when they are evaluated individually. Tumor necrosis is associated with an increased incidence of lymph node metastases and decreased survival rates,[259] but this feature is usually associated with tumors of high histologic grade.

The presence of tumor emboli in lymphatic vessels within the breast is associated with an increased risk of distant metastases.[278] Other unfavorable prognostic signs are invasion of the pectoralis muscle and of blood vessel lumina, especially when associated with axillary node metastases.[256,273]

Another important determination to be made with tissue containing breast carcinoma is the

Table 52 Relationship of size of breast cancers to frequency of nodal metastases and death after radical mastectomy*

Diameter of cancer (cm)	Number of patients in whom cancers measured	Number of cancers associated with axillary nodel metastases	Number of patients dying within 60 months after radical mastectomy
1	63	7 (11%)	6 (9%)
1-2	151	60 (40%)	43 (28%)
2-3	190	99 (52%)	72 (38%)
3-4	136	102 (75%)	70 (51%)
4-5	75	56 (74%)	47 (63%)
5-6	37	29 (78%)	30 (81%)
6-7	24	21 (87%)	19 (79%)
7-10	30	25 (83%)	24 (80%)
10+	11	8 (73%)	7 (64%)
Total	717	407 (57%)	318 (44%)

*From Butcher HR Jr: Effectiveness of radical mastectomy for mammary cancer: an analysis of mortalities by the method of probits. Ann. Surg. **154**:383-396, 1961.

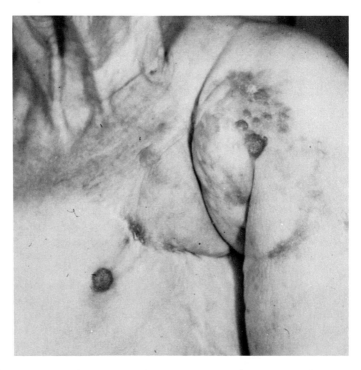

Fig. 1078 Patient with local recurrence of carcinoma twenty-seven years after original operation. (WU neg. 50-1781.)

in vitro evaluation of estrogen receptors, because this has been shown to correlate well with clinical response to hormone therapy and chemotherapy.[271a] The seminal work of Jensen and DeSombre[272b] in this field deserves widespread recognition. The fresh tissue should be deep frozen immediately after excision and submitted to the appropriate laboratory. Immunohistochemical techniques have been attempted for localization of estrogen receptors in tissue sections,[279] but so far the results have not been easily reproducible. Rosen et al.[283] and Eusebi et al.[261] have stated that lobular carcinomas are estrogen receptor–positive with a higher frequency than ductal carcinomas, but in a larger series, Rosen[281a] has not found statistical differences between the two. Several other authors have found no correlation between the histologic type of tumor and the presence of this receptor protein,[287] although there is general agreement that medullary carcinomas and the "comedo" type of intraductal carcinomas usually are negative.[274c,283b,285] Generally, estrogen receptor concentrations are lower in tumors of premenopausal women than in those of postmenopausal women.[283b] Fisher et al.[266a] found positive estrogen receptors to be significantly associated with high nuclear and low histologic grades, absence of tumor necrosis, presence of marked tumor elastosis, and older patients.

The interesting observation has been made that breast cancers with no elastosis have a lower rate of response to endocrine therapy than those with gross elastosis.[277a]

All patients with treated breast carcinoma must be followed indefinitely, because both local recurrence and distant metastases may take place many years after the original operation[256a] (Fig. 1078). Local recurrence is usually in the form of skin nodules around the mastectomy scar or subcutaneous parasternal nodules. The presence of recurrent carcinoma in these nodules as well as in supraclavicular lymph nodes should always be documented by biopsy, because the condition can be closely simulated by foreign body granulomas and infectious processes. Distant metastases are seen most commonly in the skeletal system, lungs, liver, and central nervous system. Bone marrow examination (particularly biopsy) is very efficient in documenting systemic disease,[272a,274b] but the incidence of positivity when both bone scan and roentgenograms are normal is too low (4%) to justify its routine use.

Ever since the Halsted radical mastectomy was proposed as the therapy of choice for resectable breast carcinoma, alternative operations have been advocated in an attempt to increase the survival rates and/or decrease the morbidity.[257,258] Extended radical mastectomies were devised to remove potentially involved lymph nodes that are not included in a routine radical mastectomy, particularly the internal mammary nodes. The overall incidence of involvement of these nodes in operable breast cancer is about 22%.[260] The probability of metastatic disease in this node group can be estimated according to the following formula:

Tumor in outer half and negative axillary nodes	Less than 1%
Tumor in inner half and negative axillary nodes	About 20%
Tumor in outer half and positive axillary nodes	About 30%
Tumor in inner half and positive axillary nodes	Over 50%

Because of these figures, some surgeons have recommended the removal of the internal mammary chain in conjunction with radical mastectomy for all tumors arising in the inner half and/or accompanied by positive axillary nodes.[287] However, it has never been proved that these superradical mastectomies result in better survival. Most surgeons have concluded that internal mammary metastases reflect generalized tumor spread and that local therapy directed at these nodes has a negligible influence on prognosis.[260,274] As a result, this type of operation is rarely performed at the present time. Actually, the question that has preoccupied physicians and patients the most is whether even the standard radical mastectomy might not be too extensive and multilating an operation and whether a more conservative approach might not result in similar survival figures with less morbidity and better cosmetic results. Some of the most respected surgeons in the field remain staunch advocates of the standard radical mastectomy[269]; yet, it seems to us that the evidence accumulated in recent years indicates that lesser operations may do just as well. However, the extent of the ideal procedure remains to be defined. The most extreme conservative approach consists of a local excision of the mass (so-called lumpectomy). Although this type of operation may prove adequate for the most favorable forms of breast cancers, it would seem insufficient therapy for the vast majority of the cases, because of the high frequently with which carcinoma would be left behind. Rosen at al.[282] studied this problem by performing a "local excision" with a 2 cm gross margin in specimens of radical mastectomy and studying microscopically the remainder of the breast. Of eighteen mastectomies for cancer measuring less than 1 cm, residual invasive carcinoma was found in 11% and residual in situ carcinoma in an additional 22%. A somewhat related problem is that of microscopic involvement of the nipple by breast carcinoma, since this structure would obviously be left in the patient if a local excision of the lump were carried out. Lagios et al.[274a] found such an involvement in 30.2% of a consecutive series of 149 mastectomy specimens; 94% were associated with tumors located less than 2.5 cm from the nipple.

A seemingly more logical approach has been to combine local excision with postoperative radiation therapy. This was done by Wise et al.[288] for Stages I and II cancer; their survival curves were comparable to those obtained with radical mastectomy, but the study was nonrandomized. A slight extension of this approach consists of simple mastectomy followed by radiation therapy, as advocated many years ago by McWhirter[276]; again, the results were comparable to those of radical mastectomy, but lack of randomization prevented this study from being widely accepted.

The operation known as modified radical mastectomy (better designated as total mastectomy with axillary dissection) is gaining an increasingly large number of supporters because it appears to represent the best possible compromise.[262a] This operation consists of removal of the breast and of low and mid axillary lymph nodes, with preservation of the pectoralis muscle.[252] It seems certain that this operation is preferable to radical mastectomy for Types I and II carcinomas, and there is mounting evidence that it may be just as good for most of the others.

Finally, ''radical'' radiation therapy has been used by some as the primary treatment for breast carcinoma, with or without a preoperative lumpectomy.[279a]

It is likely that the outcome in breast cancer is more dependent on the nature of the individual tumor than on the type of therapy performed. There is certainly a striking similarity in survival rates from different centers employing widely disparate therapeutic approaches.[275] A complicating factor in evaluating therapeutic results is the marked individual variations in the natural life history of the disease, which renders imperative the use of carefully randomized studies. Bloom et al.[255] provided a good baseline on which to judge the effectiveness of therapy by showing that in a series of 250 *untreated* breast cancers, the five-year survival rate after diagnosis was 18%.

The problem of comparing results and reaching an agreement on this field is well demonstrated by the data and arguments put forward in recent years.[262,271] In 1971, the National Surgical Adjuvant Breast Project implemented a well-planned and well–carried out prospective randomized clinical trial to compare the relative worth of the following therapies:

I With clinically negative axillary nodes
  1 Conventional radical mastectomy
  2 Total mastectomy with postoperative regional radiation
  3 Total mastectomy alone (followed by axillary dissection in those patients who subsequently develop positive nodes)
II With clinically positive axillary nodes
  1 Conventional radical mastectomy
  2 Total mastectomy with postoperative regional radiation

The results of this trial, presently in its sixth year, have been published.[266] So far, no significant differences in treatment failure or survival have been detected in either group.

All the evidence that is accumulating from these studies seems to challenge the traditional concepts of the biology of breast carcinoma, which led to the establishment of Halsted's radical mastectomy as the treatment of choice. These traditional concepts can be paraphrased as follows: breast cancer spreads in an orderly manner, mainly on the basis of mechanical factors; regional lymph nodes are barriers to the passage of tumor cells but, eventually, are the instigators of distant disease; the bloodstream is of little significance as a route of tumor dissemination; a tumor is autonomous of its host; operable breast cancer is a local-regional disease; and the extent and nuances of the operation are the dominant factors influencing patient outcome.

Against these time-honored concepts, Fisher et al.[266] have proposed these alternative ones: there is no orderly pattern of tumor dissemination; regional nodes are ineffective as barriers to tumor spread and, when positive, are more an indicator of a particular host-tumor relationship than the instigator of distant metastases; the bloodstream is of considerable importance in tumor dissemination; complex host-tumor interrelationships affect every facet of the disease; operable breast cancer is a systemic disease; and variations in local-regional therapy are unlikely to substantially affect survival.

REFERENCES
Method of pathologic examination

1 Davies JD, Roberts G, Richardson PJ: Technical methods. A serial whole-organ slicing technique for examining surgically resected breasts. J Clin Pathol **26**: 891-892, 1973.
2 Editorial: Hormone-receptor assays and cancer of the breast. Am J Clin Pathol **70**:719-720, 1978.

3 Fisher ER, Palekar A, Kim WS, Redmond C: The histopathology of mammographic patterns. Am J Clin Pathol **69:**421-426, 1978.

4 Fisher ER, Swamidoss S, Lee CH, Rockette H, Redmond C, Fisher B: Detection and significance of occult axillary node metastases in patients with invasive breast cancer. Cancer **42:**2025-2031, 1978.

5 Gallager HS: Breast specimen radiography. Obligatory, adjuvant and investigative. Am J Clin Pathol **64:**749-766, 1975.

6 Koehl RH, Snyder RE, Hutter RVP, Foote FW Jr: The incidence and significance of calcifications within operative breast specimens. Am J Clin Pathol **53:** 3-14, 1970.

7 McDivitt RW: Breast carcinoma. Hum Pathol **9:**3-21, 1978.

8 Monroe CW: Lymphatic spread of carcinoma of the breast. Arch Surg **57:**479-486, 1948.

9 National Cancer Institute: Standardized management of breast specimens. Recommended by Pathology Clin Pathol **60:**789-798, 1973.

10 Pickren JW: Significance of occult metastases. A study of breast cancer. Cancer **14:**1266-1273, 1961.

11 Rosen PP, Snyder RE, Robbins G: Specimen radiography for nonpalpable breast lesions found by mammography: procedures and results. Cancer **34:**2028-2033, 1974.

12 Rosen P, Snyder RE, Foote FW, Wallace, T: Detection of occult carcinoma in the apparently benign breast biopsy through specimen radiography. Cancer **26:**944-952, 1970.

13 Saphir O, Amromin GD: Obscure axillary lymph node metastasis in carcinoma of the breast, Cancer **1:** 238-241, 1948.

14 Stevens GM, Jamplis RW: Mammographically directed biopsy of nonpalpable breast lesions. Arch Surg **102:**292-295, 1971.

15 Wolfe JN: Breast patterns as an index of risk for developing breast cancer. Am J Roentgenol **126:** 1130-1139, 1976.

Cytology

16 Franzén S, Zajicek J: Aspiration biopsy in diagnosis of palpable lesions of the breast. Critical review of 3479 consecutive biopsies. Acta Radiol [Ther]

17 Hajdu DI, Melamed ME: The diagnostic value of aspiration smears. Am J Clin Pathol **59:**350-356, 1973.

18 Kline TS, Neal HS: Needle aspiration biopsy: a critical appraisal. Eight years and 3,267 specimens later. JAMA **239:**36-39, 1978.

19 Kline TS, Neal HS: Needle aspiration of the breast why bother? Acta Cytol (Baltimore) **20:**324-327, 1976. 1976.

20 Kline TS, Joshi LP, Neal HS: Fine-needle aspiration of the breast: diagnoses and pitfalls. A review of 3545 cases. Cancer **44:**1458-1464, 1979.

21 Kreuzer G, Boquoi E: Aspiration biopsy cytology, mammography and clinical exploration: a modern set up in diagnosis of tumors of the breast. Acta Cytol (Baltimore) **20:**319-323, 1976.

22 Linsk J, Kreuzer G, Zajicek J: Cytologic diagnosis of mammary tumors from aspiration biopsy smears. II. Studies on 210 fibroadenomas and 210 cases of benign dysplasia. Acta Cytol **16:**130-138, 1972.

23 McDivitt RH: Breast carcinoma. Hum Pathol **9:**3-21, 1978.

24 Rosen P, Najdu SI, Robbins G, Foote FW: Diagnosis of carcinoma of the breast by aspiration biopsy. Surg Gynecol Obstet **134:**837-838, 1972.

25 Van Bogaert LJ, Mazy G: Reliability of the cyto-radio-clinical triplet in breast pathology diagnosis. Acta Cytol (Baltimore) **21:**60-62, 1977.

26 Wilson SL, Ehrmann RL: The cytologic diagnosis of breast aspirations. Acta Cytol **22:**470-475, 1978.

27 Zajdela A, Ghossein A, Pilleron JP, Ennuyer A: The value of aspiration cytology in the diagnosis of breast cancer: experience at the Fondation Curie. Cancer **35:** 499-506, 1975.

Frozen section

28 Saltzstein SL: Histologic diagnosis of breast carcinoma with the Silverman needle biopsy. Surgery **48:**366-374, 1960.

Inflammatory lesions

29 Adair FE: Plasma cell mastitis. A lesion simulating mammary carcinoma. Arch Surg **26:**735-749, 1933.

30 Cutler M: Plasma-cell mastitis. Report of a case with bilateral involvement. Br Med J **1:**94-96, 1949.

31 Halpert B, Parker JM, Thuringer JM: Plasma cell mastitis. Arch Pathol **46:**313-319, 1948.

32 Tuttle HK, Kean BH: Circumscribed chronic suppurative mastitis simulating cancer. Surg Gynecol Obstet **84:**933-938, 1947.

Fat necrosis

33 Adair FE, Munzer JT: Fat necrosis of the female breast. Am J Surg **74:**117-128, 1947.

34 Binkley JS: Relapsing nodular nonsuppurative panniculitis. JAMA **113:**113-116, 1939.

35 Foote FW, Stewart FW; Comparative studies of cancerous vs. noncancerous breasts. Ann Surg **121:**6-79, 1945.

36 Hadfield G: Fat necrosis of the breast. Br J Surg **17:** 673-682, 1930.

37 Lee BJ, Adair FE: Traumatic fat necrosis of the female breast and its differentiation from carcinoma. Ann Surg **72:**188-195, 1920.

38 Lee BJ, Adair FE: Traumatic fat necrosis of the female breast and its differentiation from carcinoma. Ann. Surg. **80:**670-691, 1924.

Mammary duct ectasia

39 Haagensen CD: Mammary-duct ectasia. A disease that may simulate carcinoma. Cancer **4:**749-761, 1951.

40 Lepper EH, Weaver MO: Generalized distention of the ducts of the breast by fatty secretion. J Pathol Bacteriol **45:**465-467, 1937.

Fibrocystic disease

41 Ashikari R, Huvos, AG, Snyder RE, Lucas JC, Hutter RVP, McDivitt RW, Schottenfeld D: A clinicopathologic study of atypical lesions of the breast. Cancer **33:**310-317, 1974.

41a Azzopardi JG: Problems in breast pathology. Vol. 11 of Bennington JL (consulting ed): Major problems in pathology. Philadelphia, 1979, W. B. Saunders Co.

42 Bhagavan BS, Patchefsky A, Koss LG: Florid subareolar duct papillomatosis (nipple adenoma) and mammary carcinoma: report of three cases. Hum Pathol **4:**289-295, 1973.

43 Eusebi V, Azzopardi JG: Vascular infiltration in benign breast disease. J Pathol **118:**9-16, 1976.

44 Fenoglio C, Lattes R: Sclerosing papillary proliferations in the female breast. A benign lesion often mistaken for carcinoma. Cancer **33:**691-700, 1974.

45 Fisher ER, Paulson JD: Karyotypic abnormalities in

precursor lesions of human cancer of the breast. Am J Clin Pathol **69:**284-288, 1978.

46 Fisher ER, Palekar AS, Kotwal N, Lipana N: A non-encapsualted sclerosing lesion of the breast. Am J. Clin Pathol **71:**240-246, 1979.

47 Foote FW, Stewart FW: Comparative studies of cancerous vs. noncancerous breasts. Ann Surg **121:**6-79, 1945.

48 Frantz VK, Pickren JW, Melcher GW, Auchincloss H Jr: Incidence of chronic cystic disease in so-called "normal breast." Cancer **4:**762-783, 1951.

49 Golinger RC: Hormones and the pathophysiology of fibrocystic mastopathy. Surg Gynecol Obstet **146:**273-285, 1978.

50 Haagensen CD: Diseases of the breast, ed. 2, Philadephia, 1971, W. B. Saunders Co.

50a Hutchinson WB, Thomas DB, Hamlin WB, Roth GJ, Peterson AV, Williams B: Risk of breast cancer in women with benign breast disease. J Natl Cancer Inst **65:**13-20, 1980.

51 Kern WH, Brooks RN: Atypical epithelial hyperplasia associated with breast cancer and fibrocystic disease. Cancer **24:**668-675, 1969.

52 Kiaer W: Relation of fibroadenomatosis ("chronic mastitis") to cancer of the breast. Copenhagen, 1954, Munksgaard.

53 Le Gal Y, Gros CM, Bader P: L'adenomatose erosive du mamelon. Ann Acad Path (Paris) **4:**292-304, 1959.

54 McDivitt RW: Breast carcinoma. Hum Pathol **9:**3-21, 1978.

55 Minkowitz S, Hedayati H, Hiller S, Gardner B: Fibrous mastopathy: a clinical histopathologic study. Cancer **32:**913-916, 1973.

56 Perzin KH, Lattes R: Papillary adenoma of the nipple (florid papillomatosis, adenoma, adenomatosis). A clinicopathologic study. Cancer **29:**996-1009, 1972.

57 Sandison AT: An autopsy study of the adult human breast: with special reference to proliferative epithelial changes of importance in the pathology of the breast. Natl Cancer Inst Monogr **8:**1-145, 1962.

58 Steinhoff NG, Black, WC: Florid cystic disease preceding mammary cancer. Ann Surg **171:**501-508, 1970.

59 Taylor HB, Norris HJ: Epithelial invasion of nerves in benign diseases of the breast. Cancer **20:**2245-2249, 1967.

60 Taylor HB, Robertson AG: Adenomas of the nipple. Cancer **18:**995-1002, 1966.

61 Tremblay G, Buell RH, Seemayer TA; Elastosis in benign sclerosing ductal proliferation of the female breast. Am J Surg Pathol **1:**155-159, 1977.

62 Urban JA, Adair FE: Sclerosing adenosis. Cancer **2:**625-634, 1949.

Benign tumors

62a Azzopardi JG: Problems in breast pathology. Vol. 11 of Bennington JL (consulting ed): Major problems in pathology. Philadelphia, 1979, W. B. Saunders Co.

63 Bannayan GA, Hajdu SI: Gynecomastia: clinicopathologic study of 351 cases. Am J Clin Pathol **57:**431-437, 1972.

64 Buzanowski-Konakry K, Harrison EG Jr, Payne WS: Lobular carcinoma arising in fibroadenoma of the breast. Cancer **35:**450-456, 1975.

65 Carstens PHB: Ultrastructure of human fibroadenoma. Arch Pathol **98:**23-32, 1974.

66 Curran RC, Dodge OG: Sarcoma of breast, with particular reference to its origin from fibroadenoma. J Clin Pathol **15:**1-16, 1962.

66a Eusebi V, Azzopardi JG: Lobular endocrine neoplasia in fibroadenoma of the breast. Histopathology **4:**413-428, 1980.

67 Fisher ER, Creed DL: Nature of the periductal stroma in gynecomastia. Lab Invest **5:**267-275, 1956.

68 Fondo EY, Rosen PP, Fracchia AA, Urban JA: The problem of carcinoma developing in a fibroadenoma. Recent experience at Memorial Hospital. Cancer **43:**563-567, 1979.

69 Goldman RC, Friedman NB: Carcinoma of the breast arising in fibroadenomas with emphasis on lobular carcinoma. A clinicopathologic study. Cancer **23:**544-550, 1969.

70 Haagensen CD, Stout AP: Granular cell myoblastoma of the mammary gland. Ann Surg **124:**218-227, 1946.

71 Haagensen CD, Stout AP, Phillips JS: The papillary neoplasms of the breast. Ann Surg **133:**18-36, 1951.

72 Hertel BF, Zaloudek C, Kempson RL: Breast adenomas. Cancer **37:**2891-2905, 1976.

72a Kiaer HW, Kiaer WW, Linell F, Jacobsen S: Extreme duct papillomatosis of the juvenile breast. Acta Pathol Microbiol Scand [A] **87:**353-359, 1979.

73 Kraus FT, Neubecker RD: The differential diagnosis of papillary tumors of the breast. Cancer **15:**444-455, 1962.

74 Le Gal Y: Adenomas of the breast: relationship of adenofibromas to pregnancy and lactation. Am Surg **27:**14-22, 1961.

75 McDivitt RW, Holleb AI, Foote FW: Prior breast disease in patients treated for papillary carcinoma. Arch Pathol **85:**117-124, 1968.

76 McDivitt RW, Stewart FW, Farrow JH: Breast carcinoma arising in solitary fibroadenomas. Surg Gynecol Obstet **125:**572-576, 1967.

77 Madalin HE, Clagett OT, McDonald JR: Lesions of the breast associated with discharge from the nipple. Ann Surg **146:**751-763, 1957.

78 Murad TM, Swaid S, Pritchett P: Malignant and benign papillary lesions of the breast. Hum Pathol **8:**379-390, 1977.

79 Oberman HA, Nosanchuk HS, Finger JE: Periductal stromal tumors of breast with adipose metaplasia. Arch Surg **98:**384-387, 1969.

79a Rosen PP, Cantrell B, Mullen DL, DePalo A: Juvenile papillomatosis (Swiss cheese disease) of the breast. Am J Surg Pathol **4:**3-12, 1980.

80 Sirtori C, Veronesi U: Gynecomastia. A review of 218 cases. Cancer **10:**645-654, 1957.

81 Snyder WH, Chaffin L: Main duct papilloma of the breast. Arch Surg **70:**680-685, 1955.

82 Wheeler CE, Cawley EP, Curtis AC: Gynecomastia: a review and an analysis of 160 cases. Ann Intern Med **40:**985-1004, 1954.

83 Williams MJ: Gynecomastia: its incidence, recognition and host characterization in 447 autopsy cases. Am J Med **34:**103-112, 1963.

Malignant tumors
Carcinoma

84 Fisher ER: Ultrastructure of the human breast and its disorders. Am J Clin Pathol **66:**291-374, 1976.

85 Fisher ER, Gregorio R, Redmond C, Vellios F, Sommers SC, Fisher B: Pathologic findings from the National Surgical Adjuvant Breast Project (Protocol

no. 4). I. Observations concerning the multicentricity of mammary cancer. Cancer **35**:247-254, 1975.

86 Gould VE, Miller J, Jao W: Ultrastructure of medullary, intraductal, tubular and adenocystic breast carcinomas. Comparative patterns of myoepithelial differentiation and basal lamina deposition. Am J Pathol **78**:401-407, 1975.

87 King RE, Terz JJ, Lawrence W Jr: Experience with opposite breast biopsy in patients with operable breast cancer. Cancer **37**:43-45, 1976.

87a Mesa-Tejada R, Keydar I, Ramanarayanan M, Ohno T, Fenoglio C, Spiegelman S: Detection in human breast carcinomas of an antigen immunologically related to a group-specific antigen of mouse mammary tumor virus. Proc Natl Acad Sci USA **75**:1529-1533, 1978.

87b Spiegelman S, Keydar I, Mesa-Tejada R, Ohno T, Ramanarayanan M, Nayak R, Bausch J, Fenoglio C: Possible diagnostic implications of a mammary tumor virus related protein in human breast cancer. Cancer **46**:879-892, 1980.

Invasive ductal carcinoma

88 Azzopardi JG, Laurini RN: Elastosis in breast cancer. Cancer **33**:174-183, 1974.

89 Davies JD: Hyperelastosis, obliteration and fibrous plaques in major ducts of the human breast. J Pathol **110**:13-26, 1973.

90 Fisher ER, Palekar AS, Gregorio RM, Redmond C, Fisher B: Pathological findings from the National Surgical Adjuvant Breast Project (Protocol no. 4). IV. Significance of tumor necrosis. Hum Pathol **9**:523-530, 1978.

91 Hutter RVP, Kim DU: The problem of multiple lesions of the breast. Cancer **28**:1591-1607, 1971.

92 Jackson JG, Orr JW: The ducts of carcinomatous breasts, with particular reference to connective-tissue changes. J Pathol Bacteriol **74**:265-273, 1957.

93 Qualheim RE, Gall EA: Breast carcinoma with multiple sites of origin. Cancer **10**:460-468, 1957.

94 Tremblay G, Buell RH, Seemayer TA: Elastosis in benign sclerosing ductal proliferation of the female breast. Am J Surg Pathol **1**:155-159, 1977.

Intraductal carcinoma with or without invasion

95 Betsill WL, Rosen PP, Robbins GF: Intraductal carcinoma: long term follow-up after treatment by biopsy only. JAMA **239**:1863-1867, 1978.

95a Brown PW, Silverman J, Owens E, Tabor DC, Terz JJ, Lawrence W Jr: Intraductal "noninfiltrating" carcinoma of the breast. Arch Surg **111**:1063-1067, 1976.

96 Carter D, Smith RRL: Carcinoma in situ of the breast. Cancer **40**:1189-1193, 1977.

97 Fisher ER, Gregorio RM, Fisher B with assistance of Redmond C, Vellios F, Sommers SC, and cooperating investigators: The pathology of invasive breast cancer. A syllabus derived from findings of the National Surgical Adjuvant Breast Project (Protocol no. 4). Cancer **36**:1-85, 1975.

98 Frable WJ, Kay S: Carcinoma of the breasts. Histologic and clinical features of apocrine tumors. Cancer **21**:756-763, 1968.

99 Millis RR, Thynne GSJ: In situ intraduct carcinoma of the breast: a long-term follow-up study. Brit J Surg **62**:957-962, 1975.

99a Rosen PP: Axillary lymph node metastases in patients with occult noninvasive breast carcinoma. Cancer **46**:1298-1306, 1980.

99b Rosen PP, Braun DW Jr, Kinne DE: The clinical significance of pre-invasive breast carcinoma. Cancer **46**:919-925, 1980.

100 Rosen PP, Senie R, Schottenfeld D, Ashikari R: Noninvasive breast carcinoma. Ann Surg **189**:377-382, 1979.

101 Silverberg SG, Chitale AR: Assessment of significance of proportions of intraductal and infiltrating tumor growth in ductal carcinoma of the breast. Cancer **32**:830-837, 1973.

102 Westbrook KC, Gallager HS: Intraductal carcinoma of the breast. A comparative study. Am J Surg **130**:667-670, 1975.

Medullary carcinoma

103 Bloom HJG, Richardson WW, Fields JR: Host resistance and survival in carcinoma of breasts. A study of 104 cases of medullary carcinoma in a series of 1,411 cases of breast cancer followed for 20 years. Br Med J **3**:181-188, 1970.

104 Moore OS Jr, Foote FW Jr: The relatively favorable prognosis of medullary carcinoma of the breast. Cancer **2**:635-642, 1949.

105 Richardson WW: Medullary carcinoma of the breast A distinctive tumour type with a relatively good prognosis following radical mastectomy. Br J Cancer **10**:415-423, 1956.

106 Ridolfi RL, Rosen PP, Port A, Kinne D, Miké V: Medullary carcinoma of the breast. A clinicopathologic study with 10 year follow-up. Cancer **40**:1365-1385, 1977.

Paget's disease

107 Ashikari R, Park K, Huvos AG, Urban JA: Paget's disease of the breast. Cancer **26**:680-685, 1970.

108 Bussolati G, Pich A: Mammary and extramammary Paget's disease. An immunocytochemical study. Am J Pathol **80**:117-127, 1975.

109 Neubecker RD, Bradshaw RP: Mucin, melanin, and glycogen in Paget's disease of the breast. Am J Clin Pathol **36**:40-53, 1961.

110 Paget J: On disease of the mammary areola preceding cancer of the mammary gland. St Barth Hosp Rep **10**:87-89, 1874.

111 Sagebiel RW: Ultrastructural observations on epidermal cells in Paget's disease of the breast. Am J Pathol **57**:49-64, 1969.

Inflammatory carcinoma

112 Ellis DL, Teitelbaum SL: Inflammatory carcinoma of the breast. A pathological definition. Cancer **33**:1045-1047, 1974.

113 Lucas FV, Perez-Mesa C: Inflammatory carcinoma of the breast. Cancer **41**:1595-1605, 1978.

114 Saltzstein SL: Clinically occult inflammatory carcinoma of the breast. Cancer **34**:382-388, 1974.

Papillary carcinoma with or without invasion

114a Azzopardi JG: Problems in breast pathology. Vol 11 of Bennington JL (consulting ed): Major problems in pathology. Philadelphia, 1979, W. B. Saunders Co.

114b Fisher ER, Palekar AS, Redmond C, Barton B, Fisher B: Pathologic findings from the National Surgical Adjuvant Breast Project (Protocol No. 4). VI. Invasive papillary cancer. Am J Clin Pathol **73**:313-322, 1980.

115 Kraus FT, Neubecker RD: The differential diagnosis

of papillary tumors of the breast. Cancer **15**:444-455, 1962.

116 Murad TM, Swaid S, Pritchett P: Malignant and benign papillary lesions of the breast. Hum Pathol **8**: 379-380, 1977.

Mucinous carcinoma

116a Capella C, Eusebi V, Mann B, Azzopardi JG: Endocrine differentiation in mucoid carcinoma of the breast. Histopathology **4**:613-630, 1980.

116b Fisher ER, Palekar AS, NSABP collaborators: Solid and mucinous varieties of so-called mammary carcinoid tumors. Am J Clin Pathol **72**:909-916, 1979.

117 Norris HJ, Taylor HB: Prognosis of mucinous (gelatinous) carcinoma of the breast. Cancer **18**:879-885, 1965.

117a Rosen PP, Wang T-Y: Colloid carcinoma of the breast: analysis of 64 patients with long-term follow-up. Am J Clin Pathol **73**:304, 1980 (abstract).

118 Saphir O: Mucinous carcinoma of the breast. Surg Gynecol Obstet **72**:908-914, 1941.

Epidermoid carcinoma

119 Cornog JL, Mobini J, Steiger E, Enterline HT: Squamous carcinoma of the breast. Am J Clin Pathol **55**: 410-417, 1971.

120 Gersell D, Katzenstein A: Spindle cell carcinoma of the breast: a clinicopathologic and ultrastructural study. Lab Invest **40**:256, 1979 (abstract).

121 McDivitt RW, Stewart FW, Berg JW: Tumors of the breast. In Atlas of tumor pathology, 2nd series, Fasc. 2. Washington, D. C., 1968, Armed Forces Institute of Pathology.

Adenoid cystic carcinoma

122 Cavanzo FJ, Taylor HB: Adenoid cystic carcinoma of the breast. An analysis of 21 cases. Cancer **24**: 740-745, 1969.

123 Elsner B: Adenoid cystic carcinoma of the breast. Review of the literature and clinicopathologic study of seven patients. Pathol Eur **5**:357-364, 1970.

124 Harris M, Pseudoadenoid cystic carcinoma of the breast. Arch Pathol Lab Med **101**:307-309, 1977.

125 Koss LG, Brannan CD, Ashikari R: Histologic and ultrastructural features of adenoid cystic carcinoma of the breast. Cancer **26**:1271-1279, 1970.

126 Nayer HR: Cylindroma of the breast with pulmonary metastases. Dis Chest **31**:324-327, 1957

Well-differentiated (tubular) carcinoma

127 Cooper HS, Patchefsky AS, Krall RA: Tubular carcinoma of the breast. Cancer **42**:2334-2342, 1978.

128 Erlandson RA, Carstens PHB: Ultrastructure of tubular carcinoma of the breast. Cancer **29**:987-995, 1972.

128a Flotte TJ, Bell DA, Greco MA: Tubular carcinoma and sclerosing adenosis. The use of basal lamina as a differential feature. Am J Surg Pathol **4**:75-77, 1980.

129 Jao W, Recant W, Swerdlow MA: Comparative ultrastructure of tubular carcinoma and sclerosing adenosis of the breast. Cancer **38**:180-186, 1976.

129a Lagios MD, Rose MR, Margolin FR: Tubular carcinoma of the breast. Association with multicentricity, bilaterality, and family history of mammary carcinoma. Am J Clin Pathol **73**:25-30, 1980.

129b Linell F, Ljungberg O, Andersson I: Breast carcinoma. Aspects of early stages, progression and related problems. Acta Pathol Microbiol Scand [A] [Suppl] **272**:1-233, 1980.

129c Oberman HA, Fidler WJ Jr: Tubular carcinoma of the breast. Am J Surg Pathol **3**:387-395, 1979.

130 Taylor HB, Norris HJ: Well-differentiated carcinoma of the breast. Cancer **25**:687-692, 1970.

131 Tobon H, Salazar H: Tubular carcinoma of the breast. Clinical histological, and ultrastructural observations. Arch Pathol Lab Med **101**:310-316, 1977.

Lobular carcinoma

132 Andersen JA: Invasive breast carcinoma with lobular involvement. Frequency and location of lobular carcinoma in situ. Acta Pathol Microbiol Scand [A] **82**: 719-729, 1974.

133 Andersen JA: Lobular carcinoma in situ. A histological study of 52 cases. Acta Pathol Microbiol Scand [A] **82**:735-741, 1974.

134 Andersen JA: Lobular carcinoma in situ. A long-term follow-up in 52 cases. Acta Path Microbiol Scand [A] **82**:519-533, 1974.

135 Andersen JA: Lobular carcinoma in situ of the breast. An approach to rational treatment. Cancer **39**:2597-2602, 1977.

136 Andersen JA: Lobular carcinoma in situ of the breast with ductal involvement. Frequency and possible influence on prognosis. Acta Pathol Microbiol Scand [A] **82**:655-662, 1974.

137 Battifora H: Intracytoplasmic lumina in breast carcinoma. A helpful histopathologic features. Arch Pathol **99**:614-617, 1975.

138 Breslow A, Brancaccio ME: Intracellular mucin production by lobular breast carcinoma cells. Arch Pathol Lab Med **100**:620-621, 1976.

139 Eusebi V: Il carcinoma lobulare della mammella. Patologíca **67**:19-37, 1975.

139a Eusebi V, Betts CM, Bussolati G: Tubular carcinoma: a variant of secretory breast carcinoma. Histopathology **3**:407-419, 1979.

140 Eusebi V, Pich A, Macchiorlatti E, Bussolati G: Morpho-functional differentiation in lobular carcinoma of the breast. Histopathology **1**:301-314, 1977.

141 Fechner RE: Ductal carinoma involving the lobule of the breast: a source of confusion with lobular carcinoma in situ. Cancer **28**:274-281, 1971.

142 Fechner RE: Epithelial alterations in the extralobular ducts of breasts with lobular carcinoma. Arch Pathol **93**:164-171, 1972.

143 Fechner RE: Infiltrating lobular carcinoma without lobular carcinoma in situ. Cancer **29**:1539-1545, 1972.

144 Fechner RE: Histologic variants of infiltrating lobular carcinoma of the breast. Hum Pathol **6**:373-378, 1975.

145 Fisher ER, Gregorio RM, Redmond C, Fisher B: Tubulolobular invasive breast cancer: a variant of lobular invasive cancer. Hum Pathol **8**:679-683, 1977.

146 Foote FW, Stewart, FW: Lobular carcinoma in situ. Am J Pathol **17**:491-496, 1941.

147 Haagensen CD, Lane N, Lattes R: Neoplastic proliferation of the epithelium of the mammary lobules: adenosis, lobular neoplasia and small cell carcinoma. Surg Clin North Am **52**:497-524, 1972.

148 Haagensen CD, Lane N, Lattes R, Bodian C: Lobular neoplasia (so-called lobular carcinoma in situ) of the breast. Cancer **42**:737-769, 1978.

149 Hassler O: Microradiographic investigations of calcifications of the female breast. Cancer **23**:1103-1109, 1969.

149a Hull MT, Seo IS, Battersby JS, Csicsko JF: Signetring carcinoma of the breast. A clinicopathologic study of 24 cases. Am J Clin Pathol **73**:31-35, 1980.

150 Hutter RVP, Snyder RE, Lucas JC, Foote FW Jr, Farrow JH: Clinical and pathologic correlation with mammographic findings in lobular carcinoma in situ. Cancer **23:**826-839, 1969.

151 Lambird PA, Shelley WM: The spatial distribution of lobular in situ mammary carcinoma. Implications for size and site of breast biopsy. JAMA **210:** 689-693, 1969.

151a Martinez V, Azzopardi JG: Invasive lobular carcinoma of the breast: incidence and variants. Histopathology **3:**467-488, 1979.

152 Newman W: Lobular carcinoma of the female breast. Ann Surg **164:**305-314, 1966.

152a Rosen PP: Coexistent lobular carcinoma in situ and intraductal carcinoma in a single lobular-duct unit. Am J Surg Pathol **4:**241-246, 1980.

153 Rosen PP, Kosloff C, Lieberman PH, Adair F, Braun DW Jr: Lobular carcinoma in situ of the breast. Detailed analysis of 99 patients with average follow-up of 24 years. Am J Surg Pathol **2:**225-251, 1978.

154 Steinbrecher JS, Silverberg SG: Signet-ring cell carcinoma of the breast. The mucinous variant of infiltrating lobular carcinoma? Cancer **37:**828-840, 1976.

155 Tobon H, Price HM: Lobular carcinoma in situ. Some ultrastructural observations. Cancer **39:**1082-1091, 1972.

155a van Bogaert L-J, Maldague P: Infiltrating lobular carcinoma of the female breast. Deviations from the usual histopathologic appearance. Cancer **45:**979-984, 1980.

156 Warner NE: Lobular carcinoma of the breast. Cancer **23:**840-846, 1969.

157 Wheeler JE, Enterline HT: Lobular carcinoma of the breast in situ and infiltrating. Pathol Ann **11:**161-188, 1976.

158 Wheeler JE, Enterline HT, Roseman JM, Tomasulo JP, McIlraine CH, Fitts WT, Jr, Kirshenbaum J: Lobular carcinoma in situ of the breast. Long-term follow-up. Cancer **34:**554-563, 1974.

Other types

158a Agnantis NT, Rosen PP: Mammary carcinoma with osteoclast-like giant cells. A study of eight cases with follow-up data. Am J Clin Pathol **72:**383-389, 1979.

159 Cubilla AL, Woodruff JM: Primary carcinoid tumor of the breast. A report of eight patients. Am J Surg Pathol **1:**283-292, 1977.

160 Fisher ER, Gregorio R, Kim WS, Redmond C: Lipid in invasive cancer of the breast. Am J Clin Pathol **68:**558-561, 1977.

161 Harrist TJ, Kalisher L: Breast metastasis: an unusual manifestation of a malignant carcinoid tumor. Cancer **40:**3102-3106, 1977.

162 Hood CI, Front RL, Zimmerman LE: Metastatic mammary carcinoma in the eyelid, with histiocytoid appearance. Cancer **31:**793-800, 1973.

163 Kaneko H, Hōjō H, Ishikawa S, Yamanouchi H, Sumida T, Saito R: Norepinephrine-producing tumors of bilateral breasts. A case report. Cancer **41:**2002-2007, 1978.

164 Llombart-Bosch A, Peydro A: Malignant mixed osteogenic tumours of the breast. An ultrastructural study of two cases. Virchows Arch [Pathol Anat] **366:**1-14, 1975.

165 Patchefsky AS, Frauenhoffer CM, Krall RA, Cooper HS: Low-grade mucoepidermoid carcinoma of the breast. Arch Pathol Lab Med **103:**196-198, 1979.

166 Ramos CV, Taylor HB: Lipid-rich carcinoma of the breast. Cancer **33:**812-819, 1974.

167 Smith BH, Taylor HB: The occurrence of bone and cartilage in mammary tumors. Am J Clin Pathol **51:** 610-618, 1969.

Classification and grading

168 Bloom HJC, Richardson WW: Histological grading and prognosis in breast cancer. A study of 1409 cases of which 359 have been followed for 15 years. Br J Cancer **11:**359-377, 1957.

169 Fisher ER: The pathologist's role in the diagnosis and treatment of invasive breast cancer. Surg Clin North Am **58:**705-721, 1978.

170 Hultborn KA, Tornberg B: Mammary carcinoma. The biologic character of mammary carcinoma studied in 517 cases by a new form of malignancy grading. Acta Radiol [Suppl] (Stockh) **196:**1-143, 1960.

171 Kouchoukos NT, Ackerman LV, Butcher HR, Jr: Prediction of axillary nodal metastases from the morphology of primary mammary carcinomas—a guide to operative therapy. Cancer **20:**948-960, 1967.

172 Lane N, Boksel H, Salerno RA, Haagensen CD: Clinico-pathologic analysis of the surgical curability of breast cancers: a minimum ten-year study of personal series. Ann Surg **153:**483-498, 1961.

Effects of irradiation

173 Ackerman LV: An evaluation of the treatment of cancer of the breast at the University of Edinburgh (Scotland), under the direction of Dr. Robert McWhirter. Cancer **8:**883-887, 1955.

174 Guttman R: Survival and results after 2-million volt irradiation in the treatment of primary operable carcinoma of the breast with proved internal mammary and/or highest axillary node metastases. Cancer **15:** 383, 1962.

175 McWhirter R: The treatment of carcinoma of the breast. Irish J Med Sci 6th series, pp. 475-483, 1956.

Effects of steroid hormones

176 Eckert C, Aikman W, Weichselbaum TE, Elman R, Ackerman LV: Surgical oophorectomy and adrenalectomy in the management of advanced breast cancer: clinical indications and results. South Med J **49:** 437-443, 1956.

177 Emerson WJ, Kennedy BJ, Graham JN, Nathanson IT: Pathology of primary and recurrent carcinoma of the human breast after administration of steroid hormones. Cancer **6:**641-670, 1953.

178 Lemon HM: Medical treatment of cancer of the breast and prostate. Disease-a-Month, May, 1959.

Cystosarcoma phyllodes/Other stromal tumors and tumorlike conditions/Malignant lymphoma and related lesions

178a Ali M, Fayemi AO, Braun EV, Remy R: Fibromatosis of the breast. Am J Surg Pathol **3:**501-505, 1979.

178b Azzopardi JG: Problems in breast pathology. Vol. 11 of Bennington JL (consulting ed): Major problems in pathology. Philadelphia, 1979, W. B. Saunders Co.

179 Barnes L, Pietruszka M: Rhabdomyosarcoma arising within a cystosarcoma phyllodes. Case report and review of the literature. Am J Surg Pathol **2:**423-429, 1978.

180 Beltaos E, Banerjee TK: Chondrosarcoma of the breast. Report of two cases. Am J Clin Pathol **71:** 345-349, 1979.

180a Brooks JJ, Krugman DT, Damjanov I: Myeloid metaplasia presenting as a breast mass. Am J Surg Pathol **4:**281-285, 1980.

181 De Cosse JJ, Berg JW, Fracchia AA, and Farrow JH: Primary lymphosarcoma of the breast: a review of 14 cases. Cancer **15**:1264-1268, 1962.

181a Fisher ER, Palekar AS, Paulson JD, Golinger R: Pseudolymphoma of breast. Cancer **44**:258-263, 1979.

182 Gulesserian HP, Lawton RL: Angiosarcoma of the breast. Cancer **24**:1021-1026, 1969.

183 Haggitt RC, Booth JL: Bilateral fibromatosis of the breast in Gardner's syndrome. Cancer **25**:161-166, 1970.

184 Hart WR, Bauer RC, Oberman HA: Cystosarcoma phyllodes. A clinicopathologic study of twenty-six hypercellular periductal stromal tumors of the breast. Am J Clin Pathol **70**:211-216, 1978.

185 Hill RP, Stout AP: Sarcoma of the breast. Arch Surg **44**:723-759, 1942.

186 Kaplan L, Walts AE: Benign chondrolipomatous tumor of the human female breast. Arch Pathol Lab Med **101**:149-151, 1977.

187 Leder LD: Über die selektive fermentcytochemische Darstellung von neutrophilen myeloischen Zellen und Gewebsmastzellen in Paraffinschnitt. Klin Wochenschr. **42**:553, 1964.

188 Lester J, Stout AP: Cystosarcoma phyllodes. Cancer **7**:335-353, 1954.

188a Lin JJ, Farha GJ, Taylor RJ: Pseudolymphoma of the breast. I. In a study of 8,654 consecutive tylectomies and mastectomies. Cancer **45**:973-978, 1980.

189 McDivitt RW, Urban JA, Farrow JH: Cystosarcoma phyllodes. Johns Hopkins Med J **120**:33-45, 1967.

190 Mambo NC, Burke JS, Butler JJ: Primary malignant lymphomas of the breast. Cancer **39**:2033-2040, 1977.

191 Menon M, van Velthoven PCM: Liposarcoma of the breast. A case report. Arch Pathol **98**:370-372, 1974.

192 Nascimento AG, Karas M, Rosen PP, Caron AG: Leiomyoma of the nipple. Am J Surg Pathol **3**:151-154, 1979.

193 Norris HJ, Taylor HB: Relationship of histologic features to behavior of cystosarcoma phyllodes. Analysis of ninety-four cases. Cancer **20**:2090-2099, 1967.

194 Norris HJ, Taylor, HB: Sarcomas and related mesenchymal tumors of the breast. Cancer **22**:22-28, 1968.

195 Oberman HA: Cystosarcoma phyllodes of the breast. Cancer **18**:697-710, 1965.

196 Oberman HA: Primary lymphoreticular neoplasms of the breast. Surg Gynecol Obstet **123**:1047-1051, 1966.

197 Pardo-Mindan J, Garcia-Julian G, Altuna ME: Leiomyosarcoma of the breast. Report of a case. Am J Clin Pathol **62**:477-480, 1974.

198 Pascoe HR: Tumors composed of immature granulocytes occurring in the breast in chronic granulocytic leukemia. Cancer **25**:697-704, 1970.

199 Pietruszka M, Barnes L: Cystosarcoma phyllodes. A clinicopathologic analysis of 42 cases. Cancer **41**:1974-1983, 1978.

200 Rhodes RH, Frankel KA, Davis RL, Tatter D: Metastatic cystosarcoma phyllodes. A report of 2 cases presenting with neurological symptoms. Cancer **41**:1179-1187, 1978.

200a Rosen PP: Multinucleated mammary stromal giant cells. A benign lesion that simulates invasive carcinoma. Cancer **44**:1305-1308, 1979.

201 Rosen PP, Ridolfi RL: The perilobular hemangioma. A benign microscopic vascular lesion of the breast. Am J Clin Pathol **68**:21-23, 1977.

202 Rosen Y, Papasozomenos SC, Gardner B: Fibromatosis of the breast. Cancer **41**:1409-1413, 1978.

203 Smith BH, Taylor HB: The occurrence of bone and cartilage in mammary tumors. Am J Clin Pathol **51**:610-618, 1969.

204 Steingaszner LC, Enzinger, FM, Taylor HB: Hemangiosarcoma of the breast. Cancer **18**:352-361, 1965.

205 Sternby NH, Gynning I, Hogeman KE: Postmastectomy angiosarcoma. Acta Chir Scand **121**:420-432, 1961.

206 Treves N: A study of cystosarcoma phyllodes. Ann N Y Acad Sci **114**:922-936, 1964.

207 Treves N, Sunderland DA: Cystosarcoma phyllodes of the breast. Cancer **4**:1286-1332, 1951 (extensive bibliography and beautiful illustrations).

208 Wiseman C, Liao, KT: Primary lymphoma of the breast. Cancer **29**:1705-1712, 1972.

209 Woodward AH, Ivins JC, Soule, EH: Lymphangiosarcoma arising in chronic lymphedematous extremities. Cancer **30**:562-572, 1972.

Other lesions

210 Davis AB, Patchefsky AS: Basal cell carcinoma of the nipple. Case report and review of the literature. Cancer **40**:1780-1781, 1977.

211 Elsner B, Harper FB: Disseminated Wegener's granulomatosis with breast involvement. Report of a case. Arch Pathol **87**:544-547, 1969.

212 Farrow JH: Thrombophlebitis of the superficial veins of the breast and anterior chest wall (Mondor's disease). Surg Gynecol Obstet **101**:63-68, 1955.

213 Finck FM, Schwinn CP, Keasby LE: Clear cell hidradenoma of the breast. Cancer **22**:125-135, 1968.

214 Hajdu SI, Urban JA: Cancers metastatic to the breast. Cancer **22**:1691-1696, 1968.

215 Hamit HF: Implantation of plastics in the breast. Arch Surg **75**:224-229, 1957.

216 Herrmann JB: Thrombophlebitis of breast and contiguous thoracicoabdominal wall (Mondor's disease). N Y State J Med **66**:3146-3152, 1966.

217 Johnson WC, Wallrich R, Helwig EB: Superficial thrombophlebitis of the chest wall JAMA **180**:103-108, 1962.

218 Lucey JJ: Spontaneous infarction of the breast. J Clin Pathol **28**:937-943, 1975.

219 Nudelman HL, Kempson RL: Necrosis of the breast. A rare complication of anticoagulant therapy. Am J Surg **111**:728-733, 1966.

220 Rickert RR, Rajan S: Localized breast infarcts associated with pregnancy. Arch Pathol **97**:159-161, 1974.

221 Robitaille Y, Seemayer TA, Thelmo WL, Cumberlidge MC: Infarction of the mammary region mimicking carcinoma of the breast. Cancer **33**:1183-1189, 1974.

222 Sheth MT, Hathway D, Petrelli M: Pleomorphic adenoma ("mixed" tumor) of human female breast mimicking carcinoma clinico-radiologically. Cancer **41**:659-665, 1978.

223 Symmers W St C: Silicone mastitis in "topless" waitress and some other varieties of foreign-body mastitis. Br Med J **3**:19-22, 1968.

Hormone therapy and breast

224 Fechner RE: Fibroadenomas in patients receiving oral contraceptives: a clinical and pathologic study. Am J Clin Pathol **53**:857-864, 1970.

225 Fechner RE: Fibrocystic disease in women receiving oral contraceptive hormones. Cancer **25**:1332-1339, 1970.

226 Fechner RE: Breast cancer during oral contraceptive therapy. Cancer **26**:1204-1211, 1970.

227 Fechner RE: The surgical pathology of the reproductive system and breast during oral contraceptive therapy. Pathol Annu **6:**299-319, 1971.

228 Fechner RE: Influence of oral contraceptives on breast diseases. Cancer **39:**2764-2771, 1977.

229 Goldenberg VE, Wiegenstein L, Mottet NK: Florid breast fibroadenomas in patients taking hormonal oral contraceptives. Am J Clin Pathol **49:**52-59, 1968.

230 Hoover R, Gray LA, Sr, Cole P, MacMahon B: Menopausal estrogens and breast cancer. N Engl J Med **295:**401-405, 1976.

231 LiVolsi VA, Stadel BV, Kelsey JL, Holford TR, White C: Fibrocystic breast disease in oral-contraceptive users. A histopathological evaluation of epithelial atypia. N Engl J Med **299:**381-385, 1978.

232 Ory H, Cole P, MacMahon B, Hoover R: Oral contraceptives and reduced risk of benign breast diseases. N Engl J Med **294:**419-422, 1976.

Breast diseases in children and adolescents

233 Farrow JH, Ashikari H: Breast lesions in young girls. Surg Clin North Am **49:**261-269, 1969.

234 McDivitt RW, Stewart FW: Breast carcinoma in children. JAMA **195:**388-390, 1966.

235 Ramirez G, Ansfield FJ: Carcinoma of the breast in children. Arch Surg **96:**222-225, 1968.

236 Sandison AT, Walker JC: Diseases of the adolescent female breast. Br J Surg **55:**443-448, 1068.

237 Steiner MW: Enlargement of the breast during childhood. Pediatr Clin North Am **2:**575-593, 1955.

237a Tavassoli FA, Norris HJ: Secretory carcinoma of the breast. Cancer **45:**2404-2413, 1980.

Tumors of male breast

238 Benson WR: Carcinoma of the prostate with metastases to breast and testis. Cancer **10:**1235-1245, 1957.

239 El-Gazayerli M, Abdel-Aziz AS: On bilharziasis and male breast cancer in Egypt—a preliminary report and review of the literature. Br J Cancer **17:**566-571, 1963.

240 Giffler RF, Kay S: Small-cell carcinoma of the male mammary gland. A tumor resembling infiltrating lobular carcinoma. Am J Clin Pathol **66:**715-722, 1976.

240a Heller KS, Rosen PP, Schottenfeld D, Ashikari R, Kinne DW: Male breast cancer: a clinicopathologic study of 97 cases. Ann Surg **188:**60-65, 1978.

241 Hernandez FJ: Leiomyosarcoma of male breast originating in the nipple. Am J Surg Pathol **2:**299-304, 1978.

242 Jackson AW, Muldal S, Ockey CH, O'Connor PJ: Carcinoma of male breast in association with the Klinefelter syndrome. Br Med J **1:**223-225, 1965.

243 Norris HJ, Taylor HB: Carcinoma of the male breast. Cancer **23:**1428-1435, 1969.

244 O'Grady WP, McDivitt RW: Breast cancer in a man treated with diethylstilbestrol. Arch Pathol **88:**162-165, 1969.

245 Ribeiro GG: Carcinoma of the male breast: a review of 200 cases. Br J Surg **64:**381-383, 1977.

246 Tedeschi LG, McCarthy PE: Involutional mammary duct ectasia and periductal mastitis in a male. Hum Pathol **5:**232-236, 1974.

247 Treves N, Holleb AI: Cancer of the male breast. A report of 146 cases. Cancer **8:**1239-1250, 1955.

248 Visfeldt J, Scheike O: Male breast cancer, I. Histologic typing and grading of 187 Danish cases. Cancer **32:**985-990, 1973.

249 Waldo ED, Sidhu GS, Hu AW: Florid papillomatosis of the male nipple after diethylstilbestrol therapy. Arch Pathol **99:**364-366, 1975.

Clinicopathologic correlation

250 Alderson MR, Hamlin I, Staunton MD: The relative significance of prognostic factors in breast carcinoma. Br J Cancer **25:**646-655, 1971.

251 Ashikari R, Rosen PP, Urban JA, Senoo T: Breast cancer presenting as an axillary mass. Ann Surg **183:**415-417, 1976.

252 Auchincloss H, Jr: Significance of location and number of axillary metastases in carcinoma of the breast. A justification for a conservative operation. Ann Surg **158:**37-46, 1963.

253 Berg JW, Robbins GF: Factors influencing short and long-term survival of breast cancer patients. Surg Gynecol Obstet **122:**1311-1316, 1966.

254 Black MM, Barclay THC, Hankey BF: Prognosis in breast cancer utilizing histologic characteristics of the primary tumor. Cancer **36:**2048-2055, 1975.

255 Bloom HJG, Richardson WW, Harries ED; Natural history of untreated breast cancer. Comparison of untreated cases according to histological grade of malignancy. Br Med J **2:**213-221, 1962.

256 Breast Cancer Study Group: Identification of breast cancer patients with high risk of early recurrence after radical mastectomy. II. Clinical and pathological correlations. Cancer **42:**2809-2826, 1978.

256a Brinkley D, Haybittle JL: The curability of breast cancer. Lancet **2:**95-97, 1975.

257 Butcher HR Jr: Effectiveness of radical mastectomy for mammary cancer: an analysis of mortalities by the method of probits. Ann Surg **154:**383-396, 1961.

258 Butcher HR Jr: Mammary carcinoma. A discussion of therapeutic methods. Cancer **24:**1272-1279, 1969.

259 Carter D, Pipkin RD, Shepard RH, Elkins RC, Abbey H: Relationship of necrosis and tumor border to lymph node metastases and 10-year survival in carcinoma of the breast. Am J Surg Pathol **2:**39-46, 1978.

260 Donegan WL: The influence of untreated internal mammary metastases upon the course of mammary cancer. Cancer **39:**533-538, 1977.

261 Eusebi V, Pich A, Macchiorlatti E, Bussolati G: Morpho-functional differentiation in lobular carcinoma of the breast. Histopathology **1:**301-314, 1977.

262 Fisher B: Cooperative clinical trials in primary breast cancer: a critical appraisal. Cancer **31:**1271-1286, 1973.

262a Fisher B: Breast-cancer management. Alternatives to radical mastectomy. N Engl J Med **301:**326-328, 1979.

263 Fisher B, Slack NH, Bross IDJ: Cancer of the breast: size of neoplasm and prognosis. Cancer **24:**1071-1080, 1969.

264 Fisher ER, Gregorio R, Redmond C, Dekker A, Fisher B: Pathologic findings from the National Surgical Adjuvant Breast Project (Protocol no. 4). II. The significance of regional node histology other than sinus histiocytosis in invasive mammary cancer. Am J Clin Pathol **65:**21-30, 1976.

265 Fisher ER, Gregorio RM, Redmond C, Kim WS, Fisher B: Pathologic findings from the National Surgical Adjuvant Breast Project (Protocol no. 4). III. The significance of extranodal extension of axillary metastases. Am J Clin Pathol **65:**439-444, 1976.

266 Fisher B, Montague E, Redmond C, Barton B, Bor-

land D, Fisher ER, Deutsch M, Schwarz G, Margolese R, Donegan W, Volk H, Honvolinka C, Gardner B, Cohn I, Jr, Lesnick G, Cruz AB, Lawrence W, Nealon T, Butcher H, Lawton R: Comparison of radical mastectomy with alternative treatments for primary breast cancer. A first report of results from a prospective randomized clinical trial. Cancer **39**:2827-2839, 1977.

266a Fisher ER, Redmond CK, Liu H, Rockette H, Fisher B, and collaborating NSABP investigators: Correlation of estrogen receptor and pathologic characteristics of invasive breast cancer. Cancer **45**:349-353, 1980.

267 Fitts WT Jr, Steiner GC, Enterline HT: Prognosis of occult carcinoma of the breast. Am J Surg **106**:460-463, 1963.

268 Fitzpatrick TB: Human melanogenesis. Tyrosinase reaction in pigment cell neoplasms, with particular reference to the malignant melanoma: preliminary report. Arch Dermatol Syphilol **65**:379-391, 1952.

269 Haagensen CD: The choice of treatment for operable carcinoma of the breast. Surgery **76**:685-714, 1974.

270 Haagensen CD, and Stout AP: Carcinoma of the breast. Ann Surg **116**:801-815, 1942.

271 Haagensen CD, Cooley E, Kennedy CS, Miller E, Butcher HR Jr, Dahl-Iversen E, Tobiassen T, Williams IG, Curwen MP, Kaae S, Johansen H: The treatment of early mammary carcinoma. Ann Surg **157**:157-179, 1963.

271a Hawkins RA, Roberts MM, Forrest APM: Oestrogen receptors and breast cancer: current status. Br J Surg **67**:162-165, 1980.

271b Hutter RVP: The influence of pathologic factors on breast cancer management. Cancer **46**:961-976, 1980.

272 Huvos AG, Huttes RVP, Berg JW: Significance of axillary marcometastases and micrometastases in mammary cancer. Ann Surg **173**:44-46, 1971.

272a Ingle JN, Tormey DC, Tan HK: The bone marrow examination in breast cancer. Diagnostic considerations and clinical usefulness. Cancer **41**:670-674, 1978.

272b Jensen EV, DeSombre ER: Estrogen-receptor interaction. Science **182**:126-134, 1973.

273 Kister SJ, Sommers SC, Haagensen CD, Cooley E: Re-evaluation of blood vessel invasion as a prognostic factor in carcinoma of the breast. Cancer **19**:1213-1216, 1966.

274 Lacour J, Bucalossi P, Cacers E, Koszarowski T, Le M, Rumeau-Rouqueite C, Veronesi U, Jacobelli G: Radical mastectomy versus radical mastectomy plus internal mammary dissection. Five-year results of an international cooperative study. Cancer **37**:206-214, 1976.

274a Lagios MD, Gates EA, Westdahl PR, Richards V, Alpert BS: A guide to the frequency of nipple involvement in breast cancer. A study of 149 consecutive mastectomies using a serial subgross and correlated radiographic technique. Am J Surg **138**:135-142, 1979.

274b Landys K: Prognostic value of bone marrow biopsy in breast cancer. Cancer (in press).

274c Lee SH: Cancer cell estrogen receptor of human mammary carcinoma. Cancer **44**:1-12, 1979.

275 Lewison EF, Montague ACW, Kuller L: Breast cancer treated at The Johns Hopkins Hospital, 1951-1956. Review of international ten-year survival rates. Cancer **19**:1359-1368, 1966.

276 McWhirter R: The treatment of carcinoma of the breast. Irish J Med Sci 6th series, pp. 475-483, 1956.

277 Mambo NC, Gallager HS: Carcinoma of the breast. The prognostic significance of extranodal extension of axillary disease. Cancer **39**:2280-2285, 1977.

277a Masters JRW, Millis RR, King, RJB, Rubens RD: Elastosis and response to endocrine therapy in human breast cancer. Br J Cancer **39**:536-539, 1979.

277b Mesa-Tejada R, Keydar I, Ramanarayanan M, Ohno T, Fenoglio C, Spiegelman S: Detection in human breast carcinomas of an antigen immunologically related to a group-specific antigen of mouse mammary tumor virus. Proc Natl Acad Sci USA **75**:1529-1533, 1978.

277c Millis RR, Davis R, Stacey AJ: The detection and significance of calcification in the breast: a radiological and pathological study. Br J Radiol **49**:12-26, 1976.

278 Nime FA, Rosen PP, Thaler HT, Ashikari R, Urban JA: Prognostic significance of tumor emboli in intramammary lymphatics in patients with mammary carcinoma. Am J Surg Pathol **1**:25-30, 1977.

279 Pertschuk LP, Tobin EH, Brigati DJ, Kim DS, Bloom ND, Gaetjens E, Berman PJ, Carter AC, Degenschein GA: Immunofluorescent detection of estrogen receptors in breast cancer. Comparison with dextran-coated charcoal and sucrose gradient assays. Cancer **41**:907-911, 1978.

279a Pierguin B, Owen R, Maylin C, Otmezguine Y, Raynal M, Mueller W, and Hannoun S: Radical radiation therapy of breast cancer. Int J Radiat Oncol Biol Phys **6**:17-24, 1980.

280 Rodriguez HA, McGavran MH: A modified dopa reaction for the diagnosis and investigation of pigment cells. Am J Clin Pathol **52**:219-227, 1969.

281 Rosai J, Rodriguez HA: Application of electron microscopy to the differential diagnosis of tumors. Am J Clin Pathol **50**:555-562, 1968.

281a Rosen PP: Personal communication, 1980.

282 Rosen PP, Fracchia AA, Urban JA, Schattenfeld D, Robbins GF: "Residual" mammary carcinoma following simulated partial mastectomy. Cancer **35**:739-747, 1975.

283 Rosen PP, Menendez-Botet CJ, Nisselbaum JS, Urban JA, Miké V, Fracchia A, Schwartz MK: Pathological review of breast lesions analyzed for estrogen receptor protein. Cancer Res **35**:3187-3194, 1975.

283a Saigo P, Rosen PP: Prognostic factors in invasive mammary carcinomas 1.0 cm or less in diameter. Am J Clin Pathol **73**:303-304, 1980 (abstract).

283b Silfverswärd C, Gustafsson JÅ, Gustafsson SA, Humla S, Nordenskjöld B, Wallgren A, Wrange Ö: Estrogen receptor concentrations in 269 cases of histologically classified human breast cancer. Cancer **45**:2001-2005, 1980.

283c Simon N, Silverstone SM: Radiation as a cause of breast cancer. Bull NY Acad Sci **52**:741-751, 1976.

284 Smith JA III, Gamez-Araujo J, Gallager HS, White EC, McBride CM: Carcinoma of the breast. Analysis of total lymph node involvement versus level of metastasis. Cancer **39**:527-532, 1977.

284a Spiegelman S, Keydar K, Mesa-Tejada R, Ohno T, Ramanarayanan M, Nayak R, Bausch J, Fenoglio C: Possible diagnostic implications of a mammary tumor virus related protein in human breast cancer. Cancer **46**:879-892, 1980.

285 Terenius L, Johansson H, Rimsten A, Thorén L:

Malignant and benign human mammary disease: Estrogen binding in relation to clinical data. Cancer **33:** 1364-1368, 1974.

286 Tsakraklides V, Olson P, Kersey JH, Good RA: Prognostic significance of the regional lymph node histology in cancer of the breast. Cancer **34:**1259-1266, 1974.

287 Urban JA: Clinical experience and results of excision of the internal mammary lymph node chain in primary operable breast cancer. Cancer **12:**14-22, 1959.

288 Wise L, Mason AY, Ackerman LV: Local excision and irradiation: an alternative method for the treatment of early mammary cancer. Ann Surg **174:**392-401, 1971.

20 Lymph nodes

Biopsy

The microscopic interpretation of abnormal lymph nodes is extremely difficult. Probably more diagnostic errors are made on lymph nodes than on any other organ of the body. The most common mistake is the diagnosis of a benign node as malignant lymphoma. Thus, Symmers[5,6] found that of 600 cases submitted with an initial histologic diagnosis of Hodgkin's disease, the diagnosis was mistaken in 47%. The condition most commonly confused with Hodgkin's disease was chronic nonspecific lymphadenitis. Of 226 cases initially diagnosed as reticulum cell sarcoma (histiocytic lymphoma), the error was 27%. In a study carried out by the Southwestern Oncology group,[3a] a 33% discordance was noted in the classification of Hodgkin's disease between the contributing and the referring pathologists. These figures clearly indicate the need for a review of the pathologic material whenever a patient is admitted to the hospital because a lymph node biopsy done elsewhere was interpreted as malignant lymphoma.

There are several ways to mishandle a patient with lymphadenopathy. The internist requests lymph node biopsy in a patient with generalized lymphadenopathy. The surgeon, tempted by its accessibility, biopsies an inguinal node. Unfortunately, inguinal lymph nodes invariably show chronic inflammatory changes and fibrosis that obscure the presence of other pathologic processes. The surgeon should biopsy the more elusive axillary or deep cervical node rather than superficial or inguinal nodes when generalized lymphadenopathy exists. A superficial cervical lymph node may show only hyperplasia, yet a deeper node of the same group may contain metastatic carcinoma or Hodgkin's disease.[4] Similarly, the most accessible enlarged lymph node found at laparotomy may not show the pathologic process causing the intra-abdominal lymphadenopathy. Whenever possible, the largest lymph node of the region should be the one biopsied.[2]

The surgeon biopsying intra-abdominal nodes or large cervical or axillary masses should have frozen section performed to be certain that the tissue is representative—*not* to obtain a specific diagnosis at this point. This may save a second biopsy. The biopsy of a lymph node in the cervical or axillary area should be performed only by a surgeon. An inexperienced physician trying to biopsy an apparently easily accessible node may be unable to find the node or may encounter hemorrhage from adjacent large vessels.

If there is any question that the node contains something other than a tumor, an adequate sample of the biopsied lymph node must be sent directly for bacteriologic study or must be placed

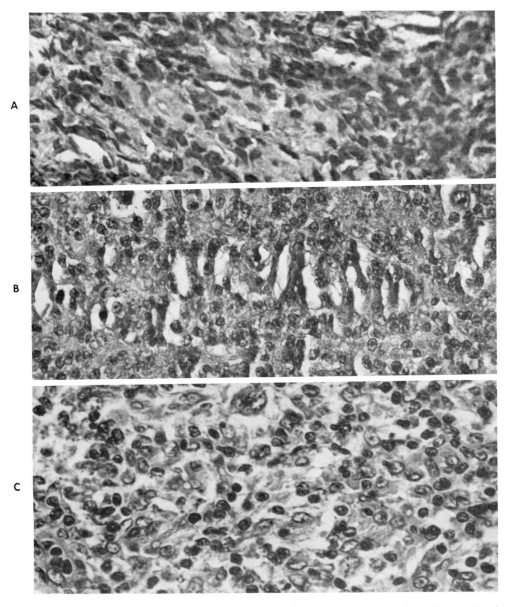

Fig. 1079 A, Hodgkin's disease. Lymph node was poorly fixed and somewhat dry before being stained. No diagnosis is possible. **B,** Section of node shown in **A** cut with dull knife. Note distortion. Diagnosis is difficult. **C,** Same node shown in **A** and **B** well fixed and stained. There is no cytologic distortion, and nuclear details are clear. (**A** to **C,** ×600; **A,** WU neg. 51-1662; **B,** WU neg. 51-1664; **C,** WU neg. 51-1661.)

in a sterile Petri dish in the refrigerator. We recommend and follow the latter procedure. If permanent sections show an inflammatory process, the material can then be taken from the refrigerator and studied bacteriologically. Furthermore, the microscopic pattern of the permanent sections may be helpful in suggesting the diagnosis to the bacteriologist. In numerous instances, the bacteriologic study is more rewarding than the microscopic study.[8] The search for acid-fast bacilli or fungi in the paraffin section often is fruitless. A technique that complements the study of tissue sections and that is too often neglected is the examination of touch preparations from the cut surface of the fresh lymph node stained with Giemsa or Wright's solution.[3,7] This is particularly useful in the evaluation of lymphoma and leukemia. Granulocytic leukemia can closely simulate histocytic lymphoma in an hematoxylin-eosin section, but an imprint will readily differentiate the two conditions. Additional techniques useful for the study of lymph node pathology are electron microscopy and immunologic markers determinations. They both require special handling at the time that the fresh lymph node is biopsied (see Appendix).

The most frequent reason for an incorrect diagnosis of a lymph node is improper preparation of the biopsied tissue. A poorly prepared slide may be produced in the following ways:

1. Fragmenting or crushing the lymph node at time of excision
2. Delaying placing the node in fixative; leaving the fresh node in a gauze and exposing it to a strong light leads to drying of the tissue, especially the periphery, and may result in uninterpretable material (Fig. 1079)
3. Running the node too quickly through the alcohols, xylene, and paraffin
4. Overheating the paraffin wax
5. Cutting the sections with a dull knife (Fig. 1079)
6. Cutting the sections too thick
7. Overstaining the sections with hematoxylin.

We make it our policy never to make a diagnosis on any poorly prepared lymph node that is sent to us. We are often amazed at the confident diagnoses that others make on such sections. Adherence to a strict technique for the preparation of lymph nodes is of paramount importance.[1] The specimen should be received fresh in the laboratory immediately after excision, be bisected as soon as it is received, and sampled for the appropriate studies. The portion to be embedded in paraffin (which should not exceed 3 mm in thickness) can be placed in 10% buffered formalin or, preferably, in Zenker's fixative or B5. In our laboratory, we use the latter. The alcohols and xylenes should be changed frequently. Sections should be cut with a sharp knife without distortion at 5μ or less. As a routine, satisfactory results can be attained with hematoxylin-eosin staining[1,1b] (Fig. 1079, C).

Needle biopsy and frozen section of a lymph node can be very useful to confirm a diagnosis of metastatic carcinoma.[1a] On the other hand, whenever a diagnosis of lymphoma is seriously considered clinically, we strongly recommend removal of the entire node, in one piece, with the capsule intact, overnight fixation, and paraffin embedding.

Microscopic examination and functional histology

In the histologic evaluation of a lymph node, more than in any other tissue, it is important that a systematic approach be used. The critical features to be assessed are as follows:

1. Capsular and pericapsular infiltration
2. Sinusoidal, follicular, interfollicular, or diffuse pattern of the proliferation
3. If the proliferation is follicular, distribution, size, shape, and cell composition of the follicles
4. Preservation or effacement of the nodal architecture
5. Phagocytosis by histiocytes
6. Vascular proliferation
7. Granulomas
8. Necrosis
9. Cell composition of the infiltrate

Whereas none of these features can be regarded as pathognomonic for a given entity, they usually allow a distinction between a benign and a malignant process to be made when all are taken into consideration.

A new dimension to the microscopic interpretation of lymph node biopsies has been added by the recently acquired knowledge of lymph node composition and structure in relation to immunologic function.[12] It is now recognized that two major subpopulations of lymphocytes exist.[10] One, known as B lymphocyte, is responsible for humoral immunity and is dependent on the presence of the bursa of Fabricius in the chicken and an as yet unidenti-

Table 53 Principal markers of human lymphocytes and histiocytes

Marker	B lym-phocytes	T lym-phocytes	Histiocytes/Monocytes
Surface Ig	+	−	−
Human B lymphocyte antigen (HBLA)	+	−	+
Sheep erythrocyte receptors (E rosette)	−	+	−
Human T lymphocyte antigen (HTLA)	−	+	−
Fc receptors (aggregated IgG or EA rosette)	+	−	+ +
Complement receptors (EAC rosette)	+	−	+
Phagocytosis	−	−	+

fied counterpart in the human being (perhaps bone marrow, fetal liver, or bowel). Upon antigenic stimulation, these cells become plasma cells through a stage of blastic transformation and secrete immunoglobulins. The other major subpopulation is made of T lymphocytes, which have acquired other properties in the thymus and are responsible for cell-mediated immunity. They also undergo blastic transformation upon the proper antigenic stimulation but eventually revert to cells with the features of small mature lymphocytes. Subdivisions within the system exist. For instance, at least three subtypes of T lymphocytes have been described, respectively named effector, suppressor, and helper lymphocytes. A close cooperation and interdependence between the B and T systems has been demonstrated. Some primitive cells lack either T or B features and are referred to as N (null) cells. Others have cell markers of both B type and T type.

Despite these complexities in this poorly understood and rapidly changing field, it is useful for operational purposes to think of T and B lymphocytes as two distinct compartments that can be identified by a set of cell surface markers[13] (Table 53; Figs. 1080 and 1081). Of all of these, the more commonly used are the surface immunoglobulin for B lymphocytes and the E rosette for T lymphocytes because of their reliability and simplicity. Determination of these parameters may be helpful in deciding whether a given lymphoid proliferation is reactive or malignant, and, if it is neoplastic, it may better define its nature.

Another important cell marker is provided by the immunocytochemical demonstration of immunoglobulin (in B lymphocytes and plasma cells) and lysozyme (in histiocytes) in routinely processed tissue with the unlabeled antibody method (Figs. 1082 and 1083).

Important information about the immunologic status of a patient also can be gained by examination of a routinely processed lymph node biopsy.[9] Changes in both architectural features and cell composition are important. The three major regions of a lymph node are the cortex, paracortex, and medulla. The cortex is situated beneath the capsule and contains the largest number of germinal centers. The medulla, close to the hilum, is rich in lymphatic sinuses, arteries, and veins but contains only a minor lymphocytic component. Both cortex and medulla represent B zones and are therefore associated with humoral types of immune response. Proliferated germinal centers are always indicative of humoral antibody production. They are usually located in the cortical portion, but under conditions of intense antigenic stimulation, they also can appear within the medullary cords. The paracortex is a T zone situated between the cortex and the medulla, in close relation to the postcapillary venules. It contains the mobile pool of lymphocytes, which are mainly responsible for cell-mediated immune responses. Its expansion is therefore suggestive of a cell-mediated immunologic reaction. The number of lymphocytes within the lumen and wall of postcapillary venules gives a rough indication of the degree of lymphocyte recirculation. Some cell types are always associated with a specific type of immune response. Proliferation of plasma cells, usually within the medullary cords, indicates the production of immunoglobulins and therefore of a humoral response. Epithelioid cells are usually an expression of a cell-mediated reaction. Large or small lymphoid cells with prominent nuclear cleaves and their neoplastic counterparts originate in the germinal centers and are of B cell derivation; they are variously referred to as large cleaved and small cleaved (cloven) cells, germinoblasts

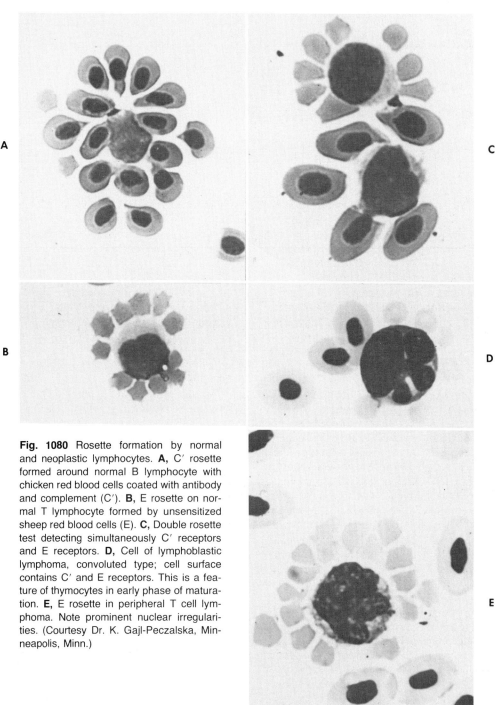

Fig. 1080 Rosette formation by normal and neoplastic lymphocytes. **A,** C′ rosette formed around normal B lymphocyte with chicken red blood cells coated with antibody and complement (C′). **B,** E rosette on normal T lymphocyte formed by unsensitized sheep red blood cells (E). **C,** Double rosette test detecting simultaneously C′ receptors and E receptors. **D,** Cell of lymphoblastic lymphoma, convoluted type; cell surface contains C′ and E receptors. This is a feature of thymocytes in early phase of maturation. **E,** E rosette in peripheral T cell lymphoma. Note prominent nuclear irregularities. (Courtesy Dr. K. Gajl-Peczalska, Minneapolis, Minn.)

and germinocytes, and centroblasts and centrocytes. Small mature lymphocytes with round dark nuclei cannot be identified on routine histologic preparations as belonging to the B or T system, although a convoluted or cerebroid shape of the nuclear contour suggests a T cell type; however, this seems to be more a feature of neoplastic rather than hyperplastic or normal T lymphocytes. Large lymphoid cells (immunoblasts; transformed lymphocytes; reticular lymphoblasts) also can be of either B or T cell type. B immunoblasts show dark basophilic or am-

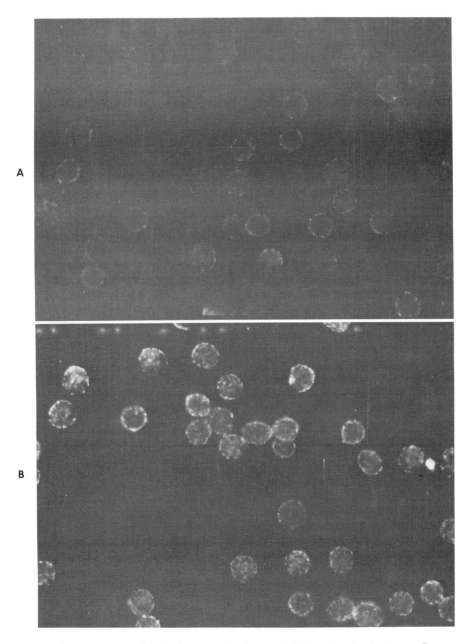

Fig. 1081 Surface immunoglobulin demonstration in neoplastic lymphocytes by immunofluorescence using antibodies against μ heavy chain. **A,** Chronic lymphocytic leukemia. Faint but definite staining may be seen in all cells. **B,** Malignant lymphoma associated with Waldenström's macroglobulinemia. Staining is more intense. Cells of nodular lymphoma stain with similar degree of intensity, although not all cells will be stained. (Courtesy Dr. K. Gajl-Peczalska, Minneapolis, Minn.)

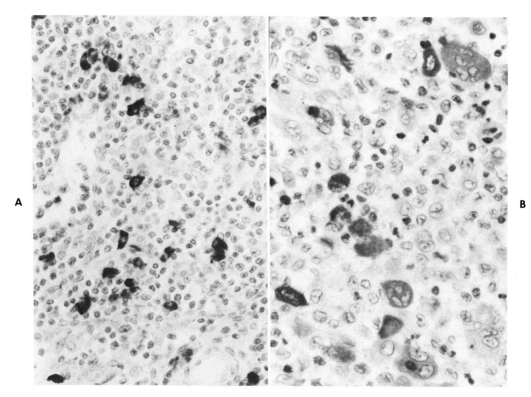

A   B

Fig. 1082 Demonstration of two useful immunocytochemical markers for study of lymphoreticular techniques shown with Sternberger's unlabeled immunoperoxidase method. **A,** Immunoglobulins in reactive plasma cells. **B,** Lysozyme in reactive histiocytes.

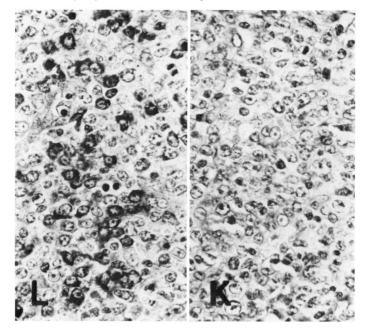

Fig. 1083 Demonstration of monoclonality in lymphocytic lymphoma with immunoperoxidase technique for immunoglobulins. Most tumor cells show intracytoplasmic content of lambda light chain, **L,** whereas stain for kappa light chain, **K,** is completely negative.

phophilic staining of the cytoplasm, prominent paranuclear hof, thick nuclear membrane, clumped chromatin, and prominent basophilic nucleolus (irregular in outline and often located adjacent to the nuclear membrane) and usually are seen accompanied by plasmacytoid elements and mature plasma cells. It is said that the T immunoblast has a scantier and lighter-staining cytoplasm, more dispersed chromatin pattern, nuclear folding, and less prominent nucleolus and that it lacks the company of plasmacytoid and plasma cells.[11] It should be pointed out that even if these subtle morphologic distinctions allow one to predict with some accuracy to which type of the immune response a certain lymphoid cell belongs, the definitive decision has to be made by employing the immunologic tests listed in Table 53, as well as others that undoubtedly will be developed in the near future in this rapidly advancing field.

Immunodeficiencies

The many varieties of primary immunodeficiencies, most of which remain unclassified at the present time, can be broadly divided in three major categories according to the type of the immunologic deficit: humoral, cell-mediated, and combined.[17,29] The diagnosis of these is based on a variety of laboratory tests, including qualitative and quantitative immunoglobulin determinations, delayed-type skin reactions, and *in vitro* stimulation of lymphocytes. Sometimes lymph nodes are biopsied in order to assess the amount and composition of the lymphoid tissue. In immune diseases of the humoral type, cortical reactive centers and medullary plasma cells are scanty or absent. In diseases of cell-mediated immunity, the thickness of the paracortical area is greatly diminished. When both humoral and cell-mediated types of immunities are defective, the lymphocyte and plasma cell content of the node is practically nil. The lymph node is reduced to a mass of connective tissue and blood vessels.[19] If an antigen such as diphtheria or tetanus toxoid is injected into the medial aspect of the thigh and an ipsilateral inguinal node is biopsied five to seven days later, its capacity to react to the antigenic stimulus can be evaluated.[18]

There is an increased incidence of malignant tumors, particularly lymphomas, in patients with primary immunodeficiencies.[22,25,27,28] Chronic antigenic stimulation—possibly by oncogenic viruses—and perhaps loss of antibody feedback inhibition of the lymphoid prolifera-tion may account for the high rate of lymphoid malignancies. The Epstein-Barr virus in particular has been repeatedly implicated.[24] In favor of this interpretation is the close morphologic similarity between some of these lymphomas and those developing in immunosuppressed organ transplant recipients. Also supportive of a possible role for the Epstein-Barr virus comes from the description by Purtilo et al.[26] of a family with an X-linked recessive lymphoproliferative syndrome, presumably resulting from an immunodeficiency to the Epstein-Barr virus. Several members of this family have developed American Burkitt's lymphoma, immunoblastic sarcoma of B cells, fatal infectious mononucleosis, and "plasmacytoma." For some types of immune deficiency, such as ataxia-telangiectasia, the pathogenesis may be related to the existence of karyotypically abnormal lymphoid clones. Patients with ataxia-telangiectasia and the Wiskott-Aldrich syndrome are particularly prone to this complication, about 10% of the reported patients having died from it. We recently reviewed the microscopic material available in the Immunodeficiency-Cancer Registry of the University of Minnesota and found a very interesting difference between the lymphomas arising in Wiskott-Aldrich syndrome and those arising in ataxia-telangiectasia. The former were all of non-Hodgkin's type (predominantly B immunoblastic sarcomas) and presented as localized extranodal masses, whereas the latter were both of Hodgkin's and non-Hodgkin's types, with a more usual organ distribution. Surprisingly for this age group, half of the cases of Hodgkin's disease belonged to the lymphocyte depletion type. Most of the non-Hodgkin's lymphomas in ataxia-telangiectasia were of the histologic types associated with the 14q+ chromosomal abnormality, i.e., the tumors designated by Lukes as large or small noncleaved follicular center cell lymphomas.[16] The microscopic diagnosis in the early cases can be extremely difficult. In three of our patients, the only diagnosis we could make was that of an atypical lymphoproliferative process.

Chronic granulomatous disease is not a disorder of either cellular or humoral immunity but rather the result of an intracellular (probably enzymatic) defect of granulocytes and monocytes. These cells ingest microorganisms but are unable to destroy them. The leukocytic abnormality can be detected by the nitro blue tetrazolium test.[14] The original description was that of a familial disease in male children, but what seems to be a closely related condition has now been observed in females.[20] The main clinical features are recurrent lymphadenitis, hepatosplenomegaly, skin rash, pulmonary infiltrates, anemia, leukocytosis, and hypergammaglobulinemia.[15] Microscopically, granulomas with necrotic purulent centers are seen in lymph nodes and other organs. They closely simulate the appearance of cat-scratch disease and lymphopathia venereum.[21] Collections of histiocytes containing a lipofuscin-like pigment also are commonly observed.[23]

Hyperplasia

Lymph nodes respond to infection by enlarging. A carcinoma of the large bowel or lung may be associated with inflammation which alone may cause regional lymph node enlargement. Regardless of the skill of the surgeon, he cannot determine by palpation whether an enlarged, firm lymph node does or does not contain cancer. On many occasions, we have been handed inflamed lymph nodes by surgeons who have told us with confidence that they were simply "checking" those nodes which they knew contained cancer. If the surgeon relies on palpation, he may be denying his patient a curative operation.

It is not generally realized how large hyperplastic nodes may be. We have seen them reaching a size of 10 cm. Probably one of the largest hyperplastic nodes on record is the one mentioned by Gall and Rappaport,[45] which measured $17 \times 12 \times 8$ cm. A hyperplastic lymph node often is firm and its cut surface homogeneously gray. Frozen section of such nodes may be very difficult to interpret.

Microscopically, the hyperplasia may be primarily located in the reactive centers, in the intervening lymphoid tissue, or within the sinuses. In the first case, the hyperplasia may simulate nodular lymphoma; in the second, diffuse lymphoma; and in the latter, metastatic carcinoma or malignant histiocytosis. Although a combination of these three patterns is not uncommon, it is useful to evaluate them separately, since the predominance of one over another may provide the clue to the specific agent involved.[36,66]

Dorfman and Warnke[36] have classified the lymph node diseases that simulate malignant lymphoma into four major categories according to the predominant pattern of growth (Table 54). Their classification includes not only the

Table 54 Lymph node diseases that simulate malignant lymphoma classified according to their predominant pattern of growth*

Follicular (nodular) pattern
  Nonspecific reactive follicular hyperplasia
  Secondary syphilis
  Rheumatoid arthritis
  (Felty's syndrome and Still's disease)
  Giant lymph node hyperplasia
  (Hyaline-vascular and plasma cell types)

Sinus pattern
  Histiocytosis X
  Sinus histiocytosis with massive lymphadenopathy
  "Lymphoma-like" Kaposi's sarcoma
  Vascular transformation of sinuses
  Lymphangiogram effect
  Metastatic carcinoma and melanoma

Diffuse pattern
  Postvaccinial lymphadenitis
  Hydantoin (Dilantin) hypersensitivity
  Viral (herpes zoster) lymphadenitis
  Immunoblastic lymphadenopathy
  Dermatopathic lymphadenopathy
  Lupus erythematosus
  Metastatic carcinoma and melanoma

Mixed patterns
  Infectious mononucleosis
  Toxoplasmosis
  Cat-scratch disease
  Lymphogranuloma inguinale
  Metastatic carcinoma and melanoma

---

*From Dorfman RF, Warnke R: Lymphadenopathy simulating the malignant lymphomas. Hum Pathol **5**:519-550, 1974.

hyperplasias, but also the granulomatous inflammatory processes and malignant neoplasms that can simulate lymphomas. These processes are discussed in different sections of this chapter according to their nature. Only those diseases that represent primarily hyperplastic processes of one or more lymph node compartments are included in this discussion of hyperplasia.

Nonspecific follicular hyperplasia

The criteria laid down by Rappaport et al.[71] remain as the most useful and reliable to distinguish reactive follicular hyperplasia from follicular (nodular) lymphoma (Table 55). In general, reactive follicles vary considerably in size and shape; their margins are sharply defined and surrounded by a mantle of small lymphocytes, often arranged circumferentially with an onion-skin pattern and sometimes con-

Table 55 Architectural and cytologic features of nodular lymphoma and of reactive follicular hyperplasia*

Nodular lymphoma	Reactive follicular hyperplasia
Architectural features	
Complete effacement of normal architecture	Preservation of nodal architecture
Even distribution of "follicles" throughout cortex and medulla	Follicles more prominent in cortical portion of lymph node
Slight or moderate variations in size and shape of "follicles"	Marked variations in size and shape of follicles with presence of elongated, angulated, and dumbbell-shaped forms
Fading of "follicles"	Sharply demarcated reaction centers
Massive infiltration of capsule and pericapsular fat with or without formation of neoplastic follicles outside capsule	No, or only moderate, infiltration of capsule and pericapsular fat tissue with inflammatory cells that may be arranged in perivascular focal aggregates (when associated with lymphadenitis)
Condensation of reticulin fibers at periphery of "follicles"	Little or no alteration of reticular framework
Cytologic features	
"Follicles" composed of neoplastic cells exhibiting cellular pleomorphism with nuclear irregularities	Centers of follicles (reaction centers) composed of reticulum cells and their histiocytic derivatives, with few or no cellular and nuclear irregularities
Lack of phagocytosis	Active phagocytosis in reaction centers
Relative paucity of mitotic figures usually without significant difference in their number inside and outside the "follicles"; occurrence of atypical mitoses	Moderate to pronounced mitotic activity in reaction centers; rare or no mitoses outside reaction centers; no atypical mitoses
Similarity of cell type inside and outside "follicles"	Infiltration of tissue between reaction centers with inflammatory cells (when associated with lymphadenitis)

*From Rappaport H, Winter WJ, Hicks EB: Follicular lymphoma. A re-evaluation of its position in the scheme of malignant lymphoma, based on a survey of 253 cases. Cancer **9**:792-821, 1956.

centrating on one pole of the follicle (supposedly on the side of the antigenic stimulation); they are composed of an *admixture* of small and large lymphoid cells with irregular (elongated and cleaved) nuclei; mitoses are numerous; and phagocytosis of nuclear debris is prominent. The lymphoid tissue present between the follicles is distinctly different from that of the follicles themselves (although this also may be true for follicular lymphoma); it is composed of a mixture of small lymphocytes, large lymphoid cells, prominent postcapillary venules, and, sometimes, an admixture of mature plasma cells.

There is a morphologic variation of reactive germinal centers that is particularly likely to be confused with the nodules of a nodular lymphoma. The name *progressively transformed* germinal centers has been applied to these formations.[70a] They usually are seen in conjunction with more typical reactive germinal cen-

ters, and they often are located more centrally within the node. They are large and contain numerous small lymphocytes, their borders are indistinct, and the interphase between the center of large lymphoid cells and the cuff of small lymphocytes is blurred. However, residual starry sky macrophages are present, together with scattered large lymphoid cells (cleaved and noncleaved), dendritic reticulum cells, and occasional epithelioid cells.[70a]

Syphilis

Generalized lymphadenopathy is a common finding in secondary syphilis, whereas localized node enlargement can be seen in the primary and tertiary stages of the disease. The former is the one more likely to be confused with malignant lymphoma.

Microscopically, the most striking changes occur in the inguinal nodes. They include capsular and pericapsular inflammation and extensive fibrosis, diffuse plasma cell proliferation, proliferation of blood vessels, with endothelium swelling and inflammatory infiltration of their wall (phlebitis and endarteritis), and follicular hyperplasia.[49] Rarely, noncaseating granulomas and abscesses are present. Spirochetes can be identified in most cases by the Warthin-Starry or Levaditi techniques or by immunofluorescence applied to imprint preparations.[31a] They are most frequently found in the wall of blood vessels. Other lymph node groups show only nonspecific follicular hyperplasia.[38]

Rheumatoid arthritis

Most patients with rheumatoid arthritis have generalized lymphadenopathy at some time during their illness.[67,74] The lymph node enlargement may precede the arthritis and raise the clinical suspicion of lymphoma.

Microscopically, the most important changes are follicular hyperplasia and plasma cell proliferation, with formation of Russell bodies.[70] Vascular proliferation is also a consistent finding. The appearance may be quite similar to that of the plasma cell type of giant lymph node hyperplasia. Small foci of necrosis and clumps of neutrophils are seen in some instances. The capsule is often infiltrated by lymphocytes. Other collagen-vascular diseases, such as lupus erythematosus, polyarteritis nodosa, and scleroderma, are usually not associated with this type of lymph node abnormality.

Giant lymph node hyperplasia

We believe that giant lymph node hyperplasia, also known as lymph nodal hamartoma and Castleman's disease, represents in most cases a peculiar type of lymph node hyperplasia rather than a neoplasm or a hamartoma. The mediastinum is by far the most common location, but this lesion also has been found in the neck, lung, axilla, mesentery, broad ligament, retroperitoneum, and soft tissues of the extremities.[85] It may reach a size of 16 cm. Grossly, it is round and well circumscribed and has a solid gray cut surface.

Microscopically, large follicles are seen scattered in a mass of lymphoid tissue. Prominent vascular proliferation and hyalinization are the most characteristic features of the subtype known as hyaline-vascular or angiofollicular, which comprises over 90% of the cases. The well-vascularized follicles have been confused with Hassall's corpuscles and with splenic red pulp, prompting in the first case a mistaken diagnosis of thymoma and in the second of ectopic spleen. There is a tight concentric layering of lymphocytes at the periphery of the follicles, resulting in an onion-skin appearance. The interfollicular stroma is also prominent, with numerous hyperplastic vessels and an admixture of plasma cells, eosinophils, and immunoblasts. In some cases (designated by Keller et al.[51] as the lymphoid subtype of the hyaline-vascular type), the follicles are composed predominantly or exclusively of small lymphocytes; only a few contain small, well-defined germinal centers. It is this variant of giant lymph node hyperplasia that is most likely to be confused with nodular lymphoma. Remnants of normal lymph node structures or early changes of similar nature in adjacent nodes are sometimes observed.

Seven of the eighty-one cases reviewed by Keller et al.,[51] designated by them as the plasma cell type, differed from the rest by virtue of a diffuse plasma cell proliferation in the interfollicular tissue, sometimes accompanied by numerous Russell bodies. The hyaline-vascular changes in the follicles are inconspicuous or absent; instead, one often encounters in the center a deposition of an amorphous acidophilic material that probably contains fibrin and immune complexes. The overall appearance is quite reminiscent of that seen in the lymph nodes from patients with rheumatoid arthritis. This group was often found associated with fever, anemia, elevated erythrosedimentation rate, hypergammaglobulinemia, and hypoalbuminemia (which rapidly regressed after excision of the mass), whereas the more common hyaline-vascular type was, in most instances, asymptomatic. Surgical excision is the treatment of choice.

The hyaline-vascular type of this disease is nearly always characterized by a large *single* mass, even if on microscopic examination one sometimes finds similar changes in the neighboring lymph nodes. Instead, the plasma cell variant may present with generalized lymphadenopathy and even involve the spleen.[44] We have recently studied ten examples of this systemic form of Castleman's disease, all of the plasma cell type. The clinical and laboratory features were remarkably similar to those of angioimmunoblastic lymphadenopathy, perhaps suggesting a related pathogenesis based on an abnormal hyperimmune response. Two patients also had Kaposi's disease. Of the ten patients, six are alive with persistent lymphadenopathy; the other four have died, one with a morphologic picture consistent with immunoblastic sarcoma and the others as a result of renal or pulmonary complications.[43]

Histiocytosis X

The terms of histiocytosis X, differentiated histiocytosis, and eosinophilic granuloma are applied to a specific, although remarkably variable, clinicopathologic entity characterized and defined by the proliferation of a highly distinctive element known as Langerhans' cell. This is presently regarded as a distinct type of histiocytic or reticular cell that is involved in the capturing of some antigens and their presentation to the lymphoid cells. Contrary to a widely held belief, these cells are not primarily phagocytic in nature, and their cytoplasmic content of lysozyme is nil or absent. Their nuclei are highly characteristic: irregular, usually elongated, with prominent grooves and folds that traverse them in all directions. The cytoplasm is abundant and acidophilic, sometimes to the point that an embryonal rhabdomyosarcoma is simulated. Most Langerhans' cells are mononuclear, but occasional ones contain several nuclei, while still maintaining the aforementioned nuclear and cytoplasmic features. Histochemically, they show rather weak acid phosphatase and nonspecific esterase activity but considerable leucyl-β-naphtylamidase activity. The cells contain receptors for the Fc fragment of IgG but no receptors for C3.[37] Electron microscopy shows that they contain a highly characteristic and apparently diagnostic organelle: Langerhans' or Birbenck's granule. This is an elongated, zipperlike cytoplasmic structure, sometimes continuous with the cell membrane.

Scattered Langerhans' cells (with their granules) are normally present in the skin, lymph node, thymus, and perhaps other organs. Therefore, the identification of one or two cells with this feature in a lymph node is not necessarily indicative that the patient has histiocytosis X.[86] Rather, the infiltrate should be composed predominantly of these cells or at least in good part before such a diagnosis is entertained. Conversely, the identification of Langerhans' cells is necessary for the diagnosis of histiocytosis X, just as the identification of Sternberg-Reed cells is necessary for the diagnosis of Hodgkin's disease. There is already too much confusion in the literature stemming from the fact that cases have been given this label only because a widespread proliferation of histiocytes was associated with a compatible clinical picture.

The most common manifestation of histiocytosis X is in the form of bone involvement, either as a monostotic or polyostotic variety; this is fully discussed in Chapter 23. Lymph node involvement can be evidence of multisystem involvement (sometimes designated with the confusing eponyms of Hand-Schüller-Christian disease and Letterer-Siwe disease) or be the only manifestation of the disease.[66a,73] Williams and Dorfman[88] studied seventeen patients in whom lymphadenopathy was the initial manifestation of histiocytosis X. The morphology was characteristic: distention of the sinuses by an infiltrate of mononuclear and multinuclear Langerhans' cells was invariably seen, admixed with a variable number of eosinophils (Fig. 1084); foci of necrosis were common, often surrounded by a rim of eosinophils (so-called eosinophilic microabscesses) but always confined to the sinuses. Follow-up showed a broad spectrum of involvement, embracing all those syndromes that have been associated with histiocytosis X. However, the prognosis was uniformly excellent. Kjeldsberg and Kim[52] described six cases as focal incidental findings in lymph nodes with malignant lymphoma: three were associated with Hodgkin's disease and three with non-Hodgkin's lymphoma.

Sinus histiocytosis with massive lymphadenopathy

Sinus histiocytosis with massive lymphadenopathy is characterized by fever, leukocytosis, elevated erythrosedimentation rate, hypergammaglobulinemia, and massive lymph node enlargement, mainly in the cervical region. The large majority of cases occur during the first or second decade of life.[57,79] Blacks are affected more than whites. A large proportion of cases has originated in Africa and the Caribbean region. In about 25%, the disease involves extranodal sites. This is usually seen in the presence of massive lymphadenopathy, and the disease is therefore easily recognized. However, in some cases these extranodal manifestations represent the predominant or even exclusive manifestation of the disease. The most important sites are the orbit,[40] upper respiratory tract,[39] skeletal system,[87] skin,[83] and central nervous system.[40a] In general, the course of the disease in these patients is similar to that in

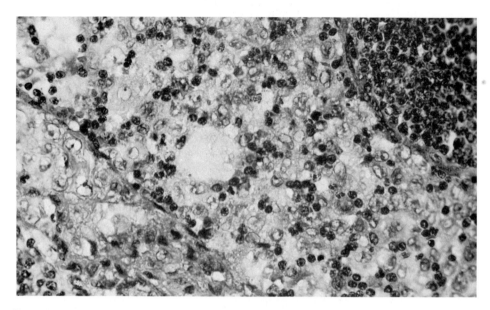

Fig. 1084 Lymph node involved by histiocytosis X. Langerhans' cells with large vesicular and grooved nuclei and abundant acidophilic cytoplasm distend peripheral sinuses. Eosinophils also are present. (×460; WU neg. 50-475; slide contributed by Dr. A. R. Crane, Philadelphia, Pa.)

those with only nodal involvement; the histology is similar to that seen in the lymph nodes, although fibrosis tends to be more accentuated.

Microscopically, the striking abnormality in the nodes is a pronounced dilatation of the lymphatic sinuses, resulting in almost complete architectural effacement (Fig. 1085). The sinuses are occupied, among other inflammatory cells, by numerous histiocytes with large vesicular nucleus and abundant clear cytoplasm. The latter often contain within their cytoplasm numerous phagocytosed lymphocytes, a feature of diagnostic significance[75] (Fig. 1085, *inset*). Plasma cells are numerous in the intersinusal tissue. Capsular and pericapsular inflammation and fibrosis are common. Electronmicroscopically, there are no microorganisms or Langerhans' granules.[79a] The disease is relatively unaffected by medical therapy and follows a protracted course leading eventually to complete recovery in the majority of the cases. The etiology is unknown.

Postvaccinial and other viral lymphadenitides

Lymph nodes draining an area of the skin subjected to smallpox vaccination can enlarge and become painful. If removed and examined microscopically, they can be easily confused with lymphoma, especially if the history of vaccination is overlooked. Of twenty cases reported by Hartsock,[48] thirteen were located in the supraclavicular region on the side of the vaccination. The largest node measured 6 cm in diameter. The interval between the vaccination and the biopsy varied between one week and three months.

Microscopically, the changes are those of a diffuse or nodular hyperplasia, with mixed cellular proliferation, consisting of eosinophils, plasma cells, and a large number of large lymphoid cells, accompanied by vascular and sinusoidal changes (Fig. 1086, *B*). According to Hartsock,[48] the most important histologic feature of postvaccinial hyperplasia is the presence of numerous large lymphoid cells (immunoblasts or reticular lymphoblasts) scattered among the lymphocytes and imparting to the lymphoid tissue a mottled appearance. He noted that follicular hyperplasia was present only in those nodes removed more than fifteen days after the vaccination. The lymph node changes of postvaccinial hyperplasia, which have been reproduced experimentally,[48] are indistinguishable from those of herpes zoster and quite similar to those of infectious mononucleosis. The latter also can result in a mixed pattern of reaction and is discussed under a separate heading. It is likely that similar morphologic changes occurring in the absence of these three

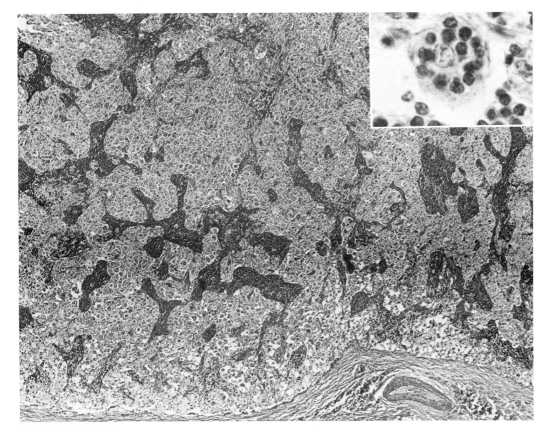

Fig. 1085 Sinus histiocytosis with massive lymphadenopathy. Note capsular fibrosis and extreme dilatation of sinuses. **Inset** illustrates phenomenon of lymphocytophagocytosis by sinus histiocytes. (×39; WU neg. 71-9685; **inset,** ×720; WU neg. 71-9690.)

clinical conditions are, in most cases, the result of some unidentified viral infection.

Prominent regional lymphadenopathy also may follow the administration of live attenuated measles virus vaccine. Microscopically, the typical multinucleated giant cell of Warthin-Finkeldey may be found[35] (Fig. 508).

Anticonvulsant therapy

Antiepileptic drugs derived from hydantoin, such as diphenylhydantoin (Dilantin) and mephenytoin (Mesantoin), can result in a hypersensitivity reaction manifested by skin rash, fever, generalized lymphadenopathy (mainly cervical), and peripheral eosinophilia. The reaction, which is quite uncommon, tends to occur within the first few months of therapy. The changes disappear if the drug is discontinued. The nodal enlargement can occur in the absence of some of the other manifestations of the drug reaction.

Microscopically, partial effacement of the architecture by a *polymorphic* cellular infiltration is seen. Histiocytes, immunoblasts, eosinophils, neutrophils, and plasma cells are all present. Some of the immunoblasts have atypical nuclear features, but Sternberg-Reed cells are absent. Foci of necrosis are common[77] (Fig. 1087). In some of the cases, the microscopic appearance is indistinguishable from that of angioimmunoblastic lymphadenopathy. The problem may simply be one of semantics: probably these cases represent angioimmunoblastic lymphadenopathy induced by the anticonvulsant therapy.

Angioimmunoblastic lymphadenopathy

Angioimmunoblastic lymphadenopathy[41] or immunoblastic lymphadenopathy[61] occurs almost exclusively in adults and elderly individuals and is characterized clinically by fever, anemia (usually hemolytic), polyclonal hyper-

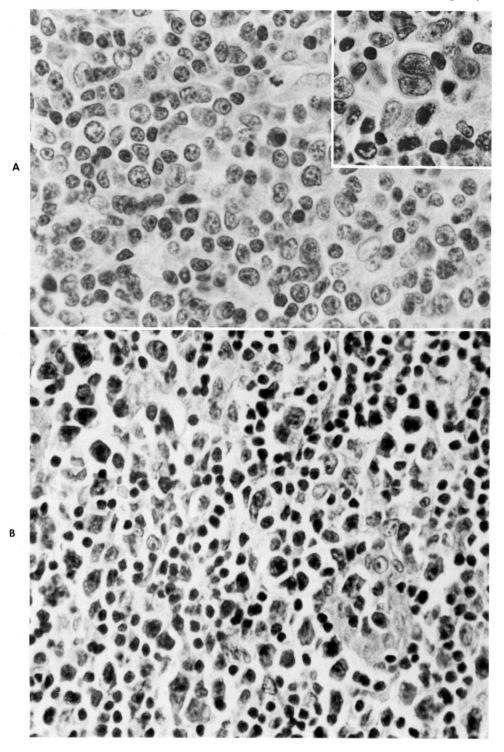

Fig. 1086 Two examples of lymphoid hyperplasia due to viruses. **A,** Tonsil from 17-year-old black woman with infectious mononucleosis. Heterophil antibody was strongly positive, and patient fully recovered. There is polymorphic infiltrate containing numerous immunoblasts, one of them binucleated **(inset).** Lymph node changes are very similar. **B,** Lymph node draining vaccination site. Note polymorphism and presence of immunoblasts. (**A,** ×480; **inset,** ×700; **B,** ×720; WU neg. 67-438.)

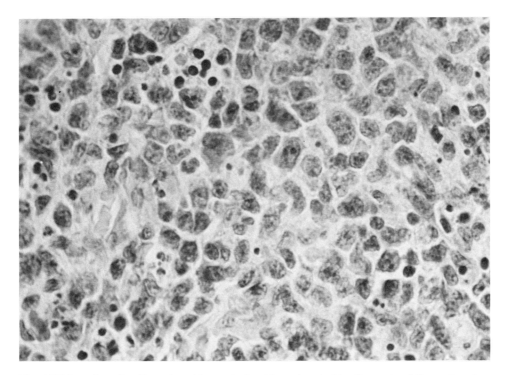

Fig. 1087 Lymph node with profound hyperplasia of large lymphoid cells, eosinophilia, and nuclear debris. Patient was child with generalized lymphadenopathy and splenomegaly and had been taking Peganone, an anticonvulsant drug. Clinically and pathologically, he was first thought to have malignant lymphoma. With discontinuance of drug, symptoms and clinical findings completely disappeared, and child recovered. (×750; WU neg. 58-1456.)

gammaglobulinemia, and generalized lymphadenopathy. Other common manifestations include hepatomegaly, splenomegaly, constitutional symptoms, and skin rash.[42,80a] In 27% of the patients studied by Lukes and Tindle,[61] the disease occurred abruptly after administration of drugs, particularly penicillin.

Microscopically, the disease is systemic, with lesions in lymph nodes, spleen, liver, bone marrow, and skin. However, only the lymph node changes can be regarded as diagnostic of the entity (Fig. 1088). They are characterized by obliteration of the nodal architecture (with focal preservation of sinuses) by a polymorphic cellular infiltrate and an extensive proliferation of finely arborizing vessels of the caliber of postcapillary venules. The cellular infiltrate is composed of small lymphocytes, plasma cells, numerous immunoblasts, frequent and sometimes abundant eosinophils, and, occasionally, multinucleated giant cells. Normal germinal centers are consistently absent; what one may find instead are germinal centers composed of loose aggregates of pale histiocytes,

rare immunoblasts, or large epithelioid cells; these are referred to as "burnt-out germinal centers" and can closely resemble the appearance of granulomas. An amorphous, eosinophilic PAS-positive intercellular material may be found scattered throughout the node. Extension of the infiltrate in the capsule and pericapsular tissue is common. Methyl green–pyronine stain shows that most of the large lymphoid cells are pyroninophilic, and immunoperoxidase stain reveals a polyclonal pattern of immunoglobulin production. Occasionally, amyloid deposition is observed.[63]

Jones et al.[50a] studied eight patients with this disorder with a variety of immunologic and pathologic techniques and thought that they could roughly divide their cases into two groups, depending upon whether B cells (associated with numerous plasma cells) or T cells (associated with numerous blast cells and eosinophils but scanty plasma cells) predominated. The clinical course was more aggressive in the second group.

According to Lukes and Tindle,[61] the basic

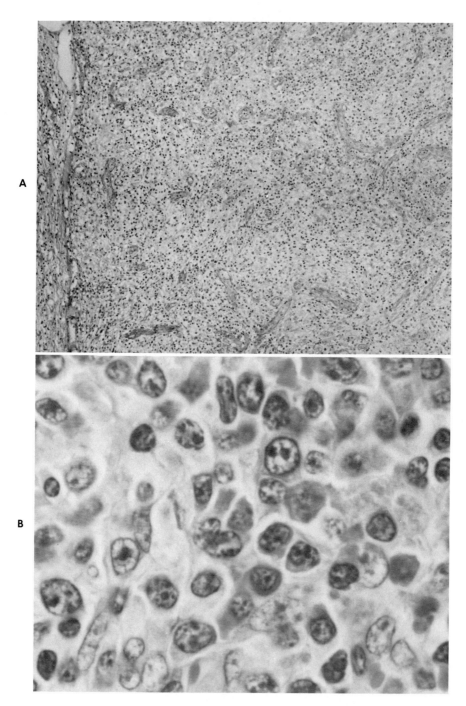

Fig. 1088 Angioimmunoblastic lymphadenopathy. **A,** There is effacement of nodal architecture by hypocellular process accompanied by marked vascular proliferation. Germinal centers are absent. Peripheral sinus is patent, but infiltrate extends beyond capsule. **B,** High-power view of infiltrate, illustrating its polymorphic composition. There are lymphocytes, plasma cells, immunoblasts, histiocytes, and plump endothelial cells. (**A,** ×120; **B,** ×1,480; **A** and **B,** courtesy Dr. G. Frizzera, Minneapolis, Minn.)

process appears to be a nonneoplastic hyper-immune proliferation of the B cell system involving an exaggerated transformation of lymphocytes to immunoblasts and plasma cells. It has been suggested that the primary abnormality might be in the T cell system[32a,54] and specifically that the disease may be the result of a loss of suppressor T cells, with consequent hyperfunction of the B lymphocyte system.[30a,69] The possibility that a viral infection might be the initiating factor for some cases of this disease has been repeatedly voiced. In this regard, it is interesting to note that Krueger et al.[55a] found rubella virus antigen by immunofluorescent techniques in the lymph node sections of eleven of fourteen patients with the morphologic changes of angioimmunoblastic lymphadenopathy.

In the series of Frizzera et al.,[42] approximately half of the patients were long-term survivors, whereas the others died in a relatively short time regardless of the treatment given. Nathwani et al.[68] identified a morphologic pattern associated with a particularly aggressive clinical course, that they designated as malignant lymphoma of the immunoblastic type. This was characterized initially by the appearance of "clones" (clusters or islands) of tightly packed immunoblasts, eventually followed by a diffuse replacement of the node by these elements. The dividing line between pure angioimmunoblastic lymphadenopathy and angioimmunoblastic lymphadenopathy with immunoblastic sarcoma is difficult to define and appears somewhat subjective; also, the true neoplastic nature of the former has yet to be conclusively proved. However, a very important practical conclusion emanates from this study; i.e., the more clumps of immunoblasts one sees in a node with this disease, the more likely the clinical course will be progressive and ultimately fatal. In this regard, angioimmunoblastic lymphadenopathy can be viewed as a somewhat arbitrarily defined portion of a wide spectrum of atypical immunoproliferative disorders (for which Lennert and Mohri[57a] have coined the term lymphogranulomatosis X), which ranges from the clearly reactive and reversible to the highly aggressive and questionably neoplastic. In retrospect, we believe that the cases that we described some years ago as malignant histiocytosis with cutaneous involvement and eosinophilia[60] belong to this general category as representatives of the more aggressive type.

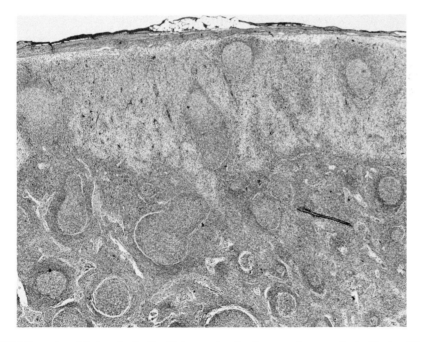

Fig. 1089 Dermatopathic lymphadenitis. Note prominent pale area of paracortical widening. There is also marked follicular hyperplasia. Lesion often contains melanin pigment. (Low power; WU neg. 49-4548.)

Dermatopathic lymphadenitis
(lipomelanosis reticularis of Pautrier)

Dermatopathic lymphadenitis is merely advanced hyperplasia associated with chronic dermatitis, particularly of the exfoliative type.[56] It may occur in any skin condition in which itching, scratching, and infection are prominent. Rarely, it may occur in the absence of clinical skin disease. In the series reported by Cooper et al.,[32] the disease was associated with malignant lymphoma in nearly 25% of the cases. The authors found no distinguishing features between this group and the rest. The lymph node may be quite large, the cut surface bulging, and the color pale yellow. Sometimes, black linear areas are seen in the periphery, representing clumps of melanin pigment and simulating the appearance of malignant melanoma.

Microscopically, the nodal architecture is preserved. The main change is represented by a marked pale widening of the thymic-dependent paracortical zone, which stands out prominently on low-power examination (Fig. 1089). The cells occupying this area are thought to be of three types: histiocytes, Langerhans' cells, and interdigitating reticulum cells.[72] Many of the histiocytes contain phagocytosed melanin and neutral fat in their cytoplasm. Plasma cell infiltration and follicular hyperplasia are often present (Fig. 1089). A scattering of eosinophils also may be seen. These nodes may be confused with Hodgkin's disease, mycosis fungoides, monocytic leukemia, or histiocytosis X.[56]

Lupus erythematosus

The lymph nodes changes in lupus erythematosus are generally of a non-specific nature and consist of some follicular hyperplasia associated with increased vascularization and scattered immunoblasts and plasma cells, some of the latter containing PAS-positive cytoplasmic bodies[65] that probably represent sites of immunoglobulin production. Occasionally, one encounters a peculiar form of necrosis characterized by the deposition of hematoxyphilic material in the stroma, in the sinuses, and on the wall of blood vessels (Fig. 1090). These have been found to be composed of DNA de-

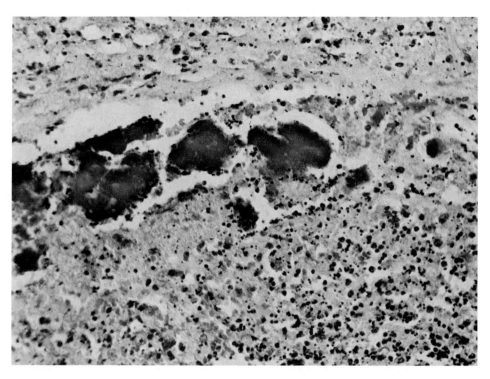

Fig. 1090 Lymph node with hematoxylin bodies in patient with disseminated lupus erythematosus. Diagnosis of this disease was made on basis of pathologic alterations in lymph node. This finding is rare in our experience. (×260; WU neg. 55-3684.)

rived from karyorrhectic nuclear material, presumably from lymphocytes.[53]

Infectious mononucleosis

It is rare for the pathologist to see a lymph node from a patient with a typical clinical picture of infectious mononucleosis, for in most instances the presumptive clinical diagnosis is confirmed by finding the characteristic cells in blood smears and an elevated heterophil antibody titer. It is in the atypical case, presenting with lymphadenopathy without fever, sore throat, or splenomegaly, that the clinician will perform a lymph node biopsy to rule out the possibility of malignant lymphoma.

Microscopically, nodes affected by infectious mononucleosis can be confused with malignant lymphoma because of the effacement of the architecture, infiltration of the trabeculae, capsule, and perinodal fat, and the marked proliferation of large lymphoid cells.[33] Features of importance in the differential diagnosis with lymphoma include predominantly sinusal distribution of the large lymphoid cells, follicular hyperplasia with marked mitotic activity and phagocytosis, increase in the number of plasma cells, and vascular proliferation[78] (Fig. 1086, *A*). Focal necrosis may be present. Another important feature is the fact that, although the nodal architecture may appear effaced, the sinusal pattern remains intact or even focally accentuated. This can be appreciated particularly well with reticulin stains. Sieracki and Fisher[81] described as a characteristic feature of this disease the presence in the sinuses of clusters or colonies of lymphocytes in graduated sizes, from the small lymphocyte to the large lymphoid cell or immunoblast. The latter cell usually has only one large vesicular nucleus with a thin nuclear membrane and one or two prominent amphophilic or basophilic nucleoli. When binucleated, it may closely resemble a Sternberg-Reed cell.[62,84] A paranuclear hof is often seen. Under the electron microscope, the large lymphoid cell bears a striking similarity to a lymphocyte transformed *in vitro* under the influence of phytohemagglutinin.[31]

Hyperplasia and malignant lymphoma

Unfortunately, there is not a single microscopic feature than can be used as an absolute criterion in the differential diagnosis between hyperplasia and malignant lymphoma.[34] Infiltration of the capsule and perinodal fat, effacement of the architecture, atypical lymphoid cells, and (exceptionally) even elements indistinguishable from Sternberg-Reed cells can all appear, alone or in combination, in a hyperplastic node. The final diagnosis should be based on a thorough evaluation of the microscopic features having a full knowledge of the clinical picture. Features favoring a diagnosis of hyperplasia include polymorphic nature of the infiltrate in the absence of Sternberg-Reed cells, presence of plasma cells, vascular proliferation, and preservation of the lymphatic sinuses. In the presence of a follicular (nodular) pattern of growth, we have found the criteria laid out by Rappaport et al.[71] extremely useful (see Table 56). In case of doubt, the pathologist must be conservative. A false positive diagnosis results in mental anguish to the patient and in treatment that usually consists of radiation therapy, often combined with some form of chemotherapy. We know of several instances in which the incorrect diagnosis of lymphoma was made and the patients died of complications of the therapy.

In some patients with apparently abnormal and even normal-appearing lymph nodes, the clinical signs and symptoms may strongly support a diagnosis of lymphoma. Further biopsies are indicated during the following months in order to establish the diagnosis. No evidence exists to suggest that a short delay in diagnosis will shorten the useful life of the patient if he is treated.[55] Of fifty-six patients in whom a nonspecific diagnosis was made initially by lymph node biopsy, the diagnosis was established in fifty-one within six months.[76] Treatment should not be instituted until a firm diagnosis is established.

The clinical information is extremely important but, like everything else, should be viewed with an open mind. We have seen unquestionable cases of malignant lymphoma in patients receiving anticonvulsivant drugs,[50] in individuals affected by rheumatoid arthritis, and in young patients with typical clinical and laboratory features of infectious mononucleosis. We also have seen lymphoma and hyperplasia coexisting in the same patient and even in the same lymph node. In the majority of the cases of lymphoma associated with a history of arthritis, anticonvulsant therapy, or vaccination, the association is probably coincidental. There is obviously no reason why a patient with malignant lymphoma could not receive a smallpox vaccination or also be affected by rheumatoid arthritis or epilepsy. On the other hand, there is a suggestion that in some instances the group of diseases resulting in nodal hyperplasia may actually induce the appearance of a malignant lymphoma, perhaps as a result of persistent immunologic stimulation. The oncogenic effect of such stimulation has been demonstrated in experimental conditions.[64,80] Reference has already been made to the alleged development of immunoblastic sarcoma in cases of angioimmunoblastic lymphadenopathy. As increased incidence of lymphoma has been reported in rheumatoid arthritis,[46] psoriatic arthritis, lupus erythematosus,[47] Sjögren's syndrome, and other connective tissue diseases.[30] Hyman and Sommers[50] found six cases of malignant lymphoma in patients on anticonvulsant therapy, and additional cases have been reported,[59] suggesting a causal relationship. A similar relationship has been suggested between Hodgkin's disease and previous infectious mononucleosis.[75a] At one institution, twenty-nine cases of infectious mononucleosis preceding Hodgkin's disease, the interval being less than one year in eight,[58,92] have been collected.

Granulomatous inflammation

The pathologist is often asked to make a definite diagnosis of a lymph node containing chronic granulomatous inflammation. Sometimes he may make such a diagnosis with fair accuracy. However, the reaction of the lymph nodes to the presence of various bacteria and fungi may be quite similar. In fact, some disease entities cause identical microscopic alterations. Often, definite diagnosis of a lymph node lesion can be made only by careful bacteriologic study.

The surgical pathologist should know the results of prior bacteriologic studies and of serologic and skin tests before attempting to interpret a granulomatous lymph node lesion. The clinical history and physical findings also may be quite helpful. Immunohistochemical techniques may provide a specific diagnosis. This can be made even from formalin-fixed and paraffin-embedded tissues for such lesions as tularemia.[134]

It is not rare for a lymph node containing a chronic granulomatous process to remain undiagnosed despite careful and extensive bacteriologic and pathologic study. It should be remembered that noncaseating granulomas in a lymph node may simply be the secondary manifestation of an underlying malignant disorder. We have seen them in lymph nodes draining carcinoma,[105,116] and in nodes involved by Hodgkin's disease and other lymphomas.[108]

Tuberculosis

Tuberculous lymph nodes often show caseation, epithelioid cells, and Langhans' giant cells. They may be adherent to each other and may form a large multinodular mass (Fig. 1091). Large, firm, tuberculous cervical nodes in the adult may be confused with metastatic cancer. We have seen radical neck dissection mistakenly performed under this circumstance. With evidence of pulmonary tuberculosis and draining sinuses in the neck, the diagnosis becomes almost certain. However, we still do not make this diagnosis unless acid-fast organisms are found. These are best demonstrated by culture.

Atypical mycobacteriosis

Atypical mycobacteria are a common cause of granulomatous lymphadenitis. A caseating granulomatous disease in a cervical lymph node of a child unaccompanied by pulmonary involvement is more likely to be caused by an atypical organism than by *Mycobacterium tuberculosis*.[112] This process typically involves lateral nodes in the midportion of the neck. Drainage may continue for months or years in the absence of specific therapy, and healing may result in scarring and contractures. Microscopically, the host reaction may be indistinguishable from that of tuberculosis, but often the granulomatous response is over-shadowed by necrotic and suppurative changes.[114,122] An acid-fast stain should be performed in every granulomatous and suppurative lymphadenitis of unknown etiology, especially if the patient is a child. The final identification of the organism rests on the cultural characteristics.

Sarcoidosis

The diagnosis of sarcoidosis is always one of exclusion. A noncaseating granulomatous inflammation in the lymph nodes or skin microscopically indistinguishable from sarcoidosis can be seen in tuberculosis, atypical mycobacteriosis (including swimming pool granuloma), fungous diseases, leprosy, syphilis, leishmaniasis, brucellosis, tularemia, chalazion, zirconium granuloma, berylliosis, Crohn's disease, Hodgkin's disease, in nodes draining a carcinoma, and in several other conditions[90,96] (Figs. 1092 and 1093). If all these possibilities have been excluded and the clini-

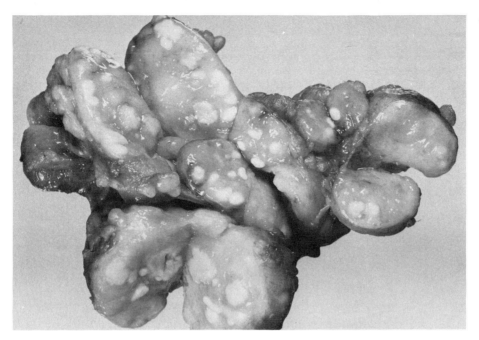

Fig. 1091 Large adherent tuberculous lymph nodes containing large zones of caseation necrosis. (WU neg. 50-3030.)

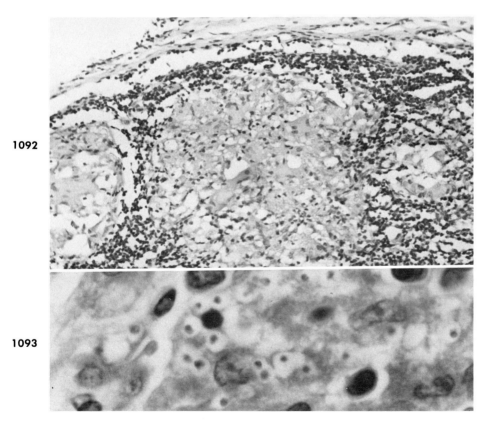

1092

1093

Fig. 1092 Noncaseating lesion in axillary lymph node. No organisms could be identified. At postmortem examination it was discovered that patient had disseminated histoplasmosis. (×200; WU neg. 50-2057.)

Fig. 1093 Histoplasmosis. Note well-defined bodies surrounded by clear area. (High power; WU neg. 47-394.)

cal picture is characteristic, there is justification in labeling a case as sarcoidosis for clinical purposes. Whether this is a specific disease or a peculiar granulomatous reaction to a variety of agents is unknown at the present time. Scandinavian countries are particularly affected.[127] In the United States, the disease is ten to fifteen times more common in blacks than in whites. Practically every organ can be in-volved, but the ones most commonly affected are the lung, lymph nodes, eyes, and skin. Erythema nodosum often precedes or accompanies the disease. Functional hypoparathyroidism is the rule, although a few cases of sarcoidosis coexisting with primary hyperparathyroidism have been reported.[97,135]

Microscopically, the basic lesion is a small granuloma mainly composed of epithelioid

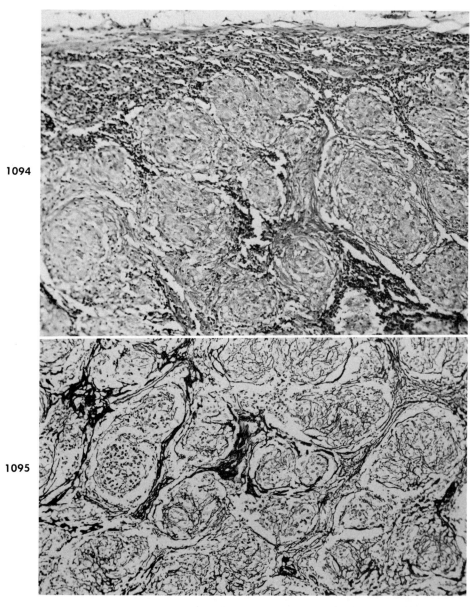

Fig. 1094 Lymph node involved by sarcoidosis demonstrating noncaseating granulomatous lesions. (Moderate enlargement; WU neg. 49-6723.)
Fig. 1095 Even distribution of reticulin in sarcoidosis. (Moderate enlargement; WU neg. 49-6724.)

cells, with scattered Langhans' giant cells and lymphocytes (Figs. 1094 and 1095). Necrosis is either absent or limited to a small central fibrinoid focus. Schaumann bodies, asteroid bodies, and calcium oxalate crystals are sometimes found in the cytoplasm of the giant cells (Fig. 1096). None of these inclusions are specific for sarcoidosis. Schaumann bodies are round, have concentric laminations, and contain iron and calcium. Azar and Lunardelli[91] have shown by electron microscopy that asteroid bodies are made of crisscrossing bundles of collagen fibrils. Peculiar Schiff-positive inclusions, sometimes designated as Wesenberg-Hamazaki bodies, have been claimed to be specific for sarcoidosis.[94,133] Histochemical and

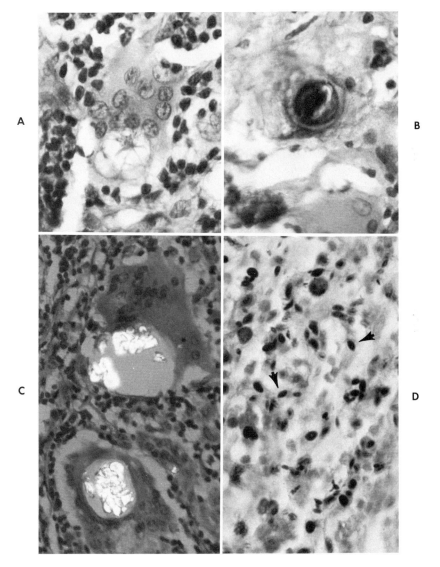

Fig. 1096 Four types of inclusions that can be found in sarcoidosis. None of them is specific for this condition. **A,** Asteroid body within cytoplasm of multinucleated giant cell. **B,** Schaumann body. Note round shape and concentric lamination. **C,** Calcium oxalate crystals seen under polarized light. **D,** So-called Wesenberg-Hamasaki bodies concentrated in perivascular location. They are of small size and have oval or needlelike configuration (arrows). All sections are from same case and originated in lymph node involved by disease. (**A,** ×600; WU neg. 73-564; **B,** ×600; WU neg. 73-563; **C,** ×350; WU neg. 73-562; **D,** acid-fast stain; ×600; WU neg. 73-681; **A-D,** AFIP; slides contributed by Dr. F. B. Johnson, Washington, D. C.)

electron microscopic studies by Sieracki and Fisher[125] have shown instead that they have no etiologic or pathogenetic significance. They probably represent large lysosomes containing hemolipofuscin material and are found in a large variety of conditions.[129a]

The Kveim skin test is positive in 60%-85% of patients with sarcoidosis. False positive results are rare. The skin should be biopsied four to six weeks after injection and examined microscopically. If positive, a granulomatous inflammation identical to that of the original disease is encountered.[115] An international Kveim trial employing a single test suspension has been completed among 2,400 subjects in thirty-seven countries on six continents.[126] The level of Kveim reactivity was similar from country to country, and the excised Kveim papules were histologically indistinguishable from one country to another, supporting the concept that sarcoidosis is the same disease the world over. Although the etiology remains elusive, mycobacterial organisms are the prime suspects. Substances like α, ϵ-diaminopimelic acid and mycolic acid, which occur in mycobacteria but are foreign to human tissue, have been identified in sarcoid lesions.[118] In several careful microscopic and cultural studies performed on supposedly typical cases of sarcoidosis, acid-fast organisms have been identified in a significant number.[113,130]

Tularemia

Tularemia causes caseation necrosis with less epithelioid cell production than in tuberculosis. Axillary lymph nodes may be enlarged. A history of handling or cleaning rabbits suggests the diagnosis. The organism may pass through the intact skin. In practically all cases, the agglutination titer is elevated.

Brucellosis

Brucellosis causes a chronic granulomatous reaction that is indistinguishable from tuberculosis. It may even suggest Hodgkin's diseases. A definitive diagnosis can be made only by bacteriologic isolation of the organism and a high agglutination titer.[132]

Fungous diseases

Fungous diseases cause a chronic granulomatous process that may or may not be associated with caseation necrosis. We have seen several cases of generalized histoplasmosis producing striking hyperplasia of the sinus histiocytes without granuloma formation. In one instance, this resulted in a mistaken diagnosis of reticuloendotheliosis. The Gomori methenamine-silver (GMS) and PAS-Gridley stains are extremely helpful in identifying organisms such as *Histoplasma capsulatum, Coccidioides,* and *Blastomyces.* In some instances, however, the number of organisms in a given section may be so small that they are not seen by the use of these stains. In such cases, only bacteriologic study can be diagnostic.

Lymphopathia venereum

The diagnosis of lymphopathia venereum usually is possible with a positive Frei test if the node involved is inguinal and the microscopic pattern is characteristic.

The earliest change in a lymph node is focal accumulation of neutrophilic leukocytes in tiny necrotic foci. These coalesce to form the classic stellate abscess (Fig. 1097). A marginal zone of epithelioid cells and fibroblasts appears with aging. This process may become confluent and be associated with cutaneous sinus tracts. In healing stages, a dense fibrous wall surrounds amorphous material.[128] This microscopic pattern is highly suggestive of this disease. However, we also have seen it with chronic tuberculosis. Smith and Custer[128] reported it with chronic tularemia.

Cat-scratch disease

Cat-scratch disease is characterized by a primary cutaneous lesion and enlargement of regional lymph nodes, usually axillary or cervical. The changes in the nodes vary with time. Early lesions have histiocytic proliferation and follicular hyperplasia, intermediate lesions have granulomatous changes, and late lesions have microscopic and macroscopic abscesses.[117,136] These abscesses are very suggestive of the diagnosis because of their pattern of central, sometimes stellate necrosis with neutrophils, surrounded by a palisading of histiocytes. However, similar abscesses can be seen in lymphopathia venereum. Another common feature of lymph nodes with cat-scratch disease is the packing of sinuses by monocytoid cells, which, together with the follicular hyperplasia, may simulate toxoplasmosis. However, clusters of perifollicular and intrafollicular epithelioid cells are absent[101] (Fig. 1098). Suppuration was present in forty-seven of 160 cases of cat-scratch disease reported by Daniels and MacMurray.[99]

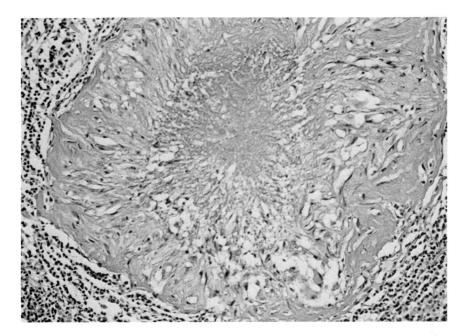

Fig. 1097 Stellate abscess in lymphopathia venereum. (×520; WU neg. 52-4494; slide contributed by Armed Forces Institute of Pathology.)

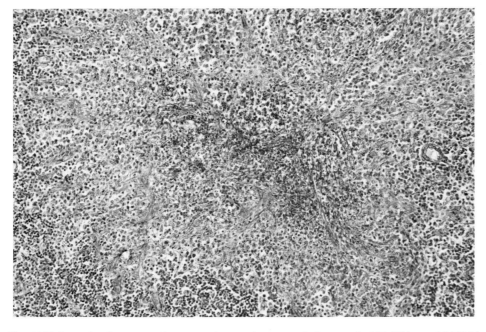

Fig. 1098 Area of stellate necrosis in proved case of cat-scratch disease. (×115; WU neg. 62-7610.)

The primary lesion is a red papule in the skin at the site of inoculation, usually appearing between seven and twelve days following contact. It may become pustular or crusted. Microscopically, there are foci of necrosis in the dermis surrounded by a mantle of histiocytes. Multinucleated giant cells, lymphocytes, and eosinophils are also present.[107] The agent is thought to be a microorganism of the psittacosis-lymphogranuloma group. The diagnosis can be confirmed by skin testing. Rare complications of the disease include granulomatous conjunctivitis ("oculoglandular syndrome of Parinaud"), thrombocytopenic purpura, and central nervous system manifestations.[93]

Toxoplasmosis

Toxoplasmosis is not the rare disease it was once thought to be.[129] There are indolent forms of this entity. The patient is often a woman, and the nodes involved are frequently the cervical[123,124] (so-called Piringer-Kuchinka lymphadenitis). These nodes feel firm, and their microscopic appearance, to those experienced with the disease, is highly suggestive of the diagnosis. Certainly, the cases of Saxen et al.,[124] which we have reviewed, had a distinctive pattern. The architecture of the lymph node is rather well preserved, and there is a striking degree of follicular hyperplasia, associated with marked mitotic activity and prominent phagocytosis of nuclear debris by histiocytes. The most characteristic feature of the disease is the presence of clusters of epithelioid cells, which encroach upon and blur the margins of the follicles[120] (Fig. 1099). They also can be seen within the germinal center itself. They may be accompanied by occasional Langhans' type giant cells, but necrosis is usually absent. Another consistent feature of toxoplasmic lymphadenitis is the focal distention of the sinuses by monocytoid cells. The medullary cords often contain an admixture of plasma cells and immunoblasts. It is extremely rare to find *Toxoplasma* organisms. However, the combination of microscopic features described correlates remarkably well with serologic studies. Of thirty-one cases studied by Dorfman and Remington,[100] the Sabin-Feldman dye test was positive in all, and the IgM immunofluorescent antibody test was positive in 97% of the cases. Some nodes with toxoplasmosis are still incorrectly diagnosed as Hodgkin's disease. Exceptionally, the two diseases can be seen together. It is likely that some of the apparent cures of Hodgkin's disease of the lymphocyte predominance type

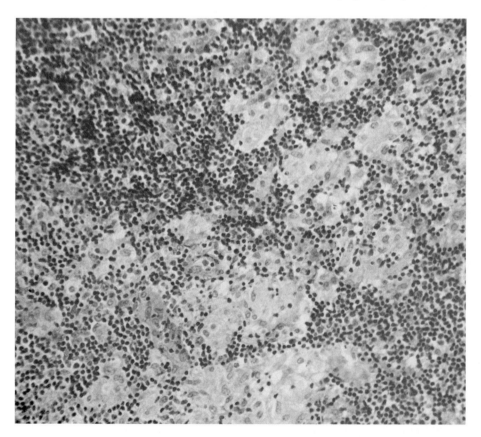

Fig. 1099 Typical collection of proliferating histiocytes in cervical lymph node of patient with proved toxoplasmosis. (×275; WU neg. 62-7377; slide contributed by Dr. E. Saxen, Helsinki, Finland.)

fall in this group. Lymph nodes involved by leishmaniasis also can exhibit a microscopic picture reminiscent of toxoplasmosis.[98] If the diagnosis of toxoplasmic lymphadenitis is suspected from the microscopic pattern, it should be confirmed serologically; it should be remembered, however, that these tests may be normal in the early stages of the disease. Kikuchi et al.[110] have suggested that toxoplasmosis may be the cause for at least some cases of necrotizing lymphadenitis, as reported mainly from Japan.[103]

Allergic granulomatosis

We have seen only four examples of allergic granulomatosis, a rare disorder which simulates Hodgkin's disease and histiocytosis X. It is characterized by nodular infiltration of the lymph node by mature histiocytes and eosinophils. Multiple foci of necrosis are seen, many of them apparently arising in a cluster of eosinophilic leukocytes. Sternberg-Reed and Langerhans' cells are absent.[104] Whether this

represents a specific entity or simply a pattern of reaction to a variety of stimuli remains to be determined.

Lipophagic granulomas

There are several conditions that result in the accumulation of phagocytosed fat within foamy histiocytes and multinucleated giant cells in the lymph node sinuses. The most common is the type seen in periportal and mesenteric nodes in asymptomatic individuals, probably the result of mineral oil ingestion.[109] Boitnott and Margolis[92] found this change in 78% of a series of forty-nine autopsied adults. Their chemical and histochemical studies showed that the oil droplets represented deposits of liquid-saturated hydrocarbons. Mineral oil is extensively used in the food processing industry, as a release agent and lubricant in capsules, tablets, bakery products, and dehydrated fruits and vegetables.

In *Whipple's disease,* the lipophagic granulomas are accompanied by collections of histiocytes containing a PAS-positive glycopro-

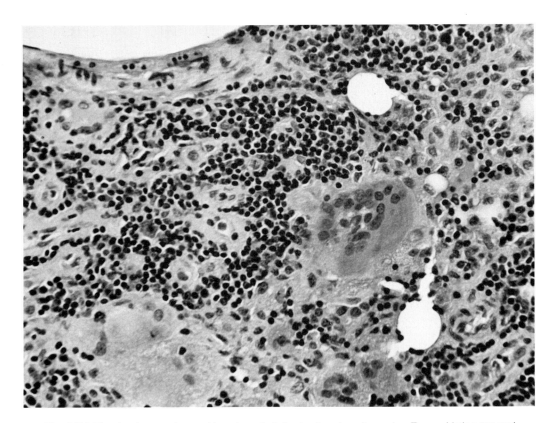

Fig. 1100 Lipophagic granuloma of lymph node following lymphangiography. Foamy histiocytes and multinucleated giant cells fill dilated sinuses. (×350; WU neg. 72-1301.)

tein.[102] Under oil immersion, and with electron microscopy, characteristic bacillary bodies may be identified.[131] The glycoprotein-containing histiocytes also can be seen in the peripheral nodes,[95] and this may be the first clue to the diagnosis in a patient with gradual weight loss, weakness, and polyarthritis. Steatorrhea, the other classical symptom of the disease, may appear only in a later stage. Unfortunately, the peripheral lymph node changes are not pathognomonic unless bacillary bodies can be demonstrated. All that the pathologist can do is to suggest the possibility and request a small bowel biopsy.

Lymphangiography, an increasingly popular technique, induces a lipophagic granulomatous reaction that may persist for several months. The sinuses are markedly distended and lined by histiocytes, many of which are multinucleated. Eosinophils may be present in appreciable numbers in the medullary cords. This is preceded by a predominantly neutrophilic infiltration[121] (Fig. 1100).

Cases of lymphadenitis characterized by a prominent component of foamy histiocytes have been described under the term *(idiopathic) xanthogranulomatosis lymphadenitis.*[95a,115a]

Mesenteric lymphadenitis

The diagnosis of mesenteric lymphadenitis (so-called Masshoff lymphadenitis) is too often made on normal or mildly hyperplastic nodes in an attempt to explain why a patient with the clinical picture of acute appendicitis has a normal appendix. This is not to say that mesenteric lymphadenitis is a myth. Cases having lymphoid hyperplasia, granuloma formation, and abscesses have been reported, sometimes accompanied by inflammation of the terminal ileum and cecum. Large pyroninophilic cells with the appearance of immunoblasts can be seen scattered throughout the node.[89] *Yersinia pseudotuberculosis* and *Yersinia enterocolitica,* two gram-negative polymorphic coccoid or ovoid motile organisms, have been isolated from many of these lesions.[106,119] Knapp[111] identified 115 cases of mesenteric lymphadenitis due to *Yersinia pseudotuberculosis* in a five-year period. The disease is benign and self-limited.

Malignant lymphoma

Malignant lymphoma is the generic term given to tumors of the lymphoreticular system that includes lymphocytes of T, B, and null

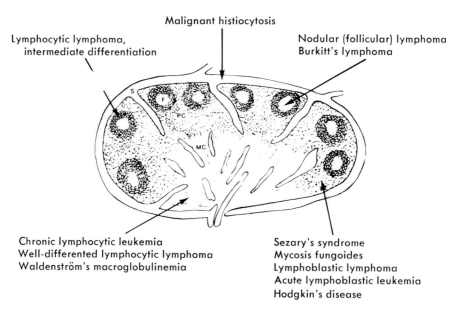

Malignant histiocytosis

Lymphocytic lymphoma, intermediate differentiation

Nodular (follicular) lymphoma
Burkitt's lymphoma

S
F
PC
MC

Chronic lymphocytic leukemia
Well-differented lymphocytic lymphoma
Waldenström's macroglobulinemia

Sezary's syndrome
Mycosis fungoides
Lymphoblastic lymphoma
Acute lymphoblastic leukemia
Hodgkin's disease

Fig. 1101 Diagram of lymph node showing anatomic and functional compartments and relating different lymphoreticular malignancies to these compartments. **S,** Sinuses. **F,** Follicles. **PC,** Paracortex. **MC,** Medullary cords. (From Mann RB, Jaffe ES, Berard CW: Malignant lymphomas—a conceptual understanding of morphologic diversity. A review. Am J Pathol **94:**105-191, 1979.)

types, histiocytes-monocytes, and reticular cells. The overwhelming majority of these tumors are of lymphocytic origin, particularly of B type.[141,142] A few seem to have the markers of histiocytes (certainly much less than the numbers of lymphomas that are currently diagnosed as histiocytic on purely morphologic grounds). The existence of neoplasms of the reticular cells (and four different types of these elements have been described in normal lymph nodes) has been postulated but not conclusively proved. Although some overlapping exists, the term *malignant lymphoma* is reserved for those neoplastic processes that initially present as localized lesions and are characterized by the formation of gross tumor nodules.[139] Neoplastic proliferations that are systemic and diffuse from their inception are called leukemias or malignant histiocytosis depending on their presumed cell of origin, which in the former case also leads to a complex subclassification.

The malignant lymphomas can be divided into two major categories, which are usually separated with ease: Hodgkin's disease and all the others, which, for lack of a better term, are known as non-Hodgkin's lymphomas.[137,138] Both categories are further subdivided into several more or less distinct subcategories. In gen-

eral, there is constancy within these groups, so that a patient with a certain type of lymphoma at a given site will have the same type at other sites and will maintain it during the entire evolution of the disease. However, on occasion one encounters two distinct types of lymphoma in the same patient, either sequentially or simultaneously, even in the same lymph node. The occurrence of two different and well-delineated varieties of lymphoma occurring in a single anatomic site or mass is known as *composite lymphoma*,[143] the most common combinations being Hodgkin's disease and non-Hodgkin's lymphoma and, among the non-Hodgkin's lymphomas, nodular poorly differentiated lymphocytic and diffuse histiocytic.[140] Some of these combinations may indeed represent the occurrence of two unrelated neoplasms, either spontaneously or as a result of the therapy given for one of them. The majority, however, are probably the expression of different biologic and morphologic manifestations of the same lesion, the more malignant one representing the undifferentiated or blastic form of the other.[144]

Non-Hodgkin's lymphoma

The classification of non-Hodgkin's lymphomas that has gained most acceptance, at least in the United States, is that proposed by Rap-

Table 56 Markers of lymphoreticular malignancies*†

	E	EAC	EA	Sig	TdT	Phago-cytosis	B-EST	ALP	AP
Well-differentiated lymphocytic lymphoma	−	±	±	+	−	−	−	−	−
Lymphocytic lymphoma, intermediate differentiation	−	+	±	+	−	−	−	±	−
Nodular lymphoma	−	+	±	+	−	−	−	± (rare)	−
Burkitt's lymphoma	−	±	±	+	−	−	−	± (rare)	−
Lymphoblastic lymphoma	+	±	−	−	+	−	−	−	+
Mycosis fungoides/Sézary's syndrome	+	−	−	−	−	−	−	−	+
Large cell lymphomas									
B cell type	−	±	±	+	−	−	−	−	−
T cell type	+	−	−	−	−	−	−	−	+
Histiocytic type	−	+	+	−	−	+	+	−	+
Null cell type	−	−	−	−	−	−	−	−	±
Malignant histiocytosis	−	+	+	−	ND	+	+	−	+
Hairy cell leukemia	−	±	+	±	−	±	−	−	+‡

*From Mann RB, Jaffe ES, Berard CW: Malignant lymphomas—a conceptual understanding of morphologic diversity. A review. Am J Pathol **94:**105-191, 1979.

†E = Rosette formation with unsensitized sheep erythrocytes; EAC = rosette formation with erythrocyte-IgM antibody-complement complexes; EA = rosette formation with erythrocyte-IgG antibody complexes; SIg = cell-synthesized membrane-bound immunoglobulin; TdT = terminal deoxynucleotidyl transferase activity; B-EST = α-naphthyl butyrate esterase activity; ALP = alkaline phosphatase activity; AP = acid phosphatase activity; ND = not determined; ‡ = tartrate-resistant.

paport[164] in 1966. This represents a modification of the classification that he and Gall presented at a Seminar of the American Society of Clinical Pathologists held in New Orleans, Louisiana, in 1963. This, in turn, was based on the classification proposed by Gall and Mallory[154] as part of their comprehensive critical study of 618 lymphomas. Rappaport's classification[164] was, of necessity, based entirely on morphologic grounds. Numerous independent clinicopathologic studies have shown its reproducibility, usefulness, and clinical relevance.[149] However, application of the remarkable advances in the field of immunology in the past few years to the study of lymphomas has shown that these can be viewed as clonal expansions of the normal anatomic and functional components of the immune system (Fig. 1101). Most of them have been studied using immunologic markers (Table 56) and, as a result, have been "typed" as to their normal counterparts, from which presumably they arose[144a,155a,161a,163] (Table 57). Electron microscopic studies have also been of great value in this regard.[166a] In addition, aggressive clinical investigations coupled with staging laparotomies have provided a wealth of new information on the sites of predilection and spread of the lymphomas according to type.[152,155,166] The results obtained with these investigations, especially the immunologic ones, have raised serious questions as to the scientific validity of

Rappaport's classification.[148,165] As a result, at least five new classifications have been proposed to remedy this situation and supposedly to take into account this new information[150,151,156-158, 161b,162] (Table 58). Needless to say, this has resulted in a confusing state of affairs, both for pathologists and clinicians. Since no evidence has yet been put forward to demonstrate that one classification is clearly superior to the others, the National Cancer Institute has sponsored a retrospective study of 1,175 cases of non-Hodgkin's lymphomas, which have been classified according to the different classifications by the investigators who proposed them, as well as by a panel of "control" pathologists. This study is now nearing completion, and some preliminary conclusions have already been made.[162a] Analysis of the data showed that all six classifications were successful in predicting the prognosis in a large number of lymphoma patients and that no classification appeared superior to any other in this respect. It also confirmed that lymphomas with a nodular pattern of growth (a feature consistently identified by all reviewers) had a more favorable prognosis than those with diffuse patterns within the same cytologic subtypes. This was true whether the nodularity was extensive or only partial. Finally, it confirmed the suspicion that within the "histiocytic lymphoma" of Rappaport there is a variety of morphologically recognizable neoplasms with

Table 57 Cell types of lymphoreticular malignancies*

Well-differentiated lymphocytic malignancies	B lymphocytic
Chronic lymphocytic leukemia (98%)	
Well-differentiated lymphocytic lymphoma	
Waldenström's macroglobulinemia	
Heavy chain diseases	
Lymphocytic lymphoma, intermediate differentiation	B lymphocytic
Nodular (follicular) lymphoma	B lymphocytic
Burkitt's lymphoma	B lymphocytic
Lymphoblastic lymphoma	T lymphocytic
Acute lymphoblastic leukemia (25%)	T lymphocytic
Chronic lymphocytic leukemia (2%)	T lymphocytic
Mycosis fungoides/Sézary's syndrome	T lymphocytic
Large cell lymphomas	Heterogeneous
"Histiocytic" lymphoma	
Undifferentiated, pleomorphic (non-Burkitt's) lymphoma	
Malignant histiocytosis	Histiocytic
Hairy cell leukemia	B lymphocytic-histiocytic
Hodgkin's disease	Not settled

*From Mann RB, Jaffe ES, Berard CW: Malignant lymphomas—a conceptual understanding of morphologic diversity. A review. Am J Pathol **94**:105-191, 1979.

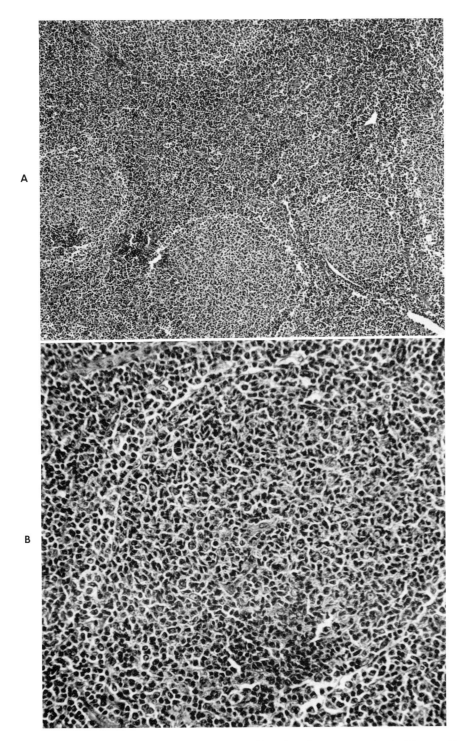

Fig. 1102 Nodular lymphoma of poorly differentiated lymphocytic type occurring in 51-year-old man with generalized lymphadenopathy. **A,** Large nodules scattered throughout. **B,** Large nodule in which cells inside are streaming outside follicle. There is no evidence of phagocytosis. (**A,** ×87; WU neg. 62-8265; **B,** ×285; WU neg. 62-8264.)

Table 58 Major recently proposed classifications of non-Hodgkin's lymphoma as modified by the respective authors for use in the National Cancer Institute–sponsored study on the subject and new International Formulation[162a]

Rappaport	Lukes and Collins	Kiel	World Health Organization
Nodular	Undefined cell type	Low-grade malignancy	Nodular lymphosarcoma
Lymphocytic, well differentiated	T cell type	Lymphocytic	Prolymphocytic
Lymphocytic, poorly differentiated	Small lymphocytic	Chronic lymphocytic leukemia	Prolymphocytic-lymphoblastic
Mixed (lymphocytic and histiocytic)	Sezary-mycosis fungoides (cerebriform)	Other	Diffuse lymphosarcoma
Histiocytic	Convoluted lymphocytic	Lymphoplasmacytoid	Lymphocytic
Diffuse	Immunoblastic sarcoma (T cell)	Centrocytic	Lymphoplasmacytic
Lymphocytic, well differentiated	B cell type	Centroblastic-centrocytic	Prolymphocytic
Without plasmacytoid features	Small lymphocytic	Follicular, without sclerosis	Prolymphocytic-lymphoblastic
With plasmacytoid features	Plasmacytoid lymphocytic	Follicular, with sclerosis	Lymphoblastic
Lymphocytic, poorly differentiated	Follicular center cell*	Follicular and diffuse, without sclerosis	Immunoblastic
Without plasmacytoid features	Small cleaved	Follicular and diffuse, with sclerosis	Burkitt's tumor
With plasmacytoid features	Large cleaved	Diffuse	Mycosis fungoides
Lymphoblastic	Small noncleaved	Unclassified	Plasmacytoma
Convoluted	Large noncleaved	High-grade malignancy	Unclassified
Nonconvoluted	Immunoblastic sarcoma (B cell)	Centroblastic	Composite
Mixed (lymphocytic and histiocytic)	Histiocytic	Lymphoblastic	
Histiocytic	Unclassified	Burkitt's type	
Without sclerosis	Composite	Convoluted cell type	
With sclerosis		Other (unclassified)	
Burkitt's tumor		Immunoblastic	
Undifferentiated		Unclassified	
Unclassified		Composite	
Composite			

Dorfman	National Lymphoma Investigation (England)	New International Formulation
Follicular (or follicular and diffuse)†	Follicular lymphoma	Low grade
Small lymphoid	Follicle cells, predominantly small	ML,‡ small lymphocytic
Mixed (small and large lymphoid)	Follicle cells, mixed small and large	Consistent with chronic lymphocytic leukemia
Large lymphoid	Follicle cells, predominantly large	Plasmacytoid
Diffuse†	Diffuse lymphoma	ML, follicular, predominantly small cleaved cell
Small lymphocytic	Lymphocytic, well differentiated (small round lym-	With diffuse areas
Without plasmacytoid differentiation	phocyte)	With sclerosis
With plasmacytoid differentiation	Lymphocytic, intermediately differentiated (small follicle	ML, follicular, mixed (small cleaved and large cell)

Atypical small lymphoid
Lymphoblastic
  Convoluted
  Nonconvoluted
Large lymphoid
  Without plasmacytoid differentiation
  With plasmacytoid differentiation
Mixed (small and large lymphoid)
Histiocytic
Burkitt's lymphoma
Lymphoepithelioid cellular
  (Lennert's lymphoma)
Mycosis fungoides
Undifferentiated
Unclassified
Composite

lymphocyte)
Lymphocytic, poorly differentiated (lymphoblast)
  Non-Burkitt
  Burkitt's tumors
  Convoluted cell mediastinal lymphoma
Lymphocytic, mixed (small lymphoid and large cell; mixed
  follicle cells)
Undifferentiated large cell (large lymphoid cell)
Histiocytic cell (mononuclear phagocytic cell)
Plasma cell (extramedullary plasma cell)
Unclassified
Subdivisions
  (1) With or without plasmacytoid differentiation
  (2) Without sclerosis; with fine sclerosis; with banded
      sclerosis

with diffuse areas
  With sclerosis
Intermediate grade
ML, follicular, predominantly large cell
  With diffuse areas
  With sclerosis
ML, diffuse, small cleaved cell
  With sclerosis
ML, diffuse, mixed (small and large cell)
  With sclerosis
  With epithelioid cell component
ML, diffuse, large cell
  Cleaved cell
  Noncleaved cell
  With sclerosis
High grade
ML, large cell, immunoblastic
  Plasmacytoid
  Clear cell
  Polymorphous
  With epithelioid cell component
ML, lymphoblastic
  Convoluted
  Nonconvoluted
ML, small noncleaved cell
  Burkitt's
  With follicular areas
Miscellaneous
  Composite
  Mycosis fungoides
  Histiocytic
  Extramedullary plasmacytoma
  Unclassifiable
  Other

*Subdivided into (1) follicular, follicular and diffuse, and diffuse and (2) without sclerosis and with sclerosis.
†Subdivided into with sclerosis and without sclerosis.
‡ML, Malignant lymphoma.

a somewhat different natural history. As a result of the analysis of these 1,175 cases, the investigators involved in this study proposed a new classification of non-Hodgkin's malignant lymphomas, based primarily upon light microscopic differences, as seen in sections stained with hematoxylin-eosin, that show a correlation with survival. Ten major types plus a miscellaneous group were identified, and these could be divided into three major prognostic groups which were of favorable, intermediate, and unfavorable prognosis, respectively (Table 58). It remains to be seen whether this new International Formulation will eventually replace the existing ones.

For the time being, it is probably wiser for the practicing pathologist to continue using the classification with which both he and the clinician are more familiar and the one that has proved more than any other its clinical relevance. For most countries, this means Rappaport's classification,[164] with some unavoidable modifications stemming from the most relevant new information. I would only add that, of all the proposed classifications, the one that offers the most novel approach is that championed by Lukes.[160] In addition to incorporating a number of entities which, at the time, were barely known but are now generally accepted, it maintains that a functional classification of lymphomas is possible on the basis of the morphologic interpretation of routinely stained sections.[159-161] Frizzera et al.[153] tested this concept independently by attempting to predict the T versus the B cell nature of sixty non-Hodgkin's lymphomas on a morphologic basis and comparing their results with those obtained from surface marker studies in the same cases. The correlation was remarkably good: 97% for nodular lymphomas and 81% for diffuse lymphomas. However, some discrepancies existed in this and in similar studies,[147] indicating that there are limitations to this morphologic approach and also that the final functional characterization of a lymphoma needs to be done with immunologic tests. This becomes particularly important in view of the suggestion that there is a difference in survival rates depending on the cell surface immunologic features for tumors of similar histology. In general, patients whose lymphomas express the markers predicted from morphology respond to therapy and/or survive significantly better than the others.[145,146] Another important approach to malignant lymphoma is through chromosomal studies of the tumor cells by the newly developed banding techniques. Abnormalities already have been found in many cases of lymphoma, and there is a suggestion that some may correlate with specific morphologic types.[153a]

The individual descriptions that follow generally employ Rappaport's terminology,[164] with some unavoidable changes stemming from recent advances in the field, and incorporate the equivalent terms in the new International Formulation.[162a]

Nodular (follicular) lymphoma

Although regarded by Rappaport et al.[181] as the result of a pattern of growth that most cytologic types of lymphoma could exhibit, it has now become evident that nodular lymphoma represents a specific type of lymphoma that arises from the follicular center cells.[170] This tumor comprises about 50% of all adult non-Hodgkin's lymphomas in the United States, but

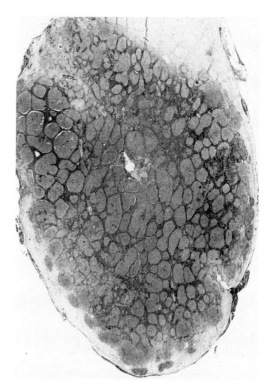

Fig. 1103 Low-power view of nodular lymphoma. Nodules of relatively uniform size and shape efface nodal architecture. (×6.5; from Mann RB, Jaffe ES, Berard CW: Malignant lymphomas—a conceptual understanding of morphologic diversity. A review. Am J Pathol **94**:105-191, 1979.)

in other countries the incidence seems to be much lower. Most cases occur in elderly individuals. As a group, it has a much better prognosis than diffuse lymphoma.[180] It is very unusual under 20 years of age and relatively uncommon in blacks.[173] Most of the cases diagnosed as nodular lymphomas in children actually represent nodular types of lymphocyte predominance Hodgkin's disease or reactive follicular hyperplasias. However, Frizzera and Murphy[171] recently reported eight well-docu-

mented cases of nodular lymphoma in patients under 15 years of age.

At low-power examination, the most distinctive feature of these tumors is the nodular pattern of growth (Figs. 1102 and 1103). Rappaport et al.[181] have carefully outlined the main differential points between these nodules and the reactive follicles of follicular hyperplasia (Table 56) (Fig. 1104). The nodules of this lymphoma actually represent neoplastic follicles, as shown by enzyme histochemical,

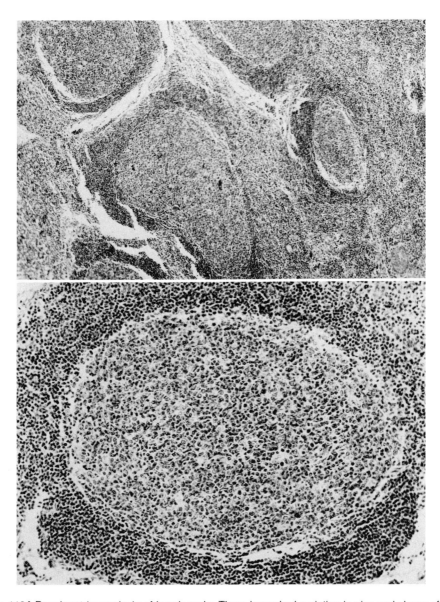

Fig. 1104 Prominent hyperplasia of lymph node. There is marked variation in size and shape of follicles. Note delimitation of hyperplastic germinal centers surrounded by mantle of lymphocytes. Germinal center has prominent phagocytes. (WU negs. 48-5750 and 48-5746.)

immunocytochemical, and electron microscopic studies.[177,178,183] The most convincing and spectacular demonstration of this fact has been obtained by identifying in frozen sections the presence of Fc receptors in the tumor cells with tagged red blood cells (better seen on dark-field examination; Fig. 1105) or by documenting with antibodies to kappa and light chains the presence of monoclonal immunoglobulin in the nodules, which are surrounded by a normal polyclonal population of lymphocytes[183] (Fig. 1106).

Therefore, these tumors could be more accurately designated as follicular, as the original proponents of the entity did. With progression of the disease, this distinct nodularity becomes blurred, and eventually most of the proliferation acquires a diffuse pattern. As long as some

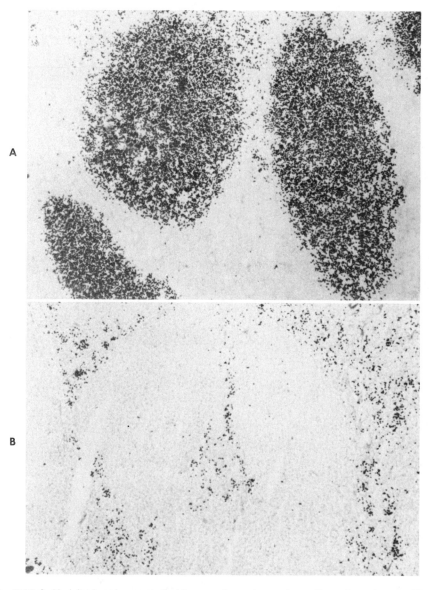

Fig. 1105 A, Nodular lymphoma studied for complement receptors with erythrocytes sensitized with IgM antibody and complement. Erythrocytes adhere to neoplastic nodules. **B,** Cryostat section from same tissue shown in **A** treated with erythrocytes sensitized with IgG antibody for Fc receptors. Neoplastic nodules are negative; there are scattered Fc-positive cells in surrounding lymphoid tissue. (Courtesy Dr. K. Gajl-Peczalska, Minneapolis, Minn.)

nodularity is evident somewhere in the node, it is recommended that the lymphoma be classified as nodular. The cytologic composition of the neoplastic nodules is characterized by a mixture in different proportion of small and large lymphoid cells, both of which resemble their normal follicular counterparts. The small cells have scanty cytoplasm and an irregular, elongated, cleaved nucleus with prominent indentations and infoldings; the size is similar or slightly larger than that of normal lymphocytes, the chromatin is coarse, and the nucle-

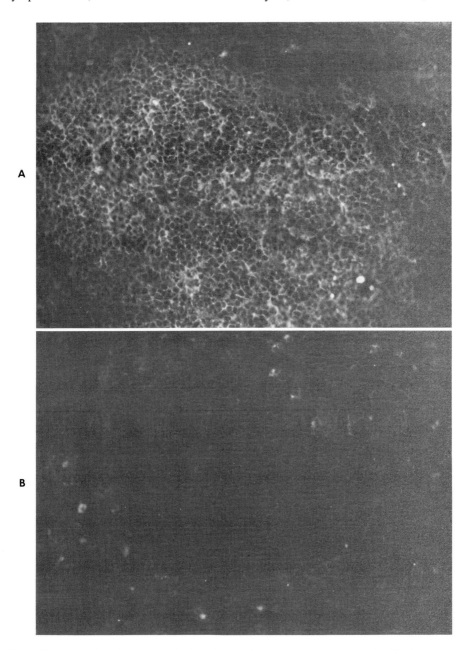

Fig. 1106 Nodular lymphoma examined by immunofluorescence for immunoglobulins in cryostat sections. **A,** Neoplastic nodule shows strong positivity for μ heavy chain, mainly at surface. Scattered cells with same specificity, probably neoplastic, are present outside nodule. **B,** Surrounding nonneoplastic lymphoid tissue stains for γ heavy chain. Nodule is completely negative. (Courtesy Dr. K. Gajl-Peczalska, Minneapolis, Minn.)

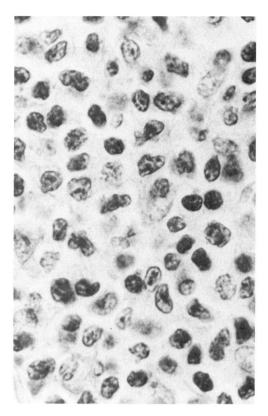

Fig. 1107 Nodular lymphoma of poorly differentiated lymphocytic type. Note cleaved and indented nuclei with coarsely clumped chromatin. Mitoses are rare. (×1,000; from Mann RB, Jaffe ES, Berard CW: Malignant lymphomas—a conceptual understanding of morphologic diversity. A review. Am J Pathol **94:**105-191, 1979.)

Depending on the relative proportion of small and large cells, nodular lymphomas are subdivided into three categories, respectively designated in the classification of Rappaport et al.[181] as follows:

1. Poorly differentiated lymphocytic, when the population of large cells in the nodules is less than 20% ("malignant lymphoma, follicular, predominantly small cleaved cells" in the new International Formulation)
2. Mixed, when the proportion of large cells is between 20%-50% ("malignant lymphoma, follicular, mixed, small cleaved and large cell" in the new International Formulation)
3. Histiocytic, when the proportion of large cells is more than 50% ("malignant lymphoma, follicular, predominantly large cell" in the new International Formulation)

In the first category, which is the most common, mitotic activity is infrequent. Conversely, the apparition of large cells is often accompanied by a parallel increase in the number of mitoses.

Several important clinical differences exist between these three groups. Patients with poorly differentiated lymphocytic lymphoma are often asymptomatic, usually have generalized disease (often involving extranodal sites, such as liver and bone marrow), and, paradoxically, have a good prognosis.[174] Histiocytic nodular lymphomas are more commonly localized at the time of presentation but run a more aggressive clinical course[173] and are more likely to lose their nodular pattern of growth to become diffuse. The prognosis of mixed nodular lymphoma is intermediate between these two but closer to the poorly differentiated type. As a matter of fact, in one series it was associated with a longer survival than the latter.[167] Another morphologic parameter that has been evaluated in this tumor is the relative degree of nodularity. Warnke et al.[184] have shown that among the poorly differentiated lymphocytic and mixed lymphomas, the survival rate is similar in patients with purely nodular tumors and those with tumors of a nodular *and* diffuse pattern. Instead, in the histiocytic lymphoma category, patients with tumors of both nodular *and* diffuse patterns have a worse prognosis than those with tumors of a pure nodular pattern. An earlier suggestion that nodular lymphomas having a prominent rim of small lym-

olus is inconspicuous (Fig. 1107). These cells have been variously referred as germinocytes, centrocytes, poorly differentiated lymphocytes, small cleaved follicular center cells, and prolymphocytes. The large cells are two or three times the size of normal lymphocytes; they have a distinct rim of cytoplasm and a vesicular nucleus with one to three nucleoli often adjacent to the nuclear membrane. These cells, which have a rapid turnover rate and probably represent the proliferating component of the tumor, are known as germinoblasts, centroblasts, histiocytes, large (cleaved or noncleaved) follicular center cells, large lymphoid cells, and lymphoblasts. Some may be binucleated and simulate Sternberg-Reed cells.[179] It is now clear that both the large and small lymphoid cells belong to a same line of B lymphocytes of follicular center origin.[172,176]

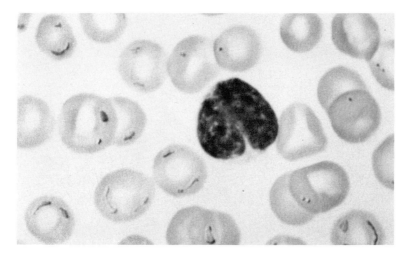

Fig. 1108 Blood smear from patient with mixed type of nodular malignant lymphoma showing so-called "notched nucleus cell" or "buttock cell." (×1,080; from Rappaport H, Winter WJ, Hicks EB: Follicular lymphoma. A reevaluation of its position in the scheme of malignant lymphoma, based on a survey of 253 cases. Cancer **9:**792-821, 1956.)

phocytes and vascular prominence between the nodules are associated with a better prognosis has not been confirmed.[168a]

The extranodal spread of nodular lymphoma is quite predictable. In the spleen, it tends to affect the B-derived lymphoid follicles located eccentrically in the white pulp. In the liver, the infiltrate is predominantly portal. The bone marrow infiltrates tend to have a paratrabecular location. In the skin, there is an extensive dermal infiltrate without particular relation to vessels or adnexa.

In some cases of nodular lymphoma (particularly in the poorly differentiated type), malignant cells are found in the peripheral blood; hematologists refer to them by the inelegant term "buttock" cells because of their prominent nuclear cleft (Fig. 1108). No prognostic significance has been assigned to this finding. A different matter is the occasional "blastic" transformation of nodular lymphoma, in which the tumor cells acquire the morphologic features of lymphoblasts; this is accompanied by a highly aggressive clinical course.[169]

Three morphologic variations in the theme of nodular lymphoma have been described. One is characterized by the presence of fine or coarse bands of fibrosis that accentuate even more the nodular character of the lesion but, in so doing, may induce confusion with carcinoma; this feature is more commonly seen in the histiocytic type and seems to be associated with a slightly improved prognosis.[168,182]

The second refers to the deposition of a proteinaceous material in the center of the nodules, similar to that seen in some reactive conditions, particularly the plasma cell variant of Castleman's disease. The material is amorphous, acellular, and brightly eosinophilic, and it may represent a mixture of fibrin and precipitated immunoglobulins. It can appear both in poorly differentiated lymphocytic and mixed nodular lymphomas and has no prognostic significance.[182] The third variation, less common and so far described only in connection with the poorly differentiated lymphocytic and mixed types, relates to the presence of large cytoplasmic eosinophilic globules (presumably immunoglobulins) that push the nucleus laterally and result in a signet-ring effect.[175]

Diffuse lymphoma

The group of diffuse lymphomas is larger, more heterogeneous, and not so well defined as that of the nodular lymphomas. It actually includes cases of nodular (follicular center cell) lymphomas in which the nodularity has been lost altogether. It comprises about half of the adult cases of non-Hodgkin's lymphoma in adults and nearly all of the cases in children.[185]

Well-differentiated lymphocytic lymphoma. Well-differentiated lymphocytic lymphoma ("malignant lymphoma, small lymphocytic" in the new International Formulation) preferentially occurs in middle-aged and elderly

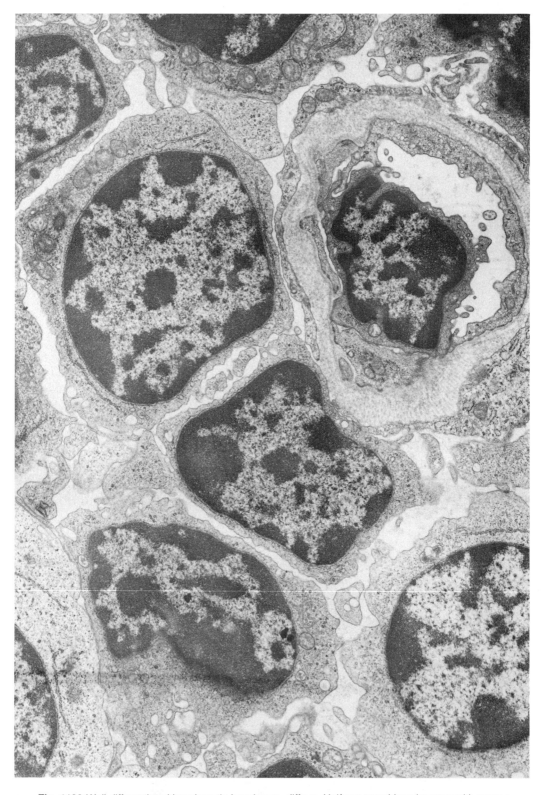

Fig. 1109 Well-differentiated lymphocytic lymphoma, diffuse. Uniform round lymphocytes with sparse mitochondria, poorly developed endoplasmic reticulum, and numerous ribosomes. Nuclei have clumped, peripherally situated chromatin. (×11,230.)

individuals. The symptoms are scanty, the evolution is prolonged, and the survival is very good. Some cases represent the tissue manifestation of chronic lymphocytic leukemia, whereas others present with lymphadenopathy without peripheral blood involvement.[193] No morphologic differences are apparent between these two groups.[187] In the large majority of the cases, the cells have the markers of B lymphocytes: monoclonal immunoglobulin, usually of the IgM type, is consistently found in their surface (Fig. 1081). They differ from the B lymphocytes of nodular lymphoma in the intensity and appearance of the reaction (brighter and more clumped in the former), as well as by their lesser content of complement receptors. In a small number of cases of chronic lymphocytic leukemia, the lymphocytes have T rather than B cell markers and differ clinically and cytologically from the rest.[188,192] The cells are somewhat larger, have numerous azurophilic granules, and contain large amounts of acid phosphatase and β-glucuronidase.

The architecture of the node in well-differentiated lymphocytic lymphoma is massively and monotonously effaced by a population of small round lymphocytes with clumped chromatin, inconspicuous nucleolis, barely visible cytoplasm, and scanty mitotic activity. Ultrastructurally, they are extremely well differentiated (Fig. 1109). In a recent study of this condition, Pangalis et al.[193] divided their cases in three categories: those with absolute lymphocytosis (i.e., chronic lymphocytic leukemia), those associated with monoclonal gammopathy (50% of which had bone marrow involvement), and those with neither; the latter were often accompanied by hypogammaglobulinemia. No statistical differences in survival between these groups was found. In the cases associated with immunoglobulin production, some or most of the neoplastic lymphocytes may exhibit morphologic signs of plasmacytoid differentiation, (as evidenced by oval shape, lateralization of the nucleus, appearance of a perinuclear halo, and pyroninophilia) and admixture of plasma cells (Fig. 1110). Effacement of the nodal architecture is usually not so complete as with the usual well-differentiated type. These cases are referred to as well-differentiated lymphocytic lymphoma with plasmacytoid differentiation and are discussed further in the section on lymphoma and dysproteinemia.

Not infrequently, cases of well-differentiated lymphocytic lymphoma with or without leu-

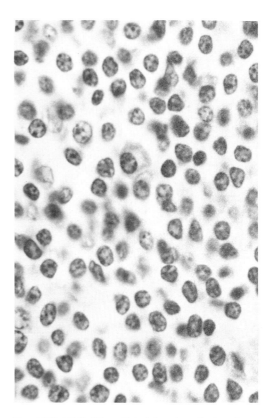

Fig. 1110 Well-differentiated lymphocytic lymphoma accompanied by Waldenström's macroglobulinemia. Proliferation is composed of lymphocytes and plasmacytoid lymphocytes. (×1,000; from Mann RB, Jaffe ES, Berard CW: Malignant lymphomas—a conceptual understanding of morphologic diversity. A review. Am J Pathol **94**:105-191, 1979.)

kemia show, in addition to the well-differentiated lymphocytes, an admixture of larger cells with vesicular nuclei and prominent nucleoli, singly or in small aggregates that simulate germinal centers[189,193] (Fig. 1111). This feature, which is apparently of no prognostic significance, should not lead to confusion with nodular mixed lymphoma or lymphocyte predominance Hodgkin's disease. Evans et al.[190] have made the interesting observation that well-differentiated lymphocytic lymphoma having a mitotic rate in excess of 30 per 20 high-power fields have a significantly poorer prognosis than those with lesser mitotic rates, independent of the number of large lymphocytes present. They propose the term "intermediate lymphocytic lymphoma" for this group, although it is not yet clear whether this represents the same lesion as the one described in the following paragraph. An even more serious development

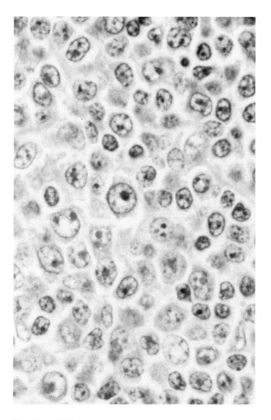

Fig. 1111 Diffuse lymphoma of well-differentiated lymphocytic type exhibiting pseudofollicular foci referred to as "growth centers." These foci contain large cells with vesicular nuclei and prominent, often central, nucleoli. Tumors exhibiting these features should not be confused with histiocytic or undifferentiated lymphoma. (×1,000; from Mann RB, Jaffe ES, Bernard CW: Malignant lymphomas—a conceptual understanding of morphologic diversity. A review. Am J Pathol **94:**105-191, 1979.)

is the transformation of a well-differentiated lymphocytic lymphoma into a "blastic" or "histiocytic" neoplasm.[186] This occurrence, when developing in the background of chronic lymphocytic leukemia, is known as Richter's syndrome[191] and is accompanied by a precipitous decline in the clinical course. Fever, increasing lymphadenopathy, weight loss, and abdominal pain are frequent,[193a] sometimes accompanied by hepatomegaly and splenomegaly. The earliest infiltrates may be detected in the lymph nodes or in the bone marrow.[190a] Cell surface studies in these cases have shown that the large cells possess the same type of immunoglobulin heavy and light chain as the preexisting small lymphocytes, indicating that

they represent dedifferentiation of the original tumor rather than a second neoplasm.

Intermediately differentiated lymphocytic lymphoma. A newly recognized type of B cell lymphoma, intermediately differentiated lymphocytic lymphoma used to be included with both the poorly differentiated and well-differentiated types. As in the latter types, it occurs in middle-aged and elderly individuals and runs an indolent course. The low-power appearance is that of a diffuse lymphoma, although there may be a suggestion of nodularity accentuated by the occasional presence of small germinal center–like structures (Fig. 1112, *A*). Most of the cells are small lymphocytes similar to those of well-differentiated lymphocytic lymphoma, but there is an admixture of cells with cleaved nuclei like those seen in poorly differentiated lymphocytic lymphoma (Fig. 1112, *B*). It has been suggested, on the basis of some histochemical features, that this tumor arises from the lymphocytes of primary follicles and/or the mantle zones of secondary follicles.[194]

Poorly differentiated lymphocytic lymphoma. In Rappaport's classification, poorly differentiated lymphocytic lymphoma includes three probably unrelated neoplasms: follicular center lymphoma, lymphoblastic lymphoma, and peripheral T cell lymphoma.

(1) *Follicular center lymphoma* ("malignant lymphoma, diffuse, small cleaved cell" in the new International Formulation) is a tumor of small cleaved cells in which the nodularity is not evident. As expected, they are of B cell type. As a matter of fact, biopsies at other sites may reveal residual nodularity not apparent in the original biopsy. In one recent series,[198] the estimated two-year survival rate was significantly lower (43%) than that seen in the nodular (or nodular *and* diffuse) lymphomas of similar microscopic type (83%).

Tolksdorf et al.[212a] maintain that diffuse lymphomas composed exclusively of poorly differentiated lymphocytes (small cleaved cells, centrocytes) represent a distinct clinicopathologic entity rather than a diffuse stage of a nodular lymphoma. This tumor is closely related to, and may be identical with, the intermediately differentiated lymphocytic lymphoma described in the preceding section.

(2) *Lymphoblastic lymphoma* ("malignant lymphoma, lymphoblastic, convoluted and/or nonconvoluted" in the new International Formulation) is seen primarily in children and adolescents, but it also occurs in adults.[210]

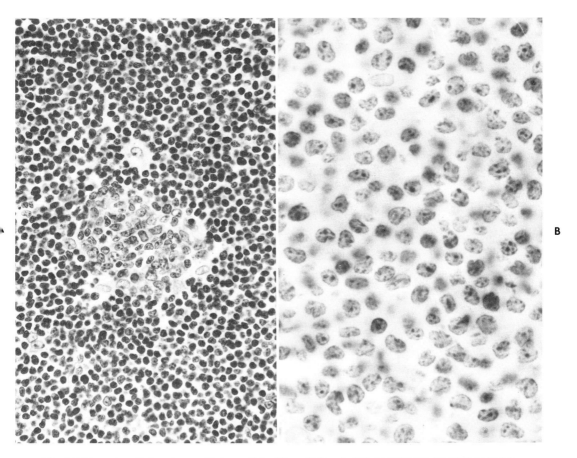

Fig. 1112 Lymphocytic lymphoma of intermediate differentiation. **A,** Diffuse infiltrate with small germinal center–like structure in center of field. **B,** High-power view of same case illustrated in **A** shows that proliferation consists of small round lymphocytes admixed with irregular lymphoid cells. (**A,** ×420; **B,** ×1,000; **A** amd **B,** from Mann RB, Jaffe ES, Berard CW: Malignant lymphomas—a conceptual understanding of morphologic diversity. A review. Am J Pathol **94:**105-191, 1979.)

It has a distinctive clinical pattern. In approximately half of the cases there is a mediastinal mass in the thymic region. The clinical course is extremely aggressive, with rapid multisystem dissemination, leukemic blood picture, and death after a few months.[205a,207] Microscopically, there is a diffuse and relatively monomorphic pattern of proliferation, broken only by a focal "starry sky" appearance. The neoplastic cells have scanty cytoplasm and a nucleus which has a round contour (instead of the angulated one typical of poorly differentiated lymphocytic lymphoma) but which shows, on close examination, the presence of delicate convolutions resulting from multiple small invaginations of the nuclear membrane. Oil-immersion examination of well-prepared, very thin sections is necessary to demonstrate this feature, which may be present in only a small percentage of the tumor cells. The chromatin is finely stippled, and nucleoli are inconspicuous. Mitotic activity is extremely high. These convoluted cells are similar to the cerebroid cells of mycosis fungoides–Sézary's syndrome (as one might assume from their confusingly similar neurologic names), but differ from the latter because the nuclear membrane is thinner, the chromatin more disperse, and the invaginations more delicate. Actually, the need for distinction between these two cell types is more theoretical than real, because of the fact that the two diseases are vastly different in their clinical presentation.

In some cases (up to 50% in the series of Nathwani et al.[207]), nuclear convolutions are not appreciated despite the fact that all the other morphologic and clinical features are the same as for the cases that exhibit them.

Remnants of thymus often are found in the mediastinal mass, and this may lead to a mistaken diagnosis of thymoma; in this regard, it should be remembered that thymoma is very infrequent in children and that, when it occurs, it is characterized by a population of small or activated lymphocytes but not convoluted ones. When lymphoblastic lymphoma spreads to lymph nodes, it preferentially involves the paracortical (thymic-dependent) zone.

The lymphocytes of this tumor have, in most cases, T cell markers.[194a,200,212] However, some hetereogeneity has been shown by these immunologic studies that is hardly predictable from morphologic examination.[196,199] Cases with positive T cell markers are usually in males, and mediastinal localization is the rule. A very interesting recent development has been the finding that many of the tumor cells have receptors for *both* sheep erythrocytes (the classic marker for T cells) and complement (usually regarded as a B cell marker).[211] The recent demonstration that this is a normal finding in fetal thymocytes[211] ties it together nicely by suggesting that lymphoblastic lymphoma may be a tumor of thymocytes (i.e., very primitive T cell precursors). Other features of this cell include the presence of acid phosphatase (focally strong in a paranuclear location, as in normal thymocytes), β-glucuronidase, α-naphthyl acetate esterase,[209b] and terminal deoxynucleotidyl transferase (TdT), another marker of thymocytes.[197,199]

The close clinical, immunologic, and morphologic relationship between lymphoblastic lymphoma and acute lymphoblastic leukemia (particularly the T cell variety) has been extensively discussed although not completely elucidated.[201,206,209]

(3) *Peripheral T cell lymphoma* is the tentative name proposed for a poorly defined group of tumors having in common the proliferation of small atypical lymphocytes in association with epithelioid histiocytes. These occur in adults and are often generalized, and constitutional symptoms are common.[213] The neoplastic lymphocytes vary a great deal in size and shape, and deep nuclear grooves are common. These cells are admixed with larger ones, which may be binucleated or multinucleated and thus simulate Hodgkin's disease. In addition, there is the already mentioned component of benign-appearing epithelioid histiocytes and a marked proliferation of small vessels with plump endothelial cells. Immunologic studies have shown

T cell markers in the tumor cells.[213] Other clinical and morphologic variants of malignant lymphomas thought to be of peripheral T cell type have been described.[208a,209a] Some of these probably correspond to the "malignant lymphoma, large cell, immunoblastic, polymorphous type" in the new International Formulation.

•　•　•

A probably related neoplasm is the so-called *Lennert's lymphoma* (lymphoepithelioid cell lymphoma).[195,205] It is similar in clinical presentation and microscopic appearance to the previously described type (Fig. 1113). In the series studied by Kim et al.,[203] 74% of the patients had Stage IV disease at presentation, and the prognosis was poor. Microscopically, it differs only in the sense that the component of large lymphoid cells is more numerous and polymorphic (in this regard, it would more properly fit the mixed category in Rappaport's classification). Plasma cells and eosinophils are also common, which adds to the diagnostic difficulty with Hodgkin's disease. The main distinguishing features (which also apply to the previous entity) are the cytologic abnormal lymphocytes and the rarity of classic Sternberg-Reed cells. The nature of Lennert's lymphoma is still unclear, partially because no large-scale immunologic studies have been carried out on this neoplasm. It would seem, though, that some cases carrying this label are simply examples of Hodgkin's disease accompanied by epithelioid cell granulomas (45%), others are non-Hodgkin's lymphomas accompanied by the same type of reaction (40%), others represent still undefined types of atypical lymphoepithelial proliferation (13%), and still others may be variants of angioimmunoblastic lymphadenopathy.[202] Important clinical and prognostic differences exist between them, and their separation is warranted. It seems likely that at least some of the cases in the group of non-Hodgkin's lymphoma represent examples of peripheral T cell lymphoma[208]; if this is confirmed, it may be preferable to reserve the term "Lennert's lymphoma" for the latter. This probably corresponds to the "malignant lymphoma, large cell, immunoblastic, polymorphous type, with epithelioid cell component" in the new International Formulation.

As in most other types of lymphocytic tumors, some cases of Lennert's lymphomas are seen to undergo a "blastic" transformation into a large cell lymphoma.[204]

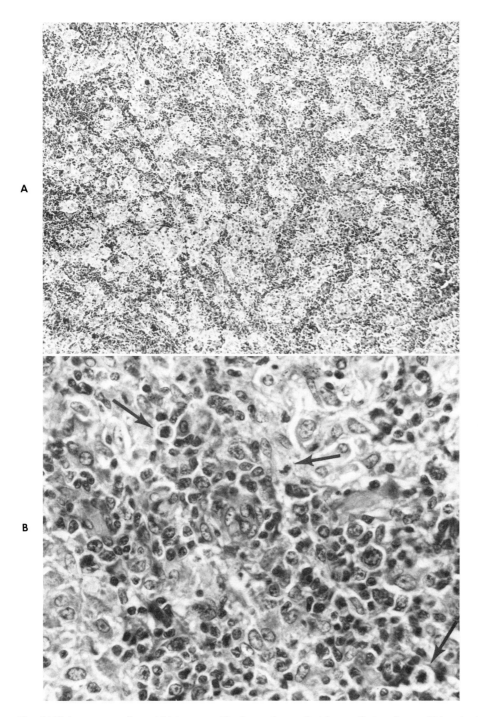

Fig. 1113 Low-power, **A,** and high-power, **B,** views of so-called Lennert's lymphoma. Extensive in-filtrate of epithelioid histiocytes may be seen closely admixed with small lymphocytes (some of them atypical) and scattered large lymphoid cells; several mitotic figures are present (arrows). (From Kim H, Jacobs C, Warnke RA, Dorfman RF: Malignant lymphoma with a high content of epithelioid histiocytes. A distinct clinicopathologic entity and a form of the so-called "Lennert's lymphoma." Cancer **41:**620-635, 1978.)

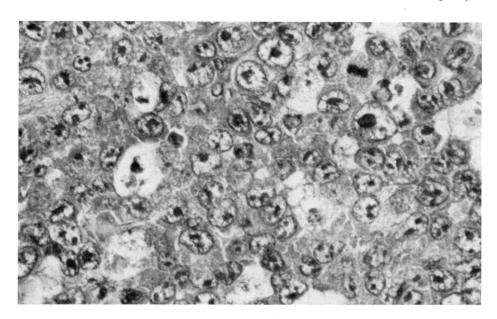

Fig. 1114 High-power view of histocytic lymphoma involving inguinal lymph node. As may rarely occur, phagocytosis was present. Individual tumor cells have large vesicular nuclei, prominent nucleoli, and abundant cytoplasm. (×720; WU neg. 52-4080.)

Mixed (lymphocytic-histiocytic) lymphoma. Most mixed (lymphocytic-histiocytic) lymphomas (''malignant lymphoma, diffuse, mixed, small and large cell'' in the new International Formulation) represent the diffuse counterpart of the nodular (or nodular *and* diffuse) variety of the same cell type combination, and the same considerations apply. The others belong to the category of Lennert's lymphoma previously described.

Histiocytic lymphoma. Histiocytic lymphoma is the most complex and heterogeneous of all the non-Hodgkin's lymphomas. It corresponds to the old reticulum cell sarcoma and is morphologically defined by the large size of the cells, their vesicular nuclei with prominent nucleoli, and their relatively abundant cytoplasm (Fig. 1114). Although the great majority of these tumors have been shown *not* to be of histiocytic origin, the term is presently retained for the practical reasons given in the introduction to the discussion of malignant lymphoma. As a group, histiocytic lymphoma occurs both in children and adults, but mostly in the latter. In comparison with other lymphomas, it has a greater tendency for extranodal presentation, for being localized at the time of presentation, and for a poor prognosis. In more than half of the cases, the tumor is limited to one side of the diaphragm (40%, as opposed to 90% for

nodular lymphoma).[215] Involvement of the bone marrow or liver is less common than in the lymphocytic tumors.[232] About 40% of the cases present in extranodal sites, such as digestive system, skin, and skeletal system.[215] When the liver or spleen is involved, it is usually in the form of scattered large tumor masses instead of the multiple smaller nodules or miliary type seen with the lymphocytic types. The involved nodes usually are markedly enlarged, homogeneous, and individualized and with little or no necrosis (Fig. 1115). Immunologic studies performed in these tumors have shown a remarkable heterogeneity.[213b,233a] This suggests that histiocytic lymphoma may not be a specific entity like the others but rather a common denominator for all the highly anaplastic or ''blastic'' lymphomas, just as large cell undifferentiated carcinoma of the lung represents the end of the spectrum for all major microscopic types of pulmonary carcinoma. About 50%-60% of the ''histiocytic'' lymphomas exhibit B cell markers, 5%-15% have T-cell markers, 5% have features consistent with true histiocytes, and as many as a third of the cases have no markers at all (''null'' lymphomas).[223] Of all the lymphomas, this is the type most likely to be confused with carcinoma, especially when the nodal involvement is focal or sinusoidal.[225a] In particularly difficult cases, enzyme histo-

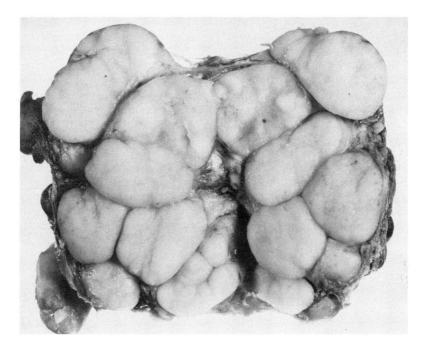

Fig. 1115 Mass of nodes in malignant lymphoma. Note separation of lymph nodes and occasional areas of necrosis. (WU neg. 49-3387.)

chemistry,[220] surface marker studies, immunoperoxidase stains for immunoglobulins,[226,231] and electron microscopic examination[213a,217,218] can be decisive. We have not found reticulin stains of much help in this differential.

Several morphologic subtypes can be recognized within the category of histiocytic lymphoma, which bear some relation to the just mentioned immunologic findings. The terminology used here is largely that proposed by Lukes,[222] because there are no equivalent terms in Rappaport's original classification.[227]

(1) *Large cleaved cell lymphoma* (''malignant lymphoma, diffuse, large cell'' in the new International Formulation, together with the large noncleaved cell lymphoma) probably represents the diffuse variety of the nodular (or nodular *and* diffuse) lymphoma composed of the corresponding cell type. When totally diffuse, the behavior of this tumor is more aggressive than when some nodularity is present.[233] Some of these cases are accompanied by marked sclerosis, and this seems to confer them an improved prognosis.[214,229]

(2) In *B cell immunoblastic sarcoma* (''malignant lymphoma, large cell, immunoblastic, plasmacytoid type'' in the new International Formulation), the predominant cell has the appearance of an immunoblast: large vesicular nucleus with prominent central nucleoli and thick nuclear membrane and deeply staining amphophilic and pyroninophilic cytoplasm with a distinct nuclear hof. Some of the cells are binucleated or multinucleated and simulate Sternberg-Reed cells. Others acquire plasmacytoid features (cartwheel chromatin, larger perinuclear hof) and others are clearly plasma cells. Immunoperoxidase staining often shows intracytoplasmic immunoglobulin. This is the most common type of lymphoma arising on the basis of natural immunodeficiency, immunosuppression, immunoproliferative states (such as angioimmunoblastic lymphadenopathy), and other immune diseases, such as Hashimoto's thyroiditis, Sjögren's disease, α-chain disease, and lupus erythematosus.[222,225] This was true for 30% of the thirty-three patients studied by Lichtenstein et al.[221] The prognosis is poor; the disease disseminates early and progresses rapidly.[228] In the series of Lichtenstein et al.,[221] the median survival was fourteen months.

We have recently reviewed a series of so-called *post-transplant malignant lymphomas*, all of them occurring in immunosuppressed renal transplant recipients.[219,224] Most of them ran a remarkably rapid clinical course, with death usually occurring a few months or even weeks after diagnosis. Clinically, the two most common forms of presentation were (1) a generalized, multisystem involvement and (2) localization of the disease to the central nervous system. Microscopically, these two types did not differ. They were all of the large cell ("histiocytic") type, and many conformed to the description of immunoblastic sarcoma. Atypia was pronounced, and mitoses were numerous. Three disconcerting facts, though, were the polymorphic nature of the infiltrate, the constant presence of a component of follicular center cells, and the polyclonal nature of the immunoglobulin secretion, as determined by immunoperoxidase stains. Even more intriguing, we have now seen two microscopically somewhat similar cases, one located in the palate and the other in the transplanted kidney, in which spontaneous regression occurred following discontinuation of the immunosuppressive therapy. Evidence of Epstein-Barr virus infection is commonly present in these patients. These facts suggest the possibility that most cases of "post-transplant lymphomas" may represent virally induced B proliferations that have become luxuriant and unrestrained because of the lack of the suppression effect of the T cell system. Some of these proliferations are polymorphic but hyperplastic and potentially reversible; we prefer to call them polymorphic diffuse B cell hyperplasias. Others are still polymorphic but with the cytologic features of malignancy; these we call polymorphic B cell lymphomas.[216a]

(3) *T cell immunoblastic sarcoma* (probably equivalent to the "malignant lymphoma, large cell, immunoblastic, clear cell type" in the new International Formulation) is not so well defined as the previous entity, and its very existence (or at least its microscopic recognition) is debatable. According to Lukes et al.,[222] the tumor cells differ from those of their more common B cell counterpart by having irregular, contorted nuclei and a pale, water-clear cytoplasm with well-defined interlocking plasma membranes, giving the tumor a cohesive appearance. The chromatin is finely dispersed, and the nucleoli are smaller. A wide size range exists among cells exhibiting these features. The neighboring cells are atypical lymphocytes, rather than plasmacytoid cells and mature plasma cells. Reactive histiocytes may be present in large numbers. Vascularity is not striking. The initial lymph node involvement is in the paracortical region.[222] In contrast to the

B cell immunoblastic sarcoma, the T cell variety is usually not preceded by an abnormal immune disorder. However, it can be superimposed on mycosis fungoides (a T cell malignancy). It may be seen in children and in adults and is usually associated with generalized lymphadenopathy and polyclonal hypergammaglobulinemia.

(4) *Large noncleaved cell lymphoma* ("malignant lymphoma, diffuse, large cell" in the new International Formulation, together with the large cleaved cell lymphoma) may be difficult to distinguish from B cell immunoblastic sarcoma. The subtle differences, according to Lukes,[222] are the lighter-staining and less pyroninophilic cytoplasm, the more peripheral location of the nucleoli, the absence of plasmacytoid differentiation, and the occasional admixture with small and large cleaved cells. Sometimes, a vaguely follicular pattern is discerned. Mitoses are numerous and a "starry sky" pattern may be present. This is a rapidly growing tumor, with quick dissemination.

Although the minor morphologic differences between these four subtypes are not easy to recognize at first glance and a good deal of overlap exists, it is becoming increasingly obvious that these differences not only are real but also can be translated to the clinical situation. The fact that there is such a dramatic difference in survival rates among patients with "histiocytic" lymphoma[216] should stimulate the pathologist to search for morphologic subtleties that may explain those differences. In the series of Strauchen et al.,[230] large cleaved lymphoma had the best prognosis, large noncleaved lymphoma an intermediate one, and immunoblastic sarcoma the worst. Instead, in the series of Armitage et al.,[213a] the best prognosis was seen with the large noncleaved lymphomas.

Undifferentiated lymphoma ("malignant lymphoma, small noncleaved cell" in the new International Formulation). The name undifferentiated lymphoma is again somewhat misleading, because most of the neoplasms have been shown to be of B cell types. Lukes refers to the tumor as lymphoma of small noncleaved cells. Two major categories exist: pleomorphic (non-Burkitt's) lymphoma and Burkitt's lymphoma.

(1) In *pleomorphic (non-Burkitt's) lymphoma*, the tumor cells are somewhat intermediate in size between those of poorly differentiated lymphocytic lymphoma and histiocytic

lymphoma. A distinct pleomorphism is evident, which sets this tumor apart from Burkitt's lymphoma. Most of the cells have a well-defined rim of cytoplasm; their nucleus contains a large, eosinophilic nucleolus. Binucleated and multinucleated cells are common, and phagocytosis of nuclear debris by reactive histiocytes is frequently observed, resulting in a "starry sky" appearance. The pattern of growth is generally diffuse, but areas of minimal nodularity may be encountered. The clinical course is aggressive, and response to chemotherapy is poor.

(2) *Burkitt's lymphoma*, a well-publicized type, has definite epidemiologic, clinical, and microscopic features. It is endemic in the equatorial strip of Africa, and it has been reported in a sporadic form throughout the world. Most cases occur in childhood. The African patients characteristically present with jaw lesions, whereas the American cases most often manifest themselves with abdominal masses (ileocecal region, ovaries, abdominal lymph nodes, and retroperitoneum). Peripheral lymphadenopathy is rare and, when present, usually limited to a single group.[235,236] Bone marrow involvement is common in the late stages of the disease, but leukemic manifestations are rare. Response to chemotherapy is good, especially in the African cases, although relapse develops in over half of the patients.[241,242] Presence of the DNA viral genome has been repeatedly demonstrated in the tumor cells, although more consistently in the African than in the American cases.[234]

Microscopically, a *monotonous* and diffuse infiltrate of small (10 μ-25 μ) round cells is seen. The nuclei are round or oval and have *several* prominent basophilic nucleoli. The chromatin is coarse and the nuclear membrane is rather thick. The cytoplasm is easily identifiable; it is amphophilic in hematoxylin-eosin preparations, and strongly pyroninophilic. Fat-containing small vacuoles are prominent; these are particularly well appreciated in touch preparations. Mitoses are numerous, and a prominent "starry sky" pattern is the rule, although by no means pathognomonic.[237] In well-fixed material, the cytoplasm of individual cells "squares off," forming acute angles in which the membranes of adjacent cells abut upon each other. Ultrastructurally, the main features are abundant ribosomes, frequent lipid inclusions, lack of glycogen particles, and presence of nuclear pockets or projections[238] (Fig. 1116). The tumor cells have B lympho-cyte markers, with IgM being the predominant surface immunoglobulin.[239,239a] Although the pattern of growth is nearly always diffuse, early nodal lesions show selective involvement of germinal centers.[240]

Other non-Hodgkin's lymphomas

Other well-defined types of non-Hodgkin's lymphoma and leukemias are discussed in other chapters, depending on the site or sites that they affect more frequently. They are (1) mycosis fungoides–Sézary syndrome (Chapter 3); (2) hairy cell leukemia (Chapters 21 and 22); (3) leukemias and myeloproliferative conditions (Chapter 22).

Lymphoma and dysproteinemia

In view of the fact that most malignant lymphomas arise from B lymphocytes (i.e., cells normally engaged in humoral immune responses[243,272]), it is not surprising that in some of them the tumor cells express their potentialities by producing immunoglobulins of one sort or another.[244,262] Ranging in between the typical malignant lymphoma without globulin abnormalities and the typical plasma cell myeloma with monoclonal peak and Bence Jones proteinuria, all types of morphologic and biochemical hybrids have been encountered. Tumors have been described that secrete completely assembled immunoglobulins of the IgG, IgA, IgM, IgD, or IgE type, with or without concomitant production of isolated light chains, isolated light chains to the almost total exclusion of complete immunoglobulin molecules, and "heavy chains" (or, more accurately, Fc fragments) of IgG, IgM, or IgA specificity. Some of these immunoglobulins have the physicochemical properties of cryoglobulins and can result in necrotizing vasculitis.[249] This remarkably diverse expression of function has led to the introduction of such names as Waldenström's macroglobulinemia, light chain disease, α-chain disease, Franklin's heavy chain disease, etc., and even to the proposal of grouping all immunoglobulin-secreting lymphoid and plasmacytic tumors under the term *immunocytoma*.[248,251,256,259]

This practice has led to considerable confusion as happens whenever morphologic and functional parameters are mixed in a common terminology. For instance, the serum picture of macroglobulinemia can be associated with a microscopic picture of lymphocytic lymphoma, lymphocytic lymphoma with plasmacytic dif-

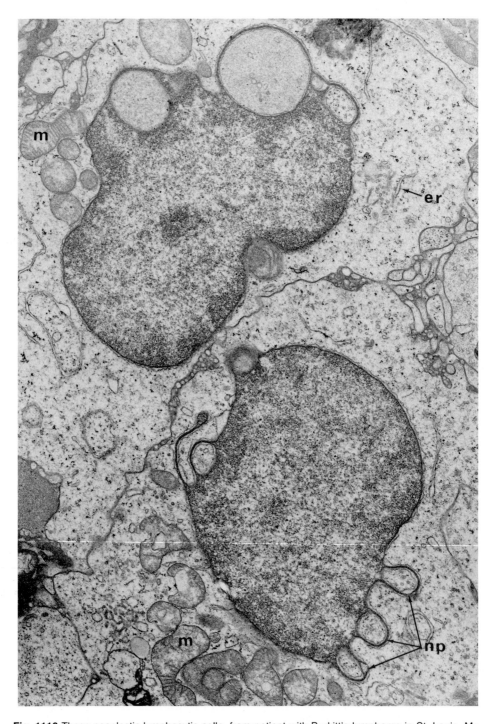

Fig. 1116 These neoplastic lymphocytic cells, from patient with Burkitt's lymphoma in St. Louis, Mo., have numerous peculiar, although not unique, nuclear projections, **np,** polar aggregates of mitochondria, **m,** sparse endoplasmic reticulum, **er,** and scattered ribosomes. (Approximately ×13,000.)

ferentiation, plasma cell myeloma, and histiocytic (large cell) lymphoma. It is obvious that by giving a tissue diagnosis "consistent with macroglobulinemia," the pathologist is not rendering an accurate account of the situation. We believe that these neoplasms should be classified according to conventional morphologic criteria rather than by the biochemical findings in the patient's serum—i.e., a well-differentiated lymphocytic lymphoma should be designated as such whether it produces macroglobulins, heavy chains, light chains, or no detectable globulins. Four main cytologic patterns are observed in these immunoglobulin-secreting neoplasms:

1 Malignant lymphomas of conventional appearance, usually of lymphocytic type, indistinguishable from those not associated with immunoglobulin abnormalities.

2 Plasma cell myelomas, in which most of the tumor cells have the characteristic light and electron microscopic features of plasma cells.

3 Tumors having the overall appearance of a malignant lymphoma of lymphocytic type, but in which a certain proportion of the tumor cells has undergone a plasmocytic differentiation, as evidenced light microscopically by lateralization of the nucleus, coarse chromatin clumping, appearance of a perinuclear clear halo, and/or increased basophilic cytoplasm and ultrastructurally by prominence of the Golgi apparatus and abundance of granular endoplasmic reticulum. Some of the tumor cells may be PAS-positive. Immunoperoxidase stains will often show monoclonal immunoglobulin in the cytoplasm of the plasmacytoid cells much more frequently than in ordinary well-differentiated lymphocytic lymphomas or chronic lymphocytic leukemias.[269,269a] We designate these lesions as malignant lymphoma, lymphocytic, with plasmacytoid differentiation and suggest that the clinician investigate for the possibility of immunoglobulin abnormalities.[246]

4 Large cell lymphoma, classified as histiocytic according to Rappaport, and composed of an admixture of immunoblasts, large plasmacytoid cells, and mature plasma cells. These cases are better designated as immunoblastic sarcomas. Some of the reported cases of primary plasmacytomas of lymph nodes[242a,255,257] belong to this

or to the previous category. If one were to use the term plasmacytoma of lymph nodes at all, it would be wise to restrict it only to those cases having typical bone marrow involvement by plasmacytoma and/or cases in which nearly all of the malignant cells have plasmacytoid rather than lymphocytoid features.

Attempts to correlate the microscopic appearance with the secretory activity of these tumors have been made by several authors. The results have been largely discouraging, although a few more or less distinctive patterns have emerged.[258,261] In general, tumors producing IgM globulin or "heavy chains" have the anatomic distribution and cytologic appearance of malignant lymphoma, whereas most of those secreting IgG globulin or a light chain are clinically and microscopically classifiable as plasma cell myeloma. There is no reliable light microscopic or fine structural criteria which allow one to predict the type of immunoglobulin secreted by a plasma cell myeloma. Not even the rare "nonsecretory" plasma cell myelomas can be separated from the others by morphology alone.[247] Presence of Russell bodies, a rare occurrence in plasma cell myeloma, correlates with lack of Bence Jones protein in the urine.[254] Intranuclear and cytoplasmic inclusions are not specific for any type of immunoglobulin. However, those composed of IgM or IgA are often PAS positive due to their high carbohydrate content, whereas those composed of IgG are not.[250,253] The immunoglobulin inclusions may appear as round eosinophilic bodies or crystals.[267] The former may be so abundant and prominent, perhaps due to a failure in secretion, as to displace the nucleus laterally, creating a signet-ring effect.[260] The same phenomenon can be seen in reactive conditions.[266] The best way to demonstrate the immunoglobulin nature of these formations in tissue sections is by immunocytochemical techniques. Sternberger's unlabeled immunoperoxidase method is particularly useful because it can be applied to formalin-fixed, paraffin-embedded material. Tumors which have been reported as secreting IgA "heavy chains" have involved the gastrointestinal tract[252,271] or, much less commonly, the respiratory tract.[270] The former is discussed in Chapter 10. Production of IgM heavy chains, an exceptionally rare event, occurs in elderly patients who present with chronic lymphocytic leukemia.[265]

Of all the anatomic varieties of malignant lymphoma, Hodgkin's disease and lymphomas with nodular pattern of growth are the least likely to be associated with immunoglobulin serum abnormalities. The more obvious the plasmacytic differentiation, the higher the chances of immunoglobulin alterations. However, it should be remembered that even fully differentiated plasma cell myelomas may sometimes be associated with complete lack of detectable immunoglobulin production. These "nonsecretory" plasma cell myelomas, as well as those that produce only light chains, seem to run an accelerated clinical course.[259]

The term *benign monoclonal gammopathy* has been applied to the presence on serum electrophoresis of a discrete, homogeneous protein ("M-protein") in the absence of clinical manifestations of plasma cell myeloma or lymphoma.[273] The incidence of this condition in the adult population is close to 1%, many times higher than that of overt myeloma.[245] Migliore and Alexanian[268] believe that its association with carcinomas of various organs is coincidental. It is possible that some of the cases of "benign monoclonal gammopathy" represent an early phase of plasma cell myeloma.[264] Kyle[263] followed 241 patients with a monoclonal protein in the serum for more than five years: myeloma, macroglobulinemia, or amyloidosis developed in 11%. He could not distinguish initially between the patients with stable benign disease and those with progressive disease and recommended periodic reexamination of patients with monoclonal gammopathy.

Bone marrow examination in these patients shows an increased number of mature plasma cells. In order to make a diagnosis of plasma cell myeloma, there should be cytologic abnormalities of the plasma cells, not just a numerical increase of them. Production of immunoglobulin fragments, suppression of normal immunoglobulin production, serum paraprotein levels higher than 1 gm/100 ml, and progressive rise in paraprotein levels all strongly suggest the malignant nature of a lymphocytic or plasmacytic proliferation.[259]

Hodgkin's disease

Hodgkin's disease lacks the monomorphic appearance of most other malignant lymphomas. Lymphocytes, eosinophils, plasma cells, and histiocytes may all be present in greater or lesser amount depending on the microscopic type. Identification of typical Sternberg-Reed

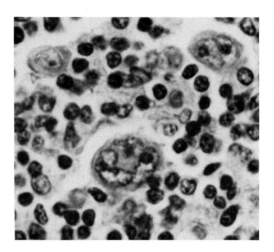

Fig. 1117 Classic Sternberg-Reed cells with multilobated nuclei and prominent nucleoli. (High power; WU neg. 48-4608.)

cells are necessary for the initial diagnosis of Hodgkin's disease. This cell is of relatively large size, its cytoplasm is abundant, either basophilic or amphophilic, and two or more vesicular nuclei are present, each having a thick nuclear membrane and a single, prominent, acidophilic or amphophilic nucleolus, surrounded by a clear halo (Fig. 1117). The origin of the Sternberg-Reed cell remains enigmatic.[280,319] It was originally thought to be the histiocyte, and there is recent evidence to suggest that this might indeed be the case.[295,300] Another proposed candidate has been the B lymphocyte, on the basis of its ultrastructural features,[287] and the demonstration by immunoperoxidase techniques that Sternberg-Reed cells contain intracytoplasmic immunoglobulin[283,284,320]; however, this could be the result of phagocytosis or passive absorption rather than production (as we have demonstrated in the histiocytes of sinus histiocytosis with massive lymphadenopathy).[292,307] Other candidates are the T lymphocyte[307] and one of the four types of reticular cells of the lymph nodes,[280,305] particularly the interdigitating reticulum cell found in T-dependent areas of the node.[289]

Cells with only one nucleus should not be designated as Sternberg-Reed cells. On the other hand, we often see patients with morphologically documented Hodgkin's disease in whom a biopsy of bone marrow, liver, or some other organ done for staging purposes shows a polymorphic infiltrate *with atypical mononuclear cells* but without identifiable Sternberg-Reed cells. Our policy in these cases has been

Table 59 Major morphologic differences between the pleomorphic immunoblast (Sternberg-Reed-like cell) of infectious mononucleosis and the Sternberg-Reed cell of Hodgkin's disease*

	Immunoblast	Sternberg-Reed cell
Nucleolus		
Staining pattern	Basophilic	Acidophilic
Contours	Irregular	Regular, with clear halo (inclusion-like)
Position	Adjacent to nuclear membrane	More centrally located
Cytoplasm		
Staining pattern	Usually amphophilic	Usually acidophilic
Pyroninophilia	Invariably strong	Variable
Paranuclear hof	Prominent	Inconspicuous
Surrounding cells	Mononuclear immunoblasts and plasmacytoid cells	Lymphocytes and histiocytes

*Compiled from data in Dorfman RF, Warnke R: Lymphadenopathy simulating the malignant lymphomas. Hum Pathol **5**:519-550, 1974.

to regard these organs as involved by Hodgkin's disease. However, a note of caution should be interjected. Atypical cells *need* to be present; an infiltrate of eosinophils, lymphocytes, and plasma cells or a collection of epithelioid granulomas is not enough. It also should be remembered that patients with Hodgkin's disease may develop, either spontaneously or as a result of therapy, non-Hodgkin's lymphoma or leukemia.[277,298]

The Sternberg-Reed cell, although necessary for the initial diagnosis of Hodgkin's disease, is not pathognomonic of this entity. Megakaryocytes can simulate it closely in hematoxylin-eosin sections, but they can be identified by the presence of a strongly PAS-positive substance in their cytoplasm.[282] Cells morphologically indistinguishable from Sternberg-Reed cells, presumably representing pleomorphic immunoblasts, can be seen in infectious mononucleosis and other viral diseases.[321] The most important morphologic differences between these two cells are summarized in Table 59; unfortunately, exceptions to most of them exist. Neoplastic cells from a variety of epithelial and mesenchymal (including lymphoreticular) tumors also can resemble Sternberg-Reed cells.[318] In all of these, the architecture and cell composition of the remaining elements were indicative of their respective nature. These findings restrict even further the diagnostic requirements of Hodgkin's disease. These can be summarized by saying that for the initial diagnosis of this disease, Sternberg-Reed cells not only need to be present but must be situated in the proper architectural and cytologic background.

The mixed cell composition and the presence of necrosis and fibrosis result in a heterogeneous gross appearance, quite dissimilar in most cases from that of the other malignant lymphomas. In the early stages, only focal involvement of a lymph node may be encountered,[314] often restricted to the paracortical region between the follicles. Some authors refer to this pattern as interfollicular Hodgkin's disease, but it is doubtful whether it represents a specific type of this disorder. Noncaseating granulomas are sometimes present in nodes and other organs involved by Hodgkin's disease.[299] They may be quite numerous and obscure the diagnostic features of the disease. In other instances, these granulomas may be seen within otherwise uninvolved organs of patients with Hodgkin's disease.[290] Their significance is unknown. Perhaps they represent an expression of delayed hypersensitivity. Their presence does not indicate involvement of that organ by Hodgkin's disease and should therefore not influence the staging criteria. Actually, it has been shown that, within a given stage, the presence of this granuloma is associated with a better prognosis.[311]

For many years, Jackson and Parker's classification of Hodgkin's disease into a granuloma, paragranuloma, and sarcoma variant[288] was used with some measure of success, the major objection being that too many of the cases (about 80%) fell into one of the categories—i.e., Hodgkin's granuloma. The concept

Table 60 Comparison between the different classifications of Hodgkin's disease*

Jackson and Parker (1947)[289]	Smetana and Cohen's modification (1956)[312]	Lukes (1963)[301]	Rye Conference (1966)[303]
Paragranuloma	Paragranuloma	Lymphocytic and histiocytic, diffuse / Lymphocytic and histiocytic, nodular	Lymphocyte predominance
	Nodular sclerosis	Nodular sclerosis	Nodular sclerosis
Granuloma	Granuloma	Mixed cellularity	Mixed cellularity
Sarcoma	Sarcoma	Diffuse fibrosis / Reticular	Lymphocyte depletion

*Note the close correspondence between Smetana and Cohen's modification of Jackson and Parker's classification and the currently used Rye classification.

of a sclerosing type of Hodgkin's disease was first introduced by Smetana and Cohen in 1956,[312] and this was incorporated into a new classification proposed by Lukes et al.[302] This basic concept, somewhat simplified and with some changes in nomenclature, was adopted by the Nomenclature Committee at the Rye Conference[303] on Hodgkin's disease and has gained widespread recognition. The relationship between these classifications is shown in Table 60.

Four major categories are accepted. In *lymphocyte predominance* Hodgkin's disease, diagnostic Sternberg-Reed cells are scanty, scattered among a large number of lymphocytes, some of which may appear immature or stimulated, and sometimes accompanied by proliferation of benign-appearing histiocytes. Most of the lymphocytes are of the B type.[308a] Postcapillary venules may be prominent.[313] The lymph node architecture is usually effaced, and the infiltrate may have a diffuse or nodular pattern of growth. The latter may be so pronounced as to simulate on low power the appearance of nodular lymphoma. Eosinophils, plasma cells, and foci of fibrosis are nil or absent. Atypical mononuclear cells and a variant of the Sternberg-Reed cell characterized by a folded and lobulated nucleus and smaller nucleolus may be abundant. Conversely, classic Sternberg-Reed cells are difficult to find. If numerous diagnostic Sternberg-Reed cells are found in a node with a lymphocyte predominance background, the case should probably be classified as one of mixed cellularity. Poppema et al.[308c] have made the intriguing and highly attractive suggestion that cases of lymphocyte predominance Hodgkin's disease having a nodular pattern of growth (the lymphocytic and histiocytic nodular type of the clas-

sification of Lukes et al.[302]) arise from B cell regions of the node and specifically from an unusual type of reactive germinal center that they designate as "progressively transformed." In accordance with this line of thought, they believe that the peculiar type of Sternberg-Reed cell seen in this condition (the lymphocytic and histiocytic variant of Lukes et al.[302]) arises from a B lymphocyte and, as such, it contains *monoclonal* immunoglobulin.[308d] On the basis of these findings plus some epidemiologic data,[308b] they propose to separate this type of Hodgkin's disease from the diffuse form of lymphocyte predominance.

In Hodgkin's disease of the *mixed cell type*, a large number of eosinophils, plasma cells, and atypical mononuclear cells are admixed with classical Sternberg-Reed cells, which tend to be numerous. Focal necrosis may be present, but fibrosis should be minimal or absent. The *lymphocyte depletion* group includes two morphologically different types, designated as "diffuse fibrosis" and "reticular" in the classification of Lukes.[301] In the diffuse fibrosis subtype, the number of lymphocytes and other cells progressively decrease as the result of heavy deposition of collagen fibers. The reticular subtype is characterized by a very large number of diagnostic Sternberg-Reed cells (many of them of bizarre configuration) among atypical mononuclear cells and other elements. Areas of necrosis are more common than in other types, although by no means exclusive. The "reticular" subtype of lymphocyte Hodgkin's disease needs to be distinguished from the pleomorphic variant of histiocytic lymphoma and the variant of nodular sclerosis Hodgkin's disease characterized by large aggregates of lacunar cells.

Nodular sclerosis, which in many recent se-

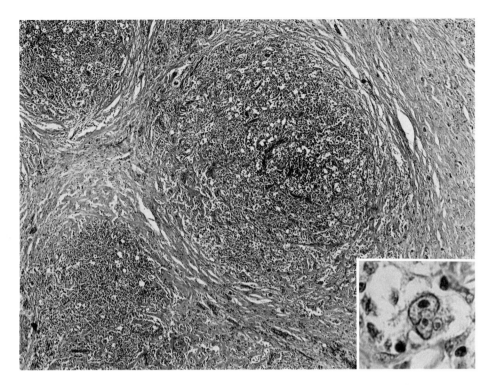

Fig. 1118 Nodular sclerosis Hodgkin's disease. Bands of collagen separate nodules. **Inset** shows lacunar Sternberg-Reed cell. (×38; WU neg. 66-13059A; **inset,** ×800; WU neg. 66-13056.)

ries has been the most common variant of Hodgkin's disease, is characterized by broad collagen bands separating the lymphoid tissue in well-defined nodules (Fig. 1118). The fibrosis often centers around blood vessels. By electron microscopy, abundant collagen fibers are seen together with myofibroblasts.[311a] It has been suggested that the latter contribute to the retraction seen in this condition. The cytologic pattern within the nodules may be one of lymphocyte predominance, lymphocyte depletion, or mixed cell type, and there is some suggestion that this may have a bearing upon prognosis. In any event, the classification of a case as nodular sclerosis takes precedence over other histologic types that may be present in the same section.[305a] Clumps of foamy macrophages are sometimes present.[322] In addition to the typical Sternberg-Reed cell, a variant designated as "cytoplasmic" or "lacunar" is seen (Fig. 1119). It is quite large (40μ-50μ in diameter), with an abundant clear cytoplasm and several nuclei having complicated infoldings and nucleoli of smaller size than those of the diagnostic Sternberg-Reed cell. This cell seems to be the result of a shrinking artifact in-

duced by formalin fixation, inasmuch as it is absent in tissues fixed in Zenker or other fluids. In some cases there is a massive concentration of these lacunar cells, particularly around areas of necrosis, to the point that a mistaken diagnosis of histiocytic lymphoma, carcinoma, or thymoma can be made. Some observers regard this peculiar variant of the Sternberg-Reed cell as more typical of this type of Hodgkin's disease than the fibrosis itself and make the diagnosis of nodular sclerosis Hodgkin's disease in their presence even if fibrosis is totally lacking.[315] This concept of a "cellular phase" of nodular sclerosis Hodgkin's disease remains controversial and should be used with caution. Lacunar cells can be seen in mixed cellularity Hodgkin's disease and even in reactive conditions.[304]

Nodular sclerosis often presents in the neck and mediastinum of young females[279]; this is the only type of Hodgkin's disease that is more common in females than in males. Cases of the nodular sclerosis type occurring in older males often exhibit abundant lacunar cells with prominent nucleoli and run a more aggressive clinical course. The long controversy over the

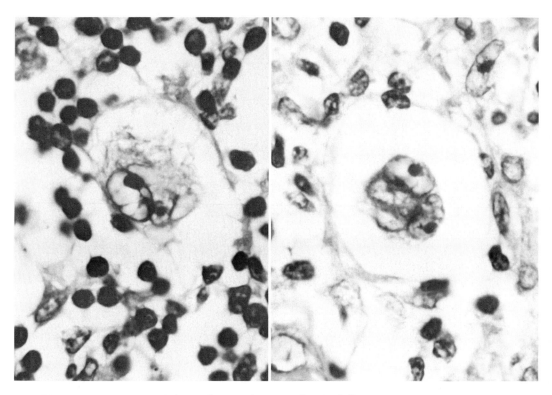

Fig. 1119 Two examples of "lacunar" type of Sternberg-Reed cell. Retraction of cytoplasm in formalin-fixed tissue creates large empty space. (WU negs. 74-5060 and 74-5062.)

nature of "granulomatous thymoma" has now been settled. It represents Hodgkin's disease of the nodular sclerosis type involving the thymus and adjacent lymph nodes and accompanied by a peculiar proliferation of the thymic epithelium.[281,296] It should be remembered that practically all types of Hodgkin's disease can exhibit some degree of fibrosis, particularly after therapy. If the pathologist is too liberal in his criteria for the diagnosis of nodular sclerosis, the clinical and prognostic connotations associated with this microscopic type will lose most of their meaning. Strum and Rappaport[315] showed that the histologic types of Hodgkin's disease remain constant over long follow-up periods in the large majority of the cases. They found this to be especially the case in the nodular sclerosis variety. When change occurred, it was usually toward a histologically more malignant form.

The microscopic typing of Hodgkin's disease should always be made on examination of a biopsy obtained prior to the institution of treatment.[305a] Radiation therapy and chemotherapy result in focal necrosis, fibrosis, and profound nuclear aberrations (Figs. 1120 and

1121)—features that may render impossible a proper pathologic evaluation. In patients who have relapses in a site *not included* in the radiation field (and who had not received chemotherapy), the same histologic appearance is often maintained in the relapse biopsies.[276a]

The currently used classification of Hodgkin's disease is a useful one, but far from ideal. Its nomenclature, for instance, is such that there is very little relation between the names given and the microscopic picture observed. A case with lymphocyte predominance or mixed cellularity will be diagnosed as nodular sclerosis if bands of fibrous tissue are present. A case with marked predominance of lymphocytes will be categorized as mixed cellularity if there are numerous Sternberg-Reed cells. In lymphocyte depletion Hodgkin's disease, lymphocytes are still the numerically more abundant cells, more so than in the mixed cellularity type.

An alternative approach has been tried by Coppleson et al.[278] and consists of evaluating individually the frequencies of the different cell types. They found that a large number of lymphocytes was associated with a good progno-

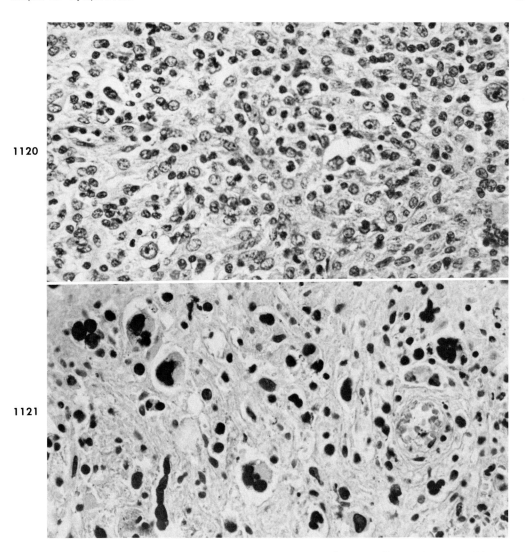

Fig. 1120 Typical Hodgkin's disease. Note pleomorphism and Sternberg-Reed cells. (×480; WU neg. 50-5996.)

Fig. 1121 Lymph node from patient who had transient response to nitrogen mustard and died. This node shows fibrosis and prominent nuclear abnormalities. Patient had not received radiation therapy. (×480; WU neg. 50-5994.)

sis, whereas malignant and benign-appearing histiocytes independently influenced the prognosis adversely. Sternberg-Reed cells had no prognostic effect independent of the malignant mononuclear cells, and eosinophils and plasma cells had no prognostic value. However, these authors concluded that the Rye classification of Hodgkin's disease furnished more prognostic information than any estimates of individual cell frequencies.

The diagnosis of Hodgkin's disease should be questioned for any lymphoma involving Waldeyer's ring, the skin and the gastrointestinal tract, especially if this happens to be the first manifestation of the disease. Most of these cases are examples of Lennert's lymphoma or pleomorphic histiocytic lymphoma with Sternberg-Reed-like cells. A diagnosis of Hodgkin's disease also should be viewed with suspicion if it presents as a complication of a natural immune deficiency (other than ataxia-telangiectasia), immunosuppression, or other immune diseases. Most of these cases actually represent immunoblastic sarcomas containing binu-

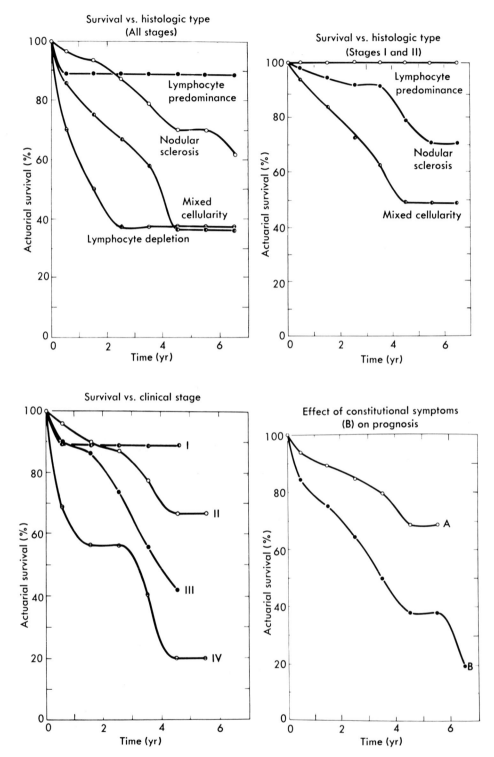

Fig. 1122 Relationships in Hodgkin's disease of microscopic typing and clinical staging with prognosis and age of onset. All these survival curves have improved in recent years because of advances in therapy. (From Keller AR, Kaplan HS, Lukes RJ, Rappaport H: Correlation of histopathology with other prognostic indicators in Hodgkin's disease. Cancer **22:**487-499, 1968.)

cleated immunoblasts morphologically similar to Sternberg-Reed cells.

Clinicopathologic correlation

The two main factors influencing the prognosis of Hodgkin's disease are the clinical staging and microscopic typing, although the spectacular advances in the therapy of this disease obtained in recent years have blurred significantly the differences among these parameters. According to Kaplan,[294,294a] who should be credited more than any other for these notable results, only Stage IV disease, lymphocyte depletion histology, constitutional symptoms, and age over 50 years continue to present serious therapeutic problems. There is a definite correlation between types and stages. Most lymphocyte predominance and nodular sclerosis cases are in Stages I and II, whereas most lymphocyte depletion cases are in Stages III and IV. However, the differences in survival rates among the different types are maintained even within clinical staging groups[297] (Fig. 1122). Lymphocytic predominance and nodular sclerosis are most favorable, mixed cellularity is intermediate, and the lymphocytic depletion type has the worst prognosis.[276] The latter type is very rare in children.[308c] Males, blacks, and patients over 40 years of age with nodular sclero-

sis Hodgkin's disease tend to do poorly. The long-term prognosis of lymphocyte predominance Hodgkin's disease is so good that some people refer to it as "the benign form" of Hodgkin's disease and others even doubt that it represents a neoplastic process.[323] The typical patient with lymphocyte predominance Hodgkin's disease is a man in his forties with involvement of the high cervical nodes. This microscopic form practically never involves spleen, liver, or bone marrow except when it changes to a more aggressive histologic pattern.[305a]

Mediastinal involvement is the rule in nodular sclerosis, inconstant in mixed cellularity, and exceptional in lymphocyte predominance. On the other hand, the risk of abdominal involvement is highest in mixed cellularity and lymphocyte predominance, as compared with nodular sclerosis. Lymphocyte depletion Hodgkin's disease may present in adults or elderly patients as a febrile illness with pancytopenia or lymphocytopenia, hepatomegaly, abnormal liver function tests, and no peripheral lymphadenopathy[306] or manifest the usual clinical presentation of Hodgkin's disease. In a series of thirty-nine patients studied by Bearman et al.,[275] the median survival was 25.1 months; eight (21%) patients survived four years or longer. No clinical or survival differences were found between the reticular and diffuse fibrosis subtypes. Mediastinal involvement was present in 36% of the cases and was found to be a favorable prognostic feature.

Most cases of Hodgkin's disease spread by

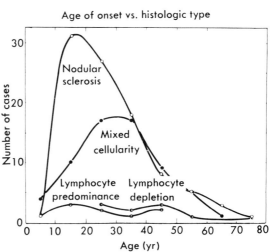

Fig. 1122 cont'd For legend, see opposite page.

involvement of adjacent lymph node groups.[293] This contiguous manner of spread is particularly common in the nodular sclerosis and lymphocytic predominance types.[297] The most common sites of extranodal involvement by Hodgkin's disease are the spleen, liver, bone marrow, lung, and skin. New important information has been acquired in regard to the frequency and significance of extranodal involvement as a result of a more aggressive diagnostic approach, particularly with the use of laparot-

omy as a routine staging procedure.[285,286,291] Of the nodes biopsied at laparotomy, the most likely to be involved are those located in the splenic hilum and retroperitoneum. Mesenteric nodes are almost always spared. A spleen weighing 400 gm or more is practically always histologically positive. The converse is not true: spleens below this weight are involved in a high proportion of cases. The focal nature of the disease calls for a careful gross examination of this organ.

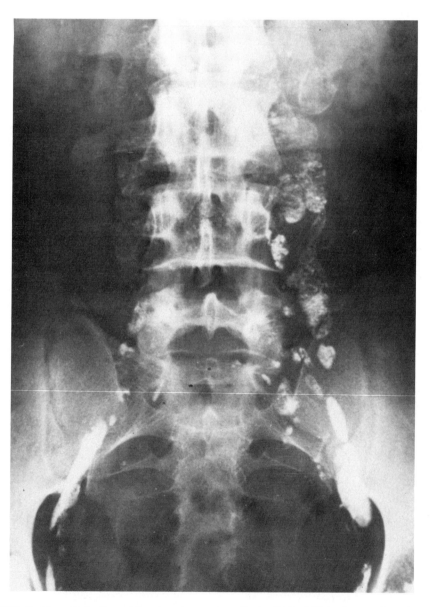

Fig. 1123 Positive retroperitoneal lymphangiogram in patient with Hodgkin's disease. Lymph nodes are enlarged and have coarse reticulated appearance.

Spleens should be sectioned throughout in thin slices, and every suspicious area should be examined microscopically. If no nodules are detected on gross inspection, the chances of finding Hodgkin's disease in random microscopic sections are negligible. Splenic involvement is thought to represent a critical stage in the spread of Hodgkin's disease and the early manifestation of blood vessel discrimination. Hepatic disease is almost invariably associated with splenic and retroperitoneal lymph node involvement and with so-called "B" symptoms. Clinical assessment of liver involvement is quite unreliable. In competent hands, lymphangiography has an overall diagnostic accuracy in excess of 90%; it is more effective in detecting involvement below the level of the second lumbar vertebra (Fig. 1123) but inconsistent for nodes situated higher in the periaortic area. About 30% of patients with negative lymphangiograms in whom the para-aortic nodes are left untreated will later demonstrate lymphoma below the diaphragm.[274] Involvement of lung or chest wall by the nodular sclerosis type often represents direct extension from mediastinal nodes and does not result in an appreciable decrease in survival[297] (Fig. 1123). Bone marrow involvement is better detected with a surgical biopsy than by the conventional smear. Elevation of serum alkaline phosphatase level is the most reliable sign of marrow disease.[310]

Vascular invasion has been detected microscopically in 6%-14% of the cases of Hodgkin's disease by the use of elastic tissue stains.[317] This finding is apparently associated with an increased incidence of extranodal organ involvement.[309]

Aggressive radiation therapy and chemotherapy are often successful in controlling Hodgkin's disease, but this does not always mean total eradication. Of nineteen autopsied patients who died after having survived Hodgkin's disease for ten years or more, Strum and Rappaport[316] found residual disease in sixteen.

The main clinical differences between Hodgkin's disease and the other malignant lymphomas are summarized in Table 61.

Malignant histiocytosis

Malignant histiocytosis is a term first proposed by Rappaport[335] for a disease characterized by a systemic, neoplastic proliferation of histologically recognizable histiocytes and their precursors. It can affect any age group, but has a predilection for children and young adults.[326,340a] Fever, lymph node enlargement, and constitutional symptoms appear early in the course. Hepatomegaly, splenomegaly, and skin involvement also are common. It is typical of the disease, although exceptions occur, that the patient is acutely ill when first seen by the physician. Common laboratory findings are anemia, leukopenia, and thrombocytopenia.[339] Microscopically, the distinctive feature in the involved lymph nodes is the proliferation of atypical lymphocytes within the subcapsular or medullary sinuses and/or within the lymphoid parenchyma. The tumor cells often surround lymphoid follicles in a concentric fashion, re-

Table 61 Clinical differences between Hodgkin's disease and other malignant lymphomas*

	Hodgkin's disease	Other malignant lymphomas
Age	Peak between 18 and 38 yr	Common at extremes of life
General condition of patient	Usually excellent	Often affected
Pruritus	May precede and fairly frequently accompanies	Usually not present
Fever	May be found in early cases	Rarely observed in early cases
Presence of lesion in upper air passages or gastrointestinal tract	Rarely involves these structures secondarily	Strong suggestion of primary lesion in these structures
Cervical lymph nodes	Often unilateral, lower cervical and jugular chains	Often bilateral, upper cervical, spinal, and jugular chains
Physical character	Often polylobated	Often voluminous, ovoid mass
Sternal lymph nodes	When involved, probably Hodgkin's disease	Practically never involved
Epitrochlear lymph nodes	Practically never involved	May be involved
Response to radiations	Marked radiosensitivity; delayed response	Great radiosensitivity; immediate response

*From del Regato JA, Spjut HJ: Ackerman and del Regato's Cancer, ed. 5. St. Louis, 1977, The C. V. Mosby Co.

sulting in a characteristic low-power appearance. A variable number of cells within the infiltrate exhibit phagocytosis (especially of red blood cells), but it is sometimes difficult to decide whether this phagocytosis is occurring in neoplastic cells or in accompanying reactive histiocytes. This feature is better demonstrated in bone marrow smears and touch preparations of lymph nodes than in tissue sections. Plasma cells are usually present in small numbers but may be abundant. Capsular invasion is rare; even when present, the peripheral sinuses tend to be preserved. The histiocytes themselves exhibit a pattern of individual cell infiltration rather than the cohesive masses of histiocytic lymphoma. Their cytoplasm is more abundant and eosinophilic, to the point that some cases that we have seen were originally misinterpreted as metastatic malignant melanoma or carcinoma. Enzyme histochemical and surface marker studies in cases of malignant histiocytosis have shown that the neoplastic cells indeed have the markers of histiocytes (in contrast to most cases of so-called histiocytic lymphoma.[329] The enzymes lysozyme (muramidase) and alpha$_1$-antichymotrypsin can be shown in the cytoplasm of the tumor cells with the immunoperoxidase technique,[333a] although poorly differentiated cells may lack them.[333b] Ultrastructurally, Lombardi et al.[331] identified histiocytes with variable degree of differentiation, some of them exhibiting active phagocytosis. Most of the cases are progressively and rapidly fatal, although recently an atypical form of the disease characterized by a chronic course and massive splenomegaly has been described[338]; this is discussed in Chapter 21. At autopsy, widespread organ involvement is found, usually without formation of large tumor masses but rather growing diffusely in the interstitium. In the skin, the infiltrate is periappendageal and perivascular, in contrast to the diffuse dermal infiltration with epidermal involvement observed in histiocytosis X. In the series of Byrne, Jr., and Rappaport,[325] two-thirds of the patients died within the first months after diagnosis.

The differential diagnosis has to be made with atypical reactive hyperplasia induced by viral and parasitic agents,[333] sinus histiocytosis with massive lymphadenopathy, histiocytosis X, Hodgkin's disease, metastatic melanoma or carcinoma, histiocytic lymphoma, and malignant fibrous histiocytoma. The latter possibility arises because some cases of malignant his-

tiocytosis have been reported exhibiting marked pleomorphism[340] and spindle cell metaplasia.[332]

The entity described by Scott and Robb-Smith[337] as *histiocytic medullary reticulosis* needs to be discussed in this context.[327] This has been described clinically as characterized by hepatosplenomegaly, jaundice, and rapidly fatal outcome and pathologically by prominent erythrophagocytosis by more or less atypical histiocytes. Probably some of these cases are equivalent to the fore described malignant histiocytosis[325]; as a matter of fact, some authors use the two terms synonymously.[339] On the other hand, Risdall et al.[336] have provided convincing evidence that viral infection (primarily herpes virus and adenovirus groups) can induce the proliferation of benign-appearing histiocytes in lymph nodes and bone marrow, accompanied by striking phagocytosis of red blood cells, platelets, and granulocytes (see Chapter 22). This important finding raises the possibility of so-called familial hemophagocytic reticulosis being a viral infection occurring in a family with an immune defect that makes them susceptible to the virus.[334] Similarly, it is possible that some of the reported cases of lymphoma, leukemia, or myeloproliferative diseases terminating in histiocytic medullary reticulosis[328,330] represent overwhelming viral infections in a compromised host.

The entity of *hairy cell leukemia* (leukemic reticuloendotheliosis) should not be equated with malignant histiocytosis because of a confusingly similar terminology. Actually, the two diseases could not be more different in clinical presentation, evolution, and microscopic appearance. Hairy cell leukemia is fully discussed in Chapters 21 and 22. Suffice it to say here that the lymph nodes can be involved by the disease and that this involvement is characterized by diffuse infiltration of the subcapsular sinuses, cortex, and medullary cords by the typical small mononuclear cells having nuclei slightly larger than those of lymphocytes, fine chromatin pattern, relatively abundant cytoplasm, and essentially no mitotic activity. Despite the extensiveness of the infiltrate, the nodal architecture is partially preserved.[324]

Metastatic tumors

Lymph nodes frequently contain unexpected malignant processes. The pathologist is often asked to decide whether the malignant cells are epithelial or mesenchymal in character and

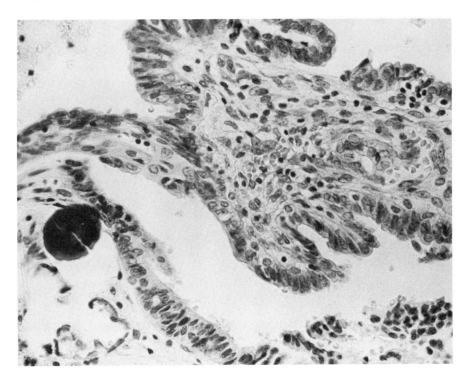

Fig. 1124 Metastatic carcinoma in cervical lymph node. Tumor is epithelial with papillary arrangement. Primary neoplasm arose from ovary. (×300; WU neg. 52-4089.)

their probable site of origin. In some instances, the microscopic changes are sufficiently diagnostic to give this information, but in others the changes warrant only a shrewd guess or a listing of possibilities in order of likelihood, based on the morphologic pattern and the exact location of the lymph node.[342,343]

A small, firm supraclavicular lymph node may contain well-differentiated papillary tumor. Tumors with this pattern, forming acini and having psammoma bodies, most commonly arise from the thyroid gland. However, if a mucin stain is positive, the tumor could not be primary in the thyroid gland. Such a papillary tumor would be unusual from the breast or lung, although the location of the metastases would be compatible with such origin. The most likely source of the primary tumor might well be the ovary (Fig. 1124). There are many cases, however, in which all the pathologist can say is that the lymph node is replaced by a highly undifferentiated malignant tumor, source unknown.

Biopsy of a peripheral lymph node may obviate a major operation. A small supraclavicular node may be biopsied and found to contain carcinoma metastatic from the breast. In such

cases, breast surgery is fruitless. When well-differentiated squamous carcinoma replaces a lymph node, central necrosis may make the node cystic (Fig. 1125). We have seen such lesions diagnosed clinically and pathologically as branchial cleft cysts (Fig. 1126). Carcinoma may be so undifferentiated that it cannot be distinguished from malignant lymphoma. Under these circumstances, the reticulin stain and the cytologic details are not helpful. By light microscopy, the pattern of tumor cells growing in small nests separated by stroma is often the *only* feature suggesting carcinoma (Fig. 1127). Electron microscopic examination of some of these nodes may be diagnostic of metastatic carcinoma by demonstrating complex desmosomes and tonofibrils.[344] Other techniques that can be very useful in order to make this differential diagnosis are touch preparations (by showing clumping of the cells in carcinoma and lack of it in lymphoma), immunoperoxidase stains for cytoplasmic immunoglobulins (which may be positive in a monoclonal fashion in lymphoma), and cell surface marker studies (which may demonstrate the lymphocytic or histiocytic nature of a tumor).

The metastatic carcinomas that most closely

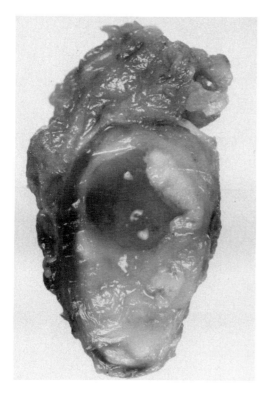

Fig. 1125 Metastatic squamous cell carcinoma in lymph node. Cavitation incident to necrosis is evident. (WU neg. 66-8430.)

simulate a malignant lymphoreticular process are nasopharyngeal "lymphoepithelioma" and lobular carcinoma of the breast. The first masquerades clinically and pathologically as Hodgkin's disease, because of its common presentation in a young adult with painless unilateral cervical lymphadenopathy and the presence of a polymorphic population (including eosinophils) on microscopic examination.[341] The second may be easily confused with histiocytic lymphoma or malignant histiocytosis.

Other lesions

Inclusions of different types of benign tissue can occur within lymph nodes. Lack of awareness of this phenomenon can lead to the mistaken diagnosis of metastatic carcinoma. Salivary gland tissue is commonly seen in high cervical nodes.[346] Thyroid follicles may be found within the marginal sinus of a midcervical node in the absence of any pathologic change of the thyroid gland.[356] Inclusions of müllerian or coelomic epithelium, regarded by some as endometriosis, are not rare in pelvic lymph nodes of females.[352] These may be difficult to distinguish from metastases originating in low-grade ovarian neoplasms, since they may grow into the peripheral sinuses, form papillae, be accompanied by psammoma bodies, and even proliferate as small sheets of cells.[349a] Mor-

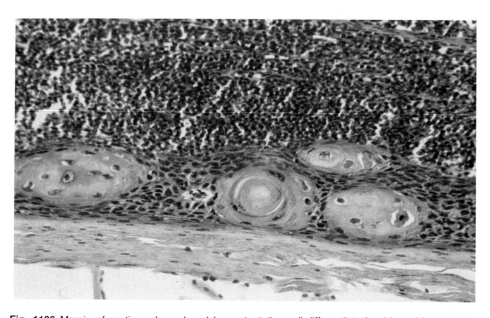

Fig. 1126 Margin of cystic node replaced by metastatic, well-differentiated epidermoid carcinoma. This pattern can easily be mistaken for branchial cleft cyst, for inner layer consists of keratin and squamous cells and next layer is composed of lymphoid tissue. (×300; WU neg. 62-8260.)

phologically similar inclusions of obscure histogenesis have been seen in para-aortic nodes of males.[354] Decidual reaction may occur within lymph nodes during pregnancy and may mimic metastatic carcinoma on frozen section[346a] (Fig. 1128).

Johnson and Helwig[351] reported six cases in which the capsule of a lymph node contained clusters of nevus cells, without involvement of the nodal parenchyma. Five of the six nodes were located in the axilla. Exceptionally, ectopic breast tissue is found in axillary lymph nodes.[349] We have seen a "benign metastasis" from a mammary intraductal papilloma to the peripheral sinus of an axillary node, probably as a result of a too energetic manipulation of the primary tumor.

Another lesion worth mentioning in this context is the *ectopic thymus* occasionally seen in supraclavicular lymph node biopsies. The pathologist unaware of this occurrence might easily interpret the Hassall's corpuscles as islands of metastatic epidermoid carcinoma.

Extensive *adipose metaplasia* of lymph nodes ("lipolymph nodes") may lead to the formation of large masses (up to 14 cm in diameter). The external iliac and obturator groups are those most commonly involved.[355a]

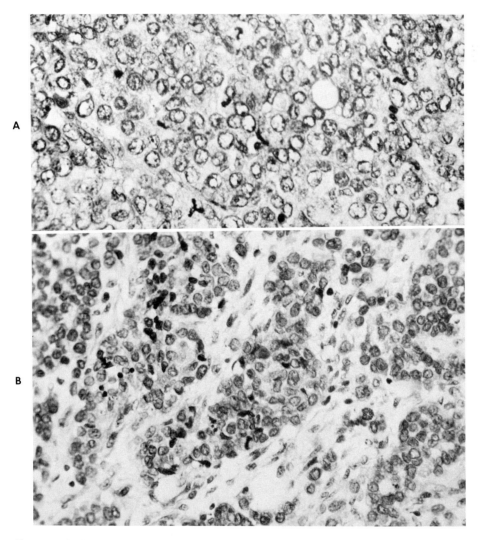

Fig. 1127 A, Area in lymph node of replacement by carcinoma which is impossible to differentiate from malignant lymphoma. **B,** Another lymph node from same patient from whom node shown in **A** was taken. Diagnosis of carcinoma can be made from this node because of carcinoma cells growing in small nests. (**A,** ×420; WU neg. 51-4668; **B,** ×300; WU neg. 51-4669.)

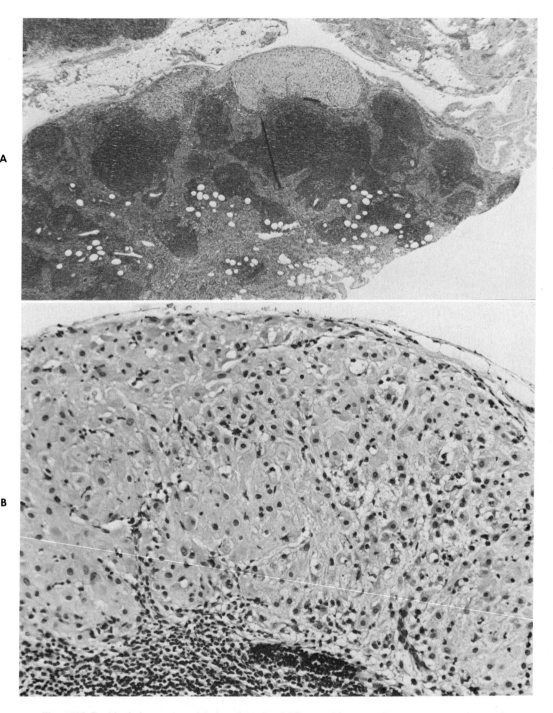

Fig. 1128 Decidual change in pelvic lymph node of 27-year-old pregnant woman operated upon for postirradiation persistence of cervical carcinoma. Subserial sections of nodes did not reveal any glandular elements. **A,** Low power. **B,** High power. (**A** and **B,** Slides courtesy Dr. R. Fechner, Charlottesville, Va.; photos by Media Services, SUNY at Stony Brook.)

Infarction of the lymph nodes presents with painful swelling, usually located in a superficial lymph node chain. Microscopically, there is extensive necrosis of medullary and cortical lymphoid cells, with marked reactive perinodal inflammation and a layer of granulation tissue. A thin rim of viable subcapsular lymphoid tissue may be present. Davies and Stansfeld[347] suggested thrombosis of veins within the substance and the hilum of the nodes as the pathogenesis. Other cases are the result of embolism.[359] It is possible that some cases actually represent necrotizing lymphadenitis of viral or toxoplasmic etiology.[345] Care should be exercised in ruling out an extensively necrotic lymphoma or metastatic carcinoma.

It is not uncommon for lymph nodes, especially those situated in the aortoiliac region, to contain wide bands of *hyaline material* among the lymphoid elements.[353] Its presence has no pathologic significance. We have seen it confused with amyloidosis and radiation effect. Three cases of what perhaps represents an extreme form of this phenomenon have been described by Osborne et al.[357] as *proteinaceous lymphadenopathy;* each patient had at least transient hypergammaglobulinemia, and the material deposited was ·markedly similar but histochemically and ultrastructurally distinct from amyloid.

Mast cells are normally present in small numbers in human lymph nodes.[353a] When markedly increased, the possibility of mastocytosis should be considered. In cases of diffuse (malignant) mastocytosis, there may be an effacement of the nodal architecture by a monotonous proliferation of round cells that may simulate malignant lymphoma.[353b] Clues as to the nature of the proliferation include the regular contours of the round or oval nucleus, the clear or granular cytoplasm, the well-defined cell outlines, and the admixture of eosinophils. Naturally, metachromatic or other stains for mast cells should be used whenever the possibility of mastocytosis exists.

Kaposi's sarcoma involving lymph nodes may be associated with the classic cutaneous involvement or be present without skin lesions.[356a] The latter occurrence is seen mainly in African children,[348] but it also has been reported in adult patients in the United States. Microscopically, the involved nodes show the typical proliferation of spindle cells separated by slitlike spaces containing red blood cells and accompanied by marked follicular hyperplasia and plasmocytic infiltration.[358] The earliest changes are seen in the subcapsular and trabecular sinuses, but eventually there is involvement of the entire node and extension into the perinodal tissues. The changes may be widespread in the node or present as discrete deposits. The degree of lymphocytic, plasmacytic, and immunoblastic proliferation may be such as to simulate a malignant lymphoma.[355] Cases of Kaposi's sarcoma have been reported in association with malignant lymphoma and leukemia,[360] and we have seen two cases in patients with the systemic form of giant lymph node hyperplasia.

Kaposi's sarcoma of the lymph nodes also needs to be distinguished from the benign condition known as *vascular transformation of the sinuses* or nodal angiomatosis.[350] This is probably the result of venous obstruction and is characterized by a vascularized sinusoidal fibrosis of the node. This alteration is not likely to be confused with malignant lymphoma, but it may be misdiagnosed as Kaposi's sarcoma.

REFERENCES
Biopsy

1 Banks PM, Long JC, Howard CA: Preparation of lymph node biopsy specimens. Hum Pathol **10**:617-621, 1979.

1a Betsill WL Jr, Hajdu SI: Percutaneous aspiration biopsy of lymph nodes. Am J Clin Pathol **73**:471-479, 1980.

1b Butler, JJ: Non-neoplastic lesions of lymph nodes of man to be differentiated from lymphomas. Nat Cancer Inst Monogr **32**:233-255, 1969.

2 Dawson PJ, Cooper RA, Rambo OM: Diagnosis of malignant lymphoma. Cancer **17**:1405-1413, 1964.

3 Moore RD, Weisberger AS, Bowerfind ES, Jr: An evaluation of lymphadenopathy in systemic disease. Arch Intern Med **99**:751-759, 1957.

3a Neiman RS: Current problems in the histopathologic diagnosis and classification of Hodgkin's disease. Pathol Annu **13**(Pt 2):289-328, 1978.

4 Slaughter DP, Economeu SG, Southwick HW: Surgical management of Hodgkin's disease. Ann Surg **148**:705-710, 1958.

5 Symmers W St C: Survey of the eventual diagnosis in 600 cases referred for a second histological opinion after an initial biopsy diagnosis of Hodgkin's disease. J Clin Pathol **21**:650-653, 1968.

6 Symmers W St C: Survey of the eventual diagnosis in 226 cases referred for a second histological opinion after an initial biopsy diagnosis of reticulum cell sarcoma. J Clin Pathol **21**:654-655, 1968.

7 Velez-Garcia E, Fradera J, Grillo AJ, Velazquez J, Maldonado N: A study of lymph node and tumor imprints and aspirations. Bol Asoc Med P R **63**:188-203, 1971.

8 Weed LA, Dahlin DC: Bacteriologic examination of tissues removed for biopsy. Am J Clin Pathol **20**:116-132, 1950.

Microscopic examination and functional histology

9 Cottier H, Turk J, Sobin L: A proposal for a standardized system of reporting human lymph node morphology in relation to immunological function. Bull WHO **47:**375-408, 1972.

10 Kersey JH, Gajl-Peczalska KJ: T and B lymphocytes in humans. A review. Am J Pathol **81:**446-457, 1975.

11 Parker JW, Taylor CR, Pattengale PK, Royston I, Tindle BH, Cain MJ, Lukes RJ: Morphologic and cytochemical comparison of human lymphoblastoid T-cell and B-cell lines: light and electron microscopy. J Natl Cancer Inst **60:**59-68, 1978.

12 Weissman IL, Warnke R, Butcher EC, Rouse R, Levy R: The lymphoid system. Its normal architecture and the potential for understanding the system through the study of lymphoproliferative diseases. Hum Pathol **9:**25-45, 1978.

13 Whiteside TL, Rowlands DT, Jr: T-cell and B-cell identification in the diagnosis of lymphoproliferative disease. A review. Am J Pathol **88:**754-790, 1977.

Immunodeficiencies

14 Baehner RL, Nathan DG: Quantitative nitroblue tetrazolium test in chronic granulomatous disease. N Engl J Med **278:**971-976, 1968.

15 Carson MJ, Chadwick DL, Brubaker CA, Cleland RS, Landing BH: Thirteen boys with progressive septic granulomatosis. Pediatrics **35:**405-412, 1965.

16 Frizzera G, Rosai J, Dehner LP, Spector BD, Kersey JH: Lymphoreticular disorders in primary immunodeficiencies. New findings based on an up-to-date histologic review of 35 cases. Cancer **46:**692-699, 1980.

17 Fudenberg H: Primary immunodeficiencies. Report of a World Health Organization Committee. Pediatrics **47:**927-946, 1971.

18 Gitlin D, Janeway CA, Apt L, Craig JM: Agammaglobulinemia. In Lawrence, H (ed): Cellular and humoral aspects of hypersensitivity states. New York, 1959, Paul B. Hoeber, Inc., pp. 375-441.

19 Heymer B, Niethammer D, Spanel R, Galle J, Kleihauer E, Haferkamp O: Pathomorphology of humoral, cellular and combined primary immunodeficiencies. Virchows Arch [Pathol Anat] **374:**87-103, 1977.

20 Holmes B, Park BH, Malawista SE, Quie, PG, Nelson DL, Good RA: Chronic granulomatous disease in females. A deficiency of leukocyte glutathione peroxidase. N Engl J Med **283:**217-221, 1970.

21 Johnston RB, McMurry JS: Chronic familial granulomatosis. Am J Dis Child **114:**370-378, 1967.

22 Kersey JH, Spector BD, Good RA: Primary immunodeficiency diseases and cancer: the immunodeficiency-Cancer Registry. Int J Cancer **12:**333-347, 1973.

23 Landing BH, Shirkey NS: A syndrome of recurrent infection and infiltration of viscera by pigmented lipid histiocytes. Pediatrics **20:**431-438, 1957.

24 Louie S, Schwartz RS: Immunodeficiency and the pathogenesis of lymphoma and leukemia. Semin Hematol **15:**117-138, 1978.

25 Lukes RJ, Collins RD: Immunologic characterization of human malignant lymphomas. Cancer **34:**1488-1503, 1974.

26 Purtilo DT, DeFlorio D Jr, Hutt LM, Bhawan J, Yang JP, Otto R, Edwards W: Variable phenotypic expression of an X-linked recessive lymphoproliferative syndrome. N Engl J Med **297:**1077-1081, 1977.

27 Spector BD, Perry GS III, Kersey, JH: Genetically determined immunodeficiency diseases (GDID) and ma-

lignancy: report from the immunodeficiency-Cancer Registry. Clin Immunol Immunopathol **11:**12-29, 1978.

28 Spector BD, Perry GS III, Good RA, Kersey JH: Immunodeficiency diseases and malignancy. In Twomey JJ, Good RA (eds): The immunopathology of lymphoreticular neoplasms. Vol 4 of Good RA, Day SB (series eds): Comprehensive immunology. New York, 1978, Plenum Medical Book Co., pp. 203-222.

29 Stiehm ER, Fulginiti VA: Immunologic disorders in infants and children. Philadelphia, 1973, W. B. Saunders Co.

Hyperplasia

30 Banks PM, Witrak GA, Conn DL: Lymphoid neoplasia following connective tissue disease. Mayo Clin Proc **54:**104-108, 1979.

30a Bluming AZ, Cohen HG, Saxon A: Angioimmunoblastic lymphadenopathy with dysproteinemia. A pathogenetic link between physiologic lymphoid proliferation and malignant lymphoma. Am J Med **67:**421-428, 1979.

31 Carter RL: Review of some recent observations on "glandular fever cells." J Clin Pathol **19:**448-455, 1966.

31a Choi YJ, Reiner L: Syphilitic lymphadenitis. Immunofluorescent identification of spirochetes from imprints. Am J Surg Pathol **3:**553-555, 1979.

32 Cooper RA, Dawson PJ, Rambo ON: Dermatopathic lymphadenopathy. A clinicopathologic analysis of lymph node biopsy over a fifteen-year period. Calif Med **106:**170-175, 1967.

32a Cullen MH, Stansfeld AG, Oliver RTD, Lister TA, Malpas JS: Angio-immunoblastic lymphadenopathy: report of ten cases and review of the literature. Q J Med **48:**151-177, 1979.

33 Custer RP, Smith EB: The pathology of infectious mononucleosis. Blood **3:**830-857, 1948.

34 Dawson PJ, Cooper RA, Rambo OM: Diagnosis of malignant lymphoma. Cancer **17:**1405-1413, 1964.

35 Dorfman RF, Herweg, JC: Live, attenuated measles virus vaccine. Inguinal lymphadenopathy complicating administration. JAMA **198:**320-321, 1966.

36 Dorfman RF, Warnke R: Lymphadenopathy simulating the malignant lymphomas. Hum Pathol **5:**519-550, 1974.

37 Elema JD, Poppema S: Infantile histiocytosis X (Letterer-Siwe disease): investigations with enzymehistochemical and sheep-erythrocyte rosetting techniques. Cancer **42:**555-565, 1978.

38 Evans N: Lymphadenitis of secondary syphilis (its resemblance to giant follicular lymphadenopathy). Arch Pathol **37:**175-179, 1944.

39 Foucar E, Rosai J, Dorfman RF: Sinus histiocytosis with massive lymphadenopathy. Ear, Nose, and throat manifestations. Arch Otolaryngol **104:**687-693, 1978.

40 Foucar E, Rosai J, Dorfman RF: The ophthalmologic manifestations of sinus histiocytosis with massive lymphadenopathy. Am J Ophthalmol **87:**354-367, 1979.

40a Foucar E, Rosai J, Dorfman RF, Brynes RK: The neurologic manifestations of sinus histiocytosis with massive lymphadenopathy. Neurology (in press).

41 Frizzera G, Moran EM, Rappaport H: Angio-immunoblastic lymphadenopathy with dysproteinaemia. Lancet **1:**1070-1073, 1974.

42 Frizzera G, Moran EM, Rappaport H: Angio-immunoblastic lymphadenopathy. Diagnosis and clinical course. Am J Med **59:**803-818, 1975.

43 Frizzera G, Rosai J, Banks PM, Bayrd ED, Massarelli G: A multicentric lymphoproliferative disorder with the morphologic features of Castleman's disease: a clinicopathologic study of ten patients. Lab Invest **42**:118, 1980 (abstract).

44 Gaba AR, Stein RS, Sweet DL, Variakojis D: Multicentric giant lymph node hyperplasia. Am J Clin Pathol **69**:86-90, 1978.

45 Gall EA, Rappaport H: Seminar on diseases of lymph nodes and spleen. In Proceedings of the 23rd Seminar of the American Society of Clinical Pathologists, Chicago, 1958, American Society of Clinical Pathologists, pp. 7-9.

46 Goldenberg GJ, Paraskevas F, Israels, LG: The association of rheumatoid arthritis with plasma cell and lymphocytic neoplasms. Arthritis Rheum **12**:569-579, 1969.

47 Green JA, Dawson AA, Walker W: Systemic lupus erythematosus and lymphoma. Lancet **2**:753-756, 1978.

48 Hartsock, RJ: Postvaccinial lymphadenitis. Hyperplasia of lymphoid tissue that simulates malignant lymphomas. Cancer **21**:632-649, 1968.

49 Hartsock RJ, Halling W, King FM: Luetic lymphadenitis: a clinical and histologic study of 20 cases. Am J Clin Pathol **53**:304-314, 1970.

50 Hyman GA, Sommers SC: The development of Hodgkin's disease and lymphoma during anticonvulsant therapy. Blood **28**:416-427, 1966.

50a Jones DB, Castleden M, Smith JL, Mepham BL, Wright DH: Immunopathology of angioimmunoblastic lymphadenopathy. Br J Cancer **37**:1053-1062, 1978.

51 Keller AR, Hochholzer L, Castleman, B: Hyaline-vascular and plasma-cell types of giant lymph node hyperplasia of mediastinum and other locations. Cancer **29**:670-683, 1972.

52 Kjeldsberg CR, Kim H: Eosinophilic granuloma as an incidental finding in malignant lymphoma. Arch Pathol Lab Med **104**:137-140, 1980.

53 Klemperer P, Boris G, Lee SL, Leuchtenberger C, Pollister AW: Cytochemical changes of acute lupus erythematosus. Arch Pathol **49**:503-516, 1950.

54 Kosmidis PA, Axelrod AR, Palacas C, Stahl M: Angioimmunoblastic lymphadenopathy. A T-cell deficiency. Cancer **42**:447-452, 1978.

55 Kreyberg L, Iversen OH: Early diagnosis of malignant conditions in lymph nodes. Br J Cancer **13**:26-32, 1959.

55a Krueger GRF, Bergholz M, Bartsch H-H, Fischer R, Schauer A: Rubella virus antigen in lymphocytes of patients with angioimmunoblastic lymphadenopathy (AIL). J Cancer Res Clin Oncol **95**:87-91, 1979.

56 Laipply TC: Lipomelanotic reticular hyperplasia of lymph nodes. Arch Intern Med **81**:19-36, 1948.

57 Lampert F, Lennert K: Sinus histiocytosis with massive lymphadenopathy. Fifteen new cases. Cancer **37**:783-789, 1976.

57a Lennert K, Mohri N: Histopathology and diagnosis of non-Hodgkin lymphoma. In Lennert, K: Malignant lymphomas other than Hodgkin's disease: histology, cytology, ultrastructure, immunology. Berlin, 1978, Springer-Verlag, p. 182.

58 Levine PH, Stevens DA, Coccia PF, Dabich L, Roland A: Infectious mononucleosis prior to acute leukemia: a possible role for the Epstein-Barr virus. Cancer **30**:1-6, 1972.

59 Li FP, Willard DR, Goodman R, Vawter G: Malignant lymphoma after diphenylhydantoin (dilantin) therapy. Cancer **36**:1359-1362, 1975.

60 Liao KT, Rosai J, Daneshbod K: Malignant histiocytosis with cutaneous involvement and eosinophilia. Am J Clin Pathol **57**:438-448, 1972.

61 Lukes RJ, and Tindle BH: Immunoblastic lymphadenopathy. A hyperimmune entity resembling Hodgkin's disease. N Engl J Med **292**:1-8, 1975.

62 McMahon NJ, Gordon HW, Rosen RB: Reed-Sternberg cells in infectious mononucleosis. Am J Dis Child **120**:148-150, 1970.

63 Madri JA, Fromowitz F: Amyloid deposition in immunoblastic lymphadenopathy. Hum Pathol **9**:157-162, 1978.

64 Metcalf D: Reticular tumours in mice subjected to prolonged antigenic stimulation. Br J Cancer **15**:769-779, 1961.

65 Moore RD, Weisberger AS, Bowerfind ES, Jr: An evaluation of lymphadenopathy in systemic disease. Arch Intern Med **99**:751-759, 1957.

66 Moragas A: Linfadenopatias benignas. Bases morfologicas de su interpretacion clinica. Medicina Clinica, Monograph # 1, 1971, pp. 1-174.

66a Motoi M, Helbron D, Kaiserling E, Lennert K: Eosinophilic granuloma of lymph nodes—a variant of histiocytosis X. Histopathology **4**:585-606, 1980.

67 Motulsky OG, Weinberg S, Saphir O, Rosenberg E: Lymph nodes in rheumatoid arthritis. Arch Intern Med **90**:660-676, 1952.

68 Nathwani BN, Rappaport H, Moran EM, Pangalis GA, Kim H: Malignant lymphoma arising in angioimmunoblastic lymphadenopathy. Cancer **41**:578-606, 1978.

69 Neiman RS, Dervan P, Haudenschild C, Jaffe R: Angioimmunoblastic lymphadenopathy. An ultrastructural and immunologic study with review of the literature. Cancer **41**:507-518, 1978.

70 Nosanchuk JS, Schnitzer B: Follicular hyperplasia in lymph nodes from patients with rheumatoid arthritis. A clinicopathologic study. Cancer **24**:343-354, 1969.

70a Poppema S, Kaiserling E, Lennert K: Hodgkin's disease with lymphocytic predominance, nodular type (nodular paragranuloma) and progressively transformed germinal centres—a cytohistological study. Histopathology **3**:295-308, 1979.

71 Rappaport H, Winter WJ, Hicks EB: Follicular lymphoma. A re-evaluation of its position in the scheme of malignant lymphoma, based on a survey of 253 cases. Cancer **9**:792-821, 1956.

72 Rausch E, Kaiserling E, Goos M: Langerhans cells and interdigitating reticulum cells in the thymus-dependent region in human dermatopathic lymphadenitis. Virchows Arch [Cell Pathol] **25**:327-343, 1977.

73 Reid H, Fox H, Whittaker JS: Eosinophilic granuloma of lymph nodes. Histopathology **1**:31-37, 1977.

74 Robertson MDJ, Hart FD, White WF, Nuki G, Boardman PL: Rheumatoid lymphadenopathy. Ann Rheum Dis **27**:253-260, 1968.

75 Rosai J, Dorfman RF: Sinus histiocytosis with massive lymphadenopathy: a pseudolymphomatous benign disorder. Analysis of 34 cases. Cancer **30**:1174-1188, 1972.

75a Rosdahl N, Larsen SO, Clemmesen J: Hodgkin's disease in patients with previous infectious mononucleosis: 30 years' experience. Br Med J **1**:253-256, 1974.

76 Saltzstein SL: The fate of patients with nondiagnostic lymph node biopsies. Surgery **58**:659-662, 1965.

77 Saltzstein SL, Ackerman LV: Lymphadenopathy induced by anticonvulsant drugs clinically and pathologically mimicking malignant lymphomas. Cancer **12:**164-182, 1959.

78 Salvador AH, Harrison EG, Kyle RA: Lymphadenopathy due to infectious mononucleosis: its confusion with malignant lymphoma. Cancer **27:**1029-1040, 1971.

79 Sanchez R, Rosai J, Dorfman RF: Sinus histiocytosis with massive lymphadenopathy: an analysis of 113 cases with special emphasis on its extranodal manifestations. Lab Invest **36:**21-22, 1977 (abstract).

79a Sanchez R, Sibley RK, Rosai J, Dorfman RF: The electron microscopic features of sinus histiocytosis with massive lymphadenopathy. A study of 11 cases. Ultrastr Pathol (in press).

80 Schwartz R, André-Schwartz J, Armstrong MYK, Beldotti L: Neoplastic sequelae of allogenic disease. I. Theoretical considerations and experimental design. Ann NY Acad Sci **129:**804-821, 1966.

80a Seehafer JR, Goldberg NC, Dicken CH, Su WPD: Cutaneous manifestations of angioimmunoblastic lymphadenopathy. Arch Dermatol **116:**41-45, 1980.

81 Sieracki JC, Fisher ER: Diagnostic problems involving nodal lymphomas. In Sommers SC (ed): Pathology annual, vol. 5. New York, 1970, Appleton-Century-Crofts, pp. 91-124.

82 Stevens DA: Infectious mononucleosis and malignant lymphoproliferative diseases. JAMA **219:**897-898, 1972.

83 Thawerani H, Sanchez RL, Rosai J, Dorfman RF: The cutaneous manifestations of sinus histiocytosis with massive lymphadenopathy. Arch Dermatol **114:**191-197, 1978.

84 Tindle BH, Parker JW, Lukes RJ: "Reed-Sternberg cells" in infectious mononucleosis? Am J Clin Pathol **58:**607-617, 1972.

85 Tung KSK, McCormack LJ: Angiomatous lymphoid hamartoma. Cancer **20:**525-536, 1967.

86 Vernon ML, Fountain L, Krebs HM, Barbosa LH, Fuccillo DA, Sever JL: Birbeck granules (Langerhan's cell granules) in human lymph nodes. Am J Clin Pathol **60:**771-779, 1973.

87 Walker PD, Rosai J, Dorfman RF: The osseous manifestations of sinus histiocytosis with massive lymphadenopathy. Am J Clin Pathol (in press).

88 Williams JW, Dorfman RF: Lymphadenopathy as the initial manifestation of histiocytosis X. Am J Surg Pathol **3:**405-421, 1979.

Granulomatous inflammation

89 Ahlqvist J, Ahvohen P, Rasanen JA, Wallgren GR: Enteric infection with yersinia enterocolitica. Large pyroninophilic cell reaction in mesenteric lymph nodes associated with early production of specific antibodies. Acta Pathol Microbiol Scand [A] **79:**109-122, 1971.

90 Anderson R, James DG, Peters PM, Thomson AD: Local sarcoid-tissue reactions. Lancet **1:**1211-1213, 1962.

91 Azar HA, Lunardelli C: Collagen nature of asteroid bodies of giant cells in sarcoidosis. Am J Pathol **57:**81-92, 1969.

92 Boitnott JK, Margolis S: Mineral oil in human tissues. II. Oil droplets in lymph nodes of the porta hepatis. Bull Hopkins Hosp. **118:**414-422, 1966.

93 Carithers HA, Carithers CM, Edwards RO, Jr.: Cat-scratch disease. Its natural history JAMA **207:**312-316, 1969.

94 Carter CJ, Gross MA, Johnson FB: The selective staining of curious bodies in lymph nodes of patients as

a means for diagnosis of sarcoid. Stain Technol **44:**1-4, 1969.

95 Chears WC Jr, Smith AG, Ruffin JM: Diagnosis of Whipple's disease by peripheral lymph node biopsy. Report of a case. Am J Med **27:**351-353, 1959.

95a Cozzutto C, Soave F: Xanthogranulomatous lymphadenitis. Virchows Arch [Pathol Anat] **385:**103-108, 1979.

96 Cunningham JA: Sarcoidosis. In Sommers SC, (ed): Pathology annual, vol. 2. New York, 1967, Appleton-Century-Crofts, pp. 31-46.

97 Cushard WG Jr, Simon AB, Caterbury JM, Reiss E: Parathyroid function in sarcoidosis. N Engl J Med **286:**395-398, 1972.

98 Daneshbod K: Localized lymphadenitis due to leishmania simulating toxoplasmosis. Value of electron microscopy for differentiation. Am J Clin Pathol **69:**462-467, 1978.

99 Daniels WB, MacMurray FG: Cat scratch disease. JAMA **154:**1247-2151, 1954.

100 Dorfman RF, Remington JS: Value of lymph-node biopsy in the diagnosis of acute acquired toxoplasmosis. N Engl J Med **289:**878-881, 1973.

101 Dorfman RF, Warnke R: Lymphadenopathy simulating the malignant lymphomas. Hum Pathol **5:**519-550, 1974.

102 Fisher ER: Whipple's disease: pathogenetic considerations. Electron microscopic and histochemical observations. JAMA **181:**396-403, 1962.

103 Fujimoto Y, Kojima Y, Yamaguchi K: Cervical subacute necrotizing lymphadenitis. Int Med **30:**920-927, 1972.

104 Gall EA, Rappaport H: Seminar on diseases of lymph nodes and spleen. In Proceedings of the 23rd Seminar of the American Society of Clinical Pathologists, Chicago, 1958, American Society of Clinical Pathologists, pp. 7-9.

105 Gorton G, Linell F: Malignant tumours and sarcoid reactions in regional lymph nodes. Acta Radiol (Stockh) **47:**381-392, 1957.

106 Jansson E, Wallgren GR, Ahvenen P: Y. enterocolitica as a cause of acute mesenteric lymphadenitis. Acta Paediatr Scand **57:**448-450, 1968.

107 Johnson WT, Helwig EB: Cat-scratch disease. Histopathologic changes in the skin. Arch Dermatol **100:**148-154, 1969.

108 Kadin ME, Donaldson SS, Dorfman RF: Isolated granulomas in Hodgkin's disease. N Engl J Med **283:**859-861, 1970.

109 Kelsall GR, Blackwell JB: The occurrence and significance of lipophage clusters in lymph nodes and spleen. Pathology **1:**211-220, 1969.

110 Kikuchi M, Yoshizumi T, Nakamura H: Necrotizing lymphadenitis: possible acute toxoplasmic infection. Virchows Arch [Pathol Anat] **376:**247-253, 1977.

111 Knapp W: Mesenteric adenitis due to Pasteurella pseudotuberculosis in young people. N Engl J Med **259:**776-778, 1958.

112 Llewelyn DM, Dorman D: Mycobacterial lymphadenitis. Aust Paediatr J **7:**97-102, 1971.

113 Määtta KT: Histological study of mediastinal lymph nodes in clinical sarcoidosis. A report of 86 cases. Ann Acad Sci Fenn [Med.] **138:**1-106, 1968.

114 Mackellar A, Hilton HB, Masters PL: Mycobacterial lymphadenitis in childhood. Arch Dis Child **42:**70-74, 1967.

115 Mitchell DN: The Kveim test. In Dyke SC (ed): Recent advances in clinical pathology, series 5.

Boston, 1968, Little, Brown and Co., chap. 4.
115a Moragas A: Linfadenopatias benignas. Bases morfologicas de su interpretacion clinica. Medicina Clinica, Monograph #1, 1971, pp. 1-174.
116 Nadel E, Ackerman LV: Lesions resembling Boeck's sarcoid Am J Clin Pathol **20**:952-957, 1952.
117 Naji AF, Carbonell F, Barker HJ: Cat scratch disease. A report of three new cases, review of the literature, and classification of the pathologic changes in the lymph nodes during various stages of the disease. Am J Clin Pathol **38**:513-521, 1962.
118 Nethercott SE, Strawbridge WG: Identification of bacterial residues in sarcoid lesions. Lancet **2**:1132, 1956.
119 Nilthn B: Studies on Yersinia enterocolitica with special reference to bacterial diagnosis and occurrence in human enteric disease. Acta Pathol Microbiol Scand [suppl] **206**:1-48, 1969.
120 Piringer-Kuchinka A, Martin I, Thalhammer O: Ueber die vorzuglich cerviconuchale Lymphadenitis mit kleinherdiger Epitheloid-zellwucherung. Virchows Arch [Pathol Anat] **331**:522-535, 1958.
121 Ravel R: Histopathology of lymph nodes after lymphangiography. Am J Clin Pathol **46**:335-355, 1966.
122 Reid JD, Wolinsky E: Histopathology of lymphadenitis caused by atypical mycobacteria. Am Rev Respir Dis **99**:8-12, 1969.
123 Saxen E, Saxen L, Grönroos P: Glandular toxoplasmosis. A report of 23 histologically diagnosed cases. Acta Pathol Microbiol Scand **44**:319-328, 1958.
124 Saxen L, Saxen E, and Tenhunen A: The significance of histological diagnosis in glandular toxoplasmosis. Acta Pathol Microbiol Scand **56**:284-294, 1962.
125 Sieracki JC, Fisher ER: The ceroid nature of the so-called "Hamazaki-Wesenberg bodies." Am J Clin Pathol **59**:248-253, 1973.
126 Siltzbach LE: Results of Kveim testing. An international Kvein test study (Proceedings of the Third International Conference on Sarcoidosis). Acta Med Scand **176**(suppl 425):178-190, 1964.
127 Siltzbach LE: Geographic aspects of sarcoidosis. Trans NY Acad. Sci **29**(Ser. II):364-374, 1967.
128 Smith EB, Custer RP: The histopathology of lymphogranuloma venereum. J Urol **63**:546-563, 1950.
129 Stansfeld AG: The histological diagnosis of toxoplasmic lymphadenitis. J Clin Pathol **14**:565-573, 1961.
129a Tudway AJC: Yellow bodies in superficial and deep lymph nodes. J Clin Pathol **32**:52-55, 1979.
130 Vaněk J, Schwarz J: Demonstration of acid-fast rods in sarcoidosis. Am Rev Respir Dis **101**:395-400, 1970.
131 Watson JH, Haubrich WS: Bacilli bodies in the lumen and epithelium of the jejunum in Whipple's disease. Lab Invest **21**:347-357, 1969.
132 Weed LA, Dahlin DC: Bacteriologic examination of tissues removed for biopsy. Am J Clin Pathol **20**:116-132, 1950.
133 Wesenberg W: Saurefeste, Spindelkorper Hamazaki bei Sarkoidose. Arch Klin Exp Med **227**:101-112, 1966.
134 White JD, McGavran, NH: Identification of Pasteurella tularensis. JAMA **194**:180-182, 1965.
135 Winnacker JL, Becker KL, Friedlander M, Higgins GA, Moore CF: Sarcoidosis and hyperparathyroidism. Am J Med **46**:305-312, 1969.
136 Winship T: Pathologic changes in so-called cat-scratch fever. Review of findings in lymph nodes of 29 patients and cutaneous lesions of 2 patients. Am J Clin Pathol **23**:1012-1018, 1953.

Malignant lymphoma

137 Banks PM, Berard CW: Histopathology of the malignant lymphomas. In Williams WJ (ed): Hematology. New York, 1977, McGraw-Hill Book Co.
138 Berard CW, Dorfman RF: Histopathology of malignant lymphomas. Clin Haematol **3**:39-76, 1974.
139 Come SE, Jaffe ES, Anderson JC, Mann RB, Johnson BL, DeVita VT, Young RC: Leukemic progression of non-Hodgkin's lymphoma: clinicopathologic features and therapeutic implications. Blood (in press).
140 Cossman J, Schnitzer B, Deegan MJ: Coexistence of two lymphomas with distinctive histologic, ultrastructural, and immunologic features. Am J Clin Pathol **70**:409-415, 1978.
141 Jaffe ES, Braylan RC, Nanba K, Frank MM, Berard CW: Functional markers: a new perspective on malignant lymphomas. Cancer Treat Rep **61**:953-962, 1977.
142 Jaffe ES, Shevach EM, Sussman EH, Frank M, Green I, Berard CW: Membrane receptor sites for the identification of lymphoreticular cells in benign and malignant conditions. Br J Cancer **31**(Suppl 2):107-120, 1975.
143 Kim H, Hendrickson MR, Dorfman RF: Composite lymphoma. Cancer **40**:959-976, 1977.
144 Woda BA, Knowles DM II: Nodular lymphocytic lymphoma eventuating into diffuse histiocytic lymphoma. Immunoperoxidase demonstration of monoclonality. Cancer **43**:303-307, 1979.

Non-Hodgkin's lymphoma

144a Aisenberg AC, Wilkes BM, Long JC, Harris NL: Cell surface phenotype in lymphoproliferative disease. Am J Med **68**:206-213, 1980.
145 Bloomfield CD, Kersey JH, Brunning RD, Gajl-Peczalska KJ: Prognostic significance of lymphocytic surface markers and histology in adult non-Hodgkin's lymphoma. Cancer Treat Rep **61**:963-970, 1977.
146 Bloomfield CD, Gajl-Peczalska KJ, Frizzera G, Kersey JH, Goldman AI: Clinical utility of lymphocyte surface markers combined with the Lukes-Collins histologic classification in adult lymphoma. N Engl J Med (**301**:512-518, 1979).
147 Bom-van Noorloos AA, Splinter TAW, van Heerde P, Van Beck AAM, Melief CJM: Surface markers and functional properties of non-Hodgkin's lymphoma cells in relation to histology. Cancer **42**:1804-1817, 1978.
148 Braylan RC, Jaffe ES, Berard CW: Malignant lymphomas: current classification and new observations. Pathology Annu **10**:213-270, 1975.
149 Byrne GE Jr: Rappaport classification of non-Hodgkin's lymphoma: histologic features and clinical significance. Cancer Treat Rep **61**:935-944, 1977.
150 Dorfman RF: Classifications of the malignant lymphomas. Am J Surg Pathol **1**:167-170, 1977.
151 Dorfman RF: Pathology of the non-Hodgkin's lymphomas: new classifications. Cancer Treat Rep **61**:945-951, 1977.
152 Dorfman RF, Kim H: Relationship of histology to site in the non–Hodgkin's lymphomata: a study based on surgical staging procedures. Br J Cancer **31**:217-220, 1975.
153 Frizzera G, Gajl-Peczalska KJ, Bloomfield CD, Kersey JH: Predictability of immunologic phenotype of malignant lymphomas by conventional morphology. A study of 60 cases. Cancer **43**:1216-1224, 1979.
153a Fukuhara S, Rowley JD, Variakojis D, Golomb

HM: Chromosome abnormalities in poorly differentiated lymphocytic lymphoma. Cancer Res **39:**3119-3128, 1979.

154 Gall EA, Mallory TB: Malignant lymphoma. A clinicopathologic survey of 618 cases. Am J Pathol **18:** 381-429, 1942.

155 Goffinet DR, Warnke R, Dunnick NR, Castellino R, Glatstein E, Nelsen TS, Dorfman RF, Rosenberg SA, Kaplan AS: Clinical and surgical (laparotomy) evaluation of patients with non-Hodgkin's lymphomas. Cancer Treat Rep **61:**981-992, 1977.

155a Habeshaw JA, Catley PF, Stansfeld AG, Brearley RL: Surface phenotyping, histology and the nature of non-Hodgkin lymphoma in 157 patients. Br J Cancer **40:**11-34, 1979.

156 Lennert K: Classification of non-Hodgkin's lymphomas. In Lennert K, Coll: Malignant lymphomas other than Hodgkin's disease. Histology, cytology, ultrastructure, immunology. Berlin, 1978, Springer-Verlag, pt 3, 1978, pp. 83-110.

157 Lennert K, Stein H, Kaiserling E: Cytological and functional criteria for the classification of malignant lymphomata. Br J Cancer **31:**29-43, 1975.

158 Lennert K, Mohri N, Stein H, Kaiserling E: The histopathology of malignant lymphoma. Br J Haematol **31** (Suppl):193-203, 1975.

159 Lukes RJ, Collins RD: Immunologic characterization of human malignant lymphomas. Cancer **34:**1488-1503, 1974.

160 Lukes RJ, Parker JW, Taylor CR, Tindle BH, Cramer AD, Lincoln TL: Immunologic approach to non-Hodgkin lymphomas and related leukemias. Analysis of the results of multiparameter studies of 425 cases. Semin Hematol **15:**322-351, 1978.

161 Lukes RJ, Taylor CR, Chir B, Parker PSW, Lincoln TL, Pattengale PK, Tindle BH: A morphologic and immunologic surface marker study of 299 cases on non-Hodgkin lymphomas and related leukemias. Am J Pathol **90:**461-485, 1978.

161a Mason DY, Bell JI, Christensson B, Biberfeld P: An immunohistological study of human lymphoma. Clin Exp Immunol **40:**235-248, 1980.

161b Nathwani BN: A critical analysis of the classifications of non-Hodgkin's lymphomas. Cancer **44:**347-384, 1979.

162 Nathwani BN, Kim H, Rappaport H, Solomon J, Fox M: Non-Hodgkin's lymphomas. A clinicopathologic study comparing two classifications. Cancer **41:**303-325, 1978.

162a National Cancer Institute: Non-Hodgkin Lymphoma Classification Study (in preparation).

163 Pinkus GS, Said JW: Characterization of non-Hodgkin's lymphomas using multiple cell markers. Immunologic, morphologic, and cytochemical studies of 72 cases. Am J Pathol **94:**349-376, 1979.

164 Rappaport H: Tumors of the hematopoietic system. In Atlas of tumor pathology, Sect. 3, Fasc. 8. Washington, D. C., 1966, Armed Forces Institute of Pathology.

165 Rilke F, Pilotti S, Carbone A, Lombardi L: Morphology of lymphatic cells and of their derived tumors. J Clin Pathol **31:**1009-1056, 1978.

166 Rosenberg SA, Dorfman RF, Kaplan HS: A summary of the results of a review of 405 patients with non-Hodgkin's lymphoma at Stanford University. Br J Cancer **31:**168-173, 1975.

166a Said JW, Hargreaves HK, Pinkus GS: Non-Hodg-

kin's lymphomas: an ultrastructural study correlating morphology with immunologic cell type. Cancer **44:**504-528, 1979.

Nodular (follicular) lymphoma

167 Anderson T, Bender RA, Fisher RI, DeVita VT, Chabner BA, Berard CW, Norton L, Young RC: Combination chemotherapy in non-Hodgkin's lymphoma: results of long-term followup. Cancer Treat Rep **61:** 1057-1066, 1977.

168 Bennett MH: Sclerosis in non-Hodgkin's lymphomata. Br J Cancer **31:**44-52, 1975.

168a Colby TV, Hoppe RT, Burke JS: Nodular lymphoma. Clinicopathologic correlations of parafollicular small lymphocytes and degree of nodularity. Cancer **45:**2364-2367, 1980.

169 Come SE, Jaffe ES, Anderson JC, Mann RB, Johnson BL, DeVita VT, Young RC: Leukemic progression of non-Hodgkin's lymphoma: Clinicopathologic features and therapeutic implications. Blood (In press)

170 Dorfman RF: Classical concepts of nodular (follicular) lymphomas. Gann Monogr Cancer Res **15:**177-188, 1973.

171 Frizzera G, Murphy SB: Follicular (nodular) lymphoma in childhood: a rare clinical-pathological entity. Report of eight cases from four cancer centers. Cancer **44:**2218-2235, 1979.

172 Jaffe ES, Shevach EM, Frank MM, Berard CW, Green I: Nodular lymphoma: evidence for origin from follicular B lymphocytes. N Engl J Med **290:**813-819, 1974.

173 Jones SE, Fuks Z, Bull M, Kadin ME, Dorfman RF, Kaplan HS, Rosenberg SA, Kim H: Non-Hodgkin's lymphomas. IV. Clinicopathologic correlation in 405 cases. Cancer **31:**806-823, 1973.

174 Kim H, Dorfman RF: Morphological studies of 84 untreated patients subjected to laparotomy for the staging of non-Hodgkin's lymphomas. Cancer **33:**657-674, 1974.

175 Kim H, Dorfman RF, Rappaport H: Signet ring cell lymphoma. A rare morphologic and functional expression of nodular (follicular) lymphoma. Am J Surg Pathol **2:**119-132, 1978.

176 Leech JH, Glick AD, Waldron JA, Flexner JM, Horn RG, Collins RD: Malignant lymphomas of follicular center cell origin in man. I. Immunologic studies. J Natl Cancer Inst **54:**11-21, 1975.

177 Lennert K: Follicular lymphoma: a tumor of the germinal centers. Malignant diseases of the hematopoietic system, Gann Monogr Cancer Res. **15:**217-231, 1973.

178 Levine GD, Dorfman RF: Nodular lymphoma: an ultrastructural study of its relationship to germinal centers and a correlation of light and electron microscopic findings. Cancer **35:**148-164, 1975.

179 McKenna RW, Brunning RD: Reed–Sternberg-like cells in nodular lymphoma involving the bone marrow. Am J Clin Pathol **63:**779-785, 1975.

180 Patchefsky AS, Brodovsky HS, Menduke H, Southard M, Brooks J, Nicklar D, Hoch WS: Non-Hodgkin's lymphomas: A clinicopathologic study of 293 cases. Cancer **34:**1173-1186, 1974.

181 Rappaport H, Winter WJ, Hicks EB: Follicular lymphoma; a re-evaluation of its position in the scheme of malignant lymphoma, based on a survey of 253 cases. Cancer **9:**792-821, 1956.

182 Rosas-Uribe A, Variakojis D, Rappaport H: Protein-

aceous precipitate in nodular (follicular) lymphomas. Cancer **31**:534-542, 1973.

183 Warnke R, Levy R: Immunopathology of follicular lymphomas. A model of B-lymphocyte homing. N Engl J Med **298**:481-486, 1978.

184 Warnke RA, Kim H, Fuks D, Dorfman RF: The coexistence of nodular and diffuse patterns in nodular non-Hodgkin's lymphomas. Significance and clinicopathologic correlation. Cancer **40**:1229-1233, 1977.

Diffuse lymphoma

185 Hausner RJ, Rosas-Uribe A, Wickstrum DA, Smith SC: Non-Hodgkin's lymphoma in the first two decades of life. A pathological study of 30 cases. Cancer **40**:1533-1547, 1977.

Well-differentiated lymphocytic lymphoma

186 Armitage JO, Dick FR, Corder MP: Diffuse histiocytic lymphoma complicating chronic lymphocytic leukemia. Cancer **41**:422-427, 1978.

187 Braylan RC, Jaffe ES, Burbach JW, Frank MM, Johnson RE, Berard CW: Similarities of surface characteristics of neoplastic well-differentiated lymphocytes from solid tissues and from peripheral blood. Cancer Res **36**:1619-1625, 1976.

188 Brouet J-C, Sasportes M, Flandrin G, Preud'Homme J-L, Seligmann M: Chronic lymphocytic leukaemia of T-cell origin: immunological and clinical evaluation in eleven patients. Lancet **2**:890-893, 1975.

189 Dick FR, Maca RD: The lymph node in chronic lymphocytic leukemia. Cancer **41**:283-292, 1978.

190 Evans HL, Butler JJ, Youness EL: Malignant lymphoma, small lymphocytic type. A clinicopathologic study of 84 cases with suggested criteria for intermediate lymphocytic lymphoma. Cancer **41**:1440-1455, 1978.

190a Foucar C, Rydell RE: Richter's syndrome in chronic lymphocytic leukemia. Cancer **46**:118-134, 1980.

191 Long JC, Aisenberg AC: Richter's syndrome. A terminal complication of chronic lymphocytic leukemia with distinct clinicopathologic features. Am J Clin Pathol **63**:786-795, 1975.

192 McKenna RW, Parkin J, Kersey JH, Gajl-Peczalska KJ, Peterson L, Brunning RD: Chronic lymphoproliferative disorder with unusual clinical, morphologic, ultrastructural and membrane surface marker characteristics. Am J Med **62**:588-596, 1977.

193 Pangalis GA, Nathwani BN, Rappaport H: Malignant lymphoma, well differentiated lymphocytic: its relationship with chronic lymphocytic leukemia and macroglobulinemia of Waldenström. Cancer **39**:999-1010, 1977.

193a Trump DL, Mann RB, Phelps R, Roberts H, Conley CL: Richter's syndrome: diffuse histiocytic lymphoma in patients with chronic lymphocytic leukemia. A report of five cases and review of the literature. Am J Med **68**:539-548, 1980.

Intermediately differentiated lymphocytic lymphoma

194 Nanba K, Jaffe ES, Braylan RC, Soban EJ, Berard CW: Alkalin phosphatase-positive malignant lymphoma: a subtype of B-cell lymphomas. Am J Clin Pathol **68**:535-542, 1977.

Poorly differentiated lymphocytic lymphoma

194a Boucheix C, Diebold J, Bernadou A, Reynes M, Tulliez M, Cadiou M, Paczynski V, Capron F, Bilski-Pasquier G: Lymphoblastic lymphoma/leukemia with

convoluted nuclei. The question of its relation to the T-cell lineage studied in 13 patients. Cancer **45**:1569-1577, 1980.

195 Burke JS, Butler JJ: Malignant lymphoma with a high content of epithelioid histiocytes (Lennert's lymphoma). Am J Clin Pathol **66**:1-9, 1976.

196 Coccia PF, Kersey JH, Gajl-Peczalska KJ, Krivit W, Nesbit ME: Prognostic significance of surface marker analysis in childhood non-Hodgkin's lymphoproliferative malignancies. Am J Hematol **1**:405-417, 1976.

197 Donlon JA, Jaffe ES, Braylan RC: Terminal deoxynucleotidyl transferase activity in malignant lymphomas. N Engl J Med **297**:461-464, 1977.

198 Ezdinli EZ, Costello W, Lenhard RE Jr, Bakemeier R, Bennett JM, Berard CW, Carbone PP: Survival of nodular versus diffuse pattern lymphocytic poorly differentiated lymphoma. Cancer **41**:1990-1996, 1978.

199 Jaffe ES, Braylan RC, Frank MM, Green I, Berard CW: Heterogeneity of immunologic markers and surface morphology in childhood lymphoblastic lymphoma. Blood **48**:213-222, 1976.

200 Kaplan J, Masfrangelo R, Peterson WD Jr: Childhood lymphoblastic lymphoma, a cancer of thymus-derived lymphocytes. Cancer Res **34**:521-525, 1974.

201 Kersey JH, Gajl-Peczalska KJ, Coccia PF, Nesbit ME: The nature of childhood leukemia and lymphoma. Am J Pathol **90**:487-495, 1978.

202 Kim H, Nathwani BN, Rappaport H: So-called "Lennert's lymphoma": is it a clinicopathologic entity? Cancer **45**:1379-1399, 1980.

203 Kim H, Jacobs C, Warnke RA, Dorfman RF: Malignant lymphoma with a high content of epithelioid histiocytes. A distinct clinicopathologic entity and a form of so-called "Lennert's lymphoma." Cancer **41**:620-635, 1978.

204 Klein MA, Jaffe R, Neiman RS: "Lennert's lymphoma" with transformation to malignant lymphoma, histiocytic type (immunoblastic sarcoma). Am J Clin Pathol **68**:601-605, 1977.

205 Lennert K, Mestdagh J: Lymphogranulomatosen mit konstant hohem Epitheloidzellgehalt. Virchows Arch [Pathol Anat] **344**:1-20, 1968.

205a Long JC, McCaffrey RP, Aisenberg AC, Marks, SM, Kung PC: Terminal deoxynucleotidyl transferase positive lymphoblastic lymphoma. A study of 15 cases. Cancer **44**:2127-2139, 1979.

206 Mann RB, Jaffe ES, Berard CW: Malignant lymphomas—a conceptual understanding of morphologic diversity. A review. Am J Pathol **94**:105-191, 1979.

207 Nathwani BN, Kim H, Rappaport H: Malignant lymphoma, lymphoblastic. Cancer **38**:964-983, 1976.

208 Palutke M, Varadachari C, Weise RW, Husain M, Tabaczka P: Lennert's lymphoma, a T-cell neoplasm [letter]. Am J Clin Pathol **69**:643-646, 1977 the editor).

208a Palutke M, Tabaczka P, Weise RW, Axelrod A, Palacas C, Margolis H, Khilanani P, Ratanatharathorn V, Piligian J, Pollard R, Husain M: T-cell lymphomas of large cell type. A variety of malignant lymphomas: "histiocytic" and mixed lymphocytic-"histiocytic." Cancer **46**:87-101, 1980.

209 Pangalis GA, Nathwani BN, Rappaport H, Rosen RB: Acute lymphoblastic leukemia. The significance of nuclear convolutions. Cancer **43**:551-557, 1979.

209a Pinkus GS, Said JW, Hargreaves H: Malignant lymphoma, T-cell type. A distinct morphologic variant with large multilobulated nuclei, with a report of four cases. Am J Clin Pathol **72:**540-550, 1979.

209b Pinkus GS, Hargreaves HK, McLeod JA, Nadler LM, Rosenthal DS, Said JW: α-Naphthyl acetate esterase activity—a cytochemical marker for T lymphocytes. Correlation with immunologic studies of normal tissues, lymphocytic leukemias, non-Hodgkin's lymphomas, Hodgkin's disease, and other lymphoproliferative disorders. Am J Pathol **97:**17-42, 1979.

210 Rosen PJ, Feinstein DI, Pattengale PK, Tindle BH, Williams AH, Cain MJ, Bonorris JB, Parker JW, Lukes RJ: Convoluted lymphocytic lymphoma in adults. A clinicopathologic entity. Ann Intern Med **89:** 319-324, 1978.

211 Stein H, Müller-Hermelink HK: Simultaneous presence of receptors for complement and sheep red blood cells on human fetal thymocytes. Br J Haematol **36:** 225-230, 1977.

212 Stein H, Petersen N, Gaedicke G, Lennert K, Landbeck G: Lymphoblastic lymphoma of convoluted or acid phosphatase type—a tumor of T precursor cells. Int J Cancer **17:**292-295, 1976.

212a Tolksdorf G, Stein H, Lennert K: Morphological and immunological definition of a malignant lymphoma derived from germinal-centre cells with cleaved nuclei (centrocytes). Br J Cancer **41:**168-182, 1980.

213 Waldron JA, Leech JH, Glick AD, Flexner JM, Collins RD: Malignant lymphoma of peripheral T-lymphocyte origin. Immunologic, pathologic, and clinical features in six patients. Cancer **40:**1604-1617, 1977.

Histiocytic lymphoma

213a Armitage JO, Dick FR, Platz CE, Corder MP, Leimert JT: Clinical usefulness and reproducibility of histologic subclassification of advanced diffuse histiocytic lymphoma. Am J Med **67:**929-934, 1979.

213b Azar HA, Jaffe ES, Berard CW, Callihan TR, Braylan RR, Cossman J, Triche TJ: Diffuse large cell lymphomas (reticulum cell sarcomas, histiocytic lymphomas). Correlation of morphologic features with functional markers. Cancer **46:**1428-1441, 1980.

214 Bennett MH: Sclerosis in non-Hodgkin's lymphomata. Br J Cancer **31:**44-52, 1975.

215 Chabner BA, Johnson RE, Young RC, Canellos GP, Hubbard SP, Johnson SK, DeVita VT Jr: Sequential nonsurgical and surgical staging of non-Hodgkin's lymphoma. Ann Intern Med **85:**149-154, 1976.

216 DeVita VT Jr, Canellos GP, Chabner B, Schein P, Hubbard SP, Young RC: Advanced diffuse histiocytic lymphoma, a potentially curable disease. Results with combination chemotherapy. Lancet **1:**248-250, 1975.

216a Frizzera G, Hanto DW, Gajl-Peczalska KJ, Rosai J, McKenna R, Sibley RK, Holahan K, Lindquist L: Lympho-proliferative disorders in renal transplant recipients. I. A morphologic and biologic spectrum. Cancer Res (in press).

217 Gillespie JJ: The ultrastructural diagnosis of diffuse large-cell ("histiocytic") lymphoma. Fine structural study of 30 cases. Am J Surg Pathol **2:**9-20, 1978.

218 Henry K: Electron microscopy in the non-Hodgkin's lymphomata. Br J Cancer **31:**73-93, 1975.

219 Hertel BF, Rosai J, Dehner LP, et al: Lymphoproliferative disorders in organ transplant recipients Lab Invest **36:**340, 1977 (abstract).

220 Li C-Y, Harrison EG Jr: Histochemical and immuno-

histochemical study of diffuse large-cell lymphomas. Am J Clin Pathol **70:**721-732, 1978.

221 Lichtenstein A, Levine AM, Lukes RJ, Cramer AD, Taylor CR, Lincoln TL, Feinstein DI: Immunoblastic sarcoma. A clinical description. Cancer **43:**343-352, 1979.

222 Lukes RJ, Parker JW, Taylor CR, Tindle BH, Cramer AD, Lincoln TL: Immunologic approach to non-Hodgkin lymphomas and related leukemias. Analysis of the results of multiparameter studies of 425 cases. Semin Hematol **15:**322-351, 1978.

223 Mann RB, Jaffe ES, Berard CW: Malignant lymphomas—a conceptual understanding of morphologic diversity. A review. Am J Pathol **94:**105-191, 1979.

224 Matas AJ, Hertel BF, Rosai J, Simmons RL, Najarian JS: Post-transplant malignant lymphoma. Distinctive morphologic features related to its pathogenesis. Am J Med **61:**716-720, 1976.

225 Michel RP, Case BW, Moinuddin M: Immunoblastic lymphosarcoma. A light, immunofluorescence, and electron microscopic study. Cancer **43:**224-236, 1979.

225a Osborne BM, Butler JJ, Mackay B: Sinusoidal large cell ("histiocytic") lymphoma. Cancer **46:**2484-2491, 1980.

226 Radaszkiewicz T, Denk H: Immunohistologic detection of immunoglobulins in malignant lymphomas and its value in histopathologic diagnosis. Virchows Arch [Pathol Anat] **381:**141-158, 1979.

227 Rappaport H: Tumors of the hematopoietic system. In Atlas of tumor pathology, Sect. 3, Fasc. 8. Washington, D. C., 1966, Armed Forces Institute of Pathology.

228 Reed RJ, Dhurandhar HN: Stem cell (immunoblastic) lymphoma. A variant of B lymphocytic lymphoma. Am J Clin Pathol **68:**8-16, 1977.

229 Rosas-Uribe A, Rappaport H: Malignant lymphoma, histiocytic type with sclerosis (sclerosing reticulum cell sarcoma). Cancer **29:**946-953, 1972.

230 Strauchen JA, Young RC, DeVita VT Jr, Anderson T, Fantone JC, Berard CW: Clinical relevance of the histopathological subclassification of diffuse "histiocytic" lymphoma. N Engl J Med **299:**1382-1387, 1978.

231 van den Tweel JG, Taylor CR, Parker JW, Lukes RJ: Immunoglobulin inclusions in non-Hodgkin's lymphomas. Am J Clin Pathol **69:**306-313, 1978.

232 Veronesi U, Musumeci R, Pizzetti F, Gennari L, Bonadonna G: The value of staging laparotomy in non-Hodgkin's lymphomas (with emphasis on the histiocytic type). Cancer **33:**446-459, 1974.

233 Warnke RA, Kim H, Fuks Z, Dorfman RE: The coexistence of nodular and diffuse patterns in nodular non-Hodgkin's lymphomas. Significance and clinicopathologic correlation. Cancer **40:**1229-1233, 1977.

233a Warnke R, Miller R, Grogan T, Pederson M, Dilley J, Levy R: Immunologic phenotype in 30 patients with diffuse large-cell lymphoma. N Engl J Med **303:** 293-300, 1980.

Undifferentiated lymphoma

234 Andersson M, Klein G, Ziegler JL, Henle W: Association of Epstein-Barr viral genomes with American Burkitt lymphoma. Nature **260:**357-359, 1976.

235 Arseneau JC, Canellos GP, Banks PM, Berard CW, Gralnick HR, DeVita VT Jr: American Burkitt's lymphoma: a clinicopathologic study of 30 cases. I. Clinical factors relating to prolonged survival. Am J Med **58:**314-321, 1975.

236 Banks PM, Arseneau JC, Gralnick HR, Cannellos GP,

DeVita VT Jr, Berard CW: American Burkitt's lymphoma: a clinicopathologic study of 30 cases. II. Pathologic correlations. Am J Med **58**:322-329, 1975.

237 Bennett JM, Berard C, Thomas, O'Conor LB: Histopathologic definition of Burkitt's tumor. Bull WHO **40**:601-608, 1969.

238 Bernhard W: Fine structure of Burkitt's lymphoma. In Burkitt DP, Wright DH (eds): Burkitt's lymphoma. Edinburgh and London, 1970, E. and S. Livingstone, pp. 103-117.

239 Binder RA, Jencks JA, Chun B, Rath CE: "B" cell origin of malignant cells in a case of American Burkitt's lymphoma: characterization of cells from a pleural effusion. Cancer **36**:161-168, 1975.

239a Gunvén P, Klein G, Klein E, Norin T, Singh S: Surface immunoglobulins on Burkitt's lymphoma biopsy cells from 91 patients. Int J Cancer **25**:711-719, 1980.

240 Mann RB, Jaffe ES, Braylan RC, Nanba K, Frank MM, Ziegler JL, Berard CW: Non-endemic Burkitt's lymphoma: a B cell tumor related to germinal centers. N Engl J Med **295**:685-691, 1976.

241 Nkrumah FK, Perkins IV: Burkitt's lymphoma. A clinical study of 100 patients. Cancer **37**:671-676, 1976.

242 Ziegler JL: Treatment results of 54 American patients with Burkitt's lymphoma are similar to the African experience. N Engl J Med **297**:75-80, 1977.

Lymphoma and dysproteinemia

242a Addis BJ, Isaacson P, Billings JA: Plasmacytoma of lymph nodes. Cancer **46**:340-346, 1980.

243 Aisenberg AC, Bloch KJ: Immunoglobulins on the surface of neoplastic lymphocytes. N Engl J Med **287**:271-276, 1972.

244 Alexanian R: Monoclonal gammopathy in lymphoma. Arch Intern Med **135**:62-66, 1975.

245 Axelsson V, Bachmann R, Hallen J: Frequency of pathological proteins (M-components) in 6995 sera from an adult population. Acta Med Scand **179**:234-247, 1966.

246 Azar HA, Hill WT, Osserman EF: Malignant lymphoma and lymphatic leukemia associated with myeloma-type serum proteins. Am J Med **23**:239-249, 1957.

247 Azar HA, Zaino EC, Pham TD, Yannopoulos K: "Non-secretory" plasma cell myeloma. Observations on seven cases with electron microscopic studies. Am J Clin Pathol **58**:618-629, 1972.

248 Ballard HS, Hamilton LM, Marcus AJ, Illes CH: A new variant of heavy-chain disease (μ-chain disease). N Engl J Med **282**:1060-1062, 1970.

249 Brouet J-C, Clauvel J-P, Danon F, Klein M, Seligmann M: Biologic and clinical significance of cryoglobulins: a report of 86 cases. Am J Med **57**:775-788, 1974.

250 Brunning RD, Parkin J: Intranuclear inclusions in plasma cells and lymphocytes from patients with monoclonal gammopathies. Am J Clin Pathol **66**:10-21, 1976.

251 Cohen RJ, Bohannon RA, Wallterstein RO: Waldenstrom's macroglobulinemia. A study of ten cases. Am J Med **41**:274, 1966.

252 Doe WF: Alpha chain disease. Clinicopathological features and relationship to so-called Mediterranean lymphoma. Br J Cancer **31**(Suppl 2):350-355, 1975.

253 Dutcher TF, Fahey JL: The histopathology of the macroglobulinemia of Waldenstrom. J Natl Cancer Inst **22**:887-917, 1959.

254 Fisher ER, Zawadski ZA: Ultrastructural features of plasma cells in patients with paraproteinemias. Am J Clin Pathol **54**:779-789, 1970.

255 Fishkin BG, Spiegelberg HL: Cervical lymph node metastasis as the first manifestation of localized extramedullary plasmacytoma. Cancer **38**:1641-1644, 1976.

256 Franklin EC, Lowenstein J, Bigelow B, Meltzer M: Heavy chain disease—a new disorder of serum gamma-globulins: report of the first case. Am J Med **37**:332-350, 1964.

257 Gaston EA, Dollinger MR, Strong EW, Hajdu SI: Primary plasmacytoma of lymph nodes. Lymphology **1**:7-15, 1969.

258 Harrison CV: The morphology of the lymph node in the macroglobulinaemia of Waldenstrom. J Clin Pathol **25**:12-16, 1972.

259 Hobbs JR: Immunocytoma o' mice an' men. Br Med J **2**:67-72, 1971.

260 Kim H, Dorfman RF, Rappaport H: Signet ring cell lymphoma. A rare morphologic and functional expression of nodular (follicular) lymphoma. Am J Surg Pathol **2**:119-132, 1978.

261 Kim H, Heller P, Rappaport H: Monoclonal gammopathies associated with lymphoproliferative disorders. A morphologic study, Am J Clin Pathol **59**:282-294, 1973.

262 Krauss S, Sokal JE: Paraproteinemia in the lymphomas. Am J Med **40**:400-413, 1966.

263 Kyle RA: Monoclonal gammopathy of undetermined significance. Natural history in 241 cases. Am J Med **64**:814-826, 1978.

264 Kyle RA, Bayrd ED: Benign monoclonal gammopathy—a potentially malignant condition? Am J Med **40**:426-430, 1966.

265 Lee SL, Rosner F, Ruberman W, Glasberg S: μ-Chain disease. Ann Intern Med **75**:407-414, 1971.

266 Lough J, Shuster J: Constipated plasma cells associated with monomeric macroglobulinemia. Hum Pathol **6**:251-255, 1975.

267 Mennemeyer R, Hammar SP, Cathey WJ: Malignant lymphoma with intracytoplasmic IgM crystalline inclusions. N Engl J Med **291**:960-963, 1974.

268 Migliore PJ, Alexanian R: Monoclonal gammopathy in human neoplasia. Cancer **21**:1127-1131, 1968.

269 Pangalis GA, Nathwani BN, Rappaport H: Detection of cytoplasmic immunoglobulin in well-differentiated lymphoproliferative diseases by the immunoperoxidase method. Cancer **45**:1334-1339, 1980.

269a Papadimitriou CS, Müller-Hermelink U, Lennert K: Histologic and immunohistochemical findings in the differential diagnosis of chronic lymphocytic leukemia of B-cell type and lymphoplasmacytic/lymphoplasmacytoid lymphoma. Virchows Arch [Pathol Anat] **384**:149-158, 1979.

270 Seligmann M: Immunochemical, clinical, and pathological features of α-chain disease. Arch Intern Med **135**:78-82, 1975.

271 Seligmann M, Danon F, Hurez D, Mihaesco E, Preud'homme J-L: Alpha-chain disease: a new immunoglobulin abnormality. Science **162**:1396-1397, 1968.

272 Stein H, Lennert K, Parwaresch MR: Malignant lymphomas of B-cell type. Lancet **2**:855-857, 1972.

273 Zawadski ZA, Edwards GA: Dysimmunoglobulinemia in the absence of clinical features of multiple myeloma and macroglobulinemia. Am J Med **42**:67-88, 1967.

Hodgkin's disease

274 Aisenberg AC: Malignant lymphoma, N Engl J Med **288**:883-890, 935-941, 1973.

275 Bearman RM, Pangalis GA, Rappaport H: Hodgkin's disease, lymphocyte depletion type. A clinicopathologic study of 39 patients. Cancer **41**:293-302, 1978.

276 Butler JJ: Relationship of histologic findings to survival in Hodgkin's disease. Gann Monogr Cancer Res **15**:275-286, 1973.

276a Colby TV, Warnke RA: The histology of the initial relapse of Hodgkin's disease. Cancer **45**:289-292, 1980.

277 Coleman CN, Williams CJ, Flint A, Glatstein EJ, Rosenberg SA, Kaplan HS: Hematologic neoplasia in patients treated for Hodgkin's disease. N Engl J Med **297**:1249-1252, 1977.

278 Coppleson LW, Rappaport H, Strum SB, Rose J: Analysis of the Rye classification of Hodgkin's disease. The prognostic significance of cellular composition. J Natl Cancer Inst **51**:379-390, 1973.

279 Cross RM: A clinicopathological study of nodular sclerosing Hodgkin's disease, J Clin Pathol **21**:303-310, 1968.

280 Curran RC, Jones EL: Hodgkin's disease: An immunohistochemical and histological study. J Pathol **125**:39-51, 1978.

281 Fechner RE: Hodgkin's disease of the thymus. Cancer **23**:16-23, 1969.

282 Fisher ER, Hazard JB: Differentiation of megakaryocyte and Reed-Sternberg cell. Lab Invest **3**:261-269, 1954.

283 Garvin AJ, Spicer SS, McKeever PE: The cytochemical demonstration of intracellular immunoglobulin. In neoplasms of lymphoreticular tissue. Am J Pathol **82**:457-472, 1976.

284 Garvin AJ, Spicer SS, Parmley RT, Munster AM: Immunohistochemical demonstration of IgG in Reed-Sternberg and other cells in Hodgkin's disease. J Exp Med **139**:1077-1083, 1974.

285 Glatstein E, Guernsey JM, Rosenberg SA, Kaplan HS: The value of laparotomy and splenectomy in the staging of Hodgkin's disease. Cancer **24**:470-718, 1969.

286 Glatstein E, Trueblood HW, Enright LP, Rosenberg SA, Kaplan HS: Surgical staging of abdominal involvement in unselected patients with Hodgkin's disease. Radiology **97**:425-432, 1970.

287 Glick AD, Leech JH, Flexner JM, Collins RD: Ultrastructural study of Reed-Sternberg cells. Comparison with transformed lymphocytes and histiocytes. Am J Pathol **85**:195-200, 1976.

288 Goldman LB, Victor AW: Hodgkin's disease, New York J Med **45**:1313-1318, 1945.

289 Kadin ME: A reappraisal of the Reed-Sternberg cell. A commentary. Blood Cells **6**:525-532, 1980.

290 Kadin ME, Donaldson SS, Dorfman RF: Isolated granulomas in Hodgkin's disease. N Engl J Med **283**:859-861, 1970.

291 Kadin ME, Glatstein E, Dorfman RF: Clinicopathologic studies of 117 untreated patients subjected to laparotomy for the staging of Hodgkin's disease. Cancer **27**:1277-1294, 1971.

292 Kadin ME, Stites DP, Levy R, Warnke R: Exogenous immunoglobulin and the macrophage origin or Reed-Sternberg cells in Hodgkin's disease. N Engl J Med **299**:1208-1214, 1978.

293 Kaplan HS: Contiguity and progression in Hodgkin's disease, Cancer Res. **31**:1811-1813, 1971.

294 Kaplan HS: Hodgkin's disease and other human malignant lymphomas: advances and prospects—G.H.A. Clowes Memorial Lecture. Cancer Res **36**:3863-3878, 1976.

294a Kaplan HS: Hodgkin's disease: unfolding concepts concerning its nature, management and prognosis. Cancer **45**:2439-2474, 1980.

295 Kaplan HS, Gartner S: "Sternberg-Reed" giant cells of Hodgkin's disease: cultivation in vitro, heterotransplantation, and characterization as neoplastic macrophages. Int J Cancer **19**:511-525, 1977.

296 Katz A, Lattes R: Granulomatous thymoma or Hodgkin's disease of thymus? A clinical and histologic study and a reevaluation. Cancer **23**:1-15, 1969.

297 Keller AR, Kaplan HS, Lukes RJ, Rappaport H: Correlation of histopathology with other prognostic indicators in Hodgkin's disease. Cancer **22**:487-499, 1968.

298 Krikorian JG, Burke JS, Rosenberg SA, Kaplan HS: Occurrence of non-Hodgkin's lymphoma after therapy for Hodgkin's disease. N Engl J Med **300**:452-458, 1979.

299 Lennert K, Mestdagh J: Lymphogranulomatosen mit konstant hohem Epitheloidzellgehalt. Virchows Arch [Pathol Anat] **344**:1-20, 1968.

300 Long JC, Zamecnik PC, Aisenberg AC, Atkins L: Tissue culture studies in Hodgkin's disease: morphologic, cytogenetic, cell surface, and enzymatic properproperties of cultures derived from splenic tumors. J Exp Med **145**:1484-1500, 1977.

301 Lukes RJ: Relationship of histologic features to clinical stages in Hodgkin's disease. Am J Roentgenol **90**:944-955, 1963.

302 Lukes RJ, Butler JJ, Hicks EB: Natural history of Hodgkin's disease as related to its pathologic picture. Cancer **19**:317-344, 1966.

303 Lukes RJ, Craver LF, Hall TC, Rappaport H, Ruben P: Report of Nomenclature Committee, Cancer Res **26**:1311, 1966.

304 Marshall AHE, Matilla A, Pollock DJ: A critique and case study of nodular sclerosing Hodgkin's disease. J Clin Pathol **29**:923-930, 1976.

305 Müller-Hermelink HK, Lennert K: The cytologic, histologic, and functional bases for a modern classification of lymphomas. In Lennert K, Coll: Malignant lymphomas other than Hodgkin's disease. histology, cytology, ultrastructure, immunology. Berlin, 1978, Springer-Verlag, pt 1, pp. 1-2.

305a Neiman RS: Current problems in the histopathologic diagnosis and classification of Hodgkin's disease. Pathol Annu **13**(Pt 2):289-328, 1978.

306 Neiman RS, Rosen PJ, Lukes RJ: Lymphocyte-depletion Hodgkin's disease. A clinicopathologic entity. N Engl J Med **288**:751-755, 1973.

307 Order SE, Hellman S: Pathogenesis of Hodgkin's disease. Lancet **1**:571-573, 1972.

308 Poppema S, Elema JD, Halie MR: The significance of intracytoplasmic proteins in Reed-Sternberg cells. Cancer **42**:1793-1803, 1978.

308a Poppema S, Elema JD, Halie MR: The localization of Hodgkin's disease in lymph nodes. A study with immunohistological, enzyme histochemical and rosetting techniques on frozen sections. Int J Cancer **24**:532-540, 1979.

308b Poppema S, Kaiserling E, Lennert K: Epidemiology of nodular paragranuloma (Hodgkin's disease with lymphocytic predominance, nodular). J Cancer Res Clin Oncol **95:**57-63, 1979.

308c Poppema S, Kaiserling E, Lennert K: Hodgkin's disease with lymphocytic predominance, nodular type (nodular paragranuloma) and progressively transformed germinal centres—a cytohistological study. Histopathology **3:**295-308, 1979.

308d Poppema S, Kaiserling E, Lennert K: Nodular paragranuloma and progressively transformed germinal centers. Ultrastructural and immunohistologic findings. Virchows Arch [Cell Pathol] **31:**211-225, 1979.

308e Poppema S, Lennert K: Hodgkin's disease in childhood. Histopathologic classification in relation to age and sex. Cancer **45:**1443-1447, 1980.

309 Rappaport H, Strum SB, Hutchison G, Allen LW: Clinical and biological significance of vascular invasion in Hodgkin's disease. Cancer Res **31:**1794-1798, 1971.

310 Rosenberg SA: Hodgkin's disease of the bone marrow. Cancer Res **31:**1733-1736, 1971.

311 Sacks EL, Donaldson SS, Gordon J, Dorfman RF: Epithelioid granulomas associated with Hodgkin's disease. Clinical correlations in 55 previously untreated patients. Cancer **41:**562-567, 1978.

311a Seemayer TA, Lagace R, Schürch W: On the pathogenesis of sclerosis and nodularity in nodular sclerosing Hodgkin's disease. Virchows Arch [Pathol Anat] **385:**283-291, 1980.

312 Smetana HF, Cohen BM: Mortality in relation to histologic type in Hodgkin's disease. Blood **11:**211-224, 1956.

313 Soderstrom N, Norberg B: Observations regarding the specific post-capillary venules of lymph nodes in malignant lymphomas. Acta Pathol Microbiol Scand [A] **82:**71-79, 1974.

314 Strum SB, Rappaport H: Significance of focal involvement of lymph nodes for the diagnosis and staging of Hodgkin's disease. Cancer **25:**1314-1319, 1970.

315 Strum SB, Rappaport H: Interrelations of the histologic types of Hodgkin's disease. Arch Pathol **91:**127-134, 1971.

316 Strum SB, Rappaport H: The persistence of Hodgkin's disease in long-term survivors. Am J Med **51:**222-240, 1971.

317 Strum SB, Hutchison GB, Park JK, Rappaport H: Further observations on the biologic significance of vascular invasion in Hodgkin's disease. Cancer **27:**1-6, 1971.

318 Strum SB, Park JK, Rappaport H: Observation of cells resembling Sternberg-Reed cells in conditions other than Hodgkin's disease. Cancer **26:**176-190, 1970.

319 Stuart .AE, Williams ARW, Habeshaw JA: Rosetting and other reactions of the Reed-Sternberg cell. J Pathol **122:**81-90, 1977.

320 Taylor CR: The nature of Reed-Sternberg cells and other malignant "reticulum" cells. Lancet **2:**802-807, 1974.

321 Tindle BH, Parker JW, Lukes RJ: "Reed-Sternberg cells" in infectious mononucleosis? Am J Clin Pathol **58:**607-617, 1972.

322 Variakojis D, Strum SB, Rappaport H: The foamy macrophages in Hodgkin's disease. Arch Pathol **93:**453-456, 1971.

323 Wright CJE: Prospects of cure in lymphocyte-predominant Hodgkin's disease. Am J Clin Pathol **67:**507-511, 1977.

Malignant histiocytosis

324 Burke JS, Byrne GE Jr, Rappaport H: Hairy cell leukemia (leukemic reticuloendotheliosis). I. A clinical pathologic study of 21 patients. Cancer **33:**1399-1410, 1974.

325 Byrne GE Jr, Rappaport H: Malignant histiocytosis. Gann Monogr Cancer Res **15:**145-162, 1973.

326 Dehner LP: Non-Hodgkin's lymphomas and malignant histiocytosis in children. Semin Oncol **4:**273-286, 1977.

327 Friedman RM, Stiegbigel NH: Histiocytic medullary reticulosis. Am J Med **28:**130-133, 1965.

328 Griffin JD, Ellman L, Long JC, Dvorak AM: Development of a histiocytic medullary reticulosis-like syndrome during the course of acute lymphocytic leukemia. Am J Med **64:**851-858, 1978.

329 Huhn D, Meister P: Malignant histiocytosis. Morphologic and cytochemical findings. Cancer **42:**1341-1349, 1978.

330 Karcher DS, Head DR, Mullins JD: Malignant histiocytosis occurring in patients with acute lymphocytic leukemia. Cancer **41:**1967-1973. 1978.

331 Lombardi L, Carbone A, Pilotti S, Rilke F: Malignant histiocytosis: a histological and ultrastructural study of lymph nodes in six cases. Histopathology **2:**315-328, 1978.

332 Macgillivray JB, Duthie JS: Malignant histiocytosis (histiocytic medullary reticulosis) with spindle cell differentiation and tumour formation. J Clin Pathol **30:**120-125, 1977.

333 Matzner Y, Behar A, Beeri E, Gunders AE, Hershko C: Systemic leishmaniasis mimicking malignant histiocytosis. Cancer **43:**398-402, 1979.

333a Meister P, Huhn D, Nathrath W: Malignant histiocytosis. Immunohistochemical characterization on paraffin embedded tissue. Virchows Arch [Pathol Anat] **385:**233-246, 1980.

333b Mendelsohn G, Eggleston JC, Mann RB: Relationship of lysozyme (muramidase) to histiocytic differentiation in malignant histiocytosis. An immunohistochemical study. Cancer **45:**273-279, 1980.

334 Perry MC, Harrison EG Jr, Burgert EO, Gilchrist GS: Familial erythrophagocytic lymphohistiocytosis. Report of two cases and clinicopathologic review. Cancer **38:**209-218, 1976.

335 Rappaport H: Tumors of the hematopoietic system. In Atlas of tumor pathology, Sect. III, Fasc. 8. Washington, D.C., 1966, Armed Forces Institute of Pathology, pp. 91-206.

336 Risdall RJ, McKenna RW, Nesbitt ME, Krivit W, Balfour HH, Simmons RL, Brunning RD: Virus associated hemophagocytic syndrome. Cancer (in press, 1979).

337 Scott RB, Robb-Smith AH: Histiocytic medullary reticulosis. Lancet **2:**194-198, 1939.

338 Vardiman JW, Byrne GE Jr, Rappaport H: Malignant histiocytosis with massive splenomegaly in asymptomatic patients: a possible chronic form of the disease. Cancer **36:**419-427, 1975.

339 Warnke RA, Kim H, Dorfman RF: Malignant histiocytosis (histiocytic medullary reticulosis). I. Clinicopathologic study of 29 cases. Cancer **35:**215-230, 1975.

340 Watanabe S, Mikata A, Toyama K, Kitamura K, Minato K: Sarcomatous variant of malignant histiocytosis. A case report and review of the literature. Acta Pathol Jpn **28:**963-978, 1978.

340a Zucker JM, Caillaux JM, Vanel D, Gerard-Marchant R: Malignant histiocytosis in childhood. Clinical study and therapeutic results in 22 cases. Cancer **45:** 2821-2829, 1980.

Metastatic tumors

341 Giffler RF, Gillespie JJ, Ayala AG, Newland JR: Lymphoepithelioma in cervical lymph nodes of children and young adults. Am J Surg Pathol **1:**293-302, 1977.

342 Kinsey DL, James AG, Bonta JA: A study of metastatic carcinoma of the neck. Ann Surg **147:**366-374, 1958.

343 Lindbergh R: Distribution of cervical lymph node metastases from squamous cell carcinoma of the upper respiratory and digestive tracts. Cancer **29:**1446-1449, 1972.

344 Rosai J, Rodriguez HA: Application of electron microscopy to the differential diagnosis of tumors. Am J Clin Pathol **50:**555-562, 1968.

Other lesions

345 Benisch BM, Howard RG: Lymph-node infarction in two young men. Am J Clin Pathol **63:**818-823, 1975.

346 Brown RB, Gaillard RA, Turner JA: The significance of aberrant or heterotopic parotid gland tissue in lymph nodes. Ann Surg **138:**850-856, 1953.

346a Covell LM, Disciullo AJ, Knapp RC: Decidual change in pelvic lymph nodes in the presence of cervical squamous cell carcinoma during pregnancy. Am J Obstet Gynecol **127:**674-676, 1977.

347 Davies JD, Stansfeld AG: Spontaneous infarction of superficial lymph nodes. J Clin Pathol **25:**689-696, 1972.

348 Davies JNP, Lothe F: Kaposi's sarcoma in African children. In Ackerman LV, Murray JF (eds): Symposium on Kaposi's sarcoma. Basel, Switzerland, 1963, S. Karger, AG, pp. 81-86.

349 Edlow DW, Carter D: Heterotopic epithelium in axillary lymph nodes. Am J Clin Pathol **59:**666-673, 1973.

349a Ehrmann RL, Federschneider JM, Knapp RC: Distinguishing lymph node metastases from benign glandular inclusions in low-grade ovarian carcinoma. Am J Obstet Gynecol **136:**737-746, 1980.

350 Fayemi AO, Toker C: Nodal angiomatosis. Arch Pathol **99:**170-172, 1975.

351 Johnson WT, Helwig EB: Benign nevus cells in the capsule of lymph nodes. Cancer **23:**747-753, 1969.

352 Karp LA, Czernobilsky B: Glandular inclusions in pelvic and abdominal paraaortic lymph nodes. Am J Clin Pathol **52:**212-218, 1969.

353 Lasersohn JT, Thomas LB, Smith RR, Ketcham AS, Dillon JS: Carcinoma of the uterine cervix. A study of surgical pathological and autopsy findings. Cancer **17:** 338-351, 1964.

353a Lennert K, Illert E: Die Häufigkeit der Gewebsmastzellen im Lymphknoten bei verschiedenen Erkrankungen. Frankf Z Pathol **70:**121-131, 1959.

353b Lennert K, Parwaresch MR: Mast cells and mast cell neoplasia: a review. Histopathology **3:**349-365, 1979.

354 Longo S: Benign lymph node inclusions. Hum Pathol **7:**349-354, 1976.

355 Lubin J, Rywlin AM: Lymphoma-like lymph node changes in Kaposi's sarcoma. Arch Pathol **92:**338-341, 1971.

355a Magrina JF, Symmonds RE, Dahlin DC: Pelvic "lipolymph nodes": a consideration in the differential diagnosis of pelvic masses. Am J Obstet Gynecol **136:**727-731, 1980.

356 Meyer JS, Steinberg LS: Microscopically benign thyroid follicles in cervical lymph nodes. Serial section study of lymph node inclusions and entire thyroid gland in 5 cases. Cancer **24:**302-311, 1969.

356a O'Connell, K. M.: Kaposi's sarcoma in lymph nodes: histological study of lesions from 16 cases in Malawi. J Clin Pathol **30:**696-703, 1977.

357 Osborne BM, Butler JJ, Mackay B: Proteinaceous lymphadenopathy with hypergammaglobulinemia. Am J Surg Pathol **3:**137-145, 1979.

358 Rywlin AM, Recher L, Hoffman E: Lymphoma-like presentation of Kaposi's sarcoma. Arch Dermatol **93:** 554-561, 1966.

359 Shah KH, Kisilevsky R: Infarction of the lymph nodes: A cause of a palisading macrophage reaction mimicking necrotizing granulomas. Hum Pathol **9:**597-599, 1978.

360 Weshler Z, Leviatan A, Krasnokuki D, Kopolovitch J: Primary Kaposi's sarcoma in lymph nodes concurrent with chronic lymphatic leukemia. Am J Clin Pathol **71:**234-237, 1979.

21 Spleen

Introduction

The spleen performs many functions, some of which only recently have been elucidated and correlated with morphologic parameters.[1-6] Following are the most important splenic functions: (1) hematopoiesis (erythrocytes, granulocytes, magakaryocytes, lymphocytes, and macrophages), (2) serving as a reservoir (storage or sequestration of platelets and other formed elements), (3) phagocytosis (removal of particulate matter, red blood cell destruction, pitting, and erythroclasis), and (4) immunity (trapping and processing of antigen, "homing" of lymphocytes, lymphocyte transformation and proliferation, antibody production).[2] The surgical pathologist often is frustrated by the lack of pathologic alterations of diagnostic value. The spleen is removed from patients with diverse clinical syndromes. If the pathologist does not know the clinical and laboratory data, particularly the hematologic findings, he may be unable to make a specific diagnosis.

Tabulation of positive pathologic changes from numerous articles and textbooks aids very little. We have tried unsuccessfully to chart the significant pathologic changes seen in each clinical syndrome. Only the changes that appear to be most significant are mentioned. Even these frequently are not diagnostic.

Biopsy and pathologic examination

In the United States, biopsy of the spleen is not done as a rule because of the technical difficulty at operation and the fear of hemorrhage after needle biopsy. When a large liver and spleen are encountered, the liver is usually biopsied, but the spleen is sacrosanct because of the danger of hemorrhage. However, biopsying both organs can produce a diagnosis that may not be made by liver biopsy alone. Certainly, splenic puncture should not be performed upon patients with bleeding tendency. However, the risk of this diagnostic procedure has been grossly exaggerated. For instance, Moeschlin[11] punctured the spleen in 300 patients and Soderström[12] in over 800 without mortality and essentially without morbidity.

The method of Block and Jacobson[7] (splenic puncture using the Vim-Silverman needle) would seem the most effective. Tissue so obtained may be fixed, cut, and stained as a conventional section. Block and Jacobson[7] and Ferris and Hargraves[9] reported a large number of splenic punctures resulting in a definitive diagnosis that was not possible by bone marrow biopsy, lymph node biopsy, or clinical data.

Surgically excised spleens obtained for diagnostic purposes should be cut in the fresh state into 1 cm slices, fixed overnight in formalin, and then sliced as thinly as possible (2-3 mm). We have used for this purpose an electrically driven meat-cutting machine with excellent results. The cut slices are then carefully examined, and all suspicious areas are submitted for microscopic examination. Farrer-Brown et al.[8] mentioned three cases of Hodgkin's disease in which the areas of involvement appeared grossly as foci of slight prominence of the malpighian corpuscles. A careful search also should be made for hilar lymph nodes.

For the evaluation of the red pulp in states associated with hypersplenism, we have found it very helpful to inject the specimen with formalin through the splenic artery. A sharp distinction between sinuses and cords is thus possible.[10] A lesser substitute for those unwilling to perform this time-consuming procedure is the examination of special stains that delineate the sinusal wall, such as periodic acid–Schiff or silver impregnation.

Rupture; splenectomy

Blunt trauma to the abdomen and surgical intervention within the abdominal cavity are the two most common factors responsible for rupture of the normal spleen.[22] In most instances,

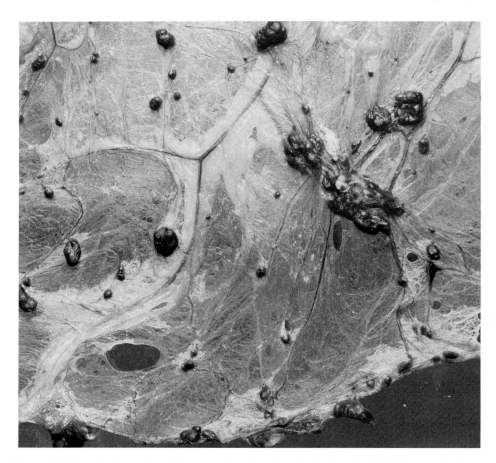

Fig. 1129 Splenosis in small nodules on peritoneal surface. Patient previously had ruptured spleen. (WU neg. 55-3599.)

hemoperitoneum is an immediate consequence, leading to an emergency splenectomy. In about 15% of the cases, the rupture is "delayed" anywhere from forty-eight hours to several months.[18] Examination of the excised spleen will reveal the ruptured area which, in many cases, is limited to a deceivingly small capsular tear. Microscopically, leukocytic infiltration often is seen along the edges of the tear.

Following traumatic rupture, splenic tissue in small nodules may grow as implants on the peritoneal surface, and even within the pleural cavity[14] (Fig. 1129). The process is known as *splenosis*. These nodules are surrounded by a capsule, but malpighian follicles with a central arteriole do not form.[13,17]

The diseases most commonly associated with *spontaneous rupture* of the spleen are infectious mononucleosis, malaria, pregnancy, typhoid fever, subacute bacterial endocarditis, splenic tumors, and leukemias.[24] In every case

of ruptured spleen without history of trauma or in which the trauma seems insignificant, a careful microscopic study should be performed in order to rule out all these possibilities. Rupture of the spleen with the resulting hemoperitoneum is the most frequent cause of death in infectious mononucleosis. This complication usually occurs from ten to twenty-one days after the onset of the disease.[23] Exceptionally, "spontaneous" rupture may occur in a perfectly normal spleen.[20]

Splenectomy performed in adults for traumatic rupture of the spleen does not seem to result in any sequelae of significance.[21] On the other hand, an increased incidence and severity of infections has been reported following splenectomy in young children.[19] Ellis and Smith[15,16] have shown that this is the result of a decrease in immunoglobulin production and phagocytic activity during transient bacteremia. Whenever splenectomy is performed for hematologic disorders, a thorough search should be made of accessory spleens for the purpose of removal. Their incidence is approximately 10%, and their most common location is the region of the hilus of the spleen and the tail of the pancreas.

Hypersplenism (dyssplenism)

The splenic red pulp acts primarily as a biologic filter for the removal of abnormal or aged blood cells and their pathologic inclusions. This mechanism operates during the transit of the cells through the splenic cords from the *penicilli* arteries to the splenic sinuses and results from a combination of mechanical, rheologic, metabolic, and immunologic factors.[60] When this normal function increases to a significant degree, the resulting condition is designated as *hypersplenism* or *dysplenism*.[25,38] Any of the cellular elements of the blood may be affected, singly or in combination. Thus, neutropenia, thrombocytopenia, hemolytic anemia, or pancytopenia may all be present. In some conditions, such as spherocytic hemolytic anemia or idiopathic thrombocytopenic purpura, the basic abnormality resides in the blood elements themselves. In others, the hypersplenism results from widening of the splenic cords with an increase in macrophages and/or connective tissue fibers and premature destruction of the normal elements of the blood. The latter phenomenon has been reproduced experimentally by the intraperitoneal injection of methyl cellulose.[46] Hypersplenism resulting from this mechanism can be seen with congestive splenomegaly, Gaucher's disease (Fig. 1130, *A*), malignant lymphoma, leukemia, histiocytosis X, hemangioma, hamartoma, angiosarcoma, and practically any condition involving more or less diffusely the splenic parenchyma.[48]

The classic studies of Harrington et al.[36] demonstrated that if small amounts of blood from a patient with *idiopathic thrombocytopenic purpura* are given to a normal person, a humoral factor will cause a precipitous fall in platelets, thus establishing an immunologic basis for the disease. Karpatkin and Siskind[39] demonstrated antiplatelet activity in the serum of 73% of patients with idiopathic thrombocytopenic purpura. Subsequent studies showed that this antiplatelet factor is a gamma G immunoglobulin reactive to antigen associated with both autologous and homologous platelets.[55,56] The spleen is an important site for the production of this antiplatelet antibody.[42,43] The anti-body-coated platelets have a short life span because they are rapidly removed by the reticuloendothelial system of the spleen and liver.[34,35] There is some evidence that the number of antibody molecules bound to the platelets may determine the main site of removal. Heavily coated platelets are removed by the liver phagocytes, whereas lightly coated platelets pass through the liver but are sequestered in the spleen.[56]

The changes found in the spleen in idiopathic thrombocytopenic purpura have been summarized well by Bowman et al.[28] The spleen is slightly to moderately enlarged with moderately dilated sinusoids and a prominent increase in the number of germinal centers, many of them containing phagocytosed nuclear debris. Large numbers of perivascular plasma cells can be seen in the marginal zone, and there is a moderate increase in megakaryocytes (but not of granulocyte precursors).

Phospholipid deposits in the histiocytes of the splenic pulp were observed by Saltzstein[53] in seven spleens removed for thrombocytopenic purpura (Fig. 1130, *B*). This material is presumably derived from the breakdown of platelets,[29] a phenomenon that can be readily appreciated ultrastructurally.[41a,58] This microscopic finding was not seen in over 700 other spleens removed for other reasons, although foamy cells with a similar appearance in routinely stained sections can be found in Gaucher's disease, Niemann-Pick disease, thalassemia,[33] hyperlipemic states,[52] the sea-blue histiocyte syndrome,[57] and follicular lipoidosis. Biochemical studies in the latter condition have demonstrated the presence of saturated hydrocarbons, thus implying ingestion of exogenous mineral oil.[40] Recent evidence suggests that the "sea-blue histiocyte" is not the morphologic expression of a specific entity but rather accompanies a wide variety of conditions, such as chronic myelocytic leukemia and various types of lipid metabolism abnormalities.[47] Histochemical techniques usually allow for a distinction among these different conditions.[50]

Splenectomy in idiopathic thrombocytopenic purpura is reserved for the patients unresponsive to steroid or immunosuppressive therapy.[27] It achieves sustained remission in 50%-80% of the cases. Unfortunately, at present there is no method that can accurately predict the effect of splenectomy.[26] Occasionally, thrombocytopenic purpura is seen as a manifestation of lupus erythematosus, viral infection, drug hy-

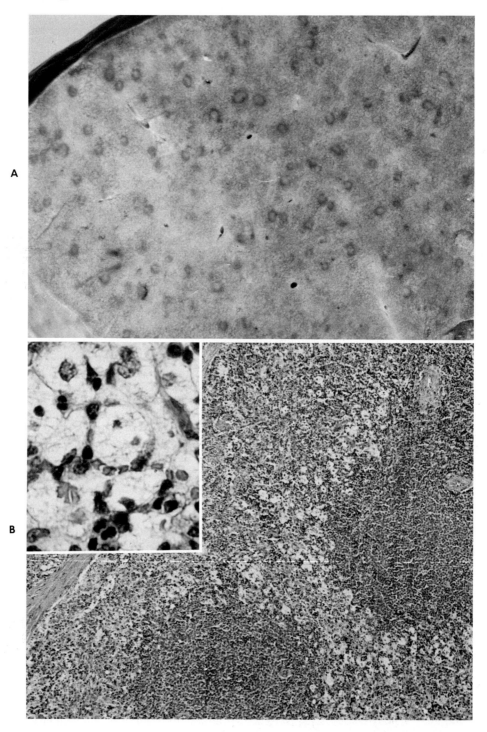

Fig. 1130 A, Huge spleen in Gaucher's disease. White pulp is widely separated by massive red pulp replaced by cells of Gaucher's disease. **B,** Idiopathic thrombocytopenic purpura. Lipid-filled macrophages in splenic white pulp immediately around malpighian corpuscles. **Inset,** high power, demonstrates foamy nature of cytoplasm. Patient had no platelets before splenectomy. (**A,** WU neg. 72-6653; **B,** ×85; WU neg. 60-4376; **inset,** WU neg. 60-4379.)

persensitivity,[26] chronic lymphocytic leukemia,[32] or Hodgkin's disease.[51]

Hereditary spherocytosis is a hemolytic disease in which the red blood cells are abnormal (spherocytes). The abnormality lies in the cell membrane of the red blood cell, but the basic biochemical disorder has not yet been elucidated.[37] The erythrocytes lack the plasticity of normal red blood cells and become trapped in the interstices of the spleen.[59] If washed normal red blood cells are given to a patient with congenital hemolytic anemia, the cells survive normally. Conversely, if spherocytes are given to a normal individual, the survival of the cells remains short, supporting the concept that the erythrocyte is defective. Furthermore, this defect persists after removal of the spleen, but hemolysis is decreased.

Acquired hemolytic anemia can be due to toxins (bacterial hemolysins), plasma lipid abnormalities, parasites that invade red blood cells, and, most importantly, immune reactions that result in deposition of immunoproteins (antibodies; complement components) on red blood cell membranes. About one-half of the cases of immune hemolytic anemias are unassociated with other significant pathologic abnormalities. The other are seen as a manifestation of a large variety of diseases, such as various forms of acute and chronic leukemia, Hodgkin's disease, sarcoidosis, lupus erythematosus, tuberculosis, and brucellosis. The Coombs test is used to distinguish between the acquired and congenital types of hemolytic anemia. The patient's washed red cells are mixed with antihuman globulin rabbit serum. If the test is positive, agglutination occurs.

The pathologic changes in the congenital and acquired types are somewhat different. In both, the spleen is enlarged (100-1,000 gm), fairly firm and deep red, has a thin capsule, and has no grossly discernible malpighian follicles. In hereditary spherocytosis, the splenic cords are congested whereas the sinusoids are relatively empty[61] (Fig. 1131). The lining cells of the sinuses are prominent, sometimes resulting in an adenoid appearance. Hemosiderin deposition and erythrophagocytosis are present

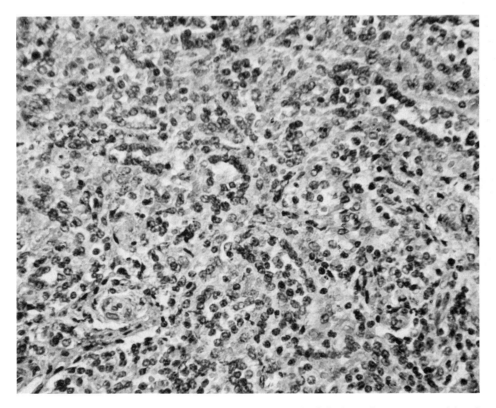

Fig. 1131 Spleen of 4-year-old girl with hereditary spherocytosis. Splenic cords are congested, but sinusoids as seen on light microscopy seem practically empty. (×350; WU neg. 67-1570.)

in both conditions but are usually more pronounced in the acquired variety. Ultrastructural studies have shown that the splenic cords are not empty but rather contain red blood cells that have lost their electron density, thus corresponding to the red cell ghosts of light microscopy.[44]

In acquired hemolytic anemia, the congestion may predominate in the cords or sinuses or be equally prominent in both. Rappaport and Crosby[49] found a high correlation between spherocytosis and increased osmotic fragility on one hand and the degree of cord congestion on the other. Foci of extramedullary hematopoiesis may be present. Splenic infarcts are found in 24% of the cases.[49]

Hereditary spherocytosis is the hematologic disease that most benefits from splenectomy. The clinical cure rate is practically 100%, although the intrinsic red cell abnormality persists.[31] In acquired hemolytic anemia, splenectomy is usually reserved for cases that cannot be controlled by steroid or immunosuppressive therapy.[41] A sustained remission rate is obtained in about 50% of the cases and an objective improvement in an additional 25%. Studies of splenic sequestration using Cr[51]-tagged red cells give a rough estimation of the benefit to be expected from splenectomy.[25] A syndrome

Table 62 Splenectomies performed at Barnes Hospital, 1947-1961*

Condition	Number of patients	Sustained remission†
Idiopathic thrombocyto-penic purpura	111	60
Acquired (autoimmune) hemolytic anemia	24	16
Hereditary spherocyto-sis	38	36
Chronic lymphocytic leukemia	29	16
Malignant lymphoma	19	6
Aplastic anemia (hypo-plastic anemia)	13	4
Agnogenic myeloid metaplasia	7	0
Hypersplenism	41	20
Disseminated lupus erythematosus	4	2
Total	286	158

*Statistics from James T. Adams, M.D., Barnes Hospital, St. Louis, Mo.
†Over two years.

of hyperplenism developing in *uremic hemodialyzed* patients has also been recognized.[45] Splenectomy resulted in a marked improvement; a striking degree of lymphoid hyperplasia was found in the spleens.

The conditions for which splenectomy is done and the results obtained at Barnes Hospital in St. Louis are indicated in Table 62.[30,31,54]

Agnogenic myeloid metaplasia (myelofibrosis)

In myeloid metaplasia, one of the myeloproliferative diseases, there is a great variation in the degree of myelofibrosis and myelosclerosis of the bone marrow.[62,75] The extramedullary hematopoiesis present in the spleen, liver, lymph nodes, and other organs was considered by some to be a compensatory mechanism and an expression of a systemic myeloproliferative disorder by others. At the present time, the latter view is almost universally accepted.[66,71,73,74] The spleens are extremely large (430-4,100 gm, averaging 2,013 gm).[69]

Microscopically, there are congestion, small and diluted follicles, and hemosiderosis.[72] Most important, all bone marrow elements are present. Large numbers of megakaryocytes, erythroid precursors, and granulocyte precursors are present in the red pulp (Figs. 1132 and 1133). The latter are made evident with von Leder's chloroacetate esterase stain. The megakaryocytes often have atypical nuclear features and can simulate closely Sternberg-Reed cells.[65] Biopsy of the liver shows extensive hematopoiesis among and within the sinusoids. Exceptionally large nodular masses of extramedullary hematopoiesis develop in the mediastinum and simulate a primary malignant tumor of this location.[67] This phenomenon also has been described in congenital spherocytosis and other types of anemia.[64,70]

Factors that serve to distinguish myelofibrosis from chronic myelocytic leukemia include a lower total white cell count, normal numbers of eosinophils and basophils, nucleated red cells in the peripheral blood, organ infiltrates consisting of several cell lines, greater marrow fibrosis with less cellular immaturity, higher values of leukocyte alkaline phosphatase, and difficulty in performing a successful marrow aspiration. Usually, the evaluation of all such factors will enable one successfully to classify a given case as either myelofibrosis or leukemia, but transitional or intermediate cases are frequent.[69]

A test of greater significance in the differential diagnosis between these two conditions is chromosome analysis. It has been shown that approximately 90% of patients with chronic myelocytic leukemia have a chromosomal abnormality known as the Philadelphia chromosome.[63] Originally this was thought to represent a deletion of part of the longer arm of this chromosome; it has now been determined that it is instead a balanced reciprocal translocation between chromosomes 9 and 22.[67a] This abnormality, which apparently is acquired, is also present in cells of the erythroid series and megakaryocytes of patients with this disease, suggesting a common stem origin for these cell lines. On the other hand, it is practically never found in agnogenic myeloid metaplasia or in other myeloproliferative diseases.[68]

Splenectomy is sometimes carried out for agnogenic myeloid metaplasia, especially when hemolytic phenomena or thrombocytopenia is severe. The results are not spectacular, but in some cases a moderate improvement has been noted.

Congestive and idiopathic splenomegaly

In *congestive splenomegaly*, there are enlargement of the spleen, signs of hypersplenism (anemia, leukopenia, and/or thrombocytopenia), and often alarming gastric hemorrhages secondary to a collateral circulation that develops between the portal and peripheral venous systems. This condition develops in the presence of increased pressure in the portal circulation as reflected through the splenic vein. The etiology can be extrahepatic or intrahepatic. If intrahepatic, it is usually some form of cirrhosis. In the extrahepatic type, there may be stenosis, thrombosis, sclerosis, or cavernous transformation of the portal vein or a major tributary. The thrombosis may be the result of inflammation, trauma, or extrinsic pressure by inflammatory or neoplastic tissue.[88] Stenotic or sclerotic changes may be the result of extension into the main portal vein of the physiologic obliterative process that takes place at birth in the umbilical vein and the ductus venosum as they empty into the left portal vein.

The portal circulation, which has no valves, carries about three-fourths of the circulation of the liver. The hepatic artery carrying oxygen supplies the other one-fourth. Both vessels have a common exit channel, the hepatic veins, which empty into the inferior vena cava. McIndoe[83] demonstrated the important fact that in advanced cirrhosis, if fluid was perfused

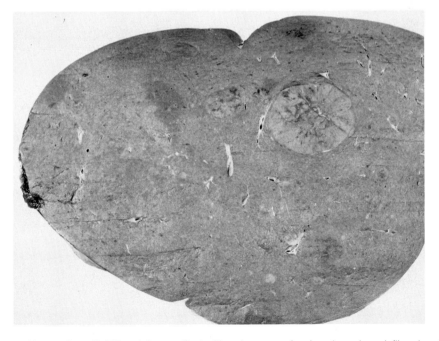

Fig. 1132 Huge spleen (3,200 gm) from patient with extreme myelosclerosis and myelofibrosis, with subsequent anemia and failure to respond to all therapeutic measures. Nodule represents area of extreme extramedullary hematopoiesis. (WU neg. 52-3980.)

through the portal circulation, all but 13% escaped through the collateral circulation. Because of this, the hepatic artery carries an increased blood flow, and when the arterial pressure falls, hepatic insufficiency occurs. The prominent increase of portal pressure leads to long-continued congestion of the spleen. The spleen enlarges, anemia develops, and collateral circulation becomes prominent. With still further time, the spleen becomes firmer and darker. Microscopically, there is marked dilatation of veins and sinuses, fibrosis of the

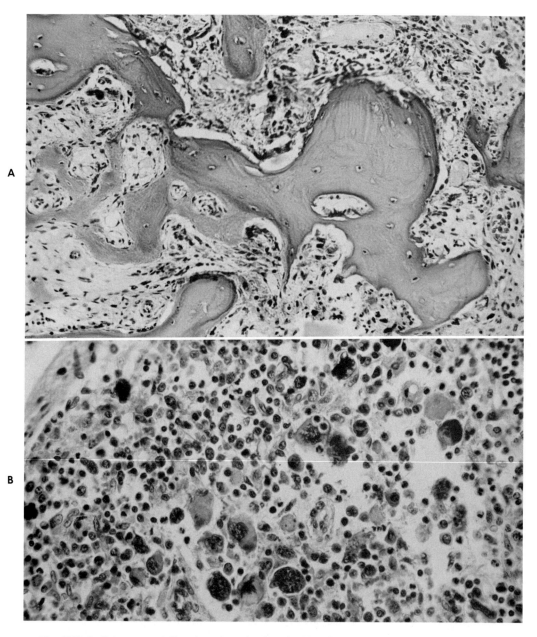

Fig. 1133 A, Extreme myelofibrosis and myelosclerosis. Note fibrosis and thickened bone trabeculae. **B,** Extensive extramedullary hematopoiesis found at postmortem examination of patient referred to in **A.** It involved practically every organ in body, including such tissues as epididymis, retroperitoneal soft tissues, and adrenal gland. This section shows large clusters of atypical megakaryocytes within lymph node. (**A,** ×200; WU neg. 52-4493; **B,** ×400; WU neg. 52-4492.)

red pulp, and accumulation of hemosiderin-containing macrophages. Lymphoid follicles are inconspicuous. Iron incrustation of the connective tissue and sclerosiderotic nodules ("Gamna-Gandy bodies") develop as a result of focal hemorrhages.

Splenectomy without shunt is successful when the coronary vein joins the portal system central the point of obstruction. Otherwise, shunt is indicated.[85] Various types have been done, including anastomosis of the splenic vein to the renal vein and anastomosis of the portal vein to the vena cava.[77] The results from these operations have been encouraging as a means of controlling repetitive hemorrhage from esophageal varices. However, such procedures do not seem to prolong life.[87]

When a similar set of functional and pathologic changes occur in the absence of an anatomic explanation for increased portal pressure, the condition is designated as *idiopathic splenomegaly.*[79] It is often impossible to differentiate on clinical and pathologic grounds whether a patient with persistent splenomegaly in the absence of an underlying disease has idiopathic splenomegaly or malignant lymphoma of the spleen. Long and Aisenberg[82] pointed out that idiopathic splenomegaly may simulate nodular lymphoma pathologically, particularly when associated with lymphocytic infiltrates in the liver and bone marrow and atypical lymphocytes in the peripheral blood. However, the follicles of idiopathic hyperplasia always show prominent germinal centers with active phagocytosis and are surrounded by a well-defined perifollicular rim of mature lymphocytes; furthermore, subendothelial lymphocytic infiltration is absent. One should be very cautious in making a diagnosis of nontropical idiopathic splenomegaly; long follow-up studies have shown that many of these cases are in reality, examples of well-differentiated lymphocytic lymphomas.[78] Bagshawe[76] compared the relative features of hypersplenism among forty-six patients with congestive splenomegaly and twenty-nine with reactive splenomegaly and found no significant differences among them. Massive splenomegaly is commonly seen in several tropical countries, such as Zaire, Malagasy Republic, Nigeria, and New Guinea.[84] Spleens removed for this "tropical splenomegaly syndrome"[80] are often extremely heavy (mean, 3,270 gm) and exhibit a uniform dark red cut surface. Microscopically, there are marked dilatation of sinuses and foci of extra-medullary hematopoiesis but no significant fibrosis or hemosiderin deposition.[84] Signs of hypersplenism are the rule. Epidemiologic and therapeutic studies suggest a causal relationship with malaria.[84,86] In this regard, it is interesting that the cases of idiopathic splenomegaly reported by Banti in 1883[81] were from an area which at the time was endemic for malaria.

Inflammation

Reactive follicular hyperplasia can be seen as an acute phenomenon as a response to a systemic infection or in a more chronic form in immune-mediated diseases, such as idiopathic thrombocytopenic purpura, acquired hemolytic anemia, rheumatoid arthritis (including Felty's syndrome), in Castleman's disease, and in hemodialyzed patients.

A more diffuse lymphoid hyperplasia, with production of immunoblasts and plasma cells, can be the result of infection (particularly viral), graft rejection, or a component of the newly described entity angioimmunoblastic lymphadenopathy (see Chapter 20). Some of the aforementioned patterns have been traditionally grouped under the rather inaccurate term of "septic spleen."

Abscess of the spleen, a vanishingly rare condition, can be the result of trauma or metastatic spread of infection from another site.[90,90a] Septic abscesses of the spleen secondary to subacute bacterial endocarditis may lead to surgical intervention.[90b]

Granulomatous inflammation is a common finding in splenectomy specimens. The granulomas can be roughly divided into three major types: large active granulomas containing epithelioid and Langhans' type giant cells, with or without central necrosis; small, widespread, sarcoidlike epithelioid granulomas with scanty giant cells and no necrosis (not to be equated with "epithelioid" germinal centers[93]); and old inactive granulomas, with fibrosis and calcification. The third type, which can be solitary or found scattered throughout the spleen, is particularly common in areas of endemic histoplasmosis.[96] We have evaluated twenty cases of splenectomy done for splenomegaly and/or hypersplenism, in which the only major pathologic finding was the presence of active granulomas of either the first or second type.[92] All of the patients were adults. Fever, weight loss, hepatosplenomegaly, and the various manifestations of hypersplenism were the most common symptoms, and these were markedly

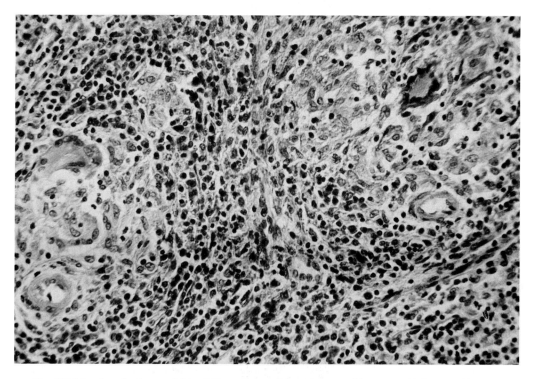

Fig. 1134 Section of spleen weighing 750 gm removed from 31-year-old woman with fever and hepato-splenomegaly. These granulomatous lesions with giant cells were proved to be reaction to *Histo-plasma capsulatum*. (×350; WU neg. 66-11901A.)

ameliorated with splenectomy. The splenic granulomas were nearly always the expression of a generalized disease, which also often involved lymph nodes, liver, and bone marrow. Despite the performance of special stains and cultures, the etiology remained unknown in all but three cases. In these, the organisms identified were *Histoplasma capsulatum,* an atypical *Mycobacterium,* and *Sporotrichum schenkii,* respectively (Fig. 1134). None of the patients developed malignant lymphoma on follow-up.

Sarcoidlike granulomas have been described in the spleen of patients with Hodgkin's disease[91] and, less commonly, non-Hodgkin's lymphoma, with or without involvement of the spleen by tumor. In three cases of non-Hodgkin's lymphomas reported by Braylan et al.,[89] the number of granulomas was such as to render the diagnosis of lymphoma quite difficult. It should be emphasized that the presence of splenic granulomas in patients with lymphoma is not per se an indication that the spleen is involved by tumor. Actually, recent evidence suggests that in patients with Hodgkin's disease, this finding is associated with an improved prognosis.[95] Neiman[94] found sarcoid-like granulomas in 24 of 412 splenectomy specimens; in addition to the conditions previously listed, he found them in chronic uremia and in a single case of IgA deficiency. He pointed out that in all cases the granulomas appeared to arise in the periarteriolar lymphoid sheath, suggesting that they are the result of abnormal or defective processing of antigen presented to the spleen.

Cysts

Approximately 75% of the nonparasitic *cysts* of the spleen are of the *false (secondary) type.*[99] Their wall is composed of dense fibrous tissue, often calcified, with no epithelial lining. The content is a mixture of blood and necrotic debris. If the cyst ruptures, massive hemoperitoneum may result. The majority of these cysts are solitary and asymptomatic. Trauma is the most likely etiologic factor, although it is possible that some represent epithelial cysts in which part or all of the lining has been destroyed (Fig. 1135). There have been about sixty reported cases of *epithelial cysts* of the spleen.[100,101] Most cases have occurred in chil-

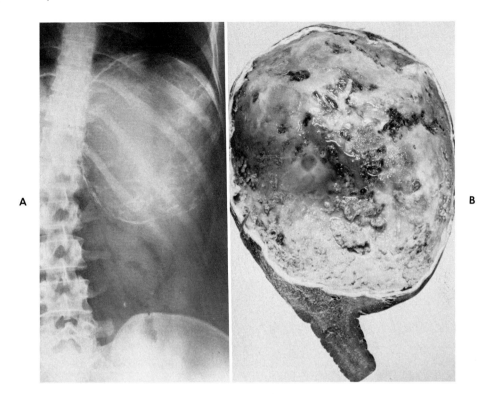

Fig. 1135 A, Large cyst of spleen. **B,** Gross specimen of lesion illustrated in **A** showing calcified cyst partially lined by stratified squamous epithelium. (**A,** WU neg. 50-3794; **B,** WU neg. 50-3542.)

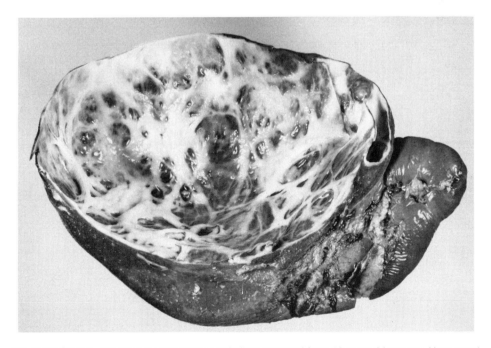

Fig. 1136 Splenic cyst lined by squamous epithelium removed from 19-year-old woman. Note prominent trabeculation. (WU neg. 70-3125.)

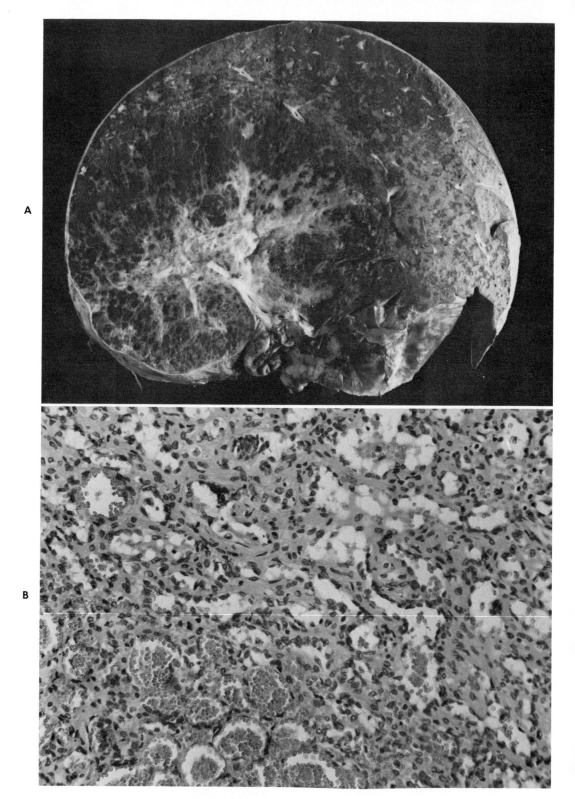

Fig. 1137 A, Large hemangioma of spleen in 44-year-old man who presented with mild anemia and leukopenia. Tumor weighed over 3,000 gm. Patient had no other vascular lesions. **B,** Microscopic appearance of same lesion. Dilated vascular channels filled with red blood cells may be seen. (Courtesy Dr. B. W. Sharpe, Jackson, Tenn.; photo by Media Services, SUNY at Stony Brook.)

dren and young adults.[97] Grossly, a glistening inner surface with marked trabeculation is often seen (Fig. 1136). Microscopically, the wall is lined by mature squamous epithelium, without skin adnexa.[98] The pathogenesis is unknown.

Tumors

Of the primary benign tumors, *hemangioma* is the most common;[116] it is often of the cavernous variety, and rupture is the commonest complication (Fig. 1137). A very large and cellular but not obviously malignant tumor of lymph vessels was reported by Hamoudi et al.[114] in a 13-year-old girl; she was well four years after splenectomy (Fig. 1138). Rappaport[121] described a *hamartoma (splenadenoma)* composed of red pulp only, resulting in marked sequestration of red cells. Five additional cases have been recently recorded.[122] A case of intrasplenic *lipoma* was reported by Easler and Dowlin.[112]

Malignant lymphoma is by far the most common malignant tumor involving the spleen[106,111] (Table 63). Although usually affected as part of a generalized process, in some cases the spleen represents the only detectable site of disease. Spleen involvement by malignant lymphoma may present as an asymptomatic splenomegaly or result in a picture of hypersplenism.[123] Ahmann et al.[102] described four gross patterns of involvement: homogeneous, miliary, multiple masses, and solitary mass (Figs. 1139 and 1140). The first two were seen with all microscopic types of lymphoma. The presence of masses, either solitary or diffuse, was encountered only in histiocytic lymphoma and Hodgkin's disease. Of their forty-eight cases, twenty-six (54%) had a nodular pattern of growth on microscopic examination. The prognosis was better for tumors composed of well-differentiated lymphocytes, for those growing in a nodular fashion, and for the Stage I (limited to the spleen) and Stage II (limited to the spleen and splenic lymph node) neoplasms. The overall five-year survival rate was 31%. In another series, more than 50% of the patients with malignant lymphoma first presenting in the spleen died within two years of the diagnosis.[118]

The microscopic diagnosis is obvious in most cases, but it may be extremely difficult with some well-differentiated lymphocytic lymphomas. The lymph nodes of the splenic hilum should be carefully dissected and examined microscopically, since they may show obvious lymphoma when the changes in the spleen are only equivocal. We have found the presence of nodular collections of lymphocytes beneath the endothelium of trabecular veins (presumably lodged in subendothelial lymphatic vessels) a helpful feature for the diagnosis of lymphocytic lymphoma or lymphocytic leukemia in the spleen[113] (Fig. 1141). The only other condition in which we have seen it in a prominent degree in an adult has been infectious mononucleosis. We have also seen this space occupied by red cell precursors in infants with erythroblastosis fetalis and (together with granulocyte precursors) in adults with myelofibrosis. The features of Hodgkin's disease involving the spleen are discussed in Chapter 20.

All types of *leukemia* can involve the spleen. Chronic lymphocytic leukemia needs to be distinguished from well-differentiated lymphocytic lymphoma (an impossible task on purely morphologic grounds) and with prolymphocytic leukemia. In the latter, the lymphocytes have larger nuclei, often indented, and distinct nucleoli.[117a]

Hairy cell leukemia (leukemic reticuloendotheliosis) is a chronic disease of insidious onset, seen only in adults and elderly persons and characterized by splenomegaly (often massive), pancytopenia, and the presence of ''hairy'' cells in the peripheral blood.[108] Grossly, the spleen shows diffuse enlargement without the formation of nodules. Microscopically, hairy cell leukemia *is a disease of the red pulp*, which shows diffuse infiltration by a monotonous population of small mononuclear cells with very

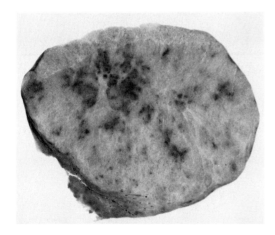

Fig. 1138 Hemangioendothelioma of spleen. This is one of many nodules that were present in organ. (Courtesy Dr. A. B. Hamoudi, Columbus, Ohio.)

scanty mitotic activity and practically no pha-gocytosis (Fig. 1142). The nuclei are small, round or oval, with irregular contour, occa-sional deep indentations, and inconspicuous nu-cleoli. The cytoplasm is usually scanty, al-though in some cells it is moderate to abun-dant and lightly stained. Pools of blood in the red pulp, lined by ''hairy'' cells and simulat-ing dilated sinuses, are commonly seen and constitute an important diagnostic feature.[119]

The ''hairy'' cells contain a virtually diag-nostic tartrate-resistant isoenzyme of acid phos-phatase, which can be demonstrated in touch preparations and tissue sections.[126] Ultrastruc-turally, the hairy projections are prominent and interdigitate to form syncytium-like aggre-

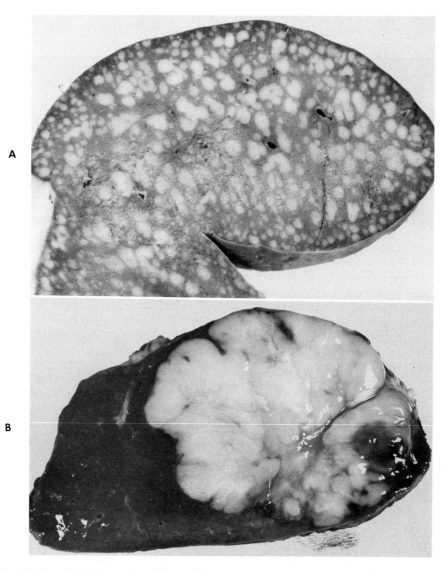

Fig. 1139 Two distinct types of splenic gross involvement by malignant lymphoma. **A,** ''Miliary'' type of involvement. Any type of lymphoma can produce this pattern. Patient was 63-year-old woman in whom only findings were splenomegaly and neutropenia. Microscopically, it was nodular lymphocytic lym-phoma. Two years after splenectomy, disseminated disease developed. **B,** Malignant lymphoma pro-ducing solitary mass. This pattern is seen only in Hodgkin's disease and histiocytic lymphoma. In this case, it was the latter. Patient, 66-year-old woman, later developed disseminated disease. (**A,** WU neg. 64-5358; **B,** WU neg. 54-3654.)

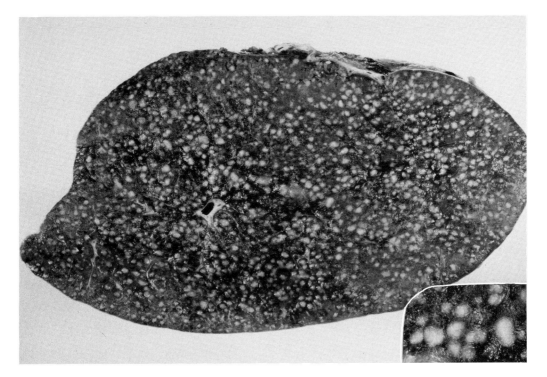

Fig. 1140 Splenic involvement by Hodgkin's disease. Innumerable white nodules are scattered throughout parenchyma. (WU neg. 72-2001.)

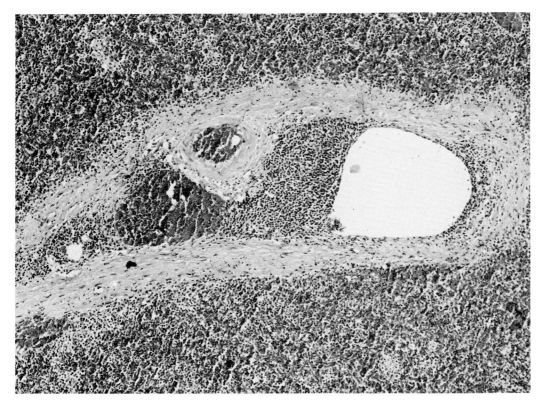

Fig. 1141 Involvement of subendothelial space of large splenic vein in well-differentiated lymphocytic lymphoma. This is important diagnostic sign. (×90; WU neg. 73-7012.)

Table 63 Differential diagnosis of some hematopoietic diseases involving spleen

	Well-differentiated lymphocytic lymphoma and chronic lymphocytic leukemia	Poorly differentiated lymphocytic lymphoma	"Histiocytic" lymphoma	Malignant histiocytosis	Hairy cell leukemia	Chronic myelocytic leukemia
Pattern of growth	White pulp	White pulp	White and red pulp	Red pulp	Red pulp	Red pulp
Area of involvement	Diffuse or nodular	Nodular (follicular)	Randomly distributed large nodules	Diffuse	Diffuse	Diffuse
Nuclei	Small and round	Angulated and cleaved	Large, vesicular and pleomorphic	Large, vesicular and pleomorphic	Small, round or oval, with irregular contours	Polymorphic infiltrate, with granulocytes at various stages of maturation (eosinophilic myelocytes may be identified in hematoxylin-eosin sections)
Chromatin	Coarsely clumped	Clumped and open	Clumped and sparse	Coarsely clumped	Finely stippled	
Nucleoli	Not visible	Usually inconspicuous	Prominent	Prominent	Usually inconspicuous	
Pleomorphism	Minimal	Minimal to moderate	Marked	Marked	Minimal	
Mitoses	Rare or absent	Rare	Abundant	Abundant	Practically absent	
Cytoplasm	Very scanty	Scanty	Abundant	Abundant	Scanty to moderate	
Phagocytosis	Absent	Absent	Rarely present	Usually present	Absent	Absent
Special techniques	Surface markers for B cells	Surface markers for B cells	Surface markers for B cells and histiocytes; methyl green–pyronine; cytoplasmic immunoglobulin (immunoperoxidase)	Surface markers for histiocytes; lysozyme (immunoperoxidase); nonspecific esterase; tartrate-labile acid phosphatase	Tartrate-resistant acid phosphatase	Chloroacetate esterase (von Leder stain)

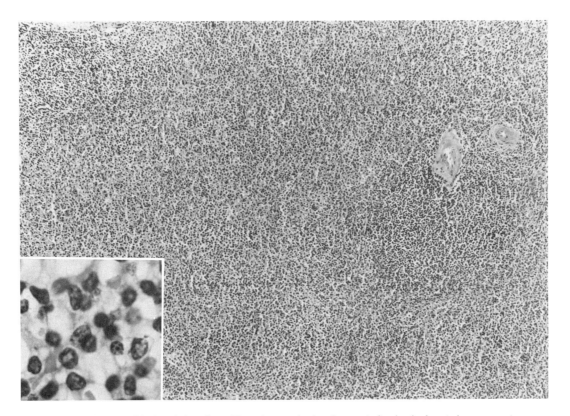

Fig. 1142 Hairy cell leukemia in spleen. There is massive involvement of red pulp. **Inset** shows monotonous cells with scanty cytoplasm and no mitoses.

gates.[109] It has not yet been ascertained whether the "hairy" cells are monocytes, B lymphocytes, or a specific subpopulation of the lymphoid system, although most evidence favors the view that these cells are related to the monocyte-histiocyte system.[107]

When the lymph nodes are involved, a paracortical pattern of permeation is seen (Fig. 1143). Bone marrow involvement often results in "dry taps." In the liver, the cells infiltrate diffusely the sinusoids. Splenectomy is the treatment of choice and long survivals are common.

Malignant lymphoma can simulate the pattern of growth of hairy cell leukemia, but the cytologic features are different.[120] Vardiman et al.[124] described four patients with massive splenomegaly resulting from a malignant process that they interpreted as a chronic form of *malignant histiocytosis;* three of these patients did eventually develop systemic symptoms of malignant histiocytosis within one year. The spleen enlargement was diffuse and, microscopically, a widespread infiltration of the splenic cords and sinuses by neoplastic histiocytes was seen. In contrast to hairy cell leukemia, the cells were large and exhibited greater cellular variation, atypia, mitotic activity, and phagocytosis.

Angiosarcoma may present as a well-defined hemorrhagic nodule or involve the spleen diffusely and may lead to spontaneous rupture of the organ[104,110] (Fig. 1144). Metastases may be widespread. The clinical course is rapid and almost invariably fatal.[103,125]

Metastatic carcinoma of the spleen is uncommon, although widely disseminated neoplasms such as *melanoma* and *mammary carcinoma* may involve this organ.[105] Herbut and Gabriel[115] reported twenty-three patients with splenic metastases. In general, metastatic carcinoma to the spleen is evidence of generalized disease.[105]

Angiographic studies can be very helpful in documenting the presence of a splenic mass and suggest its benign or malignant nature.[117]

Other lesions

Congenital absence of the spleen *(asplenia)* is associated in more than 80% of the cases with

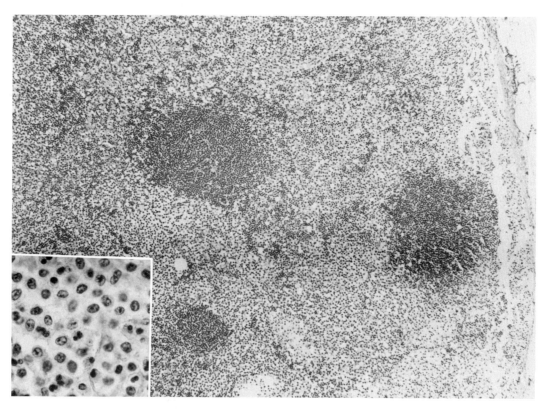

Fig. 1143 Lymph node involvement by hairy cell leukemia. T cell regions are preferentially affected. **Inset** shows uniformity of proliferation and irregular nuclear contour.

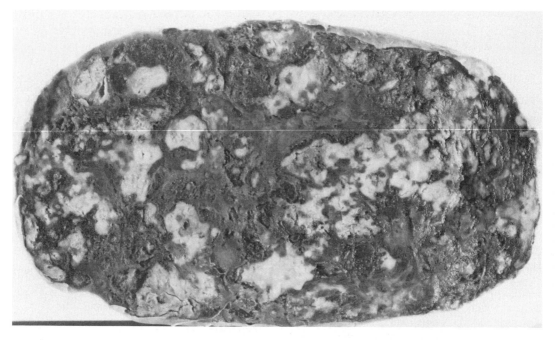

Fig. 1144 Angiosarcoma of spleen in 19-year-old woman. Weight of organ was 900 gm. There were hepatic and vertebral metastases. (Courtesy Dr. J. J. Segura, San José, Costa Rica.)

malformations of the heart, nearly always involving the atrioventricular endocardial cushion and the ventricular outflow tracts.[132] Anomalies of the blood vessels, lung, and abdominal viscera also are frequent.[128] In *polysplenia*, the cardiac anomalies are less severe and the prognosis is therefore more favorable.[134] A hereditary form of splenic *hypoplasia* has been reported.[130]

Splenic-gonadal fusion occurs in two forms. One is continuous, in which the main spleen is connected by a cord of splenic and fibrous tissue to the gonadal mesonephric structures; the other is discontinuous, in which discrete masses of splenic tissue are found fused to these same structures.[133] Of the fifty-two cases reviewed by Watson,[135] only four were in females. Eleven were associated with other congenital defects, such as peromelus and micrognathia. Various degrees of testicular ectopia and inguinal hernias are common. All of the reported cases have been on the left side.[133] A case of *spleno-hepatic fusion* was recorded by Cotelingam and Saito[127] and one of *splenorenal* fusion by Gonzalez-Crussi et al.[129]

Thrombosis of the splenic vein of unknown etiology may cause *infarction.* If the artery is tied, usually infarction does not occur. *Peliosis* of the spleen may accompany hepatic peliosis.[131]

REFERENCES

Introduction

1 Burke JS, Simon GT: Electron microscopy of the spleen. I. Anatomy and microcirculation. Am J Pathol **58:**127-155, 1970.

2 Enriquez P, Neiman RS: The pathology of the spleen. A functional approach. American Society of Clinical Pathology, 1976.

3 Lennert K, Harms D (eds): Spleen: structure, function, pathology, clinical aspects, therapy. Berlin, 1970, Springer-Verlag.

4 Li CY, Yam LT, Crosby WH: Histochemical characterization of cellular and structural elements of the human spleen. J Histochem Cytochem **20:**1049-1058, 1972.

5 Millikin PD: The nodular white pulp of the human spleen. Arch Pathol **87:**247-258, 1969.

6 Weiss L: The structure of the normal spleen. Semin Hematol **2:**205-228, 1965.

Biopsy and pathologic examination

7 Block M, Jacobson LO: Splenic puncture. JAMA **142:**641-647, 1950 (extensive bibliography).

8 Farrer-Brown G, Bennett MH, Harrison CV, Millett Y, Jelliffe AM: The diagnosis of Hodgkin's disease in surgically excised spleens. J Clin Pathol **37:**294-300, 1972.

9 Ferris DO, Hargraves MM: Splenic puncture. Arch Surg **67:**402-407, 1953.

10 Ham AW: The structure of the spleen. In Blaustein A (ed): The spleen. New York, 1963, McGraw-Hill Book Co.

11 Moeschlin S: Spleen puncture (translated from German by A. Piney). London, 1951, William Heinemann, Ltd.

12 Soderström N: Cytologie der Milz in Punktaten. In Lennert K, Harms D (eds): Die Milz. Berlin, 1970, Springer-Verlag.

Rupture; splenectomy

13 Cohen EA: Splenosis. Review and report of subcutaneous splenic implant. Arch Surg **69:**777-784, 1954.

14 Dalton ML Jr, Strange WH, Downs EA: Intrathoracic splenosis. Case report and review of the literature. Am Rev Resp Dis **103:**827-830, 1971.

15 Editorial: Infective hazards of splenectomy. Lancet **1:**1167-1168, 1976.

16 Ellis EF, Smith RT: The role of the spleen in immunity. Pediatrics **37:**111-119, 1966.

17 Fleming CR, Dickson ER, Harrison EG Jr: Splenosis: autotransplantation of splenic tissue. Am J Med **61:**414-419, 1976.

18 Foster RP: Delayed haemorrhage from the ruptured spleen. Br J Surg **57:**189-192, 1970.

19 Nordøy A: The spleenless state in man. In Lennert K, Harms D (eds): Die Milz. Berlin, 1970, Springer-Verlag.

20 Orloff MJ, Peskin GW: Spontaneous rupture of the normal spleen. A surgical enigma. Int Abstr Surg **106:**1-11, 1958.

21 Pedersen B, Videbaek A: On the late effects of removal of the normal spleen. A follow-up study of 40 persons. Acta Chir Scand **131:**89-98, 1966.

22 Pratt DB, Andersen RC, Hitchcock CR: Splenic rupture. A review of 114 cases. Minn Med **54:**177-184, 1971.

23 Rawsthorne GB, Cole TP, Kyle J: Spontaneous rupture of the spleen in infectious mononucleosis. Br J Surg **57:**396-398, 1970.

24 Stites TB, Ultmann JE: Spontaneous rupture of the spleen in chronic lymphocytic leukemia. Cancer **19:**1587-1590, 1966.

Hypersplenism (dyssplenism)

25 Amorosi EL: Hypersplenism. Semin Hematol **2:**249-285, 1965 (excellent bibliography).

26 Baldini M: Idiopathic thrombocytopenic purpura. N Engl J Med **274:**1245-1251; 1301-1306; 1360-1367, 1966.

27 Bowdler AJ: The role of the spleen and splenectomy in autoimmune hemolytic disease. Semin Hematol **13:**335-348, 1976.

28 Bowman HE, Pettit VD, Caldwell FT, Smith EB: Morphology of the spleen in idiopathic thrombocytopenic purpura. Lab Invest **4:**206-216, 1955.

29 Cohn J, Tygstrup I: Foamy histiocytosis of the spleen in patients with chronic thrombocytopenia. Scand J Hematol **16:**33-37, 1976.

30 Coller FA, Orebaugh JE: Indications for splenectomy. Surgery **37:**858-872, 1955.

31 Crosby WH: Splenectomy in hematologic disorders. N Engl J Med **286:**1252-1254, 1972.

32 Ebbe S, Wittels B, Dameshek W: Autoimmune thrombocytopenic purpura ("ITP" type) with chronic lymphocytic leukemia. Blood **19:**23-27, 1962.

33 Gupta PC Sen, Chatterjea JB, Mukherjee AM, Chat-

terji A: Observations on the foam cell in thalassemia. Blood **16:**1039-1044, 1960.

34 Harrington WJ, Arimura G: Platelet autoimmunization and thrombocytopenia. International Society of Hematology, Proceedings of Sixth Congress, 1956. New York, 1958, Grune & Stratton, Inc., p. 836.

35 Harrington WJ, Arimura G: Immune reactions of platelets. In Johnson SA, Monto RW, Rebuck JW, Horn RC Jr (eds): Blood platelets. (Henry Ford Hospital International Symposium). New York, 1961, Little, Brown and Co., pp. 659-670.

36 Harrington WJ, Minnich V, Hollingsworth JW: Demonstration of a thrombocytopenic factor in the blood of patients with thrombocytopenic purpura. J Lab Clin Med **38:**1-10, 1951.

37 Jacob HS: The defective red blood cell in hereditary spherocytosis. Annu Rev Med **20:**41-46, 1969.

38 Jacob HS: Hypersplenism: mechanisms and management. Br J Haematol **27:**1-5, 1974.

39 Karpatkin S, Siskind GW: In vitro detection of platelet antibody in patients with idiopathic thrombocytopenic purpura and systemic lupus erythematosus. Blood **33:**795-812, 1969.

40 Liber A, Rose HG: Saturated hydrocarbons in follicular lipidosis of the spleen. Arch Pathol **83:**116-122, 1967.

41 Loeb V Jr, Moore CV, Dubach R: The physiologic evaluation and management of chronic bone marrow failure. Am J Med **15:**499-517, 1953.

41a Luk SC, Musclow E, Simon GT: Platelet phagocytosis in the spleen of patients with idiopathic thrombocytopenic purpura (ITP). Histopathology **4:**127-136, 1980.

42 McMillan R, Longmire RL, Yelenosky R, Donnell RL, Armstrong S: Quantitation of platelet-binding IgG produced in vitro by spleens from patients with idiopathic thrombocytopenic purpura. N Engl J Med **291:**812-817, 1974.

43 McMillan R, Longmire RL, Yelenosky BS, Smith RS, Craddock CG: Immunoglobulin synthesis in vitro by splenic tissue in idiopathic thrombocytopenic purpura. N Engl J Med **286:**681-684, 1972.

44 Molnar Z, Rappaport H: Fine structure of the red pulp of the spleen in hereditary spherocytosis. Blood **39:**81-98, 1972.

45 Neiman R, Bischel MD, Lukes RJ: Hypersplenism in the uremic hemodialyzed patient: pathology and proposed pathophysiologic mechanisms. Am J Clin Pathol **60:**502-511, 1973.

46 Palmer JG, Eichwald EJ, Cartwright GE, Wintrobe MM: The experimental production of splenomegaly, anemia and leukopenia in Albino rats. Blood **8:**72-80, 1953.

47 Parker AC, Bain AD, Brydon WG, Harkness RA, Smith AF, Smith II, Boyd DHA: Sea-blue histiocytosis associated with hyperlipidemia. J Clin Pathol **29:**634-638, 1976.

48 Rappaport H: The pathologic anatomy of the splenic red pulp. In Lennert K, Harms D (eds): Die Milz. Berlin, 1970, Springer-Verlag.

49 Rappaport H, Crosby WH: Autoimmune hemolytic anemia. II. Morphologic observations and clinico-pathologic correlation. Am J Pathol **33:**429-458, 1957.

50 Reidbord HR, Branimir LH, Fisher ER: Splenic lipidoses: histochemical and ultrastructural differentiation with special reference to the syndrome of the sea-blue histiocyte. Arch Pathol **93:**518-524, 1972.

51 Rudders RA, Aisenberg AC, Schiller AL: Hodgkin's disease presenting as "idiopathic" thrombocytopenic purpura. Cancer **30:**220-230, 1972.

52 Rywlin AM, Lopez-Gomez A, Tachimes P, Pardo V: Ceroid histiocytosis of the spleen in hyperlipemia: relationship to the syndrome of the sea-blue histiocyte. Am J Clin Pathol **56:**572-579, 1971.

53 Saltzstein SL: Phospholipid accumulation in histiocytes of splenic pulp associated with thrombocytopenic purpura. Blood **18:**73-88, 1961.

54 Sandusky WR, Leavell BS, Burton IB: Splenectomy: indications and results in hematologic disorders. Ann Surg **159:**695-710, 1964.

55 Shulman NR, Marder V, Weinrach RA: Similarities between known antiplatelet antibodies and factor responsible for thrombocytopenia in idiopathic purpura. Ann NY Acad Sci **124:**499-542, 1965.

56 Shulman NR, Marder VJ, Hiller MC, Collier EM: Platelet and leukocyte isoantigens and their antibodies: serologic, physiologic and clinical studies. Progr Hematol **4:**222-304, 1964.

57 Silverstein MN, Ellefson RD, Ahern EJ: The syndrome of the sea-blue histiocyte. N Engl J Med **282:**1-4, 1970.

58 Tavassoli M, McMillan R: Structure of the spleen in idiopathic thrombocytopenic purpura. Am J Clin Pathol **64:**180-191, 1975.

59 Weed RI: The importance of erythrocyte deformability. Am J Med **49:**147-150, 1970.

60 Weiss L, Tavassoli M: Anatomical hazards to the passage of erythrocytes through the spleen. Semin Hematol **7:**372-380, 1970.

61 Wiland OK, Smith EB: The morphology of the spleen in congenital hemolytic anemia (hereditary spherocytosis). Am J Clin Pathol **26:**619-629, 1956.

Agnogenic myeloid metaplasia (myelofibrosis)

62 Bouroncle BA, Doan CA: Myelofibrosis. Clinical, hematologic and pathologic study of 110 patients. Am J Med Sci **243:**697-715, 1962.

63 Caspersson T, Gahrton G, Lindsten J, Zech L: Identification of the Philadelphia chromosome as a number 22 by quinacrine mustard fluorescence analysis. Exp Cell Res **63:**238-240, 1970.

64 Condon WB, Safarik LR, Elzi EP: Extramedullary hematopoiesis simulating intrathoracic tumor. Arch Surg **90:**643-648, 1965.

65 Fisher ER, Hazard JB: Differentiation of megakaryocyte and Reed-Sternberg cell. Lab Invest **3:**261-269, 1954.

66 Heller EL, Lewisohn MG, Palin WE: Aleukemic myelosis. Chronic nonleukemic myelosis, agnogenic myeloid metaplasia, osteosclerosis, leuko-erythroblastic anemia, and synonymous designations. Am J Pathol **23:**327-365, 1947.

67 Lowman RM, Bloor CM, Newcomb AW: Roentgen manifestations of thoracic extramedullary hematopoiesis. Dis Chest **44:**154-162, 1963.

67a Mayall BH, Carrano AV, Moore II DH, Rowley JD: Quantification by DNA-based cytophotometry of the 9q+/22q-chromosomal translocation associated with chronic myelogenous leukemia. Cancer Res **37:**3590-3593, 1977.

68 Nowell PC, Hungerford DA: Chromosome changes in human leukemia and a tentative assessment of their significance. Ann NY Acad Sci **113:**654-662, 1964.

69 Pitcock JA, Reinhard EH, Justus BW, Mendelsohn

RA: A clinical and pathological study of seventy cases of myelofibrosis. Ann Intern Med **57**:73-84, 1962.

70 Seidler RC, Becker JA: Intrathoracic extramedullary hematopoiesis. Radiology **83**:1057-1059, 1964.

71 Silverstein MN, Gomes MR, Re Mine WH, Elveback LR: Agnogenic myeloid metaplasia. Arch Intern Med **120**:546-550, 1967.

72 Söderström N, Bandmann U, Lundh B: Patho-anatomical features of the spleen and liver. In Videbaek A (guest ed): Polycythaemia and myelofibrosis. Clin Haematol **4**:309-329, 1975.

73 Sundberg RD: Myeloid metaplasia. In Klein H (ed): Polycythemia. Springfield, Ill., 1973, Charles C Thomas Publisher, pp. 112-180.

74 Takácsi-Nagy L, Gráf B: Definition, clinical features and diagnosis of myelofibrosis. In Videbaek A (guest ed): Polycythaemia and myelofibrosis. Clin Haematol. **4**:291-308, 1975.

75 Ward HP, Block MH: The natural history of agnogenic myeloid metaplasia (AMM) and a critical evaluation of its relationship with the myeloproliferative syndrome. Medicine **50**:357-420, 1971.

Congestive and idiopathic splenomegaly

76 Bagshawe A: A comparative study of hypersplenism in reactive and congestive splenomegaly. Br J Haematol **19**:729-737, 1970.

77 Blakemore AH, Lord JW: The technic of using Vitallium tubes in establishing portacaval shunts for portal hypertension. Ann Surg **122**:476-489, 1945.

78 Dacie JV, Galton DAG, Gordon-Smith EC, Harrison CV: Non-tropical 'idiopathic splenomegaly': a follow-up study of ten patients described in 1969. Br J Haematol **38**:185-193, 1978.

79 Dacie JV, Brain MC, Harrison CV, Lewis SM, Worlledge SM: Non-tropical idiopathic splenomegaly (primary hypersplenism): a review of ten cases and their relationship to malignant lymphomas. Br J Haematol **17**:317-333, 1969.

80 Editorial: Tropical splenomegaly syndrome. Lancet **1**:1058-1059, 1976.

81 Klemperer P: The pathologic anatomy of splenomegaly. Am J Clin Pathol **6**:99-159, 1936.

82 Long JC, Aisenberg AC: Malignant lymphoma diagnosed at splenectomy and idiopathic splenomegaly. A clinicopathologic comparison. Cancer **33**:1054-1061, 1974.

83 McIndoe AH: Vascular lesions of portal cirrhosis. Arch Pathol **5**:23-42, 1928.

84 Pitney WR: The tropical splenomegaly syndrome. Trans R Soc Trop Med Hyg **62**:717-728, 1968.

85 Rousselot LM: The late phase of congestive splenomegaly (Banti's syndrome) with hematemesis but without cirrhosis of the liver. Surgery **8**:34-42, 1940.

86 Sagoe AS: Tropical splenomegaly syndrome: long-term proguanil therapy correlated with spleen size, serum IgM, and lymphocyte transformation. Br Med J **3**:378-382, 1970.

87 Satterfield JV, Mulligan LV, Butcher HR Jr: Bleeding esophageal varices. Arch Surg **90**:667-672, 1965.

88 Whipple AO: The problem of portal hypertension in relation to the hepatosplenopathies. Ann Surg **122**:449-475, 1945 (extensive bibliography).

Inflammation

89 Braylan RC, Long J, Jaffe ES, Greco FA, Orr SL, Berard CW: Malignant lymphoma obscured by concomitant extensive epithelioid granulomas. Report of three cases with similar clinicopathologic features. Cancer **39**:1146-1155, 1977.

90 Briggs RD, Davidson AI, Fletcher BRG: Solitary abscesses of the spleen. JR Coll Surg Edinb **22**:345-347, 1977.

90a Chun CH, Raff MJ, Contreras L, Varghese R, Waterman N, Daffner R, Melo JC: Splenic abscess. Medicine **59**:50-65, 1980.

90b Hermann RE, Deltaven KE, Hawk WA: Splenectomy for the diagnosis of splenomegaly. Ann Surg **168**:896-900, 1968.

91 Kadin ME, Donaldson SS, Dorfman RF: Isolated granulomas in Hodgkin's disease. N Engl J Med **283**:859-861, 1970.

92 Kuo T, Rosai J: Granulomatous inflammation in splenectomy specimens. Clinicopathologic study of 20 cases. Arch Pathol **98**:261-268, 1974.

93 Millikin PD: Epithelioid germinal centers in the human spleen. Arch Pathol **89**:314-320, 1970.

94 Neiman RS: Incidence and importance of splenic sarcoid-like granulomas. Arch Pathol **101**:518-521, 1977.

95 Sacks EL, Donaldson SS, Gordon J, Dorfman RF: Epithelioid granulomas associated with Hodgkin's disease: clinical conditions in 55 previously untreated patients. Cancer **41**:562-567, 1978.

96 Young JM, Bills RJ, Ulrich E: Discrete splenic calcification in necropsy material. Am J Pathol **33**:189-197, 1957.

Cysts

97 Blank E, Campbell JR: Epidermoid cysts of the spleen. Pediatrics **51**:75-84, 1973.

98 Fowler RH: Nonparasitic benign cystic tumors of the spleen. Surg Gynecol Obstet **96**[Suppl]:209-227, 1953.

99 Park JY, Song KT: Splenic cyst: a case report and review of literature. Am Surg **37**:544-547, 1971.

100 Talerman A, Hart S: Epithelial cysts of the spleen. Br J Surg **57**:201-204, 1970.

101 Tsakraklikes V, Hadley TW: Epidermoid cysts of the spleen. A report of five cases. Arch Pathol **96**:251-254, 1973.

Tumors

102 Ahmann DL, Kiely JM, Harrison EG Jr, Payne S: Malignant lymphoma of the spleen. Cancer **19**:461-469, 1966.

103 Aranha GV, Gold J, Grage TB: Hemangiosarcoma of the spleen. Report of a case and review of previously reported cases. J Surg Oncol **8**:481-487, 1976.

104 Autry JR, Weitzner S: Hemangiosarcoma of spleen with spontaneous rupture. Cancer **35**:534-539, 1975.

105 Berge T: Splenic metastases. Frequencies and patterns. Acta Pathol Microbiol Scand [A] **82**:499-506, 1974.

106 Bostick WL: Primary splenic neoplasms. Am J Pathol **21**:1143-1165, 1945.

107 Braylan RC, Jaffe ES, Triche TJ, Nanba K, Fowlkes BJ, Metzger H, Frank MM, Dolan MS, Yee CL, Green I, Berard CW: Structural and functional properties of the "hairy" cells of leukemic reticuloendotheliosis. Cancer **41**:210-227, 1978.

108 Burke JS, Byrne GE Jr, Rappaport H: Hairy cell leukemia (leukemic reticuloendotheliosis). I. A clinical pathologic study of 21 patients. Cancer **33**:1399-1410, 1974.

109 Burke JS, Mackay B, Rappaport H: Hairy cell leukemia. II. Ultrastructure of the spleen. Cancer 37:
2267-2274, 1976.

110 Chen TK, Bolles J, Gilbert EF: Angiosarcoma of the
spleen. Arch Pathol Lab Med 103:122-124, 1979.

111 Das Gupta T, Coombes B, Brasfield RD: Primary malignant neoplasms of the spleen. Surg Gynecol Obstet
120:947-960, 1965.

112 Easler RE, Dowlin WM: Primary lipoma of the spleen.
Report of a case. Arch Pathol 88:557-559, 1969.

113 Goldberg GM: A study of malignant lymphomas and
leukemias. VII. Lymphogenous leukemia and lymphosarcoma involvement of the lymphatic and hemic bed,
with reference to differentiating criteria. Cancer 17:
277-287, 1964.

114 Hamoudi AB, Vassy LE, Morse TS: Multiple lym-
phangioendothelioma of the spleen in a 13-year-old
girl. Arch Pathol 99:605-606, 1975.

115 Herbut PA, Garbriel FR: Secondary cancer of the
spleen. Arch Pathol 33:917-921, 1942.

116 Husni EA: The clinical course of splenic hemangioma
with emphasis on spontaneous rupture. Arch· Surg
83:681-688, 1961.

117 Kishiwara T, Numaguchi Y, Watanabe K, Matsuura
K: Angiographic diagnosis of benign and malignant
splenic tumors. AJR 130:339-344, 1978.

117a Lampert I, Catovsky D, Marsh GW, Child JA,
Galton DAG: The histopathology of prolymphocytic
leukaemia with particular reference to the spleen. A
comparison with chronic lymphocytic leukaemia. Histopathology 4:3-19, 1980.

118 Long JC, Aisenberg AC: Malignant lymphoma diagnosed at splenectomy and idiopathic splenomegaly. A
clinicopathologic comparison. Cancer 33:1054-1061,
1974.

119 Nanba K, Soban EJ, Bowling MC, Berard CW:
Splenic pseudosinuses and hepatic angiomatous le-
sions. Distinctive features of hairy cell leukemia. Am
J Clin Pathol 67:415-426, 1977.

120 Neiman RS, Sullivan AL, Jaffe R: Malignant lymphoma simulating leukemic reticuloendotheliosis. Cancer
43:329-342, 1979.

121 Rappaport H: The pathologic anatomy of the splenic
red pulp. In Lennert K, Harms D (eds): Die Milz.
Berlin, 1970, Springer-Verlag.

122 Silverman ML, LiVolsi VA: Splenic hamartoma. Am
J Clin Pathol 70:224-229, 1978.

123 Skarin AT, Davey FR, Moloney WC: Lymphosarcoma
of the spleen. Arch Intern Med 127:259-265, 1971.

124 Vardiman JW, Byrne GE Jr, Rappaport H: Malignant
histiocytosis with massive splenomegaly in asymptomatic patients. A possible chronic form of the disease.
Cancer 36:419-427, 1975.

125 Wilkinson HA III, Lucas JC, Foote FW Jr: Primary
splenic angiosarcoma. A case report. Arch Pathol 85:
213-218, 1968.

126 Yam LT, Li CY, Lam KW: Tartrate-resistant acid
phosphatase isoenzyme in the reticulum cells of leukemic reticuloendotheliosis. N Engl J Med 284:357-
360, 1971.

Other lesions

127 Cotelingam JD, Saito R: Hepatolienal fusion: case report of an unusual lesion. Hum Pathol 9:234-236,
1978.

128 Esterly JR, Oppenheimer EH: Lymphangiectasis and
other pulmonary lesions in the asplenia syndrome.
Arch Pathol 90:553-560, 1970.

129 Gonzalez-Crussi F, Raibley S, Ballantine TVN, Gros-
feld JL: Splenorenal fusion. Heterotopia simulating a
renal neoplasm. Am J Dis Child 131:994-996, 1977.

130 Kevy SV, Tefft M, Vawter GF, Rosen FS: Hereditary
splenic hypoplasia. Pediatrics 42:752-757, 1968.

131 Lacson A, Berman LD, Neiman RS: Peliosis of the
spleen. Am J Clin Pathol 71:586-590, 1979.

132 Putschar WGJ, Manion WC: Congenital absence of the
spleen and associated anomalies. Am J Pathol 26:429-
470, 1956.

133 Putschar WGJ, Manion WC: Splenic-gonadal fusion.
Cancer 32:15-34, 1956.

134 Rose V, Izukawa T, Moës CAF: Syndromes of
asplenia and polysplenia. A review of cardiac and non-
cardiac malformations in 60 cases with special reference to diagnosis and prognosis. Br Heart J 37:840-
852, 1975.

135 Watson RJ: Splenogonadal fusion. Surgery 63:853-
858, 1968.

22 Bone marrow

Richard D. Brunning, M.D.*

*Professor of Laboratory Medicine and Pathology and Co-Director of the Division of Hematopathology, University of Minnesota Medical School, Minneapolis, Minn.

Introduction

The inclusion of a chapter on bone marrow histopathology in a textbook of surgical pathology is a reflection of the expanding role and responsibility of the pathologist in the examination of bone marrow tissue due to the increased use of the trephine bone marrow biopsy in the last decade. Although trephine biopsies utilizing several different biopsy needles have been used for many years, the merit of the procedure has been most effectively established in the staging of patients with malignant lymphomas. The efficacy of the procedure in this area of hematology and oncology has resulted in its widespread application in diagnostic hematology. The trephine biopsy should be viewed as complementary to smear preparations in the study of bone marrow tissue; it is not intended to supplant them. In many instances, however, examination of the trephine biopsy will yield definitive diagnostic information that will not be realized from examination of smear preparations.

Because of the facility of the trephine procedure with the more recently developed biopsy instruments, particularly the Jamshidi biopsy needle,[9] marrow biopsy can be accomplished with relatively minimal discomfort to the patient and is accompanied by a very low morbidity when performed by experienced individuals. The greatest utility of the procedure is in the evaluation of patients with malignant lymphomas, metastatic tumor, granulomatous disorders, myelofibrosis, aplastic anemia, and plasma cell dyscrasias.[2,3,5,6] It also serves as the most reliable method for assessing the cellularity of the bone marrow following the administration of antineoplastic drugs.

Similar to biopsy specimens from other organs, it must be recognized that the trephine specimen represents a relatively minute portion of the bone marrow tissue. Nevertheless, an extraordinary amount of information about the morphology of disorders affecting bone marrow has resulted from study of trephine sections.

The use of the plastic embedding technique

for bone marrow biopsies has been somewhat simplified by the introduction of new resins such as glycol methacrylate. Plastic embedding offers several advantages over paraffin, including excellent cytomorphology and the ability to apply numerous histochemical procedures. The technique is particularly suitable for laboratories handling large numbers of specimens from patients with leukemia or lymphoma.[11,11a]

Considerable discussion has occurred over the relative merits of the trephine biopsy of the bone marrow as opposed to sections of particles obtained by aspiration biopsy.[1,4,7,8,10] The particle section technique may yield important results in several disorders but is of limited value in processes accompanied by fibrosis, in which inadequate aspirations are frequently obtained.

The trephine biopsy should always be accompanied by a bone marrow aspiration, to be used in the preparation of smears and particle crush preparations. The smears are necessary for the detailed study of cytology and for those cytochemical studies that cannot be performed on routinely fixed tissue specimens. If particles in excess of those used for crush preparations are obtained, these can be processed for ultrastructural study or routine histologic preparation. Portions of the aspirate specimen may be used for lymphocyte membrane surface marker, chromosome, and enzymatic studies.

Biopsy procedure and processing of specimen

Several needles have been introduced for the bone marrow trephine procedure. The most satisfactory from the standpoint of safety, ease of procedure, and overall quality of specimen obtained is the Jamshidi biopsy needle.[15] This instrument is available in several sizes for both adult and pediatric patients. The 11-gauge needle is the most commonly used instrument in the United States for routine procedures in adults and older children. Difficulty is frequently encountered in obtaining satisfactory trephine specimens from patients with severe osteoporosis; in this group of patients, the 8-gauge Jamshidi needle or the Westerman-Jensen biopsy needle may prove more efficacious than the 11-gauge Jamshidi instrument. The 8-gauge needle is the preferred instrument for staging procedures in adults with lymphoma; however, difficulty may be encountered in retaining specimens with the large-bore instrument. If two or three attempts with an 8-gauge needle result in failure to obtain satisfactory

specimens, the 11-gauge needle should be substituted. Instructions for the use of the Jamshidi biopsy needle are included with the instrument, and audiovisual aids illustrating the procedure are available from the manufacturer. Individuals not acquainted with the trephine biopsy technique are advised to familiarize themselves with the procedure on cadavers.

The importance of proper technique in performing the bone marrow trephine biopsy cannot be overemphasized. Optimally, the biopsy specimen should be 1.5-2 cm in length and should be free of distortion due to crushing or other damage. Crush artifact and the deposition of fibrin in torn biopsies may render accurate interpretation difficult or impossible. In such instances, the biopsy must be repeated.

It is important that the trephine biopsy be obtained before the bone marrow aspiration; prior aspiration at the site of the biopsy will result in hemorrhage and altered architecture that may lead to interpretive difficulties with the trephine specimen. The use of multiple bone marrow biopsies in the staging of lymphomas and other malignancies and in the search for granulomatous lesions has been advocated.[11b,13] This can be accomplished by performing one or two biopsies on each posterior iliac spine. If a marrow is being evaluated solely to assess the amount of hematopoietic tissue, care must be taken to avoid sites that have been previously subjected to therapeutic doses of ionizing irradiation, since these areas may remain hypocellular for extended periods of time and may not accurately reflect the overall hematopoietic status.[14] If biopsies are being performed to detect malignant processes, biopsy of previously irradiated sites may yield positive results.

Imprint preparations should be made from the biopsy specimen immediately after it is removed from the biopsy needle. These can be used for Romanovsky's stains and special cytochemical procedures. Following the preparation of imprints, the specimen is placed in an appropriate fixative; the most satisfactory are Zenker's-acetic acid, Bouin's, B5, or 10% buffered neutral formalin.[16] In laboratories where bone marrows are processed with other tissues, buffered neutral formalin is the preferred fixative. The other fixatives require special handling of the specimen and are more suitable for laboratories dedicated to the processing of hematopoietic tissue. Details of the processing methodology, including decalcification, have been published.[12]

The biopsies should be sectioned at 4μ-5μ with a sharp knife that is checked frequently for the presence of defects. In those patients being investigated for extent of lymphomatous involvement, metastatic tumor, or granulomatous disease, the specimens should be completely sectioned and stepwise serial sections mounted for hematoxylin-eosin staining. The remaining ribbon should be retained and stored in a manner that will facilitate the ready and accurate mounting of additional sections for special diagnostic stains as deemed necessary. Most of the stains used for other fixed tissues are also applicable to bone marrow sections. Zenker's fixed tissue, however, gives unsatisfactory results with the chloracetate esterase stain.

Optimally, the pathologist, when interpreting the trephine biopsy, should avail himself of the trephine imprints, bone marrow and blood smears, and lymph node biopsy, if performed. Knowledge of the patient's clinical history, hematology profile, immunoelectrophoretic studies, and x-ray findings may be of considerable importance and greatly facilitate the interpretation of the biopsy specimen. The pathologist who ignores or avoids ancillary clinical or laboratory data does a disservice to diagnostic pathology and the patient.

Normocellular bone marrow

Assessment of marrow cellularity must take into account the age of the individual since the amount of hematopoietic tissue in bone marrow from normal individuals varies according to age.[17] In the very young, the marrow is hypercellular; in the elderly, the marrow is hypocellular. In the first decade, the mean percent of marrow occupied by hematopoietic cells is 79%; the mean value in the eighth decade is 29%. In the first three decades of life, more than half of the marrow space is comprised of hematopoietic tissue. During this period, there is a gradual decrease in the number of hematopoietic cells. From the fourth to the seventh decade, there is relative stabilization of the amount of hematopoietic cells (Fig. 1145). Beginning in the eighth decade, there is a renewed decrease in the hematopoietic tissue.

The immediate subcortical area of the bone marrow is generally more hypocellular than the deeper medullary areas. Specimens that are too superficial frequently contain a substantial amount of subcortical bone and may result in an erroneous interpretation of marrow cellularity.

Benign lymphocytic aggregates

Lymphocytic aggregates are a relatively common finding in bone marrow trephine and

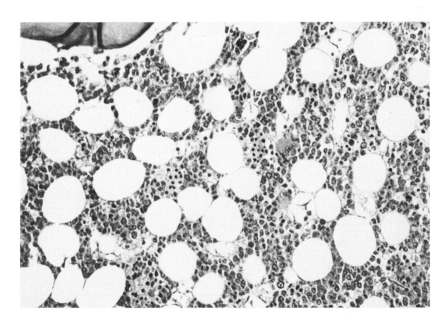

Fig. 1145 Normocellular bone marrow from 42-year-old man obtained as part of evaluation as potential donor for bone marrow transplant. Hematopoietic cells and adipose tissue are present in approximately equal quantities. (Hematoxylin-eosin; ×64.)

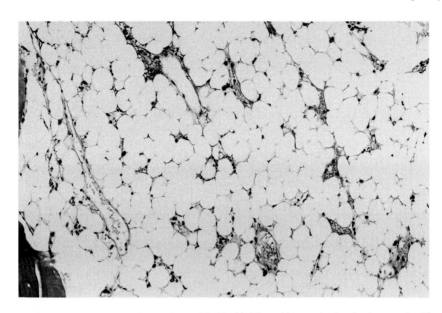

Fig. 1146 Bone marrow section from 7-year-old girl with idiopathic acquired aplastic anemia. There is almost total absence of hematopoietic cells. Sinuses and capillaries are prominent. (Hematoxylin-eosin; ×160.)

particle sections. The incidence in biopsy specimens varies from 3.3%-47%; the reported incidence in autopsy material is 26%-62%.[18-20,22] The incidence appears to increase with age and is higher in females than males. The aggregates have been noted in patients with a wide group of disorders and in patients with no recognized disease process; unusually large aggregates are sometimes found in patients with immune system diseases, such as rheumatoid arthritis. Large aggregates of lymphocytes also may be found in patients with both acute and chronic myeloproliferative disorders. The biologic significance of the aggregates in the vast majority of instances is unknown.

The number and the size of the aggregates in individual specimens vary considerably; a size range from less than 50μ to greater than $1,000\mu$ has been reported. The aggregates are usually small and well demarcated from surrounding hematopoietic tissue; the term nodular lymphoid hyperplasia has been used to describe numerous and large aggregates.[21]

The distinction between benign lymphocytic aggregates and marrow involvement by malignant lymphoma, specifically well-differentiated lymphocytic lymphoma, may be problematic. Generally, the benign aggregates are few in number, well circumscribed, and loosely structured and contain histiocytes and plasma cells in addition to lymphocytes. Vascular structures are frequently present; germinal centers are uncommonly noted but when present are evidence of a benign reaction. Neither the benign lymphocytic aggregates nor foci of well-differentiated lymphocytic lymphoma have a predilection for a paratrabecular location in contrast to the lesions of poorly differentiated lymphocytic lymphoma. If morphologic findings are equivocal, membrane marker studies may help to elucidate the monoclonal nature of a well-differentiated lymphocytic lymphoma as opposed to the polyclonal character of the cells in a benign process. In some instances, distinction between these two processes is not possible. The distinction between benign lymphocytic aggregates and the lesions of Hodgkin's disease should rest on the detection of typical Sternberg-Reed cells or their mononuclear variants in the latter disorder.

Alterations in cellularity
Aplastic anemia

Aplastic or hypoplastic anemia occurs as both acquired and congenital forms. Acquired aplastic anemia may be idiopathic or may result from exposure to drugs, chemicals, viral infections, or ionizing radiation.[23,24,28] Bone marrow aplasia also has been observed in paroxysmal nocturnal hemoglobinuria.[30] The term constitutional aplastic anemia is used collectively for all congenital forms of aplastic anemia, familial and nonfamilial, with and without malformations.[24] Fanconi's anemia is a syndrome of familial hypoplastic anemia and multiple malformations such as hypoplasia of the kidneys and absent or hypoplastic thumbs or radii occurring in the first decade of life.[26,27] An association of hypoplastic bone marrow and pancreatic dysfunction occurs as an uncommon syndrome in children.[31]

In the most severe form of aplastic anemia, the intertrabecular marrow space is occupied predominantly by adipose tissue with scattered lymphocytes, plasma cells, tissue mast cells, and hemosiderin-laden macrophages (Fig. 1146). In less severe processes, there is an increased amount of adipose tissue and scattered small collections of erythroblasts, granulocytes, and megakaryocytes. The blood picture is characterized by varying degrees of pancytopenia.

The utilization of bone marrow transplantation as a therapeutic approach to aplastic anemia is gaining wide acceptance. Evidence of marrow reconstitution will usually be present in biopsies obtained one to three weeks following transplantation and consists of foci or islands of hematopoietic cells, predominantly erythroid precursors.[29] Sequential marrow biopsies in the subsequent five-week to ten-week period contain increasing numbers of erythroid precursors, granulocytes, and megakaryocytes in those patients with successful engraftment. Impending rejection of engraftment may be heralded by a decrease in erythroid precursors. Immunosuppressive and antibiotic therapy may influence the morphology of the proliferating engrafted cells, and evidence of dyserythropoiesis may be present. At times, a maturation arrest of the proliferating neutrophil precursors at the promyelocyte stage may occur as a result of antibiotic or other drug therapy.

Serous degeneration

In patients who are extremely malnourished for a variety of reasons, the bone marrow may show hypocellularity and serous degeneration of the adipose tissue. The fat cells decrease in size, and serous fluid accumulates in the interstices. The serous fluid stains lightly eosinophilic and has a fine granular appearance in sections stained with hematoxylin-eosin; it is pale pink with the PAS stain. In patients with

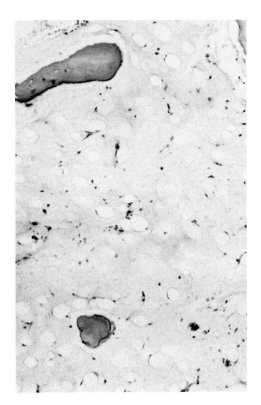

Fig. 1147 Bone marrow section from 27-year-old woman with anorexia nervosa and severe weight loss showing marked serous degeneration (gelatinous transformation). There is striking reduction in hematopoietic and fat cells with accumulation of amorphous, eosinophilic substance in interstices. (Hematoxylin-cosin; ×40.)

recent and rapid weight loss, the changes may be present with intervening areas of normal myelopoiesis; in patients with more dramatic and long-standing weight loss, virtually the entire marrow biopsy may manifest the changes of serous degeneration (Fig. 1147). These changes also have been described as gelatinous transformation of the marrow.[32] Studies have indicated that the intercellular substance is primarily hyaluronic acid.

Postchemotherapy bone marrow aplasia

Bone marrow necrosis and aplasia occur with the use of many of the antineoplastic drugs, particularly the antileukemic agents. The sequence of histopathologic events is marked initially by nuclear karyorrhexis, which is succeeded by karyolysis. The cells eventually are replaced by a granular, eosinophilic debris. This stage is followed by the beginning pro-

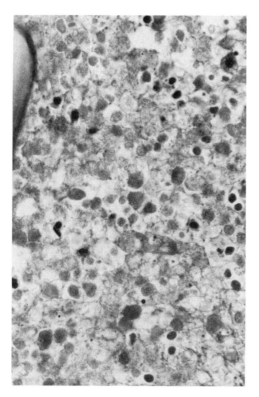

Fig. 1148 Bone marrow infarction. Section is from black patient in sickle cell crisis. Majority of cells manifest karyorrhexis characteristic of early stage of infarction. (Hematoxylin-eosin; ×160.)

liferation of cellular elements; the marrow develops a somewhat irregular, loosely structured appearance with scattered fat cells, vessels, stromal elements, and hematopoietic cells. The erythroid cells are usually the first myeloid elements to recover and frequently manifest megaloblastic changes due to the effects of chemotherapeutic drugs.[25] The regeneration of the erythroid series is followed in sequence by the granulocyte and megakaryocyte precursors in the successfully treated patient.

Reactive hyperplasia

A hypercellular bone marrow may be found in several hematopoietic disorders, both benign and neoplastic. The benign disorders characterized by hypercellularity are the cellular maturation defects such as the megaloblastic and sideroblastic anemias or the disorders attended by increased rates of destruction or utilization of the various cellular elements in which the hypercellularity is due to a compensatory hyperplasia. The hemolytic anemias are gen-

erally characterized by a striking erythroid hyperplasia. In autoimmune or drug-induced thrombocytopenia, the megakaryocytes are normal to increased in number.

Bone marrow infarction

Bone marrow infarction and necrosis uncommonly occur in patients with acute leukemia, primarily lymphoblastic[36]; it also has been observed in patients with sickle cell anemia, infectious processes, systemic lupus erythematosus, caisson disease, and megaloblastic anemias complicated by infection[33-35] (Fig. 1148). The process of infarction may be accompanied by very severe and generalized bone pain.

The marrow specimens from these patients may have a gelatinous-like consistency. The microscopic picture in the trephine section reflects the stage of necrosis. In the early stages, the nuclei show pyknosis and karyorrhexis and the cells have a granular appearance. This is followed by karyolysis; the cell outlines can be appreciated, but the cells are faintly and uniformly eosinophilic. In advanced stages, all cell outlines disappear and the medullary cavity is replaced by an amorphous, granular, eosinophilic debris. The trabeculae may be involved in the process and show loss of osteocytes.[36]

Inflammatory disorders
Granulomatous inflammation

The inflammatory diseases that may be detected in bone marrow biopsies are primarily the granulomatous disorders. The etiologic basis for these lesions varies and includes fungi, *Mycobacterium tuberculosis,* sarcoidosis, *Mycoplasma pneumoniae,* and viral infections, such as infectious mononucleosis.[37,40,42] Noninfectious granulomas also may be found in patients with Hodgkin's disease and non-Hodgkin's lymphomas.[41] Perivascular granulomas may be noted in some of the vasculitides. In approximately 80% of bone marrow granulomas, there is no etiologic basis established for the lesions.[42]

The appearance of granulomas in the bone marrow is similar to that in other tissues. A single granuloma may be found or the marrow in virtually the entire biopsy specimen may be replaced (Fig. 1149). Occasionally, the granulomas are surrounded by a collection of well-differentiated lymphocytes. The granulomas found in association with infectious mononucleosis are usually small and composed only of epithelioid cells. Cells with prominent intra-

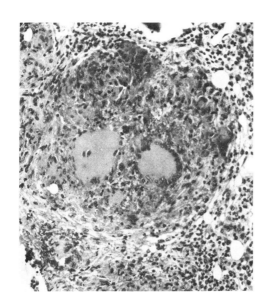

Fig. 1149 Granuloma in bone marrow section from patient being treated for acute lymphoblastic leukemia. No organisms were identified in special stains or culture specimens. (Hematoxylin-eosin; ×51.)

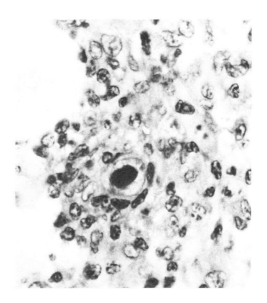

Fig. 1150 Cytomegalovirus inclusion in bone marrow cell of renal transplant patient with serologically documented cytomegalovirus infection. (Hematoxylin-eosin; ×400.)

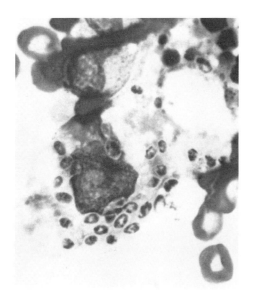

Fig. 1151 Macrophage with *Histoplasma* organisms in bone marrow smear of patient with disseminated histoplasmosis. (Wright's-Giemsa; ×400.)

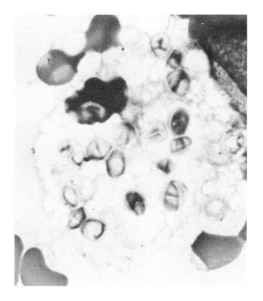

Fig. 1152 Macrophage with numerous cryptococci in bone marrow smear from patient with poorly differentiated lymphocytic lymphoma being investigated for fever. Numerous granulomas were present in marrow sections. (Wright's-Giemsa; ×400.)

nuclear inclusions may be found in patients with cytomegalovirus infection (Fig. 1150).

An unusual granulomatous lesion referred to as "doughnut type" has been noted in the bone marrow from some patients with Q fever. The appearance of these lesions varies from fat globules encircled by a rim of fibrinoid material and polymorphonuclear leukocytes to a typical granuloma.[41a] The specificity of this lesion for Q fever has been questioned.[42a]

As with other tissues, stains for acid-fast bacilli and fungi should be performed in all cases of bone marrow granulomas. The need for culture of a portion of the bone marrow aspirate for acid-fast bacilli and fungi should be anticipated in all patients suspected of having a granulomatous disorder or being investigated for a fever of undetermined etiology.

The presence of infectious granulomas in the bone marrow sections may occasionally be predicted by the presence of macrophages containing microorganisms in the bone marrow smears or trephine imprints. The morphology of the organisms in these preparations is frequently adequate to establish a diagnosis (Figs. 1151 and 1152).

Bone marrow biopsies performed on patients receiving chemotherapy for malignant disorders should always be thoroughly examined for granulomas because of the possibility of opportunistic infections occurring as a result of immunosuppression. Typical granulomas may not be present in the marrow of immunosuppressed patients with disseminated histoplasmosis; the organisms may be identified in macrophages scattered diffusely or occurring in small aggregates in biopsy sections.

Lipid granulomas in the bone marrow are similar to those found in the liver, spleen, and lymph nodes.[43] These granulomas range from 0.2μ-0.8μ in size and usually are associated with a lymphocytic aggregate or sinusoid. They contain fat vacuoles of varying size occurring either in macrophages or extracellularly (Fig. 1153). The lesions also contain lymphocytes, plasma cells, and eosinophils; giant cells are found in approximately 5% of the lesions. Some of the granulomas resemble those found in sarcoidosis. A relationship of the lipid granulomas to mineral oil ingestion has been suggested.[43]

Nonspecific inflammatory reactions

Nonspecific inflammatory alterations in the bone marrow may be noted in patients with a variety of disorders, including acute infectious processes, malignant lymphomas, and connective tissue disorders. These changes generally are characterized by changes in both the vascular structures and the parenchyma. The term "tumor myelopathy" has been applied to the nonspecific marrow changes that are observed in a high percentage of patients with malignant lymphoma.[39] These changes include swelling of the vessel walls, plasma cell and mast cell proliferations in the adventitia, protein deposits adjacent to the vessels, patchy edema of the marrow, depressed erythropoiesis, and increased granulopoiesis and megakaryocytopoiesis. Areas of acute necrosis of bone marrow tissue may be found in patients with tuberculosis and typhoid fever[38] (Fig. 1154).

Oxalosis

An unusual form of granulomatous reaction can be found in the bone marrow in the genetic

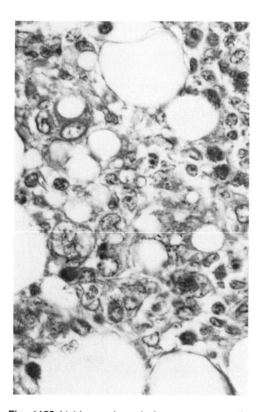

Fig. 1153 Lipid granuloma in bone marrow section. Several fat vacuoles are present both intracellularly in macrophages and extracellularly. This granuloma is associated with small aggregate of well-differentiated lymphocytes. (Hematoxylin-eosin; ×160.)

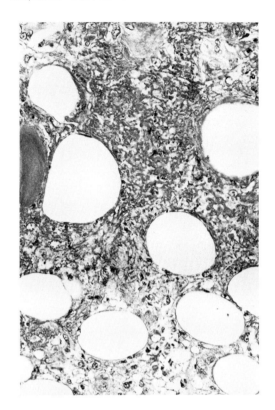

Fig. 1154 Acute fibrinoid necrosis in bone marrow section from patient with disseminated tuberculosis. No typical granulomatous lesions were found. Stains and culture for acid-fast bacilli were negative. (Hematoxylin-eosin; ×400.)

disorder of glyoxalate metabolism, primary hyperoxaluria.[44,45] The granulomatous reaction is secondary to the deposition of calcium oxalate crystals. The crystals, which have a slightly yellowish tinge and form a radial pattern, are encircled by epithelioid and giant cells and are doubly refractile with polarized light (Fig. 1155). Substantial portions of the marrow biopsy may be replaced by these lesions, which are similar to those found in the kidneys and other tissues.

Amyloidosis

Amyloid in the bone marrow is usually detected in biopsies of patients being evaluated for Bence Jones proteinuria or some other form of monoclonal gammopathy; rarely it will be found in marrows of patients without any clinical indication of the disorder. Marrow involvement may manifest either as small focal lesions or as extensive marrow replacement.[46] Early involvement is characterized by focal deposits of amyloid in the medullary vessels; these range from small deposits in the media to large accumulations that greatly thicken the walls, resulting in narrowing of the vessel lumen (Fig. 1156). With more extensive involvement, the accumulation of amyloid will be present in the perivascular tissue and marrow substance. Confluence of deposits results in large masses of amyloid with hematopoietic cells in the interstices. An increase in plasma cells is usually present. Stains for amyloid should be used to confirm the diagnosis.

Leukemias and related disorders
Acute leukemia

The diagnosis and classification of the acute leukemias are established from examination of Romanovsky-stained blood and bone marrow smears in conjunction with appropriate cytochemical techniques.[47,48] The trephine biopsy primarily provides a means for evaluating marrow cellularity. This is of considerable importance in monitoring changes resulting from chemotherapy.

In the majority of patients with acute leukemia, either myeloid or lymphocytic (both children and adults), the marrow sections will be moderately to markedly hypercellular due to an increase in leukemic cells; normal marrow elements are decreased. In some older individuals with subacute or smoldering myeloid leukemia, the marrow sections may be normocellular and occasionally moderately hypocellular, suggesting the diagnosis of aplastic anemia; the diagnosis of leukemia is established from the observation of an increased number of myeloblasts in the blood and marrow smears and the frequently accompanying maturational abnormalities in the developing myeloid cells.

Myelofibrosis may occur in the initial or late stages of the acute leukemias; it is more common in acute lymphoblastic leukemia than in acute myelogenous leukemia[53] (Fig. 1157). The presence of myelofibrosis in acute leukemia may result in difficult and inadequate marrow aspiration and an erroneous diagnosis of aplastic anemia if sections are not available. This problem is more prevalent in pediatric than adult medicine and emphasizes the importance of obtaining adequate tissue sections in aplastic anemia. The long-held view that difficult aspirations in acute leukemia are due to "packed" marrows has little basis in fact. The vast majority of hypercellular marrows in acute leukemia are readily aspirated. If difficulty in

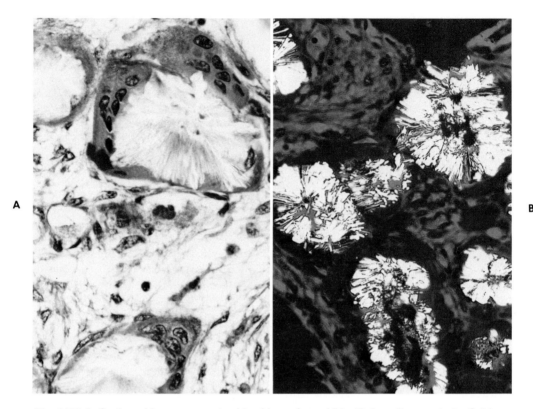

Fig. 1155 A, Section of bone marrow trephine biopsy from child with hereditary oxalosis. Calcium oxalate crystals form radial pattern and appear to be encircled by giant cells. **B,** Calcium oxalate crystals are doubly refractile in polarized light. (**A** and **B,** Hematoxylin-eosin; **A,** ×400; **B,** ×205.)

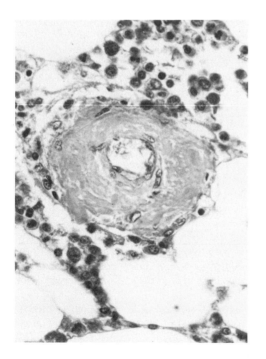

aspiration is encountered, it is probably due to poor technique or an increase in reticulin fibers in the marrow.

Granulocytic sarcoma (chloroma)

An unusual variant of myeloid malignancy characterized by a tumor mass composed of myeloblasts or myeloblasts and neutrophil promyelocytes is the granulocytic sarcoma.[51,52,58,60] In earlier literature, the term chloroma was applied to this lesion because of the green appearance of the freshly cut surface.[52] The green color, which is due to the presence of peroxidase in the leukemic cells, is not present in all tumors of this type and the less specific designation of granulocytic sarcoma is preferred for this lesion.[57] The green color fades after exposure to air but may be

Fig. 1156 Marrow vessel with amyloid accumulation in media. Specimen is from patient with primary amyloidosis. (Hematoxylin-eosin; ×128.)

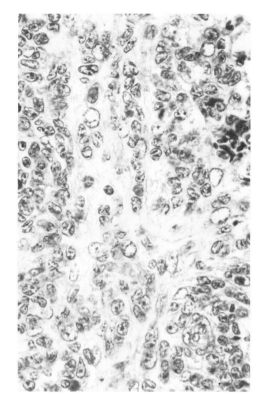

Fig. 1157 Bone marrow section from child with acute lymphoblastic leukemia showing moderate amount of fibrosis associated with leukemic proliferation. (Hematoxylin-eosin; ×160.)

temporarily restored after the application of hydrogen peroxide to the cut surface.

The granulocytic sarcomas are more frequent in children than in adults and are most commonly associated with bone structures; the bones most frequently involved are the skull, paranasal sinuses, sternum, ribs, vertebrae, and pelvis. Orbital masses leading to proptosis or spinal canal lesions resulting in neurologic manifestations are two of the clinical presentations associated with this tumor. A high incidence of granulocytic sarcomas involving the orbit has been reported in Turkish children with acute myelomonocytic leukemia.[49] Granulocytic sarcomas may also occur in nonosseous tissues. The tumor may occur simultaneously with a typical blood and bone marrow pattern of acute myelogenous leukemia or may antedate leukemia by many months or, rarely, years.[56] A granulocytic sarcoma may be the first evidence of relapse in a patient with acute myeloblastic leukemia on chemotherapy and may be the only evidence of recurrence.

Histologically, the tumor is composed of a relatively uniform population of immature cells and is frequently misdiagnosed as one of the poorly differentiated malignant lymphomas. Occasionally, the presence of immature eosinophils and differentiating neutrophils may indicate the true nature of the lesion. The chloracetate esterase stain, which stains granulocytic cells in formalin-fixed tissue, will confirm the diagnosis.[54] Imprint preparations may be extremely valuable in clarifying the myeloid nature of the cells. Auer rods may be found, and the myeloblasts may show intense myeloperoxidase activity.

Local tumor masses occurring in the absence of blood or marrow involvement may respond to local radiation therapy. Eventually the process will evolve into acute myelogenous leukemia that may be associated with additional tumor masses in other sites.

Granulocytic sarcomas may occur during the blastic transformation of chronic myelogenous leukemia and may represent the initial manifestation of the blast crisis.[50,61] Chromosome studies of the cells from these lesions will show a Philadelphia chromosome or one of the chromosome abnormalities associated with the blast crisis phase of chronic myeloid leukemia, such as a double Philadelphia chromosome,[59] an isochromosome for the long arm of chromosome 17, or a trisomy 8.

Tumor masses of monoblasts may occur and may resemble histiocytic lymphomas. The nature of these lesions is most readily appreciated from imprint preparations; the monoblasts will be variably positive with the nonspecific esterase reaction.[55] The chloroacetate esterase stain will be negative or only very slightly positive. These tumors may evolve into acute monoblastic leukemia.

Chronic myelogenous leukemia

Chronic myelogenous leukemia is generally characterized by an elevated leukocyte count with basophilia, decreased neutrophil alkaline phosphatase, and the detection of the Philadelphia chromosome. The number of myeloblasts in the blood and marrow smears in the chronic phase does not usually exceed 5%. The trephine sections are markedly hypercellular, due primarily to an increase in the granulocytes and megakaryocytes. Gaucher-like cells, usually occurring singly, may be present in the bone marrow smears and sections.

The natural history of chronic myelogenous

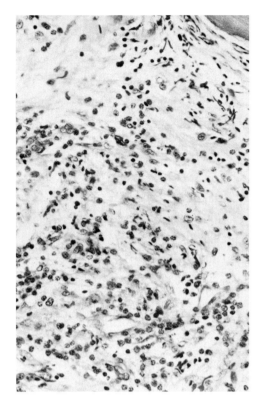

Fig. 1158 Bone marrow section from patient with chronic myelogenous leukemia in myelofibrotic stage. There is marked increase in connective tissue; hematopoietic cells are scattered throughout connective tissue. (Hematoxylin-eosin; ×100.)

leukemia is to evolve into an accelerated phase that is characterized by a progressive increase in blast cells,[62,64] basophils, or myelofibrosis (Fig. 1158). These changes may occur independently or concurrently. In some patients, the blast transformation may be initially manifest in the bone marrow sections as large, irregular, focal collections of blast cells. In approximately 25% of the blast transformations of chronic myelogenous leukemia, the immature cells will resemble the lymphoblasts of acute lymphoblastic leukemia and will contain the nuclear enzyme terminal deoxynucleotidyl transferase.[62a] The development of myelofibrosis in patients with chronic myelogenous leukemia usually occurs late in the disease process and is generally attended by a rapid clinical course,[63] in contrast to the myelofibrosis occurring in agnogenic myeloid metaplasia, which is present in some form from the outset of the disease and usually is accompanied by a prolonged clinical course, although exceptions to this generaliza-

tion have been reported.[62b] Unusually, myelofibrosis may occur in the early stages of chronic myeloid leukemia with the same prognostic implications as when it occurs late in the disease.

Polycythemia vera

Polycythemia vera is generally classified with the myeloproliferative syndromes[66]; it is characterized by an increased red cell mass and, frequently, splenomegaly. There is usually some degree of leukocytosis and thrombocytosis. The neutrophil alkaline phosphatase is elevated or at the upper range of normal in most patients. Criteria for the diagnosis have been established by the Polycythemia Study Group.[77] The bone marrow sections are usually markedly hypercellular and manifest a panhyperplasia.[67,68] Megakaryocytic hyperplasia may be striking, and many unusually large megakaryocytes may be present (Fig. 1159). A slight increase in the number of reticulin fibers may be evident at the outset of the disease. The increase in reticulin corresponds, in general, to the increase in the cellularity of the specimen.[67] Stains for iron will usually show diminished to absent hemosiderin deposits. The evolution of the disease is frequently marked by the development of myelofibrosis, which may closely resemble idiopathic myelofibrosis; the incidence varies from 15%-20%.[73-75] An additional complication in some patients with polycythemia vera is the development of acute myelogenous leukemia. The incidence in different studies has varied considerably, and some controversy has existed as to the relationship of the leukemic process to the therapy employed in polycythemia.[65,69,70,72,76]

Idiopathic thrombocythemia is a myeloproliferative disorder that is closely related to polycythemia vera. The bone marrow findings of increased and large megakaryocytes are similar to those found in polycythemia.[71]

Myelofibrosis

Myelofibrosis is an accompaniment of several of the diseases that involve bone marrow tissue[78,82]; the most common causes are metastatic tumor and malignant lymphoma. Marrow fibrosis also occurs relatively frequently in the evolution of some of the myeloproliferative disorders, such as chronic myelogenous leukemia and polycythemia vera. In these various diseases, the myelofibrosis is related to the underlying disease process and may be referred to

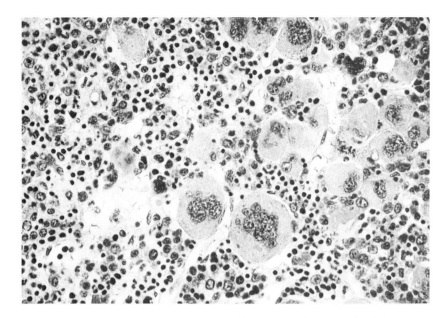

Fig. 1159 Hyperplastic bone marrow from patient with polycythemia vera. All cellular elements are increased. Prominent megakaryocytes show considerable variation in size; many are unusually large. (Hematoxylin-eosin; ×100.)

as secondary myelofibrosis. The etiologic basis for the myelofibrosis in these instances usually can be identified in the marrow biopsy or established from the clinical history.

Idiopathic or primary myelofibrosis is a disease of undetermined etiology; both benign and neoplastic origins have been proposed.[81,83,84,86,88] It occurs primarily in adults; the average age at diagnosis is approximately 60 years.[88] Rare cases have been reported in the pediatric population.[87] The marrow fibrosis in this disorder is usually accompanied by some degree of detectable hepatosplenomegaly due to extramedullary hematopoiesis. A commonly recognized term for this combination of findings is agnogenic myeloid metaplasia. Idiopathic myelofibrosis may, at times, be confused with chronic myelogenous leukemia; the important differentiating clinical and laboratory findings have been described in detail.[88] An important distinguishing feature is the presence of the Philadelphia chromosome in the myeloid cells in approximately 80%-90% of the patients with chronic myelogenous leukemia and its absence in the myeloid cells of patients with primary myelofibrosis. In addition, the neutrophil alkaline phosphatase is decreased in approximately 90% of the patients with chronic myeloid leukemia and is normal or increased in the majority of patients with agnogenic myeloid meta-

plasia. Marrow fibrosis in chronic myeloid leukemia is generally a late occurrence, and its onset usually heralds a more malignant course, unlike agnogenic myeloid metaplasia, where marrow fibrosis is present from the inception and is generally associated with a prolonged clinical course.

In primary myelofibrosis, the medullary space is hypercellular with varying proportions of connective tissue elements and hematopoietic cells. In the early stages, the marrow is characterized by an increase in myeloid cells, arterial vascular structures, and connective tissue.[80,88] The increase in connective tissue elements may be very slight, and an appreciation of the increase in reticulin fibers may be discerned only with the use of special stains; however, difficulty in aspirating bone marrow may be noted even in this early phase. In later stages of the disease, there may be a striking distortion of the marrow due to the deposition of dense fibrous connective tissue. Megakaryocytes are increased in number, show pronounced variation in size, and may occur in clusters. A reduction in the number of erythroid and granulocyte elements is evident. In advanced myelofibrosis, the marrow space appears to be almost totally replaced by connective tissue with scattered foci of hematopoiesis (Fig. 1160, *A*). Attempts at aspiration at this stage are almost uni-

Fig. 1160 A, Trephine biopsy from patient with seven-year history of idiopathic myelofibrosis (agnogenic myeloid metaplasia). There is extensive marrow fibrosis with marked reduction in hematopoietic tissue. **B,** Reticulin stain of specimen illustrated in **A** shows marked increase in reticulin fibers, which are thickened and have wavy pattern. (**A,** Hematoxylin-eosin; ×100; **B,** Wilder's reticulin; ×100.)

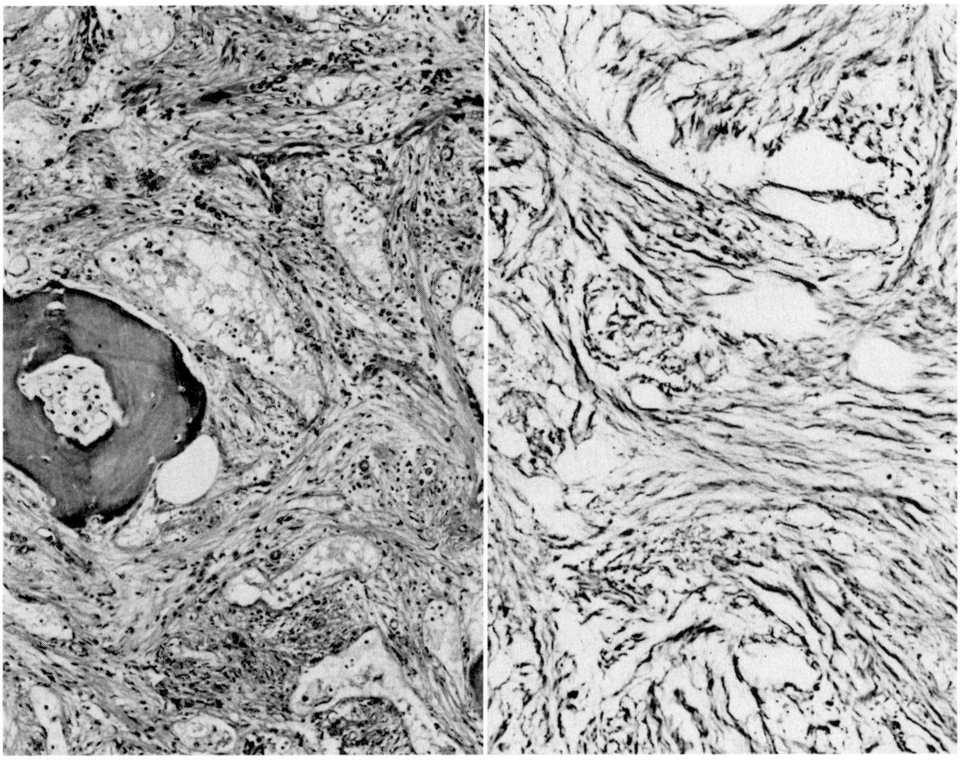

formly unsuccessful. Special stains for collagen frequently show only slight positivity; stains for reticulin show a marked increase in dense reticulin fibers, which may have a wavy pattern (Fig. 1160, *B*). The increase in connective tissue elements in the medullary portion of the marrow may be accompanied by an increase in the size of the bone trabeculae due to membranous bone formation.[88] This stage is referred to as myelosclerosis or osteosclerosis. The findings at this stage are in contrast to the myelofibrosis associated with chronic myelogenous leukemia and polycythemia vera, in which abnormal medullary bone formation is unusual. In approximately 40% of the patients with agnogenic myeloid metaplasia, osteosclerotic changes can be demonstrated by x-ray examination, most notably in the bones of the axial skeleton and the proximal portions of the long bones.[88]

The majority of patients with primary myelofibrosis have a relatively long clinical course

with an estimated median survival of approximately ten years from the onset of disease. A minor population of patients with this disorder have a more rapid course, with a median survival of approximately two years. The term "malignant myelosclerosis" has been used to describe patients with the more aggressive form of this disease.[79,85]

Chronic lymphocytic leukemia

Chronic lymphocytic leukemia is characterized by an increase in well-differentiated lymphocytes in the blood and marrow.[97,98] The absolute blood lymphocyte count generally exceeds 15,000,[101] although the diagnosis should be suspected in adults with a persistent absolute lymphocyte count exceeding 5,000. It is primarily a disorder of B cells, although the lymphocytes from approximately 1% of patients with chronic lymphocytic leukemia have T cell membrane surface markers.[91] The disease frequently is accompanied by some degree of

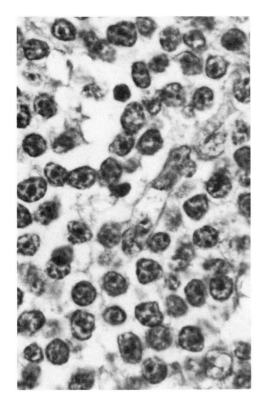

Fig. 1161 Lymphocytes in this bone marrow section from patient with chronic lymphocytic leukemia have clumped nuclear chromatin, absent or indistinct nucleoli, and regular nuclear outline. (Hematoxylin-eosin; ×400.)

lymphadenopathy and hepatosplenomegaly. The morphology of the proliferating cells in chronic lymphocytic leukemia and well-differentiated lymphocytic lymphoma is similar.

The cytology of the lymphocytes in chronic lymphocytic leukemia may be somewhat heterogeneous from case to case and within a case, and this heterogeneity is reflected in the section material.[97,98] In the majority of patients, the predominating cell is small with a sparse amount of cytoplasm (Fig. 1161). The nuclear chromatin is clumped and nucleoli are absent or indistinct. In a minority of patients, the lymphocytes will possess a moderate amount of cytoplasm and the nucleus will show less clumping. Nucleoli may be present and occasionally prominent.

The lymphocytic infiltration in the bone marrow in chronic lymphocytic leukemia may be focal or diffuse or a combination of these patterns. The diffuse distribution is more common. When the increase in blood lymphocytes is modest, the degree of marrow infiltration may vary considerably. In some instances, there may be only minimal replacement of marrow tissue by the well-differentiated lymphocytes with considerable sparing of normal marrow elements. In other cases, the marrow may appear to be entirely replaced. In patients with a very high absolute lymphocyte count, the marrow generally manifests extensive replacement. Even in patients with extensive infiltration, there may be evidence of normal marrow function as reflected by a normal hemoglobin, platelet count, and neutrophil count. Biopsies from approximately 25% of the patients with chronic lymphocytic leukemia will demonstrate an increase in reticulin fibers.

In some patients with chronic lymphocytic leukemia, there will be a dedifferentiation of the proliferating cell type; this usually occurs late in the course of the disease in approximately 5% of the patients and has been referred to as "prolymphocytoid" transformation.[93a] In this group, the marrow infiltration may contain foci of more immature lymphocytes, prolymphocytes, and precursors. These foci may be circumscribed by more well-differentiated lymphocytes. These cells have a moderate amount of basophilic to amphophilic cytoplasm, coarsely reticular nuclear chromatin, and relatively prominent nucleoli. These foci are similar to the immature foci noted in the lymph nodes of some patients with this disorder[93,98] (Fig. 1162).

The prolymphocytic variant of chronic lymphocytic leukemia, described by Galton et al.,[94] is an unusual form of the disease occurring primarily in older individuals and is characterized by a primary proliferation of more immature lymphocytes referred to as prolymphocytes (Figs. 1163 and 1164). The lymphocyte count is markedly elevated; the patients have massive splenomegaly without prominent peripheral lymphadenopathy. The bone marrow sections show an infiltration by lymphocytes that have the cytologic characteristics of the prolymphocytes found in the immature foci that may occur in lymph nodes from patients with chronic lymphocytic leukemia.[93,98] The marrow pattern may be characterized by foci of prolymphocytes surrounded by well-differentiated lymphocytes. This variant is usually marked by an aggressive clinical course.

Difficulties may occur in distinguishing immature foci in chronic lymphocytic leukemia from poorly differentiated lymphocytic lym-

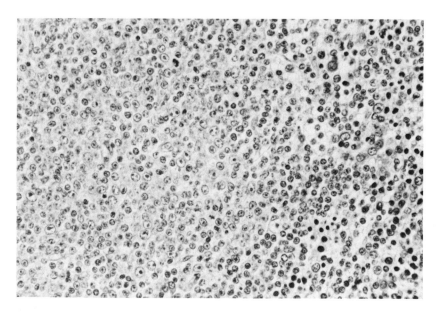

Fig. 1162 Immature focus in bone marrow section from patient with four-year history of chronic lymphocytic leukemia. Cells on left are large and have prominent nucleoli in contrast to well-differentiated lymphocytes on right, which are more typical of chronic lymphocytic leukemia. Blood smear from this patient contained numerous prolymphocytes. Patient survived for four months after this biopsy. (Hematoxylin-eosin; ×100.)

phoma. An important feature in chronic lymphocytic leukemia is the differentiation of the more immature-appearing cells to well-differentiated lymphocytes. Examination of the blood and marrow smears will aid considerably in distinguishing these two disorders.

The distinction between chronic lymphocytic leukemia and well-differentiated lymphocytic lymphoma in the marrow is based on arbitrary criteria. If the absolute lymphocyte count exceeds 5,000, the designation chronic lymphocytic leukemia is preferred.

Richter's syndrome

Richter's syndrome has been used to describe the rare occurrence of a plemorphic lymphoma in a patient with a prior history of chronic lymphocytic leukemia.[95,96,99] The syndrome is characterized by an abrupt change in the patient's clinical course with manifestations of fever, weight loss, localized adenopathy, lymphocytopenia, dysglobulinemia, and histopathologic demonstration of a pleomorphic malignant lymphoma containing multinucleated giant cells. Evidence of chronic lymphocytic leukemia is usually present in bone marrow or lymph node. The disorder is usually marked by an aggressive clinical course and rapid deterioration. The term "Richter's transformation" has been used to describe a somewhat broader spectrum of pathologic findings in patients with chronic lymphocytic leukemia who present with a similar clinical evolution.[93b] The occurrence of a diffuse histiocytic lymphoma in patients with a prior history of chronic lymphocytic leukemia, who do not manifest the findings of Richter's syndrome, has been reported.[89]

The biologic events resulting in the terminal lymphoma are not completely understood, but a dedifferentiation or transformation of the cells of the chronic lymphocytic leukemia has been suggested.[100] This concept is supported by membrane surface marker studies that have shown similar surface markers on the cells of the original CLL cells and of the subsequent lymphoma cells.[90] A similar biologic evolution has been suggested for Waldenström's macroglobulinemia.[92] One instance in which the cells of the leukemic process and the cells of the pleomorphic lymphoma had dissimilar membrane light-chain markers has been described.[102]

The bone marrow in the Richter transformation (Fig. 1165) may be involved by the pleomorphic lymphoma; the lymphocytes of chronic lymphocytic leukemia and the pleomorphic

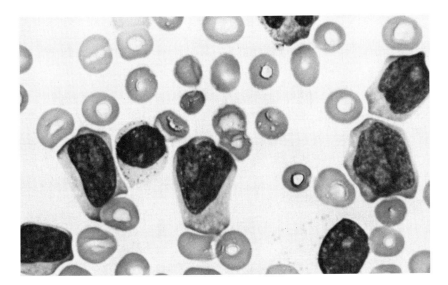

Fig. 1163 Blood smear from 91-year-old male with prolymphocytic variant of chronic lymphocytic leukemia. Prolymphocytes have abundant blue cytoplasm and reticular nuclei with very prominent nucleoli. Well-differentiated lymphocytes are also present. (Wright's-Giemsa; ×400.)

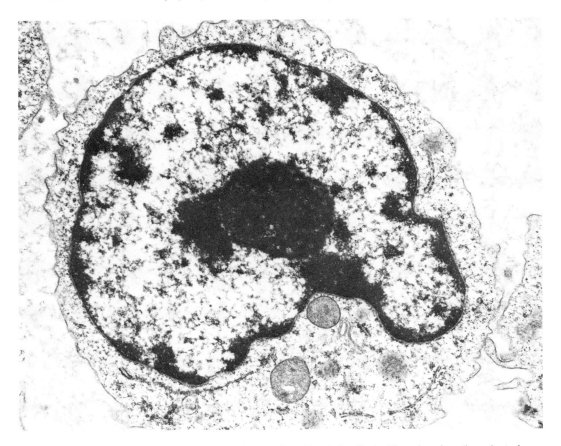

Fig. 1164 Electron micrograph of prolymphocyte from blood of patient with prolymphocytic variant of chronic lymphocytic leukemia. Chromatin is finely distributed and nucleolus is very prominent. (Uranyl acetate–lead citrate; ×15,000.)

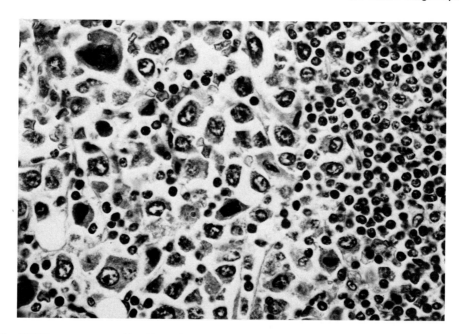

Fig. 1165 Bone marrow trephine biopsy from a patient with history of chronic lymphocytic leukemia who developed pleomorphic lymphoma and clinical picture of Richter's syndrome. Biopsy contains two distinct cell populations, small lymphocytes and large pleomorphic cells, some of which are multinucleated. (Hematoxylin-eosin; ×205.)

lymphoma may be present in the same marrow biopsy. The blood usually shows no involvement by the pleomorphic cells.

Hairy cell leukemia (leukemic reticuloendotheliosis)

Hairy cell leukemia is a disease of apparent B cell origin that is initially diagnosed from blood and bone marrow specimens.[104-106,111-115,116a,117] It has a male predominance and the age range is from 20-80 years, with a median of approximately 50 years.[106,115] The patients generally have cytopenias or pancytopenia and splenomegaly without prominent peripheral lymphadenopathy. The disorder may, on occasion, be confused with other lymphoproliferative disorders, both clinically and morphologically. The disease in the majority of patients follows a chronic course. Splenectomy may be therapeutically beneficial in a substantial number of patients, particularly those with marked thrombocytopenia and neutropenia.

In the majority of patients with leukopenia, only occasional leukemic cells may be found in the peripheral blood. In the 5%-10% of the patients who have white cell counts exceeding 10,000, the hairy cells may comprise the majority of the leukocytes. They typical hairy

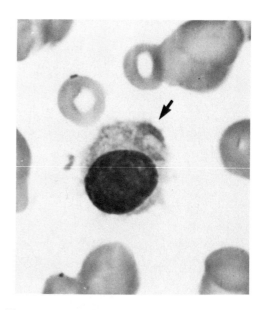

Fig. 1166 Leukemic cell in blood smear of patient with hairy cell leukemia. Cytoplasm is marked by delicate projections, and several ribosome lamella complexes are noted in one area of cytoplasm (arrow). (Wright's-Giemsa; ×400.)

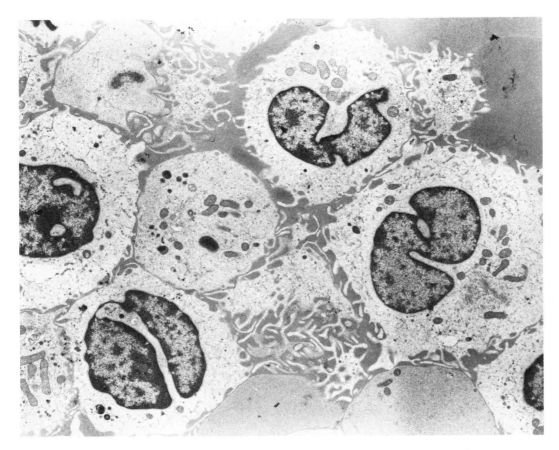

Fig. 1167 Electron micrograph of several cells from blood of patient with hairy cell leukemia. Numerous delicate cytoplasmic projections emanate from cell surfaces. Nuclei are irregular in outline and show margination of chromatin. Nucleoli are relatively inconspicuous. (Uranyl acetate–lead citrate; ×5,000.)

cell measures 10μ-14μ and has an oval, folded, or indented nucleus that has coarsely reticular chromatin and an indistinct nucleolus. The cytoplasm is clear to pale blue with numerous delicate and broad projections (Fig. 1166). These projections have a hairlike appearance on phase microscopy and ultrastructural examination (Fig. 1167). Vacuoles may be present in the cytoplasm. Morphologic variations of the hairy cell have been described.[114]

Difficulty may be encountered in aspirating bone marrow from patients with hairy cell leukemia and "dry taps" occur in 30-50% of the cases.[106] The leukemic infiltrate may be manifest as diffuse or partial involvement; the diffuse type is more common. In the marrows with partial involvement, the lesions of the leukemic process are irregular in outline with a poorly defined line of demarcation from the normal marrow tissue. In very early stages of the disease, the partial involvement may take the form of

relatively small, indistinctly outlined foci of leukemic cells. An important histopathologic feature of hairy cell leukemia is the loose arrangement of the leukemic cells (Fig. 1168, A). In formalin-fixed tissue, artifactual changes resulting in retraction of the cytoplasm of the leukemic cells may create a halo effect around the nucleus. These findings are in contrast to the infiltrates in the poorly differentiated and well-differentiated lymphocytic lymphomas in which the cells are in close apposition. The nuclear chromatin of the hairy cells is relatively fine; nucleoli are not usually prominent. Mitotic figures are infrequently noted. The sparse eosinophilic cytoplasm is irregularly distributed around the nucleus (Fig. 1168, B). A reticulin stain will show increased deposition of thickened reticulin fibers in the areas of the infiltrates (Fig. 1168, C). Marrow uninvolved by the leukemic process is frequently hypocellular; this hypocellularity may, in part, be age related.

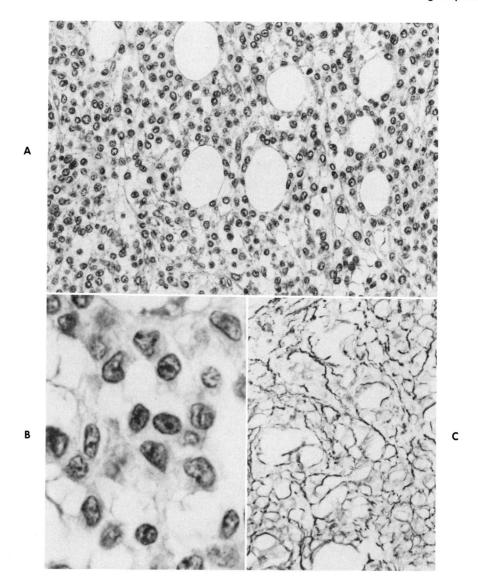

Fig. 1168 A, Bone marrow section from patient with hairy cell leukemia illustrating loosely structured arrangement of leukemic cells characteristic of this disorder. **B,** High magnification of bone marrow section from patient with hairy cell leukemia. Cytoplasm of leukemic cells is sparse, and many of nuclei are folded or irregular in outline. Nucleoli are inconspicuous. Halo effect around nucleus, characteristic of formalin-fixed tissue, is not prominent in this specimen fixed with Zenker's fluid. Mitotic figures are infrequent. **C,** Reticulin stain of bone marrow section from patient with hairy cell leukemia. Thickened and increased reticulin fibers are very irregular in configuration and appear to partially outline individual cells. (**A** and **B,** Hematoxylin-eosin; **A,** ×64; **B,** ×400; **C,** Wilder's reticulin; ×160.)

In some patients with partial involvement, the uninvolved marrow may be hypercellular due primarily to an erythroid hyperplasia.

An important diagnostic procedure in hairy cell leukemia is the demonstration of tartrate-resistant acid phosphatase activity in the leukemic cells.[108,110,116] Other lymphoproliferative disorders in which the proliferating cells have tartrate-resistant acid phosphatase activity have been described[107,110a]; however, these cases are uncommon and do not negate the diagnostic importance of tartrate-resistant acid phosphatase staining in the cells of hairy cell leukemia. Nonspecific esterase positivity also has been demonstrated in the leukemic cells of hairy cell leukemia, utilizing alpha-napthyl acetate and

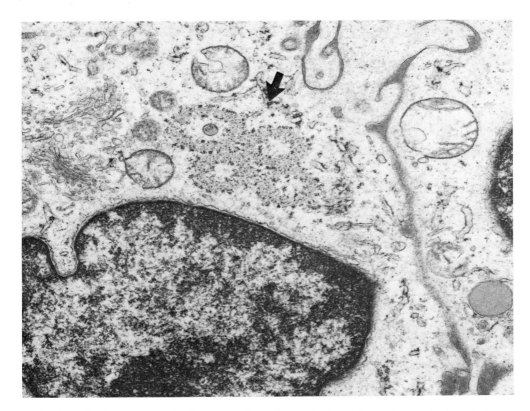

Fig. 1169 Electron micrograph of specimen illustrated in Fig. 1165. Several ribosome-lamella complexes are present in cytoplasm of leukemic cell (arrow). (Uranyl acetate–lead citrate; ×21,000.)

alpha-napthyl butyrate as substrates.[106a,114a] The enzyme activity is inhibited by fluoride when alpha-napthyl acetate is used as a substrate and is fluoride resistant when alpha-napthyl butyrate is used.

An unusual configuration of ribosomes and lamellae, the ribosome lamella complex, has been observed on ultrastructural examination of the cells of leukemic reticuloendotheliosis[109,113] (Fig. 1169). This structure occurs in a varying percentage of hairy cells in approximately 50% of the patients[106]; rarely it may be observed in hairy cells in routinely stained smears (Fig. 1166). The ribosome lamella complex has been observed in the cells of other hematopoietic disorders and lacks diagnostic specificity.[103]

Non-Hodgkin's lymphomas

The value of the bone marrow trephine biopsy in the initial staging of the non-Hodgkin's lymphomas in adults has been amply demonstrated in several studies.[129,133,134,139,154,157] Because marrow involvement constitutes evidence of Stage IV disease, obviates the need for exploratory laparotomy, and contraindicates radiotherapy as a curative procedure, the detection of lymphoma in the marrow has important procedural and therapeutic implications for the patient. The most extensive studies of marrow involvement in the non-Hodgkin's lymphomas in adults have utilized the Rappaport lymph node classification of these tumors.[152] One study utilizing the Lukes-Collins classification has been reported.[137a] The demonstration of marrow involvement at the time of initial diagnosis varies with the different subtypes; the incidence for the subclasses in aggregate is approximately 40% in most of the larger studies.[134,154] In contrast to the experience with adults, the yield of positive trephine biopsies in children with non-Hodgkin's lymphoma in one study was reported to be 3.8%.[148]

Well-differentiated lymphocytic lymphoma

The well-differentiated lymphocytic lymphoma represents a proliferation of the mature or well-differentiated lymphocyte; some observers consider this type of lymphoma as the tissue counterpart of chronic lymphocytic leuke-

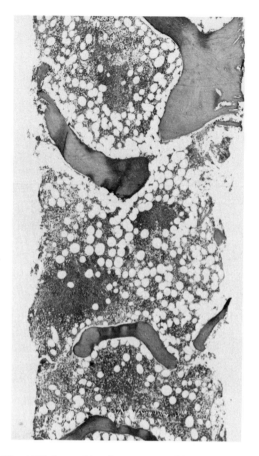

Fig. 1170 Several focal aggregates of lymphocytes in marrow of patient with well-differentiated lymphocytic lymphoma. Foci of lymphocytes are variable in size and have irregular, poorly circumscribed outline. (Hematoxylin-eosin; ×10.)

mia.[140] However, it has been demonstrated that well-differentiated lymphocytic lymphoma may exist as an entity distinct from chronic lymphocytic leukemia and may be associated with the production of a monoclonal immunoglobulin.[151] Because of the cytologic similarity of well-differentiated lymphocytic lymphoma and chronic lymphocytic leukemia, the distinction of these two disorders is based on arbitrary criteria. If the marrow manifests a proliferation of well-differentiated lymphocytes in the absence of a blood lymphocytosis greater than 5,000, the diagnosis of well-differentiated lymphocytic lymphoma is preferred to chronic lymphocytic leukemia. Chronic lymphocytic leukemia is frequently accompanied by hypogammaglobulin; this finding is uncommon in patients with well-differentiated lymphocytic lymphoma.[151] In both chronic lymphocytic leukemia

and well-differentiated lymphocytic lymphoma, the proliferative lymphocyte in the vast majority of instances appears to be of B cell origin.[118,122,128]

In trephine sections, the well-differentiated lymphocytic lymphoma may occur in either a focal or diffuse distribution. The focal aggregates may be irregular in size and outline, and very large aggregates may be present. The aggregates are frequently poorly circumscribed (Fig. 1170). Careful examination of the marrow, exclusive of the focal deposits, will usually reveal an infiltration of the apparently normal tissue by varying numbers of well-differentiated lymphocytes. When the focal aggregates are extremely numerous or very large, they tend to become confluent and resemble a diffuse pattern of involvement. In contrast to some of the poorly differentiated lymphocytic lymphomas, there appears to be no predilection for a paratrabecular distribution of the focal lesions in the well-differentiated lymphocytic lymphomas.

The cells in the well-differentiated lymphocytic lymphomas in sections and smears are characterized by a clumped nuclear chromatin and indistinct or absent nucleoli. The nuclear outlines are uniformly regular; there is no cleavage or folding. A sparse rim of cytoplasm may be present. Some of the well-differentiated lymphocytic lymphomas will contain varying numbers of cells with plasmacytoid characteristics and plasma cells. These may be associated with a monoclonal gammopathy, primarily of the IgM class.[151]

Poorly differentiated lymphocytic lymphoma

The poorly differentiated lymphocytic lymphomas encompass a heterogenous biologic group of lymphomas; this heterogeneity is reflected in the cytology, membrane surface marker characteristics, and clinical evolution.[122,123,126] The nodular lymphocytic lymphomas appear to have more biologic unity than their diffuse counterparts.[140] Marrow involvement in the poorly differentiated lymphocytic lymphomas may occur in a focal or diffuse pattern. It is important to recognize that the characterization of marrow involvement as focal or diffuse bears no relationship to the lymph node pattern of nodular or diffuse lymphoma. Lymphomas of both nodular and diffuse lymph node patterns may manifest as focal or diffuse involvement of the marrow.

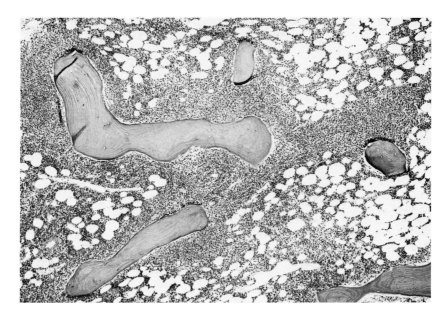

Fig. 1171 Bone marrow section from patient with nodular poorly differentiated lymphocytic lymphoma illustrating prominent paratrabecular distribution of infiltrate. (Hematoxylin-eosin; ×40.)

The incidence of demonstrable marrow involvement in nodular poorly differentiated lymphocytic lymphomas at time of initial diagnosis is approximately 55%-60%.[134,145,157] Both lower and higher percentages of involvement have been reported. In one prospective study, 85% of the patients with nodular poorly differentiated lymphocytic lymphoma had marrow involvement.[154] The reported incidence of marrow involvement for the diffuse poorly differentiated lymphocytic lymphomas at the time of initial diagnosis varies from 30%-60% in different studies.[129,133,134] Bone marrow involvement was observed in approximately 50% of nineteen cases of Lennert's lymphoma.[139a]

The focal marrow lesions in the poorly differentiated lymphocytic lymphomas frequently have a paratrabecular distribution (Fig. 1171), although lesions unrelated to trabeculae are found. The predilection for the paratrabecular location appears to be a more prominent feature in the nodular poorly differentiated lymphocytic lymphomas than in the diffuse poorly differentiated lymphocytic lymphomas. In certain instances the trabeculae appear to serve as a demarcation between large areas of focal marrow involvement and normal marrow. The focal lesions in nodular lymphoma may mimic germinal centers (Fig. 1172). In the marrows with diffuse involvement, the entire marrow space is replaced by tumor, although islands of normal hematopoiesis may be scattered among the lymphoma cells. Increased reticulin fibers can be demonstrated in both focal and diffuse lesions.

The cytology of the lesions in the bone marrow sections generally mimics that of the lesions in the lymph node; occasionally, there will not be exact correspondence. The nodular poorly differentiated lymphocytic lymphomas frequently manifest a spectrum from small, relatively well-differentiated lymphocytes to large, histiocytic-appearing cells.[145] In occasional patients with this type of lymphoma, cells closely resembling Sternberg-Reed cells and their mononuclear variants may be identified[144] (Fig. 1173). This finding appears to be more common in patients with a long history of the disease and in those treated with chemotherapy. These immature cells are usually present in foci scattered among more differentiated cells and may resemble the immature foci of chronic lymphocytic leukemia (Fig. 1174). In a small number of patients, the bone marrow lesions of poorly differentiated lymphocytic lymphoma may contain very large numbers of epithelioid-type histiocytes (Fig. 1175). These may be observed in both the nodular and diffuse types; the arrangement of the histiocytes may, in certain instances, impart a granulomatoid appearance to the lesions. A similar granulomatous appearance characterizes the

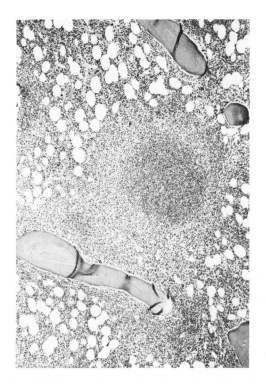

Fig. 1172 Focus of tumor in marrow of patient with nodular poorly differentiated lymphocytic lymphoma that mimics germinal center. Central portion of focus is occupied by more well-differentiated lymphocytes. Peripheral portion has fewer well-differentiated cells. (Hematoxylin-eosin; ×40.)

marrow lesions of Lennert's lymphoma which is frequently multifocal in distribution.[139a] Both benign lymphocytic aggregates and granulomas may occur as incidental findings in the bone marrow of patients with poorly differentiated lymphocytic lymphoma with or without marrow involvement by the lymphoma. The amorphous proteinaceous material described in the lymph node lesions of nodular poorly differentiated lymphocytic lymphoma also may be observed in bone marrow sections.[153]

Peripheral blood involvement may occur in any of the poorly differentiated lymphocytic lymphomas. Although this usually occurs late in the course of the disease, it may be present at initial diagnosis. Uncommonly, it represents the first recognized manifestation of the disease. Patients with nodular poorly differentiated lymphocytic lymphoma may present with marked leukocytosis and a peripheral blood picture resembling chronic lymphocytic leukemia.[145,156] A characteristic cell type, the small nodular lymphoma cell or notched nuclear cell, helps to distinguish these cases from the latter disorder (Figs. 1176 and 1177). A small number of patients with nodular poorly differentiated lymphocytic lymphoma present with a leukemic blood picture marked by a predominance of immature cells and only occasional more dif-

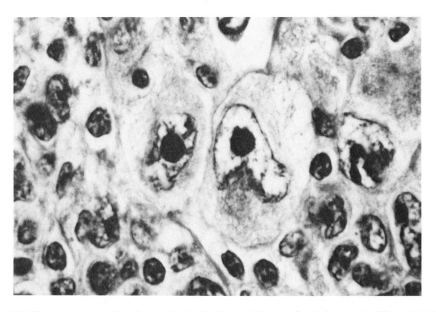

Fig. 1173 Bone marrow section from patient with six-year history of nodular poorly differentiated lymphocytic lymphoma. Two large cells resembling Sternberg-Reed mononuclear variants are present. (Hematoxylin-eosin; ×400.)

ferentiated cells. The accompanying hematologic picture may vary considerably; the hemoglobin, platelet count, and neutrophil count may be normal or markedly decreased, depending upon the degree of marrow replacement.

Lymphoma cells may be found in blood and marrow smears in the absence of obvious infiltration of the sections. These situations are very unusual, and considerable caution must be exercised in the disposition of these cases. In children, normal and reactive marrows may con-

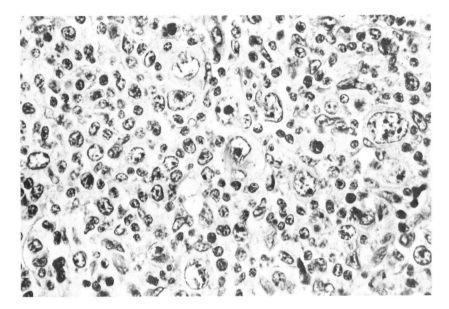

Fig. 1174 Focus of large poorly differentiated cells in marrow of patient with nodular poorly differentiated lymphocytic lymphoma. Numerous smaller cells, more typical of this lesion, are present in this field. (Hematoxylin-eosin; ×160.)

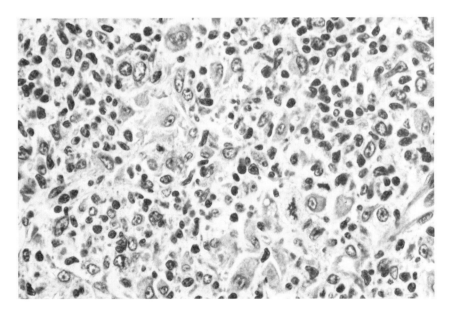

Fig. 1175 Marrow lesions in this patient with nodular poorly differentiated lymphocytic lymphoma contain numerous epithelioid-type histiocytes. (Hematoxylin-eosin; ×100.)

tain increased numbers of ''hematogones,'' normal marrow lymphoid cells that may be mistaken for lymphoma cells.[145]

''Peripheralizing poorly differentiated lymphocytic lymphoma'' or ''lymphosarcoma cell leukemia'' are diagnostic terms frequently misapplied by pathologists and clinicians to cases of acute lymphoblastic leukemia in which the lymphoblasts manifest some degree of nuclear clefting or contortion; the terms are frequently used in the absence of a lymph node biopsy. Although it may not always be possible to distinguish cases of acute lymphoblastic leukemia from poorly differentiated lymphocytic lymphoma with marrow and blood involvement, diffuse infiltration of the marrow accompanied by substantial numbers of blasts in the blood is more compatible with acute lymphoblastic leukemia than lymphoma. The presence of focal lymphadenopathy and tissue masses and evidence of sparing of marrow function as reflected by normal platelet and neutrophil counts and hemoglobin level are more suggestive of lymphoma. If a lymphoma is suspected, the diagnosis should be established from biopsy of a lymph node or tissue mass. In the absence of an extramedullary lesion, the diagnosis of leukemia is preferred.

Histiocytic lymphoma

As noted in the chapter on lymph nodes, the cell type in histiocytic lymphoma in the vast majority of instances probably represents a transformed lymphocyte or immunoblast. Whatever the true biology of the cell classified as a histiocyte, the occurrence of marrow involvement in the lymphomas of this classification is relatively uncommon and, in most series, is the type with the lowest incidence of marrow involvement, approximately 10%.[129,133,157] Two types of involvement have been described in diffuse histiocytic lymphoma, a well-demarcated proliferation of histiocytes in a matrix of increased fibrous tissue and a diffuse infiltration of histiocytes with minimal disruption of the marrow architectural pattern.[133]

The cells of histiocytic lymphoma in the marrow sections resemble the cells in the lymph node tissue (Fig. 1178). The cells, which are of true histiocyte origin as determined by membrane surface markers and positive reactivity with the nonspecific esterase stain, are large and have abundant amounts of eosinophilic cytoplasm and a nucleus that is vesicular in appearance. Nucleoli are frequently very prominent. In imprint and smear preparations, the cells measure approximately 30μ-40μ and have

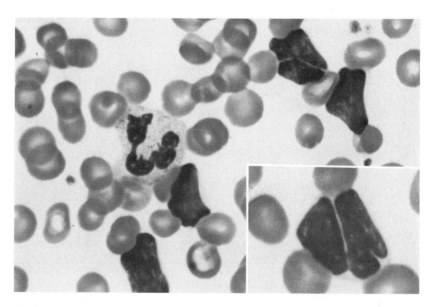

Fig. 1176 Blood smear from patient with nodular poorly differentiated lymphocytic lymphoma presenting with leukocyte count of 34,000 and 70% small nodular lymphoma cells. Blood smear resembles chronic lymphocytic leukemia but is distinguished from that disorder by high percentage of cells with markedly hyperchromatic, clefted nuclei. **Inset,** Higher magnification of small nodular lymphoma cell illustrating marked nuclear clefting that may occur in these cells. (Wright's-Giemsa; ×400; **inset,** Wright's-Giemsa; ×512.)

abundant cytoplasm that is frequently deeply basophilic and contains numerous sharply defined vacuoles. The nuclei may be round or contorted and have nucleoli of varying prominence. Many cells have delicate azurophilic cytoplasmic granules.

Burkitt's lymphoma

Approximately 16% of the patients with the African form of Burkitt's lymphoma[125,131] have evidence of marrow involvement at some time during the course of their illness; this finding has been associated with a relatively poor prognosis.[127] The American form of the Burkitt's lymphoma, although cytologically similar to the African type, appears to have a higher incidence of bone marrow and abdominal involvement.[119,120,132,135,150] Approximately 20% of the patients with the American form of Burkitt's tumor have marrow involvement at the time of

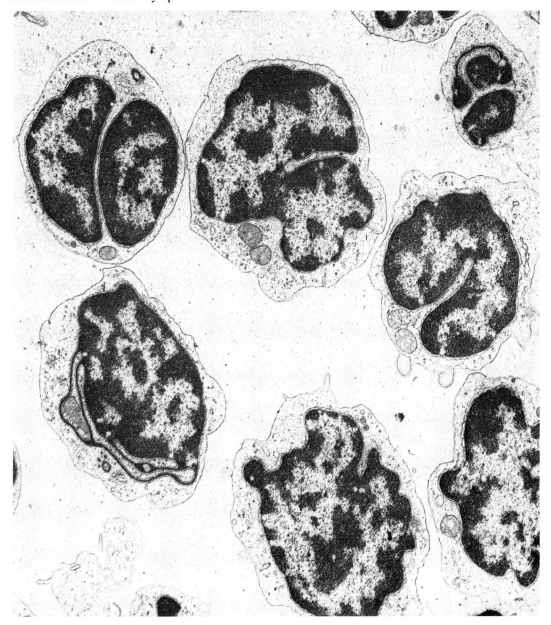

Fig. 1177 Electron micrograph of blood specimen illustrated in Fig. 1175. Many of lymphoma cells show deep nuclear clefts or total bisection of nucleus. (Uranyl acetate-lead citrate; ×9,500).

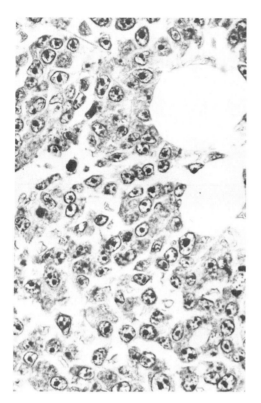

Fig. 1178 Bone marrow section from patient with lymph node diagnosis of histiocytic lymphoma. Tumor cells are large and have abundant cytoplasm and prominent nucleoli. Nuclear rim is very prominent in many cells. (Hematoxylin-eosin; ×160.)

initial diagnosis, and an additional 10% develop marrow involvement during the course of their illness.[119,120]

The marrow biopsy in the involved cases frequently manifests extensive replacement of the hematopoietic cells. The lymphoma cells show a characteristic uniformity in appearance; the nuclei are round or ovoid with no clefting or convolution. A distinct rim of cytoplasm is noted. The large macrophages that lend the "starry sky" appearance to this tumor in lymph nodes are not usually found in the bone marrow sections.

The bone marrow smears and imprints show the characteristic cytology of Burkitt's cells, regularly shaped nuclei, and deeply basophilic cytoplasm that contains several sharply demarcated vacuoles. Small numbers of the lymphoma cells may be present in the peripheral blood, but frankly leukemic pictures are uncommon except as a terminal event. Despite the apparent extensive marrow replacement, evidence of bone marrow sparing, as reflected

by normal platelet and neutrophil counts and hemoglobin, may be present. Survival from the time of marrow involvement is generally brief; a median survival of 2.5 months is reported in one series.[130] A small number of cases of acute leukemia with the typical cytomorphology and B cell membrane surface marker characteristics of Burkitt's tumor cells have been reported[137]; this cytologic type of leukemia is designated L3 in the French-American-British classification of the acute leukemias.[124]

Lymphoblastic lymphoma

Malignant lymphoma, lymphoblastic, is a type of diffuse lymphoma that is distinguished histologically from poorly differentiated lymphocytic lymphoma by a high mitotic index and the cytologic similarity of the lymphoma cells to the lymphoblasts and prolymphocytes of acute lymphoblastic leukemia.[149] Lymphoblastic lymphoma has a high incidence of mediastinal mass and a tendency for early bone marrow and blood involvement and is most frequently observed in male children and young adults. The bone marrow involvement may be present at the time of initial diagnosis, and the distinction between a leukemic process and lymphoma may be difficult. The presence of a tissue mass and evidence of sparing of bone marrow function as indicated by a normal platelet count and normal numbers of neutrophils in the blood are suggestive of a lymphoma, as opposed to leukemia.

The marrow infiltration pattern in lymphoblastic lymphoma is generally diffuse with extensive replacement of myeloid cells. There may be some residual hematopoietic tissue; scattered megakaryocytes and islands of normoblasts and neutrophils may be present. In some instances, less than 50% of the marrow is replaced by tumor; the lymphoma cells are diffusely scattered among the normal hematopoietic elements.

Cytologically, this lymphoma is divided into the convoluted and nonconvoluted types. The cells of the nonconvoluted type have a round or ovoid nucleus. There is a maturation progression from the lymphoblast to the prolymphocyte, a cell characterized by a more condensed nuclear chromatin and less distinct nucleoli than the lymphoblast. The cells of the convoluted nucleus type are smaller than the nonconvoluted nucleus type and manifest a higher incidence of prolymphocytic differentiation. Only a proportion of the cells may show nuclear convolution. Both cytologic types are characterized by

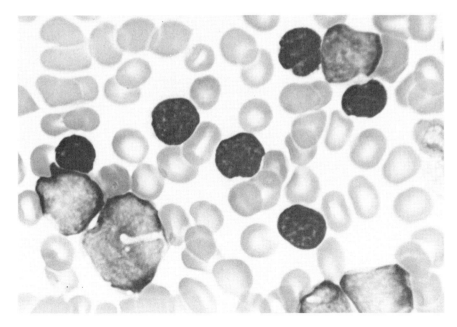

Fig. 1179 Peripheral blood smear from patient with lymphoblastic lymphoma, T cell type, with mediastinal mass diagnosed three months previously. Lymphoma cells consist of lymphoblasts (larger cells) and prolymphocytes (smaller cells). (Wright's-Giemsa; ×400.)

a high mitotic index. Peripheral blood and marrow involvement may be present at the time of diagnosis or may occur later in the course of the disease (Fig. 1179).

A malignant lymphoma of convoluted lymphocytes of probable T cell origin with a high incidence of blood and marrow involvement and clinical findings similar to lymphoblastic lymphoma has been proposed as a distinct clinical morphologic entity.[121] Cases with these morphologic and clinical features have also been described under the term of Sternberg sarcoma.[155]

Although the term lymphoblastic lymphoma was proposed because of the cytologic similarity of the cells in this lesion to the lymphoblasts and prolymphocytes of acute lymphoblastic leukemia, there is a limited biologic similarity of the processes. Lymphoblastic lymphoma is generally marked by a fairly rapid clinical course in contrast to the majority of cases of acute lymphoblastic leukemia, which have a very prolonged clinical course. The clinical course of this lymphoma, however, is similar to that of the approximately 20% of the cases of acute lymphoblastic leukemias that are of T cell type. The lymphoblasts and prolymphocytes in the majority of patients with T cell acute lymphoblastic leukemia manifest

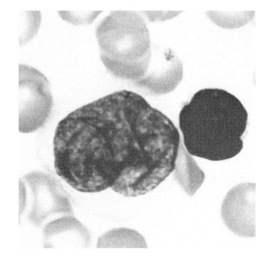

Fig. 1180 Large Sézary cell with "cerebriform" nucleus in peripheral blood of patient with erythroderma. Nucleus of this Sézary cell shows striking degree of convolution. Smaller lymphocyte also has convoluted nucleus. (Wright's-Giemsa; ×400.)

morphologic and cytochemical features that distinguish them from the lymphoblasts and prolymphocytes of the majority of patients with non-T, non-B (null cell) acute lymphoblastic leukemias.[146,147]

Sézary syndrome

The Sézary syndrome is characterized by erythroderma and abnormal lymphoid cells of T cell origin in the peripheral blood[136,142,158,160]; this disorder is closely related to mycosis fungoides and is considered by some observers to be the peripheral blood manifestation of that disease.[138,159]

The leukocyte count may be normal or slightly elevated with a high percentage of Sézary cells. This cell, as represented in Romanovsky-stained blood smears, has distinctive features. The nucleus frequently has an unusual configuration that has been characterized as cerebriform (Fig. 1180). Cytoplasmic vacuoles, which stain positively with the periodic acid–Schiff reaction, may be present in a perinuclear location. This finding is not so frequently noted as the unusual nuclear configuration. Large and small cell variants of the Sézary cell have been described.[143] Ultrastructurally, the cells are similar to those found in the skin in mycosis fungoides[141,159] (Fig. 1181). The bone marrow sections in the majority of patients are normal. Uncommonly, infiltrations similar to those observed in chronic lymphocytic leukemia may be present.[136]

Hodgkin's disease

The incidence of bone marrow involvement in Hodgkin's disease varies from 2%-29% in reported series of previously untreated patients.[161,162,167,168,170,172,174] The demonstration of marrow involvement in Hodgkin's disease appears, in part, to be related to the amount of tissue obtained at biopsy. Accord-

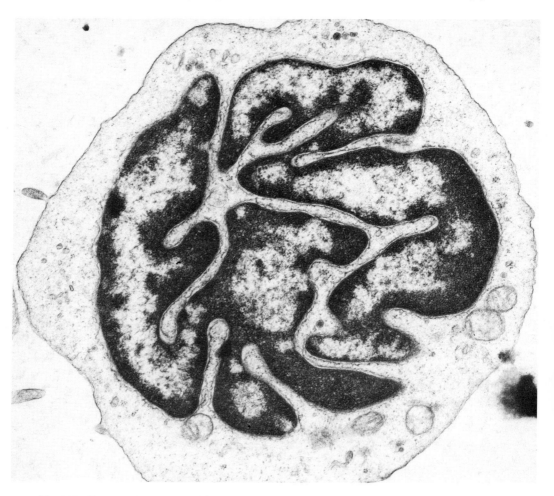

Fig. 1181 Electron micrograph of Sézary cell from peripheral blood of patient with Sézary syndrome. Extreme convolution of nucleus is characteristic ultrastructural feature of Sézary cell. (Uranyl acetate–lead citrate; ×22,000.)

ingly, the performance of multiple biopsies may result in a higher yield of positive cases than if a single biopsy is performed. Marrow involvement may be by virtue of direct extension from contiguously involved lymph nodes or as a result of widely disseminated disease. The latter type of involvement is most common and constitutes Stage IV disease.

The majority of patients with Hodgkin's dis-

ease in the bone marrow at the time of diagnosis have mixed cellularity or nodular sclerosis type; the lymphocyte depletion type is accompanied by a high incidence of marrow involvement but is an uncommon form of Hodgkin's disease.[169] Marrow involvement is most unusual in lymphocyte predominant type.

The histopathologic classification of Hodgkin's disease should not be based on bone mar-

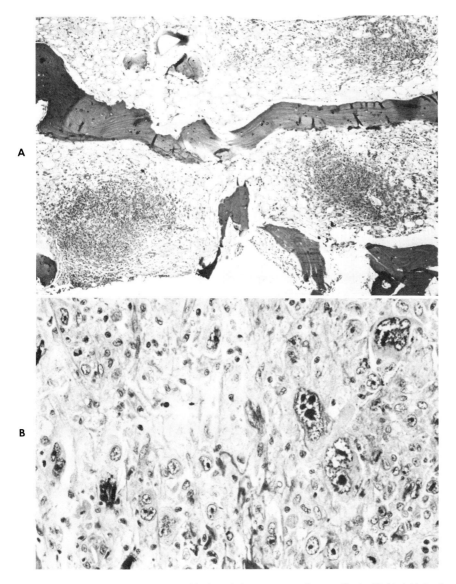

Fig. 1182 A, Three densely cellular focal lesions in bone marrow from patient with Hodgkin's disease. Marrow exclusive of focal lesions is markedly hypocellular, with evidence of serous degeneration. **B,** Bone marrow biopsy from patient with mixed cellularity Hodgkin's disease. Several unusually large Sternberg-Reed-like cells and several mononuclear variants are present. Scattered lymphocytes, plasma cells, histiocytes, and fibroblasts are present. (**A,** Hematoxylin-eosin; ×16; **B,** hematoxylin-eosin; ×160.)

row biopsies because of the difference in manifestations of the disease in lymph node and bone marrow tissue.

Definitive histopathologic criteria for the diagnosis of marrow involvement in Hodgkin's disease have been established.[163,165,171] Involvement may be diagnosed when typical Sternberg-Reed cells are found in a cellular environment characteristic of Hodgkin's disease: fibrous connective tissue containing lymphocytes, eosinophils, plasma cells, and histiocytes. If typical Sternberg-Reed cells cannot be found, the presence of mononuclear variants in a typical Hodgkin's environment will suffice if typical Sternberg-Reed cells have been previously identified in biopsy tissue. The presence of atypical cells in a characteristic Hodgkin's environment in a patient with histopathologically proved disease should be considered suspicious. The presence of fibrosis in the absence of Sternberg-Reed cells or mononuclear variants in a patient with an established diagnosis of Hodgkin's disease should be viewed as suspicious but is not, in itself, sufficient evidence for a definitive diagnosis of marrow involvement.

Hodgkin's lesions in the marrow may be diffuse or focal. The diffuse pattern is found in approximately 70%-80% of the positive cases.[170] In this form, the Hodgkin's tissue replaces the entire area between trabeculae. In the focal pattern, the Hodgkin's tissue is distributed in small isolated lesions that are surrounded by normal hematopoietic tissue. Diffuse and focal involvement may be present in the same specimen. The extent of marrow involvement in different patients may range from a single, small focal lesion to complete replacement of multiple biopsy specimens. The small focal lesions tend to be markedly cellular (Fig. 1182, *A*). The diffuse lesions manifest two types of cellularity: a moderately to markedly hypocellular pattern with a fairly even distribution of cells and variably sized, focally hypercellular areas in a background of loose, sparsely cellular connective tissue in which the predominant cells are lymphocytes or plasma cells, or both. The cellular composition of the focally cellular areas varies; some are polycellular with varying numbers of lymphocytes, plasma cells, eosinophils, neutrophils, histiocytes, and Sternberg-Reed cells or their mononuclear variants (Fig. 1182, *B*). Other infiltrates are predominantly of one cell type, such as lymphocytes, atypical histiocytes, or Sternberg-Reed cells and mononuclear variants. Areas of necrosis, at times extensive, may be present with large areas of fibrin deposition. Stains for reticulin will show an increased number of thickened reticulin fibers in the Hodgkin's lesions.

The identification of Sternberg-Reed cells or their mononuclear variants is of critical impor-

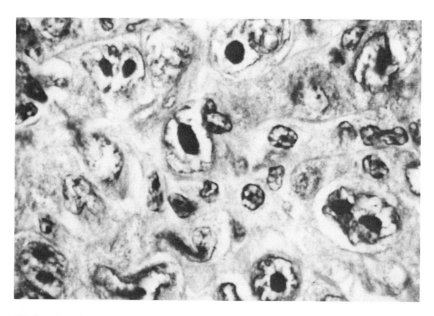

Fig. 1183 Sternberg-Reed cell and mononuclear variants in bone marrow section of patient with nodular sclerosis type of Hodgkin's disease. (Hematoxylin-eosin; ×400.)

tance to the recognition of Hodgkin's disease in the marrow, and the diagnosis should not be established without the demonstration of these cell types in the appropriate milieu for the disease (Fig. 1183). Several serial sections of the marrow biopsies may have to be examined before satisfactory Sternberg-Reed cells or mononuclear variants are identified. Sternberg-Reed cells will not be located in normal hematopoietic tissue, and it is important not to misinterpret megakaryocytes as forms of Sternberg-Reed cells. Although Sternberg-Reed-like cells have been reported in the marrow of patients with nodular lymphoma,[166] the clinical history, membrane marker studies, and characteristic tissue changes of Hodgkin's disease should aid in distinguishing these two disorders.

Bone marrow tissue from patients with Hodgkin's disease that is not involved by the disease process may show nonspecific alterations such as stromal damage, inflammatory infiltration, and disturbed hematopoiesis.[173] These alterations may occur singly or in combination.

Similar to the spleen, liver, and lymph node, benign granulomatous lesions may be found in the bone marrow in cases of Hodgkin's disease.[170] The bone marrow is the least likely organ in this group to contain the granulomas, but their presence may lead to diagnostic difficulty. The granulomas may occur in the ab-

sence of bone marrow involvement by Hodgkin's disease and by themselves do not constitute evidence of the disease.[164,170]

Benign lymphocytic aggregates also may be found in the marrow in the absence of Hodgkin's involvement.

Plasma cell dyscrasias
Multiple myeloma

Multiple myeloma is characterized by a neoplastic proliferation of plasma cells and the production of a monoclonal immunoglobulin detectable in the serum or urine.[175,182,183,188] The distribution of the plasma cells in the marrow in multiple myeloma may be focal in character, and the percentage of these cells may vary considerably in aspirates from different sites. In trephine sections, the plasma cells may be diffusely scattered among the hematopoietic cells or occur in large solid aggregates (Fig. 1184). Because of the possibility of a focal distribution of the plasma cells, it may be necessary to biopsy more than one site in this disorder. Uncommonly, patients with multiple myeloma present with a large number of plasma cells in the peripheral blood (Fig. 1185). The term plasma cell leukemia is used when the plasma cells exceed 20% of the blood leukocytes and the absolute plasma cell count exceeds 2,000.[184] Although this finding is frequently associated with an unfavorable progno-

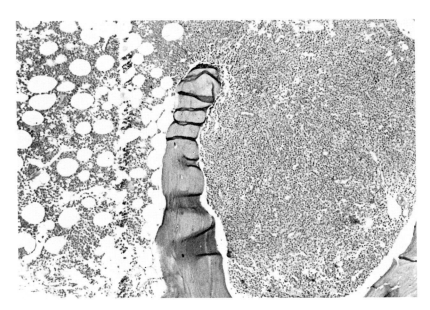

Fig. 1184 Bone marrow section from patient with multiple myeloma illustrating dense focal collection of myeloma cells that appears to be partially demarcated by bone trabeculum. (Hematoxylin-eosin; ×26.)

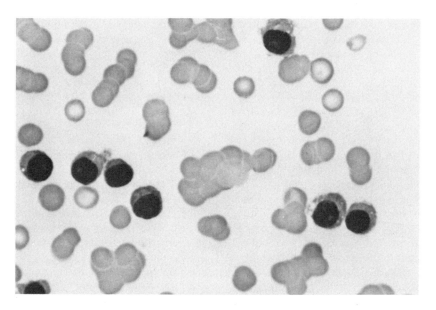

Fig. 1185 Blood smear from patient with IgA monoclonal gammopathy and leukocyte count of 60,000 with 70% plasma cells. This is referred to as plasma cell leukemia. Bone marrow was totally replaced by plasma cells. (Wright's-Giemsa; ×256.)

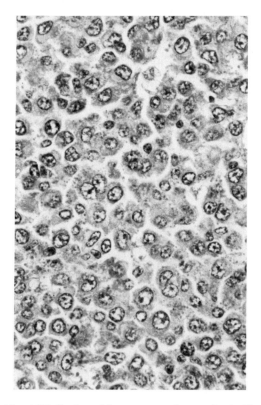

Fig. 1186 Section of bone marrow from patient with IgG myeloma. Myeloma cells have abundant cytoplasm and large nuclei with fine chromatin pattern. (Hematoxylin-eosin; ×160.)

sis,[189a] it should be considered as a variant of myeloma and not as a separate entity. The term should be reserved for those patients who present initially with this finding; plasma cells are frequently detected in the blood in the terminal stages of multiple myeloma. The first two reported cases of IgE myeloma presented as plasma cell leukemia.

In sections stained with hematoxylin-eosin, the myeloma cells are generally relatively similar in appearance, although considerable variation in size may be present in some patients. The cytoplasm is amphophilic to eosinophilic. The nucleus in the more differentiated myeloma cells is eccentric in location (Fig. 1186). In the more immature myeloma cells, the nucleus may be more centrally located and the infiltrate may resemble a leukemic process. Nucleoli may be strikingly prominent with perinucleolar halos. Multinucleated cells may be present and at times may resemble Sternberg-Reed cells or mononuclear variants. In some patients with myeloma, the proliferative cell may more nearly resemble a lymphocyte type of cell, although definite plasmacytic features are usually present. Intranuclear inclusions of various types may be noted.[177] A low percentage of patients with multiple myeloma will manifest marrow fibrosis.

Uncommonly, a patient with the clinical, x-ray, and histopathologic features of multiple

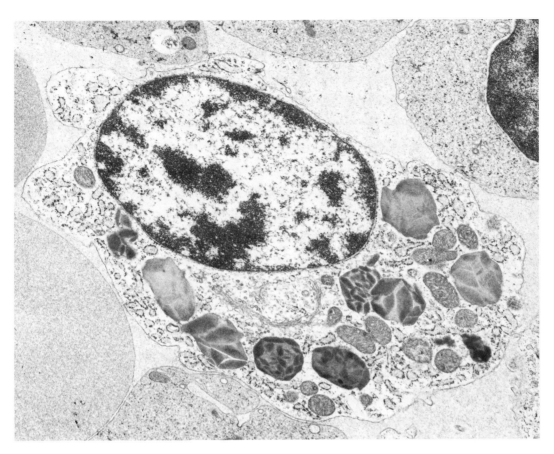

Fig. 1187 Electron micrograph of myeloma cell from marrow of patient with Fanconi's syndrome and Bence Jones variant of multiple myeloma. Cytoplasm contains several inclusions composed of crystalline structures. (Uranyl acetate–lead citrate; ×12,000.)

myeloma will not demonstrate evidence of monoclonal immunoglobulin production in the serum or urine. These cases have been referred to as "nonsecretory" myeloma.[176] Considerable caution should be exercised in the use of this term since striking reactive plasmacytosis may be observed with nonmyelomatous neoplasms and in several nonmalignant conditions, including liver disease, connective tissue disorders, chronic granulomatous disorders, hypersensitivity states, and agranulocytosis.[179,181] When a nonsecretory myeloma is suspected, the monoclonal character of the proliferating plasma cells should be confirmed by immunofluorescent or immunoperoxidase techniques that will demonstrate monoclonal intracellular immunoglobulin.[178,187]

Multiple myeloma or amyloidosis may occur in patients with the adult Fanconi's syndrome; the renal abnormalities may precede the overt manifestations of the plasma cell dyscrasia for several years. Bence Jones proteinuria of k light chain type is a common finding. A high percentage of the patients with this variant of myeloma manifest crystalline inclusions in the cytoplasm of the proliferating plasma cells and renal tubular cells[183,185] (Fig. 1187).

An increasing number of marrow biopsies are being performed on patients with monoclonal gammopathy occurring in the absence of other evidence of a plasma cell dyscrasia. The bone marrow in these patients may be entirely normal or manifest a slight increase in mature-appearing plasma cells. Occasionally, a small number of abnormal plasma cells may be present. The pathologist should exercise a conservative approach to these problems. Some of these cases represent incipient myeloma, but others continue for several years without undergoing an obvious neoplastic evolution.[183] The term benign monoclonal gammopathy is used to describe the latter group of patients. If the morphologic findings are suggestive but not diagnostic of myeloma, the patient should be followed with marrow examination at six-month intervals for approximately two years. An increase in the number of abnormal plasma cells and an increase in the amount of immunoglobulin portend a neoplastic process. A stable immunoglobulin level and plasma cell percentage is probably reflective of a benign monoclonal gammopathy.

The distinction between multiple myeloma and a focal tumor mass of myeloma cells in bone, the solitary plasmacytoma of bone, depends on the absence of bone marrow aspirate and x-ray and immunoelectrophoretic evidence of myeloma in the latter condition.[183] If a monoclonal protein is present in a patient with an apparent solitary plasmacytoma, the disappearance of the immunoelectrophoretic abnormality following tumoricidal radiation to the lesion confirms the diagnosis. If the monoclonal

protein persists, the diagnosis of multiple myeloma is more likely than solitary plasmacytoma. Although occasional patients with a plasmacytoma are apparently cured by radiation, most eventually develop multiple myeloma.[186] This evolution is delayed for many years in the majority of patients.[189] A syndrome of plasmacytoma, polyneuropathy, and endocrine abnormalities has been reported in a small number of Japanese.[180]

Waldenström's macroglobulinemia

Waldenström's macroglobulinemia is a form of plasma cell dyscrasia characterized by the production of an IgM immunoglobulin and the proliferation of a cell that usually has the characteristics of a well-differentiated lymphocyte or a lymphocyte with plasmacytoid features.[198,202] The disease has a slight male predominance with a median age of onset of approximately 60 years.[197] Hepatosplenomegaly,

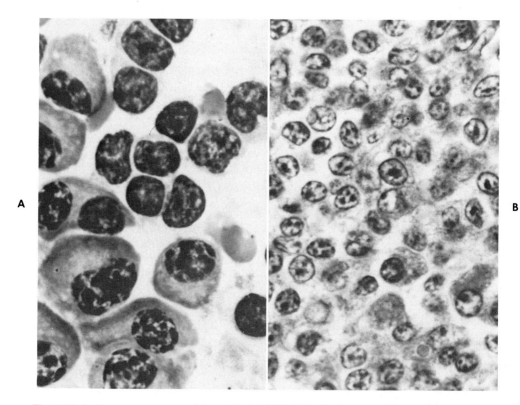

Fig. 1188 A, Bone marrow smear from patient with Waldenström's macroglobulinemia. Lymphocytic cells have characteristics of well-differentiated lymphocytes. Plasma cells have clumped nuclear chromatin without prominent nucleoli. There are no apparent transitional cells. **B,** Section of bone marrow from same patient whose bone marrow smear is illustrated in **A.** Majority of cells in section are well-differentiated lymphocytes; occasional plasma cells can be identified. (**A,** Wright's-Giemsa; ×400; **B,** hematoxylin-eosin; ×400.)

lymphadenopathy, and neurologic abnormalities are frequent clinical findings; anemia and hyperviscosity are commonly noted laboratory abnormalities. The clinical and pathologic features of Waldenström's macroglobulinemia also have been observed in patients with monoclonal immunoglobulins of IgG and IgA heavy-chain type.[201]

The peripheral blood in Waldenström's macroglobulinemia is characterized by a relative or absolute lymphocytosis in the majority of patients. The bone marrow smears usually show a predominating pattern of well-differentiated lymphocytes and plasmacytoid lymphocytes (Fig. 1188, *A*). In some instances, the lymphocytes have abundant, pale cytoplasm. Mature plasma cells, tissue mast cells, and histiocytes may be increased in number. In the bone marrow sections, the infiltration by the lymphocytes may be focal or diffuse; the latter is more commonly observed. The marrow replacement is frequently extensive with a marked decrease in the normal marrow elements. Reflecting their appearance in the smears, the lymphocytes in the sections have the features of mature, well-differentiated lymphocytes (Fig. 1188, *B*). Cells intermediate in appearance to mature lymphocytes and plasma cells may be found; these appear to be lymphocytes with abundant cytoplasm. Intranuclear inclusions that stain variably positive with the PAS reaction may be present in some cells[195] (Fig. 1189). This finding is not specific for macroglobulinemia and has been found in myelomas of various immunoglobulin classes and in reactive immunocyte proliferations.[192,193]

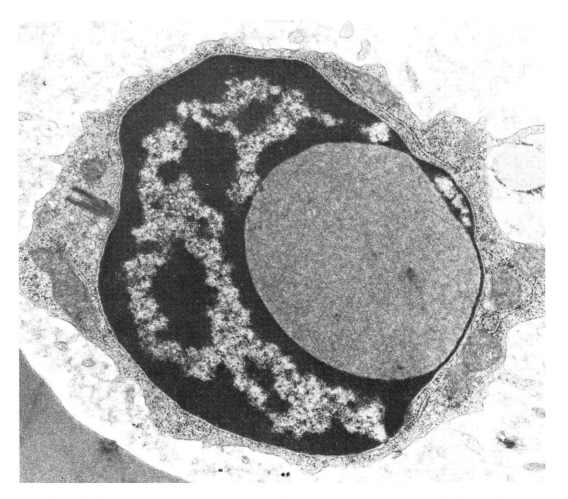

Fig. 1189 Electron micrograph of lymphocytic cell from bone marrow of patient with Waldenström's macroglobulinemia. Large "intranuclear" inclusion is present. (Uranyl acetate-lead citrate; ×22,000.)

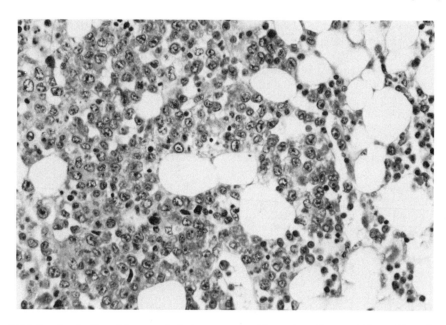

Fig. 1190 Focal collection of tumor cells in bone marrow biopsy from 3-year-old boy with malignant histiocytosis. Tumor cells are large and have abundant, slightly basophilic cytoplasm and nuclei that are frequently irregular in outline. Nucleoli are variably prominent. (Hematoxylin-eosin; ×100.)

An IgM monoclonal protein may be found in patients without the classic laboratory and clinical findings of Waldenström's macroglobulinemia. The histopathologic spectrum of disorders that may be found includes chronic lymphocytic leukemia, lymphocytic lymphomas, and multiple myeloma.[190,191,196,199,200] The occurrence of a Richter's syndrome-like evolution has been reported in Waldenström's macroglobulinemia.[194]

Heavy-chain disease

The heavy-chain diseases are clinical syndromes that are associated with the production of heavy-chain fragments.[203]

Gamma-chain disease has more of the features of a malignant lymphoma than of multiple myeloma. There is frequently anemia, leukopenia, and thrombocytopenia. Atypical lymphocytes and plasma cells may be found in the peripheral blood. The bone marrow is usually abnormal and shows an increase in lymphocytes, plasma cells, or both. There is frequently an accompanying eosinophilia. There are no significant changes in the bone marrow in alpha-chain disease.[206] Most of the reported cases of mu-chain disease have had long histories of chronic lymphocytic leukemia.[203,204] In several of the patients reported, the marrow contained vacuolated plasma cells. The occur-

rence of tumors composed of undifferentiated lymphoid cells in patients with heavy-chain disease has been reported.[205,207]

Histiocytic disorders
Malignant histiocytosis

The term malignant histiocytosis was introduced by Rappaport[212] to describe a disorder characterized by a systemic, neoplastic proliferation of histiocytes and their precursors.[208,210-212,214] The cells of malignant histiocytosis may be detected in bone marrow material at the time of initial diagnosis or subsequently. The smears of the bone marrow aspirate have been found to have more utility than the bone marrow sections by some observers.[210,214] Occasional malignant cells may be identified in the blood smears of some patients in the late stages of the disease.

In marrow sections, the infiltration may be focal or diffuse (Fig. 1190). Bone marrow involvement may be extremely difficult to recognize in section material that contains only scattered malignant cells. Marrow involvement, as detected in Romanovsky-stained smears, is characterized by malignant cells occurring singly or in small groups scattered among the normal hematopoietic cells or at the edges of the smears. This contrasts with acute monoblastic leukemia in which the bone marrow ex-

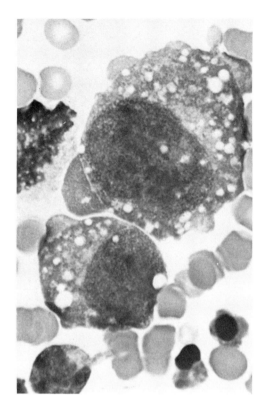

Fig. 1191 Two malignant cells in bone marrow smear from patient with malignant histiocytosis. Abundant, basophilic cytoplasm is characterized by pseudopod formation and numerous vacuoles. Nucleoli are indistinct in these two cells. (Wright's-Giemsa; ×400.)

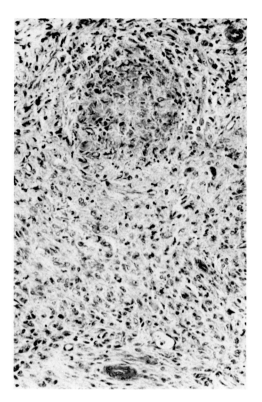

Fig. 1192 Bone marrow section from child with histiocytosis X. Large portion of marrow is replaced by differentiated histiocytes that assume granuloma-like arrangement. (Hematoxylin-eosin; ×51.)

hibits extensive replacement of the normal hematopoietic elements by the leukemic cells. The malignant histiocyte varies in size; cells up to 40μ-50μ may be found (Fig. 1191). The cytoplasm of the smaller cells is usually intensely basophilic and vacuolated. The cytoplasm of the larger cells is less basophilic with numerous small vacuoles. The cytoplasm may be abundant with evidence of pseudopod formation and fragmentation. Very small azurophilic granules may be found in the cytoplasm of some of the larger cells. Although occasional malignant histiocytes may show evidence of phagocytosis, prominent hemophagocytosis is a relatively uncommon finding in unequivocally malignant-appearing histiocytes. The nucleus may be round or contorted; the larger cells generally have more contorted nuclei. The nuclear chromatin is coarsely reticular. Nucleoli may be very prominent or almost indistinct. Stains for nonspecific esterase and acid phosphatase are positive.

Histiocytosis X

Histiocytosis X (chronic differentiated histiocytosis)[212] may be detected in random bone marrow trephine biopsies. The lesions are generally focal and have a granulomatous appearance (Fig. 1192). Confluent lesions may replace substantial portions of the medullary space. The cells have a low nuclear:cytoplasmic ratio and mature nuclei without prominent nucleoli.

Virus-associated hemophagocytic syndrome

An association has been reported between virus infection, primarily herpesvirus and adenovirus groups, and the proliferation of benign-appearing histiocytes in lymph node and bone marrow tissue.[213] The blood picture is generally characterized by pancytopenia. The marrow smears may contain an extraorindarily large number of histiocytes manifesting marked phagocytosis of erythroid cells, platelets, and

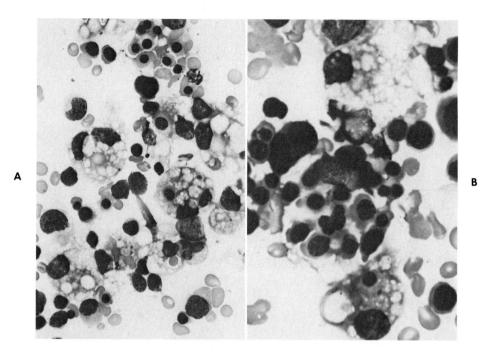

Fig. 1193 A, Bone marrow smear from patient with virus-associated hemophagocytic syndrome. Numerous macrophages with ingested red cells and erythroblasts are present. **B,** High magnification of marrow smear illustrated in **A.** One of macrophages contains numerous erythroblasts. (**A** and **B,** Wright's-Giemsa; **A,** ×250; **B,** ×400.)

granulocytes (Fig. 1193). There is frequently an accompanying depression of erythroid precursors, granulocytic precursors, or both; megakaryocytes are usually normal or increased in number. The lymph node may show lymphocyte depletion with increased histiocytes in the sinusoidal spaces. Evidence of multisystem involvement is usually present, and the clinical course is often fulminant. A high percentage of patients have coagulation abnormalities. The disorder occurs in a spontaneous form, primarily in children, or in patients on immunosuppressive drugs. The course of the disease in the majority of patients follows a viral infection by two to six weeks and is of two to three weeks' duration. In infants, the disease may be particularly severe, and there is a high mortality in this age group. This disorder is frequently misdiagnosed as histiocytic medullary reticulosis, another term for malignant histiocytosis.[214] Antineoplastic drugs appear to be contraindicated. Treatment is directed toward supportive therapy and withdrawal of immunosuppressive drugs. A similar constellation of clinical and laboratory findings has been reported in tuberculosis.[209]

Angioimmunoblastic lymphadenopathy

Angioimmunoblastic lymphadenopathy or immunoblastic lymphadenopathy is viewed primarily as a disorder of lymph nodes in that all patients have either focal or diffuse lymphadenopathy.[215-217] However, the disease is manifest in both blood and bone marrow specimens in a relatively high percentage of patients, and the bone marrow biopsy may be virtually diagnostic of the disorder.[218]

Immunocytes in varying stages of development may be found in both the blood and the marrow; occasionally the blood may contain an extraordinarily high number of these cells. In contrast, there is commonly a lymphocytopenia.

The lesions of angioimmunoblastic lymphadenopathy in bone marrow sections may be either focal or diffuse and extensively involve the marrow in some patients (Fig. 1194). A paratrabecular distribution of the lesion has been noted frequently. The focal lesions show collections of lymphocytes, plasma cells, histiocytes, and, rarely, large immunoblasts. Special stains for reticulin show an increase in reticulin fibers in the lesions. In the more ex-

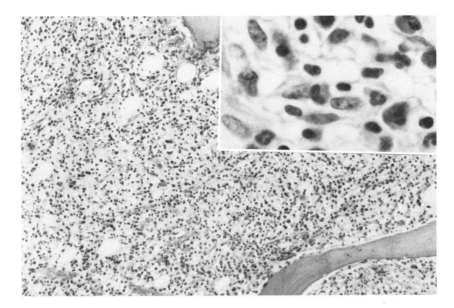

Fig. 1194 Bone marrow biopsy from patient with angioimmunoblastic lymphadenopathy. Marrow is diffusely involved by process. **Inset,** Heterogeneous cell population is loosely distributed. Numerous fibroblasts and endothelial cells are present. (Hematoxylin-eosin; ×40; **inset,** hematoxylin-eosin; ×400.)

tensive lesions, the areas of involvement appear hypocellular with collections of lymphocytes, plasma cells, and histiocytes. Numerous collections of eosinophils also may be present. Fibroblastic cells with spindle-shaped nuclei are often prominent (Fig. 1194). Vascular proliferation is present in approximately half of the marrow lesions; endothelial cells are found in a higher percentage.

The marrow exclusive of the angioimmunoblastic lesion is usually hypercellular. The hypercellularity may be due to an erythroid hyperplasia secondary to hemolytic anemia, which is a frequent occurrence, or there may be a generalized increase in all marrow elements.

Systemic mastocytosis

The marrow lesions of systemic mastocytosis may be found as a direct result of search in a patient with urticaria pigmentosa or may be detected in a biopsy performed for some reason unrelated to suspected mastocytosis.[219,220,224,226] In the latter instance, when there is no clinical suggestion of mastocytosis, the lesions of mast cell disease frequently are overlooked or misinterpreted because of the difficulty of identifying mast cells in routine sections and the changes inherent in the mast cells in this disease. Smears obtained by bone mar-

row aspirate may suggest the diagnosis of mastocytosis if large numbers of mast cells are present; the number should exceed 7%, since up to that percentage has been reported in patients without mast cell disease.[224] In many instances, the mast cells in the marrow in mastocytosis are associated with an increase in reticulin fibers and are not readily aspirated. As a result, the pathologist is not alerted to the possibility of mast cell disease from the smears.

The marrow infiltration in mastocytosis may be diffuse or focal.[221] The focal lesions may take several forms: mast cell aggregates, fibrotic foci associated with mast cells, lymphocytic aggregates surrounded by a collar of mast cells (Fig. 1195), or a focus of mast cells surrounded by a collar of lymphocytes (Fig. 1196). Fibrotic foci may be found in a paratrabecular location (Fig. 1197), and nodular granulomatous foci may be present. A prominent perivascular arrangement of mast cells is sometimes noted; hyperplasia of the vessel wall and perivascular collagenous fibrosis may occur. Eosinophilia is usually prominent in the area of the mast cell aggregates and may be the most conspicuous morphologic finding. The bone trabeculae frequently show sclerotic thickening; osteoporosis may occur. Blood eosinophilia and hypocholesterolemia frequently are associated laboratory findings.

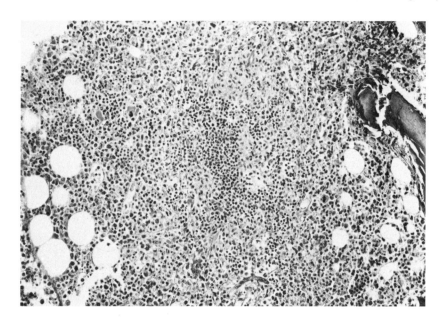

Fig. 1195 Lesion in bone marrow from patient with systemic mastocytosis. Central collection of well-differentiated lymphocytes is surrounded by lighter-staining mast cells. Contrast this with Fig. 1196. (Hematoxylin-eosin; ×40.)

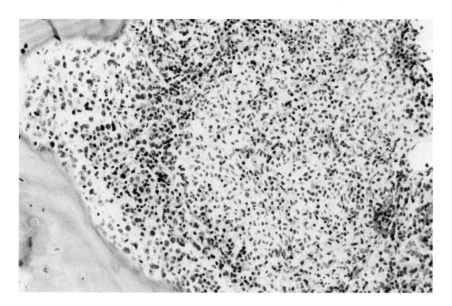

Fig. 1196 Bone marrow from patient with systemic mastocytosis. There is focal lesion with central group of lighter-staining mast cells partially surrounded by denser-staining well-differentiated lymphocytes. Numerous eosinophils are also scattered among lymphocytes. (Hematoxylin-eosin; ×100.)

A major difficulty in the diagnosis of mast cell lesions results from the frequently abnormal morphology of the mast cells in this disorder. The cells often resemble histiocytes in that they possess abundant eosinophilic cytoplasm (Fig. 1198). The granules are difficult to identify even when the true nature of the lesion is suspected. In the fibrotic foci, the mast cells may have a spindly appearance and resemble fibroblasts. Large fibrotic lesions may be misinterpreted as idiopathic myelofibrosis. The identification of the mast cells is best accomplished with the Giemsa or toluidine blue 0 stains (Fig. 1199) or electron microscopy (Fig.

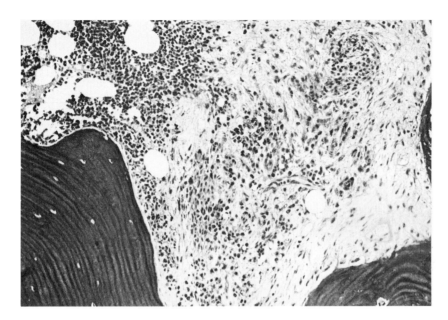

Fig. 1197 Paratrabecular fibrosis in marrow of patient with systemic mastocytosis. Numerous mast cells, occurring in groups and singly, are enmeshed in fibrous connective tissue. Many of mast cells are elongated and have histiocytic appearance. (Hematoxylin-eosin; ×40.)

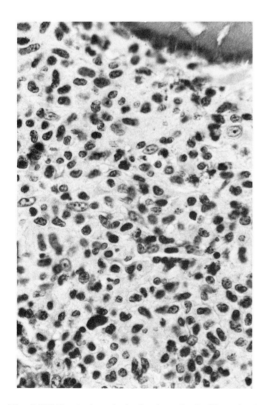

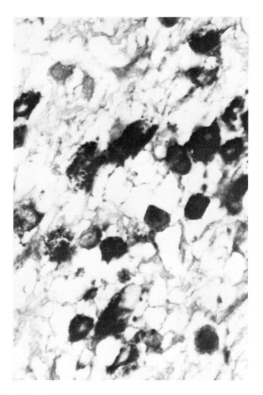

Fig. 1198 Paratrabecular lesion in patient with systemic mastocytosis. Mast cells have round or slightly contorted nuclei and pale cytoplasm. Because of inconspicuous granulation, mast cells resemble histiocytes. (Hematoxylin-eosin; ×160.)

Fig. 1199 Granules of mast cells of specimen illustrated in Fig. 1197 are intensely metachromatic with toluidine blue 0 stain. (Toluidine blue 0; ×400.)

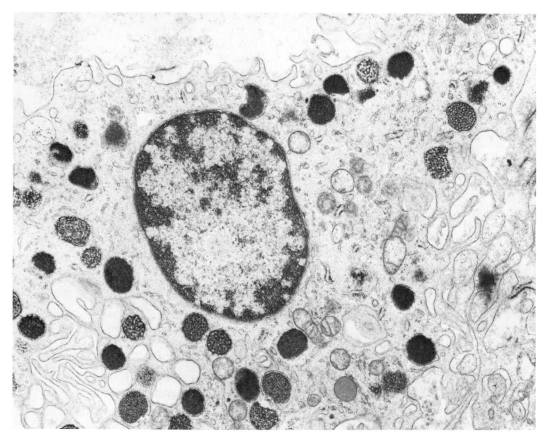

Fig. 1200 Electron micrograph of mast cell in bone marrow aspirate from patient with systemic masto-cytosis. Abundant cytoplasm is irregularly distributed around nucleus and has several cytoplasmic projections. Granules vary in density; subunits in some of granules have honeycomb appearance. (Uranyl acetate–lead citrate; ×17,000.)

1200). With the toluidine blue 0 stain, the mast cell granules appear reddish purple; the staining of the granules can be enhanced in decalcified tissue by treatment of the section with potassium permanganate followed by oxalic acid prior to the staining procedure.[219,223] The mast cells will react with the chloracetate esterase stain, but this reaction is less specific than the toluidine blue 0 stain.

"Malignant mastocytosis" has been distinguished from "benign systemic mastocytosis" on the basis of the cytologic and cytochemical features of the mast cells in the two disorders. The mast cells in the malignant variant have larger nuclei, often manifest mitotic activity, and may be poorly granulated. Proliferation is present in various organs. Most patients with the malignant disorder die within two years of diagnosis; mast cell leukemia develops in about 15% of these patients.[219a]

The marrow lesions in systemic mastocytosis resemble some of the changes described under the term eosinophilic fibrohistiocytic lesion.[222,225]

Metastatic tumor

Bone marrow biopsies frequently are used for the staging of patients with known primary malignancies[227,229,231,232]; they also may be performed on patients with suspected malignancy in an attempt to obtain material for a histologic diagnosis. The tumors most frequently detected in bone marrow biopsies in the adult population are carcinoma of the breast, prostate, lung, stomach, colon, kidney, and thyroid gland. The incidence of positive marrow biopsies in patients with oat cell carcinomas of the lung is notably high in some studies.[230] Sarcomas have a relatively low incidence of marrow metastasis in adults. In the pediatric age group, neuroblastoma is the most common metastatic lesion, followed by rhabdo-

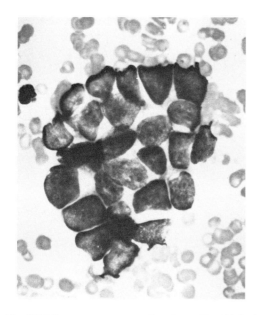

Fig. 1201 Bone marrow smear from 8-month-old infant with diagnosis of neuroblastoma showing cluster of metastatic tumor cells. Cohesive character of tumor cells in this illustration would be unusual for malignant hematopoietic tumor cells. (Wright's-Giemsa; ×256.)

myosarcoma, Ewing's sarcoma, and retinoblastoma. Wilm's tumor metastatic to marrow is rare.[228]

Tumor cells may be detected in bone marrow smears, particle sections, trephine imprints, or trephine biopsies. The relative merits of these techniques for detecting tumor have been the subject of considerable discussion. The yield of positive results has probably increased with the performance of multiple trephine biopsies and the biopsy of specific radiologic lesions.

In smears, the tumor cells frequently occur in clusters. This may be an important diagnostic feature, since tumors of hematopoietic origin generally do not occur in groups and are usually evenly distributed throughout the smear. The cells of metastatic neuroblastoma may be present both in clusters and as individual cells (Fig. 1201). In trephine sections, the metastatic tumor may occur as small focal lesions surrounded by hematopoietic cells or replace the entire specimen. In focal lesions or those occupying only a portion of the biopsy, the tumor is usually sharply demarcated from the adjacent hematopoietic tissue. Many tumors, most notably breast and prostate, may be associated with a marked desmoplastic reaction and attempts at aspiration may be unsuccessful (Fig. 1202). These tumors also may be accompanied

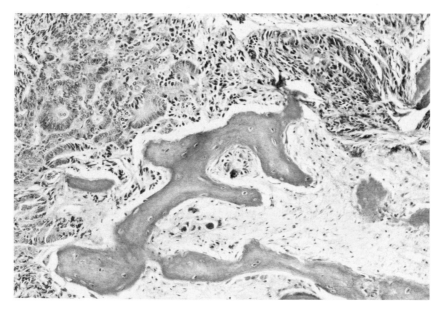

Fig. 1202 Bone marrow involved by metastatic adenocarcinoma from prostate gland. This marrow illustrates variable pattern that may be manifest in marrow lesions of metastatic tumor. Portion of marrow is densely fibrotic with small number of scattered tumor cells. Upper left portion of field shows recognizable glandular structures. (Hematoxylin-eosin; ×40.)

by an increase in new bone formation. In general, the morphology of the metastatic lesions mimics the primary tumor. The approach to determination of the site of origin of a metastatic tumor in a patient without a known primary lesion should be the same as for metastatic lesions in other sites; this includes the use of all pertinent cytochemical techniques and electron microscopy, if available.

Lipid storage diseases
Gaucher's disease

Gaucher's disease is an autosomal recessive sphingolipid storage disorder caused by the accumulation of glucocerebroside in the organs and tissues.[233] It occurs in three forms:

Type I—chronic nonneuropathic (adult) type
Type II—acute neuropathic type
Type III—subacute neuropathic (juvenile) type

The characteristic diagnostic feature of the disorder is the presence of Gaucher's cell in bone marrow, spleen, liver, and lymph node.

In the bone marrow sections, Gaucher's cells may be found in small focal accumulations or may replace large areas of the intertrabecular structure. There is an associated increase in reticulir fibers. In imprint and smear preparations, Gaucher's cell is large, measures 20μ-100μ in diameter, and has one or more centrally or eccentrically located nuclei.[235] The cytoplasm has a characteristic fibrillary or striated pattern and is pale blue-gray in color. In sections stained with hematoxylin-eosin, the cytoplasm is slightly eosinophilic; a fibrillary pattern may be very prominent (Fig. 1203). The Gaucher cells are variably, and often intensely, positive with the periodic acid–Schiff stain. The cells also react positively for iron. Cells similar to Gaucher's cells may be found in the marrow of some patients with chronic myelogenous leukemia,[237-239] type II congenital dyserythropoietic anemia,[243] and thalassemia.[244] A monoclonal gammopathy may be present in patients with chronic Gaucher's disease and may be associated with a marrow plasmacytosis.[240]

Niemann-Pick disease

Niemann-Pick disease comprises a group of autosomal recessive disorders characterized by the accumulation of sphingomyelin and other lipids throughout the body.[234] Five distinct clinical types are recognized. The foam cell as seen in hematopoietic tissue in Niemann-Pick disease is not a diagnostically specific cell and may be found in other disorders of lipid metabolism, such as hypercholesterolemia and Tangier disease.[235] In Romanovsky-stained smears, the cell measures 20μ-50μ; the cytoplasm is filled with varying sized clear vacuoles. In sections, the cytoplasm appears clear to finely granular.

Fabry's disease

Fabry's disease is an X-linked inborn error of glycosphingolipid metabolism.[236] The characteristic storage cells in bone marrow specimens in this disease are filled with small globular inclusions that stain blue in Romanovsky-stained smears and lightly eosinophilic in sections stained with hematoxylin-eosin. The cytoplasmic substance reacts intensely with the periodic acid–Schiff and Sudan black B stains.

Sea-blue histiocyte syndrome

The macrophages of the sea-blue histiocyte syndrome[241,242] contain a substance that stains

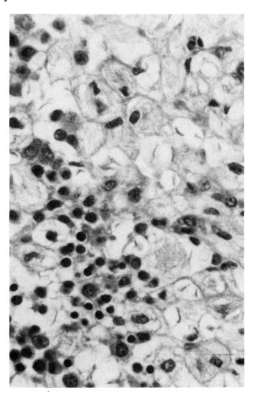

Fig. 1203 Bone marrow section from adult with Gaucher's disease. Cytoplasm of many of Gaucher's cells has fibrillary or granular appearance. Nuclei are small and usually eccentric in location. Group of erythroblasts is present. (Hematoxylin-eosin; ×160.)

blue in Romanovsky-stained smears and yellow to tan in sections stained with hematoxylin-eosin. Positive reactions occur with the periodic acid–Schiff and Sudan black B stains. In some instances, the substance appears to be ceroid; in others the material has not been well characterized. Macrophages containing blue pigment may be observed in several unrelated disorders and lack diagnostic specificity.

REFERENCES

Introduction

1 Block M: Bone marrow examination: aspiration or core biopsy, smear or section, hematoxylin-eosin or Romanowsky stain–which combination? Arch Pathol Lab Med **100**:454-456, 1976.
2 Brunning RD, Bloomfield CD, McKenna RW, Peterson L: Bilateral trephine bone marrow biopsies in lymphoma and other neoplastic diseases. Ann Int Med **82**:365-366, 1975.
3 Contreras E, Ellis LD, Lee RE: Value of the bone marrow biopsy in the diagnosis of metastatic carcinoma. Cancer **29**:778-783, 1972.
4 Dee JW, Valdivieso M, Drewinko B: Comparison of the efficacies of closed trephine needle biopsy, aspirated paraffin-embedded clot section, and smear preparation in the diagnosis of bone marrow involvement by lymphoma. Am J Clin Pathol **65**:183-194, 1976.
5 Ellman L: Bone marrow biopsy in the evaluation of lymphoma, carcinoma and granulomatous disorders. Am J Med **60**:1-7, 1976.
6 Garrett TJ, Gee TS, Leiberman PH, McKenzie S, Clarkson BD: The role of bone marrow aspiration and biopsy in detecting marrow involvement by nonhematologic malignancies. Cancer **38**:2401-2403, 1976.
7 Grann V, Pool JL, Mayer K: Comparative study of bone marrow aspiration and biopsy in patients with neoplastic disease. Cancer **19**:1898-1900, 1966.
8 Gruppo RA, Lampkin BC, Granger S: Bone marrow cellularity determination: comparison of the biopsy, aspirate and buffy coat. Blood **49**:29-31, 1977.
9 Jamshidi K, Swaim WR: Bone marrow biopsy with unaltered architecture: a new biopsy device. J Lab Clin Med **77**:335-342, 1971.
10 Liao KT: The superiority of histologic sections of aspirated bone marrow in malignant lymphomas. Cancer **27**:618-628, 1971.

Biopsy procedure and processing of specimen

11 Beckstead JH, Bainton DF: Enzyme histochemistry on bone marrow biopsies: reactions useful in the differential diagnosis of leukemia and lymphoma applied to 2-micron plastic sections. Blood **55**:386-394, 1980.
11a Brinn NT, Pickett JP: Glycol methacrylate for routine, special stains, histochemistry, enzyme histochemistry and immunohistochemistry. A simplified method for surgical biopsy tissue. J Histotechnol **2**:125-130, 1979.
11b Brunning RD, Bloomfield CD, McKenna RW, Peterson L: Bilateral trephine bone marrow biopsies in lymphoma and other neoplastic diseases. Ann Int Med **82**:365-366, 1975.
12 Brynes RK, McKenna RW, Sundberg RD: Bone marrow aspiration and trephine biopsy. Am J Clin Pathol **70**:753-759, 1978.

13 Ellman L: Bone marrow biopsy in the evaluation of lymphoma, carcinoma and granulomatous disorders. Am J Med **60**:1-7, 1976.
14 Goswitz FA, Andrews GA, Kniseley RM: Effects of local irradiation (Co^{60} teletherapy) on the peripheral blood and bone marrow. Blood **21**:605-619, 1963.
15 Jamshidi K, Swaim WR: Bone marrow biopsy with unaltered architecture: a new biopsy device. J Lab Clin Med **77**:335-342, 1971.
16 Luna LG (ed): Manual of histologic staining methods of the Armed Forces Institute of Pathology, ed. 3. New York, 1968, McGraw-Hill Book Co.

Normocellular bone marrow
Benign lymphocytic aggregates

17 Hartsock RJ, Smith EB, Petty CS: Normal variations with aging of the amount of hematopoietic tissue in bone marrow from the anterior iliac crest. Am J Clin Pathol **43**:326-331, 1965.
18 Hashimoto H, Hashimoto N: The occurrence of lymph nodules in human bone marrow with particular reference to their number. Kyusha J Med Sci **14**:343-354, 1963.
19 Hashimoto M, Higuchi M, Saito T: Lymph nodules in human bone marrow. Acta Pathol Jpn **7**:33-52, 1957.
20 Maeda K, Hyun BH, Rebuck JW: Lymphoid follicles in bone marrow aspirates. Am J Clin Pathol **67**:41-48, 1977.
21 Rywlin AM, Ortega RS, Dominguez CJ: Lymphoid nodules of bone marrow: normal and abnormal. Blood **43**:389-400, 1974.
22 Williams RJ: The lymphoid nodules of human bone marrow. Am J Pathol **15**:377-384, 1939.

Alterations in cellularity

23 Ajlouni K, Doeblin T: The syndrome of hepatitis and aplastic anemia. Br J Haematol **27**:345-355, 1974.
24 Alter BP, Potter NU, Li FP: Classification and aetiology of the aplastic anemias. Clin Haematol **7**:431-465, 1978.
25 Brunning R: The effects of leukemia and lymphoma therapy on hematopoietic cells. Am J Med Tech **39**:165-174, 1973.
26 Dawson JP: Congenital pancytopenia associated with multiple congenital anomalies (Fanconi type). Review of the literature and report of a 20-year-old female with a 10-year follow-up and apparently good response to splenectomy. Pediatrics **15**:325-333, 1955.
27 Estren S, Dameshek W: Familial hypoplastic anemia of childhood. Am J Dis Child **73**:671-687, 1947.
28 Haak HL, Hartgrink-Groeneveld CA, Eernisse JG, Speck B, Van Rood JJ: Acquired aplastic anemia in adults. Acta Hematol **58**:257-277, 1977.
29 Naeim F, Smith GS, Gale RP: Morphologic aspects of bone marrow transplantation in patients with aplastic anemia. Hum Pathol **9**:295-308, 1978.
30 Rosse WF: Paroxysmal nocturnal hemoglobinuria in aplastic anemia. Clin Haematol **7**:541-553, 1978.
31 Schwachman H, Diamond LK, Oski FA, Khaw KT: The syndrome of pancreatic insufficiency and bone marrow dysfunction. J Pediatr **65**:645-663, 1964.
32 Seaman JP, Kjeldsberg CR, Linker A: Gelatinous transformation of the bone marrow. Hum Pathol **9**:685-692, 1978.

Bone marrow infarction

33 Brown CH: Bone marrow necrosis. A study of seventy cases. Johns Hopkins Med J **131:**189-203, 1972.

33a Diggs LW: Sickle cell crises. Am J Clin Pathol **44:** 1-19, 1965.

34 Goodall HB: Atypical changes in the bone marrow in acute infections. In Clark WJ, Howard EB, Hachett PL (eds): Myeloproliferative disorders of animal and man. Oak Ridge, Tenn., 1970, United States Atomic Energy Commission, pp. 314-339.

35 Kahlstron SC, Burton CC, Phemister DB: Infarction of bones in Caisson disease. Surg Gynecol Obstet **68:** 129-146, 1939.

36 Kundel DW, Brecher G, Bodey GP, Brittin GM: Reticulin fibrosis and bone infarction in acute leukemia. Implications for prognosis. Blood **23:**526-544, 1964.

Inflammatory disorders

37 Browne PM, Sharma OP, Salkin D: Bone marrow sarcoidosis. JAMA **240:**2654-2655, 1978.

38 Custer RP: An atlas of the blood and bone marrow. Philadelphia, 1974, W. B. Saunders Co., pp. 276-279.

39 Georgii A, Vykoupil KF: Unspecific mesenchymal reaction in bone marrow in patients with Hodgkin's disease. Recent Results Cancer Res **46:**39-44, 1974.

40 Hovde RF, Sundberg RD: Granulomatous lesions in the bone marrow in infectious mononucleosis: a comparison of the changes in the bone marrow of infectious mononucleosis with those in brucellosis, tuberculosis, sarcoidosis and lymphatic leukemia. Blood **5:**209-232, 1950.

41 Kadin ME, Donaldson SS, Dorfman RF: Isolated granulomas in Hodgkin's disease. N Engl J Med **283:**859-861, 1970.

41a Okun DB, Sun NCJ, Tanaka KR: Bone marrow granulomas in Q fever. Am J Clin Pathol **71:**117-121, 1979.

42 Pease GL: Granulomatous lesions in bone marrow. Blood **11:**720-734, 1956.

42a Rywlin AM: A pathologist's view of the bone marrow. J Fla Med Assoc **67:**121-124, 1980.

43 Rywlin AM, Ortega R: Lipid granulomas of the bone marrow. Am J Clin Pathol **57:**457-462, 1972.

Oxalosis

44 McKenna RW, Dehner LP: Oxalosis: an unusual cause of myelophthisis in childhood. Am J Clin Pathol **66:** 991-997, 1976.

45 Williams HE, Smith LH Jr: Primary hyperoxaluria. In Stanbury JB, Wyngaarden JB, Fredrickson DS (eds): The metabolic basis of inherited disease. New York, 1978, McGraw-Hill Book Co., pp. 184-204.

Amyloidosis

46 Conn RB Jr, Sundberg RD: Amyloid disease of the bone marrow. Am J Pathol **38:**61-71, 1961.

Leukemias and related disorders
Acute leukemias/Granulocytic sarcoma (chloroma)

47 Bennett JM, Catovsky D, Daniel MT, Sultan C, Flandrin G, Galton DAG, Gralnick HR: Proposals for the classification of the acute leukemias. Br J Haematol **33:**451-458, 1976.

48 Bloomfield CD, Brunning RD: Prognostic implications of cytology in acute leukemia in the adult. Hum Pathol **5:**641-659, 1974.

49 Cavdar AO, Arcasoy A, Babacan E, Gözdasoğlu S,

Topuz Ü, Fraumeni JF: Ocular granulocytic sarcoma (chloroma) with acute myelomonocytic leukemia in Turkish children. Cancer **41:**1606-1609, 1978.

50 Garfinkle LS, Bennet DE: Extramedullary myeloblastic transformation in chronic myelocytic leukemia simulating a coexistent malignant lymphoma. Am J Clin Pathol **51:**638-645, 1969.

51 Gralnick HR, Dittmar K: Development of myeloblastoma with massive breast and ovarian involvement during remission in acute leukemia. Cancer **24:**746-749, 1969.

52 Kandel EV: Chloroma. Review of the literature from 1926 to 1936 and report of three cases. Arch Int Med **59:**691-704, 1937.

53 Kundel DW, Brecher G, Bodey GP, Brittin GM: Reticulin fibrosis and bone infarction in acute leukemia. Implications for prognosis. Blood **23:**526-544, 1964.

54 Leder LD: The selective enzymochemical demonstration of neutrophilic myeloid cells and tissue mast cells in paraffin sections. Klin Wochenschr **42:**553, 1964.

55 McKenna RW, Bloomfield CD, Dick F, Nesbit ME, Brunning RD: Acute monoblastic leukemia: diagnosis and treatment of ten cases. Blood **46:**481-494, 1975.

56 Mason TE, Damaree R, Margolis CI: Granulocytic sarcoma (chloroma) two years preceding myelogenous leukemia. Cancer **31:**423-432, 1973.

57 Rappaport H: Tumors of the hematopoietic system. In Atlas of tumor pathology, Sect. III, Fasc. 8. Washington, D.C., 1966, Armed Forces Institute of Pathology.

58 Reardon G, Moloney WC: Chloroma and related myeloblastic neoplasms. Arch Int Med **108:**864-871, 1961.

59 Rowley JD: Chromosomes in leukemia and lymphoma. Semin Hematol **14:**301-319, 1978.

60 Wiernik PH, Serpick AA: Granulocytic sarcoma (chloroma). Blood **35:**361-369, 1970.

61 Woodson DL, Bennett DE, Sears DA: Extramedullary myeloblastic transformation of chronic myelocytic leukemia. Arch Int Med **134:**523-526, 1974.

Chronic myeloid leukemia

62 Barton JC, Conrad M: Current status of blastic transformation in chronic myelogenous leukemia. Am J Hematol **4:**281-291, 1978.

62a Brunning RD: Philadelphia chromosome positive leukemia. Hum Pathol **11:**307-309, 1980.

62b Clough V, Geary CG, Hashmi K, Davson J, Knowlson T: Myelofibrosis in chronic granulocytic leukaemia. Br J Haematol **42:**515-526, 1979.

63 Gralnick HR, Harbor J, Vogel C: Myelofibrosis in chronic granulocytic leukemia. Blood **37:**152-162, 1971.

64 Peterson LC, Bloomfield CD, Brunning RD: Blast crisis as an initial or terminal manifestation of chronic myeloid leukemia. Am J Med **60:**209-220, 1976.

Polycythemia vera

65 Bloomfield CD, Brunning RD: Acute leukemia as a terminal event in nonleukemic hematopoietic disorders. Semin Oncol **3:**297-317, 1976.

66 Dameshek W: Some speculations on the myeloproliferative syndromes. Blood **6:**372-375, 1951.

67 Ellis JT, Silver RT, Coleman M, Geller SA: The bone marrow in polycythemia vera. Semin Hematol **12:**433-444, 1975.

68 Klein H: Morphology of the hematopoietic tissue. In Klein H (ed): Polycythemia, theory and management.

Springfield, Ill., 1973, Charles C Thomas, Publisher, pp. 201-208.
69 Landau SA: Acute leukemia in polycythemia vera. Semin Hematol **13**:33-48, 1976.
70 Lawrence JH, Winchell HS, Donald WG: Leukemia in polycythemia vera: relationship to splenic myeloid metaplasia and therapeutic radiation dose. Ann Int Med **70**:763-771, 1969.
71 Lazlo J: Myeloproliferative disorders (MPD): myelofibrosis, myelosclerosis, extramedullary hematopoiesis, undifferentiated MPD and hemorrhagic thrombocythemia. Semin Hematol **12**:409-432, 1975.
72 Modan B, Lilienfeld AM: Polycythemia vera and leukemia–the role of radiation treatment. Medicine (Baltimore) **44**:305-344, 1965.
73 Roberts BE, Miles DW, Woods CG: Polycythaemia vera and myelosclerosis: a bone marrow study. Br J Haematol **16**:75-85, 1969.
74 Silverstein MN: Post-polycythemia myeloid metaplasia. Arch Int Med **134**:113-115, 1974.
75 Silverstein MN: The evolution into and the treatment of late stage polycythemia vera. Semin Hematol **13**:79-84, 1976.
76 Szur L, Lewis SM: The haematological complications of polycythaemia vera and treatment with radioactive phosphorus. Br J Radiol **39**:122-130, 1966.
77 Wasserman LR: The management of polycythemia vera. Br J Haematol **21**:371-376, 1971.

Myelofibrosis

78 Bauermeister DE: Quantitation of bone marrow reticulin—a normal range. Am J Clin Pathol **56**:24-31, 1971.
79 Bearman RM, Gerassimas A, Pangalis A, Rappaport H: Acute (''malignant'') myelosclerosis. Cancer **43**:279-293, 1979.
80 Block M, Burkhardt R, Chelloul N, Demmler K, Duhamel G, Georgii A, Kirsten WH, Lennert K, Nezelof C, TeVelde J: Myelofibrosis-osteosclerosis syndrome—pathology and morphology (working paper). Adv Biosciences **16**:219-240, 1974.
81 Burkhardt R, Bartl R, Beil E, Demmler K, Hoffman E, Kronseder A, Irrgang U, Ulrich M, Wiemann H, Langecker H, Saar U: Myelofibrosis-osteosclerosis syndrome—review of literature and histomorphology. Adv Biosciences **16**:1-56, 1974.
82 Burston J, Pinniger JL: The reticulin content of bone marrow in hematological disorders. Br J Haematol **9**:172-184, 1963.
83 Dameshek W: Some speculations on the myeloproliferative syndromes. Blood **6**:372-375, 1951.
84 Dameshek W: The myeloproliferative disorders. In Clark WJ, Howard EB, Hackett DL (eds): Myeloproliferative disorders of animal and man, Oak Ridge, Tenn., 1970, United States Atomic Energy Commission, pp. 413-420.
85 Lubin J, Rozen S, Rywlin AM: Malignant myelosclerosis. Arch Int Med **136**:141-145, 1976.
86 Nelson B, Knisely RM: Marrow fibrosis in myeloproliferative disorders. In Clark WJ, Howard EB, Hackett DL (eds): Myeloproliferative disorders of animal and man, Oak Ridge, Tenn., 1970, United States Atomic Energy Commission, pp. 533-555.
87 Tobin MS, Tan C, Argano SAP: Myelofibrosis in pediatric age group. NY State J Med **69**:1080-1083, 1969.
88 Ward HP, Block MH: The natural history of agnogenic myeloid metaplasia (AMM) and a critical evaluation of

its relationship with the myeloproliferative syndrome. Medicine **50**:357-420, 1971.

Chronic lymphocytic leukemia/Richter's syndrome

89 Armitage JO, Dick FR, Corder M: Diffuse histiocytic lymphoma complicating chronic lymphocytic leukemia. Cancer **41**:422-427, 1978.
90 Brouet JC, Preud'Homme JL, Seligmann M, Bernard J: Blast cells with monoclonal surface immunoglobulin in two cases of acute blast crisis supervening on chronic lymphocytic leukaemia. Br Med J **4**:23-24, 1973.
91 Brouet JC, Flandrin G, Sasportes M, Preud'Homme JL, Seligmann M: Chronic lymphocytic leukemia of T-cell origin. Lancet **2**:890-893, 1975.
92 Case records of the Massachusetts General Hospital (Case 6-1978). N Engl J Med **298**:387-396, 1978.
93 Dick FR, Maca RD: The lymph node in chronic lymphocytic leukemia. Cancer **41**:283-292, 1978.
93a Enno A, Catovsky D, O'Brien M, Cherchi M, Kumaran TO, Galton DAG: ''Prolymphocytoid'' transformation of chronic lymphocytic leukaemia. Br J Haematol **41**:9-18, 1979.
93b Foucar K, Rydell RE: Richter's syndrome in chronic lymphocytic leukemia. Cancer **46**:118-134, 1980.
94 Galton DAG, Goldman JM, Wiltshaw E, Catovsky D, Henry K, Goldenberg GJ: Prolymphocytic leukaemia. Br J Haematol **27**:7-23, 1974.
95 Goldstein J, Baden J: Richter's syndrome. South Med J **70**:1381-1382, 1977.
96 Long JC, Aisenberg AC: Richter's syndrome: a terminal complication of chronic lymphocytic leukemia with distinct clinicopathologic features. Am J Clin Pathol **63**:786-795, 1975.
97 Peterson LC, Bloomfield CD, Sundberg RD, Gajl-Peczalska KJ, Brunning RD: Morphology of chronic lymphocytic leukemia and its relationship to survival. Am J Med **59**:316-324, 1975.
98 Rausig A: Lymphocytic leukemia and malignant lymphoma in the adult. Acta Med Scand [Suppl] **595**:1-270, 1976.
99 Richter MN: Generalized reticular cell sarcoma of lymph nodes associated with lymphatic leukemia. Am J Pathol **4**:285-292, 1928.
100 Seligmann M, Preud-Homme JL, Brouet JC: Membrane markers in human lymphoid malignancies: clinicopathological correlations and insights into the differentiation of normal and neoplastic cells. In Clarkson B, Marks P, Till JR (eds): Differentiation of normal and neoplastic hematopoietic cells, Cold Spring Harbor, N. Y., 1978, Cold Spring Harbor Laboratory, pp. 859-876.
101 Silver RT, Sawitsky A, Rai K, Holland JF, Glidewell O: Guidelines for protocol studies in chronic lymphocytic leukemia. Am J Hematol **4**:343-358, 1978.
102 Splinter TA, Bom-van Noorloos A, Van Heerde P: CLL and diffuse histiocytic lymphoma in one patient. Clonal proliferation of two different cells. Scand J Haematol **20**:29-36, 1978.

Hairy cell leukemia (leukemic reticuloendotheliosis)

103 Brunning RD, Parkin J: Ribosome-lamella complexes in neoplastic hematopoietic cells. Am J Pathol **79**:565-578, 1975.
104 Burke JS: The value of the bone marrow biopsy in the diagnosis of hairy cell leukemia. Am J Clin Pathol **70**:876-884, 1978.

105 Burke JS, Byrne GE Jr, Rappaport H: Hairy cell leukemia (leukemic reticuloendotheliosis). I. A clinical pathologic study of 21 patients. Cancer 33:1399-1410, 1974.

106 Golomb HM, Catovsky D, Golde DW: Hairy cell leukemia: a clinical review based on 71 cases. Ann Int Med 89:677-683, 1978.

106a Higby KE, Burns GF, Hayhoe FGJ: Identification of the hairy cells of leukemic reticuloendotheliosis by an esterase method. Br J Haematol 38:99-106, 1978.

107 Huhn D, Rodt H, Thiel E: Acid phosphatase in acute lymphocytic leukemia. In Thierfelder S, Rodt H, Thiel E (eds): Immunologic diagnosis of leukemias and lymphomas, New York, 1977, Springer-Verlag New York, Inc., pp. 169-170.

108 Janckila AJ, Li CY, Lam KW, Yam LT: The cytochemistry of tartrate resistant acid phosphatase. Technical considerations. Am J Clin Pathol 70:45-55, 1978.

109 Katayama I, Schneider GB: Further ultrastructural characterization of hairy cells of leukemic reticuloendotheliosis. Am J Pathol 86:163-182, 1977.

110 Katayama I, Yang JPS: Reassessment of a cytochemical test for differential diagnosis of leukemic reticuloendotheliosis. Am J Clin Pathol 68:268-282, 1977.

110a Katayama I, Motohiko A, Pechet L, Sullivan JL, Roberts P, Humphreys RE: B-Lineage prolymphocytic leukemia as a distinct clinicopathologic entity. Am J Pathol 99:399-412, 1980.

111 Naeim F, Smith GS: Leukemic reticuloendotheliosis. Cancer 34:1813-1821, 1974.

112 Rieber EP, Linke RP, Hadam M, Saal JG, Riethmüller G, v Heyden HW, Waller HD, Schwarz H: Hairy cell leukemia: simultaneous demonstration of autochthonous surface-Ig and monocytic functions of hairy cells. In Thierfelder S, Rodt H, Thiel E (eds): Immunologic diagnosis of leukemias and lymphomas, New York, 1977, Springer-Verlag New York, Inc., pp. 157-161.

113 Schnitzer B, Kass L: Hairy cell leukemia: clinicopathologic and ultrastructural study. Am J Clin Pathol 61:176-187, 1974.

114 Turner A, Kjeldsberg CR: Hairy cell leukemia: a review. Medicine 57:477-499, 1978.

114a Variakojis D, Vardiman JW, Golomb HM: Cytochemistry of hairy cells. Cancer 45:72-77, 1980.

115 Vykoupil KF, Thiele J, Georgii A: Hairy cell leukemia: bone marrow findings in 24 patients. Virchows Arch [Pathol Anat] 370:273-289, 1976.

116 Yam LT, Li CY, Lam KW: Tartrate-resistant acid phosphatase isoenzymes in the reticulum cells of leukemic reticuloendotheliosis. N Engl J Med 284:357-360, 1971.

116a Yanovich S, Marks SM, Rosenthal DS, Moloney WC, Schlossman SF: Cell-surface characteristics of hairy cell leukemia in seven patients. Cancer 43:2348-2351, 1979.

117 Zidar BL, Winkelstein A, Whiteside TL, Bellingham AJ, Walker S: Hairy cell leukemia: seven cases with probable B-lymphocytic origin. Br J Haematol 37:455-465, 1977.

Non-Hodgkin's lymphomas

118 Aisenberg AC, Wilkes B: Lymphosarcoma cell leukemia: the contribution of cell surface study to diagnosis. Blood 48:707-715, 1976.

119 Arseneau JG, Canellos GP, Banks PM, Berard CW, Gralnick HR, DeVita VT: American Burkitt's lymphoma: a clinicopathologic study of 30 cases. I. Clinical factors relating to prolonged survival. Am J Med 58:314-321, 1975.

120 Banks PM, Arseneau JG, Gralnick HR, Canellos GP, DeVita VT, Berard CW: American Burkitt's lymphoma: a clinicopathologic study of 30 cases. II. Pathologic correlations. Am J Med 58:322-329, 1975.

121 Barcos MP, Lukes RJ: Malignant lymphomas of convoluted lymphocytes—a new entity of possible T-cell type. In Sinks LR, Godden JO (eds): Conflicts in childhood cancer: an evaluation of current management, vol. 4. New York, 1975, Alan R. Liss, Inc., pp. 147-178.

122 Belpomme D, Borella L, Braylan R, Greaves M, Herberman R, Hitzis W, Kersey J, Petrov R, Ritts R, Seligmann M, Sobin L, Thierfelder S, Torrigiani G: Immunologic diagnosis of leukemia and lymphoma: A World Health Organization/International Union of Immunological Societies technical report. Br J Haematol 38:85-97, 1978.

123 Belpomme D, Lelarge M, Mathe G, Davies AJS: Etiological, clinical and prognostic significance of the T-B immunological classification of primary acute lymphoid leukemias and non-Hodgkin's lymphomas. In Thierfelder S, Rodt H, Thiel B (eds): Immunological diagnosis of leukemias and lymphoma, New York, 1977, Springer-Verlag New York, Inc., pp. 33-45.

124 Bennett JM, Catovsky D, Daniel MT, Flandrin G, Galton DAG, Gralnick HR, Sultan C: Proposals for the classification of the acute leukemias. Br J Haematol 33:451-458, 1976.

125 Berard CW, O'Conor GT, Thomas LB, Torloni H: Histopathological definition of Burkitt's tumor. Bull WHO 40:601-607, 1969.

126 Bloomfield CD, Kersey JH, Brunning RD, Gajl-Peczalska KJ: Prognostic significance of lymphocyte surface markers in adult non-Hodgkin's lymphomas. Lancet 2:1330-1333, 1976.

127 Bluming AZ, Ziegler JL, Carbone PP: Bone marrow involvement in Burkitt's lymphoma: results of a prospective study. Br J Haematol 22:369-376, 1972.

128 Braylan RC, Jaffe ES, Burbach JW, Frank MM, Johnson RE, Berard CW: Similarities of surface characteristics of neoplastic well-differentiated lymphocytes from solid tissues and from peripheral blood. Cancer Res 36:1619-1625, 1976.

129 Brunning RD: Bone marrow and peripheral blood involvement in non-Hodgkin's lymphomas. Geriatrics 30:75-80, 1975.

130 Brunning RD, McKenna RW, Bloomfield CD, Coccia P, Gajl-Peczalska KJ: Bone marrow involvement in Burkitt's lymphoma. Cancer 40:1771-1779, 1977.

131 Burkitt D, Hutt MSR, Wright DH: The African lymphoma: preliminary observations on response to therapy. Cancer 18:399-410, 1965.

132 Cohen MH, Bennett JM, Berard CW, Ziegler JL, Vogel CL, Sheagren JN, Carbone PP: Burkitt's tumor in the United States. Cancer 23:1259-1272, 1969.

133 Coller BS, Chabner BA, Gralnick HR: Frequencies and patterns of bone marrow involvement in non-Hodgkin's lymphomas: observations on the value of bilateral biopsies. Am J Hematol 3:105-119, 1977.

134 Dick F, Bloomfield CD, Brunning RD: Incidence, cytology and histopathology of non-Hodgkin's lympho-

mas in the bone marrow. Cancer **33**:1382-1398, 1974.

135 Dorfman RF: Childhood lymphosarcoma in St. Louis, Missouri, clinically and histologically resembling Burkitt's tumor. Cancer **18**:418-430, 1965.

136 Flandrin G, and Brouet J: The Sezary cell: cytologic, cytochemical and immunologic studies. Mayo Clin Proc **49**:575-583, 1974.

137 Flandrin G, Brouet JC, Daniel MT, Preud'homme JL: Acute leukemia with Burkitt's tumor cells: a study of six cases with special reference to lymphocyte surface markers. Blood **45**:183-188, 1975.

137a Foucar K, McKenna RW, Frizzera G, Brunning RD: Incidence and patterns of bone marrow and blood involvement by lymphoma in relationship to the Lukes-Collins classification. Blood **54**:1417-1422, 1979.

138 Glendenning WE, Brecher G, van Scott EL: Mycosis fungoides: relationship to malignant cutaneous reticulosis and the Sezary syndrome. Arch Dermatol **89**: 785-792, 1964.

139 Hennekeuser HH: Bone marrow biopsy in malignant lymphoma. Recent Results Cancer Res **46**:133-140, 1974.

139a Kim H, Jacobs C, Warnke R, Dorfman RF: Malignant lymphoma with a high content of epithelioid histiocytes: a distinct clinicopathologic entity and a form of so-called "Lennert's lymphoma." Cancer **41**:620-635, 1978.

140 Lukes RJ, Collins RD: A functional classification of malignant lymphomas. In Rebuck JW, Berard CW, Abell MW (eds): The reticuloendothelial system, Baltimore, 1975, The Williams & Wilkins Co., pp. 213-242.

141 Lutzner MA, Jordan HW: The ultrastructure of an abnormal cell in Sezary's syndrome. Blood **31**:719-726, 1968.

142 Lutzner MA, Edelson RS, Smith RW, Shevach EM, Green I: Two varieties of Sezary syndrome, both bearing T-cell markers. Lancet **2**:207, 1973.

143 Lutzner MA, Emerit I, Durepaire R, Flandrin G, Grupper Ch, Prunieras M: Cytogenetic, cytophotometric and ultrastructural study of large cerebriform cells of the Sezary syndrome and description of a small cell variant. J Natl Cancer Inst USA **50**:1145-1162, 1973.

144 McKenna RW, Brunning RD: Reed-Sternberg-like cells in nodular lymphoma involving the bone marrow. Am J Clin Pathol **63**:779-785, 1975.

145 McKenna RW, Bloomfield CD, Brunning RD: Nodular lymphoma: bone marrow and blood manifestations. Cancer **36**:428-440, 1975.

146 McKenna R, Parkin J, Brunning R: Morphological and ultrastructural characteristics of T cell acute lymphoblastic leukemia. Cancer **44**:1290-1297, 1979.

147 McKenna RW, Brynes R, Nesbit M, Bloomfield CD, Kersey JH, Spanjers E, Brunning RD: Cytochemical profiles in acute lymphoblastic leukemia. Am J Pediatr Hematol Oncol **1**:263-275, 1979.

148 Murphy SB, Caces J: Limited utility of bone marrow biopsy in staging children with non-Hodgkin's lymphoma (NHL). Blood **52** [Suppl]:265, 1978.

149 Nathwani BN, Kim H, Rappaport H: Malignant lymphoma, lymphoblastic. Cancer **38**:964-983, 1976.

150 O'Conor GT, Rappaport H, Smith EB: Childhood lymphoma resembling "Burkitt tumor" in the United States. Cancer **18**:411-417, 1978.

151 Pangalis GA, Nathwani BN, Rappaport H: Malignant lymphoma, well differentiated lymphocytic: its relationship with chronic lymphocytic leukemia and macroglobulinemia of Waldenstrom. Cancer **39**:999-1010, 1977.

152 Rappaport H: Tumors of the hematopoietic system. In Atlas of tumor pathology, Sect. III, Fasc. 8. Washington D. C., 1966, Armed Forces Institute of Pathology.

153 Rosas-Uribe A, Variakojis D, Rappaport H: Proteinaceous precipitate in nodular (follicular) lymphomas. Cancer **31**:534-542, 1973.

154 Rosenberg SA: Bone marrow involvement in the non-Hodgkin's lymphomata. Br J Cancer **31** [Suppl II]: 261-264, 1975.

155 Smith JL, Barker CR, Clein GP, Collins RD: Characteristics of malignant mediastinal lymphoid neoplasm (Sternberg sarcoma) as thymic in origin. Lancet **1**:74-77, 1973.

156 Spiro S, Galton DAG, Wiltshaw E, Lohmann RC: Follicular lymphoma: a study of 75 cases with special reference to the syndrome resembling chronic lymphocytic leukaemia. Br J Cancer **31** [Suppl II]:60-72, 1975.

157 Stein RS, Ultmann JE, Byrne GE Jr, Moran EM, Golomb HM, Oetzel N: Bone marrow involvement in non-Hodgkin's lymphoma. Implications for staging and therapy. Cancer **37**:629-636, 1976.

158 Taswell HF, Winkelman RK: Sezary syndrome: a malignant reticulemic erythroderma. JAMA **177**:465-472, 1961.

159 Variakojis D, Rosas-Uribe A, Rappaport H: Mycosis fungoides: pathologic findings in staging laparotomies. Cancer **33**:1589-1600, 1974.

160 Zucker-Franklin D, Melton JW, Quagliata F: Ultrastructural, immunologic and functional studies on Sezary cells. A neoplastic variant of thymus-derived (T) lymphocytes. Proc Natl Acad Sci USA **71**: 1877-1881, 1974.

Hodgkin's disease

161 Bartl R, Burkhardt R, Lengsfeld H, Huhn D: Die Bedeutang der histologischen knockenmarks Beunterlung bie Morbus Hodgkin. Klin Wochenschr **54**:1061-1074, 1976.

162 Bennett JM, Gralnick HR: Bone marrow biopsy in Hodgkin's disease. N Engl J Med **278**:1179, 1968.

163 Dorfman RF: In discussion of Lukes RJ: Criteria for involvement of lymph node, bone marrow, spleen and liver in Hodgkin's disease. Cancer Res **31**:1768-1769, 1971.

164 Koene-Bogman J: Granulomas and the diagnosis of Hodgkin's disease. N Engl J Med **299**:533, 1978.

165 Lukes RJ: Criteria for involvement of lymph node, bone marrow, spleen and liver in Hodgkin's disease. Cancer Res **31**:1755-1767, 1971.

166 McKenna RW, Brunning RD: Reed-Sternberg-like cells in nodular lymphoma involving the bone marrow. Am J Clin Pathol **63**:779-785, 1975.

167 Meyers CE, Chabner BA, DeVita VT, Gralnick HR: Bone marrow involvement in Hodgkin's disease: pathology and response to MOPP chemotherapy. Blood **44**:197-204, 1974.

168 Musshoff K: Prognostic and therapeutic implications of staging in extranodal Hodgkin's disease. Cancer Res **31**:1814-1821, 1971.

169 Neiman RS, Rosen PJ, Lukes RJ: Lymphocyte-depletion Hodgkin's disease. A clinicopathological entity. N Engl J Med **288**:751-755, 1973.

170 O'Carroll DI, McKenna RW, Brunning RD: Bone marrow manifestations of Hodgkin's disease. Cancer **38:**1717-1728, 1976.

171 Rappaport H, Berard CW, Butler JJ, Dorfman RF, Lukes RJ, Thomas LB: Report of the Committee on histopathological criteria contributing to staging of Hodgkin's disease. Cancer Res **31:**1864-1865, 1971.

172 Rosenberg SA: Hodgkin's disease of the bone marrow. Cancer Res **31:**1733-1736, 1971.

173 Te Velde J, Den Ottolander GJ, Spaander PJ, Van den Berg C, Hartgrink-Groeneveld CA: The bone marrow in Hodgkin's disease: the non-involved marrow. Histopathology **2:**31-46, 1978.

174 Webb DI, Ubogy G, Silver RT: Importance of bone marrow biopsy in the clinical staging of Hodgkin's disease. Cancer **26:**313-317, 1970.

Plasma cell dyscrasias
Multiple myeloma

175 Azar HA: Plasma cell myelomatosis and other monoclonal gammopathies. Pathol Annu **7:**1-17, 1977.

176 Azar HA, Zaino EC, Pham TD, Yannopoulos K: Nonsecretory plasma cell myeloma; observations on seven cases with electron microscopic studies. Am J Clin Pathol **58:**618-629, 1972.

177 Brunning R, Parkin J: Intranuclear inclusions in plasma cells and lymphocytes from patients with monoclonal gammopathies. Am J Clin Pathol **66:**10-21, 1976.

178 Hurez D, Preud'Homme JL, Seligmann M: Intracellular "monoclonal" immunoglobulin in non-secretory human myeloma. J Immunol **104:**263-264, 1970.

179 Hyun BK, Kwa D, Gabaldon H, Ashton JK: Reactive plasmacytic lesions of the bone marrow. Am J Clin Pathol **65:**921-928, 1976.

180 Imawari M, Akatsuka N, Ishibachi M, Beppu H, Suzuki H, Yoshitoshi Y: Syndrome of plasma cell dyscrasia, polyneuropathy, and endocrine disturbances. Ann Int Med **81:**490-493, 1974.

181 Klein H, Block M: Bone marrow plasmacytosis: a review of 60 cases. Blood **8:**1034-1041, 1953.

182 Kyle RA: Multiple myeloma: review of 869 cases. Mayo Clin Proc **50:**29-40, 1975.

183 Kyle RA, Greipp PR: The laboratory investigation of monoclonal gammopathies. Mayo Clin Proc **53:**719-739, 1978.

184 Kyle RA, Maldonado JE, Baryd ED: Plasma cell leukemia: report on 17 cases. Arch Int Med **133:**813-818, 1974.

185 Maldonado J, Velosa JA, Kyle RA, Wagoner RD, Holley KE, Salassa RM: Fanconi syndrome in adults. A manifestation of a latent form of myeloma. Am J Med **58:**354-364, 1975.

186 Meyer JE, Schulz MD: "Solitary" myeloma of bone: a review of 12 cases. Cancer **34:**438-440, 1974.

187 Preud'Homme JL, Hurez D, Danon F, Brouet JC, Seligmann M: Intracytoplasmic and surface-bound immunoglobulines in "nonsecretory" and Bence-Jones myeloma. Clin Exp Immunol **25:**428-436, 1976.

188 Snapper I, Kahn A: Myelomatosis. Baltimore, 1971, University Park Press.

189 Wiltshaw E: The natural history of extramedullary plasmacytoma and its relation to solitary myeloma of bone and myelomatosis. Medicine (Baltimore) **55:**217-238, 1976.

189a Woodruf RK, Malpas JS, Paxton AM, Lister TA: Plasma cell leukemia (PCL): a report on 15 patients. Blood **52:**839-845, 1978.

Waldenström's macroglobulinemia

190 Alexanian R: Monoclonal gammopathy in lymphoma. Arch Int Med **135:**62-66, 1975.

191 Berman HH: Waldenstrom's macroglobulinemia with bone lesions and plasma-cell morphology. Am J Clin Pathol **63:**397-402, 1975.

192 Brittin G, Tanaka Y, Brecher G: Intranuclear inclusions in multiple myeloma and macroglobulinemia. Blood **21:**335-351, 1963.

193 Brunning R, Parkin J: Intranuclear inclusions in plasma cells and lymphocytes from patients with monoclonal gammopathies. Am J Clin Pathol **66:**10-21, 1976.

194 Case records of the Massachusetts General Hospital (Case 6-1978). N Engl J Med **298:**387-396, 1978.

195 Dutcher TF, Fahey JL: The histopathology of the macroglobulinemia of Waldenstrom. J Natl Cancer Inst USA **22:**887-917, 1959.

196 Kim H, Heller P, Rappaport H: Monoclonal gammopathies associated with lymphoproliferative disorders. Am J Clin Pathol **59:**282-294, 1973.

197 MacKenzie MR, Fudenberg HH: Macroglobulinemia, an analysis for forty patients. Blood **39:**874-889, 1972.

198 McCallister BD, Bayrd ED, Harrison EG Jr, McGuckin WF: Primary macroglobulinemia: review with a report on 31 cases and notes on the value of continuous chlorambucil therapy. Am J Med **43:**394-434, 1967.

199 Rywlin AW, Civantos F, Ortega RS, Dominguez CJ: Bone marrow histology in monoclonal macroglobulinemia. Am J Clin Pathol **63:**769-778, 1975.

200 Tubbs RR, Hoffman GC, Deodhar SD, Hewlett JS: IgM monoclonal gammopathy: histopathologic and clinical spectrum. Cleve Clin Q **43:**217-235, 1976.

201 Tursz T, Brouet J, Flandrin G, Danon F, Clauvel JP, Seligmann M: Clinical and pathologic features of Waldenstrom's macroglobulinemia in seven patients with serum monoclonal IgG or IgA. Am J Med **63:**499-502, 1977.

202 Waldenstrom J: Incipient myelomatosis or "essential" hypergammaglobulinemia with fibrinogenopenia: a new syndrome? Acta Med Scand **117:**216-247, 1944.

Heavy-chain disease

203 Frangione B, Franklin ED: Heavy chain diseases: clinical features and molecular significance of the disordered immunoglobulin structure. Semin Hematol **10:**53-64, 1973.

204 Franklin EC: Mu-Chain disease. Arch Int Med **135:**71-72, 1975.

205 Jønsson V, Videbaek A, Axelsen NH, Harboe M: Mu-chain disease in a case of chronic lymphocytic leukemia and malignant histiocytoma. I. Clinical aspects. Scand J Haematol **16:**209-217, 1976.

206 Seligmann M: Immunochemical, clinical and pathologic features of alpha-chain disease. Arch Int Med **135:**78-82, 1975.

207 Seligmann M, Preud'Homme JL, Brouet JC: Membrane markers in human lymphoid malignancies. Clinicopathological correlations and insights into the differentiation of normal and neoplastic cells. In Clarkson B, Marks P, Till JR (eds): Differentiation of normal and neoplastic hematopoietic cells. Cold Spring Harbor, N. Y., 1978, Cold Spring Harbor Laboratory, pp. 859-876.

Histiocytic disorders

208 Byrne GE, Rappaport H: Malignant histiocytosis. Gann Monogr Cancer Res **15**:145-162, 1973.

209 Chandra P, Chaudhery SA, Rosner F, Kagen M: Transient histiocytosis with strinking phagocytosis of platelets, leukocytes and erythrocytes. Arch Int Med **135**: 989-991, 1975.

210 Chih-Fei Y, Chung-Hang T, Huai-Teh H, Teh-Ts-Ung T, Hsi-Lien K, Ch'Iu-T'Ang Y, Chieh L: Histiocytic medullary reticulosis. Chin Med J [Engl] **80**:466-474, 1960.

211 Lampert IA, Catovsky D, Bergier M: Malignant histiocytosis: a clinicopathological study of 12 cases. Brit J Haematol **40**:65-77, 1978.

212 Rappaport H: Tumors of the hematopoietic system. In Atlas of tumor pathology, Sect. III, Fasc. 8. Washington D. C., 1966, Armed Forces Institute of Pathology.

213 Risdall RJ, McKenna RW, Nesbitt ME, Kriuit W, Balfour HH, Simmons RL, Brunning RD: Virus associated hemophagocytic syndrome. Cancer **44**:993-1002, 1979.

214 Warnke RA, Kim H, Dorfman RF: Malignant histiocytosis (histiocytic medullary reticulosis) I. Clinicopathologic study of 29 cases. Cancer **35**:215-230, 1975.

Angioimmunoblastic lymphadenopathy

215 Frizzera G, Moran EM, Rappaport H: Angio-immunoblastic lymphadenopathy with dysproteinaemia. Lancet **1**:1070-1073, 1974.

216 Frizzera G, Moran EM, Rappaport H: Angio-immunoblastic lymphadenopathy. Diagnosis and clinical course. Am J Med **59**:803-818, 1975.

217 Lukes RJ, Tindle BH: Immunoblastic lymphadenopathy. A hyperimmune entity resembling Hodgkin's disease. N Engl J Med **292**:1-8, 1975.

218 Pangalis GA, Moran EM, Rappaport H: Blood and bone marrow findings in angio-immunoblastic lymphadenopathy. Blood **51**:71-83, 1978.

Systemic mastocytosis

219 Johnstone JM: The appearance and significance of tissue mast cells in human bone marrow. J Clin Pathol **7**:275-280, 1954.

219a Lennert K, Parwaresch MR: Mast cells and mast cell neoplasia: a review. Histopathology **3**:349-365, 1979.

220 Parker C, Jost RG, Bauer E, Haddad J, Garza R: In Cryer PE, and Kissane JM (eds): Clinicopathologic conference: systemic mastocytosis. Am J Med **61**: 671-680, 1976.

221 Rappaport H: Tumors of the hematopoietic system. In Atlas of tumor pathology, Sect. III, Fasc. 8, Washington D. C., 1966, Armed Forces Institute of Pathology.

222 Rywlin AM, Hoffman EP, Ortega RS: Eosinophilic fibrohistiocytic lesion of bone marrow: a distinctive new morphologic finding, probably related to drug hypersensitivity. Blood **40**:464-472, 1972.

223 Sagher F, Even-Paz Z: Mastocytosis and the mast cell. Chicago, 1967, Year Book Medical Publishers, Inc.,

224 Szweda JA, Abraham JP, Fine G, Nixon RK, Rupe CE: Systemic mast cell disease: a review and report of three cases. Am J Med **32**:227-239, 1962.

225 TeVelde J, Vismans FJFE, Leenheers-Binnendijk L, Vos CJ, Smecnk D, Bijvoet OLM: The eosinophilic fibrohistiocytic lesion of the bone marrow. A mastocellular lesion in bone disease. Virchows Arch [Pathol Anat] **377**:277-284, 1978.

226 Woessner S, LaFuente R, Pardo P, Rosell R, Rozman C, Sans-Sabrafen J: Systemic mastocytosis: a case report. Acta Hematol **58**:321-331, 1977.

Metastatic tumor

227 Anner RM, Drewinko B: Frequency and significance of bone marrow involvement by metastatic solid tumors. Cancer **39**:1337-1344, 1977.

228 Finkelstein JZ, Ekert H, Isaacs H, Higgins G: Bone marrow metastases in children with solid tumors. Am J Dis Child **119**:49-52, 1976.

229 Hansen HH, Muggia FM, Selawry OS: Bone-marrow examination in 100 consecutive patients with broncogenic carcinoma. Lancet **2**:443-445, 1971.

230 Hirsch F, Hansen HH, Dombernowsky P, Hainau B: Bone-marrow examination in the staging of small-cell anaplastic carcinoma of the lung with special reference to subtying. Cancer **39**:2563-2567, 1977.

231 Ingle JN, Tormey DC, Tan HK: The bone marrow examination in breast cancer. Diagnostic considerations and clinical usefullness. Cancer **41**:670-674, 1978.

232 Singh G, Krause JR, and Breitfeld V: Bone marrow examination for metastatic tumor, aspiration and biopsy. Cancer **40**:2317-2321, 1977.

Lipid storage diseases

233 Brady RO: Glucosyl ceramide lipidosis: Gaucher's disease. In Stanbury JB, Wyngaarden JB, Frederickson DS (eds): The metabolic basis of inherited disease. New York, 1978, McGraw-Hill Book Co., pp. 747-769.

234 Brady RO: Sphingomyelin lipidosis: Niemann-Pick disease. In Stanbury JB, Wyngaarden JB, Frederickson DS (eds): The metabolic basis of inherited disease. New York, 1978, McGraw-Hill Book Co., pp. 718-730.

235 Brunning RD: Morphologic alterations in nucleated blood and marrow cells in genetic disorders. Hum Pathol **1**:99-124, 1970.

236 Desnick RJ, Klionsky B, Sweeley CC: Fabry's disease (α galactosidase A deficiency). In Stanbury JB, Wyngaarden JB, Frederickson DS (eds): The metabolic basis of inherited disease. New York, 1978, McGraw-Hill Book Co., pp. 810-840.

237 Dosik H, Rosner F, Sawitsky A: Acquired lipidosis: Gaucher-like cells and "blue cells" in chronic granulocytic leukemia. Semin Hematol **9**:309-316, 1972.

238 Gerdes J, Marathe RL, Bloodworth JMB, MacKinney AA: Gaucher cells in chronic granulocytic leukemia. Arch Pathol **88**:194, 1969.

239 Kattlove HE, Williams JC, Gaynor E, Spivack M, Brady B, Brady R: Gaucher cells in chronic myelocytic leukemia: an acquired abnormality. Blood **33**: 379-390, 1969.

240 Pratt PW, Estren S, Kochwa S: Immunoglobulin abnormalities in Gaucher's disease: Report of 16 cases. Blood **31**:633-640, 1968.

241 Silverstein MN, Ellefson RD: The syndrome of the sea-blue histiocyte. Semin Hematol **9**:299-307, 1972.

242 Silverstein MN, Ellefson RD, Ahern EF: The syndrome of the sea-blue histiocyte. N Engl J Med **282**: 1-4, 1970.

243 Van Dorpe A, Broeckaert-Van Orshoven A, Desmet V, Verwilghen RL: Gaucher-like cells and congenital dyserythropoietic anaemia, type II (HEMPAS). Br J Haematol **25**:165-170, 1973.

244 Zaino EC, Rossi MB, Pham TD, Azar H: Gaucher's cells in thalassemia. Blood **38**:457-462, 1971.

23 Bone and joints

Introduction

The European pathologists have studied bone thoroughly, their knowledge for the most part having come from thorough postmortem study of osseous lesions. The student need only examine classic German books of pathology such as Henke-Lubarsch's work to realize how extensive has been their study. Bone examination at autopsy in the United States is considered thorough if small segments of femur, vertebra, and sternum are removed. In most instances, only a fragment of vertebra is examined. Even this specimen may not be studied microscopically.

American pathologists should study bone more thoroughly. The routine removal at autopsy of rib, the anterior half of the vertebral column, femur, and even humerus would prove worthwhile. The correlation of roentgenographic and microscopic findings in large sections of bone would add to the understanding of osseous pathologic processes. Excellent books on osseous pathology are available to guide the student in this endeavor.[1,4,5,8,9,11]

Primary neoplasms of bone are rare.[14] Their rarity plus the technical difficulty of section preparation have made the diagnosis and proper treatment of bone tumors fraught with error. There are only a few centers in the United

States where much orthopedic pathology is seen. Consequently, many pathologists and radiologists have little firsthand knowledge of these tumors. Before making a diagnosis, it is imperative that the clinical history be complete, that x-ray examination be adequate, and that the pathologic material be well prepared and representative of the lesion.

In most instances, the clinical story is helpful but not diagnostic. The radiologic pattern may be diagnostic in some, but there are many exceptions.[3] Often roentgenograms of other bones are necessary.

Too often, poorly prepared and incorrectly diagnosed slides are referred for diagnosis by experienced pathologists. The reasons are obvious. Many technicians do not know how to prepare and stain bone sections properly, and many surgeons submit inadequate biopsies for microscopic examination. The surgical pathologist must have all clinical and roentgenographic data before attempting a microscopic diagnosis. We have established in our laboratory the policy of never rendering a pathologic diagnosis on a bone tumor in the absence of roentgenograms. Failure to adhere to this policy may lead to diagnosing an exuberant callus as osteosarcoma. Furthermore, since the frequency of most tumors and tumorlike conditions of bone is closely related to the patient's age, specific bone, and area of the bone involved, knowledge of these data will help the pathologist immeasurably in his differential diagnosis. As an example, let us consider a lesion located in the diaphyseal area of the tibia in a 13-year-old boy. It is an eccentric, sharply delineated lesion. There are no other lesions in other bones. The configuration of the lesion is not that of a solitary bone cyst. The patient is too young to have giant cell tumor. In fact, there is only one lesion that will fit in this case—a metaphyseal fibrous defect (Fig. 1282). This diagnostic approach should be used for all bone lesions. In many instances, it will resolve the problem without difficulty. It is also imperative for the pathologist to acquire a thorough knowledge of the histology and development of bones.[2] He must realize that osseous reactions to injury, tumors, and metabolic conditions are limited and that they vary merely in degree. Once he has established the fundamental properties of bone clearly in his mind, he can help the orthopedic surgeon select representative material for biopsy, decalcify the specimen with care, stain the sections properly, and cor-

relate the microscopic findings with the clinical history and roentgenograms.[12]

Brief descriptions of the most important components and changes of bone as they relate to surgical pathology are given in the following paragraphs.

The *diaphysis* of the bone is its shaft. The *epiphysis* represents the ends of a long bone and is partially covered by articular cartilage. Endochondral ossification occurs at the epiphyseal plate in a growing bone. Longitudinal, regularly spaced columns of vascularized cartilage are replaced by bone. When the bone has reached its adult length, this process ends and the epiphysis "closes" by becoming calcified and ossified. The *metaphysis* is defined as the region of bone adjacent to the epiphyseal disk, consisting of spongy bone and containing the growth zone. It is a very important area in bone pathology, because it is by far the most common site for the occurrence of most primary bone tumors.

The time of closure of the epiphysis differs in various bones and in the sexes. Whether the epiphysis is closed or open influences the extension of pathologic processes. For instance, cartilage is often at least a partial barrier to spreading osteosarcoma. If the epiphysis is closed and cartilage is no longer present, this area is more easily invaded.[6]

The periosteum is closely applied to bone. It is a specialized layer of connective tissue with the capacity to form bone. This property can be nicely demonstrated by transplanting a fragment of periosteum beneath the capsule of a kidney of an experimental animal.[10] Nerve filaments are present in the periosteum and carry proprioceptive and sensory impulses. Small nerve filaments also may pass with the nutrient vessels into the medullary canal.

The periosteum may become detached and elevated from the bone in such pathologic processes as trauma, infection, and primary or secondary malignant tumors. Whenever this happens, new bone formation between the elevated periosteum and the bone will occur. This appears by roentgenographic examination as fine spicules placed perpendicular to the long axis of the bone. This finding is often considered a manifestation of a primary malignant neoplasm, particularly osteosarcoma and Ewing's sarcoma. However, periosteal bone proliferation also can occur in syphilis, tuberculosis, metastatic carcinoma, and subperiosteal hematoma (Fig. 1204). In some lesions, such

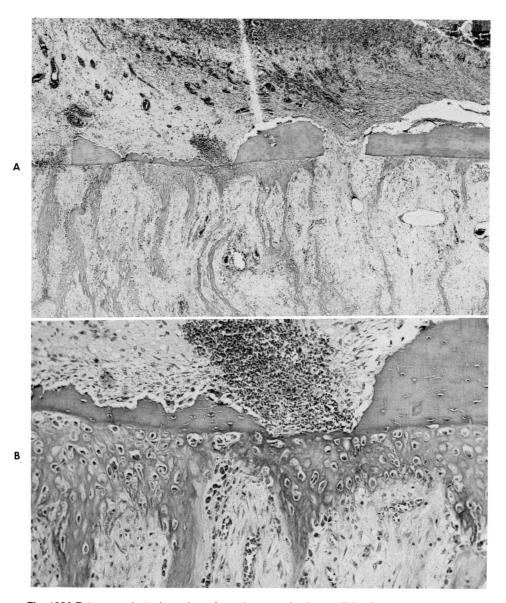

Fig. 1204 Extreme periosteal new bone formation occurring in mandible after hematoma had almost completely destroyed bone through interference with blood supply. Only fragments of dead mandible remain, but exuberant periosteal bone proliferation is extending from periosteum in long columns. (**A,** Low power; WU neg. 52-3874; B, ×150; WU neg. 52-3873.)

as plasma cell myeloma, the periosteum may be destroyed or encroached upon so that no roentgenographic changes occur.

An understanding of the blood supply of bone helps to explain spread and limitation of infection, the healing of fractures, and the involvement of bone by primary or secondary neoplasms. The metaphysis is supplied by nutrient end arteries entering from the diaphysis.

These vessels terminate at the epiphyseal plate. Vessels also enter from the periphery. The epiphyses receive their blood supply from widely anastomosing vessels. Diaphyseal cortex is supplied by vessels that enter through Volkmann's canals and communicate with the haversian system. A nutrient artery enters the medullary canal at about the center of the shaft, divides, and extends both distally and proximal-

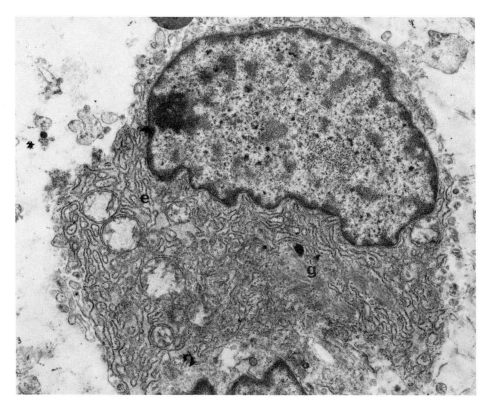

Fig. 1205 Osteoblast in ossifying fibroma showing prominent Golgi apparatus, **g,** and much ergasto-plasm, **e.** These are features that correlate with osteoid (collagen) synthesis. (Approximately ×9,000.)

ly. The metabolic exchange of calcium and phosphorus occurs primarily in the metaphysis.

Osteoblasts are the bone-producing cells. They have a plump appearance and often exhibit a perinuclear halo that given them a resemblance to plasma cells. They have a high cytoplasmic content of alkaline phosphatase. Ultrastructurally, they resemble fibroblasts by virtue of a well-developed rough endoplasmic reticulum and Golgi apparatus (Fig. 1205).

Osteoclasts are multinucleated giant cells involved in bone resorption. As such, they often are found adjacent to dead or viable bone trabeculae with ragged edges. They contain abundant acid phosphatase. Ultrastructurally, the cytoplasm has a very large number of mitochondria and scanty lysosomes; a ruffled edge is present in the area of the cell membrane that is in process of bone resorption.

Osteoid is the unmineralized organic precursor matrix of bone. It is composed of a mixture of collagen and acid mucopolysaccharides; it is not a homogeneous mass but rather shows a constant sequence of maturation and organiza-

tion patterns.[7] It has acidophilic properties in hematoxylin-eosin sections, and it may be difficult to differentiate from hyalinized collagen. When osteoid becomes calcified, *bone* is formed.

In *woven bone* (fiber bone), there is a haphazard arrangement of collagen fibers within the matrix, which is best appreciated with polarized light. Formation of woven bone is the key feature for the diagnosis of fibrous dysplasia, but it also appears in the callus of a healing fracture, osteitis fibrosa cystica, and other processes. The difference resides in the fact that in the latter group the woven bone eventually becomes *lamellar bone,* whereas in fibrous dysplasia it remains as woven bone throughout. Lamellar bone is characterized by concentric parallel lamellae as seen with polarizing lenses.

Bone necrosis can be recognized by the staining reaction of the dead bone. It stains a deeper blue than does normal bone. Lacunar cells are absent, and the margins of the bone are ragged (Fig. 1206). The presence of osteoclasts on

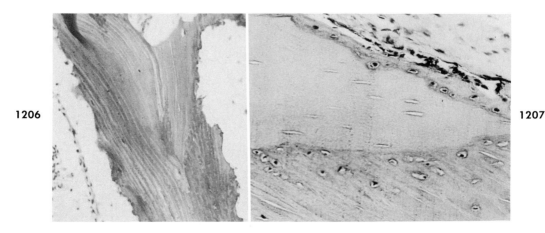

Fig. 1206 Dead bone with empty lacunae and ragged bone margins. (×270; WU neg. 49-5373.)
Fig. 1207 Appositional bone growth proceeding on surface of spicule of dead bone. Living bone is sharply demarcated, and its lacunae contain nuclei. (×300; WU neg. 49-5640.)

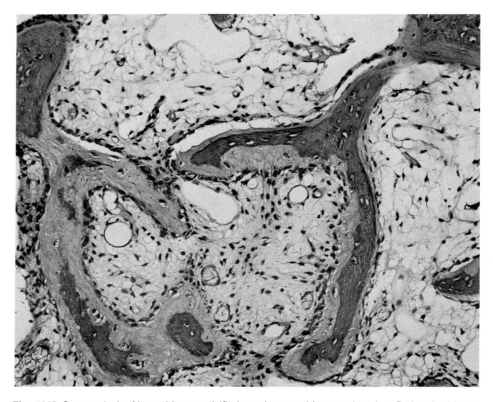

Fig. 1208 Osteomalacia. Note wide noncalcified matrix around bone trabeculae. Patient had hyperparathyroidism of long duration with profound renal insufficiency. (×140; WU neg. 61-7452.)

these margins indicates that the bone is already being reabsorbed.

Bone production can be recognized by the presence of well-stained small spicules of bone with cells in their lacunae and osteoblasts along their margins (Fig. 1207). New bone formation can be studied in a variety of physiologic and pathologic processes, such as a healing fracture, Paget's disease, metaplastic ossification, myositis ossificans, and osteitis fibrosa cystica.

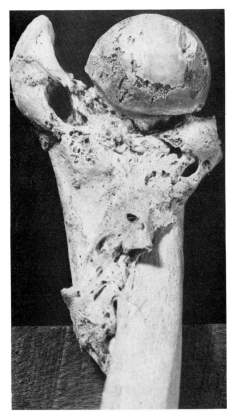

Fig. 1209 Exuberant callus formation following fracture.

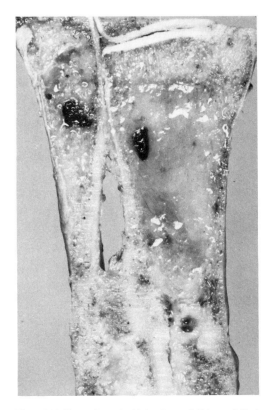

Fig. 1210 Nonunion of old fracture of tibia and fibula in 53-year-old white man. Multiple fractures had occurred two years previously and necessitated bone grafting. (WU neg. 62-3316.)

Bone destruction can be recognized by the presence of numerous osteoclasts in the ragged margins and in Howship's lacunae.

Metabolic bone diseases

Metabolic bone disease is outside the scope of this chapter. Some metabolic bone diseases will be mentioned briefly, but there are entire books, monographs, and excellent articles written on the problem.[15,16,21-26,28,30-35] If one considers only osteoporosis and osteomalacia, it becomes apparent that these two processes are not well understood.

Osteoporosis develops when an individual is unable to repair and maintain the mass of bone tissue that has been acquired throughout growth and maturation.[36] Jowsey et al.[27] have demonstrated by quantitative microradiographic studies that the main difference between the bone in most forms of osteoporosis and normal bone is an increase in the amount of resorption, bone formation levels being generally normal. Osteoporosis occurs frequently after the meno-

pause, perhaps related to estrogen deficiency.[20] The causes for osteoporosis are multiple. Fluoride consumption is probably important in its prevention.[18]

A good biopsy from the iliac crest corresponds well with changes in the spine.[17] However, roentgenographic examination of the spine is not reliable, for the changes have to be advanced before they can be seen. Studies made at autopsy by Caldwell[19] have helped to clarify the pathology. For instance, he showed that vertebral biconcavity is not a reliable index of osteoporosis.

Osteomalacia (comparable to rickets in a young person in whom the epiphyses are not yet closed) may result from a wide spectrum of congenital and acquired metabolic abnormalities which result in sufficient decrease in serum calcium, phosphorus, or both to impair mineralization of the skeleton and epiphyseal growth.[27b] Some cases have been seen secondary to bone and soft tissue neoplasms, particularly of vascular origin.[27a] In osteomalacia, the bone matrix is formed, but its calcification is incomplete, and this gives rise to a noncalcified matrix around the bone tra-beculae[37] (Fig. 1208). These changes can be demonstrated in adequate biopsies from long bones and iliac crests with preparation of non-decalcified specimens and examination with the bright-field and phase-contrast microscopes.

Sophisticated methods of investigating these metabolic bone processes have been devised, and many of them are difficult to institute in the usual pathology laboratory.[29,36]

Fractures

Fractures are breaks in the continuity of bone usually with severance of periosteum, blood

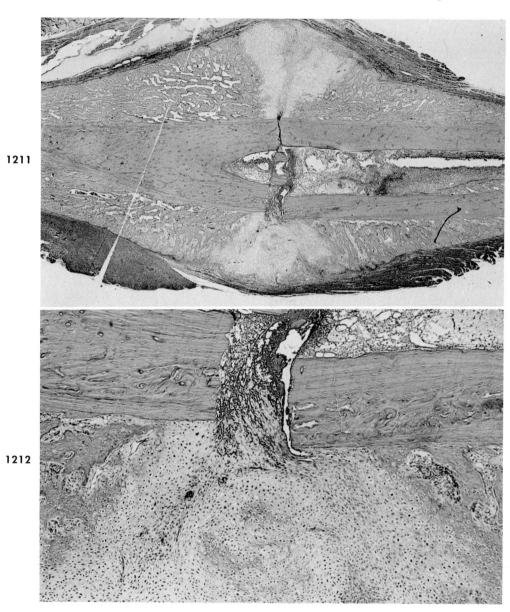

1211

1212

Fig. 1211 Healing fracture of long bone in rat at seven days. Note intact periosteum and intramem-branous bone formation. (Low power; WU neg. 52-4346.)
Fig. 1212 Detailed view of point of fracture shown in Fig. 1211. Granulation tissue has been re-placed with cartilage, and new bone is gradually replacing this cartilage. Fragment of dead bone with-in marrow cavity is being reabsorbed. (Low power; WU neg. 52-4344.)

vessels, and perhaps muscles. The return of bone to normal following fracture depends upon factors such as treatment, age of the patient, severity of the fracture, vascularity of the area, and nutrition of the patient (Fig. 1209). Fractures fail to heal because of improper immobilization, complete devascularization of segments of the fractured bone, persistent infec-

tion, and the interposition of soft tissue between the ends of the bone (Fig. 1210). A hematoma forms between the two severed ends of bone. Organization of this hematoma begins with the ingrowth of young capillaries. After about three days, the devitalized bone fragments begin to be reabsorbed. Intramembranous bone growth makes its appearance from the cambium layer

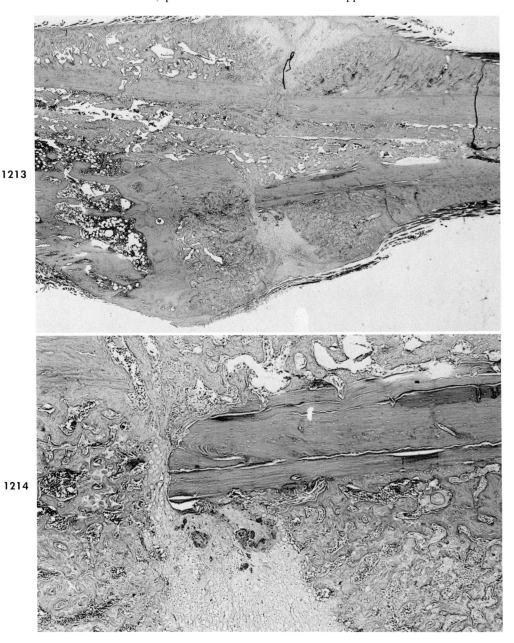

Fig. 1213 Healing fracture of long bone in rat at three weeks. (Low power; WU neg. 52-4345.)
Fig. 1214 Detailed view of fracture site shown in Fig. 1213. Bone has almost completely bridged gap. Small amount of cartilage can still be seen near dead bone fragments. (Low power; WU neg. 52-4344.)

of the periosteum, both proximal and distal to the fracture site (Figs. 1211 and 1212). The newly formed trabeculae begin to calcify as the cartilage is replaced by bone.[41,43,44] This process on each side of the fracture meets at the fracture site to form the primary callus. The periosteum is composed of an outer fibrous layer and an inner osteogenic layer.[42] This inner osteogenic layer and the endosteum contribute to the formation of callus. "Lines of stress through the fracture site do not dictate the alignment of trabeculae in the primary callus"* The secondary callus is made up of mature lamellar bone. The primary callus is absorbed. The new bone is laid down predominantly along lines of stress (Figs. 1213 and 1214). The formation and persistence of cartilage is largely dependent upon mechanical factors.[45]

The early reduction of fractures promotes rapid healing.[46] With proper reduction of the fracture, adequate blood supply, no infection,

*From Luck JV: Bone and joint diseases. Springfield, Ill., 1950, Charles C Thomas, Publisher.

and normal metabolism, the fracture heals rapidly with little visible callus. Exuberant callus usually means slow fracture healing (Fig. 1209). In children, even with prominent angulation or deformity, the bone remodels itself to an astonishing degree.[38,47] For this reason, open reduction and internal fixation of fractures in children are seldom justified. Shortening of a long bone due to overriding of fragments will nearly always correct itself in children by overgrowth of bone.

The sequence of events in a rapidly forming primary callus such as the formation of exuberant cartilage and disorderly membranous bone may produce a bewildering microscopic pattern. Such callus formation may be excessive in osteogenesis imperfecta.[48] The microscopic picture may be difficult to differentiate from osteosarcoma.

Changes in bone produced by nails, screws, and other prostheses

When a noncorrosive nail, such as a Jewett or Massie nail, is driven into a bone to immobilize a fracture, it eventually becomes complete-

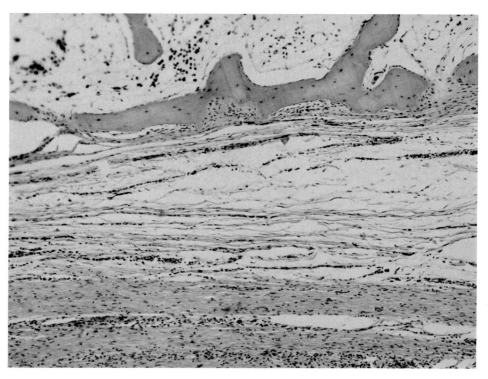

Fig. 1215 Sequestration within nail tract. Lower margin shows fibrous tissue next to nail tract which is continuous with periosteum. Layer of bone above fibrous tissue is continuous with cortical bone. (Low power; WU neg. 58-4088.)

ly isolated from the bone.[40] The nail is separated from the medullary cavity by fibrous tissue that is continuous with the periosteum. Bone similar to cortical bone forms adjacent to the fibrous tissue (Fig. 1215). This cortical bone, in turn, forms an uninterrupted continuity with the cortex of the bone. No foreign body giant cell reaction is observed.[39]

Osteomyelitis

Osteomyelitis may be caused by a large variety of microorganisms. About 70% to 90% of the cases are due to the coagulase-positive staphylococci.[58a] Other organisms such as *Klebsiella, Aerobacter, Proteus, Pseudomonas,* streptococcus, pneumococcus, gonococcus, and meningococcus and rare organisms

such as *Brucella, Histoplasma capsulatum,* and *Actinomyces* also cause it.[55] Recovery of several organisms in the culture is not unusual. Patients with abnormal hemoglobin disease, particularly sickle cell disease, are prone to develop osteomyelitis due to *Salmonella* infection.[57] Osteomyelitis may follow compound fractures. Hematogenous infections of bone occur most often in patients under 20 years of age. About 75% of cases occur in the lower extremity. The changes in the bone are conditioned by the bone involved, virulence of the organism, resistance of the host, and age of the patient.

Trueta[58] has shown that the involvement of the bone varies with the age of the patient and the vascular supply of the bone. In the infant

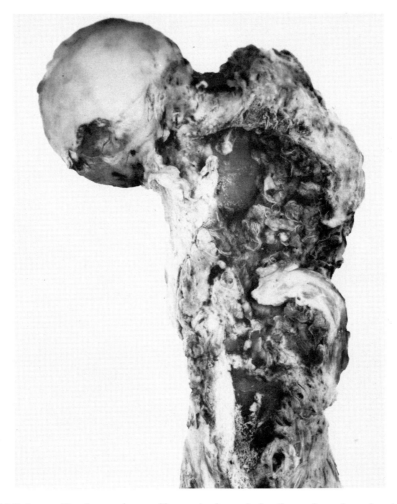

Fig. 1216 Osteomyelitis of upper femur with massive bone destruction and reactive sclerosis. (Courtesy Dr. H. Rodriguez-Martinez, Mexico City, Mexico.)

under 1 year of age, permanent epiphyseal damage and joint infection occur with little damage to the shaft and metaphysis. In children over 1 year of age, there is extensive cortical damage with involucrum formation. Permanent damage to cartilage and joints is rare. Usually with treatment, chronicity is absent.

Acute osteomyelitis of the long bones in the adult is infrequent. When it occurs, joint infection develops, and the cortex is often absorbed without formation of a sequestrum. The entire bone is involved. Chronicity is more likely to occur. Subacute and chronic osteomyelitis can closely simulate clinically and roentgenographically a malignant bone tumor (particularly Ewing's sarcoma, malignant lymphoma, and osteosarcoma) by virtue of the com-

bination of destructive and regenerative bone changes[50] (Fig. 1216).

The introduction of the strong antimicrobial drugs led initially to the treatment of acute hematogenous osteomyelitis without open drainage or saucerization. The mortality and morbidity dropped precipitously after the use of these drugs. The saucerization and drainage that were later instituted in combination with antibiotics in the treatment of acute osteomyelitis resulted in further inprovement of results. The frequency of late recrudescence of osseous infection has been much less. Combined surgical and drug therapy has also proved much more effective in treating the staphylococcal infections that are partially or totally resistant to antibiotic therapy. Infections of

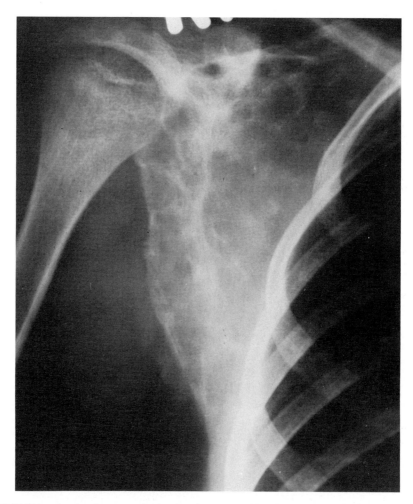

Fig. 1217 Extensive involvement of scapula of osteomyelitis of staphylococcal origin in 8-year-old child. This was apparently the only bone involved. (WU neg. 62-8972; courtesy Dr. P. Flynn, Redding, Calif.)

the latter type appear to be increasing in frequency (Fig. 1217). Hematogenous pyogenic vertebral osteomyelitis is frequently not diagnosed because of the subtle nature of the disease.[53]

If the infection is massive in the child, the inflammatory process in the metaphyseal area is often complicated by infected thrombi, leading to infarction and subsequent destruction of bone. The infectious material invades the cortex through the vessels of Volkmann's canals. The infection may spread along the medullary canal, through the cortex, or into the joint space. If pus develops beneath the periosteum, perforation through it usually takes place. With the process tending to localize, the cambium layer of the periosteum responds to the presence of dead bone (the sequestrum) by forming new bone (the involucrum). The involucrum eventually extends around the entire bone (Figs.

1218 and 1219). The sequestrum, if not too large, may be extruded through cutaneous sinuses. Chronic osteomyelitis may show prominent periosteal bone proliferation (Fig. 1220).

Osteomyelitic sinuses in the adult may become lined by squamous epithelium that may extend deeply into the bone and become discontinuous with the cutaneous surface. Despite apparent healing of the overlying skin, large epidermal inclusion cysts slowly develop in the underlying bone. These are filled with keratin-containing debris similar to that in epidermal inclusion cysts of the skin. Rarely, after a long period, squamous carcinoma develops within these sinuses. Pain and increasingly malodorous discharge heralds the development of carcinoma in such sinuses.[52,54]

The chronic osteomyelitis persists as long as infected dead bone remains. The dead bone is surrounded by granulation tissue that attacks

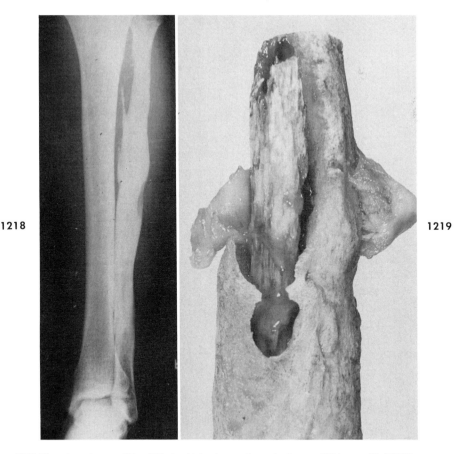

1218   1219

Fig. 1218 Chronic osteomyelitis of fibula. Note dense, irregular bone. (WU neg. 50-1493.)
Fig. 1219 Resected fibula showing dense outer involucrum surrounding loosened sequestrum with its pitted surface. (WU neg. 50-652.)

the sequestrum, making it pitted on the surface next to the marrow cavity. The cortical surface remains smooth. Operative removal of the sequestrum at the proper time usually allows the osteomyelitis to heal. The osteomyelitis may recur many years later if bacteria remain within the scar.

Tuberculous osteomyelitis as a hematogenous infection usually seen in young adults or children. Wherever pasteurization of milk is mandatory, the incidence of bone tuberculosis is low. The bones most often infected are the vertebrae and bones of the hip, knee, ankle, elbow, and wrist. Tuberculosis usually involves the metaphyseal area, the epiphysis, and the synovium.[49] There has been considerable controversy concerning the area primarily involved.

Metaphyseal infection is common in children and epiphyseal infection common in adults. This does not have too much significance, for all zones eventually become involved (Fig. 1221). Tuberculous granulation tissue forming in the synovia destroys the synovial attachments. The cartilage, no longer nourished from the synovia, undergoes progressive destruction, allowing tuberculous granulation tissue to extend into the epiphysis and finally into the metaphyseal area. If the process begins in the epiphysis, the tuberculous granulation tissue extends into the adjacent joint. When the process begins in the metaphyseal area, extension into the joint may be heralded by the development of fluid in it. Cutaneous sinuses may occur in advanced tuberculosis. These sinuses allow entry of secondary bacterial infection which modifies the pathologic changes. When the tuberculous process begins to heal, fusion of the joint may be associated with complete or partial denudation of cartilage and "kissing sequestra." Sequestra are cortical in pyogenic processes, but in tuberculous disease they are

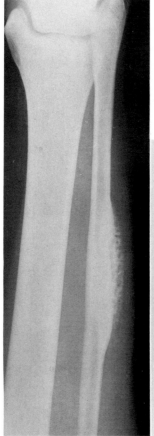

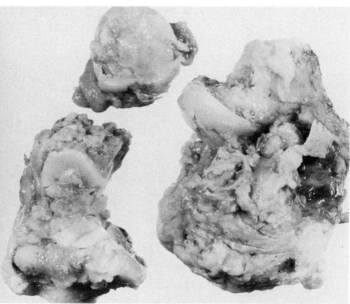

1220   1221

Fig. 1220 Prominent periosteal bone proliferation in chronic osteomyelitis. (WU neg. 51-1883.)
Fig. 1221 Extensive involvement of synovium of elbow joint by tuberculous granulation tissue (WU neg. 49-978.)

cancellous. Tuberculosis of the diaphysis also occurs.[51]

The pathologic changes in tuberculosis of bone have been greatly modified by antimyco-bacterial drugs. Tuberculous tenosynovitis of the hand may form multiple soft tissue masses that are mistaken for neoplasm.[56]

Tertiary syphilis may involve the bone and cause both osseous destruction and production. It frequently is associated with conspicuous periosteal bone proliferation[59] (Fig. 1222). The necrotic, well-defined defects are mainly cortical and periosteal and are surrounded by sclerotic bone.

These lesions may be in the vertebrae, flat bones of the hands and feet, and the diaphysis of the long tubular bones. If a single x-ray film is taken, a diagnosis of osteosarcoma may be made. Biopsy will show a granulomatous process with bone destruction and production. The diagnosis usually will be apparent if multiple films of the bones are studied. In single or isolated lesions, the diagnosis may be difficult. The presence of a positive serology does not eliminate the possibility of osteosarcoma. In such instances, a biopsy is required to make an exact diagnosis.

Bone necrosis
Infarct

Bone infarct can be the result of a large number of etiologic factors (Table 64). Roentgenographically, the changes depend on the age of the lesion and the degree of repair. During the first one or two weeks, no abnormalities are detected. Resorption of the dead bone will result in areas of decreased density, whereas new bone formation growing in apposition to dead trabeculae (so called ''creeping apposition'') will lead to an increase in bone density. The process of reossification is often irregular, and the combination of incomplete resorption of dead bone and focal deposition of new bone results in a mottled and irregular appearance in the roentgenograms (Fig. 1223).

An increased incidence of primary malignant bone tumors has been seen in association with large bone infarcts of long bones. Most of the reported cases have occurred in the medulla of the femur or tibia of male adults and have been diagnosed as malignant fibrous histiocytoma, osteosarcoma, and fibrosarcoma.[61,65]

Aseptic (avascular) bone necrosis

Osseous aseptic necrosis is an important orthopedic pathologic abnormality that has been reported in practically every secondary epiphysis and in many primary epiphyses (Figs. 1224 and 1225). Unfortunately, each site has been described independently and often given individual names such as the following:

Tibial tubercle (Osgood-Schlatter disease) (Osgood, 1903)
Patella—primary epiphysis (Kohler, 1908)
Tarsal navicular (Kohler, 1908)
Capital epiphysis femur (osteochondritis deformans juvenilis; Legg-Perthes' disease) (Legg, 1909)
Head of humerus (Lewin, 1930)

The etiology of many cases is unknown and is thought possibly to be traumatic or related to endocrine imbalance. In some, etiology is related to obliteration of the epiphyseal blood supply because of fracture or dislocation.[60]

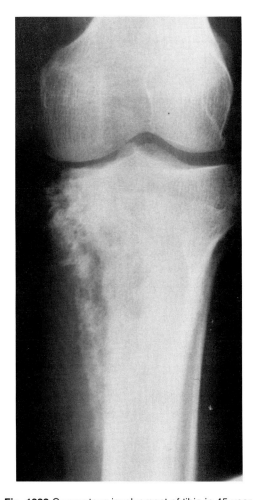

Fig. 1222 Gummatous involvement of tibia in 45-year-old woman. (Courtesy Dr. R. J. Reed, New Orleans, La.)

Table 64 Conditions associated with bone infarct*

Diaphyso-metaphyseal infarctions	Epiphyso-metaphyseal infarctions
Caisson disease (decompression sickness)	Thrombosis
Gaucher's disease	Sickle cell anemia (SS and SC hemoglobin)
Sickle cell anemia	Corticosteroids
Sickle cell trait	Thromboembolic disease
Pancreatic disease	Disease of arterial wall
Acute	Lupus erythematosus
Chronic	Rheumatoid arthritis
Occlusive vascular disease	Boeck's sarcoid
Arteriosclerosis	Arteriosclerosis
Thromboembolic disease	Disease of adjacent bone
Periarteritis nodosa (vasculitis)	Histiocytosis X
Pheochromocytoma	Gaucher's disease
Infection	Osteomyelitis
Idiopathic	Caisson disease
	Traumatic and idiopathic
	Fractures and dislocations
	Osteochrondroses

*From Libshitz HI, Osborne RL Jr: The diagnosis of bone infarction. Ann Clin Lab Sci **5:**272-275, 1975.

Phemister[66] clarified the pathogenesis of femoral head avascular necrosis secondary to complete interruption of blood supply occurring in fractures of the femoral neck.

The sequence of events implies death of the epiphysis which, in time, becomes more clearly seen roentgenographically. This death of bone is followed by hyperemia of the neighboring tissues. The overlying cartilage of the epiphysis may or may not remain viable, for it receives nourishment from the overlying synovium. The dead bone gradually undergoes resorption. There may be osteoclasis on one side of necrotic trabeculae, with osteoblastic activity on the other.[63] This bone is gradually replaced by "creeping substitution." This replacement of the dead epiphysis by new bone is a slow process, taking months or even years. This is illustrated by the sclerosis that is seen after fractures of the neck of the femur. The dense appearance of the femoral head is often incident to new bone formation upon the dead trabecular bone.[60] The new soft bone may flatten because of pressure. If this change occurs, degenerative joint disease soon follows. Aseptic necrosis of the femoral head may occur in sickle cell disease.[62]

Osteochondritis dissecans

Osteochondritis dissecans results from a small area of necrosis involving the articular cartilage and subchondral bone that totally or partially separates from adjacent structures. The etiology is uncertain but is probably related to trauma in the large majority of the cases.[64] It occurs most frequently on the lateral aspect of the medial femoral condyle, near the intercondylar notch[63] (Fig. 1226). Microscopically, a portion of articular cartilage is always present, often exhibiting secondary calcification; in addition, a fragment of subchondral bone is found in approximately half of the cases.[64] If an osteochondromatous body remains attached to the joint surface or synovium, both components remain viable. If, however, such a body becomes completely detached, its osseous portion dies but the cartilage remains alive, apparently through nutrients obtained from the synovial fluid. Patients with bilateral symmetrical involvement and cases with familial incidence have been described.

Radiation necrosis

Damage to the underlying bone can be a major complication of radiation therapy. Radiation changes resulting in serious complications have been reported in the jaw, ribs, pelvis, spine, humerus, and other bones. In cases of radiation necrosis of the pelvis and femoral neck, the changes usually occur within three years of the therapy. Microscopically, there are dead bone, fibrosis of the bone marrow, and

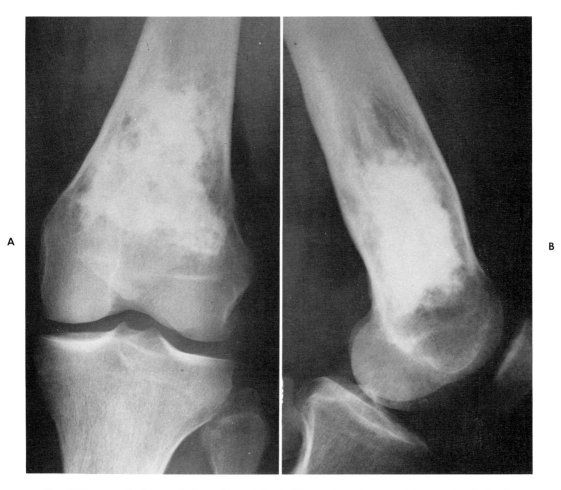

Fig. 1223 Large diaphysometaphyseal bone infarct of femur. Irregular area of increased radiodensity is indicative of new bone production superimposed on necrosis. (**A**, WU neg. 59-4049; **B**, WU neg. 59-4050; **A** and **B**, courtesy Dr. H. Danziger, Welland, Ontario.)

neovascularization. The presence of irregular, heavily staining cement lines may lead to confusion with Paget's disease.

Paget's disease

About 90% of the patients with Paget's disease are over 55 years of age. The disease is rare before the age of 40 years and uncommon between the ages of 40 and 55 years,[70] although several cases of precocious onset are on record.[70a] It affects men slightly more often than women (4:3). It has a very peculiar geographic distribution. The highest incidence is in England, Australia, and the Western European plain.[67] Collins[68] reported that at autopsy about one of every thirty patients over 40 years of age had Paget's disease in one of several locations. The most common sites are the lumbo-sacral spine, the pelvis, and the skull. It may occur in the femur, tibia, clavicle (Fig. 1227), radius, ulna, and fibula but is extremely rare in the ribs. The process may involve only a portion of a single bone. The etiology is unknown; the suggestion that it might be of viral origin has been raised by the consistent finding of nuclear inclusions resembling viral nucleocapsids of the measles type in the osteoclasts of this disease.[71a]

Initially, this lesion is osteoclastic.[69] Abnormal hyperplasia soon follows, as evidenced by primitive coarse-fibered bone in discontinuous trabeculae. Later, massive, thick trabeculae with disjointed lamellar patterns occur. Reticulin stains are often very helpful in studying the pattern of growth. The use of polarized light is less instructive. When lamellar bone

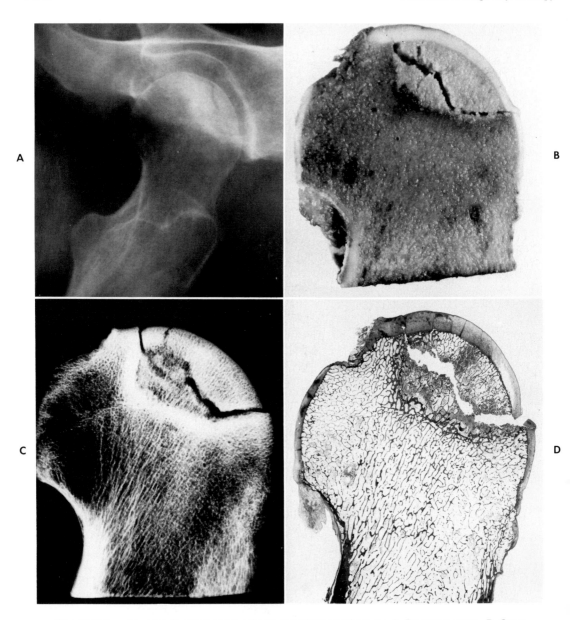

Fig. 1224 Aseptic necrosis of femoral head with superimposed fracture. **A,** Roentgenogram. **B,** Cross section of excised specimen. **C,** Roentgenogram of slice of same specimen, emphasizing peripheral eburnation. **D,** Whole-mount specimen showing well-delimited focus of necrosis. (**A,** WU neg. 73-4617; **B,** WU neg. 73-4420; **C,** WU neg. 73-5609; **D,** WU neg. 73-7722.)

becomes disorganized, a mosaic of cement lines appears. This is caused by the abrupt interruptions and changes in direction of bone lamellae and fibers resulting from resorption and regeneration of masses of bone during the course of the disease. These lines are outlined clearly by Erhlich's acid hematoxylin.

Collins[68] stressed the fact that the incidence of superimposed osteosarcoma is quite low

if one considers the frequency of Paget's disease. The complications of fracture and sarcoma in Paget's disease, however, represent a significant number of clinical problems because of the frequency of the disease. Fractures in Paget's disease usually are transverse.[71] In addition to osteosarcoma, Paget's disease may rarely be complicated by the development of chondrosarcoma, fibrosarcoma, or giant cell

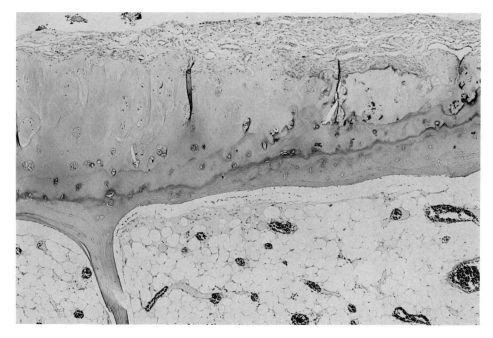

Fig. 1225 Aseptic bone necrosis in head of femur. Note fibrillation and almost complete absence of cartilage. Subchondral bone is dead with empty lacunae. (Low power; WU neg. 52-4090.)

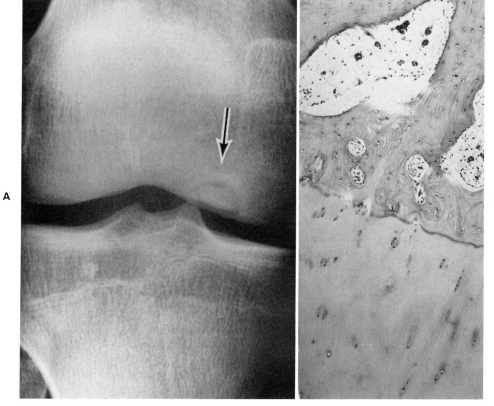

A

B

Fig. 1226 A, Sharply delimited area of osteochrondritis dissecans of medial condyle (arrow). This was easily enucleated. **B,** Same lesion shown in **A** demonstrating viability of bone removed from defect. Bone was alive because of its loose attachment to normal adjacent osseous tissue. (**A,** WU neg. 62-7783; B, WU neg. 62-8266.)

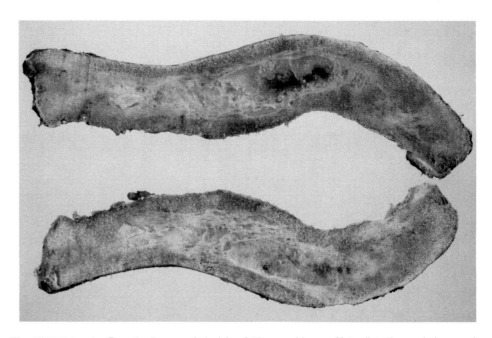

Fig. 1227 Extensive Paget's disease of clavicle of 60-year-old man. Note distortion and changes in cortex. (WU neg. 66-2557.)

tumor.[72] Instances of familial or geographic clustering of this complication have been seen. The most common location of sarcomas arising in Paget's disease are the femur, humerus, innominate bone, tibia, and skull.

Rarely, Paget's disease is predominantly a monostotic process in a long bone.[75] We have seen it in an apparent monostotic form in the maxilla, in the mandible, and in a collapsed vertebra. Under these conditions, the alkaline phosphatase level may be normal (Figs. 1228 and 1229).

The key to the microscopic pattern of the disease is the mosaic of numerous and scalloped cement lines.[74] There are many pathologic processes that undergo active reparative change accompanied by new bone formation with cement lines. If careful attention is given to the pattern of these normal cement lines which are orderly and structurally well oriented, these processes will not be confused with the microscopic appearance of Paget's disease. These lesions include irradiation effect, chronic osteomyelitis, reactive bone surrounding metastatic cancer, and polyostotic fibrous dysplasia. Uehlinger[76] pointed out that eccentric atrophy of the cortical bone is invariably present in polyostotic fibrous dysplasia but absent in Paget's disease. Rapid dissolution of bone sub-

stance may occur if a patient with Paget's disease of a long bone is immobilized because of fracture.[73]

Treatment of Paget's disease with calcitonin has led to some spectacular, although not always consistent, results.[70b]

Melorheostosis

Melorheostosis is a term derived from Greek words meaning flowing limb. The proliferation of ivorylike bone may be periosteal or endosteal. Osseous tissue also is deposited in soft tissues in the region of joints. In five biopsied lesions, the trabeculae were compact, the haversian canals were normally outlined, and the marrow was fibrotic.[77]

The excessive bone may cause locking of joints and bowing of long bones.[78] Associated soft tissue calcification is frequent.

Mastocytosis

Most cases of mast cell disease are restricted to the skin in the form of urticaria pigmentosa. In systemic mastocytosis, however, bone lesions are common. In the advanced case, they present as lytic and blastic areas involving numerous bones and simulating a metastatic carcinoma[79] (Fig. 1230). Microscopically, the diagnosis is often missed. The early lesion is in ill-defined peritrabecular nodule in which mononuclear cells of round and spindle shape alternate with eosinophils and abundant collagen fibers. Many of these mononuclear cells are mast cells, but this is not easily apparent on routinely stained sections. Special stains for metachromatic granules need to be used, although even these may be difficult to demonstrate in decalcified sections. It is likely that the lesion described by Rywlin et al.[80] as "eosinophilic fibrohistocytic lesion of the bone marrow" represents focal mastocytosis (see Chapter 22).

Tumors
Classification and distribution

The classification of bone tumors and tumorlike lesions and terminology we use are largely

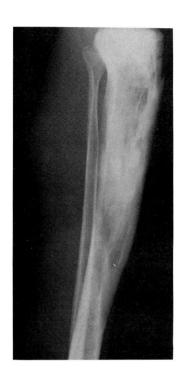

Fig. 1228 Monostotic Paget's disease of tibia with both bone destruction and bone formation. Nature of process was obscrue until biopsy. (WU neg. 51-3657.)

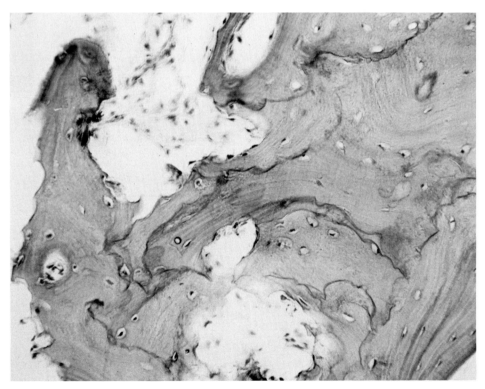

Fig. 1229 Paget's disease. Note numerous irregular but well-defined mosaic patterns of cement lines. (×275; WU neg. 66-9183.)

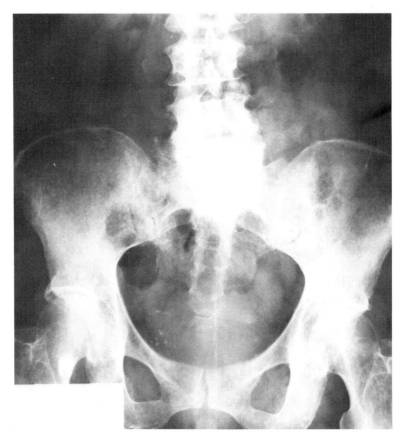

Fig. 1230 Extensive blastic and lytic lesions involving spine, iliac bones, and femurs in case of systemic mastocytosis. Roentgenographic pattern resembles that of metastatic carcinoma.

those recommended by the WHO International Reference Center for the Histological Definition and Classification of Bone Tumours[81]*:

Bone-forming tumors
  Benign
    Osteoma
    Osteoid osteoma and osteoblastoma
  Malignant
    Osteosarcoma
    Juxtacortical (parosteal) osteosarcoma
Cartilage-forming tumors
  Benign
    Chondroma
    Osteochondroma
    Chondroblastoma
    Chondromyxoid fibroma

  Malignant
    Chondrosarcoma
    Mesenchymal chondrosarcoma
Giant cell tumor
Marrow tumors
  Ewing's sarcoma
  Malignant lymphoma
  Plasma cell myeloma
Vascular tumors
  Benign
    Hemangioma
    Lymphangioma
    Glomus tumor
  Malignant
    Angiosarcoma, low grade
    Angiosarcoma, high grade
Other connective tissue tumors
  Benign
    Desmoplastic fibroma
    Lipoma
  Malignant
    Fibrosarcoma
    Malignant fibrous histiocytoma
    Leiomyosarcoma

*Adapted, with minor modifications, from Schajowicz F, Ackerman LV, Sissons HA: Histological typing of bone tumours. International Histological Classification of Tumours, No. 6. Geneva, 1972, World Health Organization.

Liposarcoma
Malignant mesenchymoma
Undifferentiated sarcoma
Other primary tumors
Chordoma
''Adamantinoma'' of long bones
Neurilemoma
Metastatic tumors
Unclassified tumors
Tumorlike lesions
Solitary bone cyst
Aneurysmal bone cyst
Ganglion cyst of bone
Metaphyseal fibrous defect (nonossifying fibroma)
Fibrous dysplasia
Myositis ossificans
Osteitis fibrosa cystica (discussed in Chapter 9)
Histiocytosis X (eosinophilic granuloma, Hand-Schüller-Christian disease, and Letterer-Siwe disease)

In this classification, most benign neoplasms are classified as benign or malignant. Although a sharp separation between these two categories is feasible in most of them, some neoplasms (such as giant cell tumors and some examples of osteoblastomas and chondroblastomas) exhibit borderline or intermediate characteristics. Most malignant bone tumors arise *de novo,* but there is a large number of benign bone lesions that predispose to the development of skeletal malignancies.[80a]

Tumors of the skeletal system, more than tumors arising anywhere else in the body, are relatively constant in their pattern of presentation. The five basic parameters in this regard are age of the patient, bone involved, specific area within the bone (epiphysis, metaphysis, or diaphysis; cortex, medulla, or periosteum), roentgenographic appearance, and microscopic appearance. The pathologist should be fully aware of the first four before trying to evaluate the fifth. Otherwise, serious mistakes will inevitably occur. Table 65 should help in providing a quick orientation to the pathologist confronted with a bone neoplasm.

Bone-forming tumors
Osteoma

It is doubtful whether osteoma is a true neoplasm. It is seen almost exclusively in the bones of the skull and face and is always benign. It may protrude inside a paranasal sinus, particularly the frontal and ethmoid, and block the normal drainage from these sinuses.[83] Microscopically, it is composed of dense, mature, predominantly lamellar bone. Patients with

Gardner's syndrome (intestinal polyposis and soft tissue tumors) may have multiple osteomas and other bone abnormalities.[82]

Osteoid osteoma and osteoblastoma

Osteoid osteoma is a benign neoplasm of bone occurring in men about twice as often as in women.[87] It is found most frequently in patients between 10 and 30 years of age.[89c] This lesion should not be confused with a local area of chronic osteomyelitis,[84] as it has been in the past. It has been reported in practically every bone but occurs most frequently in the femur, tibia, humerus, bones of hands and feet, vertebrae, and fibula. Lesions in the spine may lead to scoliosis.[87a] Lesions of long bones are usually metaphyseal; vertebral lesions often occur in the pedicle or in the arch.[89] Osteoid osteoma usually begins in the cortex (85%), but it also may be located in the spongiosa (13%) or subperiosteal tissues (2%).[90]

The central nidus of this tumor seldom is larger than 1.5 cm and is surrounded by an area of dense bone (Fig. 1231). When the lesion appears in the cortex, the area of reaction may extend for several centimeters along the bone as well as around it. The nidus itself is radiolucent with or without a dense center (Fig. 1232).

Microscopically, the lesion is sharply delineated and made up of more or less calcified osteoid growing within highly vascular osteoblastic connective tissue and surrounded by dense bone (Figs. 1233 and 1234). There is no evidence of inflammation. If the lesion is removed piecemeal, it can still be diagnosed because of the characteristics of the nidus (Fig. 1234).

The most prominent symptom is increasing pain, often well localized. Clinical and laboratory evidence of infection is lacking. If the lesion is in the cortex of the bone, a diagnosis of Garré's osteomyelitis may be incorrectly made because of the adjacent bone reaction. Removal of the lesion relieves symptoms.

Osteoblastoma (benign osteoblastoma; giant osteoid osteoma) is a tumor closely related to osteoid osteoma.[85] Microscopically and ultrastructurally, the two lesions are quite similar.[91] Osteoblastoma is distinguished by the larger size of the nidus, the absence or inconspicuousness of a surrounding area of reactive bone formation, and the lack of intense pain.[86,88] Most cases arise in the spongiosa of the bone, but cortical and subperiosteal forms also oc-

Table 65 Usual age and sex of patient and location and behavior of most common primary bone tumors and tumorlike lesions*

Tumor or tumorlike lesion	Age (yr)	Sex M:F	Bones more commonly affected (in order of frequency)	Usual location within long bone	Behavior
Osteoma	40-50	2:1	Skull and facial bones	—	Benign
Osteoid osteoma	10-30	2:1	Femur, tibia, humerus, hands and feet, vertebrae, fibula	Cortex of metaphysis	Benign
Osteoblastoma	10-30	2:1	Vertebrae, tibia, femur, humerus, pelvis, ribs	Medulla of metaphysis	Benign
Osteosarcoma	10-25	3:2	Femur, tibia, humerus, pelvis, jaw, fibula	Medulla of metaphysis	Malignant; 20% 5-yr survival rate
Juxtacortical (parosteal) osteosarcoma	30/60	1:1	Femur, tibia, humerus	Juxtacortical area of metaphysis	Malignant; 80% 5-yr survival rate
Chondroma	10-40	1:1	Hands and feet, ribs, femur, humerus	Medulla of diaphysis	Benign
Osteochondroma	10-30	1:1	Femur, tibia, humerus, pelvis	Cortex of metaphysis	Benign
Chondroblastoma	10-25	2:1	Femur, humerus, tibia, feet, pelvis, scapula	Epiphysis, adjacent to cartilage plate	Practically always benign
Chondromyxoid fibroma	10-25	1:1	Tibia, femur, feet, pelvis	Metaphysis	Benign
Chondrosarcoma	30-60	3:1	Pelvis, ribs, femur, humerus, vertebrae	Central—medulla of diaphysis Peripheral—cortex or periosteum of metaphysis	Malignant; 5-yr survival rate—low grade, 78%; moderate grade, 53%; high grade, 22%
Mesenchymal chondrosarcoma	20-60	1:1	Ribs, skull and jaw, vertebrae, pelvis, soft tissues	Medulla or cortex of diaphysis	Malignant; extremely poor prognosis
Giant cell tumor	20-40	4:5	Femur, tibia, radius	Epiphysis and metaphysis	Potentially malignant; 50% recur; 10% metastasize

	Age	Ratio	Bones involved	Site in bone	Behavior and prognosis
Ewing's sarcoma	5-20	1:2	Femur, pelvis, tibia, humerus, ribs, fibula	Medulla of diaphysis or metaphysis	Highly malignant; 20%-30% 5-yr survival rate in recent series
Malignant lymphoma, histiocytic (reticulum cell sarcoma) and mixed cell types	30-60	1:1	Femur, pelvis, vertebrae, tibia, humerus, jaw, skull, ribs	Medulla of diaphysis or metaphysis	Malignant; 22%-50% 5-yr survival rate
Plasma cell myeloma	40-60	2:1	Vertebrae, pelvis, ribs, sternum, skull	Medulla of diaphysis, metaphysis, or epiphysis	Malignant; diffuse form uniformly fatal, localized form often controlled with radiation therapy
Hemangioma	20-50	1:1	Skull, vertebrae, jaw	Medulla	Benign
Desmoplastic fibroma	20-30	1:1	Humerus, tibia, pelvis, jaw, femur, scapula	Metaphysis	Benign
Fibrosarcoma	20-60	1:1	Femur, tibia, jaw, humerus	Medulla of metaphysis	Malignant; 28% 5-yr survival rate
Chordoma	40-60	2:1	Sacrococcygeal, spheno-occipital, cervical vertebrae	—	Malignant; slow course; locally invasive; 48% distant metastases
Solitary bone cyst	10-20	3:1	Humerus, femur	Medulla of metaphysis	Benign
Aneurysmal bone cyst	10-20	1:1	Vertebrae, flat bones, femur, tibia	Metaphysis	Benign; sometimes secondary to another bone lesion
Metaphyseal fibrous defect	10-20	1:1	Tibia, femur, fibula	Metaphysis	Benign
Fibrous dysplasia	10-30	3:2	Ribs, femur, tibia, jaw, skull	Medulla of diaphysis or metaphysis	Locally aggressive; rarely complicated by sarcoma
Eosinophilic granuloma	5-15	3:2	Skull, jaw, humerus, rib, femur	Metaphysis or diaphysis	Benign

*It should be emphasized that these data correspond to the typical case and that they should not be taken in an absolute sense. Isolated exceptions to practically every one of these statements have occurred.

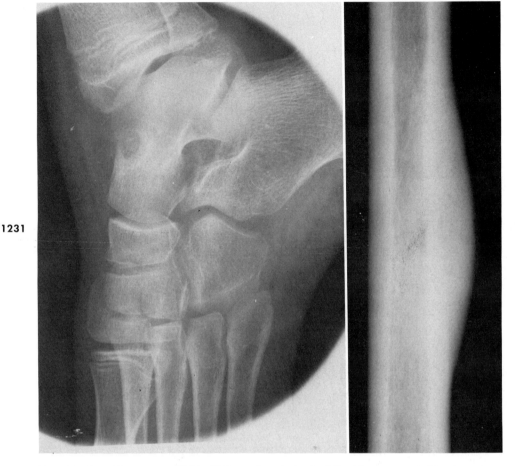

1231

1232

Fig. 1231 Osteoid osteoma of talus. Note small central osteolytic nidus surrounded by dense bone. (WU neg. 48-3921.)

Fig. 1232 Osteoid osteoma of femur obscured by area of reacting bone extending up, as well as around, bone. In past, such lesions were often diagnosed as Garré's osteomyelitis. (WU neg. 50-1910.)

cur.[90] The majority of the cases are located in the spine or major bones of the lower extremity.[89b] Osteomalacia can be seen as a complication of the tumor.[91a]

The differential diagnosis between osteoblastoma and osteosarcoma can be extremely difficult, because the latter may be very well differentiated and the former is sometimes accompanied by mild cytologic atypia and the presence of scattered bizarre tumor cells. These are probably of a degenerative nature and perhaps equivalent to those seen in atypical uterine leiomyomas. As is the case in many other bone tumors, the roentgenographic pattern is of great assistance in this differential diagnosis. However, in about one-fourth of the cases of osteoblastoma, the roentgenographic picture is consistent with a malignant neoplasm.[89a]

Cases of logically aggressive but not metastasizing osteoblastomas have been described as aggressive osteoblastomas, malignant osteoblastomas,[90a] or low-grade osteosarcomas. According to Dorfman, the differential histologic features are the presence of epithelioid osteoblasts, trabecular (sheetlike) rather than lacelike osteoid, low mitotic rate with no atypical forms, prominent osteoclastic activity, and absence of cartilage formations.[86a]

Osteosarcoma

Osteosarcoma is the most frequent primary malignant bone tumor.[98] It usually occurs in patients between 10 and 25 years of age, being exceptionally rare in preschool children.[110] Another peak age incidence occurs after 40, with most of the patients being men in whom osteosarcoma is superimposed on Paget's dis-

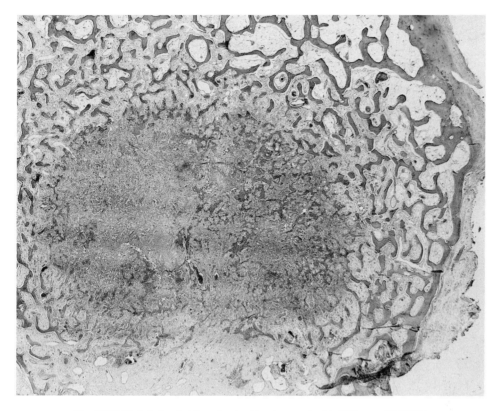

Fig. 1233 Well-defined nidus of osteoid osteoma. (×13; WU neg. 54-5990.)

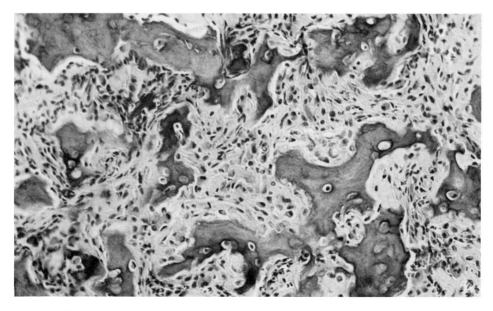

Fig. 1234 Variably calcified osteoid growing within highly vascular osteoblastic connective tissue. These changes are typical of osteoid osteoma. (Moderate enlargement; WU neg. 52-4539.)

ease. The latter is not infrequently multicentric. Rarely, multiple foci of origin appear without antecedent Paget's disease, particularly in children.[92,111]

Osteosarcoma may be seen as a complication of radiation therapy in both adults and children.[95,100,115a] Martland and Humphries[104] reported the development of osteosarcoma in factory workers who moistened brushes in their mouths when applying radium paint to luminous numerals on watches.[95a] Thorotrast administration also can lead to the development of osteosarcoma.[113]

Trauma, as far as is known, does not cause bone tumors.[99a] If it did, one would expect to find bone tumors arising after fractures, the trauma of various orthopedic procedures, bullet wounds, or other severe injuries. Trauma usually only calls attention to an already present advanced bone tumor.

Some immunologic studies have suggested the presence of an infectious agent, probably a virus, in association with human osteosarcoma,[106,108] but its pathogenetic role, if any, remains to be determined.

Osteosarcomas develop for the most part in the medullary cavity of the metaphyseal area of the long bones, particularly the lower end of the femur, the upper end of the tibia, and the upper end of the humerus.[96] The vertebral column also can be involved.[94a] When superimposed on Paget's disease, the most common sites are femur, humerus (Fig. 1235), innominate bone, tibia, and skull.

Grossly, these tumors vary in vascular, fibrous, cartilaginous, and osseous content. As they grow, they extend along the marrow cavity (Fig. 1236) and elevate or perforate the periosteum. If they elevate the periosteum, they may produce the roentgenographic picture designated as Codman's triangle (a nonspecific finding). This angle is formed by the elevated periosteum and the underlying bone (Fig. 1237). If the epiphysis is closed, the tumor often extends into the epiphysis. It may do so, although not so commonly, also in skeletally immature individuals.[112a] Rarely following fractures or extension through the periosteum, the tumor may break into the joint. Satellite nodules independent from the main tumor mass are rarely found proximal to the primary lesion, both in the same bone and transarticularly. These have been called "skip" metastases by Enneking and Kagan[99] and may be responsible for an increased incidence of local recurrences and subsequent metastases. Osteosarcoma practically never ulcerates through the skin or in-

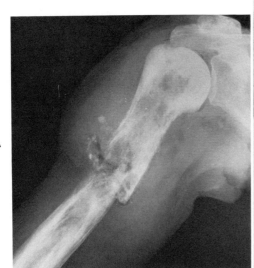

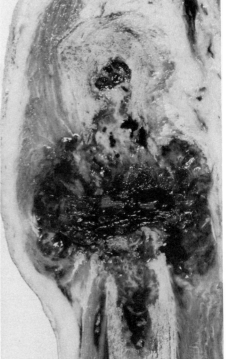

Fig. 1235 A, Osteosarcoma of upper end of humerus associated with fracture and Paget's disease. **B,** Point of fracture in humerus shown in **A** demonstrating extension of hemorrhagic neoplasm up shaft and out into soft tissues. Note porous, thickened cortical bone of Paget's disease. (**A,** WU neg. 48-6536; **B,** WU neg. 48-5008.)

volves regional lymph nodes. In a rather wide experience, we have seen involvement of lymph nodes in only three instances. On the other hand, metastases through the bloodstream to distant sites, particularly the lung, are common. In an autopsy series of fifty-four cases, the four main sites of metastases were lung (98%), other bones (37%), pleura (33%), and heart (20%); metastases appear sooner after excision of the primary tumor in children and young adults than in older individuals.[115]

Microscopically, the basic pattern is that of a sarcoma with osteoid production, recognized by its faint eosinophilic and glassy appearance, but several morphologic variants exist.[97,109] They range from extremely well-differentiated tissue with abundant bone production to highly anaplastic lesions (Figs. 1238 and 1239). Some cases are composed of small uniform cells and simulate the appearance of Ewing's sarcoma.[112] Scattered osteoclast-like giant cells are present in about one-fourth of the cases. The preexisting bone trabeculae are either destroyed by the growing tumor or enveloped by it. Biopsy of an undifferentiated osteosarcoma may show a highly vascular lesion with tumor cells of greatly variable size and shape growing between and lining blood vessels without evi-

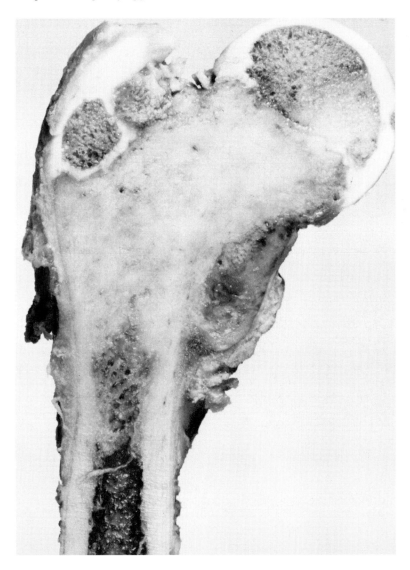

Fig. 1236 Osteosarcoma of proximal femur in 10-year-old boy. There are massive involvement of medullary cavity, invasion of cortex and soft tissues, and periosteal elevation. Note how tumor growth is partially restrained by epiphyseal cartilage. (WU neg. 68-6392.)

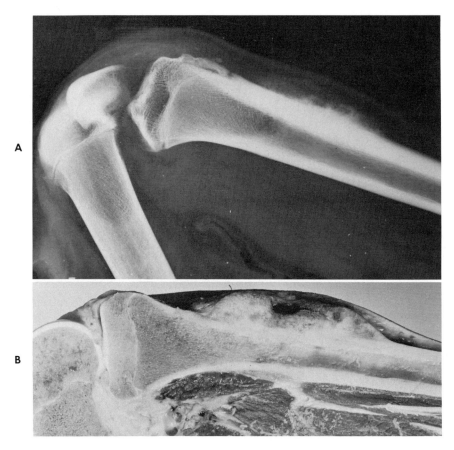

Fig. 1237 A, Osteosarcoma of upper end of tibia demonstrating prominent periosteal bone proliferation. **B,** Same tumor shown in **A** demonstrating elevation of periosteum in metaphyseal and diaphyseal
areas. (**A,** WU neg. 48-6537; **B,** WU neg. 48-5884.)

dence of osteoid formation. These telangiectatic osteosarcomas may mimic aneurysmal
bone cysts roentgenographically and pathologically, although their arteriographic patterns are
usually diagnostic. The diagnosis can be made
if the pathologist pays attention to the anaplastic
cells and infrequent atypical osteoid in the septa
of these sarcomas (Fig. 1240). The prognosis
of these telangiectatic tumors seems to be worse
than for the conventional osteosarcoma.[105]

By contrast, a tumor may produce a disorderly arrangement of well-differentiated bone
and large amounts of osteoid (Figs. 1238 and
1241). Unni et al.[114] reported a group of patients with intraosseous osteosarcoma in whom
the tumor was so well differentiated as to be
confused with a benign lesion. Most patients
were adults, and the femur and tibia were the
two most common sites. Microscopically, spindle cells with minimal cytologic atypia and

scanty mitotic figures were admixed with abundant osteoid. Thus, their appearance was similar to that of juxtacortical osteosarcoma. Recurrences were common, but metastatic spread
was unusual. The most important differential
diagnosis is with fibrous dysplasia; roentgenographically the latter lacks areas of cortical
destruction, and microscopically it does not
show atypia.

Wide areas of neoplastic cartilage occur in
some osteosarcomas, a feature that may prompt
a mistaken diagnosis of chondrosarcoma. By
definition, a malignant tumor in which osteoid
and bone are being formed by the sarcomatous
cells is an osteosarcoma, whether or not there
is tumor cartilage production in other areas.
Conversely, a cartilage-forming malignant
tumor lacking the former feature should be
designated as chondrosarcoma whether or not
the malignant cartilage is being partially re-

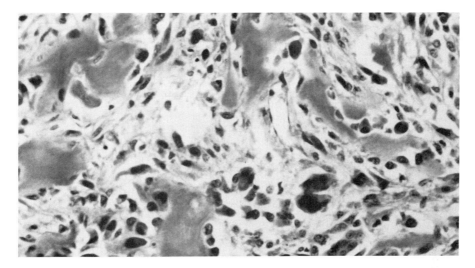

Fig. 1238 Osteosarcoma producing large amounts of neoplastic osteoid and sarcomatous stroma. (High power.)

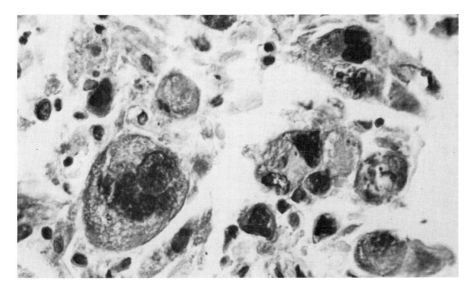

Fig. 1239 Osteosarcoma with bizarre tumor giant cells. (×600; WU neg. 52-4081.)

placed by nonneoplastic bone through a mechanism of endochondral ossification. The demonstration of alkaline phosphatase activity may help in identifying as osteosarcoma an apparently undifferentiated neoplasm or in distinguishing tumor bone from hyaline fibrous tissue or cartilage. Ultrastructurally, the neoplastic osteoblasts resemble the normal parent cells by having abundant dilated cisternae of granular endoplasmic reticulum and sparse mitochondria.[116] Other cells present are osteo-

cytes, chondroblasts, undifferentiated cells, and myofibroblasts.[108a]

The lesions mistaken for osteosarcoma include any in which there is rapid bone growth. We have seen slides of exuberant callus formation misdiagnosed because they were examined without knowledge of an antecedent fracture. The callus may be secondary to a pathologic fracture in a benign localized lesion (such as metaphyseal fibrous defect or aneurysmal bone cyst), in a metastatic carcinoma, or in osteo-

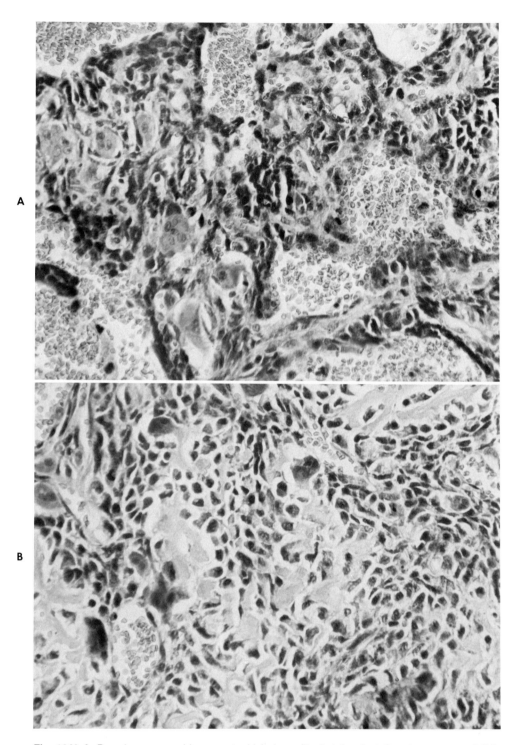

Fig. 1240 A, Pseudoaneurysmal bone cyst which, in reality, is telangiectatic osteosarcoma of tibia. This area would be almost impossible to distinguish from aneurysmal bone cyst. **B,** Same lesion shown in **A** demonstrating atypical osteoid growing in sarcomatous stroma. This finding makes the diagnosis of osteosarcoma. Patient died of disseminated disease. (**A,** ×300; WU neg. 67-1946; **B,** ×350; WU neg. 67-1945A.)

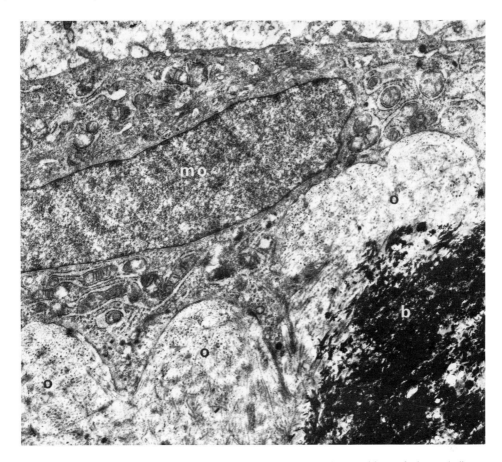

Fig. 1241 In this osteosarcoma, malignant osteoblast, **mo**, osteoid, **o**, and bone, **b**, have similar relationship as they normally do. (Approximately ×9,000.)

genesis imperfecta.[94,101] On several occasions, the highly proliferative lesions of soft tissue designated as myositis ossificans have been diagnosed by competent authorities as osteosarcoma. Lichtenstein[102] cited an instance of gumma of the bone that was diagnosed incorrectly as osteosarcoma.

The prognosis for patients with osteosarcoma is poor. Once lesions such as chondrosarcoma, fibrosarcoma, juxtacortical osteosarcoma, and osteosarcoma of the jaw (which have a better prognosis) are excluded, the five-year survival approaches 20%.[103] Whether the addition of multidrug chemotherapy will result in significant increases of survival times remains to be seen; some preliminary results are certainly encouraging.[108b] Sex, microscopic type (whether osteoblastic, chondroblastic, or fibroblastic), and grading bear no significant relationship with prognosis.[96,107] Osteosarcomas arising on the basis of Paget's disease are usually highly malignant. Osteosarcomas located below elbows and knees have a slightly better prognosis than those situated more centrally[96,107a] There is a suggestion that tumors accompanied by elevated levels of serum alkaline phosphatase have a greatly increased metastatic rate.[101a] In the series of twenty-eight radiation-induced osteosarcomas reported by Arlen et al.,[93] the prognosis was slightly better than for those arising de novo; an overall five-year survival rate of 28% was achieved.

Juxtacortical (parosteal) osteosarcoma

Juxtacortical (parosteal) osteosarcoma is an infrequent primary, slowly growing malignant tumor of bone that occurs in a slightly older group of patients than conventional osteosarcoma.[123] It arises in a juxtacortical position in the metaphyses of long bones (usually the posterior aspect of the lower femoral shaft) and may have a life history of ten to fifteen years.[121]

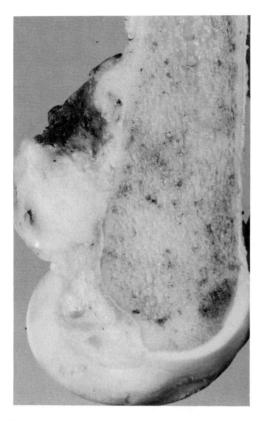

Fig. 1242 Classic juxtacortical osteosarcoma occurring in 57-year-old man. Patient remains well over ten years following amputation. (WU neg. 68-473.)

It forms a large lobulated mass and has a tendency to encircle the bone (Fig. 1242). Later in the evolution, it may penetrate into the medullary cavity, a feature associated with decreased survival. Satellite nodules may be present. The diagnosis is strongly suggested by the roentgenographic picture[124] (Fig. 1243, A).

Microscopically, there is a disorderly pattern of well-formed bone, osteoid, occasional cartilage, and a highly fibrous spindle cell stroma (Fig. 1243, B). The cytologic signs of malignancy in the fibrous stroma are often subtle, thus accounting for the great frequency of misdiagnoses made in this tumor type. Of ten cases of juxtacortical osteosarcoma we reviewed as a group, in only two was the initial histologic diagnosis correct.[119] This lesion has to be differentiated from myositis ossificans, which has an orderly pattern of bone formation without a sarcomatous stroma. With adequate treatment, the prognosis in juxtacortical osteosarcoma is excellent.[118] Occasionally, local ex-

cision is possible. Some tumors having the roentgenographic and gross features of juxtacortical osteosarcoma have highly malignant cytologic features—equivalent to those of the conventional osteosarcoma. These may be seen throughout the tumor[120] or as high-grade foci in an otherwise microscopically typical parosteal osteosarcoma.[123] Both forms are associated with a poor prognosis.[117]

Unni et al.[122] separated from the parosteal osteosarcoma another rare variant of osteosarcoma that grows on the bone surface and designated it as *periosteal osteosarcoma*. Most cases were located in the upper tibial shaft or femur and presented as small lucent lesions on the bone surface, accompanied by the presence of bone spicules arranged perpendicularly to the shaft. The lesions are limited to the cortex, without invasion of the medullary cavity.[117a] Microscopically, the tumors were relatively high-grade osteosaromas, with a *prominent cartilaginous component*. The prognosis is better than for conventional osteosarcoma.[121a,122] This entity is closely related to, if not identical with, the juxtacortical (periosteal) chondrosarcoma (see p. 1346).

Cartilage-forming tumors
Chondroma

Chondroma is a common benign cartilaginous tumor that occurs most frequently in the small bones of the hands and feet, particularly the proximal phalanges. Most cases begin in the central portion of the diaphysis (enchondromas), from which they expand and thin the cortex. Chondromas of the thumb and terminal phalanges are distinctly uncommon. In Takigawa's series[131] of 110 cases, thirty-five were multiple. Multiple enchondromas having a predominantly unilateral distribution are referred to as Ollier's disease. The association of multiple enchondromas with soft tissue hemangiomas is known as Maffucci's syndrome[128] (Fig. 1244). In both conditions, there is a significant risk of malignant transformation in the form of chondrosarcoma.[125,126] Enchondromas of the rib and long bones are distinctly unusual, although we have seen several examples. A variant of the latter, presenting in the metaphysis of long bones, is characterized by massive calcification within the neoplasm[127] (Fig. 1245). Rarely, chondromas arise in a juxtacortical (periosteal) area of a long bone or a small bone of the hand and foot.[129] They characteristically erode and induce sclerosis of the

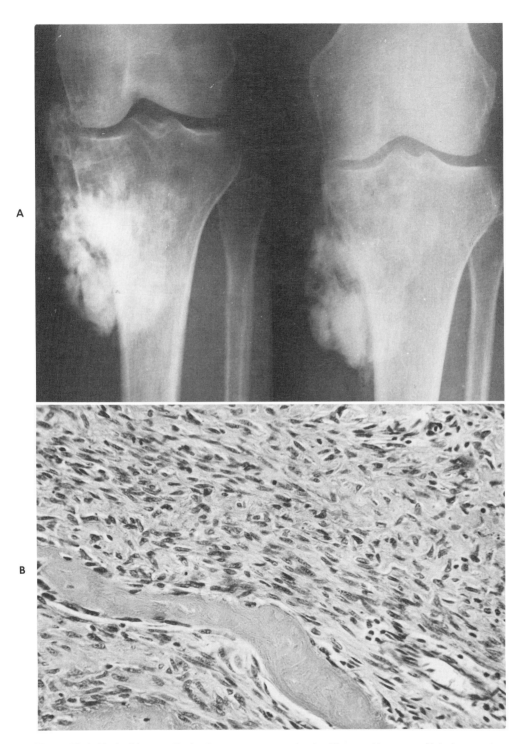

Fig. 1243 A, Typical juxtacortical osteosarcoma occurring in 40-year-old woman. Note large extra-cortical component. **B,** Same lesion shown in **A** demonstrating well-differentiated character of sar-comatous stroma. This lesion had been present for several years. (**A,** WU neg. 57-5271; **B,** WU neg. 58-3094.)

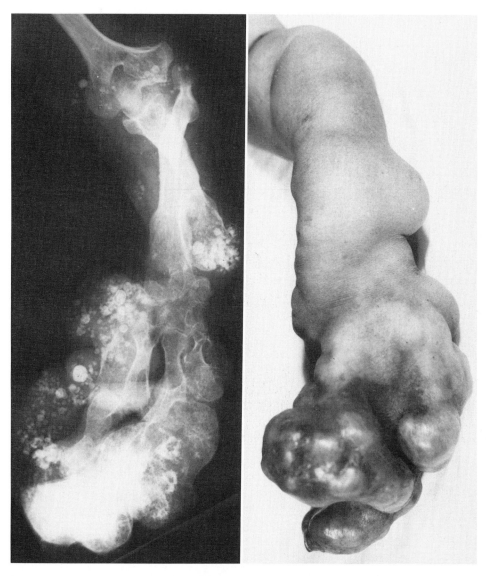

Fig. 1244 Arm of patient affected by Maffucci's syndrome. Innumerable chondromas are seen concentrated in distal aspect of extremity. Patient developed chondrosarcoma in innominate bone, with pulmonary metastases. (Courtesy Dr. O. Urteaga A., Lima, Peru.)

contiguous cortex. Recurrence may follow incomplete excision.[130]

Chondromas are composed of lobules of hyaline cartilage that microscopically appear mature. Foci of necrosis, myxoid degeneration, calcification, and endochondral ossification are common. Juxtacortical chondroma tends to be more cellular than its medullary counterpart and may contain occasional plump or double nuclei.

Osteochondroma

The *osteochondroma* is the most frequent benign bone tumor. It is usually asymptomatic, but it may lead to deformity or interfere with the function of adjacent structures such as tendons and blood vessels.[132a] The most common locations are the lower femur, upper tibia, upper humerus, and pelvis. In forty cases studied at Washington University, the average age of the patient at onset was 10.9 years. In thirty-

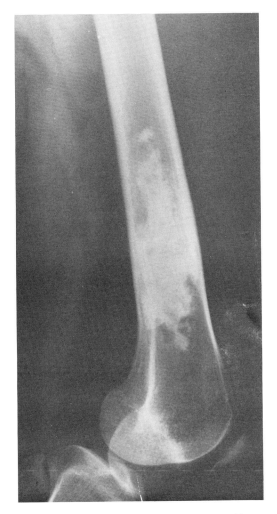

Fig. 1245 Large asymptomatic enchondroma of femur in 42-year-old woman. Tumor is extensively calcified.

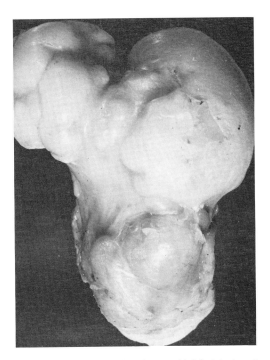

Fig. 1246 Large osteochondroma with lobulated cartilaginous cap. (WU neg. 51-3690.)

six cases, the tumor appeared before the patients were 20 years old. The average greatest dimension was 3.7 cm, and the largest tumor measured 8.5 cm. The smaller tumors were sessile and the larger ones pedunculated. All had a cap of cartilage covered by a fibrous membrane continuous with the periosteum of the adjacent bone. The average thickness of the cartilage cap was 0.6 cm (0.1-3 cm). In only seven cases was the cap thicker than 1 cm. The cartilaginous cap tended to be lobulated in large tumors (Fig. 1246). The gross and microscopic appearance of a single lesion of the familial condition known as osteochondromatosis or multiple cartilaginous exostoses (Ehrenfried's hereditary deforming chondro-dysplasia; diaphyseal aclasis) cannot be distinguished from osteochondroma.[132,133] A very small proportion of the solitary tumors evolve into chondrosarcomas,[132] but the incidence reaches 10% in the cases of multiple exostoses.[132c]

Subungual exostoses, usually located on the great toe, are different from osteochondromas but also are composed of a proliferating cartilaginous cap that merges into mature trabecular bone at its base. They may recur but are invariably benign.[132b]

Chondroblastoma

Chondroblastoma of bone is often confused with giant cell tumor and chondrosarcoma but is much rarer and bears no relation to these lesions.[138] It was classified in the past as the chondromatous variant of giant cell tumor.[134]

This tumor occurs predominantly in male individuals under 20 years of age. It arises in the epiphyseal end of long bones before epiphyseal cartilage has disappeared, particularly in the femur, humerus, and tibia (Figs. 1247 and 1248). Exceptionally, it is found in a metaphyseal location.[133a] We also have seen it involve small bones of the feet.

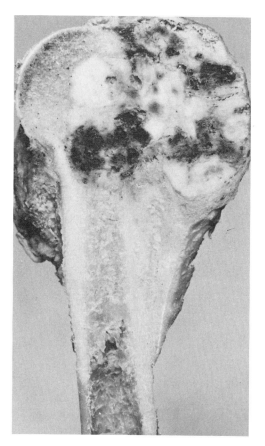

Fig. 1247 Well-outlined chondroblastoma involving epiphysis of humerus in young adult. (WU neg. 57-863; gross specimen contributed by Dr. A. J. Ramos, Manila, Philippines.)

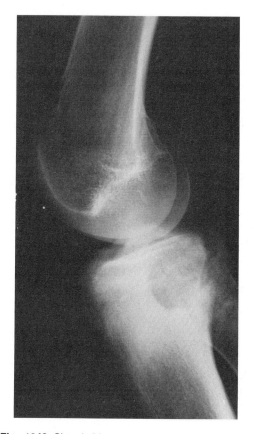

Fig. 1248 Chondroblastoma of epiphysis of tibia in young man. (WU neg. 59-3188.)

Roentgenographically, the tumor usually is fairly well delimited, contains areas of rarefaction, and may extend from the epiphysis into the metaphyseal areas. Transarticular spread occurred in two of the patients reported by Valls et al.[143]

Microscopically, this lesion often is confusing because of its extreme cellularity and variability. The occasional scattered collections of giant cells may lead to an erroneous diagnosis of giant cell tumor. The basic cell is an embryonic chondroblast without sufficient differentiation to produce intercellular chondroid.[136] The shape is usually polyhedral, although spindle elements also can be present. The cell membrane is thick and sharply defined. The nuclei vary in shape from round to indented and lobulated, a feature emphasized by Levine and Bensch.[140] Mitoses are exceptional. Intracytoplasmic glycogen granules are present,

sometimes in large numbers. Reticulin fibers surround each individual cell. Recurrent lesions may show some degree of atypia, a feature that needs not to be interpreted as a sign of malignant change.

A distinctive microscopic change is the presence of small zones of focal calcification (Fig. 1249). These zones range from faintly discernible bluish areas to obvious deposits surrounded by giant cells. This lesion can be distinguished from giant cell tumor by these focal areas of calcification and the absence of the characteristic stroma of giant cell tumors. By electron microscopy, the cells of chondroblastoma closely resemble those of normal epiphyseal cartilage cells grown in tissue culture.[142,144] They often have a prominent "fibrous lamina" lying against the inner aspect of the nuclear membrane, this resulting in the membrane thickening seen by light microscopy.[137] A por-

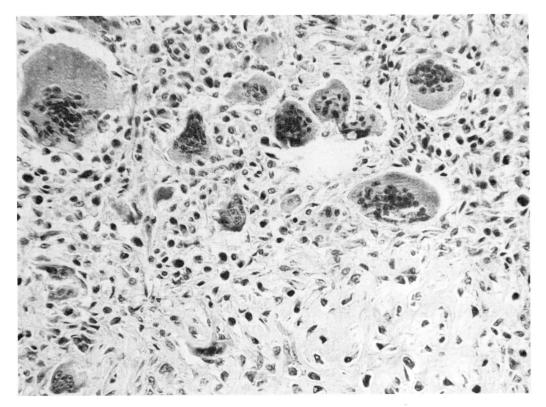

Fig. 1249 Chondroblastoma showing small cuboidal tumor cells, osteoclasts, and areas of chondroid differentiation. (WU neg. 66-9185.)

tion of a chondroblastoma cell from the humerus showing scattered glycogen particles and sparse cytoplasmic organelles is illustrated in Fig. 1250. In 24% of the cases reported by Huvos et al.,[137] areas resembling aneurysmal bone cyst were seen engrafted on the primary bone lesion. In patients with recurrent lesions, the incidence rose to 50%.

Levine and Bensch[140] have provided convincing histochemical and ultrastructural support for the truly cartilaginous nature of the basic tumor cells of chondroblastoma.

Clinically, patients with this lesion have pain that may become severe. Curettement is the indicated treatment, although local recurrence may supervene.[135] We have now seen several cases of chondroblastoma behaving locally in an aggressive fashion, invading the soft tissues and developing tumor thrombi in lymphatic channels. Most of them were located in the innominate bone.[140a] In addition, we have seen a chondroblastoma of the femur resulting in widespread visceral metastases.[139] Two instances of malignant change in chondroblastoma were recorded by Schajowicz and Gal-

lardo.[141] Careful study of the primary lesion in our cases failed to show any characteristics that would premit them to be differentiated from other ordinary chondroblastomas.

Chondromyxoid fibroma

Chondromyxoid fibroma of bone is an unusual benign tumor of cartilaginous origin, often confused with chondrosarcoma.[146] The tumors usually occur in young adults, often in a long bone, but they also have been reported in the small bones of the hands and feet, pelvis, ribs, and vertebrae.

This lesion may become large and roentgenographically is sharply defined (Fig. 1251). It is solid, has a yellowish white or tan color, replaces bone, and thins the cortex. It is highly cellular, has a myxoid matrix, and contains areas suggesting cartilage and often giant cells (Fig. 1252). A lobular pattern can be discerned grossly and microscopically. It is formed by intersecting bands of fibrous tissue lined on the sides by an increased concentration of tumor cells. The occasional presence of large pleomorphic cells may result in an erroneous diag-

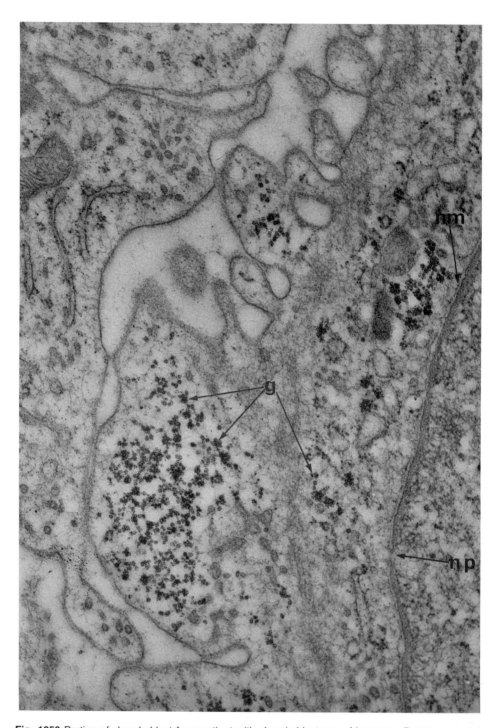

Fig. 1250 Portion of chondroblast from patient with chondroblastoma of humerus. Dense particulate material in cytoplasm is glycogen, **g.** Abnormal density is present beneath inner nuclear membrane, **nm,** and nuclear pore, **np,** can be readily seen at tip of arrow. (Lead stained; ×38,000; courtesy Dr. H. J. Spjut, Houston, Texas.)

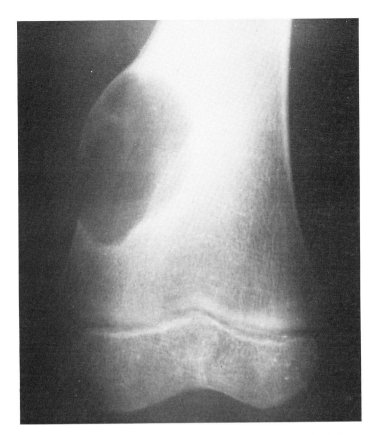

Fig. 1251 Sharply delimited chondromyxoid fibroma of lower femoral metaphysis in young boy. (WU neg. 65-779.)

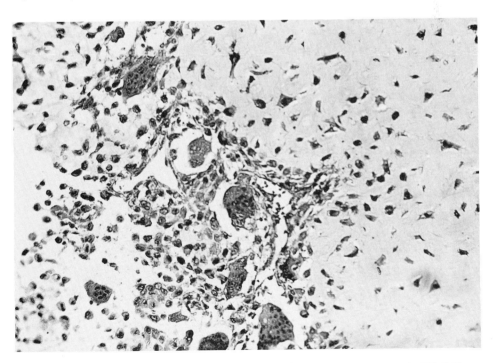

Fig. 1252 Chondromyxoid fibroma showing giant cells, cartilage, and cellular zones. (×200; WU neg. 54-1345.)

nosis of chondrosarcoma.[149] However, mitotic figures are exceptional. We have seen several tumors showing a combination of the features of chondroblastoma and chondromyxoid fibroma.[145]

Local recurrence follows curettage in about 25% of the cases. Because of this, en bloc ex-whenever possible. Soft tissue extension or implantation may occur,[146a] but we have never seen instances of distant metastases (Fig. 1253).

A tumor probably representing a variant of chondromyxoid fibroma occurring in older in-

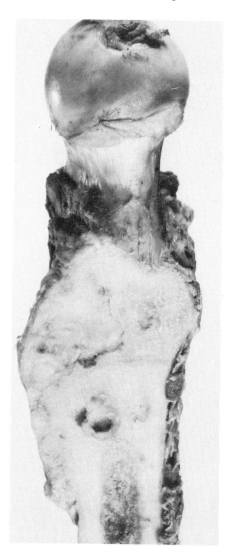

Fig. 1253 Chondromyxoid fibroma of proximal femur extending into soft tissue. This rare event should not be regarded as evidence of malignancy. (WU neg. 72-6210.)

dividuals was designated as *fibromyxoma* by Marcove et al.[148] McClure and Dahlin[147] have described three cases of primary *myxoma* of long bones; they remarked on their expansile roentgenographic appearance, distal location, benign clinical behavior, and microscopic similarities to soft tissue myxoma.

Chondrosarcoma

Chondrosarcoma is differentiated from osteosarcoma by the lack of osteoid or bone formation by the tumor cells. Bone can be present in a bona fide chondrosarcoma, but this is non-neoplastic and probably originates from reabsorption of the tumor cartilage by a mechanism of endochondral ossification. The distinction is important not only because of distinctive gross and microscopic differences, but also because of their better prognosis. The majority of the patients are between 30 and 60 years of age. Chondrosarcoma in childhood is distinctly uncommon. Most malignant bone tumors in this age group exhibiting cartilage formation are actually osteosarcomas with a predominant cartilaginous component. Chondrosarcomas are divided according to location into central, peripheral, and juxtacortical (periosteal) forms.[150a] Most chondrosarcomas are located in the central portion of a bone (Fig. 1254). Roentgenographically, they present a rather characteristic picture of an osteolytic lesion with splotchy calcification (Fig. 1255). Ill-defined margins, fusiform thickening of the shaft, and perforation of the cortex are three important diagnostic signs.[150] In advanced stages, they may break through the cortex but only rarely grow beyond the periosteum. The pelvic bones, ribs (usually at the costochondral junction), and shoulder girdle are the commonest locations. Chondrosarcomas of the small bones of the hands and feet are exceptional but have been described by several authors, particularly those involving the os calcis.[154,159]

Peripheral chondrosarcomas may arise de novo or from the cartilaginous cap of a pre-existing osteochondroma. Multiple osteochondromatosis is particularly prone to this complication (three out of twenty-eight patients reported by Jaffe[157] and three out of seven patients seen by us). In the 212 cases of chondrosarcoma reported by Dahlin and Henderson,[153] nineteen apparently arose from osteochondroma. The risk of malignant transformation in a solitary osteochondroma is less than 5%. The signs of malignancy in an osteo-

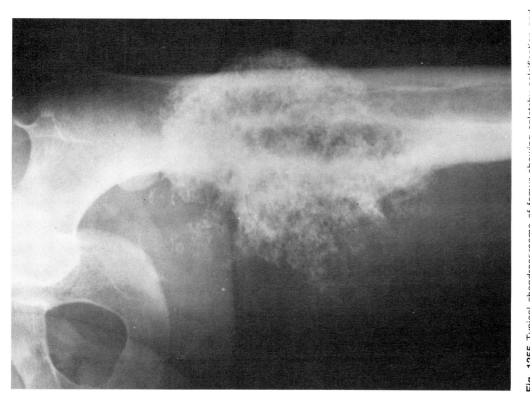

Fig. 1255 Typical chondrosarcoma of femur showing splotchy calcification and extensive cortical destruction. (WU neg. 61-6356.)

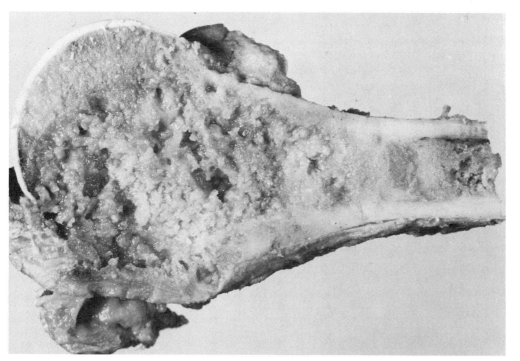

Fig. 1254 Chondrosarcoma of head of humerus. (WU neg. 54-5003.)

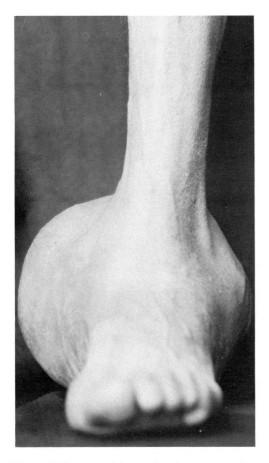

Fig. 1256 Large peripheral chondrosarcoma of os calcis in 36-year-old man. Tumor was of long duration. Patient finally came to clinic because he could no longer put on shoe.

chondroma include increased growth during adolescence, a diameter over 8 cm, and a cartilaginous cap thicker than 3 cm. The average thickness of the caps of benign osteochondromas examined at Barnes Hospital was 0.6 cm, the thickest measuring 3 cm. Conversely, and with only one exception, the caps of chondrosarcomas were all thicker than 2 cm. The greatest diameter of the peripheral chondrosarcomas examined by us varied from 8-25 cm (Fig. 1256). Roentgenographically, peripheral chondrosarcomas present as large tumors, with a heavily calcified center surrounded by a lesser denser periphery with splotchy calcification (Fig. 1257).

Juxtacortical (periosteal) chondrosarcoma involves the shaft of a long bone (most often the femur) and is characterized by a cartilaginous lobular pattern with areas of spotty calcification and endochondral ossification.[166c] This tumor is closely related to, if not identical with, the entity reported as periosteal osteosarcoma (see p. 1336).

The diagnosis of well-differentiated chondrosarcoma may be missed for such reasons as a long history of growth, lack of follow-up, and the failure of the pathologist to recognize the subtle microscopic changes that indicate a malignant cartilaginous tumor.

The microscopic diagnosis rests on the identification of abnormal nuclei in cartilage cells.[160] The nuclei are plump, atypical, and at times multinucleated (Fig. 1258). Areas near the growing edge are particularly diagnostic. Histochemically, well-differentiated chondrosarcomas have a staining reaction similar to that of adult cartilage, whereas poorly differentiated tumors resemble fetal cartilage.[158] Biochemically, a marked variability in composition has been observed.[160a,160b] Ultrastructurally, the cells of well-differentiated tumors show cytoplasmic accumulation of glycogen, lipid droplets, and dilated cisternae of granular endoplasmic reticulum.[155]

Rarely, a poorly differentiated spindle cell component resembling fibrosarcoma, osteosarcoma, or other high-grade malignancy is seen at the periphery of otherwise typical low-grade chondrosarcomas. This change can occur in the primary lesion, or more commonly, in the recurrent tissue. Dahlin and Beabout[152] found this phenomenon, which they call "dedifferentiation," in thirty-three of 370 well-differentiated chondrosarcomas that they examined. The prognosis is considerably worse than in the tumors lacking this component.[161,164a]

Two other morphologic variants of chondrosarcoma have been described. One is characterized by an abundant clear cytoplasm of the tumor cells, which may be confused with chondroblastoma.[166e] Most of the cases have involved the proximal part of the femur or humerus. The other, which may be found in long bones or soft tissues, closely resembles chordoma[164] It has been reported as chordoid sarcoma and extraskeletal myxoid chondrosarcoma (see Chapter 24). Whether the tumor reported by Dabska[151] as parachordoma is histogenetically related to the foregoing remains to be determined.

Frequently the statement is made that a benign central cartilaginous tumor became malignant or that it recurred. We have had the opportunity of examining tissue on two or more

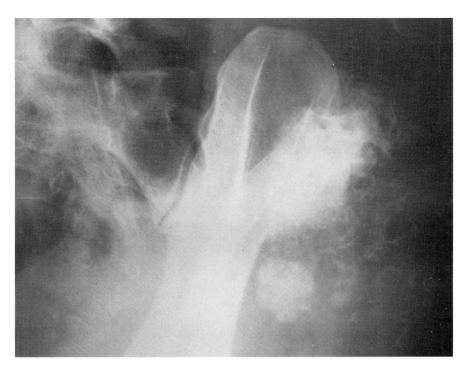

Fig. 1257 Typical roentgenographic appearance of peripheral chondrosarcoma of innominate bone. (WU neg. 66-766; courtesy Dr. W. T. Hill, Houston, Texas.)

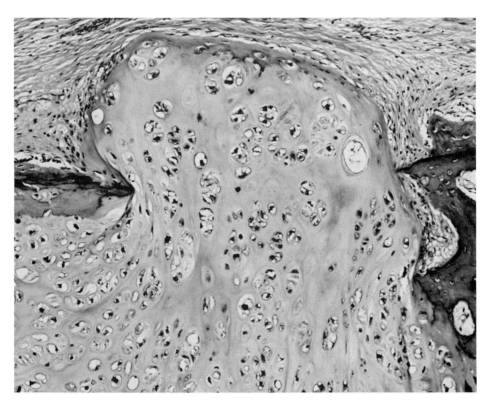

Fig. 1258 Bizarre and "plump" nuclei in rather well-differentiated chondrosarcoma from pelvis. This histologic section also shows tumor protruding through cortical bone into surrounding soft tissues. This pattern and lobular pattern seen grossly illustrate danger of enucleating these tumors. Persistent tumor is almost inevitable. (×125; WU neg. 58-3091; courtesy Dr. M. Ernest, Moose Jaw, Saskatchewan, Canada.)

occasions over periods of five months to twelve years from sixteen patients subjected to repeated operations for recurrences. *In none of these was the initial tumor clearly benign.* We believe, therefore, that in these instances the pathologist diagnosed the initial tumor incorrectly.

There is good correlation between poor differentiation, rapid growth rate, and metastases. The poorly differentiated tumors and those with elevated mitotic count metastasize early, usually to the lungs. Bloodstream invasion is particularly ominous. We have seen lymph node metastases (axillary) on only one occasion.

The correlation of the microscopic features with the clinical and roentgenographic findings is important in all bone tumors, but in the case of the cartilaginous neoplasms *it is essential.* Large tumors of long bones or ribs or those that begin to grow rapidly over adolescence and reach a size of 8 cm or more are almost invariably malignant.[163] Minor degrees of atypia in the cartilaginous cells under these circumstances justify a diagnosis of chondrosarcoma, whereas similar or even greater atypical changes in cartilaginous tumors of the hands and feet, osteochondromas, synovial osteochondromatosis, and soft tissue neoplasms are much less significant.[160] It also should be noted that the minor atypical changes on which the diagnosis of malignancy are based are often focal, a point to remember when examining a small sample of a cartilaginous neoplasm.

Soft tissue implantation following biopsy is a well known property of chondrosarcoma. Therefore, if a large cartilaginous tumor is so located that the biopsy site cannot be entirely excised, the initial surgery should be radical. If an extremely large tumor involves the pelvic bone, wide block excision or even hemipelvectomy is justified without prior histologic diagnosis. About 90% of the patients cured by hemipelvectomy had the operation for chondrosarcoma.[166] Chondrosarcomas of the rib should be excised radically, with removal of adjacent uninvolved ribs and the pleura en bloc with the lesion.[163,165] Some well-differentiated chondrosarcomas of the extremities are amenable to conservative therapy in the form of segmental resection.[166d]

In contrast to what is seen in osteosarcoma, microscopic grading of chondrosarcomas is of value in predicting the final outcome. In the series reported by McKenna et al.,[162] the five-year survival rates were 78%, 53%, and 22% for low-grade, moderate-grade, and high-grade tumors, respectively. In three more recent series, the survival figures were generally better, but the differential between the three grade was still obvious.[156,166a,166b]

Mesenchymal chondrosarcoma

A specific variant of chondrosarcoma, mesenchymal chondrosarcoma is characterized microscopically by a dimorphic pattern, areas of well-differentiated cartilage alternating with undifferentiated stroma[167,171] (Fig. 1259). The boundaries between the two components are usually abrupt. The undifferentiated element can be confused with malignant lymphoma and hemangiopericytoma. It should be noted that despite the apparently undifferentiated nature of this component both at the light and electron microscopic level,[172] pleomorphism and mitotic activity are remarkably inconspicuous.[171] The flat bones are those most commonly affected. A good number of these neoplasms involve extraosseous structures, such as the orbit, paraspinal region, meninges, or soft tissues of extremities.[168,169] The prognosis is generally poor, although there is great variability in the clinical course.[171] Jacobson[170] believes that mesenchymal chondrosarcoma is simply one morphologic type of the bone tumor that he proposes to call *polyhistioma.* He defines it as a malignant neoplasm whose basic cells are small and round, like those of Ewing's sarcoma, but which differentiate into various mesenchymal structures, such as bone and cartilage, and sometimes even into epithelial tissues. We find the term unsatisfactory but the proposal quite interesting and certainly worthy of confirmation by independent studies.

Giant cell tumor

Giant cell tumor is usually seen in patients over 20 years of age.[174a,178] It is more common in women than in men. The classical location is the epiphysis of a long bone, from which it may spread into the metaphyseal area, break through the cortex, invade intermuscular septa, or even cross a joint space.[186] The sites most commonly affected, in order of frequency, are the lower end of the femur, the upper end of the tibia, and the lower end of the radius. Naturally, exceptions occur. For instance, we have seen giant cell tumors in the metaphysis of the radius in two children in the absence of epiphyseal involvement, and similar cases

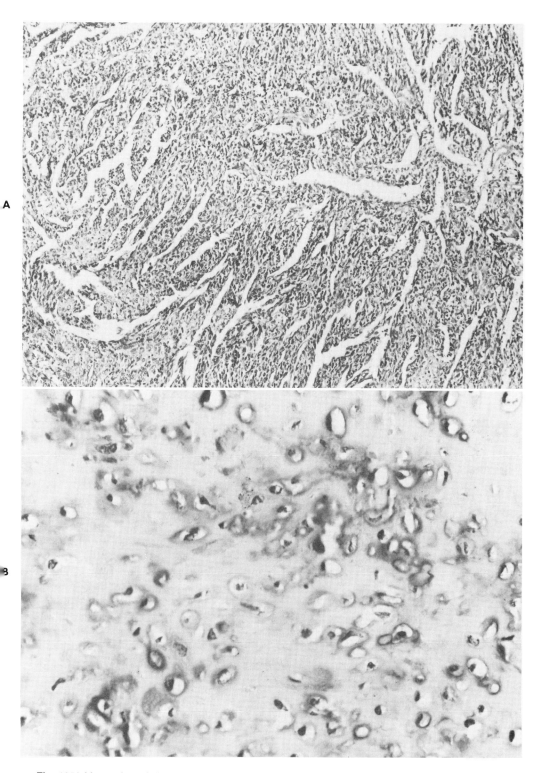

Fig. 1259 Mesenchymal chondrosarcoma. **A** illustrates cellular, hemangiopericytoma-like component. **B** shows well-differentiated cartilaginous elements.

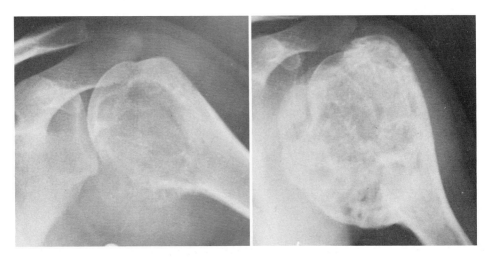

Fig. 1260 Giant cell tumor of upper end of humerus in 20-year-old girl who refused treatment. There was interval of nineteen months between x-ray films. (WU negs. 48-6970 and 48-6971.)

have been reported.[180c] We also have seen giant cell tumors in the patella, fibula, humerus, and sphenoid bone[176] (Fig. 1260). Involvement of the bones of the hands and feet, jaw, and vertebrae (other than sacrum) is distinctly unusual.

Giant cell tumors thin the cortex of the bone but only rarely produce periosteal bone formation. On section, they contain loculated spaces transversed by fibrous trabeculae (Fig. 1261). Areas of hemorrhage are frequent within them. They may be small or large. If they become large in long bones, fractures may follow.

X-ray examinations often show changes purported to be diagnostic. However, we have seen lesions diagnosed as giant cell tumors that proved to be plasma cell myeloma, fibrosarcoma, or chondrosarcoma. Whether a giant cell tumor is benign or malignant cannot be determined roentgenographically.

Microscopically, the giant cell tumor is mainly composed of two components, stromal cells and giant cells. Osteoid or bone, apparently of a reactive nature, is seen in one-third of the cases. The giant cells often are large and have many nuclei (twenty or thirty are usual) that frequently occupy the center of the cell. The prominence of the giant cells gives the tumor its name. However, it is likely that they and their mononuclear precursors are nonneoplastic and that the so-called stromal cells are the basic tumor elements.[179a] It is their relative number and appearance that correlate with the clinical evolution, not those of the giant cells. Therefore, the microscopic evaluation of a

given giant cell tumor depends on careful study of the stromal cells. In the obvious malignant tumor, the stroma shows increased cellularity and mitotic activity.[180a,183]

It is imperative that several sections of curettings be examined. We have had a giant cell tumor in which the original sections of the curettings showed no malignant tumor, but in time this tumor recurred, invaded the soft tissue, and metastasized to the lungs as a fibrosarcoma. Only two sections had been made of the initial curettings. Further sections of them showed malignant tumor in the primary lesion (Fig. 1262). Unfortunately, this lesion may appear to be entirely benign histologically, yet metastasize and kill.[175] The metastases in these instances may also appear to be cytologically benign. Except for the obviously sarcomatous (Grade III) lesions, microscopic grading of these neoplasms is of little practical value. Instead, we regard all giant cell tumors as potentially malignant in view of the fact that as many as 50% of them recur after curettage and approximately 10% give rise to distant metastases.

Many benign pathologic lesions with giant cells have been called giant cell tumors in the past. These lesions include such diverse entities as metaphyseal fibrous defect, chondromyxoid fibroma, chondroblastoma, eosinophilic granuloma, solitary bone cyst, osteitis fibrosa cystica of hyperparathyroidism, aneurysmal bone cyst, and osteoid osteoma. So-called giant cell tumors of tendon sheath are not related to giant cell tumors of bone. One of the main

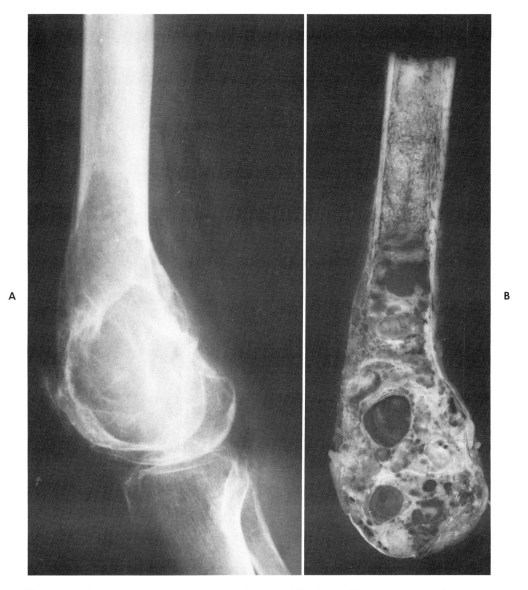

Fig. 1261 A, Typical roentgenogram of giant cell tumor of distal end of femur involving epiphysis and metaphyseal area. Lesion was resected surgically. **B,** Gross specimen that faithfully reproduces roentgenographic changes. (From Sissons HA: Malignant tumours of bone and cartilage. In Raven RW, ed: Cancer, vol. 2. London, 1958, Butterworth & Co., Ltd.)

microscopic differences between true giant cell tumor and these so-called variants resides in the spatial relationship between giant and stromal cells. They tend to be distributed regularly and uniformly in giant cell tumor, whereas in the lesions that simulate it, foci of numerous, clumped giant cells alternate with large areas completely lacking this component. Although giant cell tumors can be multiple,[184] most giant cell–containing lesions involving several bones

represent some other disease. The inclusion of the aforementioned entities has been responsible for the high cure rates reported in the past. Histochemical studies unfortunately are of no aid in differentiating giant cell tumor from its so-called variants.[181]

Willis[185] and many of the English school proposed that these tumors be designated as osteoclastomas. Electron microscopic and histochemical studies have indeed confirmed the

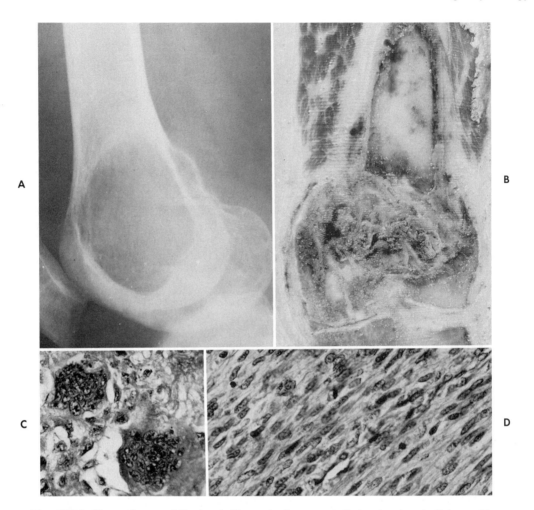

Fig. 1262 A, Giant cell tumor of distal end of femur. Lesion was curetted and replaced with bone chips. **B,** Giant cell tumor shown in **A** recurred, necessitating amputation. Gross specimen demonstrates bone chips still in place with tumor replacing femur. Review of original sections showed benign giant cell tumor, but recuts of curetted material demonstrated malignant stroma. **C,** Original section of curettings referred to in **B** showing areas of rather innocuous-appearing stroma with typical multinucleated giant cells. These changes were called benign. **D,** Later tissue section of malignant giant cell tumor referred to in **B** and **C** that has appearance of fibrosarcoma. There was no evidence of osteoid formation. Patient died of pulmonary metastases. (**A,** WU neg. 49-5963; **B,** WU neg. 50-663; **C,** high power; WU neg. 51-1535; **D,** ×460; WU neg. 50-3550.)

close similarity, if not identity, between the giant cell of this tumor and the osteoclast.[177,182] On the other hand, the ultrastructural appearance of the stromal cells is suggestive of either a fibroblastic or osteoblastic derivation.[173,174] If a giant cell lesion occurs in the maxilla or mandible or in some atypical location such as the small bones of the hand, a parathyroid adenoma must be suspected. We have seen three patients with functioning parathyroid adenomas seek medical care initially for giant cell lesions

in the small bones of the fingers. In most reported series, the incidence of clinical malignancy in giant cell tumors is in the range of 10%.[175,180] The incidence of recurrence within the bone after curettage is much higher. Therefore, whenever technically feasible, we recommend excision en bloc of the entire lesion with replacement with allograft or artificial materials as the treatment of choice.[179b,180b] Special care should be taken to prevent implantation of the tumor into the adjoining soft

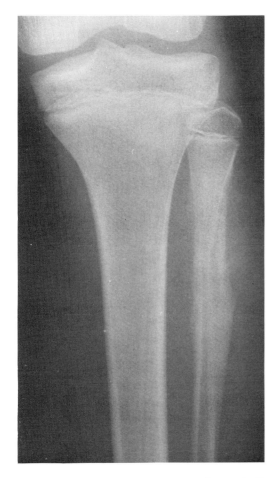

Fig. 1263 Ewing's sarcoma of fibula. Growth is ill-defined and accompanied by prominent periosteal reaction.

tissues.[179] Radiation therapy is indicated for giant cell tumors located in areas not amenable to resection.

Marrow tumors
Ewing's sarcoma

Ewing's tumor of bone occurs in children and in adults under 30 years of age, most patients being between the ages of 5 and 20 years.[191] This tumor occurs most often in the long bones (femur, tibia, humerus, and fibula) and in bones of the pelvis, rib, vertebra, mandible, and clavicle. It arises in the medullary canal of the shaft, from which it permeates the cortex and invades the soft tissues (Fig. 1263). We have seen several cases of Ewing's sarcoma presenting clinically as soft tissue neoplasms with a normal roentgenographic ap-

pearance of the underlying bone. Microscopic examination of these cases revealed that the tumor originated in the medullary canal and had diffusely permeated the marrow spaces to extend outside the bone without destroying a significant amount of bone trabeculae and thus remaining undetectable by conventional roentgenographic examination. This possibility should always be investigated before making a diagnosis of primary extraskeletal Ewing's sarcoma.

The roentgenographic changes are cortical thickening and widening of the medullary canal. With progress of the lesion, reactive periosteal bone may be deposited in layers parallel to the cortex (onion-skin appearance) or at right angles to it (sun-ray appearance)[197] (Fig. 1264). The roentgenographic appearance is not diagnostic.

Microscopically, Ewing's sarcoma consists of solid sheets of cells divided into irregular masses by fibrous strands. Individual cells are small and uniform, with round nuclei having frequent indentations and small nucleoli and inconspicuous cytoplasmic outlines (Fig. 1265). The tumor is fairly well vascularized. It often contains cellular areas with necrosis, and the tumor cells may arrange circumferentially in a rosette-like fashion, with or without a central vessel. Occasional tumors have larger, more pleomorphic cells, often with conspicuous nucleoli.[193a] One of the most important diagnostic features is the nearly constant presence of glycogen granules in the cytoplasm of the tumor cells, well demonstrated by a PAS stain with a diastase control or by electron microscopy (Fig. 1266). Although exceptions occur,[199,200a] metastatic neuroblastoma and histiocytic lymphoma are, as a rule, devoid of cytoplasmic glycogen.[196] The only other tumor which enters in the differential diagnosis with Ewing's sarcoma and which also often contains abundant glycogen is embryonal rhabdomyosarcoma. In general, the diagnosis of Ewing's sarcoma in a bone biopsy should be made with great caution, if at all, when the PAS reaction is negative. In cases of this sort, electron microscopic examination is indicated.[193,199]

The histogenesis of Ewing's sarcoma is still undecided. Several tissue culture and ultrastructural studies favor an origin from primitive marrow elements.[188-190,192,193]

Willis[200] correctly pointed out that metastatic neuroblastoma may easily be confused with primary Ewing's tumor both roentgeno-

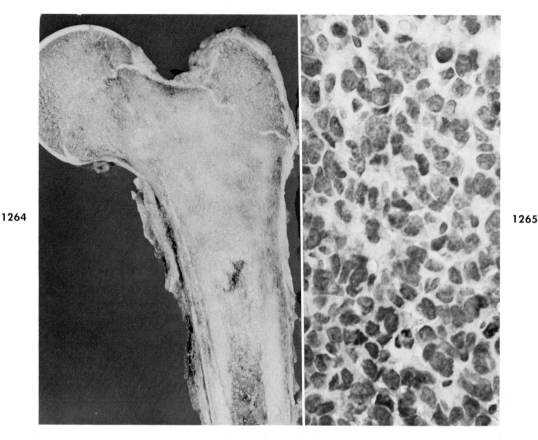

1264

1265

Fig. 1264 Resected end of femur involved by Ewing's sarcoma. Note complete replacement of marrow cavity and prominent cortical thickening. Microscopically, destruction and invasion of epiphysis were present. (WU neg. 50-1409.)

Fig. 1265 Ewing's sarcoma with uniform cells, inconspicuous cytoplasm, and no osteoid. (×600; WU neg. 51-294.)

graphically and microscopically. Features that can be used for the differential diagnosis between these two neoplasms are indicated in Table 66.

Ewing's tumor also can be confused with undifferentiated carcinoma, malignant lymphoma, or even eosinophilic granuloma.

Clinically, Ewing's sarcoma in a young adult may simulate osteomyelitis because of the pain, disability, fever, and leukocytosis. The spread of this tumor is to the lungs and pleura, other bones (particularly skull), central nervous system, and regional lymph nodes. About 25% of the patients have multiple bone and/or visceral lesions at the time of presentation.[189a] Following therapy, increased pleomorphism and bizarre giant cells may appear.[198]

Conventional treatment with surgery or radiation therapy resulted in the past in five-year survival rates of 5%-8%. Recent series in which adjuvant therapy was employed have dramatically improved this gloomy outlook. High-dose irradiation followed by multidrug chemotherapy is being presently used. The local control achieved is over 85%,[194,194a] and the actuarial five-year disease-free survival rate is 75%.[187,195]

Malignant lymphoma

Malignant lymphoma of bone is a definite entity.[201,205] About 60% of the patients are over 30 years of age, although the tumors do occur in younger persons. The sex distribution is about equal.

Grossly, this tumor involves the shaft or metaphysis of the bone, producing cortical and medullary destruction. The destruction within the bone is patchy and associated with

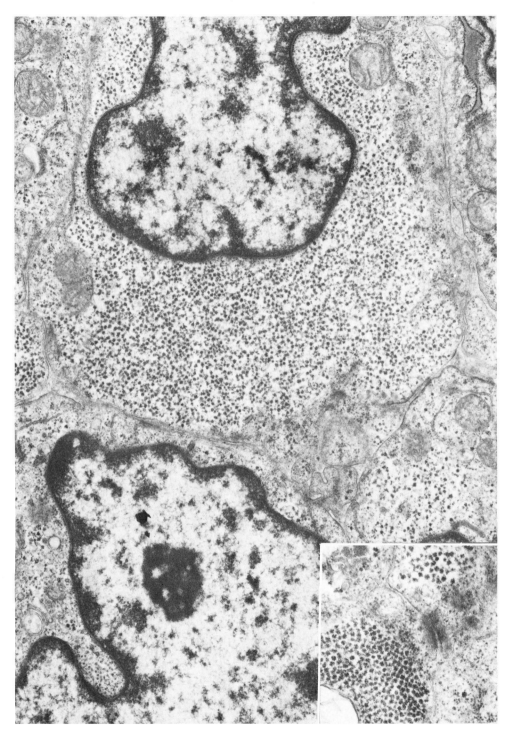

Fig. 1266 Ewing's sarcoma of bone. Cells are attached by primitive junctions and contain large amounts of particulate glycogen. In **inset** note zonula adherens-type intercellular junction and glycogen. (×16,850; **inset,** ×25,270.)

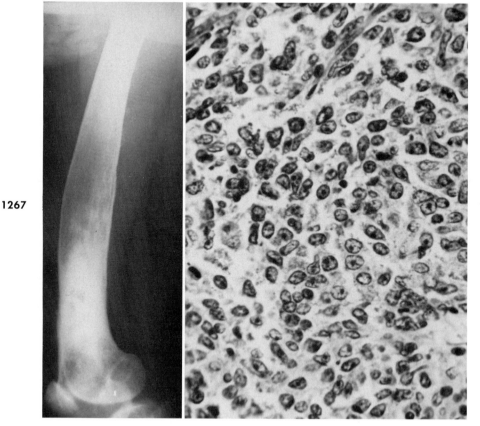

1267

1268

Fig. 1267 Malignant lymphoma involving lower end of femur demonstrating bone destruction and bone production. Such lesions are often erroneously diagnosed as chronic osteomyelitis. (WU neg. 49-4628.)

Fig. 1268 Malignant lymphoma of histiocytic type. Note large cells with prominent nucleoli. Reticulin was present. (×600; WU neg. 50-3840.)

Table 66 Differential features between Ewing's sarcoma and metastatic neuroblastoma

	Ewing's sarcoma	**Metastatic neuroblastoma**
Age	Most patients between 5 and 20 yr	Most patients under 3 yr
Number of lesions when first seen	Usually solitary	Usually multiple
Glycogen	Present; often abundant	Usually absent
Tissue culture	Grows as undifferentiated cells	Grows neurites in 24-48 hr
Electron microscopy	Undifferentiated cells; abundant glycogen	Neural processes; junctional complexes; neurosecretory granules
Urinary catecholamine derivatives	Normal	Almost always elevated

minimal to moderate periosteal reaction, usually of the lamellated type. The tumor is pinkish gray and granular, and it frequently extends into the soft tissues and invades the muscle.

Roentgenographically, a combination of bone production and bone destruction often involves a wide area of a long bone (Fig. 1267). This combination of changes is very suggestive of the diagnosis.[206] However, osteosarcoma and chronic osteomyelitis may result in a very similar appearance.

Microscopically, most malignant lymphomas presenting as primary bone tumors are of the histiocytic type (reticulum cell sarcoma) or mixed cell (histiocytic-lymphocytic) type.[204a,205a] The main source of difficulty resides in their separation from Ewing's sarcoma. The cells of malignant lymphoma are usually larger. The nuclei are somewhat pleomorphic; many are indented or horseshoe-shaped. They usually have prominent nucleoli, unlike the fine nucleoli of Ewing's sarcoma (Fig. 1268). Cytoplasmic outlines of histiocytic lymphoma are well defined, whereas those of Ewing's tumor are indistinct. The cytoplasm is more abundant and often eosinophilic. Reticulin is between individual cells and groups of cells, whereas in Ewing's sarcoma it is mainly restricted to the perivascular areas. Ultrastructurally, the features are analogous to those of nodal and other extranodal lymphomas.[204a] Classically, malignant lymphoma of bone has been regarded as a tumor of better prognosis than Ewing's sarcoma, five-year survival rates for localized tumors varying from 22%-50% in several series.[204,207,210] With recent improvements in the treatment of Ewing's sarcoma, this difference has narrowed considerably. The work-up of these patients should include skeletal survey, sternal marrow aspiration, and lymphangiogram. Radiation is the therapy of choice, supplemented by chemotherapy if indicated.

Hodgkin's disease produces roentgenographically detectable bone lesions in approximately 15% of the cases. In Horan's series,[203] the involvement was multifocal in 60%. The most frequent sites were the vertebrae, pelvis, ribs, sternum, and femur. The osseous lesions of Hodgkin's disease are often asymptomatic and in 50% of the cases are not demonstrable roentgenographically. When they become apparent in the x-ray film, the foci may be osteolytic, mixed, or purely osteoblastic. The latter appearance is particularly common in vertebrae.

Acute leukemia of childhood is associated with roentgenographic abnormalities in the skeletal system in 70%-90% of the cases.[209] In the large majority of the instances, the changes are widespread and therefore unlikely to be confused with a primary bone neoplasm.[208] In contrast, destructive bone lesions are extremely rare in the chronic leukemias. Chabner et al.[202] reported six cases in a series of 205 patients with chronic granulocytic leukemia. In three of the patients, the bone

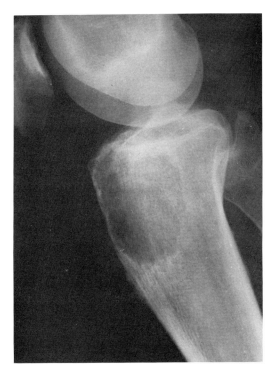

Fig. 1269 Osteolytic lesion of upper end of tibia due to localized lesion of plasma cell myeloma. Such lesion has osteolytic appearance of metastatic carcinoma. (WU neg. 50-417.)

lesion appeared at the time of blastic transformation.

Plasma cell myeloma

The pathologic expressions of plasma cell tumors are many.[211] Disseminated myeloma is the most frequent. It occurs slightly more often in men than in women. It usually occurs between 40 and 60 years of age, rarely before the age of 30 years. The tumor, when disseminated, produces osteolytic lesions in the vertebrae, pelvis, ribs, sternum, and skull. Under these circumstances, the life expectancy is usually less than two years, although occasional patients will have an extremely prolonged clinical course.[217a] In advanced disease, extraskeletal spread may be seen. Most of the cases are confined to the soft tissues adjacent to bones involved by myeloma, but distant metastases to the spleen, liver, lymph nodes, and kidney also can occur.[220] Exceptionally, the bone lesions of plasma cell meyloma will appear as osteosclerotic rather than osteolytic.[215a]

Solitary plasma cell tumors of bone may involve long or flat bones (Fig. 1269). We

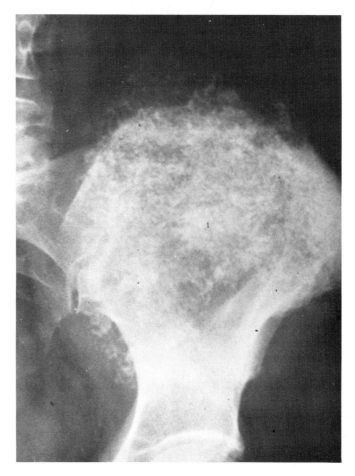

Fig. 1270 Plasma cell tumor of iliac bone simulating chondrosarcoma roentgenographically. Microscopically, there was abundant amyloid formation, which was heavily calcified. (Case contributed by Dr. R. C. Newberry, Texarkana, Ark.)

have seen a case associated with abundant amyloid formation that simulated a chondrosarcoma roentgenographically (Fig. 1270).

Plasma cell tumors may first appear clinically in the soft tissue. The most frequent extraosseous locations are the nasopharynx, nose, and tonsil. We have seen these tumors in such areas as the mediastinum, skin, and lymph nodes. Rarely, plasma cell tumors occur with the clinical and hematologic manifestations of a leukemia.[219]

The majority of the lesions initially of soft tissue eventually become disseminated in bone. Christopherson and Miller[214] collected all the apparently localized cases of plasma cell tumors. Only five of the entire group still had localized disease after a ten-year follow-up. Of the ninety-two tumors reported by Carson et al.,[213] only one could be considered to be possibly localized. Kotner and Wang[217] analyzed twenty cases of plasmacytomas of the upper air and food passages, most of which had been treated aggressively by radiation therapy. They remarked that if systemic disease develops in a patient with soft tissue plasmacytoma, it may occur many years later and even then run a prolonged course. Others have confirmed this observation.[215,222]

Bones involved by plasma cell tumors often fracture. The tissue is hemorrhagic and cellular. The focal, slowly growing tumor may have a fairly well-defined border, is grayish yellow, homogeneous, and firm.

Microscopically, an obvious well-differentiated plasma cell tumor grows in sheets separated by fine trabeculae that are seen well

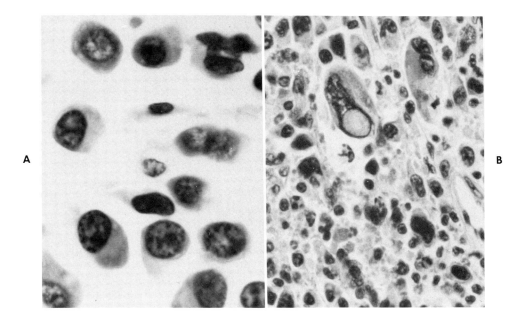

Fig. 1271 A, Well-differentiated plasma cell tumor showing plasma cells with eccentric nuclei and characteristic arrangement of chromatin. **B,** Highly undifferentiated plasma cell tumor with tumor giant cells. (**A,** High power; WU neg. 50-228; **B,** ×600; WU neg. 50-3224.)

by reticulin stain. We agree with Lichtenstein and Jaffe[218] that myeloma should not be divided into subvarieties and that the neoplasm arises from a single cell type, the plasma cell and its precursors.

Plasma cells are commonly found in chronic inflammatory conditions. They are particularly common within the oral cavity. The mere presence of large numbers of plasma cells should not be diagnosed as plasma cell tumor. The plasma cells of a granulomatous process are well differentiated and often contain Russell bodies (aggregates of eosinophilic material in the cytoplasm.) Other chronic inflammatory cells will be interspersed between the abundant plasma cells. Such plasma cell granulomas may become large enough to be mistaken for a true neoplasm. Certainly, most plasma cell–containing lesions of the conjunctiva are granulomas, and we have seen other plasmacytic granulomas in the oral cavity, mediastinum, lung, stomach, kidney, testis, and bone. The importance of the distinction of this granuloma from plasma cell myeloma is obvious.

Plasma cell tumors may be highly undifferentiated and difficult to identify. In areas, they may be difficult to distinguish from histiocytic malignant lymphoma (Fig. 1271). However, careful examination of many fields will

reveal collections of recognizable neoplastic plasma cells. The well-differentiated plasma cell has an eccentric nucleus, a cartwheel arrangement of the chromatin, and often two nuclei. Electron microscopic study may provide the diagnosis in controversial cases.[221] There seems to be no correlation between the ultrastructural appearance of the tumor cells and the type of immunoglobulin being secreted.[216]

Thorough study of a patient with an apparently single lesion of bone often demonstrates it to be only a localized manifestation of a disseminated process. Trephine biopsy of the sternal marrow is particularly important, for it may show increased plasma cells in the marrow. This finding often is present in the face of otherwise normal skeletal series, serum proteins, electrophoretic pattern of serum proteins, and absence of Bence-Jones protein. Long-time follow-up, particularly of all localized lesions, is mandatory. In the patient referred to in Fig. 1269, the local lesion was treated and sterilized by irradiation and the defect replaced by bone chips. At that time, all laboratory and x-ray examinations were normal except for slight elevation of the plasma cells in the sternal marrow. The patient was still working eight years later but had disseminated disease evidenced by massive replacement of the sternal marrow by plasma cells. This patient illustrates the effectiveness of radiation therapy in controlling localized lesions as well as the fact that patients with myeloma may live well over five years.

In a series of 112 patients studied by Carbone et al.,[212] 87% had a detectable protein abnormality. IgG proteins were found in 61%, IgA is 18%, and light chains only (Bence Jones protein) in 9%. Of the ninety patients with abnormal serum proteins, 69% had type kappa and 31% type lambda proteins. No association between the presence or type of immunoglobulin abnormality and the survival was encountered.

For a discussion on the clinicopathologic features of tumors associated with dysproteinemia, see Chapter 20.

Patients with disseminated multiple myeloma due to extensive involvement of the vertebrae and ribs develop a typical hunchback deformity. Rib fractures are frequent, anemia is prominent, and death occurs rather quickly. In one series, death occurred in fifty-seven of sixty patients with disseminated myeloma in the first two years. Thirty-one of these patients died within three months of initial diagnosis.[213] Radiation therapy may sterilize or operation may eradicate localized lesions of bone. Chlorambucil occasionally gives striking palliation.

Vascular tumors

Hemangiomas of bone are often reported in the vertebra as a postmortem finding. In 2,154 autopsies studied by Töpfer,[231] hemangiomas occurred in 11.9%. They were multiple in 34%. These lesions should probably be regarded as vascular malformations rather than true neoplasms. The most common locations of clinically significant osseous hemangiomas are the skull, vertebrae, and jawbones.[232]

Hemangiomas in the long bones are extremely rare.[223] We have seen cavernous hemangiomas of the clavicle and ribs and have observed a lesion of the fibula causing irregular bone destruction in the shaft that was incorrectly diagnosed as Ewing's tumor. When a lesion involves the flat bones (particularly the skull), sunburst trabeculation occurs because of elevation of the periosteum. On section, they often have a currant jelly appearance. They do not undergo malignant change. Microscopically, the appearance is characteristic, with a thick-walled latticelike pattern of endothelial-lined cavernous spaces filled with blood. Bone hemangiomas may be multiple. This rare condition, mainly seen in children, is associated in about half of the cases with cutaneous, soft tissue, or visceral hemangiomas.[229]

Massive osteolysis (Gorham's disease) is probably not a vascular neoplasm but is included in this discussion because of its microscopic similarities with skeletal angiomatosis. It has a destructive character that the latter lacks. It results in reabsorption of a whole bone or several bones and the filling of the residual spaces by a heavily vascularized fibrous tissue.[225,226]

Lymphangiomas are exceptional. Most cases have multiple osseous involvement and are associated with soft tissue tumors of similar appearance. The cases with multiple involvement are also termed cystic angiomatosis or hamartous hemolymphangiomatosis.[228b]

Glomus tumor of the subungual soft tissues may erode the underlying bone. Much rarer is the occurrence of a purely intraosseous glomus tumor involving the terminal phalanx.[227]

Malignant vascular tumors, which we prefer to designate as *angiosarcomas*, exhibit obvious atypia of the tumor cells, formation of solid areas alternating with others with anastomosing vascular channels, and foci of necrosis and hemorrhage.[224,226a,228] Ultrastructurally, the large majority of the cells have the appearance of endothelial cells, with only an occasional admixture of pericytes.[230] Multicentric examples occur. Distant metastases are common, particularly to the lungs. Before making a diagnosis of angiosarcoma in a bone lesion, the more common possibilities of well-vascularized osteosarcoma and metastatic carcinoma (particularly of renal origin) should be ruled out.[232]

Another vascular tumor of bone occurs, sometimes designated as hemangioendothelioma and often grouped with the aforedescribed angiosarcoma, that we believe represents a distinct entity, comparable to similar lesions of the skin, soft tissue, heart, blood vessels, and other organs. These tumors, which we designate as *histiocytoid hemangiomas*,[228a] are characterized by histiocytoid-looking endothelial cells with abundant acidophilic cytoplasm (often vacuolated) and large vesicular nuclei, scanty mitotic activity, inconspicuousness of anastomosing channels or hemorrhage, and an inconstant inflammatory component rich in eosinophils. These lesions can be locally destructive and multicentric; their clinical course is prolonged, and they can often be cured by conservative surgery. We believe that many of the cases interpreted as Grade I (and perhaps Grade II) hemangioendotheliomas of bone in some series[223a] belong to this category.

Other connective tissue tumors
Desmoplastic fibroma

A rare neoplasm, desmoplastic fibroma is formed by mature fibroblasts separated by abundant collagen.[246] Pleomorphism, necrosis, and mitotic activity are lacking. Ultrastructurally, the predominant cells are myofibroblasts, with a lesser component of fibroblasts and primitive mesenchymal cells.[240a] This lesion probably represents the osseous counterpart of soft tissue fibromatosis. Local recurrences are common, but metastases do not occur.[244]

Fibrosarcoma

Fibrosarcomas of bone often arise in the metaphyseal area of long bones.[234,237] Approximately 50% of these occur in the distal segment of the femur or proximal portion of the tibia.[242] The majority of these osteolytic tumors arise in the medullary portion, from where they destroy the cortex and often extend into the soft tissues. A less common location is the periosteum. The diagnosis of this tumor is seldom made roentgenographically. Only a diagnosis of malignant bone neoplasm is suggested.

Microscopically, this tumor is a fibroblastic neoplasm similar to soft tissue fibrosarcomas (Figs. 1272 and 1273). This tumor is distinct from other bone tumors. We have seen examples in which numerous sections of the primary tumor and its metastases showed no osteoid formation.

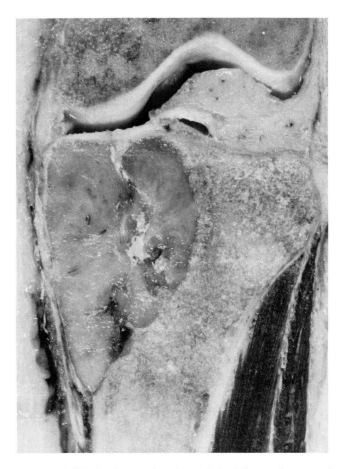

Fig. 1272 Fibrosarcoma of tibia. Lesion produced osteolytic defect and was confused roentgenographically with giant cell tumor. (WU neg. 57-789.)

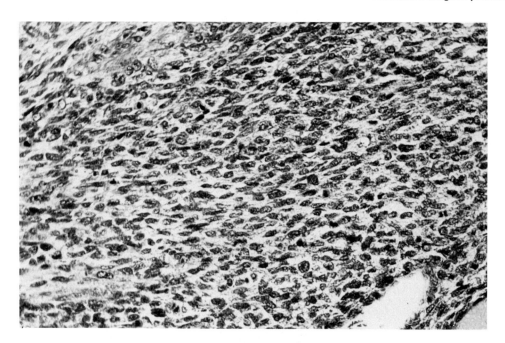

Fig. 1273 Histologic pattern of this cellular, poorly differentiated fibrosarcoma, primary in right femur, is similar to fibrosarcoma of soft tissues. (×275; WU neg. 53-623.)

Extremely well-differentiated fibrosarcomas may be misdiagnosed as benign lesions of fibrous tissue, but invariably the roentgenographic appearance suggests its malignant nature. Microscopically, the presence of cellular areas, mitotic figures, hyperchromatism, and pleomorphism are all features that favor a diagnosis of fibrosarcoma over one of desmoplastic fibroma. Fibrosarcoma also should be differentiated from the variety of osteosarcoma mainly composed of fibroblastic elements.[235] Wide local excision and amputation are the two choices of therapy, depending on the location, size, and microscopic grade of the tumor. In one recent series, the overall five-year survival rate was 34%.[239] Exceptionally, fibrosarcoma can present as a multicentric process involving numerous bones.[238] Before making this diagnosis, the possibility of metastatic sarcomatoid carcinoma (particularly from the kidney) should be ruled out.

Malignant fibrous histiocytoma

A tumor with a microscopic appearance similar to the (pleomorphic) malignant fibrous histiocytoma of the soft tissues (see Chapter 24) can appear in bone.[240,241,245] Most cases were located in long bones, and one of them was multicentric.[233] The histogenesis and differential diagnosis of this tumor when involving bone remain controversial. As Dahlin et al.[236] have pointed out, areas indistinguishable from those of malignant fibrous histiocytoma can be found in otherwise typical examples of osteosarcoma, fibrosarcoma, and chondrosarcoma and regarded as foci of anaplasia. Only when thorough sampling of the tumor reveals no areas suggestive of these lesions may a diagnosis of malignant fibrous histiocytoma of bone be justified. Even under these circumstances, we are not sure that we are confronted with a real entity or whether we are simply dealing with an undifferentiated sarcoma. The latter alternative would explain why their prognosis is so poor, at least in some series.[245]

Leiomyosarcoma

Malignant smooth muscle tumor of bone are very rare. The few reported cases have occurred in long bones, particularly the femur.[232a,243]

Liposarcoma

Primary liposarcomas of bone are exceptional.[240b] It is likely that many of the cases reported as such in the past would be reclassified today as malignant fibrous histiocytomas.

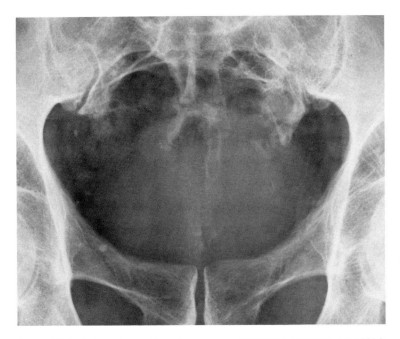

Fig. 1274 Osteolytic destruction of sacrum by chordoma. (WU neg. 52-2398.)

Other primary tumors
Chordoma

Chordoma, a malignant tumor, arises from the remnants of the fetal notochord, which is situated within the vertebral bodies and intervertebral discs and, rarely, in the presacral soft tissues.[248] Most chordomas arise from notochordal remnants in bone rather than from those located inside the discs. They are more frequent in the fifth and sixth decades but occur at all ages, and in both sexes.[251] They grow slowly, the duration of the symptoms before diagnosis usually being over five years. Fifty percent arise in the sacrococcygeal area, 35% in the spheno-occipital area, and the remaining along the cervicothoracolumbar spine.[252] The sacrococcygeal tumors are more common in the fifth and sixth decades of life, whereas many of the spheno-occipital neoplasms occur in children. In the former, a portion of the sacrum is seen destroyed by an osteolytic or rarely an osteoblastic process (Fig. 1274). If the tumor encroaches upon the spine, symptoms of spinal cord compression arise. The retroperitoneal space is often involved by direct extension. The tumor may grow large enough to narrow the lumen of the large bowel or impinge upon the bladder. It can be felt as a firm extrarectal mass. Spheno-occipital chordomas may present with a nasal, paranasal, or naso-pharyngeal mass, multiple cranial nerve involvement, and destruction of bone.[248a,256]

Grossly, the chordoma is gelatinous and soft and contains areas of hemorrhage. Microscopically, it closely resembles normal notochord tissue in its different stages of development.[247] It grows in cell cords and lobules separated by a variable amount of mucoid intercellular tissue (Fig. 1275). Some of the tumor cells are extremely large with vacuolated cytoplasm and prominent vesicular nucleus. They are sometimes designated as physaliferous. Some of the vacuoles contain glycogen.[249,257] Other tumor cells are small, with small nuclei and no visible nucleoli. Mitotic figures are scanty or absent. Areas of cartilage and bone may be present.[254] In some areas, the tumor may simulate carcinoma or spindle cell sarcoma. The microscopic differential diagnosis has to be made with chondrosarcoma, rectal signet-cell adenocarcinoma, and myxopapillary ependymoma. Erlandson et al.[250] examined three chordomas by electron microscopy and found in each case peculiar mitochondrial-endoplasmic reticulum complexes, an interesting even if nonspecific feature.

The natural history of chordoma is characterized by repeated episodes of local recurrence and an almost uniformly fatal outcome. Recurrences may develop ten years or longer after

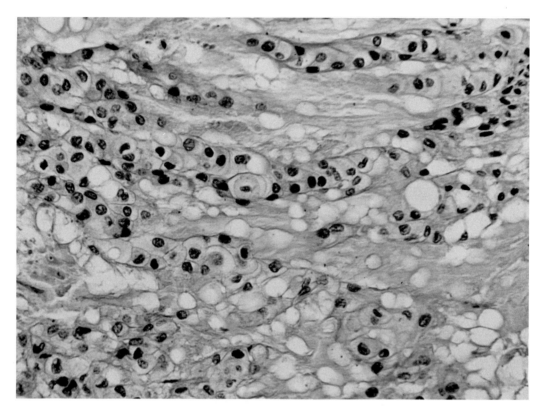

Fig. 1275 Chordoma of spheno-occipital region. Cuboidal and polyhedral cells of central nucleus form rows and nests among abundant myxoid matrix. (×350; WU neg. 73-2685; courtesy Dr. J. E. Olvera-Rabiela, Mexico City, Mexico.)

the initial therapy.[247a] Distant metastases are usually late in the evolution of the disease. The most common sites are skin and bone; the latter may be histologically misdiagnosed as mixed tumors of the skin.[248b] Distant metastases occurred in 43% of a series of patients reviewed by Higinbotham et al.[253] Total surgical excision is usually impossible. Thus radiation therapy remains as the only practical treatment.[255] Heffelfinger et al.[252] identified a morphologic variant of chordoma that they designated as *chordoid chordoma* because of an abundant cartilaginous component in addition to more typical chordoma areas. This type occurred in the spheno-occipital region and had a much better prognosis than ordinary chordoma.

"Adamantinoma" of long bones

A locally aggressive neoplasm, "adamantinoma" occurs predominantly in the tibia but has been reported in other long bones, such as the femur, ulna, and fibula.[259,261] Occasionally,

an adamantinoma of the tibia is seen also involving the adjacent fibula.[264] It may arise in the shaft or in the metaphyseal area of the bone.[260] Microscopically, several patterns of growth have been described. The most common is one formed by solid nests of basaloid cells with palisading at the periphery and sometimes a stellate configuration in the center. Less frequent forms are a "squamoid" pattern with keratinization and an "angioblastic" pattern. A fibrous dysplasia–like lesion is often seen accompanying the tumor nests; it has been interpreted by Weiss and Dorfman[265] as focal mesenchymal differentiation by the tumor. Electron microscopic studies of this tumor type have confirmed the epithelial nature of the cells.[258,262,266]

What epithelium is doing inside a long bone remains a mystery. A possible explanation is that these tumors originate in deep-seated (very deep seated!) sweat glands. Other tumors reported in the literature as adamantinomas have an altogether different appearance, some resembling vascular neoplasms and other synovial tissues. It is possible, as Schajowicz and Gallardo[263] suggest, that the term adamantinoma is often applied to loosely to probably unrelated tumors of the tibia having a similar clinicoradiographic appearance.

Bona fide adamantinoma is best treated by amputation, for local redrudescence and even distant metastases may develop.

Neurogenic tumors

Over thirty cases of intraosseous neurilemoma have been reported.[267] A strong predilection for the mandible has been noted, and origin from the mandibular nerve sometimes has been demonstrated.[269] Although Recklinghausen's disease often results in several types of skeletal abnormalities (such as scoliosis, bowing, pseudoarthrosis, and other disorders of growth),[268] intraosseous neurofibromas are virtually nonexistent.

Metastatic tumors

The incidence of osseous metastases varies with the primary neoplasm and the thoroughness of postmortem examination. We are concerned chiefly with those metastatic lesions that may be confused clinically with primary benign or malignant osseous lesions. In most instances of bone metastases, the primary tumor is known. Excluding these, metastatic tumors are still the most frequent of all malignant neoplasms of bone. These lesions are usually osteolytic but may be osteoblastic or mixed. Tumors with a tendency to produce pure osteoblastic metastases are prostatic carcinoma and carcinoid tumor.[274] The bone or bones involved and the character of the changes seen roentgenographically are helpful in predicting the site of the primary neoplasm. Certain occult primary carcinomas (carcinoma of the thyroid gland and kidney) may develop only a single bone metastasis. They also may manifest single bone metastases many years after removal of the primary neoplasm.

Thyroid carcinoma usually metastasizes to the bones of the shoulder girdle, skull, ribs, and sternum. Carcinoma of the kidney may involve the skull, sternum, flat bones of the pelvis, and upper end of the femur. Both thyroid carcinoma and carcinoma of the kidney produce osteolytic defects. If the tumor extends through the bone into soft tissue, pulsating masses may be present. Carcinomas of almost every organ may produce an apparently single

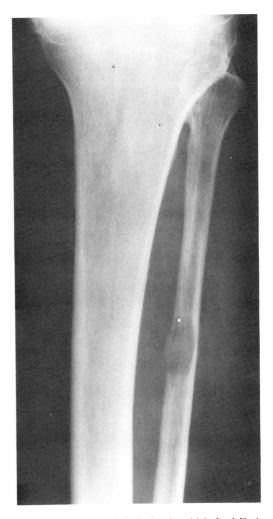

Fig. 1276 Ill-defined lytic lesion in midshaft of fibula produced by metastasis of lung carcinoma.

metastasis to bone (Fig. 1276). The area involved in the long bones is usually the metaphyseal region.

It is often stated that metastases do not occur below the knees or elbows. However, numerous exceptions occur. We have seen metastatic epidermoid carcinoma of the lung in a terminal phalanx, carcinoma of the breast in the small bones of the feet, and carcinoma of the cervix appearing as a poorly defined cyst in the lower end of the tibia.

Periosteal bone proliferation may accompany a metastatic lesion.[272] This is likely to occur in certain sclerosing metastatic lesions such as those of the prostate. However, these metastases are usually multiple and often in ribs. We have seen a single metastasis in a long bone produce excessive periosteal proliferation simulating primary osteosarcoma.[271] Such changes are unusual but have occurred in metastatic rectal, pancreatic, and lung carcinoma (Fig. 1277).

It is imperative that such metastatic lesions be biopsied in order to avoid treatment designed for primary malignant bone tumors. Once a biopsy is available, the microscopic recognition usually is simple. The source of the bone metastasis may be suggested microscopically, particularly if carcinoma of the kidney, thyroid gland, or large bowel exists. If the tumor is squamous carcinoma in a thoracic vertebra and the patient is a man in the sixth decade, metastatic carcinoma of the lung is likely.

Sarcomas of soft tissue origin do not frequently involve bone except by direct invasion. The outstanding exception is embryonal rhabdomyosarcoma of childhood, which is complicated by blood-borne bone marrow metastases in a high percentage of cases.[270]

Most metastatic bone lesions cause pain. Treatment is for its relief. Radiation therapy of localized lesions is the treatment of choice. When a pathologic fracture supervenes, internal fixation and radiation therapy provide the best results.[273] Palliative measures such as estrogen therapy and/or orchiectomy may afford relief in patients with disseminated metastases from carcinoma of the prostate. The pain of metastatic carcinoma from the breast is commonly relieved by testosterone. Occasionally, striking objective improvement in the condition of the bone is obtained. Other types of hormonal therapy than testosterone are thought less effective in the palliation of generalized bone metastases. In a few rare instances, a single metastatic focus, particularly from the thyroid gland and kidney, may be excised with benefit.

Laboratory findings

Elevation of acid phosphatase in serum is usually evidence of metastatic carcinoma arising from the prostate (a rare exception in infarction of the prostate).

Elevation of the alkaline phosphatase level is merely an expression of bone production and is nonspecific. It can be elevated in bone-producing lesions such as osteosarcoma, hyperparathyroidism, Paget's disease, and metastatic carcinoma of the breast or prostate as well as incident to hepatic metastases. The alkaline phosphatase level is normal in many processes that predominantly destroy bone, such as osteolytic osteosarcoma, metastatic carcinoma from the kidney, and plasma cell myeloma.

Plasma cell myeloma is practically the only other tumor in which there are laboratory findings that lend weight to the diagnosis. However, these findings occur only when the process is disseminated. When a localized plasmacytoma of bone exists, all laboratory findings, including bone marrow, are usually normal. In disseminated multiple myeloma, the serum protein concentration frequently is elevated (as high as 20 gm%). This elevation involves mainly the globulin fraction. The electrophoretic pattern of the serum proteins may be diagnostic, but in certain instances of apparently localized plasma cell myeloma it is normal.

Bence Jones protein is present in about half the cases. Serum calcium and phosphorus levels may be elevated because bone is being destroyed so fast that the kidneys do not

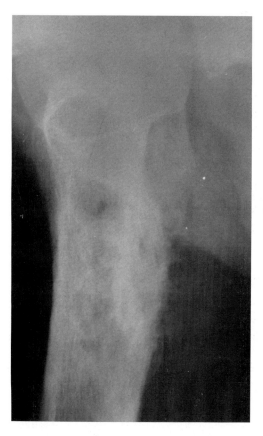

Fig. 1277 Metastatic carcinoma in femur, with extensive callus formation, which simulated osteosarcoma both roentgenographically and microscopically. Primary tumor was probably in lung. (WU neg. 67-9392.)

have time to excrete it. The uric acid may be increased through catabolism of nucleoproteins derived from myeloma cells.[275] Elevation of the sedimentation rate may be the first evidence of recurrence of Ewing's tumor.

Biopsy and frozen section

The therapy of malignant tumors of bone often implies amputation in a young person. Before such a procedure, it is imperative that the pathologic diagnosis be correct.

The surgeon must obtain adequate material for pathologic diagnosis even though the lesion is confined entirely within the bone. If possible, he should excise a segment of bone that includes both involved and uninvolved areas. He should avoid excessive trauma to the tumor while securing a biopsy and should so place the biopsy incision that it may be entirely removed if subsequent radical operation is indicated. Theoretically, the use of a tourniquet proximal to bone lesions in the extremities while securing the biopsy may reduce the possibility of distant spread. There is no evidence that the performance of a biopsy affects survival in patients with osteosarcoma or other malignant bone tumors.[275a]

If there is any question of infection, the material obtained at biopsy must be properly studied bacteriologically.

Aspiration biopsy of bone tumors has been performed extensively at the Memorial Hospital for Cancer and Allied Diseases. Snyder and Coley[280] reported 385 cases, of which 67.5% were definitely and specifically diagnostic. In no case did a false aspiration diagnosis lead to amputation for a benign process. We believe that aspiration biopsy after preparation of paraffin sections is similar to a small biopsy and is particularly valuable in lesions that are deeply located.[279] Needle biopsy of bony lesions is often diagnostic.[276-278]

Frozen section diagnosis may be technically difficult. On the other hand, osseous lesions that extend into the soft tissue are easily diagnosed by frozen section. On some occasions, a frozen section may lead to an unexpected diagnosis. An osteolytic lesion of the pelvis was thought to be a primary malignant bone tumor, and hemipelvectomy was contemplated. Frozen section, however, demonstrated metastatic carcinoma. An osteolytic lesion of the femur with extension into the soft tissue was considered Ewing's tumor but proved to be eosinophilic granuloma.

At times, an exact diagnosis cannot be made, but the pathologist can usually say whether the lesion is benign or malignant.

Tumorlike lesions
Solitary bone cyst

Solitary (unicameral) bone cysts usually occur in long bones, most often in the upper portion of the shaft of the humerus and femur[282] (Fig. 1278). They also may be seen in short bones, particularly the calcaneus.[284a] Most cases are in males (fourteen out of nineteen patients in Jaffe and Lichtenstein's series[281]), and almost all occur in patients under 20 years of age.

These lesions usually are advanced when first seen. They are usually metaphyseal in position and do not involve the epiphysis. In time, they tend to migrate away from the epiphysis.[285] The cortex is thinned, and periosteal bone proliferation does not take place except in areas of fracture. Bones affected by these lesions often fracture, usually in the proximal portion of the cystic area.[281]

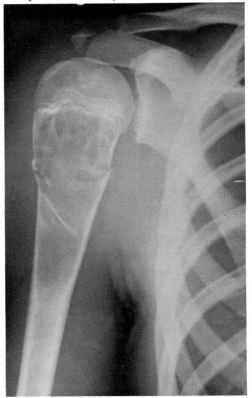

Fig. 1278 Typical solitary bone cyst of upper end of humerus abutting against epiphyseal plate in 13-year-old boy. (WU neg. 49-5897.)

The cyst contains a clear or yellow fluid and is lined by a smooth connective tissue membrane that may be brown. The fluid may be hemorrhagic if a previous fracture has occurred. Microscopically, vascular connective tissue, hemosiderin (often within phagocytes), and cholesterol clefts are frequent. The diagnosis may be difficult in the presence of reparative changes following fracture, recurrence after bone grafting, and when articular cartilage is included in the curettings. The diagnosis becomes clear if the history and the x-ray films are available.

Pommer[284] believes that these cysts develop after mild trauma without fracture but with intramedullary hemorrhage. Conversely, von Mikulicz[283] believes that this lesion has its basis in a local disorder of development and bone growth. The latter theory is the more widely accepted.

The treatment of choice is currettement and replacement of the cyst with bone chips. Treatment of these cysts may be correlated with their activity. Good results are obtained when the cyst has migrated away from the epiphyseal line. Recurrences may appear if the cyst treated is lying close to the epiphyseal line.[285]

Aneurysmal bone cyst

Aneurysmal bone cyst is a rare lesion that may be mistaken for a giant cell tumor, a hemangioma, or even an osteosarcoma.[287,292] This large cystic lesion occurs usually in patients between 10 and 20 years of age. It occurs mainly in the vertebra and flat bones but can arise in the shaft of long bones.[288] Multiple involvement of the vertebrae was observed in seven of fifteen cases studied by Tillman et al.[294]

Roentgenographically, the lesion shows an eccentric expansion of the bone, erosion and destruction of the cortex, and a small border area of periosteal bone formation (Fig. 1279). Grossly, it forms a spongy hemorrhagic mass that may extend into the soft tissues and be covered by a thin shell of reactive bone. Microscopically, large spaces filled with blood often are accompanied by numerous giant cells. The septa contained osteoid[288] (Fig. 1280).

The differential diagnosis has to be made with solitary bone cyst, giant cell tumor, with "telangiectatic" osteosarcoma, and, for the lesions located in the jaw, giant cell reparative granuloma.

The pathogenesis of aneurysmal bone cyst remains elusive. In a few cases, the lesion was preceded by trauma with subperiosteal hematoma but no fracture. In others, it seems to arise in some preexisting bone lesion as a result of changed hemodynamics.[286,291,291b] We have seen areas grossly and microscopically indistinguishable from aneurysmal bone cyst in chondroblastoma, giant cell tumor, fibrous

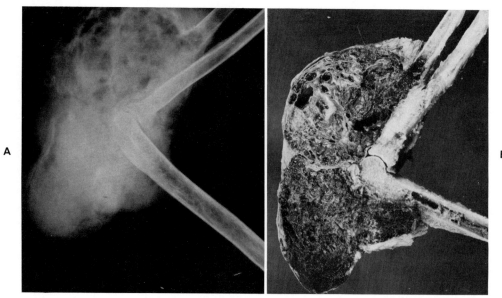

A   **B**

Fig. 1279 A, Aneurysmal bone cyst in region of elbow. Functional disability forced resection. **B,** Cyst shown in **A.** (Courtesy Dr. L. Litchtenstein, San Francisco, Calif.)

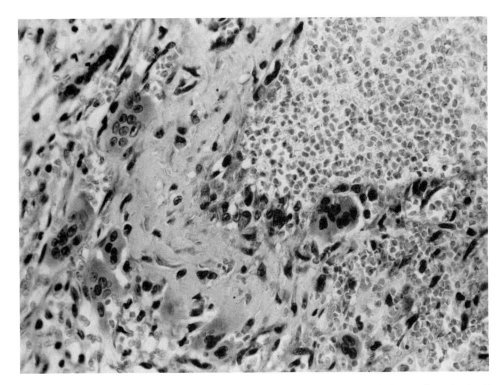

Fig. 1280 Aneurysmal bone cyst showing characteristic septum covered with giant cells and osteoid within its substance. (×400; WU neg. 54-5987.)

dysplasia, osteoblastoma, and osteosarcoma. McCarthy and Dorfman[292a] reported three aneurysmal bone cysts of the rib in infants engrafted on vascular and cartilaginous hamartomas. On the other hand, in most of the aneurysmal bone cysts that we and others have examined, an underlying lesion was not encountered.[286a,294] Naturally, this might have been the result of sampling or the fact that the aneurysmal bone cyst destroyed all evidence of the preexisting lesion. Careful morphologic studies of such cases are needed to evaluate this interesting possibility. Recurrence supervenes in approximately one-third of the cases treated by curettage alone due to incompleteness of surgical excision.[293] En bloc resection or curettage with bone grafting affords better results.[291a]

Exceptionally, lesions resembling aneurys-

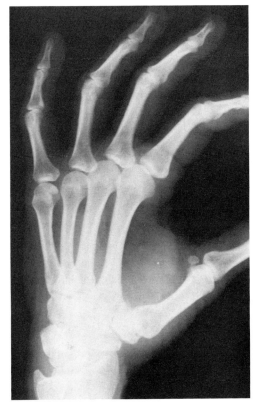

Fig. 1281 Intraosseous ganglion cyst involving base of first metacarpal. It was associated with larger ganglion of adjacent soft tissue, which is also apparent in roentgenogram. (WU neg. 71-6934; courtesy Dr. G. Davis, St. Louis, Mo.)

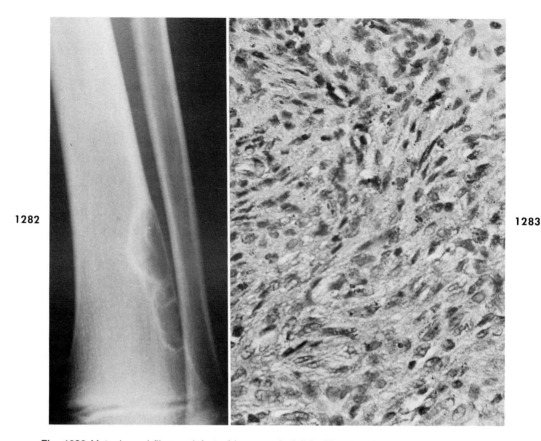

1282   1283

Fig. 1282 Metaphyseal fibrous defect of lower end of tibia. Note its sharp delineation and sclerotic margins. (WU neg. 52-3782.)

Fig. 1283 Area of metaphyseal fibrous defect demonstrating cellular whorllike masses of fibrous tissue. (×400; WU neg. 52-3453.)

mal bone cysts in most regards but lacking the blood-filled cavities are encountered. These have been reported in the small bones of the hands[289] and in the sacrum.[290] Like aneurysmal bone cysts, they probably represent exuberant reactive changes rather than true neoplasms.

Ganglion cyst of bone

On rare occasions, ganglion cysts, morphologically indistinguishable from those commonly seen in the periarticular soft tissue, are found in an intraosseous location, always close to a joint space[295] (Fig. 1281).

The cyst is surrounded by a zone of condensed bone, often multiloculated, and has a gelatinous content and a wall of attenuated fibrous tissue. The bones of the ankle, particularly the tibia, are those most commonly affected.[296] Intraosseous ganglia need to be dis-

tinguished from solitary (unicameral) bone cysts and the periarticular cysts seen in association with degenerative joint diseases.

Metaphyseal fibrous defect (nonossifying fibroma)

Metaphyseal fibrous defects are distinctive lesions of bone that occur in adolescents, most often in long tubular bones, particularly the upper or lower tibia or the lower femur.[297,299] They are eccentric, sharply delimited lesions not too distant from the epiphysis (Fig. 1282). They may involve the entire width of the bone (Fig. 1284). Fourteen of forty-five patients reported by Hatcher[298] had concomitant epiphyseal disorders. Because of this association, he doubts that this lesion is a true neoplasm. Furthermore, several facts indicate that the lesion arises as the result of some developmental aberration at the epiphyseal plate:

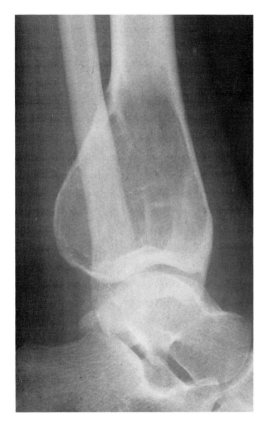

Fig. 1284 Large metaphyseal fibrous defect expanding lower tibial metaphysis. Lesions of this size are sometimes called nonossifying fibroma. (WU neg. 59-3916.)

1 It has been found only in the metaphysis of a bone.
2 It migrates (relatively) away from the epiphysis as the bone grows in length.
3 It tends to be elongated in the longitudinal axis of the bone, as though the abnormal development had occurred over a period of time.
4 Ponsetti and Friedman[300] illustrated three successive lesions arising from the same area of the epiphyseal plate, indicating that the factors producing the defects may act intermittently.
5 No evidence of malignant transformation or unusual mitotic activity has been noted.*

Grossly, the lesion is granular and brown or dark red in color. Microscopically, it consists of cellular masses of fibrous tissue often arranged in a storiform pattern (Fig. 1283). Scattered giant cells and small collections of foam cells may be seen. The microscopic appearance is very reminiscent of a benign fibrous histiocytoma (xanthogranuloma type) and is

---

*From Cunningham JB, Ackerman LV: Metaphyseal fibrous defects. J Bone Joint Surg [Am] **38:**797-808, 1956.

regarded as such by some authors. It differs from fibrous dysplasia because it does not form bone. We have seen it diagnosed incorrectly as fibrosarcoma.

Clinically, there are few or no symptoms except pain. The lesion is usually found incidentally on x-ray examination. We have seen several fractures occurring through the thinned cortex.

Fibrous dysplasia

Fibrous dysplasia, a nonneoplastic condition, can be divided into two types: monostotic and polyostotic.[307] The monostotic variety occurs frequently in older children and young adults and most commonly affects the rib, femur, and tibia. The polyostotic type (an unusual variant) usually is associated with endocrine dysfunction, precocious puberty in female individuals, and areas of cutaneous hyperpigmentation.[301] There is frequently a unilateral distribution of these lesions. Schlumberger[309] believed that the two types of fibrous dysplasia are unrelated, although they cannot be separated by examination of a single bone grossly or microscopically.

Roentgenograms of these lesions in the rib show a fusiform, expanded mass with thinning of the cortex. In the tibia, a lobulated, sharply delimited lesion of the shaft is formed (Fig. 1285). This lesion may produce a multilocular appearance because of endosteal cortical scalloping. Comparable lesions in membranous bone, particularly in the maxilla or the mandible, may show an overgrowth of dense bone.

The tissue cuts with a gritty consistency and is grayish yellow (Fig. 1286). The cortical bone often is thinned and expanded

Microscopically, narrow, curved misshaped bone trabeculae often having a characteristic fishhook configuration, are interspersed with fibrous tissue of variable cellularity (Fig. 1287). Harris et al.[303] and Reed[308] emphasized that fibrous dysplasia represents a maturation defect. Coarse fiber bone never becomes transformed to lamellar bone. Rows of cuboidal appositional osteoblasts do not appear on the surface of the trabeculae except as a pattern of reaction following local trauma. Silver stains are helpful in showing failure of maturation. If a lesion of fibrous dysplasia is biopsied over a period of years, maturation is still absent. This fundamental histologic abnormality makes it possible to differentiate fibrous dysplasia from many lesions which, in the past, were con-

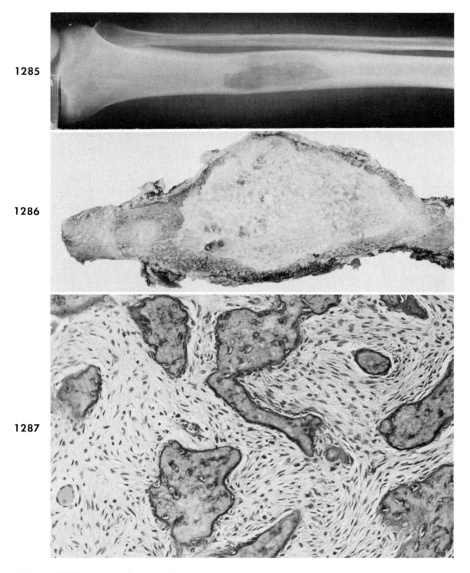

Fig. 1285 Fibrous dysplasia of tibia forming sharply delimited lesion. (WU neg. 49-5849.)

Fig. 1286 Fibrous dysplasia of rib forming fusiform, expanded mass that is grayish yellow. (WU neg. 49-4574.)

Fig. 1287 Typical fibrous dysplasia of rib demonstrating spicules of new bone formation with intervening cellular fibrous tissue. Trabeculae are not oriented along lines of stress. They form odd geometric patterns and have no osteoblasts on their surfaces. There is no maturation of this coarse fiber bone. (×140; WU neg. 52-333.)

fused with it. Kempson described as "ossifying fibroma of long bones"[305] a lesion similar in many ways to fibrous dysplasia but distinguished from it *microscopically* by the osteoblastic rimming of the bone trabeculae and *clinically* by its cortical rather than medullary location and its marked tendency to recur. We have found this distinction often difficult to make and tend to believe, like others, that these two diseases represent different expressions of the same basic process.[302]

Highly cellular areas of fibrous dysplasia may be diagnosed incorrectly as sarcoma. The osseous metaplasia is close to preexisting bone. Focal areas of hyaline cartilage[306] and small cystic areas may be present. The former are more common in the polyostotic variety and can dominate the microscopic picture to a de-

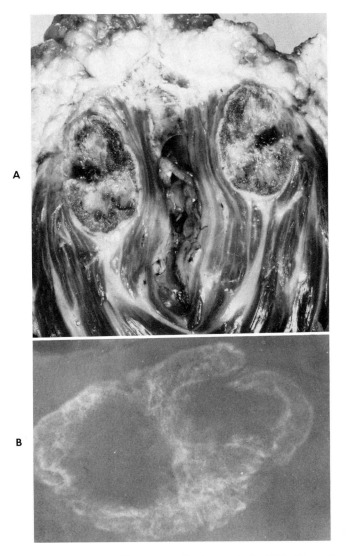

Fig. 1200 A, Well-defined myositis ossificans occurring in muscle. **B,** Same lesion shown in **A** illustrating bone formation in periphery. (**A,** WU neg. 56-6193; **B,** WU neg. 55-6190; **A** and **B,** from Ackerman LV: Extraosseous localized nonneoplastic bone and cartilage formation (so-called myositis ossificans). J Bone Joint Surg [Am] **40:**279-298, 1958.)

gree that a mistaken diagnosis of a cartilaginous tumor can be made.[307a] The transition of normal to abnormal bone is often abrupt. This is helpful in differentiating it roentgenographically from osteitis fibrosa cystica due to hyperparathyroidism. Huvos et al.[304] reported twelve cases of fibrous dysplasia associated with primary bone sarcoma. Eight of the tumors were osteosarcomas, two were chondrosarcomas, and two were labeled as spindle cell sarcomas. In half of the cases, the fibrous dysplasia was monostotic.

Resection cures fibrous dysplasia in bones such as the rib. Curettement is adequate in long bones such as the tibia. Indeed, in the maxilla, where some deformity may exist, partial removal of the lesion is all that is necessary.

Myositis ossificans

Myositis ossificans is a reactive condition that is sometimes mistaken microscopically for osteosarcoma.[312,313] The term is inaccurate because the muscle may not be involved, and inflammation is virtually absent. A history of trauma is obtained in only half of the patients. The most common locations are the flexor muscles of the upper arm (especially the brachialis anticus), the quadriceps femoris, the adductor muscles of the thigh, the gluteal muscles, and the soft tissues of the hand.[313] Roentgenograms show periosteal reaction and faint soft tissue calcification within three to six weeks of the injury; these are gradually replaced by mature heterotopic bone by ten to twelve weeks (Fig. 1288). Arteriography done during the active stage of the disease shows numerous fine vessels followed by a dense, poorly defined stain in the mass.[313a]

Microscopically, there is a highly cellular stroma associated with new bone and, less commonly, cartilage formation. In an early lesion, the centrally placed areas may be very difficult to distinguish from osteosarcoma because of their extreme cellularity. As the process evolves, osteoid appears in an orderly pattern at the periphery of this mass and subsequently matures into well-developed bone. The most important diagnostic feature is provided by this maturation pattern ("zonal phenomenon"), characterized by a central cellular area, an intermediate zone of osteoid formation, and a peripheral shell of highly organized bone[310] (Figs. 1289 and 1290). Ultrastructurally, cells with features of myofibroblasts are prominent, as befits a reactive condition of mesenchymal tissues.[312a]

The most important differential diagnosis is

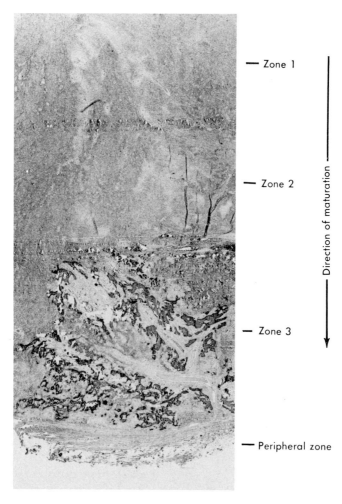

Fig. 1289 Schematic representation of zonal phenomena in myositis ossificans. (WU neg. 57-1317; from Ackerman LV: Extraosseous localized nonneoplastic bone and cartilage formation (so-called myositis ossificans). J Bone Joint Surg [Am] **40:**279-298, 1958.)

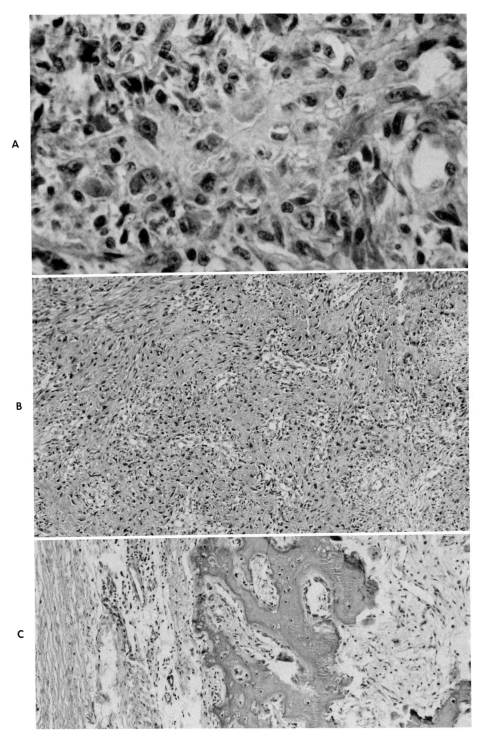

Fig. 1290 Zonal phenomena. **A,** Undifferentiated in pattern. **B,** Attempts at orientation of osteoid. **C,** Excellent bone formation at periphery. (**A** to **C,** ×450; **A,** WU neg. 55-6881; **B,** WU neg. 55-6880; **C,** WU neg. 55-6879; from Ackerman LV: Extraosseous localized nonneoplastic bone and cartilage formation [so-called myositis ossificans]. J Bone Joint Surg [Am] **40:**279-298, 1958.)

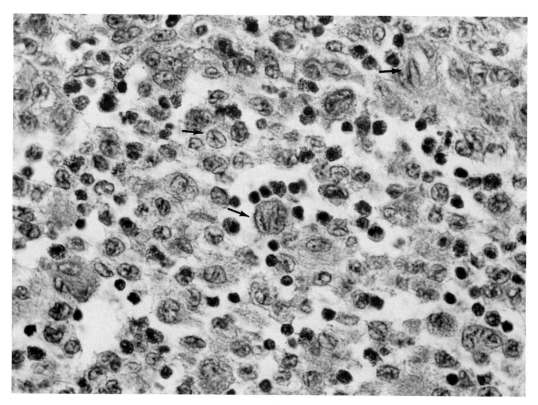

Fig. 1291 Eosinophilic granuloma of bone. Infiltrate is composed of histiocytes, lymphocytes, and eosinophils. Note lobulation and grooves in nuclei of many histiocytes (arrows). (×720; WU neg. 73-3404.)

with extraosseous osteosarcoma and juxta-cortical osteosarcoma. In the former condition, clearly sarcomatous areas are present, and the zonal phenomenon does not occur.[311] We seriously doubt whether myositis ossificans ever develops into osteosarcoma. We believe that many of the reported cases of this complication actually represent misdiagnosed instances of juxtacortical or extraosseous osteosarcoma.

Histiocytosis X (eosinophilic granuloma, Hand-Schüller-Christian disease, and Letterer-Siwe disease)

The unifying feature of the group of conditions designated as histiocytosis X or differentiated histiocytosis is an infiltration by a specific cell of the lymphoreticular system known as Langerhans' cell, accompanied by a variable admixture of eosinophils, giant cells, neutrophils, foamy cells, and areas of fibrosis. The former, which lack the cytologic stigmata of malignancy, have a characteristic appearance[321] (Fig. 1291). Their nuclei often are

lobulated or indented, sometimes with a longitudinal grove; their cytoplasm is, for the most part, distinctly acidophilic. A specific intra-cytoplasmic organelle, known as Langerhans' or Birbenck's granule, is regularly present on electron microscopic examination[314] (Fig. 1292). Scattered Langerhans' cells are normally present in the skin, lymph nodes, thymus, and other organs. It is only when they proliferate in an abnormal fashion that a diagnosis of histiocytosis X is justified. *Histiocytic proliferations with immature or undifferentiated cells should not be included in this category.* This is a mistake that has been made too frequently in the past.

The group of conditions designated as histiocytosis X can be divided into three major categories on the basis of type and extent of the organ involvement:

1 Solitary bone involvement
2 Multiple bone involvement (with or without skin involvement)
3 Multiple organ involvement (bone, liver, spleen, etc.)

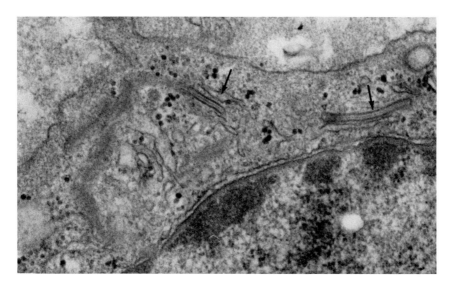

Fig. 1292 This histiocyte from eosinophilic granuloma of bone contains several Langerhans' granules (arrows). This is constant feature of histiocytes in this group of diseases. (Uranyl acetate–lead citrate; ×43,200.)

The cases with *solitary bone involvement*, which represent the most common variety, are usually referred to as *eosinophilic granuloma*.[316,318,323] Young adults are most commonly affected.[320] Any bone can be involved, with the possible exception of the hands and feet. The most common sites are the cranial vault, jaw, humerus, rib, and femur.[318] Roentgenographically, they present as an osteolytic lesion often in the metaphyseal area of long bones, sometimes associated with periosteal bone proliferation.[317] It can be confused roentgenographically with metastatic carcinoma (Fig. 1293) or Ewing's sarcoma (Fig. 1294). After fracture, this process may extend into adjacent soft tissues.[323] We have seen two recurrences in soft tissue after operation that disappeared with radiation. These lesions may spontaneously regress but are radiosensitive and radiocurable with small amounts of radiation. All of our patients remained well. None of them developed other bone lesions or involvement of other organs.

Cases of *multiple bone involvement* are better designated as multiple or polyostotic eosinophilic granulomas.[315,319] When strategically located, the bony infiltration may result in proptosis, diabetes insipidus, or chronic otitis media or a combination of these conditions. The eponym of Hand-Schüller-Christian disease has been applied to this variety. Since the circumstances on which this designation is based are fortuitous and erratic, it would probably be better to drop the term entirely. This form is characterized by a prolonged clinical course, often marked by alternating episodes of regressions and recrudescences. The eventual outcome is favorable in most cases.

This type of histiocytosis X blends imperceptibly with the form having *multiple organ involvement*. Following the skeletal system, the skin and the lungs are the two most common sites affected. It is difficult to predict the outcome of the disease in a particular case, but there are several parameters that can be used as useful guidelines. Poor prognostic factors are young age (under 18 months) at the time of diagnosis, hepatomegaly, anemia and/or thrombocytopenia, bone marrow involvement, nad hemorrhagic skin lesions. Features not associated with a poor prognosis are seborrhea-like skin lesions, diabetes insipidus, and pulmonary lesions.[321a] Microscopically, it is very difficult to separate the aggressive (Letterer-Siwe disease) from the more indolent forms. In a typical case of the former, the infiltrate will be more monomorphic, with more mitoses and necrosis and fewer giant cells and eosinophils that in a typical case of the latter,[322] but in our experience the overlap has been too great to rely on these features alone.

Articular and periarticular diseases
Ganglia; cystic meniscus

Ganglia occur about joints and rarely about tendon sheaths. They are annoying deformities that may cause some pain, weakness, partial disability of the joint, and bone changes.[325] Ganglia located in the popliteal space can produce pain or foot drop as result of compression of the common peroneal nerve.[328] Individuals

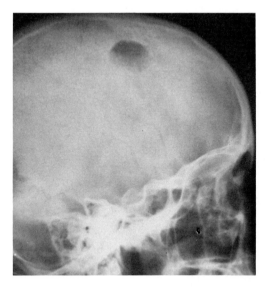

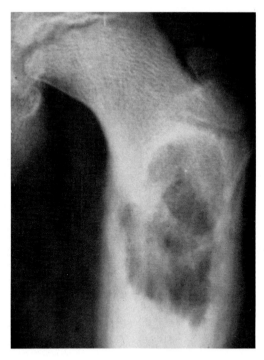

Fig. 1293 Osteolytic lesion of skull in 25-year-old woman. Roentgenographically, lesion was thought to be metastatic carcinoma but proved to be solitary lesion of eosinophilic granuloma. (WU neg. 48-4331.)

Fig. 1294 Osteolytic lesion of femur in 12-year-old boy. This was thought to be Ewing's sarcoma but proved microscopically to be eosinophilic granuloma. (WU neg. 48-6045.)

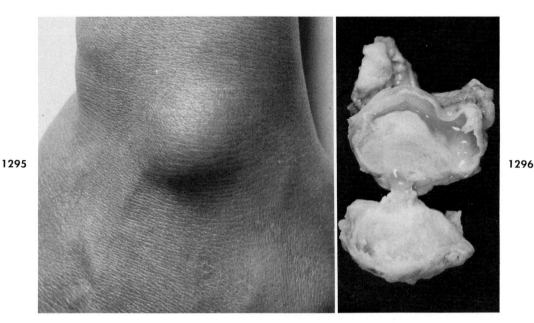

1295

1296

Fig. 1295 Typical location and appearance of ganglion. (WU neg. 49-1173.)
Fig. 1296 Ganglion illustrating mucoid appearance and poorly defined capsule. (WU neg. 50-3032.)

using the wrist and fingers (pianists, typists) are prone to this condition. A history of injury preceding ganglion formation may exist.

Ganglia develop by myxoid degeneration and cystic softening of the connective tissue of the joint capsule or tendon sheath.[326,327] The theory of a rent in the synovial membrane of a joint leading to the collection of synovial fluid and the formation of a false capsule[324] can seldom be substantiated.

The most common location is on the dorsal carpal area of the hand where the cystic lesion pushes its way toward the surface between the tendons of the extensor indices proprius and the extensor carpi radials (Fig. 1295). The second most frequent location is the volar surface of the wrist, superficial and medial to the radial artery. Ganglia also arise of the volar surfaces of the fingers just distal to the metacarpophalangeal joints, in the dorsum of the foot, and around the ankle and knee. Ganglia are not lined by synovia and do not communicate with the joint cavity, two points distinguishing them from Baker's cysts (Fig. 1296).

A lesion microscopically similar to soft tissue ganglion may occur in the menisci of the knee and is referred to simply as *cystic meniscus.* The most common site is the peripheral portion of the middle third of the lateral miniscus. It may remain confined to the meniscus or extend extracapsularly. A traumatic etiology is favored.

Bursae; Baker's cyst

Bursae are found where muscles, tendons, and skin glide over bony prominences. They are subject to all the diseases that occur in large joint spaces. Inflammation may be associated with the formation of cysts, fluid, and loose bodies (Fig. 1297). The incomplete removal of loose bodies may be followed by the disappearance of the remaining ones from the bursa.

A related lesion is subdeltoid bursitis associated with calcareous tendonitis. This entity is primarily a degeneration of a tendon or muscle in the rotator cuff of the shoulder followed by deposition of calcium in necrotic collagenous tissue. This calcific material stimulates a secondary inflammatory reaction.[330]

Baker's cyst occurs in the popliteal space from herniation of the synovial membrane through the posterior part of the capsule or from escape of joint fluid through normal anatomic connections of the knee joint with the semimembraneous bursa[329] (Fig. 1298). The cyst is lined by true synovium and may have cartilage in its wall. Any joint disease leading to increased intra-articular pressure, such as degenerative joint disease, neuropathic arthrop-

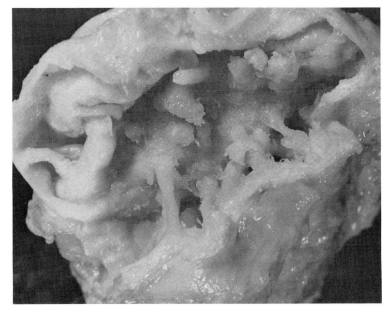

Fig. 1297 Bursal cyst of prepatellar area. Cyst contained fluid. There is extensive proliferation of synovia. (WU neg. 51-40.)

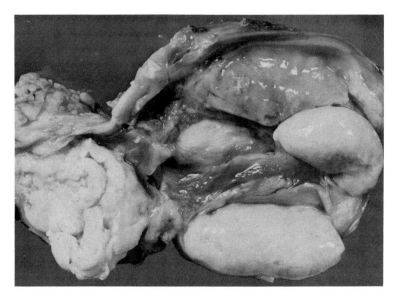

Fig. 1298 Large Baker's cyst. Synovial membrane is chronically inflamed, and loose bodies are present. (WU neg. 47-4094.)

athy, and rheumatoid arthritis, may result in the formation of Baker's cyst.[331]

Carpal tunnel syndrome

The carpal tunnel is the space between the flexor retinaculum or transverse carpal ligament and the carpal bones. The medial nerve courses through this tunnel, and its compression in this location by a variety of causes produces the symptoms of the "carpal tunnel syndrome."[333,334] These include bony deformity following trauma, masses within the canal (i.e., hemangiomas, lipomas, ganglia), rheumatoid arthritis, and amyloidosis.[332] Often, no specific etiology can be demonstrated.

Fibrous histiocytoma of tendon sheath (nodular tenosynovitis)

Fibrous histiocytoma of the tendon sheath (also called giant cell tumor of the tendon sheath, xanthogranuloma, myeloplaxoma, and benign synovioma) is a common lesion that occurs more frequently in women than men, usually appearing in young and middle-aged persons. It is practically always distributed between the wrist and fingertips and between the ankle and toetips. It is more often proximal than distal on both the hands and feet and occurs most frequently on their flexor surfaces.

This tumor is a single lesion usually measuring 1-3 cm in diameter. It has a fairly well-defined capsule, may be somewhat lobulated, and varies in color from whitish gray to yellowish brown. It arises from the inner layer of the tendon sheath.

Microscopically, this lesion contains closely packed polyhedral cells that have phagocytic properties. Giant cells containing fat and hemosiderin often are present (Fig. 1299). Cells in zones of active proliferation may show mitotic figures. Focal zones of hyalinization constitute the more quiescent areas. Sometimes, the whole lesion adopts a hypocellular fibrohyalinized appearance. We believe that the cases reported as tendon sheath fibromas[335a] are histogenetically related to fibrous histiocytoma. Their location, clinical presentation, and recurrence rate are certainly comparable. Ultrastructural studies of fibrous histiocytomas of tendon sheath have shown cells with the features of synovial cells alternating with fibroblastic elements, histiocytes, and lymphocytes.[335]

The great cellularity of this tumor, its variable pattern, and the presence of mitotic figures may lead to an erroneous diagnosis of sarcoma. However, these tumors are nearly always benign. They may erode contiguous bone by pressure. If incompletely removed, they may recur locally. New lesions also possibly develop after excision.[336,337]

The nature of this lesion is still controversial, Jaffe et al.[336] consider it a reactive process—

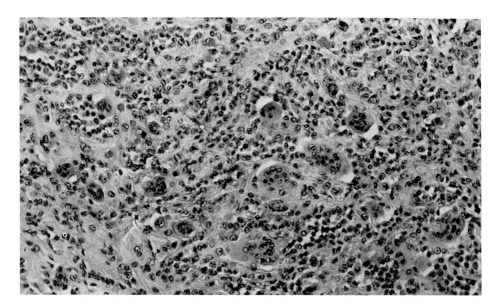

Fig. 1299 Rather cellular fibrous histiocytoma of tendon sheath origin. Giant cells are prominent, and mitotic figures are rare. (×200; WU neg. 50-1422.)

hence the name of nodular tenosynovitis. We are impressed by the close similarities with other soft tissue lesions collectively called fibrous histiocytoma and believe that they may represent their tendon sheath counterpart. A malignant counterpart of this lesion has been described as "large cell sarcoma of tendon sheath," an entity which is probably related to epithelioid sarcoma (Chapter 24).

Pigmented villonodular synovitis and bursitis

Pigmented villonodular synovitis tends to occur in young adults.[340a,341] Although the knee joint is the usual site,[338] the process may involve the ankle, hip, shoulder, or even the elbow joint. Usually only one articulation is affected, only one well-documented case of bilateral knee involvement having been reported.[340] Occasionally, the lesion may penetrate within the underlying bone.[342]

The synovitis may be focal or diffuse. When diffuse, it is made up of brownish yellow spongy tissue. Its appearance depends upon the content of hemosiderin pigment. Large amounts of tissue often are present, and complete removal may be impossible (Fig. 1300). Microscopically, the cellular component is similar to that of nodular tenosynovitis, but in addition there are papillary projections made up of foamy cells and hemosiderin-containing phagocytes (Fig. 1301).

This disease can be treated by excision. It may recur locally because complete removal is often impossible.[339] If it recurs locally, radiation therapy may be helpful. In our experience, this lesion has not become malignant. Extensively recurrent lesions, however, have been misdiagnosed as fibrosarcoma and synovial sarcoma.

Synovial osteochondromatosis and chondrosarcoma

Synovial osteochondromatosis is an infrequent disease of unknown etiology associated with the formation of osteocartilaginous bodies in the synovial membrane. This condition most often is monoarticular, affecting the knee or hip and communicating bursae. It is aggravated by infection and trauma.

Grossly, the osteocartilaginous bodies may remain confined to the synovium or be extruded within the joint cavity. They usually are partially calcified (Fig. 1302). Innumerable small bodies can be seen grossly in the resected lesion (Figs. 1303 and 1304). A single nodule beneath thinned synovium contains hyaline cartilage and at times bone (Fig. 1305). The disease seems to follow this sequence: (1) active intrasynovial disease with no loose bodies; (2) intrasynovial proliferation and free loose bodies; (3) multiple free osteochondral bodies with no demonstrable intrasynovial disease.[344a]

In order to make a diagnosis of synovial osteochondromatosis, one should find cartilaginous or osteocartilaginous bodies attached to the synovial membrane in addition to those free in the joint spaces. The latter also can occur in degenerative joint disease, neuropathic arthropathy, and osteochondritis dissecans, and the process is referred to as secondary synovial chondrometaplasia.[345a] Microscopically, the cartilage cells of primary synovial osteochondromatosis may show some degree of atypia and even binucleated forms, but this does not necessarily indicate malignancy.[345] Local recrudescence after treatment may supervene.

Synovial osteochondromatosis needs to be differentiated from the exceptionally rare synovial chondrosarcoma, which it may closely resemble roentgenographically and grossly.[343] The distinction, which may be quite difficult, is made by the presence in the chondrosarcoma of obvious cytologic features of malignancy in the cartilaginous cells.[344]

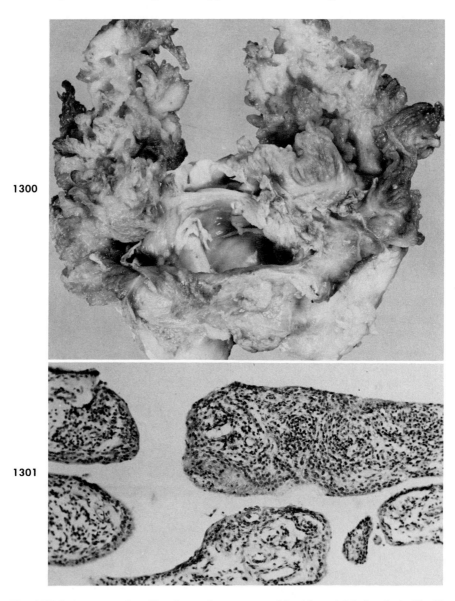

1300

1301

Fig. 1300 Large mass of papillary brown tissue removed from knee joint of patient with villonodular synovitis. (WU neg. 50-3300.)
Fig. 1301 Papillary projections in pigmented villonodular synovitis. (×120; WU neg. 50-3948.)

1302   1303

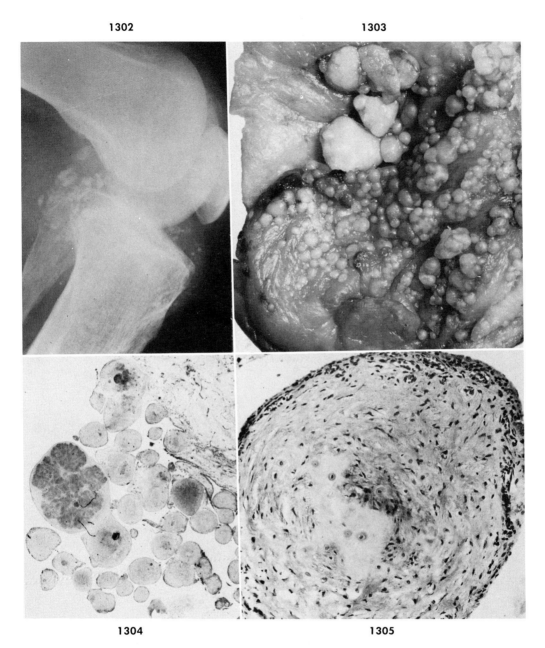

1304   1305

Fig. 1302 Synovial osteochondromatosis. Nodules can be seen clearly in joint space. (WU neg. 49-4113.)

Fig. 1303 Extensive involvement of synovium of knee joint by osteochondromatosis. (WU neg. 48-3983.)

Fig. 1304 Pattern and formation of synovial osteochondromatosis. (Low power; WU neg. 48-3981.)

Fig. 1305 Single nodule of osteochondromatosis forming beneath intact synovium. Note cartilage formation in center of this nodule. (High power; WU neg. 48-3972.)

Arthritis
Synovial biopsy

Needle biopsy of the synovium, particularly of the knee joint, is of aid in the assessment of synovial inflammatory conditions.[351] The procedure is safe, simple, and easily repeated. It is indicated for inflammatory joint diseases when the etiology remains in doubt, particularly when only one joint is affected. Examination of the synovial fluid should always be performed before biopsy. It is possible to diagnose tuberculosis and other specific granulomatous lesions by this method.[347-350,352] Other diagnosable diseases are pigmented villonodular synovitis, amyloidosis, Whipple's disease, hemochromatosis, metastatic disease, and gout. A heavy neutrophilic infiltrate is highly characteristic of infectious arthritis, although it also may be seen in Behçet's disease and familial Mediterranean fever. Unfortunately, the histologic findings in the most common rheumatic diseases are often nonspecific,[346] although the presence of prominent lymphoid follicles and marked hyperplasia of synovial cells are highly suggestive of rheumatoid arthritis. By the use of a small-caliber synovial biopsy needle (Parker-Pearson technique), Schumacher and Kulka[349] were able to obtain sufficient synovial tissue for diagnosis in 92% of the 109 joint biopsies they performed. Histologic examination proved to be of direct diagnostic value in thirty-eight cases.

Degenerative joint disease (osteoarthritis)

Surgical pathology specimens of legs amputated for traumatic reasons or because of gangrene secondary to vascular disease offer the unique opportunity for study of degenerative joint disease. The term osteoarthritis is inaccurate because this type of joint disease is degenerative and not inflammatory. The pathologic changes are related directly to age and are conditioned by use and occupation of the patient.[363,370] Both Bennett et al.[354] and Collins[355] described and illustrated these changes in the knee joint beautifully. No less can be said of the work of Hirsch et al.[359] on similar changes in the cervical spine. The classic monograph by Nichols and Richardson[366] in 1909 described the pathologic alteration so well that we have little to add today. Bauer and Bennett[353] summarized their classic description as follows:

In degenerative arthritis, the earliest and primary change in the joints is a gradual and uneven degeneration of the hyaline cartilage of the articular surfaces. This is first detected as a fibrillation of the cartilaginous matrix which generally begins near the articular surface and is associated with a disappearance of the spindle-cell perichondrium. As a result of this fibrillation, which takes place usually at right angles to the articular surface, the neighboring cartilage cells are set free and finally disintegrate and disappear. Also, the original smooth articular surface takes on a papillary appearance. At times this fibrillation is responsible for the freeing of minute masses of cartilage and fibrillated matrix. The depth to which this fibrillation extends varies. Sometimes it extends entirely through the cartilage down to the zone of provisional calcification so that masses of cartilage may be peeled away, exposing either the zone of provisional calcification or the underlying bone to the attrition of joint motion. [Fig. 1306.] Occasionally, only a portion of the articular cartilage undergoes degeneration, fibrillation, and destruction [Fig. 1307.] This leads to thinning of the cartilage over a circumscribed area. To meet this erosion and depression, an overgrowth occurs on the opposite joint surface. This is brought about by increased activity of the perichondrium. As a result, an irregular or somewhat toothed joint line is formed, and finally, with ultimate disappearance of the entire articular cartilage, the two bony surfaces are brought into contact. Since this change takes place gradually and is at first confined only to a portion of the joint, motion is continued with the result that the exposed bone undergoes marked thickening of the trabeculae and narrowing of the marrow spaces until an extremely dense bony structure has been produced. The friction of continued joint motion produces a high degree of polish on the exposed condensed bone which then acquires an appearance closely resembling ivory; hence the term "eburnation of bone."

While this process of fibrillation and destruction of cartilage with erosion is taking place in one portion of the joint and a corresponding overgrowth is occurring on the opposite joint surface, secondary changes in the joint may be produced. Changes in the shape of the joint surface may gradually, over a period of months or years, lead to more or less extensive subluxations. As a result, the amount of joint motion may be diminished, or, in certain instances, the joint surfaces may become interlocked, producing "ankylosis by deformity." There is no true ankylosis in this type of joint disease. Common among these imperfectly understood secondary changes is an increased activity of the perichondrium at the periphery of the joint where the cartilage and capsule come together. This results in the new formation of cartilage which may be transformed into bone and thus causes an increase in the size of the bone end. As a rule this increase in circumference is not uniform, but is irregular and the contour is nodular, as exemplified by Heberden's node. Since this deposit of new bone is usually within the attach-

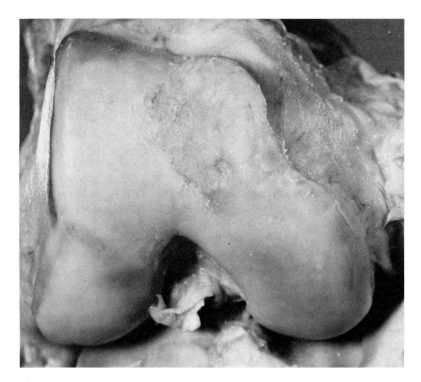

Fig. 1306 Pronounced degenerative joint disease in 55-year-old man. Note degeneration and destruction of cartilage over wide area. (WU neg. 52-3896.)

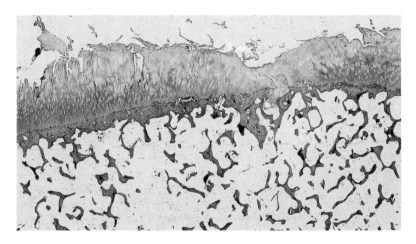

Fig. 1307 Section taken through zone shown in Fig. 1306 demonstrating fragmentation and fibrillation of thinned cartilage. (Low power; WU neg. 52-4490.)

ment of the joint capsule, it may in some cases lead to filling up of the original joint cavity, thus producing partial or complete dislocation.

As a rule, no great increase in the thickness of the joint capsules of these joints is observed, and, in many instances, the synovial membrane appears normal. However, in some cases, there is marked thickening of the synovial membrane with the production of papillary or pedunculated masses of connective tissue which may be converted by metaplasia into cartilage or bone or, in some cases, into fat tissue. Detachment of these pedunculated masses may give rise to loose bodies, the so-called joint mice. The breaking off of an osteophyte is another cause of loose-body formation. As a rule, in this type of joint disease there is very little tendency for the synovial membrane to extend over the articular surfaces and in no case does fibrous ankylosis occur.*

Nichols and Richardson[366] also called attention to the fact that there is no evidence of

*From Bauer W, and Bennett GA: Experimental and pathologic studies in the degenerative type of arthritis. J Bone Joint Surg **18:**1-18, 1936.

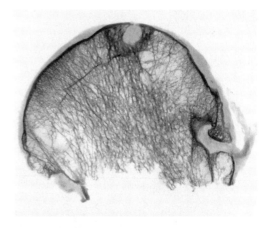

Fig. 1308 Specimen roentgenogram of femoral head with osteoarthrosis. Note irregular thinning of articular cartilage and formation of subchondral cyst surrounded by sclerotized bone.

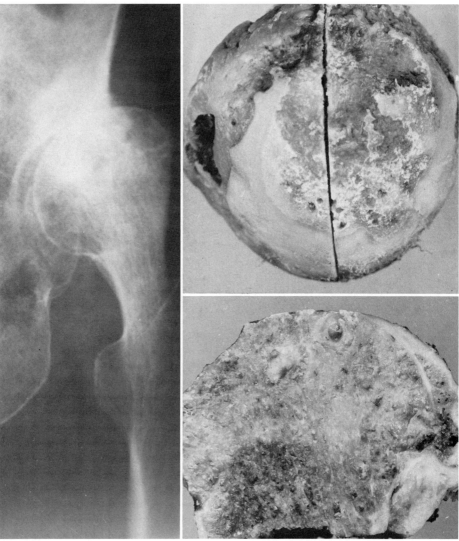

Fig. 1309 Head of femur demonstrating advanced osteoarthritic changes. There is loss of cartilage and cyst formation. (WU negs. 54-1439, 54-1273, and 54-1274.)

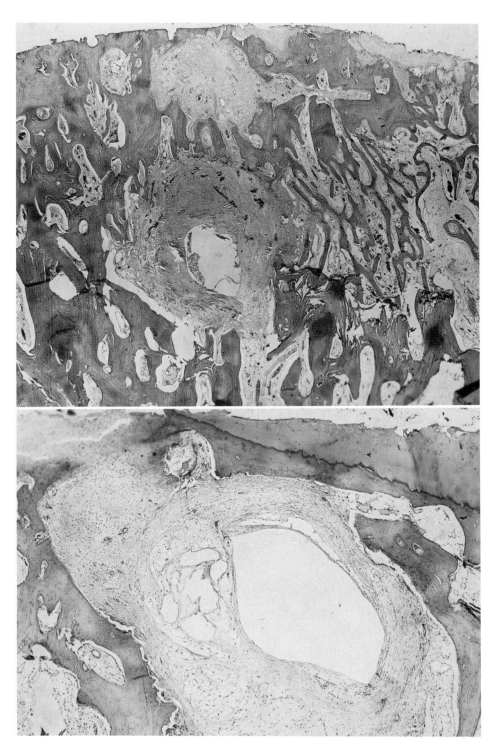

Fig. 1310 Loss of cartilage, eburnation, and cyst formation illustrated in Fig. 1309. (Low power; WU negs. 54-1493 and 55-34.)

inflammatory exudation in early degenerative joint disease. On the other hand, some degree of synovial hyperplasia with hyperemia and lymphocytic infiltration can be seen in advanced stages, especially with osteoarthritis of the hip. This change should not be confused with rheumatoid arthritis.

The cartilage is the key to the changes in osteoarthrosis.[370a] Its capacity for repair is feeble. Cartilaginous degeneration takes place in certain areas of the hip joint not exposed to pressure or friction,[358] although these changes occur most often on the joint surface exposed to friction, weight bearing, or movement.[356] There is loss of chondroitin sulfate matrix in the cartilage in advance of actual mechanical attrition.[365] With degeneration of cartilage, the stability of the chondro-osseous junction is lost. Narrowing of the joint space is, in fact, loss of cartilage thickness. If the osteoarthritic head of a femur is examined, cysts frequently are found close to the surface, where they may communicate with the joint and are surrounded by dense bone[361,364,369] (Fig. 1308). The cyst may be replaced by fibrous tissue or may contain fluid[358] (Figs. 1309 and 1310).

Neuropathic arthropathy (Charcot's joint) is a particularly destructive variant of degenerative joint disease (Fig. 1311). The process is usually slowly progressive, although on rare occasions it may have an extremely rapid evolution.[367] Particles of dead bone and cartilage often are seen in large amounts embedded in the synovial membrane.[360] However, they are not specific for this condition.

Chondromalacia patella is the name given to a condition of obscure etiology characterized by softening, fibrillation, fissuring, and erosion of the articular cartilage of the patella.[368] Microscopically, the changes are indistinguishable from those of degenerative joint disease.[357,362]

Rheumatoid arthritis

Rheumatoid arthritis is a chronic polyarticular arthritis of unknown etiology.[397a] It is most common in women during the second and third decades of life. The joints of the feet and hands are nearly always involved. Other joints frequently affected are the elbows, knees, wrists, ankles, hips, spine, and temporomandibular articulations.

Experimental studies carried out have in-

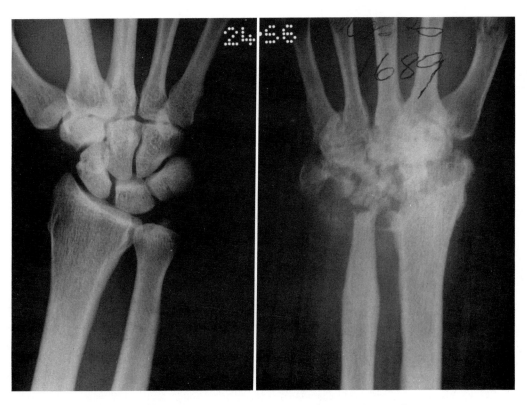

Fig. 1311 Neuropathic changes in wrist secondary to syringomyelia.

dicated that lysosomes are one of the mediators of the inflammatory reaction seen in this disease and in other joint diseases.[400] The earliest morphologic changes occur in the synovial membrane. Hyperemia of the synovium is followed by proliferation of the synovial lining cells and infiltration by plasma cells and lymphocytes[371] (Fig. 1312). Lymphoid follicles are often present. The small synovial blood vessels are lined by plump endothelial cells, and fibrin deposits often are seen close to the synovial lining or within the stroma. Sokoloff[397] and Sherman[396] remarked that these changes, although certainly supporting a diagnosis of rheumatoid arthritis in a clinically compatible case, are not pathognomonic of this entity. Two additional microscopic features, which are also nonspecific, include the presence of synovial giant cells and of bone and cartilage fragments within the actual synovial membrane. Muirden[391] found synovial giant cells in one-third of the 100 biopsies he examined. They need to be distinguished from multinucleated plasma cells, foreign body cells, and Touton giant cells that can also occur in joints with rheumatoid arthritis. Grimley and Sokoloff[381]

found them only in patients with active, seropositive disease, although they found no correlation with the serologic titer. On the other hand, Bhan and Roy[377] found them in seropositive and in seronegative cases, as well as in tuberculosis, traumatic arthritis, and villonodular synovitis. The cartilage and bone fragments tend to occur in joints with advanced disease. They appear to arise as a result of the erosive destructive process of the articular surface and can be distinguished by virtue of their position and clear demarcation from the metaplastic cartilage and bone that sometimes arises from synovial cells. They also have been seen in synovial membranes of osteoarthritis, osteochondritis dissecans, chondromalacia patella, and particularly in neuropathic joints[385,391] (Fig. 1313).

In the second phase, granulation tissue grows into the subchondral marrow of the bone.[388] Osteoporosis occurs early and may result in spontaneous fractures of long bones (particularly the femoral neck) and the pelvis.[399] Prominent pannus is formed over the articular cartilage (Fig. 1314). Cartilage and even bone form in this pannus. The granulation tissue

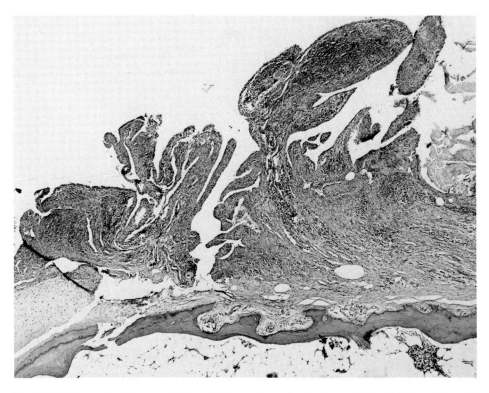

Fig. 1312 Exuberant papillary projections of inflamed synovium in rheumatoid arthritis involving wrist. (WU neg. 70-5932.)

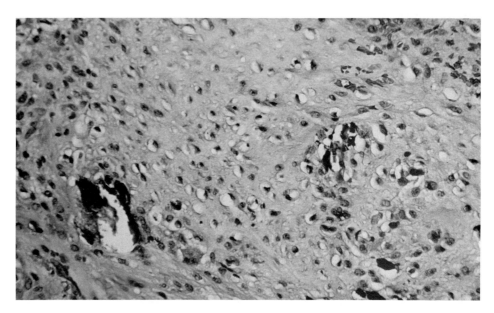

Fig. 1313 Calcific debris embedded in synovial membrane of Charcot's joint. (×250; WU neg. 62-9047.)

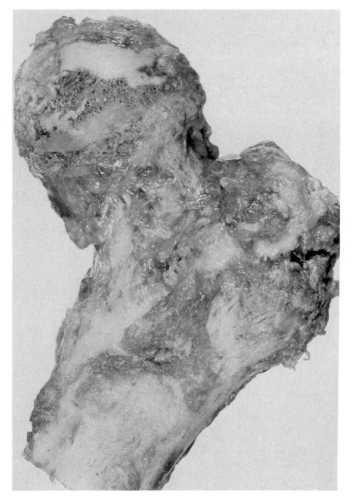

Fig. 1314 Advanced rheumatoid arthritis involving femur. There is prominent proliferation of synovium and almost complete destruction of overlying articular cartilage. (WU neg. 49-5578.)

of the subchondral area and the pannus within the joint attack the cartilage.[378] Its destruction may be followed by fibrous ankylosis and eventually bony ankylosis. Mitchell and Shepard[389] have described the early changes seen by electron microscopy in the articular cartilage. Different pathologic stages of the process occur in different joints at the same time.[393] Increased articular pressure may lead to bursting of the joint capsule and acute joint rupture,[379] bone cysts (''rheumatoid geodes''),[392] or herniation of the capsule into the soft tissues.[386] The bone cysts are roentgenographically similar to those seen in association with degenerative joint disease, but in rheumatoid arthritis they contain granulation tissue instead of fluid or myxoid material.

Rheumatoid arthritis is now generally regarded as the expression of a systemic disease.[383,384] Tenosynovitis and ''rheumatoid nodules'' are the two most common extraarticular manifestations. The latter, which are seen in approximately 20% of the patients, occur most often in tendons and tendon sheaths and periarticular subcutaneous tissue but also have been seen in the heart and large vessels, lung and pleura, kidney, meninges, and in the synovial membrane itself.[372,387,394] In exceptional instances, they have occurred systemically and have been responsible for the patient's death.[376] Microscopically, they are composed of a necrotic center impregnated with fibrin, surrounded by a predominantly histiocytic inflammatory reaction often arranged in a palisading fashion (Fig. 1315). They are not specific of rheumatoid arthritis. Nodules morphologically indistinguishable can occur in rheumatic fever, systemic lupus erythematosus, and, in children, in the absence of any apparent disease.[373,374,382] Berardinelli et al.[375] followed ten cases of the latter and found rheumatoid factor two to sixteen years after the appearance of the nodules.

Sokoloff et al.[398] found nonnecrotizing arteritis in 10% of patients with rheumatoid arthritis. Necrotizing arteritis also has been described.[390,395] Polyneuritis can be observed.[380]

The pulmonary manifestations of rheumatoid arthritis have been discussed in Chapter 6 and the lymph node changes in Chapter 20.

Amyloidosis is a significant complication of the disease. In the United States, rheumatoid arthritis has displaced tuberculosis as the most common underlying disorder associated with amyloid deposition.

Infectious arthritis

Bacterial, fungous, and parasitic infections can reach the joints either by hematogenous

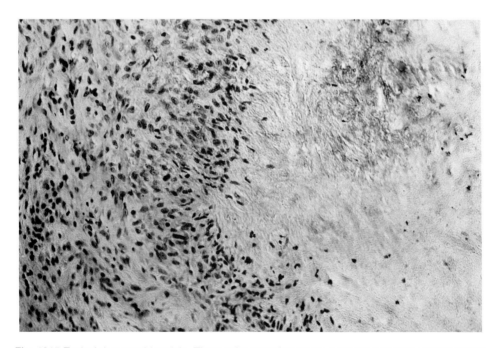

Fig. 1315 Typical rheumatoid nodule. There exist central necrosis, palisading of cells around margin of this area, and chronic inflammatory cells. (×200; WU neg. 49-4145.)

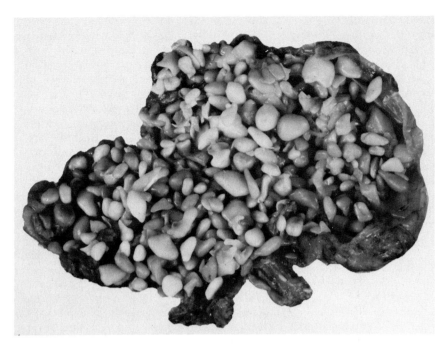

Fig. 1316 Tuberculous bursitis with innumerable "rice bodies." Latter are mainly composed of fibrin and have no diagnostic significance. (Courtesy Dr. E. F. Lascano, Buenos Aires, Argentina.)

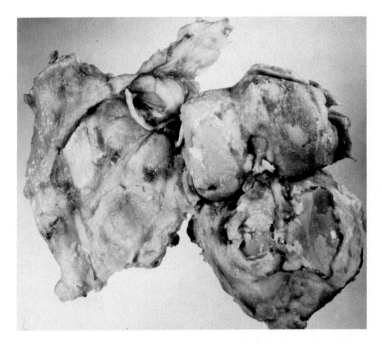

Fig. 1317 Extensive involvement of knee joint and synovium by gout. In some areas, cartilage of condyles is completely missing and there is involvement of semilunar cartilages as well. Grayish white plaques represent deposits of uric acid crystals. Patient, 83-year-old woman, had leg amputated because of arterial insufficiency, and finding of gout was unexpected. (WU neg. 59-5916.)

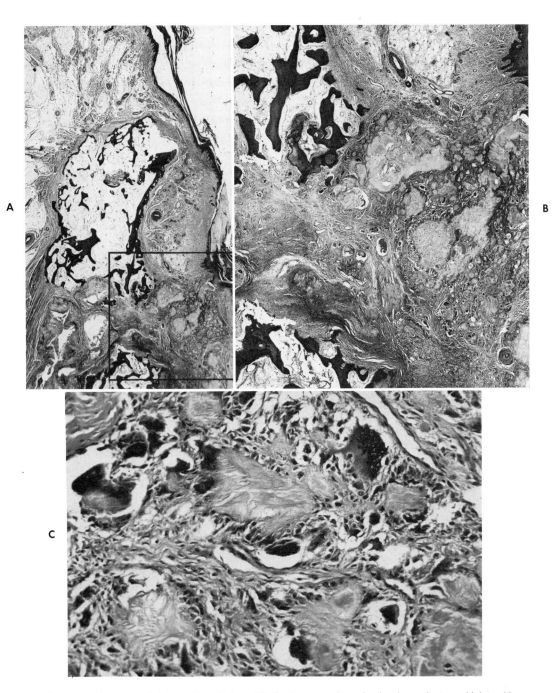

Fig. 1318 Characteristic lesion of gout. **A** and **B,** Tophaceous deposits that have destroyed joint, with complete destruction of cartilage and extension out into soft tissue and growth just beneath epidermis. **C,** Urate deposits surrounded by characteristic giant cells. Latter demonstrates characteristic picture of gout. Patient's trouble began in great toe. (**A,** ×10; WU neg. 63-73; **B,** ×40; WU neg. 63-72; **C,** ×275, WU neg. 63-74.)

spread or by contiguous extension from a neighboring osteomyelitis (Fig. 1316).

Gout

About 2%-5% of chronic joint disease is caused by gout. It may occur in families but is not restricted to man and has been reported in reptiles by Appleby.[401] The metatarsophalangeal joints are often the first to be involved, but other joints of the hands and feet are rather frequently involved, too. We also have seen gout involve the joints of the long bones.

Calcification and even ossification of tophi occur not infrequently.[404] The urate deposits progressively destroy the cartilage and may cause osteolytic, irregular destruction of subchondral bone (Fig. 1317). These deposits may extend out from a joint into the soft tissue and cause destruction of the ligaments. This destruction eventually leads to subcutaneous deposits that may erode through the skin. The microscopic pattern of gout is unmistakable. Fixation in alcohol is important for the preservation of sodium urate monohydrate deposits that appear as needle-shaped, doubly refractile crystals. The deGalantha stain is particularly suited for their demonstration.[403] Even if alcohol fixation is not done, the appearance of tophi is usually diagnostic because of the typical granulomatous response that they elicit (Fig. 1318). Histiocytes and foreign body giant cells predominate in the infiltrate. Palisading of the histiocytes sometimes occurs and may be a source of confusion with rheumatoid nodules.

Gout should be differentiated from chondrocalcinosis (pseudogout syndrome), a rare condition in which the symptoms result from diffuse deposition of calcium pyrophosphate crystals in the articular cartilage.[402,405]

Other articular and periarticular diseases

Scleroderma (progressive systemic sclerosis) is often accompanied by arthralgia or arthritis, and sometimes these dominate the clinical picture. The main microscopic changes in the synovial membrane are superficial deposition of fibrin, mild mononuclear infiltrate, *minimal* hyperplasia of synovial lining cells, proliferation of collagen fibers, and focal obliteration of small vessels.[407]

In *lupus erythematosus*, the microscopic changes in the synovium can be indistinguishable from those of rheumatoid arthritis. As a rule, however, there is a more intense surface fibrin deposition and a lesser degree of proliferation of synovial cells.[406]

REFERENCES
Introduction

1 Aegerter E, Kirkpatrick JA Jr: Orthopedic diseases, ed. 3. Philadelphia, 1968, W. B. Saunders Co.
2 Bloom W, Fawcett DW: Textbook of histology, ed. 10. Philadelphia, 1975, W. B. Saunders Co.
3 Brailsford, JF: The serious limitations and erroneous indications of biopsy in the diagnosis of tumours of bones. P R Soc Med **41:**225-236, 1948.
4 Collins DH: Pathology of bone, London, 1966, Butterworth & Co., Ltd
5 Dahlin DC: Bone tumors, ed. 3. Springfield, Ill., 1978, Charles C Thomas, Publisher.
6 Enneking WF, Kagan A.: Transepiphyseal extension of osteosarcoma: incidence, mechanism, and implications. Cancer **41:**1526-1537, 1978.
7 Fornasier VL: Osteoid: an ultrastructural study. Hum Pathol **8:**243-254, 1977.
8 Jaffe HL: Tumors and tumorous conditions of the bones and joints. Philadelphia, 1958, Lea & Febiger.
9 Jaffe HL: Metabolic, degenerative and inflammatory diseases of bones and joints. Philadelphia, 1972, Lea & Febiger.
10 La Croix P: The organization of bones. Philadelphia, 1951, The Blakiston Co.
11 Lichtenstein L: Bone tumors, ed. 5. St. Louis, 1977, The C. V. Mosby Co.
12 Luck JV: Bone and joint diseases. Springfield, Ill., 1950, Charles C Thomas, Publisher.
13 Morse A: Formic acid-sodium citrate decalcification and butyl alcohol dehydration of teeth and bones for sectioning in paraffin. J Dent Res **24:**143-153, 1945.
14 Spjut HJ, Dorfman HD, Fechner RE, Ackerman LV: Tumors of bone and cartilage. In Atlas of tumor pathology, Sect. II, Fasc. 5, Washington, D. C., 1971, Armed Forces Institute of Pathology.

Metabolic bone diseases

15 Avioli LV, Krane SM (eds): Metabolic bone disease, vol. I. New York, 1977, Academic Press, Inc.
16 Avioli LV, Teitelbaum SL: The renal osteodystrophies. In Brenner BM, Rector FC (eds): The kidney, Philadelphia, 1976, W. B. Saunders Co., pp. 1542-1591.
17 Beck JS, Nordin BEC: Histological assessment of osteoporosis by iliac crest biopsy. J Pathol Bacteriol **80:**391-397, 1960.
18 Bernstein DS, Sadowsky N, Hegsted DM, Guri CD, Stare FJ: Prevalence of osteoporosis in high- and low-fluoride areas in North Dakota. JAMA **198:**499-504, 1966.
19 Caldwell RA: Observations on the incidence, aetiology and pathology of senile osteoporosis. J Clin Pathol **15:** 421-431, 1962.
20 Davis ME, Strandjord NM, Lanzl LH: Estrogens and the aging process. JAMA **196:**219-224, 1966.
21 Dent CE, Harris H: Hereditary forms of rickets and osteomalacia. J Bone Joint Surg [Br] **38:**204, 1956.
22 Falvo KA, Bullough PG: Osteogenesis imperfecta: a histometric analysis. J Bone Joint Surg [Am] **55:**275, 1973.
23 Fourman P: Calcium metabolism and the bone, ed. 2. Philadelphia, 1968, F. A. Davis Co.

24 Frost HM: A unique histological feature of vitamin D resistant rickets observed in four cases. Acta Orthop Scand **33:**220, 1963.

25 Frost HM: Tetracycline-based histological analysis of bone remodeling. Calcif Tissue Res **3:**211-237, 1969.

26 Garn SM, Rohmann CG, Wagner B: Bone loss as a general phenomenon in man. Fed Proc **26:**1729, 1967.

27 Jowsey J, Kelly PJ, Riggs BL, Bianco AJ Jr, Scholz DA, Gershon-Cohen J: Quantitative microradiographic studies of normal and osteoporotic bone. J Bone Joint Surg [Am] **47:**785-806, 1965.

27a Linovitz RJ, Resnick D, Keissling P, Kondon JJ, Sehler B, Nejdl RJ, Rowe JH, Deftos LJ: Tumor-induced osteomalacia and rickets: a surgically curable syndrome. Report of two cases. J Bone Joint Surg [Am] **58:**419-423, 1976.

27b Mankin HJ: Rickets, osteomalacia, and renal osteodystrophy. Part II. J Bone Joint Surg [Am] **56:**352-386, 1974.

28 Merz WA, Schenk RK: Quantitative structural analysis of human cancellous bone. Acta Anat **75:**54, 1970.

29 Mignani G, Thurner J, Marchetti PG, Hussl B: Microradiographic investigations of various forms of bone disease (Paget's osteitis deformans, osteomalacia, Engel-Recklinghausen disease and Möller-Barlow disease). Frankfurt Z Pathol **70:**606-620, 1960.

30 Nagant de Deuxchaisnes C, Krane SM: Paget's disease of bone: clinical and metabolic observations. Medicine **43:**233-266, 1964.

30a Sillence DO, Horton WA, Rimoin DL: Morphologic studies in the skeletal dysplasias. A review. Am J Pathol **96:**811-870, 1979.

31 Steendijk R: Metabolic bone disease in children. Clin Orthop **77:**247-275, 1971.

32 Teitelbaum SL: Metabolic and other nontumorous disorders of the bone. In Anderson WAD, Kissane JM (eds): Pathology, ed. 7. St. Louis, 1977, The C. V. Mosby Co., pp. 1905-1977.

33 Teitelbaum SL, Bullough PG: The pathophysiology of bone and joint disease. Am J Pathol **96:**283-354, 1979.

34 Teitelbaum SL, Nichols SH: Tetracycline-based morphometric analysis of trabecular bone kinetics. In Meunier P (ed): Bone histomorphometry. Second International Workshop on Bone Morphology. Lyon, France, 1976, Armour Co., pp. 311-319.

35 Teitelbaum SL, Hruska KA, Shieber W, Debnam JW, Nichols SH: Tetracycline fluorescence in uremic and primary hyperparathyroid bone. Kidney Int **12:**366-372, 1977.

36 Urist MR, Zaccalini PS, MacDonald NS, Skoog WA: New approaches to the problem of osteoporosis. J Bone Joint Surg [Br] **44:**464-484, 1962.

37 Van Buchem FSP: Osteomalacia—pathogenesis and treatment. Br Med J **1:**933-938, 1959.

Fractures

38 Blount WP, Schaefer AA, Johnson JH: Fractures of the forearm in children. JAMA **120:**111-116, 1942.

39 Collins DH: Structural changes around nails and screws in human bones. J Pathol Bacteriol **65:**109-121, 1953.

40 Collins DH: Tissue changes in human femurs containing plastic appliances. J Bone Joint Surg [Br] **36:**458-563, 1954.

41 Ham AW: A histologic study of the early phases of bone repair. J Bone Joint Surg **12:**827-844, 1930.

42 Ham AW: Histology, ed. 7. Philadelphia, 1974, J. B. Lippincott Co.

43 Ham AW, Gordon S: The origin of bone that forms in association with cancellous chips transplanted into muscle. Br J Plast Surg **5:**154-160, 1952.

44 Ham AW, Harris WR: Repair and transplantation of bone. In Bourne GH (ed): The biochemistry and physiology of bone, ed. 2. New York, 1956, Academic Press, Inc., vol. 3, pp. 338-379.

45 Mindell ER, Rodbard S, Kwasman BG: Chondrogenesis in bone repair. A study of the healing fractures callus in the rat. Clin Orthop **79:**187-196, 1971.

46 Murray CR: Healing of fractures. Its influence on the choice of methods of treatment. Arch Surg **29:**446-464, 1934.

47 Odell RT, Leydig SM: The conservative treatment of fractures in children. Surg Gynecol Obstet **92:**69-74, 1951.

48 Schwarz E: Hypercallosis in osteogenesis imperfecta. Am J Roentgenol Radium Ther Nucl Med **85:**645-648, 1961.

Osteomyelitis

49 Berney S, Goldstein M, Bishko F: Clinical and diagnostic features of tuberculous arthritis. Am J Med **53:**36-42, 1972.

50 Cabanela ME, Sim FH, Beabout JW, Dahlin DC: Osteomyelitis appearing as neoplasms. A diagnostic problem. Arch Surg **109:**68-72, 1974.

51 Carrell WB, Childress HM: Tuberculosis of the large long bones of the extremities. J Bone Joint Surg **22:**569-588, 1940.

52 Farrow R, Cureton RJR: Carcinomatous invasion of bone in osteomyelitis, Br J Surg **50:**107-109, 1962.

53 Garcia A Jr, Grantham SA: Hematogenous pyogenic vertebral osteomyelitis. J Bone Joint Surg [Am] **42:**429-436, 1960.

54 Johnson LL, Kempson RL: Epidermoid carcinoma in chronic osteomyelitis: diagnostic problems and management. J Bone Joint Surg [Am] **47:**133-145, 1965.

55 Lewis P, Sutter VL, Finegold M: Bone infections involving anaerobic bacteria. Medicine (Baltimore) **57:**279-305, 1978.

56 Mason ML: Tuberculous tenosynovitis of the hand. Surg Gynecol Obstet **59:**363-396, 1934.

57 Silver HK, Simon JL, Clement DH: Salmonella osteomyelitis and abnormal hemoglobin disease. Pediatrics **20:**439-447, 1957.

58 Trueta J: The three types of acute haematogenous osteomyelitis. J Bone Joint Surg [Br] **41:**671-680, 1959.

58a Waldvogel FA, Vasey H: Osteomyelitis: the past decade. N Engl J Med **300:**360-370, 1980.

59 Westermark N, Hellerström S: Zwei Fälle von Osteitis luetica, osteogenes Sarkom vortäuschend. Acta Radiol **18:**422-427, 1937.

Bone necrosis

60 Bohr H, Larsen EJ: On necrosis of the femoral head after fracture of the neck of the femur. J Bone Joint Surg [Br] **47:**330-338, 1965.

61 Galli SJ, Weintraub HP, Proppe KH: Malignant fibrous histiocytoma and pleomorphic sarcoma in association with medullary bone infarcts. Cancer **41:**607-619, 1978.

62 Golding JSR, Maciver JF, Went LN: The bone changes in sickle-cell anaemia and its genetic variants. J Bone Joint Surg [Br] **41:**711-718, 1959.

63 Luck JV: Bone and joint diseases. Springfield, Ill., 1950, Charles C Thomas, Publisher.

64 Milgram JW: Radiological and pathological manifestations of osteochondritis dissecans of the distal femur. A study of 50 cases. Radiology 126:305-311, 1978.

65 Mirra JM, Bullough PG, Marcove RC, Jacobs B, Huvos AG: Malignant fibrous histiocytoma and osteosarcoma in association with bone infarcts. Report of four cases, two in caisson workers. J Bone Joint Surg [Am] 56:932-940, 1974.

66 Phemister DB: Repair of bone in the presence of aseptic necrosis resulting from fractures, transplantations, and vascular obstruction. J Bone Joint Surg 12:769-787, 1930.

66a Sengupta S, Prathap K: Radiation necrosis of the humerus. A report of three cases. Acta Radiol 12:313-320, 1973.

Paget's disease

67 Barry HC: Paget's disease of bone. Edinburgh, 1969, E. & S. Livingstone, Ltd.

68 Collins DH: Paget's disease of bone. Incidence and subclinical forms. Lancet 2:51-57, 1956.

69 Collins DH, Winn JM: Focal Paget's disease of the skull (osteoporosis circumscripta). J Pathol Bacteriol 69:1-9, 1955.

70 Dickson DD, Camp JD, Ghormley RK: Osteitis deformans. Paget's disease of the bone. Radiology 44:449-470, 1945.

70a Greenspan A, Norman A, Sterling AP: Precocious onset of Paget's disease—a report of three cases and review of the literature. J Can Assoc Radiol 28:69-72, 1977.

70b Kanis JA, Horn DB, Scott RDM, Strong JA: Treatment of Paget's disease of bone with synthetic salmon calcitonin. Br Med J 3:727-731, 1974.

71 Lake ME: The pathology of fracture in Paget's disease. Aust N Z J Surg 27:307-312, 1958.

71a Mills BG, Singer FR: Nuclear inclusions in Paget's disease of bone. Science 194:201-202, 1976.

72 Price CHG, Goldie W: Paget's sarcoma of bone. A study of 80 cases from the Bristol and the Leeds bone tumour Registries. J Bone Joint Surg [Br] 51:205-224, 1969.

73 Reifenstein EC Jr, Albright F: Paget's disease: its pathologic physiology and the importance of this in the complications arising from fracture and immobilization. N Engl J Med 231:343-355, 1944.

74 Schmorl G: Ueber Ostitis deformans Paget. Virchows Arch [Pathol Anat] 283:694-751, 1931.

75 Seaman WB: The roentgen appearance of early Paget's disease. Am J Roentgenol Radium Ther Nucl Med 66:587-594, 1951.

76 Uehlinger E: Osteofibrosis deformans juvenilis (Polyostotische fibröse Dysplasia Jaffe-Lichtenstein). Virchows Arch [Pathol Anat] 306:255-299, 1940.

Melorheostosis

77 Franklin EL, Matheson I: Melorheostosis. Br J Radiol 15:185-191, 1942.

78 Kirby SV: Melorheostosis; with report of a case. Radiology 37:62-67, 1948.

Mastocytosis

79 Barer M, Peterson LFA, Dahlin DC, Winkelmann RK, Stewart JR: Mastocytosis with osseous lesions re-

sembling metastatic malignant lesions in bone. J Bone Joint Surg [Am] 50:142-152, 1968.

80 Rywlin AM, Hoffman EP, Ortega RS: Eosinophilic fibrohistiocytic lesion of bone marrow: a distinctive new morphologic finding, probably related to drug hypersensitivity. Blood 40:464-472, 1972.

Tumors
Classification and distribution

80a Dorfman HD: Malignant transformation of benign bone lesions. In Proceedings of the Seventh National Cancer Conference, vol. 7. Philadelphia, 1973, J. B. Lippincott Co., pp. 901-913.

81 Schajowicz F, Ackerman LV, Sissons HA: Histologic typing of bone tumours. International Histological Classification of Tumours, No. 6. Geneva, 1972, World Health Organization.

Bone-forming tumors
Osteoma

82 Chang CHJ, Piatt ED, Thomas KE, Watne AL: Bone abnormalities in Gardner's syndrome. Am J Roentgenol Radium Ther Nucl Med 103:645-652, 1968.

83 Hallberg OE, Begley JW Jr: Origin and treatment of osteomas of the paranasal sinuses. Arch Otolaryngol 51:750-760, 1950.

Osteoid osteoma and osteoblastoma

84 Brown RC, Ghormley RK: Solitary eccentric (cortical) abscess in bone. Surg 14:541-553, 1943.

85 Byers PD: Solitary benign osteoblastic lesions of bone—osteoid osteoma and benign osteoblastoma. Cancer 22:43-57, 1968.

86 Dahlin DC, Johnson EW: Giant osteoid osteoma. J Bone Joint Surg [Am] 36:559-572, 1954.

86a Dorfman HD: Discussion of case records of the Massachusetts General Hospital (Case 40-1980). N Engl J Med 303:866-873, 1980.

87 Jaffe HL: Osteoid-osteoma of bone. Radiology 45:319-334, 1945.

87a Keim HA, Reina EG: Osteoid-osteoma as a cause of scoliosis. J Bone Joint Surg [Am] 57:159-163, 1975.

88 Lichtenstein L: Benign osteoblastoma. J Bone Joint Surg [Am] 46:755-765, 1964.

89 MacLennan, DI, Wilson FC Jr: Osteoid osteoma of the spine. A review of the literature and report of six new cases. J Bone Joint Surg [Am] 49:111-121, 1967.

89a McLeod RA, Dahlin DC, Beabout JW: The spectrum of osteoblastoma. Am J Roentgenol 126:321-335, 1976.

89b Marsh BW, Bonfiglio M, Brady LP, Enneking WF: Benign osteoblastoma: range of manifestations. J Bone Joint Surg [Am] 57:1-9, 1975.

89c Rigault P, Mouterde P, Padovani JP, Jaubert F, Guyonvarch G: Ostéome ostéoïde chez l'enfant. A propos de 29 cas. Rev Chir Orthop 61:627-646, 1975.

90 Schajowicz F, Lemos C: Osteoid osteoma and osteoblastoma. Acta Orthop Scand 41:272-291, 1970.

90a Schajowicz F, Lemos C: Malignant osteoblastoma. J Bone Joint Surg [Br] 58:202-211, 1976.

91 Steiner GC: Ultrastructure of osteoid osteoma. Hum Pathol 7:309-325, 1976.

91a Yoshikawa S, Nakamura T, Takagi M, Imamura T, Okano K, Sasaki S: Benign osteoblastoma as a cause of osteomalacia. A report of two cases. J Bone Joint Surg [Br] 59:279-286, 1977.

Osteosarcoma

92 Amstutz HC: Multiple osteogenic sarcomata—metastatic or multicentric? Report of two cases and review of literature. Cancer **24:**923-931, 1969.

93 Arlen M, Higinbotham NL, Huvos AG, Marcove RC, Miller T, Shah IC: Radiation-induced sarcoma of bone. Cancer **28:**1087-1099, 1971.

94 Banta JV, Schreiber RR, Kulik, WJ: Hyperplastic callus formation in osteogenesis imperfecta simulating osteosarcoma. J Bone Joint Surg [Am] **53:**115-122, 1971.

94a Barwick KW, Huvos AG, Smith J: Primary osteogenic sarcoma of the vertebral column. A clinicopathologic correlation of ten patients. Cancer **46:**595-604, 1980.

95 Cahan WG, Woodard HQ, Higinbotham NL, Stewart FW, Coley BL: Sarcoma arising in irradiated bone. Cancer **1:**3-29, 1948.

95a Campanacci M, Cervellati G: Osteosarcoma. A review of 345 cases. Ital J Orthop Traumatol **1:**5-22, 1975.

96 Dahlin DC, Coventry MB: Osteogenic sarcoma. A study of 600 cases, J Bone Joint Surg [Am] **49:**101-110, 1967.

97 Dahlin DC, Unni KK: Osteosarcoma of bone and its important recognizable varieties. Am J Surg Pathol **1:**61-72, 1977.

98 Enneking WF (ed): Osteosarcoma. Symposium. Clin Orthop **111:**1-104, 1975.

99 Enneking WF, Kagan A: "Skip" metastases in osteosarcoma. Cancer **36:**2192-2205, 1975.

99a Frentzel-Beyme R, Wagner G: Malignant bone tumours: status of aetiological knowledge and needs of epidemiological research. Arch Orthop Trauma Surg **94:**81-89, 1979.

100 Hatcher CH: The development of sarcoma in bone subjected to roentgen or radium irradiation. J Bone Joint Surg **27:**179-195, 1945.

101 Kahn LB, Wood FW, Ackerman LV: Fracture callus associated with benign and malignant bone lesions and mimicking osteosarcoma. Am J Clin Pathol **52:**14-24, 1969.

101a Levine AM, Resenberg SA: Alkaline phosphatase levels in osteosarcoma tissue are related to prognosis. Cancer **44:**2291-2293, 1979.

102 Lichtenstein L: Bone tumors, ed. 5. St. Louis, 1977, The C. V. Mosby Co.

103 Lindbom A, Soderberg G, Spjut HJ: Osteosarcoma. A review of 96 cases. Acta Radiol **56:**1019, 1961.

104 Martland HS, Humphries RE: Osteogenic sarcoma in dial painters using luminous paint. Arch Pathol **7:**406-417, 1929.

105 Matsuno T, Unni KK, McLeod RA, Dahlin DC: Telangiectatic osteogenic sarcoma. Cancer **38:**2538-2547, 1976.

106 Morton DL, Malmgren RA: Human osteosarcomas: immunologic evidence suggesting an associated infectious agent. Science **162:**1279-1281, 1968.

107 O'Hara JM, Hutter RVP, Foote FW Jr, Miller T, Woodard HQ: An analysis of 30 patients surviving longer than ten years after treatment for osteogenic sarcoma. J Bone Joint Surg [Am] **50:**335-354, 1968.

107a Polednak AP: Bone cancer among female radium dial workers. Latency periods and incidence rates by time after exposure: brief communication. J Natl Cancer Inst **60:**77-82, 1978.

108 Pritchard DJ, Finkel MP, Reilly CA Jr: The etiology of osteosarcoma. A review of current considerations. Clin Orthop **111:**14-22, 1975.

108a Reddick RL, Michelitch HJ, Levine AM, Triche TJ: Osteogenic sarcoma. A study of the ultrastructure. Cancer **45:**64-71, 1980.

108b Rosen G, Marcove RC, Caparros B, Nirenberg A, Kosloff C, Huvos AG: Primary osteogenic sarcoma. The rationale for preoperative chemotherapy and delayed surgery. Cancer **43:**2163-2177, 1979.

109 Scranton PE, DeCicco FA, Totten RS, Yunis EJ: Prognostic factors in osteosarcoma. A review of 20 years' experience at the University of Pittsburgh Health Center Hospitals. Cancer **36:**2179-2191, 1975.

110 Siegal GP, Dahlin DC, Sim FH: Osteoblastic osteogenic sarcoma in a 35-month-old girl. Report of a case. Am J Clin Pathol **63:**886-890, 1975.

111 Silverman G: Multiple osteogenic sarcoma. Arch Pathol **21:**88-95, 1936.

112 Sim FH, Unni KK, Beabout JW, Dahlin DC: Osteosarcoma with small cells simulating Ewing's tumor. J Bone Joint Surg [Am] **61:**207-215, 1979.

112a Simon MA, Bos GD: Epiphyseal extension of metaphyseal osteosarcoma in skeletally immature individuals. J Bone Joint Surg [Am] **62:**195-204, 1980.

113 Sindelar WF, Costa J, Ketcham AS: Osteosarcoma associated with Thorotrast administration. Cancer **42:**2604-2609, 1978.

114 Unni KK, Dahlin DC, McLeod RA, Pritchard DJ: Intraosseous well-differentiated osteosarcoma. Cancer **40:**1337-1347, 1977.

115 Uribe-Botero G, Russell WO, Sutow WW, Martin RG: Primary osteosarcoma of bone. A clinicopathologic investigation of 243 cases, with necropsy studies in 54. Am J Clin Pathol **67:**427-435, 1977.

115a Varela-Duran J, Dehner LP: Postirradiation osteosarcoma in childhood. A clinicopathologic study of three cases and review of the literature. Am J Pediatr Hematol/Oncol **2:**263-271, 1980.

116 Williams AH, Schwinn CP, Parker JW: The ultrastructure of osteosarcoma. A review of twenty cases. Cancer **37:**1293-1301, 1976.

Juxtacortical (parosteal) osteosarcoma

117 Ahuja SC, Villacin AB, Smith J, Bullough PG, Huvos AG, Marcove RC: Juxtacortical (parosteal) osteogenic sarcoma. Histologic grading and prognosis. J Bone Joint Surg [Am] **59:**632-647, 1977.

117a de Santos LA, Murray JA, Finklestein JB, Spjut HJ, Ayala AG: The radiographic spectrum of periosteal osteosarcoma. Radiology **127:**123-129, 1978.

118 Dwinnell LA, Dahlin DC, Ghormley RK: Parosteal (juxtacortical) osteogenic sarcoma. J Bone Joint Surg [Am] **36:**732-744, 1954.

119 Edeiken J, Farrell C, Ackerman LV, Spjut H: Parosteal sarcoma. Am J Roentgenol Radium Ther Nucl Med **111:**579-583, 1971.

120 Farr GH, Huvos AG: Juxtacortical osteogenic sarcoma. J Bone Joint Surg [Am] **51:**1205-1216, 1972.

121 Scaglietti O, Calandriello B: Ossifying parosteal sarcoma. J Bone Joint Surg [Am] **44:**635-647, 1962.

121a Spjut HJ, Ayala AG, de Santos LA, Murray JA: Periosteal osteosarcoma. In Management of primary bone and soft tissue tumors, M. D. Anderson Hospital and Tumor Institute. Chicago, 1977, Year Book Medical Publishers, Inc., pp. 79-95.

122 Unni KK, Dahlin DC, Beabout JW: Periosteal osteogenic sarcoma. Cancer **37:**2476-2485, 1976.
123 Unni KK, Dahlin DC, Beabout JW, Ivins JC: Parosteal
osteogenic sarcoma. Cancer **37:**2466-2475, 1976.
124 Van der Heul RO, Von Ronnen JR: Juxtacortical
osteosarcoma. Diagnosis, differential diagnosis, treatment, and an analysis of eighty cases. J Bone Joint
Surg [Am] **49:**415-439, 1967.

Cartilage-forming tumors
Chondroma

125 Anderson IF: Maffucci's syndrome. Report of a case
with a review of the literature. S Afr Med J **39:**1066-
1070, 1965.
126 Cowan WK: Malignant change and multiple metastases in Ollier's disease. J Clin Pathol **18:**650-653,
1965.
127 Laurence W, Franklin EL: Calcifying enchondroma
of long bones. J Bone Joint Surg [Br] **35:**224-228,
1953.
128 Lewis RJ, Ketcham AS: Maffucci's syndrome: functional and neoplastic significance. Case report and
review of the literature. J Bone Joint Surg [Am] **55:**
1465-1479, 1973.
129 Lichtenstein L, Hall JE: Periosteal chondroma. A
distinctive benign cartilage tumor. J Bone Joint Surg
[Am] **34:**691-697, 1952.
130 Nosanchuk JS, Kaufer H: Recurrent periosteal chondroma. Report of two cases and a review of the literature. J Bone Joint Surg [Am] **51:**375-380, 1969.
131 Takigawa K: Chondroma of the bones of the hand. J
Bone Joint Surg [Am] **53:**1591-1600, 1971.

Osteochondroma

132 Fairbank HAT: An atlas of general affections of
the skeleton. Edinburgh, 1951, E. & S. Livingstone,
Ltd.
132a Han SK, Henein HG, Novin N, Giargiana FA Jr:
An unusual arterial complication seen with a solitary
osteochondroma. Am Surg **43:**471-472, 1977.
132b Landon GC, Johnson KA, Dahlin DC: Subungual
exostosis. J Bone Joint Surg [Am] **61:**256-259, 1979.
132c Ochsner PE: Zum problem der neoplastischen Entar-
tung bei multiplen kartilaginären Exostosen. Z Orthop
116:369-378, 1978.
133 Unni KK, Dahlin DC: Premalignant tumors and conditions of bone. Am J Surg Pathol **3:**47-60, 1979.

Chondroblastoma

133a Aronsohn RS, Hart WR, Martel W: Metaphyseal
chondroblastoma of bone. Am J Roentgenol **127:**686-
688, 1976.
134 Codman EA: Epiphyseal chondromatous giant cell
tumors of the upper end of the humerus. Surg Gynecol
Obstet **52:**543-548, 1931.
135 Coleman SS: Benign chondroblastoma with recurrent
soft-tissue and intra-articular lesions. J Bone Joint
Surg [Am] **48:**1554-1560, 1966.
136 Hatcher CH, Campbell JC: Benign chondroblastoma
of bone: its histologic variations and a report of late
sarcoma in the site of one. Bull Hosp Joint Dis **12:**
411-430, 1951.
137 Huvos AG, Marcove RC, Erlandson RA, Mike V:
Chondroblastoma of bone. A clinico-pathologic and
electron microscopic study. Cancer **29:**760-771, 1972.
138 Jaffe HL, Lichtenstein L: Benign chondroblastoma of
bone. A reinterpretation of the so-called calcifying or

chondromatous giant cell tumor. Am J Pathol **18:**969-
991, 1942.
139 Kahn LB, Wood FM, Ackerman LV: Malignant chondroblastoma. Report of two cases and review of the
literature. Arch Pathol **88:**371-376, 1969.
140 Levine GD, Bensch KG: Chondroblastoma—the nature of the basic cell. A study by means of histochemistry, tissue culture, electron microscopy, and auto-
radiography. Cancer **29:**1546-1562, 1972.
140a Reyes CV, Kathuria S: Recurrent and aggressive
chondroblastoma of the pelvis with late malignant neoplastic changes. Am J Surg Pathol **3:**449-455, 1979.
141 Schajowicz F, Gallardo H: Epiphysial chondroblastoma of bone. A clinico-pathological study of sixty-
nine cases. J Bone Joint Surg [Br] **52:**205-226, 1970.
142 Steiner GC: Ultrastructure of benign cartilaginous tumors of intraosseous origin. Hum Pathol **10:**71-86,
1979.
143 Valls J, Ottolenghi CE, Schajowicz F: Epiphyseal
chondroblastoma of bone. J Bone Joint Surg [Am]**33:**
997-1009, 1951.
144 Welsh RA, Meyer AT: A histogenetic study of chondroblastoma. Cancer **17:**578-589, 1964.

Chondromyxoid fibroma

145 Dahlin DC: Chondromyxoid fibroma of bone, with
emphasis on its morphological relationship to benign
chondroblastoma. Cancer **9:**195-203, 1956.
146 Jaffe HL, Lichtenstein L: Chondromyxoid fibroma of
bone. A distinctive benign tumor likely to be mistaken especially for chondrosarcoma. Arch Pathol
45:541-551, 1948.
146a Kyriakos M: Soft tissue implantation of chondromyxoid fibroma. Am J Surg Pathol **3:**363-372, 1979.
147 McClure DK, Dahlin DC: Myxoma of bone. Report of
three cases. Mayo Clin Proc **52:**249-253, 1977.
148 Marcove RC, Kambolis C, Bullough PG, Jaffe HL:
Fibromyxoma of bone. Cancer **17:**1209-1213, 1964.
149 Schajowicz F, Gallardo H: Chondromyxoid fibroma
(fibromyxoid chondroma) of bone. A clinico-pathological study of thirty-two cases. J Bone Joint Surg
[Br] **53:**198-216, 1971.

Chondrosarcoma

150 Barnes R, Catto M: Chondrosarcoma of bone. J Bone
Joint Surg [Br] **48:**729-764, 1966.
150a Campanacci M, Guernelli N, Leonessa C, Boni A:
Chondrosarcoma. A study of 133 cases, 80 with long
term follow up. Ital J Orthop Traumatol **1:**387-414,
1975.
151 Dabska M: Parachordoma. A new clinicopathologic
entity. Cancer **40:**1586-1592, 1977.
152 Dahlin DC, Beabout JW: Dedifferentiation of low-
grade chondrosarcomas. Cancer **28:**461-466, 1971.
153 Dahlin DC, Henderson ED: Chondrosarcoma, a surgical and pathological problem. J Bone Joint Surg
[Am] **38:**1025-1038, 1956.
154 Dahlin DC, Salvador AH: Chondrosarcomas of bones
of the hands and feet. A study of 30 cases. Cancer
34:755-760, 1974.
155 Erlandson RA, Huvos AG: Chondrosarcoma: a light
and electron microscopic study. Cancer **34:**1642-1652,
1974.
156 Evans HL, Ayala AG, Romsdahl MM: Prognostic
factors in chondrosarcoma of bone. A clinicopatho-

logic analysis with emphasis on histologic grading. Cancer **40:**818-831, 1977.

157 Jaffe HL: Hereditary multiple exostoses. Arch Pathol **36:**335-357, 1943.

158 Kindblom L, Angervall L: Histochemical characterization of mucosubstances in bone and soft tissue tumors. Cancer **36:**985-994, 1975.

159 Lansche WE, Spjut HJ: Chondrosarcoma of the small bones of the hand. J Bone Joint Surg [Am] **40:**1139-1149, 1958.

160 Lichtenstein L, Jaffe HL: Chondrosarcoma of bone. Am J Pathol **19:**553-589, 1943.

160a Mankin HJ, Cantley KP, Lippiello L, Schiller AL, Campbell CJ: The biology of human chondrosarcoma. I. Description of the cases, grading, and biochemical analyses. J Bone Joint Surg [Am] **62:**160-176, 1980.

160b Mankin HJ, Cantley KP, Schiller AL, Lippiello L: The biology of human chondrosarcoma. II. Variation in chemical composition among types and subtypes of benign and malignant cartilage tumors. J Bone Joint Surg [Am] **62:**176-188, 1980.

161 McFarland GB, McKinley LM, Reed RJ: Dedifferentiation of low grade chondrosarcomas. Clin Orthop **122:**157-164, 1977.

162 McKenna RJ, Schwinn CP, Soong KY, Higinbotham NL: Sarcomata of the osteogenic series (osteosarcoma, fibrosarcoma, chondrosarcoma, parosteal osteogenic sarcoma, and sarcomata arising in abnormal bone). J Bone Joint Surg [Am] **48:**1-26, 1966.

163 Marcove RC, Huvos AG: Cartilaginous tumors of the ribs. Cancer **27:**794-801, 1971.

164 Martin RF, Melnick PJ, Warner NE, Terry R, Bullock WK, Schwinn CP: Chordoid sarcoma. Am J Clin Pathol **59:**623-635, 1972.

164a Mirra JM, Marcove RC: Fibrosarcomatous dedifferentiation of primary and secondary chondrosarcoma. Review of five cases. J Bone Joint Surg [Am] **56:**285-296, 1974.

165 O'Neal LW, Ackerman LV: Cartilaginous tumors of ribs and sternum. J Thorac Surg **21:**71-108, 1951 (extensive bibliography).

166 O'Neal LW, Ackerman LV: Chondrosarcoma of bone. Cancer **5:**551-577, 1952 (extensive bibliography).

166a Pritchard DJ, Lunke RJ, Taylor WF, Dahlin DC, Medley BE: Chondrosarcoma: a clinicopathologic and statistical analysis. Cancer **45:**149-157, 1980.

166b Sanerkin NG, Gallagher P: A review of the behaviour of chondrosarcoma of bone. J Bone Joint Surg [Br] **61:**395-400, 1979.

166c Schajowicz F: Juxtacortical chondrosarcoma. J Bone Joint Surg [Br] **59:**473-480, 1977.

166d Smith WS, Simon MA: Segmental resection for chondrosarcoma. J Bone Joint Surg [Am] **57:**1097-1103, 1975.

166e Unni KK, Dahlin DC, Beabout JW, Sim FH: Chondrosarcoma: clear-cell variant. A report of sixteen cases. J Bone Joint Surg [Am] **58:**676-683, 1976.

Mesenchymal chondrosarcoma

167 Dowling EA: Mesenchymal chondrosarcoma. J Bone Joint Surg [Am] **46:**747-754, 1964.

168 Goldman RL: "Mesenchymal" chondrosarcoma, a rare malignant chondroid tumor usually primary in bone. Report of a case arising in extraskeletal soft tissue. Cancer **20:**1494-1498, 1967.

169 Guccion JG, Font RL, Enzinger FM, Zimmerman LE: Extraskeletal mesenchymal chondrosarcoma. Arch Pathol **95:**336-340, 1973.

170 Jacobson SA: Polyhistioma. A malignant tumor of bone and extraskeletal tissues. Cancer **40:**2116-2130, 1977.

171 Salvador AH, Beabout JW, Dahlin DC: Mesenchymal chondrosarcoma. Observations on 30 new cases. Cancer **28:**605-615, 1971.

172 Steiner GC, Mirra JM, Bullough PG: Mesenchymal chondrosarcoma. A study of the ultrastructure. Cancer **32:**926-939, 1973.

Giant cell tumor

173 Aparisi T: Giant cell tumor of bone. Acta Orthop Scand [Suppl] (173):1-38, 1978.

174 Aparisi T, Arborgh B, Ericsson JLE: Giant cell tumor of bone. Virchows Arch [Pathol Anat] **381:**159-178, 1979.

174a Campanacci M, Giunti A, Olmi R: Giant-cell tumours of bone. A study of 209 cases with long-term follow-up in 130. Ital J Orthop Traumatol **1:**249-277, 1975.

175 Dahlin DC, Cupps RE, Johnson EW Jr: Giant-cell tumor. A study of 195 cases. Cancer **25:**1061-1070, 1970.

176 Emley WE: Giant cell tumor of the sphenoid bone. A case report and review of the literature. Arch Otolaryngol **94:**369-374, 1971.

177 Hanaoka H, Friedman B, Mack RP: Ultrastructure and histogenesis of giant-cell tumor of bone. Cancer **25:**1408-1423, 1970.

178 Jaffe HL, Lichtenstein L, Portis RB: Giant cell tumor of bone. Arch Pathol **30:**993-1031, 1940.

179 Joynt GHC, Ortved WE: The accidental operative transplantation of benign giant cell tumor. Ann Surg **127:**1232-1239, 1948.

179a Kasahara K, Yamamuro T, Kasahara A: Giant-cell tumour of bone: cytological studies. Br J Cancer **40:** 201-209, 1979.

179b Mankin HJ, Fogelson FS, Thrasher AZ, Jaffer F: Massive resection and allograft transplantation in the treatment of malignant bone tumors. N Engl J Med **294:**1247-1255, 1976.

180 Murphy WR, Ackerman LV: Benign and malignant giant-cell tumors of bone. Cancer **9:**317-339, 1956.

180a Nascimento AG, Huvos AG, Marcove RC: Primary malignant giant cell tumor of bone. A study of eight cases and review of the literature. Cancer **44:**1393-1402, 1979.

180b Parrish FF: Allograft replacement of all or part of the end of a long bone following excision of a tumor. Report of twenty-one cases. J Bone Joint Surg [Am] **55:**1-22, 1973.

180c Peison B, Feigenbaum J: Metaphyseal giant-cell tumor in a girl of 14. Radiology **118:**145-146, 1976.

181 Schajowicz F: Giant-cell tumors of bone (osteoclastoma). A pathological and histochemical study. J Bone Joint Surg [Am] **43:**1-29, 1961.

182 Steiner GC, Ghosh L, Dorfman HD: Ultrastructure of giant cell tumors of bone. Hum Pathol **3:**569-586, 1972.

183 Stewart FW, Coley BL, Farrow JH: Malignant giant cell tumor of bone. Am J Pathol **14:**515-535, 1938.

184 Sybrandy S, de la Fuente, AA: Multiple giant tumour of bone. Report of a case. J Bone Joint Surg [Br] **55:**350-356, 1973.

185 Willis RA: Pathology of tumours, ed. 4. New York, 1967, Appleton-Century-Crofts.

186 Windeyer BW, Woodyatt PB: Osteoclastoma: a study of thirty-eight cases. J Bone Joint Surg [Br] **31:**252-267, 1949.

Marrow tumors
Ewing's sarcoma

187 Chan RC, Sutow W, Lindberg D, Samuels ML, Murray JA, Johnston DA: Management and results of localized Ewing's sarcoma. Cancer **43:**1001-1006, 1979.
188 Friedman B, Gold H: Ultrastructure of Ewing's sarcoma of bone. Cancer **22:**307-322, 1968.
189 Friedman B, Hanaoka H: Round-cell sarcomas of bone. A light and electron microscopic study. J Bone Joint Surg [Am] **53:**1118-1136, 1971.
189a Gasparini M, Barni S, Lattuada A, Musumeci R, Bonadonna G, Fossati-Bellani F: Ten years experience with Ewing's sarcoma. Tumori **63:**77-90, 1977.
190 Kadin ME, Bensch KG: On the origin of Ewing's tumor. Cancer **27:**257-273, 1971.
191 Kissane JM, Askin FB, Nesbit M, Vietti T, Burgert EO Jr, Cangir A, Gehan EA, Perez CA, Pritchard DJ, Tefft M: Sarcomas of bone in childhood. Pathologic aspects. In Glicksmann A, Tefft M (eds): Bone and soft tissue sarcomas. J Natl Cancer Inst Monograph 57 (in press, 1981).
192 Llombart-Bosch A, Blache R, Peydro-Olaya A: Ultrastructural study of 28 cases of Ewing's sarcoma: typical and atypical forms. Cancer **41:**1362-1373, 1978.
193 Mahoney JP, Alexander RW: Ewing's sarcoma: a light and electron microscopic study of 21 cases. Am J Surg Pathol **2:**283-298, 1978.
193a Nascimento AG, Unni KK, Pritchard DJ, Cooper KL, Dahlin DC: A clinicopathologic study of 20 cases of large-cell (atypical) Ewing's sarcoma of bone. Am J Surg Pathol **4:**29-36, 1980.
194 Perez CA, Razek A, Tefft M, Nesbit M, Burgert EO, Kissane J, Vietti T, Gehan EA: Analysis of local tumor control in Ewing's sarcoma. Cancer **40:**2864-2873, 1977.
194a Razek A, Perez CA, Tefft M, Nesbit M, Vietti T, Burgert EO Jr, Kissane J, Pritchard DJ, Gehan EA: Intergroup Ewing's sarcoma study. Local control related to radiation dose, volume, and site of primary lesion in Ewing's sarcoma. Cancer **46:**516-521, 1980.
195 Rosen G, Caparros B, Mosende C, McCormick B, Huvos AG, Marcove RC: Curability of Ewing's sarcoma and considerations for future therapeutic trials. Cancer **41:**888-899, 1978.
196 Schajowicz F: Ewing's sarcoma and reticulum-cell sarcoma of bone. With special reference to the histochemical demonstration of glycogen as an aid to differential diagnosis. J Bone Joint Surg [Am] **41:**349-356, 1959.
197 Swenson PC: The roentgenological aspects of Ewing's tumor of bone marrow. Am J Roentgenol Radium Ther Nucl Med **50:**343-353, 1943.
198 Telles NC, Rabson AS, Pomeroy TC: Ewing's sarcoma: an autopsy study. Cancer **41:**2321-2329, 1978.
199 Triche TJ, Ross WE: Glycogen-containing neuroblastoma with clinical and histopathologic features of Ewing's sarcoma. Cancer **41:**1425-1432, 1978.
200 Willis RA: Pathology of tumours, ed 4. New York, 1967, Appleton-Century-Crofts.
200a Yunis EJ, Agostini RM Jr, Walpusk JA, Hubbard JD: Glycogen in neuroblastomas. A light- and electron-microscopic study of 40 cases. Am J Surg Pathol **3:**313-323, 1979.

Malignant lymphoma

201 Boston HC, Dahlin DC, Ivins JC, Cupps RE: Malignant lymphoma (so-called reticulum cell sarcoma) of bone. Cancer **34:**1131-1137, 1974.
202 Chabner BA, Haskell CM, Canellos GP: Destructive bone lesions in chronic granulocytic leukemia. Medicine (Baltimore) **48:**401-410, 1969.
203 Horan FT: Bone involvement in Hodgkin's disease. Br J Surg **56:**277-281, 1969.
204 Ivins JC: Reticulum-cell sarcoma of bone. J Bone Joint Surg [Am] **35:**835-842, 1953.
204a Mahoney JP, Alexander RW: Primary histiocytic lymphoma of bone. A light and ultrastructural study of four cases. Am J Surg Pathol **4:**149-161, 1980.
205 Parker F Jr, Jackson H Jr: Primary reticulum cell sarcoma of bone. Surg Gynecol Obstet **68:**45-53, 1939.
205a Reimer RR, Chabner BA, Young RC, Reddick R, Johnson RE: Lymphoma presenting in bone. Results of histopathology, staging, and therapy. Ann Intern Med **87:**50-55, 1977.
206 Sherman RS, Snyder RE: The roentgen appearance of primary reticulum cell sarcoma of bone. Am J Roentgenol **58:**291-306, 1947.
207 Shoji H, Miller TR: Primary reticulum cell sarcoma of bone. Significance of clinical features upon the prognosis. Cancer **28:**1234-1244, 1971.
208 Simmons CR, Harle TS, Singleton EB: The osseous manifestations of leukemia in children. Radiol Clin North Am **6:**115-129, 1968.
209 Thomas LB, Forkner CE, Frei E, Besse BE, Stabenau JR: The skeletal lesions of acute leukemia. Cancer **14:**608-621, 1961.
210 Wang CC, Fleischli DJ: Primary reticulum cell sarcoma of bone, with emphasis on radiation therapy. Cancer **22:**994-998, 1968.

Plasma cell myeloma

211 Azar HA: Plasma cell myelomatosis and other monoclonal gammapathies. Pathol Annu **7:**1-17, 1972.
212 Carbone PP, Kellerhouse LE, Gehan EA: Plasmacytic myeloma. A study of the relationship of survival to various clinical manifestations and anomalous protein type in 112 patients. Am J Med **42:**937-948, 1967.
213 Carson CP, Ackerman LV, Maltby JD: Plasma cell myeloma. Am J Clin Pathol **25:**849-888, 1955.
214 Christopherson WM, Miller AJ: A reevaluation of solitary plasma cell myeloma of bone. Cancer **3:**240-252, 1950.
215 Corwin J, Lindberg RD: Solitary plasmacytoma of bone vs. extramedullary plasmacytoma and their relationship to multiple myeloma. Cancer **43:**1007-1013, 1979.
215a Driedger H, Pruzanski W: Plasma cell neoplasia with osteosclerotic lesions. A study of five cases and a review of the literature. Arch Intern Med **139:**892-896, 1979.
216 Fisher ER, Zawadzki A: Ultrastructural features of plasma cells in patients with paraproteinemias. Am J Clin Pathol **54:**779-789, 1970.
217 Kotner LM, Wang CC: Plasmacytoma of the upper air and food passages. Cancer **30:**414-418, 1972.
217a Kyle RA, Greipp PR: Smoldering multiple myeloma. N Engl J Med **302:**1347-1349, 1980.

218 Lichtenstein L, Jaffe HL: Multiple myeloma. Arch Pathol **44**:207-246, 1947.

219 Moss W, Ackerman LV: Plasma cell leukemia. Blood **1**:396-406, 1946.

220 Pasmantier MW, Azar HA: Extraskeletal spread in multiple plasma cell myeloma. A review of 57 autopsied cases. Cancer **23**:167-174, 1969.

221 Rosai J, Rodriguez HA: Application of electron microscopy to the differential diagnosis of tumors. Am J Clin Pathol **50**:555-562, 1968.

222 Wiltshaw E: The natural history of extramedullary plasmacytoma and its relation to solitary myeloma of bone and myelomatosis. Medicine (Baltimore) **55**:217-238, 1976.

Vascular tumors

223 Bucy PC, Capp CS: Primary hemangioma of bone. With special reference to roentgenologic diagnosis. Am J Roentgenol **23**:1-33, 1930.

223a Campanacci M, Boriani S, Giunti A: Hemangioendothelioma of bone: a study of 29 cases. Cancer **46**:804-814, 1980.

224 Dorfman HD, Steiner GC, Jaffe HL: Vascular tumors of bone. Hum Pathol **2**:349-376, 1971.

225 Gorham LW, Stout AP: Massive osteolysis (acute spontaneous absorption of bone, phantom bone, disappearing bone). Its relation to hemangiomatosis. J Bone Joint Surg [Am] **37**:985-1004, 1955.

226 Halliday DR, Dahlin DC, Pugh DG, Young HH: Massive osteolysis and angiomatosis. Radiology **82**:627-644, 1964.

226a Larsson S-E, Lorentzon R, Boquist L: Malignant hemangioendothelioma of bone. J Bone Joint Surg [Am] **57**:84-89, 1975.

227 Mackenzie DH: Intraosseous glomus tumors. Report of two cases. J Bone Joint Surg [Br] **44**:648-651, 1962.

228 Otis J, Hutter RVP, Foote FW Jr, Marcove RC, Stewart FW: Hemangioendothelioma of bone. Surg Gynecol Obstet **127**:295-305, 1968.

228a Rosai J, Gold J, Landy R: The histiocytoid hemangiomas. A unifying concept embracing several previously described entities of skin, soft tissue, large vessels, bone, and heart. Hum Pathol **10**:707-730, 1979.

228b Schajowicz F, Aiello CL, Francone MV, Giannini RE: Cystic angiomatosis (hamartous haemolymphangiomatosis) of bone. A clinicopathological study of three cases. J Bone Joint Surg [Br] **60**:100-106, 1978.

229 Spjut HJ, Lindbom Å: Skeletal angiomatosis. Report of two cases, Acta Pathol Microbiol Scand **55**:49-58, 1962.

230 Steiner GC, Dorfman HD: Ultrastructure of hemangioendothelial sarcoma of bone. Cancer **29**:122-135, 1972.

231 Töpfer DI: Ueber ein infiltrierend wachsendes Hämangiom der Haut und multiple Kapillarektasien der Haut und innergen Organe. II. Zur Kenntnis der Wirbelangiome. Frankfurt Z Pathol **36**:337-345, 1928.

232 Unni KK, Ivins JC, Beabout JW, Dahlin DC: Hemangioma, hemangiopericytoma, and hemangioendothelioma (angiosarcoma) of bone. Cancer **27**:1403-1414, 1971.

Other connective tissue tumors

232a Angervall L, Berlin Ö, Kindblom L-G, Stener B: Primary leiomyosarcoma of bone: a study of five cases. Cancer **46**:1270-1279, 1980.

233 Chen TK: Multiple fibroxanthosarcoma of bone. Cancer **42**:770-773, 1978.

234 Cunningham MP, Arlen M: Medullary fibrosarcoma of bone. Cancer **21**:31-37, 1968.

235 Dahlin DC, Ivins JC: Fibrosarcoma of bone. A study of 114 cases. Cancer **23**:35-41, 1969.

236 Dahlin DC, Unni KK, Matsuno T: Malignant (fibrous) histiocytoma of bone—fact or fancy? Cancer **39**:1508-1516, 1977.

237 Gilmer WS Jr, MacEwen GD: Central (medullary) fibrosarcoma of bone. J Bone Joint Surg [Am] **40**:121-141, 1958.

238 Hernandez FJ, Fernandez BB: Multiple diffuse fibrosarcoma of bone. Cancer **37**:939-945, 1976.

239 Huvos AG, Higinbotham NL: Primary fibrosarcoma of bone. A clinicopathologic study of 130 patients. Cancer **35**:837-847, 1975.

240 Kahn LB, Webber B, Mills E, Anstey L, Heselson NG: Malignant fibrous histiocytoma (malignant fibrous xanthoma: Xanthosarcoma) of bone. Cancer **42**:640-651, 1978.

240a Lagacé R, Bouchard H-Ls, Delage C, Seemayer TA: Desmoplastic fibroma of bone. An ultrastructural study. Am J Surg Pathol **3**:423-430, 1979.

240b Mandard JC, Mandard AM, Le Gal Y: Les liposarcomes primitifs de l'os. A propos de 5 cas revue de la littérature. Ann Anat Pathol (Paris) **18**:329-346, 1973.

241 McCarthy EF, Matsuno T, Dorfman HD: Malignant fibrous histiocytoma of bone: a study of 35 cases. Hum Pathol **10**:57-70, 1979.

242 McLeod JJ, Dahlin DC, Ivins JC: Fibrosarcoma of bone. Am J Surg **94**:431-437, 1957.

243 Overgaard J, Frederiksen P, Helmig O, Jensen OM: Primary leiomyosarcoma of bone. Cancer **39**:1664-1671, 1977.

244 Rabhan WN, Rosai J: Desmoplastic fibroma. Report of ten cases and review of the literature. J Bone Joint Surg [Am] **50**:487-502, 1968.

245 Spanier SS, Enneking WF, Enriquez P: Primary malignant fibrous histiocytoma of bone. Cancer **36**:2084-2098, 1975.

246 Whitesides TE, Ackerman LV: Desmoplastic fibroma. A report of three cases. J Bone Joint Surg [Am] **42**:1143-1150, 1960.

Other primary tumors
Chordoma

247 Alezais H, Peyron A: Sur l'histogenèse et l'origine des chordomes. C R Acad Sci (Paris) **174**:419-421, 1922.

247a Ariel IM, Verdu C: Chordoma: an analysis of twenty cases treated over a twenty-year span. J Surg Oncol **7**:27-44, 1975.

248 Berard L, Dunet CL, Peyron A: Les chordomes de la region sarcococcygienne et leur histogenese. Bull Assoc Franc Cancer **11**:28-66, 1922.

248a Campbell WM, McDonald TJ, Unni KK, Laws ER Jr: Nasal and paranasal presentations of chordomas. Laryngoscope **90**:612-618, 1980.

248b Chambers PW, Schwinn CP: Chordoma. A clinicopathologic study of metastasis. Am J Clin Pathol **72**:765-776, 1979.

249 Crawford T: The staining reactions of chordoma. J Clin Pathol **11**:110-113, 1958.

250 Erlandson RA, Tandler B, Lieberman PH, Higinbotham NL: Ultrastructure of human chordoma. Cancer Res **28**:2115-2125, 1968.

251 Gentil F, Coley BL: Sacrococcygeal chordoma. Ann Surg 127:432-455, 1948.
252 Heffelfinger MJ, Dahlin DC, MacCarty CS, Beabout JW: Chordomas and cartilaginous tumors at the skull base. Cancer 32:410-420, 1973.
253 Higinbotham NL, Phillips RF, Farr HW, Hustu O: Chordoma; thirty-five-year study at Memorial Hospital. Cancer 20:1841-1850, 1967.
254 Mabrey RE: Chordoma. Am J Cancer 25:501-517, 1935.
255 Pearlman AW, Friedman M: Radical radiation therapy of chordoma. Am J Roentgenol Radium Ther Nucl Med 108:333-341, 1970.
256 Richter HJ, Batsakis JG, Boles R: Chordomas: nasopharyngeal presentation and atypical long survival. Ann Otol Rhinol Laryngol 84:327-332, 1975.
257 Stewart MJ, Morin JE: Chordoma: a review with report of a new sacrococcygeal case. J Pathol Bacteriol 29:41-60, 1926.

"Adamantinoma" of long bones

258 Albores-Saavedra J, Diaz Gutierrez D, Altamirano Dimas M: Adamantinoma de la tibia. Observaciones ultraestructurales. Rev Med Hosp Gral Mex 31:241-252, 1968.
259 Baker PL, Dockerty MB, Coventry MB: Adamantinoma (so-called) of the long bones. J Bone Joint Surg [Am] 36:704-720, 1954.
260 Cohen DM, Dahlin DC, Pugh DG: Fibrous dysplasia associated with adamantinoma of the long bones. Cancer 15:515-521, 1961.
261 Moon NF: Adamantinoma of the appendicular skeleton. A statistical review of reported cases and inclusion of 10 new cases. Clin Orthop 43:189-213, 1965.
262 Rosai J: Adamantinoma of the tibia. Electron microscopic evidence of its epithelial origin. Am J Clin Pathol 51:786-792, 1969.
263 Schajowicz F, Gallardo H: Adamantinoma de tibia. Revisión bibliográfica y consideración de un nuevo caso. Rev Ortoped Traumatol Lat-Am 12:105-118, 1967.
264 Unni KK, Dahlin DC, Beabout JW, Ivins JC: Adamantinomas of long bones. Cancer 34:1796-1805, 1974.
265 Weiss SW, Dorfman HD: Adamantinoma of long bone. An analysis of nine new cases with emphasis on metastasizing lesions and fibrous dysplasia—like changes. Hum Pathol 8:141-153, 1977.
266 Yoneyama T, Winter WG, Milsow L: Tibial adamantinoma: its histogenesis from ultrastructural studies. Cancer 40:1138-1142, 1977.

Neurogenic tumors

267 Fawcett KJ, Dahlin DC: Neurilemoma of bone. Am J Clin Pathol 47:759-766, 1967.
268 Hunt JC, Pugh DG: Skeletal lesions in nuerofibromatosis. Radiology 76:1-19, 1961.
269 Wirth WA, Bray CB: Intra-osseous neurilemoma. Case report and review of thirty-one cases from the literature. J Bone Joint Surg [Am] 59:252-255, 1977.

Metastatic tumors

270 Caffey J, Andersen DH: Metastatic embryonal rhabdomyosarcoma in the growing skeleton: clinical, radiographic, and microscopic features. Am J Dis Child 95:581-600, 1958.
271 Kahn LB, Wood FW, Ackerman LV: Fracture callus

associated with benign and malignant bone lesions and mimicking osteosarcoma. Am J Clin Pathol 52:14-24, 1969.
272 Norman A, Ulin R: A comparative study of periosteal new-bone response in metastatic bone tumors (solitary) and primary bone sarcomas. Radiology 92:705-708, 1969.
273 Perez CA, Bradfield JS, Morgan HC: Management of pathologic fractures. Cancer 29:1027-1037, 1972.
274 Thomas BM: Three unusual carcinoid tumours, with particular reference to osteoblastic bone metastases. Clin Radiol 19:221-225, 1968.

Laboratory findings

275 Stewart A, Weber FP: Myelomatosis. Q J Med 7:211-228, 1938.

Biopsy and frozen section

275a Broström L-A, Harris MA, Simon MA, Cooperman DR, Nilsonne U: The effect of biopsy on survival of patients with osteosarcoma. J Bone Joint Surg [Br] 61:209-212, 1979.
276 deSantos LA, Murray JA, Ayala AG: The value of percutaneous needle biopsy in the management of primary bone tumors. Cancer 43:735-744, 1979.
277 Ottolenghi CE: Diagnosis of orthopaedic lesions by aspiration biopsy. Results of 1,061 punctures. J Bone Joint Surg [Am] 37:443-464, 1955.
278 Schajowicz F, Derqui JC: Puncture biopsy in lesions of the locomotor system. Review of results in 4,050 cases, including 941 vertebral punctures. Cancer 21:531-548, 1968.
279 Sirsat MV: Interpretation and evaluation of aspiration biopsy in sixty-six cases of bone tumors. J Postgrad Med 2:32-36, 1956.
280 Snyder RE, Coley BL: Further studies on the diagnosis of bone tumors by aspiration biopsy. Surg Gynecol Obstet 80:517-522, 1945.

Tumorlike lesions
Solitary bone cyst

281 Jaffe HL, Lichtenstein L: Solitary unicameral bone cyst. Arch Surg 44:1004-1025, 1942.
282 James AG, Coley BL, Higinbotham NL: Solitary (unicameral) bone cyst. Arch Surg 57:137-147, 1948.
283 von Mikulicz J: Ueber cystische Degeneration der Knochen. Verh Ges Deutsch Naturf Aerzte 76:107, 1906.
284 Pommer G: Zur Kenntnis der progressiven Hämatom- and Phlegmasieveränderungen der Röhrenknochen. Arch Orthop Unfallchir 17:17, 1920.
284a Smith RW, Smith CF: Solitary unicameral bone cyst of the calcaneus. A review of twenty cases. J Bone Joint Surg [Am] 56:49-56, 1974.
285 Stewart MJ, Hamel HA: Solitary bone cyst. South Med J 43:926-936, 1950.

Aneurysmal bone cyst

286 Buraczewski J, Dabska M: Pathogenesis of aneurysmal bone cyst. Relationship between the aneurysmal bone cyst and fibrous dysplasia of bone. Cancer 28:597-604, 1971.
286a Clough JR, Price CHG: Aneurysmal bone cyst: pathogenesis and long term results of treatment. Clin Orthop 97:52-63, 1973.
287 Dabska M, Buraczewski J: Aneurysmal bone cyst. Pathology, clinical course and radiologic appearances. Cancer 23:371-389, 1969.

288 Dahlin DC, Besse BE, Pugh DG, Ghormley RK: Aneurysmal bone cysts. Radiology **64:**56-65, 1955.
289 D'Alonzo RT, Pitcock JA, Milford LW: Giant cell reaction of bone; report of two cases. J Bone Joint Surg [Am] **54:**1267-1271, 1972.
290 Dehner LP, Risdall RJ, L'Heureux P: Giant cell containing "fibrous" lesion of the sacrum. Am J Surg Pathol **2:**55-70, 1978.
291 Edling NPG: Is the aneurysmal bone cyst a true entity? Cancer **18:**1127-1130, 1965.
291a Koskinen EVS, Visuri TI, Holmström T, Roukkula MA: Aneurysmal bone cyst. Evaluation of resection and of curettage in 20 cases. Clin Orthop **118:**136-146, 1976.
291b Levy WM, Miller AS, Bonakdarpour A, Aegerter E: Aneurysmal bone cyst secondary to other osseous lesions. Report of 57 cases. Am J Clin Pathol **63:**1-8, 1975.
292 Lichtenstein L: Aneurysmal bone cyst. Observations on fifty cases. J Bone Joint Surg [Am] **39:**873-882, 1957.
292a McCarthy EF, Dorfman HD: Vascular and cartilaginous hamartoma of the ribs in infancy with secondary aneurysmal bone cyst formation. Am J Surg Pathol **4:**247-253, 1980.
293 Ruiter DJ, van Rijssel ThG, van der Velde EA: Aneurysmal bone cysts. A clinicopathological study of 105 cases. Cancer **39:**2231-2239, 1977.
294 Tillman BP, Dahlin DC, Lipscomb PR, Stewart JR: Aneurysmal bone cyst: an analysis of 95 cases. Mayo Clin Proc **43:**478-495, 1968.

Ganglion cyst of bone

295 Schajowicz F, Sainz MC, Slullitel JA: Juxta-articular bone cysts (intra-osseous ganglia). J Bone Joint Surg [Br] **61:**107-116, 1979.
296 Sim FH, Dahlin DC: Ganglion cysts of bone. Mayo Clin Proc **46:**484-488, 1971.

Metaphyseal fibrous defect (nonossifying fibroma)

297 Cunningham JB, Ackerman LV: Metaphyseal fibrous defects. J Bone Joint Surg [Am] **38:**797-808, 1956.
298 Hatcher CH: Pathogenesis of localized fibrous lesion in the metaphyses of long bones. Ann Surg **122:**1016-1030, 1945.
299 Jaffe HL, Lichtenstein L: Nonosteogenic fibroma of bone. Am J Pathol **18:**205-221, 1942.
300 Ponsettl IV, Friedman B: Evolution of metaphyseal fibrous defects. J Bone Joint Surg [Am] **31:**582-585, 1949.

Fibrous dysplasia

301 Albright F, Butler AM, Hampton AO, Smith P: Syndrome characterized by osteitis fibrosa disseminata, areas of pigmentation and endocrine dysfunction with precocious puberty in females. N Engl J Med **216:**727-746, 1937.
302 Campanacci M: Osteofibrous dysplasia of long bones. A new clinical entity. Ital J Orthopaed Traumatol **2:**221-237, 1976.
303 Harris WH, Dudley HR, Barry RJ: The natural history of fibrous dysplasia. J Bone Joint Surg [Am] **44:**207-233, 1962.
304 Huvos AG, Higinbotham NL, Miller TR: Bone sarcomas arising in fibrous dysplasia. J Bone Joint Surg [Am] **54:**1047-1056, 1972.

305 Kempson RL: Ossifying fibroma of the long bones. Arch Pathol **82:**218-233, 1966.
306 Lichtenstein L: Polyostotic fibrous dysplasia. Arch Surg **36:**874-898, 1938.
307 Lichtenstein L, Jaffe HL: Fibrous dysplasia of bone. Arch Pathol **33:**777-816, 1942 (extensive bibliography).
307a Pelzmann KS, Nagel DZ, Salyer WR: Case report 114: Polyostotic fibrous dysplasia and fibrochondrodysplasia. Skeletal Radiol **5:**116-118, 1980.
308 Reed RJ: Fibrous dysplasia of bone. A review of 25 cases. Arch Pathol **75:**480-495, 1963.
309 Schlumberger HG: Fibrous dysplasia of single bones (monostotic fibrous dysplasia). Milit Surg **99:**504-527, 1946.

Myositis ossificans

310 Ackerman LV: Extraosseous localized nonneoplastic bone and cartilage formation (so-called myostitis ossificans). J Bone Joint Surg [Am] **40:**279-298, 1958.
311 Fine G, Stout AP: Osteogenic sarcoma of the extraskeletal soft tissues. Cancer **9:**1027-1043, 1956.
312 Lewis D: Myositis ossificans. JAMA **80:**1281-1287, 1923.
312a Povýšil C, Matějovský Z: Ultrastructural evidence of myofibroblasts in pseudomalignant myositis ossificans. Virchows Arch [Pathol Anat] **381:**189-203, 1979.
313 Strauss: Cited by Lewis D: Myositis ossificans. JAMA **80:**1281-1287, 1923.
313a Yaghmai I: Myositis ossificans: diagnostic value of arteriography. AJR **128:**811-816, 1977.

Histiocytosis X (eosinophilic granuloma, Hand-Schüller-Christian disease, and Letterer-Siwe disease)

314 Basset F, Escaig J, LeCrom M: A cytoplasmic membranous complex in histiocytosis X. Cancer **29:**1380-1386, 1972.
315 Daneshbod K, Kissane JM: Histiocytosis. The prognosis of polyostotic eosinophilic granuloma. Am J Clin Pathol **65:**601-611, 1976.
316 Green WT, Farber S: "Eosinophilic or solitary granuloma" of bone. J Bone Joint Surg **24:**499-526, 1942.
317 Hatcher CH: Eosinophilic granuloma of bone. Arch Pathol **30:**828-829, 1940.
318 Jaffe HL, Lichtenstein L: Eosinophilic granuloma of bone. Arch Pathol **37:**99-118, 1944 (extensive bibliography).
319 Lieberman PH, Jones CR, Dargeon HWK, Begg CF: A reappraisal of eosinophilic granuloma of bone, Hand-Schüller-Christian syndrome and Letterer-Siwe syndrome. Medicine (Baltimore) **48:**375-400, 1969.
320 McGavran MH, Spady HA: Eosinophilic granuloma of bone. A study of 28 cases. J Bone Joint Surg [Am] **42:**979-992, 1960.
321 Nezelof C, Basset F, Rousseau MF: Histiocytosis X. Histogenetic arguments for a Langerhans cell origin. Biomed **18:**365-371, 1973.
321a Nezelof C, Frileux-Herbet F, Cronier-Sachot J: Disseminated histiocytosis X. Analysis of prognostic factors based on a retrospective study of 50 cases. Cancer **44:**1824-1838, 1979.
322 Newton WA, Hamoudi AB: Histiocytosis: a histologic classification with clinical correlation. Persp Ped Pathol **1:**251-283, 1973.
323 Otani S, Ehrlich JC: Solitary granuloma of bone

simulating primary neoplasm. Am J Pathol **16**:479-490, 1940.

Articular and periarticular diseases
Ganglia; cystic meniscus

324 Doyle RW: Ganglia and superficial tumours. Practitioner **156**:267-277, 1946.
325 Fisk GR: Bone concavity caused by a ganglion. J Bone Joint Surg [Br] **31**:220-221, 1949.
326 Lichtenstein L: Tumors of synovial joints, bursae, and tendon sheaths. Cancer **8**:816-830, 1955.
327 McEvedy BV: Simple ganglia. Br J Surg **49**:585-594, 1962.
328 Stack RE, Bianco AH Jr, MacCarthy CS: Compression of the common peroneal nerve by ganglion cyst. Report of nine cases. J Bone Joint Surg [Am] **47**:773-778, 1965.

Bursae; Baker's cyst

329 Meyerding HW, Van Denmark RE: Posterior hernia of the knee. JAMA **122**:858-861, 1943.
330 Pederson HE, Key JA: Pathology of calcareous tendinitis and subdeltoid bursitis. Arch Surg **62**:50-63, 1951.
331 Wagner T, Abgarowicz T: Microscopic appearance of Baker's cyst in cases of rheumatoid arthritis. Rheumatologia **8**:21-26, 1970.

Carpal tunnel syndrome

332 Bastian FO: Amloidosis and the carpal tunnel syndrome. Am J Clin Pathol **61**:711-717, 1974.
333 Entin MA: Carpal tunnel syndrome and its variants. Surg Clin North Am **48**:1097-1112, 1968.
334 Phalen GS: The carpal-tunnel syndrome: seventeen years' experience in diagnosis and treatment of six hundred, fifty-four hands. J Bone Joint Surg [Am] **48**:211-228, 1966.

Fibrous histiocytoma of tendon sheath (nodular tenosynovitis)

335 Alguacil-Garcia A, Unni KK, Goellner JR: Giant cell tumor of tendon sheath and pigmented villonodular synovitis. An ultrastructural study. Am J Clin Pathol **69**:6-17, 1978.
335a Chung EB, Enzinger FM: Fibroma of tendon sheath. Cancer **44**:1945-1954, 1979.
336 Jaffe HL, Lichtenstein L, Sutro CJ: Pigmented villonodular synovitis, bursitis, and tenosynovitis. Arch Pathol **31**:731-765, 1941.
337 Wright CJE: Benign giant cell synovioma. An investigation of 85 cases. Br J Surg **38**:257-271, 1951.

Pigmented villonodular synovitis and bursitis

338 Atmore WG, Dahlin DC, Ghormley RK: Pigmented villonodular synovitis. A clinical and pathologic study. Minn Med **39**:196-202, 1956.
339 Byers PD, Cotton RE, Deacon OW, Lowy M, Newman PH, Sissons HA, Thomson AD: The diagnosis and treatment of pigmented villonodular synovitis. J Bone Joint Surg [Br] **50**:290-305, 1968.
340 Greenfield MM, Wallace KM: Pigmented villonodular synovitis. Radiology **54**:350-356, 1950.
340a Myers BW, Masi AT: Pigmented villonodular synovitis and tenosynovitis: a clinical epidemiologic study of 166 cases and literature review. Medicine **59**:223-238, 1980.

341 Nilsonne U, Moberger G: Pigmented villonodular synovitis of joints. Histological and clinical problems in diagnosis. Acta Orthop Scand **40**:448-460, 1969.
342 Scott FM: Bone lesions in pigmented villonodular synovitis. J Bone Joint Surg [Br] **50**:306-311, 1968.

Synovial osteochondromatosis and chondrosarcoma

343 Goldman RL, Lichtenstein L: Synovial chondrosarcoma. Cancer **12**:1233-1240, 1964.
344 King JW, Spjut HJ, Fechner RE, Vanderpool DW: Synovial chondrosarcoma of the knee joint. J Bone Joint Surg [Am] **49**:1389-1396, 1967.
344a Milgram JW: Synovial osteochondromatosis. A histopathological study of thirty cases. J Bone Joint Surg [Am] **59**:792-801, 1977.
345 Murphy FP, Dahlin DC, Sullivan CR: Articular synovial chondromatosis. J Bone Joint Surg [Am] **44**:77-86, 1962.
345a Villacin AB, Brigham LN, Bullough PG: Primary and secondary synovial chondrometaplasia. Histopathologic and clinicoradiologic differences. Hum Pathol **10**:439-451, 1979.

Arthritis
Synovial biopsy

346 Goldenberg DL, Cohen AS: Synovial membrane histopathology in the differential diagnosis of rheumatoid arthritis, gout, pseudogout, systemic lupus erythematosus, infectious arthritis and degenerative joint disease. Medicine **57**:239-252, 1978.
347 Polley HF, Bickel WH: Experiences with an instrument for punch biopsy of synovial membrane. Mayo Clin Proc **26**:273-281, 1951.
348 Rodnan GP, Yunis EJ, Totten RS: Experience with punch biopsy of synovium in the study of joint disease. Ann Intern Med **53**:319-331, 1960.
349 Schumacher HR, Kulka JP: Needle biopsy of the synovial membrane; experience with the Parker-Pearson technic. N Engl J Med **286**:416-419, 1972.
350 Schwartz S, Cooper N: Synovial membrane punch biopsy. Arch Intern Med **108**:400-406, 1961.
351 Soren A: Histodiagnosis and clinical correlation of rheumatoid and other synovitis. Philadelphia, 1978, J. B. Lippincott Co.
352 Zevely HA, French AJ, Mikkelsen WM, Duff IF: Synovial specimens obtained by knee joint punch biopsy. Histologic study in joint diseases. Am J Med **20**:510-519, 1956.

Degenerative joint disease (osteoarthritis)

353 Bauer W, Bennett GA: Experimental and pathological studies in the degenerative type of arthritis. J Bone Joint Surg **18**:1-18, 1936.
354 Bennett GA, Waine H, Bauer W: Changes in the knee joint at various ages. New York, 1942, Commonwealth Fund.
355 Collins DH: The pathology of articular and spinal diseases. London, 1949, Edward Arnold & Co. (an excellent reference book).
356 Collins DH: Recent advances in the pathology of chronic arthritis and rheumatic disorders. Postgrad Med J **31**:602-608, 1955.
357 Haliburton RA, Sullivan CR: The patella in degenerative joint disease. A clinicopathologic study. Arch Surg **77**:677-683, 1958.

358 Harrison MHM, Schajowicz F, Tureta J: Osteoarthritis of the hip: a study of the nature and evolution of the disease. J Bone Joint Surg [Br] 35:598-626, 1953.

359 Hirsch C, Schajowicz F, Galante J: Structural changes in the cervical spine. A study on autopsy specimens in different age groups. Acta Orthop Scand [Suppl] 109:7-77, 1967.

360 Horwitz T: Bone and cartilage debris in the synovial membrane. Its significance in the early diagnosis of neuro-arthropathy. J Bone Joint Surg [Am] 30:579-588, 1948.

361 Jayson MI, Rubenstein D, Dixon AS: Intra-articular pressure and rheumatoid geodes (bone 'cysts'). Ann Rheum Dis 29:496-502, 1970.

362 Karlson S: Chondromalacia patellae. Acta Chir Scand 83:347-381, 1940.

363 Keefer C: The etiology of chronic arthritis. N Engl J Med 213:644-653, 1935.

364 Mankin HJ: The reaction of articular cartilage to injury and osteoarthritis. N Engl J Med 291:1285-1292, 1335-1340, 1974.

365 Matthews BF: Composition of articular cartilage in osteoarthritis. Changes in collagen/chondroitin-sulphate ratio. Br Med J 2:660-661, 1953.

366 Nichols EH, Richardson FL: Arthritis deformans. J Med Res 16:149-221, 1909.

367 Norman A, Robbins H, Milgram JE: The acute neuropathic arthropathy. A rapid, severely disorganizing form of arthritis. Radiology 90:1159-1164, 1968.

368 Outerbridge RE: The etiology of chondromalacia patellae. J Bone Joint Surg [Br] 43:752-757, 1961.

369 Rhaney K, Lamb DW: The cysts of osteoarthritis of the hip. A radiological and pathological study. J Bone Joint Surg [Br] 37:663-675, 1955.

370 Silverberg M, Frank EL, Jarrett SR, Silberberg R: Aging and osteoarthritis of the human sternoclavicular joint. Am J Pathol 35:851-865, 1959.

370a Sokoloff L: Pathology and pathogenesis of osteoarthritis. In McCarty DJ (ed): Arthritis and applied conditions, ed. 9. Philadelphia, 1979, Lea & Febiger, pp. 1135-1153.

Rheumatoid arthritis

371 Allison N, Ghormley RK: Diagnosis in joint disease. A clinical and pathological study of arthritis. New York, 1931, William Wood & Co.

372 Baggenstoss AH, Rosenberg EF: Cardiac lesions in chronic infections (rheumatoid) arthritis. Am J Pathol 16:693-695, 1940.

373 Beatty EC Jr: Rheumatic-like nodules occurring in nonrheumatic children. Arch Pathol 68:154-159, 1959.

374 Bennett GA, Zeller JW, Bauer W: Subcutaneous nodules of rheumatoid arthritis and rheumatic fever. Arch Pathol 30:70-89, 1940.

375 Berardinelli JL, Hyman CJ, Campbell EE, Fireman P: Presence of rheumatoid factor in ten children with isolated rheumatoid-like nodules. J Pediatr 81:751-757, 1972.

376 Bevans M, Nadell J, Dmartius F, Ragan C: The systemic lesions of malignant arthritis. Am J Med 16:197-211, 1954.

377 Bhan AK, Roy S: Synovial giant cells in rheumatoid arthritis and other joint diseases. Ann Rheum Dis 30:294-298, 1971.

378 Cooper NS: Pathology of rheumatoid arthritis. Med Clin North Am 52:607-621, 1968.

379 Dixon AStJ, Grant C: Acute synovial rupture in rheumatoid arthritis. Clinical and experimental observations. Lancet 1:742-745, 1964.

380 Freund HA, Steiner G, Leichtentritt B, Price AE: Peripheral nerves in chronic atrophic arthritis. Am J Pathol 18:865-893, 1942.

381 Grimley PM, Sokoloff L: Synovial giant cells in rheumatoid arthritis. Am J Pathol 49:931-954, 1966.

382 Hahn BH, Yardley JH, Stevens MB: "Rheumatoid" nodules in systemic lupus erythematosus. Ann Intern Med 72:49-58, 1970.

383 Hart FD: Rheumatoid arthritis: extra-articular manifestations. Br Med J 3:131-136, 1969.

384 Hart FD: Rheumatoid arthritis: extra-articular manifestations. Part II. Br Med J 2:747-752, 1970.

385 Horwitz T: Bone and cartilage debris in the synovial membrane. Its significance in the early diagnosis of neuro-arthropathy. J Bone Joint Surg [Am] 30:579-588, 1948.

386 Jayson MI, Dixon AS, Kates A, Pinder I, Coomes EN: Popliteal and calf cysts in rheumatoid arthritis. Treatment by anterior synovectomy. Ann Rheum Dis 31:9-15, 1972.

387 Kellgren JH: Some concepts of rheumatic disease. Br Med J 1:1152-1157, 1952.

388 Luck JV: Bone and joint diseases. Springfield, Ill., 1950, Charles C Thomas, Publisher.

389 Mitchell N, Shepard N: The ultrastructure of articular cartilage in rheumatoid arthritis. A preliminary report. J Bone Joint Surg [Am] 52:1405-1423, 1970.

390 Mongan ES, Cass RM, Jacox RF, Vaughan JH: A study of the relation of seronegative and seropositive rheumatoid arthritis to each other and to necrotizing vasculitis. Am J Med 47:23-25, 1969.

391 Muirden KD: Giant cells, cartilage and bone fragments within rheumatoid synovial membrane. Clinicopathological correlations. Aust Ann Med 2:105-110, 1970.

392 Palmer DG: Synovial cysts in rheumatoid disease. Ann Intern Med 70:61-68, 1969.

393 Pirani CR, Bennett GA: Rheumatoid arthritis: a report of three cases progressing from childhood and emphasizing certain systemic manifestations. Bull Hosp Joint Dis 12:335-367, 1951.

394 Roberts WC, Kehol JA, Carpenter DF, Golden A: Cardiac valvular lesions in rheumatoid arthritis. Arch Intern Med 122:141-146, 1968.

395 Schmid FR, Cooper NS, Ziff M, McEwen C: Arteritis in rheumatoid arthritis. Am J Med 30:56-83, 1961.

396 Sherman MS: The non-specificity of synovial reactions. Bull Hosp Joint Dis 12:335-367, 1951.

397 Sokoloff L: Biopsy in rheumatic diseases. Med Clin North Am 45:1171-1180, 1961.

397a Sokoloff L: Pathology of rheumatoid arthritis and allied disorders. In McCarty DJ (ed): Arthritis and applied conditions, ed. 9. Philadelphia, 1979, Lea & Febiger, pp. 429-447.

398 Sokoloff L, Wilens SL, Bunim JJ: Arthritis of striated muscle in rheumatoid arthritis. Am J Pathol 27:157-173, 1951.

399 Taylor RT, Huskisson EC, Whitehouse GH, Hart FD: Spontaneous fractures of pelvis in rheumatoid arthritis. Br Med J 4:663-664, 1971.

400 Weissmann G: Lysosomal mechanisms of tissue injury in arthritis. N Engl J Med 286:141-146, 1972.

Gout

401 Appleby EC: Some cases of gout in reptiles. J Pathol Bacteriol **80:**427-430, 1960.

402 Chaplin AJ: Calcium pryophosphate. Histological characterization of crystals in pseudogout. Arch Pathol Lab Med **100:**12-15, 1976.

403 deGalantha E: Technic for preservation and microscopic demonstration of nodules in gout. Am J Clin Pathol **5:**165-166, 1935.

404 Lichtenstein L, Scott HW, Levin MH: Pathologic changes in gout—survey of eleven necropsied cases. Am J Pathol **32:**871-895, 1956.

405 Moskowitz RW, Katz D: Chondrocalcinosis and chondrocalsynovitis (pseudo-gout syndrome). Analysis of 24 cases. Am J Med **43:**322-334, 1967.

Other articular and periarticular diseases

406 Goldenberg DL, Cohen AS: Synovial membrane histopathology in the differential diagnosis of rheumatoid arthritis, gout, pseudogout, systemic lupus erythematosus, infectious arthritis and degenerative joint disease. Medicine (Baltimore) **57:**239-252, 1978.

407 Rodnan GP, Medsger TA: The rheumatic manifestations of progressive systemic sclerosis (scleroderma). Clin Orthop **57:**81-93, 1968.

24 Soft tissues

Infections

Infections of subcutaneous tissues occur secondary to cutaneous, visceral, or osseous infections and trauma or as a complication of operations. Rarely, such infections may be hematogenous.

The severity of the inflammatory reaction and the type of tissue response observed pathologically depend upon the type, dose, and virulence of the infecting organism, the resistance of the host tissues, the presence or absence of necrotic tissue, hematoma, foreign body, and the anatomy of the infected area.

Clinical types of infectious processes such as hemolytic streptococcal gangrene, necrotizing fasciitis, and Meleney's synergistic gangrene must be diagnosed by clinical appearance and bacteriologic study. All advanced pyogenic and necrotizing infections produce acute inflammatory tissue reactions indistinguishable microscopically. However, in some instances the diagnosis of granulomatous infection may be made by proper staining and careful search of tissue sections for characteristic organisms (such as actinomycosis, blastomycosis, coccidioidomycosis, and sporotrichosis).

Tuberculosis also may be suspected histologically, but proof of the significance of the occasional acid-fast bacillus seen in tissue sections rests with culture and guinea pig inoculation. Certain granulomatous and chronic pyogenic infections, as well as encysted hematomas, mimic soft tissue tumors[1,2] (Fig. 1319).

Pilonidal disease

Pilonidal sinuses appear as small openings in the intergluteal fold about 3.5 cm to 5 cm posterior to the anal orifice. Hairs are sometimes

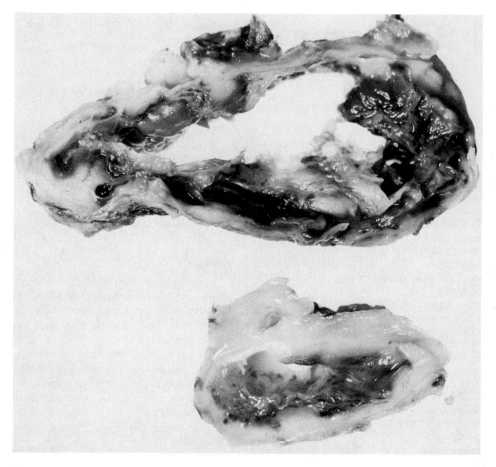

Fig. 1319 Cystic hematoma of left scapular region excised from 45-year-old black woman two weeks following injury. (WU neg. 55-4576.)

seen protruding from them. The opening is continued by a sinus tract, which is directed upward in 93% of the cases.[5] The disease is most often seen in young white males with dark, straight hair. Although congenital anomalies related to the closure of the neural canal can certainly occur in this area, it is now believed that the large majority of pilonidal sinuses have an acquired pathogenesis.[4] Hairs penetrate areas of inflammation from without, lodge in the dermis, and elicit a foreign body type of reaction (Fig. 1320). The sinus is lined by granulation tissue. In approximately 25% of the cases, hairs are not found within the lesion.

Pilonidal sinuses also have been described in other areas where skin folds are prominent, such as the axilla, umbilicus, clitoris, and axilla.[3] A further observation favoring the theory of the acquired origin is the fact that barbers and hairdressers occasionally develop a disease equivalent to pilonidal sinus between their fingers, the sinuses containing somebody else's hairs!

Tumors
Introduction

The tumors of the soft tissue are a large heterogeneous group.[8] A marked difference in age distribution is seen among the different microscopic types. As a whole, a large proportion of soft tissue sarcomas affects children[7] and may even be present at birth. Kauffman and Stout[6] remarked that congenital soft tissue tumors rarely behave malignantly, even when this behavior was to be expected from their microscopic appearance. The most common soft tissue sarcomas are liposarcoma and malignant fibrous histiocytoma in adults and rhabdomyosarcoma in children. These tumors often are badly treated. Such poor treatment is caused

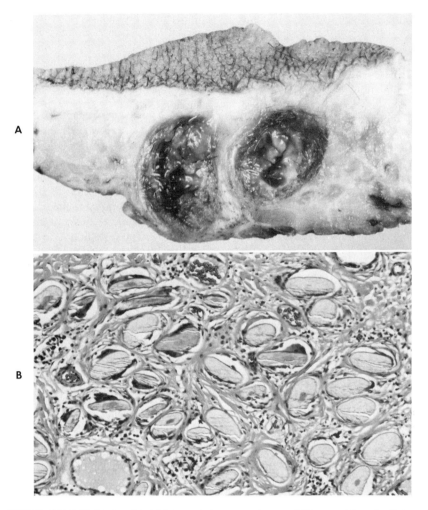

Fig. 1320 A, Pilonidal sinus removed from sacrococcygeal area of 19-year-old youth. Hair-containing cystic structures in dermis are characteristic. They communicated with each other in another plane of section. **B,** Microscopic appearance of pilonidal disease. Numerous hair shafts penetrate into dermis and elicit foreign body giant cell reaction. (**A,** WU neg. 73,1477; **B,** ×100; WU neg. 73-2073.)

by ignorance of their natural history as it relates to their pathology.

The soft tissue lesions discussed herewith exclude those of the mediastinum, retroperitoneum, and soft tissues of the visceral organs and those primarily involving the dermis, such as Kaposi's sarcoma and mycosis fungoides.

Etiology

Much has been written in the medical and legal literature on the possible relationship between trauma and soft tissue sarcoma; suffice it to say, no convincing evidence has been provided as to a definite cause-to-effect relationship between the two.[11] Individuals sub-jected to repeated serious trauma (such as football players) do not have an increased incidence of soft tissue tumors. In the overwhelming majority of the cases in which a relation between tumor and trauma seems to exist, careful review of the evidence and doubling rates studies will show that the tumor antedated the trauma and that the latter simply called the attention of the patient to its presence (so called traumatic determinism).

The large majority of soft tissue sarcomas arise *de novo* rather than from malignant degeneration of preexisting benign tumors. Although the latter phenomenon may occur (as in neurofibromas), in most cases in which a given benign tumor is said to have become malignant, review of the original material will show that it was malignant from its inception.

Convincing evidence has accumulated that a variety of soft tissue sarcoma can arise as a complication of radiation therapy.[9] Over 200 such cases are now in record, twenty-four of them following irradiation of breast carcinoma.[10] Fibrosarcomas, malignant fibrous histiocytomas, and soft tissue osteosarcomas are the most common types. The average latent period is about ten years, and the prognosis is poor.

Diagnosis and therapy

The relatively untrained surgeon confronted by a soft tissue mass boldly excises or enucleates it, invariably inadequately. He is surprised to find it malignant. Because of poor primary treatment, the extent of the corrective operation may result in deformity or sacrifice of an extremity. The proper initial procedure is careful incisional biopsy. After accurate classification of the tumor, it can then be treated intelligently.

Treatment may vary from a conservative surgical excision to a radical procedure such as amputation or disarticulation. For many years it has been thought that amputation was the best therapy for most soft tissues of the extremities. This concept has been challenged on several grounds.[11a] It has been shown for several types of soft tissue sarcomas (such as fibrosarcoma and synovial sarcoma) that a wide local excision offers as good a chance of survival as an amputation, especially if supplemented by other types of therapy. Suit et al.[9] have produced the most promising results along this line by combining limited (even incomplete) surgery with radical dose radiation therapy (6,300-7,000 rads over six and one-half to seven and one-half weeks). By using this technique, they obtained local control of the tumor in 87 of 100 patients during a follow-up of 2-12 years. They found that histologic grade correlated well with incidence of local recurrence and disease-free survival.[15] This has led to the proposal that all soft tissue sarcomas be graded microscopically in addition to being assigned, if possible, to a specific histologic type.[14] This grading is supposedly based on the relative degree of cellularity, pleomorphism, and mitotic activity as opposed to the deposition of extracellular substances, such as collagen or mucosubstances. Although it has been conclusively demonstrated that tumor grading

is of definite prognostic value in some specific types of soft tissue sarcoma (such as fibrosarsoma and liposarcoma), we believe it is too simplistic and even misleading to overemphasize grading independent of the specific microscopic type of the sarcoma and the circumstances in which it occurs. For instance, a "congenital fibrosarcoma" or a superficially located pleomorphic malignant fibrous histiocytoma may both be regarded as Grade III tumors, yet their incidence of metastatic spread is extremely low; conversely, a synovial sarcoma may receive a Grade I classification because of the uniformity of the proliferation and low mitotic count, yet it will usually behave in a fairly aggressive fashion.

Adjuvant chemotherapy has proved of great value for several types of soft tissue sarcomas in children, and there is preliminary evidence that it also may be of benefit in sarcomas of adults.[13]

Biopsy is not dangerous and does not cause metastases. Indeed, incisional biopsy followed by adequate treatment is associated with a lower incidence of local recurrence than is primary excision of the malignant soft tissue tumor when the latter is performed without prior biopsy[12] (Table 67). At the definitive operation, the area of the biopsy should be excised in continuity with the tumor. Occasionally, aspiration or needle biopsy of a soft tissue neoplasm may be diagnostic. We have not hesitated to use frozen section. If a definite diagnosis can be made, the lesion may be treated immediately.

Of course, diagnosis by aspiration biopsy and/or frozen section may not be definitive. In these instances, treatment must be delayed until diagnosis from the permanent tissue sections can be made. The importance of this concept is evident in the following three cases.

A young ballet dancer noted a soft tissue tumor of the popliteal space. If was fairly firm and ap-

Table 67 Clinical evaluation of preliminary biopsy of soft tissue masses*

	Cases	Local recurrences
Without biopsy	27	21 (78.8%)
With biopsy	12	2 (16.6%)
Total	39	23 (59.9%)

*From Lieberman Z, Ackerman LV: Principles in management of soft tissue sarcomas. Surgery 35:350-365, 1954.

peared to be deeply attached. The tumor was not biopsied before its attempted removal. The surgeon found the tumor apparently infiltrating the deeper tissues and amputated the leg. Microscopic examination showed a fibrous tissue tumor of the desmoid type that could have been cured without amputation.

A young male patient with a soft tissue tumor in the region of the upper arm had careful incisional biopsy that showed desmoid tumor. The tumor was excised locally without sacrificing the arm. The patient is alive and well ten years later.

A young male patient had an apparently encapsulated soft tissue tumor on the upper, inner thigh enucleated without biopsy. The lesion was liposarcoma. It quickly recurred locally and required hemipelvectomy to encompass the recurrence. A primary diagnosis by incisional biopsy and a radical local excision might well have saved the lower extremity.

Many malignant soft tissue sarcomas appear grossly to be encapsulated. This encapsulation is false (Fig. 1321). Therefore, attempts to enucleate fail. This pseudoencapsulation occurs often with fibrosarcoma, liposarcoma, leiomyosarcoma, and synovial sarcoma.

The pathologist who studies these lesions should make every attempt to classify them accurately, for this classification has proved extremely useful from the standpoint of treatment and prognosis. He must know the orientation of the specimen and the tissue sections so that he can state with certainty whether or not the lesion was adequately excised.

Special stains may help in the classification of these tumors. Some examples are reticulin stain for vascular tumors and synovial sarcomas, periodic acid–Schiff for alveolar soft part sarcomas (for the demonstration of intracytoplasmic crystals), phosphotungstic acid–hematoxylin or Masson's trichrome for tumors of striated muscle, and mucin stains for synovial sarcomas and myxoid tumors in general. Electron microscopy also can be extremely helpful. Fibroblasts, smooth and striated muscle cells, Schwann's cells, endothelial cells, pericytes, and the cells of granular cell tumor and alveolar soft part sarcoma have distinctive ultrastructural features that often provide a specific diagnosis. Finally, immunohistochemistry for tissue-specific markers (such as myoglobin or Factor VIII) also has proved of value for this purpose.

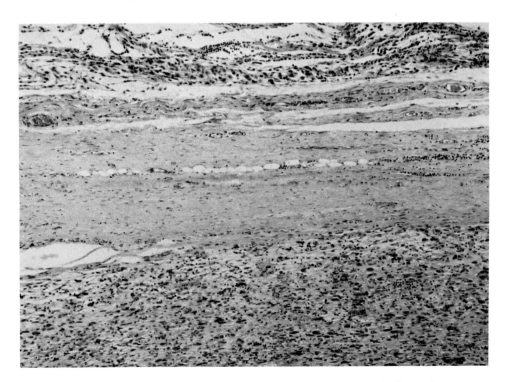

Fig. 1321 Liposarcoma. In center is broad band of connective tissue capsule. Tumor is present on both sides of capsule. Surgeon believed that he had excised neoplasm adequately. However, plane of dissection was close to capsule and through tumor. Therefore, lesion recurred locally. (×90; WU neg. 57-198.)

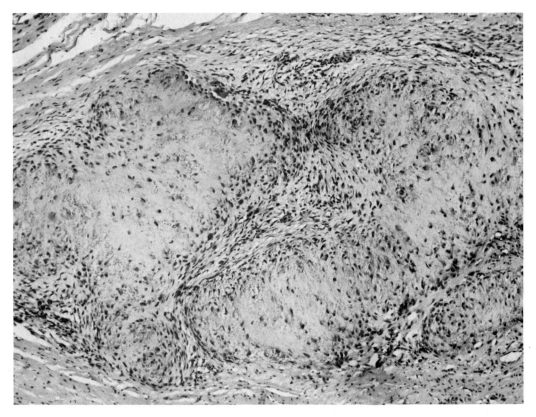

Fig. 1322 Localized nodular type of "juvenile aponeurotic fibroma" in 44-year-old man. It appeared as nodule on dorsal surface of wrist. Proliferating cells are cartilaginous in origin. (×90; WU neg. 67-1167; slide contributed by Dr. C. P. Schwinn, Los Angeles, Calif.)

Tumors and tumorlike conditions of fibrous tissue

Juvenile aponeurotic fibroma

A distinctive microscopic lesion, juvenile aponeurotic fibroma was described by Keasbey[18] in 1953. The classical presentation is that of a soft tissue mass in the hand or wrist of a child or an adolescent. At surgery, it may appear as a nodule or as an ill-defined infiltrating mass in the subcutaneous tissue or attached to a tendon. Sometimes, foci of calcification may be detected on gross inspection.

Microscopically, the lesion is characterized by a diffuse fibroblastic growth in which spotty calcification occurs (Fig. 1322). Infiltration of fat and striated muscle is often seen at the periphery. Mitoses are scarce, and atypical cytologic features are absent. Scattered osteoclast-like giant cells are frequently seen. The cells inside and surrounding the calcified foci have a strong resemblance to chondrocytes. It is this feature that led Lichtenstein and Goldman[19] to postulate that this lesion is basically of cartilaginous origin and that it represents the cartilaginous analogue of fibromatosis. We basically agree with this view.[17]

Juvenile aponeurotic fibroma can be confused with rheumatoid nodule, neurilemoma, and fibromatosis. Local recurrence is common, especially in young children. However, distant metastases do not occur.[16]

Nodular and proliferative fasciitis

The term *nodular fasciitis* is currently accepted for the condition originally designated as subcutaneous pseudosarcomatous fibromatosis.[25] It is a distinctive lesion and a very important one because of its ability to simulate a malignant process.[20] In the past, it was usually mislabeled as fibrosarcoma, liposarcoma, or rhabdomyosarcoma. Individuals in their fourth decade of life are most commonly affected. The most common locations are the upper extremities (particularly the flexor aspect

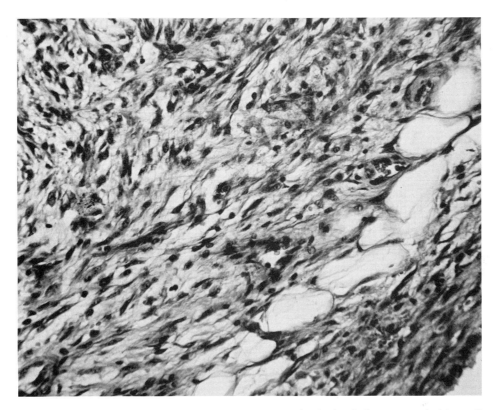

Fig. 1323 Typical nodular fasciitis in 47-year-old woman who had soft tissue mass just beneath skin in deltopectoral group which measured 3 cm × 2 cm × 1 cm and had been present for only two weeks. It is highly cellular and vascular and can easily be confused with fibrosarcoma. It infiltrates on its periphery and may show evidence of maturation. (×250; WU neg. 62-7387.)

of the forearms), trunk, and neck. A specific variant, seen in children and characterized by involvement of the skull with erosion of the underlying cranium, is referred to as *cranial fasciitis of childhood* by Lauer and Enzinger.[25a] Two important clinical features of nodular fasciitis are the history of rapid growth (usually a few weeks) and the small size. It usually extends above the fascia, but it may grow beneath it or be limited to the fascia itself.[26] Like most soft tissue growths of fibrous tissue origin, it has infiltrative margins.

Microscopically, the lesion is characterized by a cellular fibroblastic growth set in a loosely textured mucoid matrix (Fig. 1323). Vascular proliferation and chronic inflammatory cells also are present. Focal metaplastic bone formation may be present, thus establishing a link between nodular fasciitis and myositis ossificans.[22] Occasionally, involvement of the wall and lumen of medium-sized veins and arteries is seen, a change designated as *intravascular fasciitis*.[26a] The high cellularity of the lesion

and the presence of mitotic figures and of occasional cells with bizarre nuclei are responsible for the frequent confusion of this lesion with sarcoma. However, follow-up studies have conclusively shown that it is perfectly benign.[23,24,27] Ultrastructurally, many of the proliferating spindle cells have features of myofibroblasts.[28]

In *proliferative fasciitis*, the location of the lesion, rapidity of growth, and self-limited nature are the same as those of nodular fasciitis, but the presence of large basophilic cells resembling ganglion cells indicates a link with proliferative myositis (see below). Like the latter, it affects adults and follows a benign clinical course.[21]

Focal and proliferative myositis

Focal myositis is a benign inflammatory pseudotumor of skeletal muscle that affects children and adults and typically evolves over a period of a few weeks as a localized painful swelling in the soft tissues.[30] Most cases have

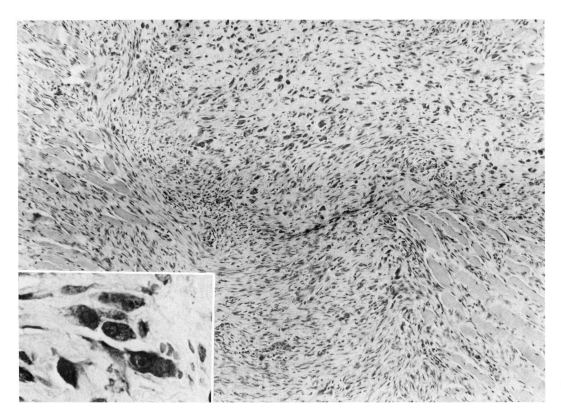

Fig. 1324 Proliferative myositis. A cellular proliferation accompanied by collagen deposition infiltrates skeletal muscle fibers. **Inset,** Large cells with prominent nuclei and nucleoli are present. Some resemble ganglion cells.

occurred in the lower extremities. Both clinically and at operation, the impression is often of a neoplasm. Grossly, the lesion is pale and ill-defined. Microscopically, degeneration and regeneration of muscle fibers are seen in association with interstitial inflammation and fibrosis. The lesion is solitary and self-limited and should be distinguished from polymyositis. Enzyme histochemical and electron microscopic studies suggested that the disease may be the result of a denervation process.[29a]

Proliferative myositis can be confused with sarcoma not only clinically and at surgery, but also microscopically.[31] The skeletal muscles of the shoulder, thorax, and thigh are those most commonly affected. Most patients are over the age of 45 years. Grossly, the lesion does not look like a sarcoma but rather as an ill-defined scarlike induration of the muscle. Microscopically, a cellular proliferation rich in fibroblasts is seen surrounding individual fibers. The hallmark of the lesion is the presence of extremely large basophilic cells with

vesicular nuclei and very prominent nucleolis, closely resembling ganglion cells or rhabdomyoblasts (Fig. 1324). Conservative surgery is curative.[29]

Elastofibroma

Elastofibroma is a benign, poorly circumscribed tumorlike condition involving almost exclusively the subscapular region of elderly individuals, although isolated cases have been seen in the deltoid muscle, hip, and thigh. There is often a history of hard manual labor. At surgery, the lesions usually are found at the apex of the scapula, beneath the rhomboid and latissimus dorsi muscles. The right side is affected more commonly than the left. Bilaterality is not infrequent.

Microscopically, collagen bundles alternate with numerous acidophilic, refractive cylinders often containing a central dense core, both of which stain strongly with elastic stains. Ultrastructurally, the cylinders are made up of immature amorphous elastic tissue, whereas the central core contains mature fibers.[32,34] Elastase digestion fully removes this material.[32] We agree with Järvi et al.[33] that this lesion is not a true neoplasm but rather a degenerative process probably produced by friction of the scapula against the rib cage. Surgery is curative.

Fibromatosis

The generic term *fibromatosis*[35] was proposed by Stout[65] for a group of related conditions having in common the following features:
1 Proliferation of well-differentiated fibroblasts
2 Infiltrative pattern of growth
3 Presence of a variable (but usually abundant) amount of collagen between the proliferating cells
4 Lack of cytologic features of malignancy and scanty or absent mitotic activity
5 Aggressive clinical behavior, characterized by repeated local recurrences, but without the capacity to produce distant metastases

Grossly, these lesions are often large, firm, and whitish, with ill-defined outlines and an irregularly whorled cut surface (Figs. 1325 and 1326). They often arise in a muscular fascia. Microscopically, the fibroblastic nature of the cells is usually quite obvious. However, in some actively proliferating types, the plump nuclei with blunted ends can closely resemble those of smooth muscle cells. In these instances, the use of trichrome stains or electron microscopy can be decisive in the differential diagnosis. In an ultrastructural study of fibromatosis, Welsh[66] described intracytoplasmic collagen formation, probably representing a pathologic process in the course of collagen synthesis. A similar change was detected by Levine et al.[57] in a variety of soft tissue sarcomas, indicating its nonspecificity.

Some pathologists add the adjective *aggressive* to some forms of fibromatosis to emphasize the biologic behavior. We do not use the term, since we regard it as redundant; most fibromatoses are potentially aggressive. Besides, there is very little correlation between the cellularity or other microscopic features of these lesions and their biologic behavior. Other authors have gone even further and have used *differentiated fibrosarcoma* as a synonym for the histologically more cellular or clinically more aggressive types of fibromatosis.[65] We are opposed to this terminology, because the designation of sarcoma endows this

lesion in the mind of many surgeons with a metastasizing potential that is does not possess. Although we recognize the difficulties involved, we always attempt to make a distinction between fibromatosis and well-differentiated fibrosarcoma, reserving the latter term for tumors showing atypical cytologic features and/or a significant number of mitotic figures (more than one per high-power field). As Enzinger[48] remarked, it is usually not possible on the basis of the histologic examination to predict whether or not a fibromatosis will recur, but it is possible to predict whether a fibrous tumor is or is not capable of metastases.

Most soft tissue fibromatoses are in intimate contact with skeletal muscles—hence their designation as *musculoaponeurotic fibromatosis*.[49] This is certainly preferable to the obsolete *desmoid tumor*, traditionally regarded as a neoplasm of the abdominal wall appearing in women during or following pregnancy, although in our experience it is almost as common in men and in other locations, such as the shoulder girdle, head and neck area, and thigh.[43,52,58] Enzinger and Shiraki[49] analyzed thirty cases located in the shoulder girdle that had been followed for a minimum of ten years. In 57% of the patients, the tumor recurred one or more times. However, at the end of the follow-up period, *all patients* were living without any evidence of continuing tumor growth. A higher incidence of recurrence was seen in young individuals and in those patients with tumors of large size.

The treatment of choice is a prompt radical excision, including a wide margin of involved tissue.[43] However, it should not sacrifice major blood vessels, nerves, or an extremity, even if recurrence is thought likely. Recurrences may still be treated by local excision with chance of control. In our experience, the incidence of local recurrence is lower in fibromatoses of the abdominal wall than in those located elsewhere.[52] Some of the latter have recurred as many as five or six times. Only rarely, however, has local aggressiveness forced amputation. Actually, cessation of attempts to excise persistent tissue locally may be followed by failure of the lesion to enlarge further.

The name *juvenile fibromatosis* has often been applied to examples of fibromatosis occurring in children and adolescents[51] (Table 68). Congenital cases also have been reported,

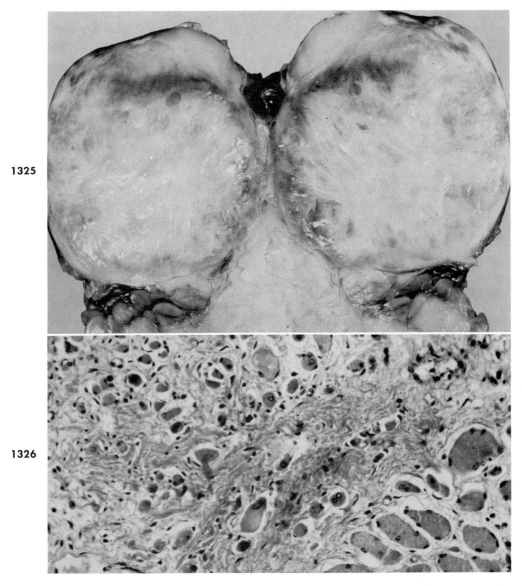

Fig. 1325 Large fibromatosis of abdominal wall. Note lack of circumscription and almost complete replacement of muscle. (WU neg. 50-5320.)
Fig. 1326 Fibromatosis with adult fibrous tissue growing between muscle bundles. (Low power.)

some of them presenting as multiple tumors.[40a] Except for their greater frequency in this age group and, in some specific instances, their greater propensity for local recurrence, there is very little either on clinical or microscopic grounds that differentiates fibromatosis in children from that occurring in other age groups.[47] We know of only two exceptions to this statement—i.e., two variants of fibromatosis apparently restricted to childhood and presenting a distinctive clinicopathologic picture: fibroma-tosis colli (congenital torticollis) and infantile digital fibromatosis.

Fibromatosis colli (congenital torticollis) is a type of fibromatosis affecting the lower third of the sternomastoid muscle and appearing at birth or shortly thereafter. Bilateral forms have been observed. Fibromatosis colli is frequently associated with various congenital anomalies. Thus, Iwahara and Ikeda[54] found congenital (usually ipsilateral) dislocations of the hip in 14% of their patients. An associa-

Table 68 Anatomic sites of fibrous tissue proliferations*

Site	Cases
Hands and feet	20
Neck	15
Shoulder and adjacent areas	14
Buttocks—thigh and leg	12
Scalp	3
Abdominal muscles	2
Ear	1
Eyelid	1
Suprapubic and perineal areas	1
Lung	1
Mesentery	1
Generalized	3

*From Stout AP: Juvenile fibromatoses. Cancer **7**:953-978, 1954.

tion between complicated deliveries (particularly breech deliveries) and fibromatosis colli has been established.[44] Although some instances of spontaneous disappearance have been recorded, this condition usually necessitates resection of the muscle. Microscopically, the cellularity of the fibrous tissue depends upon the age of the process. This condition has been considered due to birth injury, but we have never seen evidence of previous hemorrhage.[41]

The so-called *infantile digital fibromatosis* is also a form of fibromatosis restricted to childhood.[60] The typical location is the exterior surface of the end phalanges of the fingers and toes. The lesions are often multiple and either are present at birth or appear during the first two years of life. The component cells are myofibroblasts.[39] A distinctive microscopic feature, not observed in the other forms of fibromatosis, is the presence of peculilar eosinophilic cytoplasmic inclusions. These have been examined ultrastructurally and found to be composed of compact massses of granules and filaments without a limiting membrane.[37,42] Their significance is obscure, although their similarity with the "virus factories" seen in cells with certain viruses has been remarked. This disease has a high tendency for local recurrence.[61]

Generalized fibromatosis may be present as multiple nodules limited to the superficial soft tissue or be associated with internal organ involvement.[38,62] The latter form, which is usually congenital, can be fatal. Familial cases have been described.[45]

Fibromatosis hyalinica multiplex is a morphologically distinctive type of familial multiple fibromatosis probably resulting from an inborn error of metabolism and characterized microscopically by a conspicuous hyalinization of the connective tissue of the skin, oral cavity, articular capsule, and bone. It affects children but is not present at birth.[53,67]

Some forms of fibromatosis derive their names from their particular location—i.e., *palmar fibromatosis* (Dupuytren's contracture), *plantar fibromatosis* (Ledderhose's disease), and *penile fibromatosis* (Peyronie's disease).[56,63] The latter condition is discussed in Chapter 17. Both palmar and plantar fibromatosis can be extremely cellular.[59,63] We have seen them confused with fibrosarcoma (Fig. 1327). It is well to remember that fibrosarcoma of the palmar and plantar areas is exceptional.[36] The differential diagnosis of a cellular spindle cell tumor of the sole is usually between fibromatosis, synovial sarcoma, malignant melanoma, and Kaposi's sarcoma. The palmar and plantar forms of fibromatosis occur predominantly in adults. Contracture of the fingers or toes is the leading clinical manifestation. In an excellent electron microscopic study, Gabbiani and Majno[50] found nuclear deformations such as are found in contracted cells (retrospectively identified by light microscopy as cross-banded nuclei) and a cytoplasmic fibrillary system similar to that found in smooth muscle cells. They suggested that the proliferating fibroblasts had modulated toward a contractile cell and that this was responsible for the contracture evident clinically. This cell is now known as the myofibroblast, and it has been found to be implicated in a large number of reactive conditions and benign and malignant neoplasms.[46] Multiple lesions involving the palmar as well as the plantar areas are frequently observed. Bilaterality is also common. The plantar form of the disease tends to be more localized than its palmar counterpart.

Fibromatoses also have been named according to the presumed inciting cause, such as *cicatricial fibromatosis* and *postirradiation fibromatosis*. The cicatricial form may follow accidental trauma or arise in the scar of surgical procedures. Postirradiation fibromatosis differs from the other forms by virtue of the common occurrence of bizarre cells with large hyperchromatic nuclei. This feature, which in the absence of radiation exposure would be strong evidence of malignancy, should be inter-

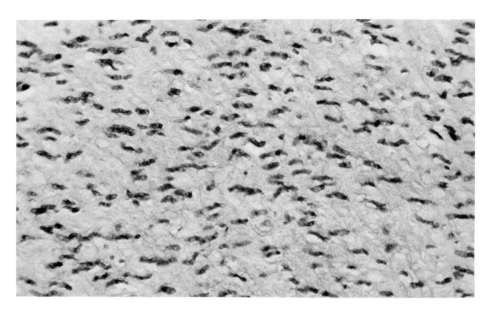

Fig. 1327 Cellular area in plantar fibromatosis, often incorrectly diagnosed as fibrosarcoma. Note uniformity of nuclei. Mitotic figures are exceptional. (×400; WU neg. 52-3448.)

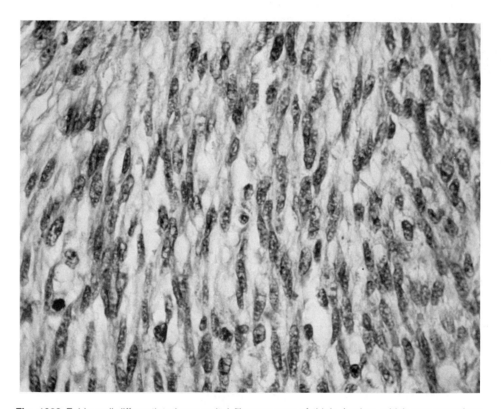

Fig. 1328 Fairly well-differentiated congenital fibrosarcoma of thigh. Lesion, which was pseudoen-capsulated mass, was locally excised and patient is living five years after operation. Patients with such tumor may have an unexpectedly good prognosis. (×600; WU neg. 62-7379.)

preted much more conservatively under these circumstances.

The association of soft tissue tumors, usually of the fibromatosis type, with multiple colonic polyposis and occasionally multiple osteomas is known as *Gardner's syndrome*.[40,64] In this condition, the fibromatosis has a particular tendency to involve intra-abdominal structures, such as omentum and mesentery.[55]

Fibrosarcoma

Fibrosarcomas are commonly tumors of adults, although they can occur in any age group and even present as congenital neoplasms[68,71a,75] (Fig. 1328). They arise from superficial and deep connective tissues such as fascia, tendon, periosteum, and scar, grow slowly or rapidly, and often appear well circumscribed (Fig. 1329). They usually are soft

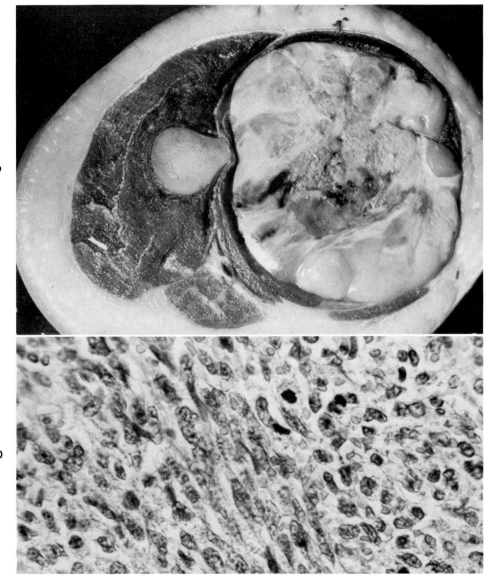

1329

1330

Fig. 1329 Moderately differentiated fibrosarcoma of thigh. Apparent encapsulation is in contrast to lack of circumscription in fibromatosis. (WU neg. 46-2006.)
Fig. 1330 Well-differentiated fibrosarcoma showing fibroblasts with occasional mitotic figures. (×600; WU neg. 52-3454.)

and cellular and may contain areas of necrosis and hemorrhage.

Microscopically, the well-differentiated tumors are easily recognized as fibroblastic (Fig. 1330). The individual cells resemble fibroblasts, and a Wilder stain demonstrates abundant reticulin *wrapped around each cell*.[74] Phosphotungstic acid–hematoxylin demstrates abundant fibroglia fibrils. The fibroblastic nature is more difficult to recognize in the undifferentiated tumors. It should be remembered that many other soft tissue tumors, particularly synovial sarcoma, liposarcoma, malignant fibrous histiocytoma, and malignant schwannoma often contain areas closely resembling fibrosarcoma. Only careful examination of different blocks of the tumor will provide the correct diagnosis in these instances. The presence of tumor giant cells in a malignant soft tissue sarcoma usually means that it is not fibrosarcoma but more probably rhabdomyosarcoma, liposarcoma, or malignant fibrous histiocytoma. Ultrastructurally, most of the tumor cells recapitulate the morphology of normal fibroblasts, whereas others have features of myofibroblasts.[69] The myofibroblast has been defined as a modified fibroblast that has acquired some morphologic and functional features of a smooth muscle cell.[71] It characteristically occurs in areas of active fibroblastic growth, such as healing wounds, nodular fasciitis, and fibromatosis. It also is seen in malignant tumors with fibroblastic differentiation, such as fibrosarcoma and malignant fibrous histiocytoma.[69] It has even been proposed to regard cases in which these cells predominate as an entity under the designation of "myofibroblastic sarcoma"; we seriously doubt whether this is justified and prefer to regard them as a morphologic variation of a fibroblastic growth.

In contrast to the fibromatoses, fibrosarcomas are capable of distant metastases. Generally, the more superficial and differentiated the tumor, the better the prognosis. Increased mitotic activity and marked cellularity (as expressed by a grading system) are associated with an increased incidence of metastases. In two large series,[72,76] fibrosarcomas in children under 5 years of age at the time of diagnosis were shown to have a high recurrence rate but an incidence of distant metastases of only 7%-8%; congenital fibrosarcomas were particularly reluctant to metastasize despite their extreme cellularity, very rapid growth,

and extensive local invasion.[70] Conversely, fibrosarcomas occurring in children 10 years old or older had a metastatic rate close to that of adult patients; i.e., 50%[73] The treatment of choice is radical excision.

Tumors of probable histiocytic origin

There has been in recent years a drastic reappraisal in the interpretation of soft tissue tumors of presumed histiocytic origin, largely initiated by the work of Stout and his colleagues at Columbia-Presbyterian Hospital.[82,90,91,102,107]

Lesions belonging to this category have been regarded by some authors as of reactive nature. We agree with Fisher and Hellstrom[83] that "the recognition that in some instances they may exhibit more aggressive growth, local recurrence and rarely metastasize would appear as ample evidence attesting to their neoplastic nature."[*] They are composed, wholly or in part, of cells with light microscopic, ultrastructural, and tissue cultural characteristics of histiocytes.[84,86a,99,102,103] In addition, many of these tumors exhibit a more or less prominent fibroblastic component. Three hypotheses have been advanced to explain this mixed composition:

1 The tumors originate from primitive mesenchymal cells with a capacity for dual differentiation toward histiocytes and fibroblasts.[77,86]

2 These are tumors of fibroblastic origin, some of the fibroblasts having the capacity to "transform" into histiocytes.

3 These are purely histiocytic neoplasms, some of the histiocytes becoming "facultative fibroblasts," a property also ascribed to Schwann's cells, smooth muscle cells, and other mesenchymal cells.

The first theory is difficult to accept in view of the different histogenetic derivation of fibroblasts and histiocytes. Similarly, there is no good evidence in support of the second hypothesis. The third possibility is the one presently favored,[107] although in our opinion and that of others[108] the interpretation of many of the morphologic and tissue culture data given as supportive evidence[89,104,110] is open to serious questions. For instance, Hashimoto et al.[87] have shown quite convincingly that the cells of

---

*From Fisher ER, Hellstrom HR: Dermatofibrosarcoma with metastases simulating Hodgkin's disease and reticulum cell sarcoma. Cancer **19:**1165-1171, 1966.

dermatofibrosarcoma protuberans often exhibit features suggestive of a neurogenic derivation. The storiform pattern often regarded as indicative of a histiocytic derivation also can appear in a variety of mesenchymal, epithelial, and neural tumors. Patterns indistinguishable from those of malignant fibrous histiocytoma can be seen in otherwise typical mesenchymal tumors of various well-defined types. The enzyme *lysozyme*, a very sensitive marker for histiocytes, has been absent in tumors of this type that we have examined. There is no question that if one were to apply the rigid criteria presently required to prove that a given malignant lymphoma is of histiocytic origin, none of the soft tissue tumors described in this section would pass the test.

Having expressed these reservations about the whole concept of soft tissue tumors of histiocytic origin, we will proceed to describe them using the current terminology for the sake of consistency (Table 69). Tumors in which most or all of the cells have the appearance of histiocytes and in which the fibroblastic-like component is meager or absent are designated as *histiocytomas.* Tumors having a conspicuous fibroblastic element in addition to the histiocytes are referred to as *fibrous histiocytomas (fibrous xanthomas).*[98] The name of *pleomorphic fibrous histiocytoma (pleomorphic fibrous xanthomas)* is proposed for a variant of the latter in which mononucleated or multinucleated bizzare cells of malignant appearance are added to the histiocytic and fibroblastic background.

Approximately twenty "entities" described in the literature can be made to fit into one or another of these three major categories. It should be noted that the only criteria used for this classification are the presence or absence of a fibroblastic-like component and the presence or absence of bizarre atypical cells. Foamy cells, multinucleated cells of innocuous cytologic appearance (Touton's giant cells, osteoclast-like cells, etc.), fibrosis, and hemosiderin are not significant in this regard. We prefer the designation "histiocytoma" over that of "xanthoma," since the term "xanthoma" merely refers to the morphologic appearance resulting from accumulation of cytoplasmic fat, which

Table 69 Classification of soft tissue tumors of probable histiocytic origin

Type	Biologic behavior	Lesions included in this category
Histiocytoma	Benign	Juvenile xanthogranuloma (nevoxanthoendothelioma; nevoid histiocytoma) Reticulohistiocytoma (reticulohistiocytic granuloma; multicentric reticulohistiocytosis; lipoid dermatoarthritis) Generalized eruptive histiocytoma
	Malignant	
Fibrous histiocytoma (fibrous xanthoma)	Benign	Subepidermal nodular fibrosis (fibrous xanthoma of skin; sclerosing hemangioma; dermatofibroma; histiocytoma) Giant cell tumor of tendon sheath (fibrous xanthoma of tendon sheath; nodular tenosynovitis) Pigmented villonodular synovitis Xanthogranuloma
	Malignant	Dermatofibrosarcoma protuberans (progressive and recurring dermatofibroma; storiform fibrous xanthoma)
Pleomorphic fibrous histiocytoma (pleomorphic fibrous xanthoma)	"Benign"	Atypical fibroxanthoma of skin (paradoxical fibrosarcoma; pseudosarcomatous dermatofibroma; pseudosarcomatous reticulohistiocytoma) Postirradiation pseudosarcoma
	Malignant	Fibroxanthosarcoma (mixed storiform and giant cell fibrous xanthoma) ? Malignant giant cell tumor of soft parts ? Epithelioid sarcoma

is a secondary and inconstant feature. Whenever possible, a label of benign or malignant should be added to tumors belonging to each one of these three major groups. Pure xanthomas, with or without accompanying serum lipid abnormalities, are regarded as nonneoplastic conditions and are excluded from this discussion.

Histiocytoma

The typical histiocytoma is made up of closely packed polygonal cells with little or no intervening stroma.[90] The cytoplasm is eosinophilic and may contain lipid droplets. Inflammatory cells are frequent. Fibrosis may be present in the older lesions; this should be differentiated from the active fibroblastic proliferation of fibrous histiocytomas. The benign tumors greatly predominate over those exhibiting a malignant behavior. The differential diagnosis between them may be difficult. Histiocytomas with clinical and/or pathologic features that single them out from the rest are juvenile xanthogranuloma, reticulohistiocytoma and generalized eruptive histiocytoma, all of which are benign. Most of these varieties are discussed in Chapter 3.

Fibrous histiocytoma (fibrous xanthoma)

Well-defined examples of the benign variant of fibrous histiocytoma include subepidermal nodular fibrosis, the so-called giant cell tumor to tendon sheath, and pigmented villonodular synovitis. The microscopic diagnosis is usually simple. A variable admixture of histiocytes (some foamy, other multinucleated, still others containing hemosiderin) and fibroblast-like cells is always present.[79,100] Some lesions can be extremely cellular, but there is no atypia nor high mitotic activity.

The malignant variant differs microscopically from the former by virtue of a more monomorphic appearance, nuclear hyperchromasia, higher mitotic activity, and most of all, the presence of what has been called a *storiform* pattern of growth. The latter can be succinctly described as a peculiar arrangement of the tumor cells about a central point, producing radiating "spokes" grouped at right angles to each other. Tridimensional reconstruction studies suggest that this structure develops at the periphery of adjacent proliferating cell groups.[98a] Although it can rarely occur in benign fibrous histiocytomas, its presence should be regarded as a probable sign of malignancy. The best example of malignant fibrous histiocytoma is the tumor traditionally known as dermatofibrosarcoma protuberans.[80] Its typical location is the dermis, but it also can occur in deeper soft tissues. The malignancy of this neoplasm is of low grade, mainly manifested by local recurrence. Distant metastases are exceptional, but they are well documented.[83,109]

We believe that most of the retroperitoneal and mediastinal lesions called *xanthogranulomas*[101] are examples of fibrous histiocytomas, either benign or malignant, whereas others probably represent idiopathic mediastinal or retroperitoneal fibrosis or even malakoplakia.[81] Therefore, we suggest that this term be dropped entirely.

Pleomorphic fibrous histiocytoma (pleomorphic fibrous xanthoma)

Bizarre tumor cells, mononucleated or multinucleated, are the hallmark of this tumor type, which otherwise resembles the group just described (Fig. 1331). Although we regard all tumors in this category at least as potentially malignant, we still divide them, for prognostic and therapeutic purposes, into a "benign" and a malignant variety. The "benign" form, generally known as atypical fibroxanthoma, typically presents as a small nodule in sun-exposed skin of elderly individuals.[93,95] Less commonly, it appears as a larger mass in the trunk and limbs of younger patients.[85] We have seen it in areas previously subjected to radiation therapy and adjacent to other skin tumors such as epidermoid carcinoma and sweat gland neoplasms.[105] The storiform pattern is usually absent. The large majority of these lesions are cured by local excision.[85,88]

The malignant type, which is also known as fibroxanthosarcoma, xanthosarcoma, or simply malignant fibrous histiocytoma, tends to occur in deeper structures, such as deep fascia and skeletal muscle.[92,112] We have seen it in the soft tissues of the extremities, mediastinum, retroperitoneum, and breast and within bones (Fig. 1332). It differs from the "benign" variety mainly by its different location and the presence of a storiform pattern of growth. Metaplastic bone formation may be present focally. This tumor is prone to local recurrence and has the capacity to metastasize to distant sites, especially the lungs and regional lymph nodes.[106] The most important prognostic factor is the depth of location, followed by size.[91a] In

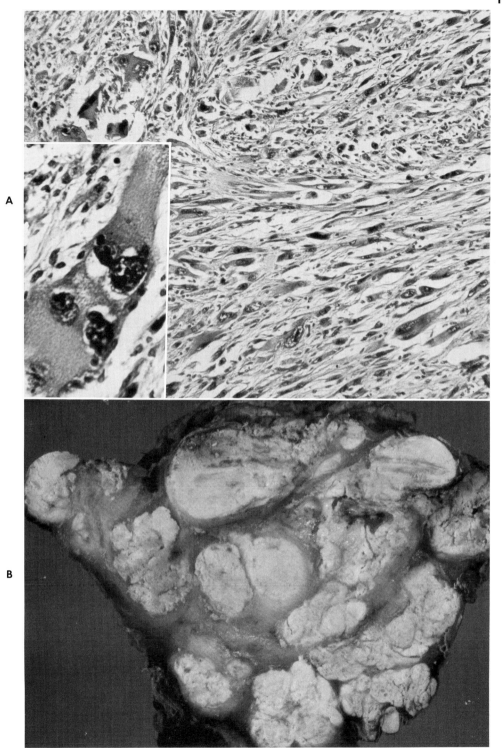

Fig. 1331 A, Malignant pleomorphic fibrous histiocytoma (fibroxanthosarcoma) of thigh (21 cm × 21 cm) excised from 38-year-old man. It recurred one year later. Note bizarre tumor giant cell, **inset,** and characteristic highly malignant spindle cell stroma. **B,** Tumoral calcinosis removed from buttock. Note nodularity with calcification. (**A,** ×150; WU neg. 68-6295; **inset,** WU neg. 68-6306; **B,** WU neg. 65-3865.)

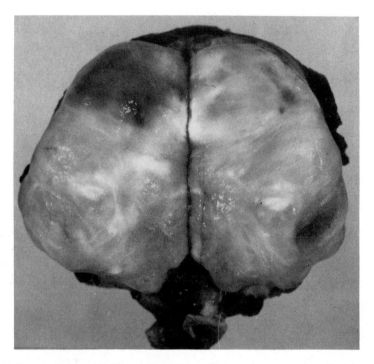

Fig. 1332 Malignant pleomorphic fibrous histiocytoma (fibroxanthosarcoma) excised from soft tissue of thigh in 27-year-old man. Lighter areas, which were yellow, are due to accumulation of foamy cells. (Courtesy Dr. M. R. Beck, San Francisco, Calif.)

a series of 200 cases reported by Weiss and Enzinger,[112] tumors that were small or superficially located or had a prominent inflammatory component (other than neutrophilic) metastasized only rarely. The malignant potential is higher than that of the ordinary malignant fibrous histiocytoma but lower than that of other soft tissue sarcomas that it resembles microscopically, such as pleomorphic liposarcoma.[107] Weiss and Enzinger[111] have reported eighty cases of tumors that they interpreted as *myxoid fibrous histiocytomas.* This is probably the same process that has been reported by Angervall et al. as myxofibrosarcoma.[78,94] Most of them arose in the extremities of adults and usually were attached to the fascia or within a major muscle and had a better prognosis than the ordinary malignant fibrous histiocytoma. Grossly, they were mucoid and resembled myxoid liposarcomas. Microscopically, they also resembled liposarcoma by virtue of an abundant matrix of acid mucopolysaccharides, high vascularity, and presence of cells resembling lipoblasts. The authors separated them from liposarcoma because of the presence (elsewhere in the tumor or in recurrences) of areas

of "typical malignant fibrous histiocytoma" and the absence of true lipoblasts (which should contain neutral fat in their cytoplasmic vacuoles rather than acid mucopolysaccharides). In our opinion, it is questionable whether it is histogenetically sound or pragmatically important to separate this tumor from the poorly differentiated type of myxoid liposarcoma. The electron microscopic features of this tumor have been described by Lagacé et al.[97]

Kyriakos and Kempson[96] have described as *inflammatory fibrous histiocytoma* a malignant soft tissue tumor in which the neoplastic cells (some of bland appearance and others bizarre and anaplastic) were admixed with, and even obscured by, an intense inflammatory infiltrate rich in neutrophils (Fig. 1333). Some of the tumor cells contained phagocytosed neutrophils in their cytoplasm. A storiform pattern, collections of foamy cells, and areas of tissue necrosis were also consistently present. The authors interpreted this lesion as a specific subgroup of malignant fibrous histiocytoma and remarked on its aggressive behavior. We have seen a very similar pattern

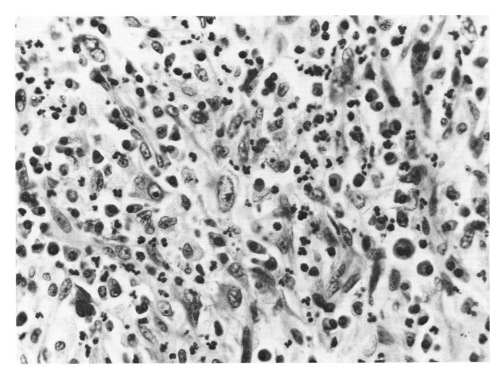

Fig. 1333 Inflammatory variant of malignant fibrous histiocytoma. Atypical cells of histiocytic appearance are seen scattered among dense inflammatory infiltrate rich in neutrophils and plasma cells.

(intense neutrophilic infiltration in pleomorphic tumors associated with phagocytosis of neutrophils by the tumor cells) in an otherwise typical myxoid liposarcoma, in an irradiated osteosarcoma, and in metastatic carcinomas from the kidney and adrenal gland. Perhaps the neutrophilic infiltration is simply a tissue response to the production and release of (? biochemically abnormal) lipid by the tumor cells.

Yet another morphologic variation in the theme recently has been described by Enzinger[81a] as *angiomatoid malignant fibrous histiocytoma*. This lesion usually presents in the extremities of children and young adults as a circumscribed, multinodular or multicystic hemorrhagic mass. Microscopically, the usual features of fibrous histiocytoma are admixed with focal areas of hemorrhagic cystlike spaces and large aggregates of chronic inflammatory cells. These lesions can simulate primary vascular neoplasms or lymph node metastases. Of twenty-four patients with follow-up information, twelve had developed recurrence and five showed distant metastases. It is important to recognize that perfectly benign dermal fibrous histiocytomas (so-called dermatofibromas) also

can be accompanied by hemorrhagic foci and that this does not endow them with any particular aggressive behavior[105a] (see Chapter 3).

It has been suggested that epithelioid sarcomas and malignant giant cell tumors of soft parts also represent malignant tumors of histiocytes. However, and until more definite evidence for this is obtained, we prefer to discuss them under the category of tumors of uncertain origin.

The microscopic appearance of benign and malignant fibrous histiocytoma can be closely simulated by a number of conditions, including malakoplakia,[81] silica reaction,[113] histioid leprosy, and metastatic carcinoma (particularly renal cell carcinoma).

Tumors and tumorlike conditions of peripheral nerves

There are four distinct lesions of the peripheral nerves: *neuroma*, a benign nonneoplastic overgrowth of nerve fibers and Schwann's cells; *neurilemoma* and *neurofibroma*, two benign neoplasms; and *malignant schwannoma*, formerly designated as neurofibrosarcoma. De-

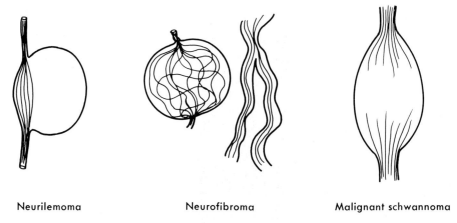

Neurilemoma   Neurofibroma   Malignant schwannoma

Fig. 1334 Schematic drawing emphasizing main differences between typical cases of three types of peripheral nerve tumors. Note diameter of nerve involved and behavior of neurites (thin black lines) in relation to neoplasm.

spite the fact that these lesions may coexist, it is important to make a distinction among them in view of their markedly different natural history. For a discussion of the features of neurilemoma and neurofibroma in the mediastinum or retroperitoneal area, see Chapters 7 and 25, respectively.

Neuroma

The large majority of neuromas follow trauma—hence their designation of *traumatic neuromas.* When a peripheral nerve is severed or crushed, the proximal end regenerates and, if it fails to meet the distal end, a tangled mass of nerve fibers results. Microscopically, all the elements of a nerve can be recognized; neurites, Schwann's cells, and perineurial fibroblasts. In addition, scar tissue is often present. Not surprisingly, this lesion is often exquisitely painful. *Amputation neuroma,* a term made popular during World War I, is merely a type of traumatic neuroma in which the original trauma involved the loss of an extremity.

Morton's neuroma (Morton's metatarsalgia) can be regarded as a specific variant of traumatic neuroma. Its typical location is the interdigital plantar nerve between the third and fourth toes. The lesion is more common in female adults. Microscopically, the affected nerve is markedly distorted. There is extensive perineurial fibrosis often arranged in a concentric fashion. The arterioles are thickened and sometimes occluded by thrombi.[139,143] It is likely that the disease is secondary to repeated mild traumas to the region.[125b]

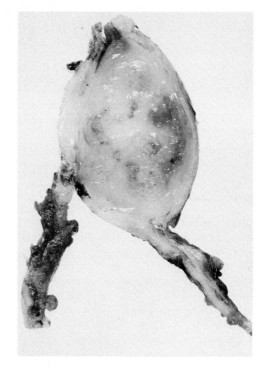

Fig. 1335 Encapsulated neurilemoma with small nerve entering its periphery. (WU neg. 52-1170.)

Neurilemoma

Neurilemoma is one of the few *truly encapsulated* neoplasms of the human body. It is almost always solitary and, for practical purposes, it never becomes malignant. The most common locations are the flexor surfaces of the extremities, neck, mediastinum, retroperi-

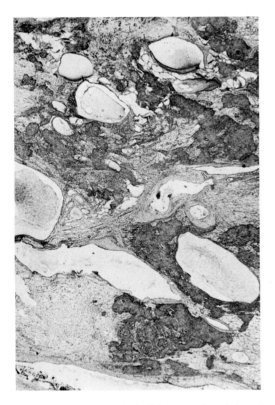

Fig. 1336 Antoni type A (cellular areas) and Antoni type B (cystic areas) tissue in neurilemoma. (Low power; WU neg. 50-438.)

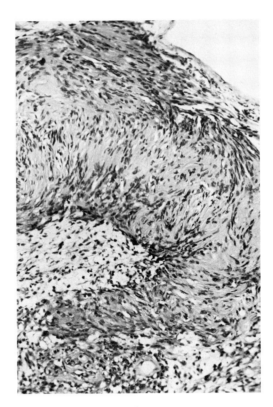

Fig. 1337 Area of Antoni type A tissue with palisading of cells. (×210; WU neg. 50-439.)

toneum, posterior spinal roots, and cerebellopontine angle.[136] The nerve of origin often can be demonstrated in the periphery, flattened along the capsule but not penetrating the substance of the tumor (Figs. 1334 and 1335). Since this is a benign neoplasm that only rarely recurs locally, every attempt should be made to preserve the nerve, if this is of any clinical significance (e.g., facial nerve or vagus nerve).

Grossly, the larger neurilemomas often contain cystic areas. The microscopic appearance is distinctive. Two different patterns usually can be recognized, designated by Antoni as A and B. The type A areas, which in small tumors comprise almost their entirety, are quite cellular, composed of spindle cells often arranged in a palisading fashion or in an organoid arrangement (Verocay's bodies) (Figs. 1336 and 1337). In type B areas, the tumor cells are separated by abundant edematous fluid that may form cystic spaces (Fig. 1336). Occasionally, isolated cells with bizarre hyperchromatic nuclei are observed. They are of no particular significance. Mitoses are absent or extreme-

ly scanty. The diagnosis of neurilemoma should be doubted if they are present more than occasionally. Blood vessels can be of such prominence as to simulate a vascular neoplasm. By electron microscopy, they have been found to be of the fenestrated type, a rather surprising feature.[127] Thrombosis and hyaline thickening of the adventitia are common. Palisading of nuclei is not unique for this neoplasm. We have seen it in leiomyoma, leiomyosarcoma, fibrous histiocytoma, juvenile aponeurotic fibroma, and even nonneoplastic smooth muscle of the appendiceal wall. Neurites are not present, except in the portion of the capsule where the nerve is attached. Collections of foamy macrophages are sometimes seen, especially in the larger neoplasms.

It is generally agreed that this neoplasm originates from Schwann's cells. By electron microscopy, the cells of neurilemoma have a continuous basal lamina, numerous extremely thin cytoplasmic processes, and aggregates of intracytoplasmic microfibrils.[147] (Fig. 1338). However, they lack what is probably the only patho-

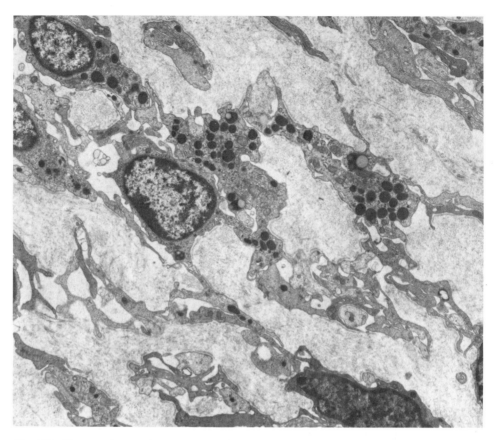

Fig. 1338 Electron microscopic appearance of neurilemoma of retroperitoneum. Elongated cells with narrow processes are partially covered by basal lamina. Cells contain lipid of varied densities. (×7,450.)

gnomonic feature of normal Schwann's cells: mesoaxons. In this respect, they resemble the so-called *perineurial cell* of normal peripheral nerve, a cell whose possible participation in the development of neurilemoma and neurofibroma deserves further investigations. Peripheral nerve tumors composed almost exclusively of cells with the ultrastructural features of perineurial cells ("perineuriomas") actually have been described; their identification depends on electron microscopic examination, inasmuch as their light microscopic appearance is that of a neurofibroma or pacinian neurofibroma.[132] "Long-spaced collagen" is frequently seen in the intercellular space of neurilemomas, but its presence is not specific for this neoplasm.[122]

Neurofibroma

The gross, microscopic, and ultrastructural features of neurofibroma, as well as its natural history, are distinct from those of neurilemoma. Therefore, it is important to distinguish between the two types of benign neoplasms.[145]

The fact that in some instances the differential diagnosis may be difficult or that in isolated cases features of both lesions may coexist does not justify lumping them together.

Neurofibromas can be solitary or multiple, the latter form being known as neurofibromatosis or Recklinghausen's disease.[119] The gross appearance varies a great deal from lesion to lesion. As a rule, the tumors are not encapsulated and have a softer consistency than neurilemoma. The more superficial tumors appear as small, soft, pedunculated nodules protruding from the skin ("molluscum pendulum"). Deeper tumors grow larger. They may result in diffuse tortuous enlargement of peripheral nerves and are then designated as plexiform neurofibromas (Fig. 1339). The diffuse involvement of the nerves may make a complete resection impossible. This particular form of neurofibromatosis is more commonly seen in the orbit, neck, back, and inguinal region.

Microscopically, neurofibromas are formed

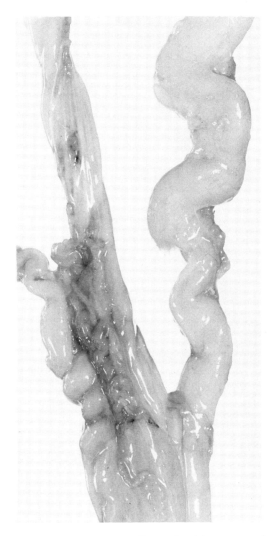

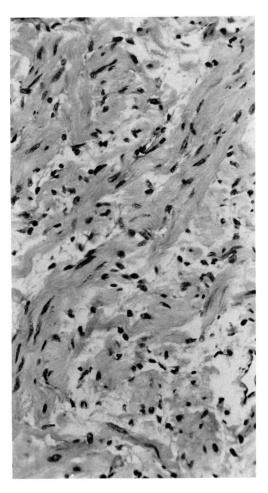

Fig. 1339 Plexiform neurofibroma involving nerves of lower extremity of young boy. Note enlargement and tortuosity of nerve bundles. (WU neg. 52-4785.)

Fig. 1340 Typical neurofibroma. Note disorderly pattern of fibers. (×400; WU neg. 52-3602.)

by a combined proliferation of all the elements of a peripheral nerve: neurites, Schwann's cells, fibroblasts, and probably perineurial cells. The former can be demonstrated by silver stains. Schwann cells usually predominate. They usually have markedly elongated nuclei, with a wavy, serpentine configuration and pointed ends (Fig. 1340). Electron microscopically, they are seen to enclose axons in plasmalemmal invaginations (mesoaxons).[147] Acetylcholinesterase activity can be demonstrated in the nerve fibers of this tumor.[130] Mucinous changes in the stroma may be prominent and result in a mistaken diagnosis of myxoma or myxoid liposarcoma. Mitoses are ex-

ceptional. Their presence should arouse the suspicion of malignant degeneration. On the other hand, occasional cellular pleomorphism is of no significance by itself (Fig. 1341). Numerous mast cells are present in the stroma.[137] Distorted organoid structures resembling Wagner-Meissner corpuscles are sometimes seen. Tumors in which these formations are particularly prominent have been sometimes been designated as *tumors of tactile end-organs*.[126,141] On the other hand, Verocay's bodies, palisading of nuclei, and hyaline thickening of the vessel wall are almost always absent. Sometimes, otherwise typical neurofibromas are seen to contain melanin, a feature

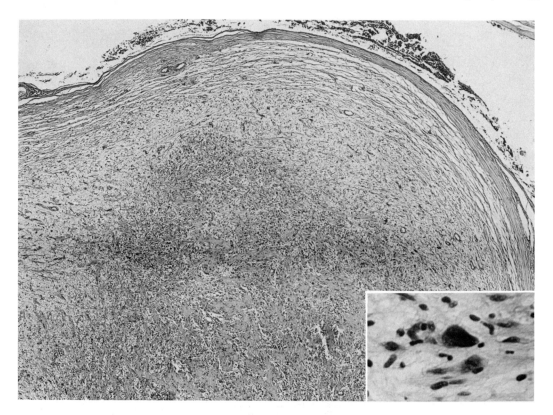

Fig. 1341 Neurofibroma excised from superficial soft tissues of arm in 38-year-old man. Focus of marked cellularity can be seen in center, surrounded by more typical areas. **Inset,** Cellular center contains scattered giant tumor cells with bizarre, hyperchromatic nuclei. This finding per se is not indication of malignant transformation. There were no mitoses. (×33; WU neg. 73-2072; **inset,** ×350; WU neg. 73-2076.)

not unexpected in view of the embryologic relationship between Schwann's cells and melanocytes.[115,117] These tumors should be differentiated from blue nevi and malignant melanomas.

In Recklinghausen's disease, neurofibromas may occur in every conceivable site: axilla, thigh, buttocks, deep-lying soft tissue, orbit, mediastinum, retroperitoneum, tongue, gastrointestinal tract, etc.[138] Plexiform neurofibromas may result in massive enlargement of a limb or some other part of the body ("elephantiasis neuromatosa") (Fig. 1342). In addition to neurofibromas, patients with Recklinghausen's disease often have many other associated lesions, the most common being the *café au lait spot.* This consists microscopically of an increase in the amount of melanin in the epidermal basal layer and is sometimes seen overlying a neurofibroma. It can be distinguished from the pigmented spots associated with Albright's syndrome by virtue of its distribution

and smooth, delicate margins.[116] Solitary café au lait spots are common in normal individuals. Only when they are present in a number of five or more can a significant association with neurofibromatosis be detected.[150] Other lesions sometimes seen in patients with Recklinghausen's disease include congenital malformations of various types,[128] megacolon, various types of vascular lesions,[140] fibrosing alveolitis,[148] neurilemoma (frequently multiple), meningioma and other intracranial neoplasms, lipoma, pheochromocytoma, medullary carcinoma of the thyroid gland, neuroblastoma,[152] ganglioneuroma,[118,133] and *Wilms' tumor.*[144] Increased activity of the protein "nerve growth factor" in the serum of patients with disseminated neurofibromatosis has been reported.[142]

A small proportion of patients with Recklinghausen's disease develop malignant schwannoma. The incidence usually given is in the range of 13%[129] but is probably much lower. The malignant tumors arise practically always in

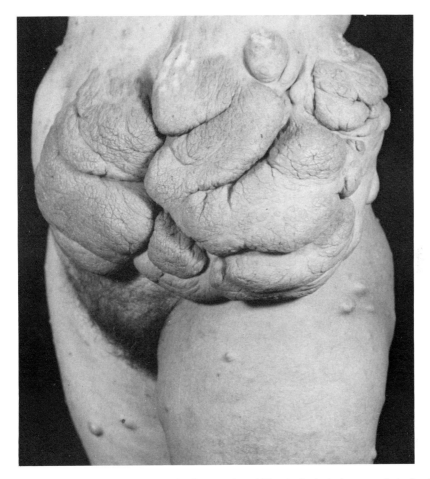

Fig. 1342 Florid case of Recklinghausen's disease. In addition to typical changes of elephantiasis in lower abdomen, multiple small neurofibromas of chest and extremities are evident. (WU neg. 64-5119.)

large nerve trunks of the neck or extremities. For practical purposes, peripheral superficial neurofibromas never become malignant, and the only reasons for surgical removal are size and unsightliness (Fig. 1343).

A syndrome of multiple **mucosal neuromas**, pheochromocytoma, and medullary carcinoma of the thyroid gland has been described[125,151] as multiple endocrine adenomatosis Type IIb or III and is more fully discussed in Chapter 8. The neuromas usually involve the tongue, lips, and conjunctiva. Despite their morphologic similarities with traumatic neuromas, they should probably be regarded as a morphologic variant of neurofibroma.

Malignant schwannoma

The term malignant schwannoma is the preferred name for a tumor also designated as neurogenic sarcoma and neurofibrosarcoma[123] (Figs. 1344 and 1345). It is the malignant counterpart of neurofibroma and *not* of neurilemoma. Because of its difficult microscopic recognition, diagnostic errors are often made, more often than not by calling malignant schwannoma some other type of soft tissue sarcoma. We know of only two circumstances in which the diagnosis of malignant schwannoma should be the primary consideration in the presence of a malignant tumor of soft tissues composed of spindle cells: (1) when the tumor develops in a patient with Recklinghausen's disease and (2) when the tumor is obviously arising within the anatomic compartment of a major nerve or in continuity with an unquestionable neurofibroma.[120] In the absence of these circumstances, the microscopic diagnosis of malignant schwannoma can rarely be more than presump-

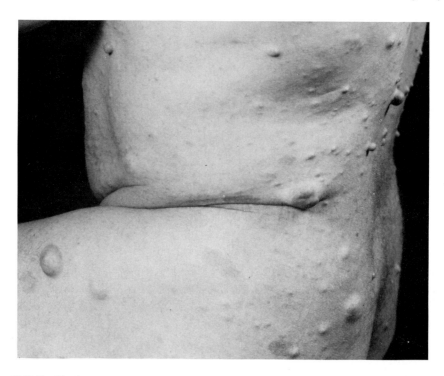

Fig. 1343 Recklinghausen's disease showing innumerable nodules and café au lait spots. (WU neg. 49-6545.)

tive. It is true that in some tumors features suggestive of nerve sheath origin can be identified, such as serpentine cells, arrangement in palisades or whorls, or large gaping vascular spaces, but none of these features is pathognomonic.[125a] In most areas, the appearance is that of an extremely cellular spindle cell neoplasm. Mitoses are usually in abundance. Although most tumors are quite monomorphic, some can be extremely bizarre. Metaplastic cartilage, bone, and skeletal muscle have been described.[154] Occasionally, even foci of glandular differentiation may be present. Woodruff[153] reported five cases associated with mucin production, three of them occurring in patients with Recklinghausen's disease. In general, any peripheral nerve tumor should be suspected of being malignant if it contains epithelial glandular structures, no matter how well differentiated they are.

The belief that these malignant neoplasms originate in Schwann's cells is largely based on circumstantial evidence, the reasoning being that if these tumors represent the malignant counterpart of neurofibromas and the latter arise primarily from Schwann's cells, then the former also must have that origin. Some

of the microscopic features just mentioned and tissue culture studies[146] favor this hypothesis, which also is supported by the electron microscopic description of infoldings of the cell membrane with lamellar configuration, presence of discontinuous basal lamina material, conspicuous intercellular junctions, and occasional dense-core granules.[118a,146b]

A large majority of malignant schwannomas arise in adults. The most common locations are the neck, forearm, lower leg, and buttock. Grossly, the finding of a large mass producing fusiform enlargement of a major nerve is characteristic (Fig. 1334).

The clinical evolution is that of a highly malignant neoplasm, despite the relatively slow growth rate of some cases.[124,144a] Local recurrence (often in the cut nerve ends) and distant metastases are frequent. In the series reported by D'Agostino et al.,[121] of thirteen patients with Recklinghausen's disease in whom malignant schwannoma occurred, nine died of tumor. This was also the case in nine of fifteen patients reported by White.[149] There is little correlation between microscopic grading and prognosis.[146a]

Exceptionally, malignant tumors are found

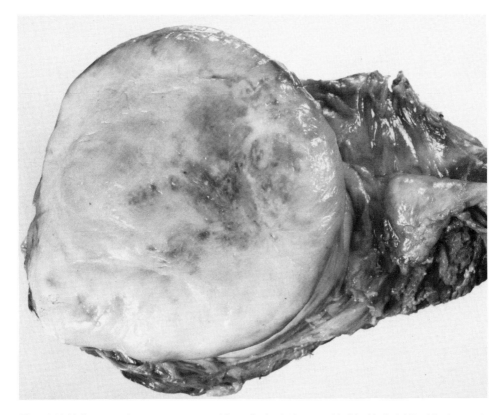

Fig. 1344 Malignant schwannoma removed from flank of 16-year-old girl with florid Recklinghausen's disease. (WU neg. 64-9254.)

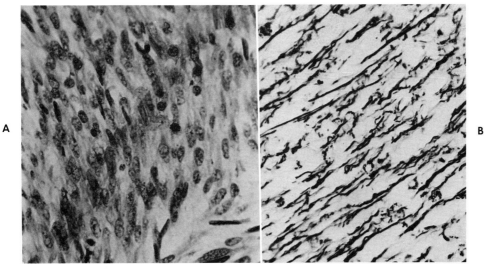

Fig. 1345 A, Fairly well-differentiated malignant schwannoma of chest wall. **B,** Same lesion shown in **A** stained for reticulin demonstrating thick, wiry fibers running in long parallel lines between tumor cells. (**A,** ×400; WU neg. 50-5445; **B,** ×400; WU neg. 50-5446.)

in major peripheral nerves or elsewhere in the soft tissue having a light and electron microscopic appearance suggestive of primitive neuroectodermal origin. These tumors are composed of small cells resembling neuroblasts, many of which form well-developed rosettes without a central lumen. Tumors of this type have been variously designated peripheral *neuroepithelioma*[131] and peripheral or adult *neuroblastoma*,[134] but these probably represent variations of the same theme. Melanin granules may be present in the tumor cells.[135] Ultrastructurally, neural differentiation in the form of neurosecretory granules, cell junctions, and dendritic processes is evident.[134] Both local recurrences and distant metastases (particularly to regional lymph nodes) are common.

The differential diagnosis needs to be made with metastatic neuroblastoma from the adrenal gland (seen in a younger age group and almost always accompanied by elevation of catecholamine metabolites), Ewing's sarcoma (lacking neural differentiation and usually containing abundant cytoplasmic glycogen), embryonal rhabdomyosarcoma, malignant lymphoma, and metastatic small cell carcinoma. We have recently studied several cases of an undifferentiated small cell tumor characteristically involving the chest wall and/or lung of children and adolescents that seems to constitute a definite clinicopathologic entity; the presence of rosettes in some of the cases and their ultrastructural features suggest a neuroepithelial derivation and therefore a probable relation to the group of tumors just described.[114]

Tumors of adipose tissue
Lipoma

Benign fatty tumors can arise in any location in which fat is normally present. The majority occur in the upper half of the body, particularly the trunk and neck. Paarlberg et al.[170] reviewed twenty-nine lipomas located in the hand. Although these tumors may be in the deep tissues, they are usually subcutaneous. In Pack and Pierson's series,[171] there were about 120 lipomas to 1 liposarcoma. Most patients are in the fifth or sixth decade of life. Children are only exceptionally affected.

Lipomas may be single or multiple. Patients with neurofibromatosis and multiple endocrine adenomatosis have an increased incidence of multiple lipomas. In *diffuse lipomatosis*, massive enlargement of a limb may be seen as a result of diffuse proliferation of mature adipose tissue. This rare condition is seen most exclusively in children.

Lipomas grow to large size and are usually encapsulated when located in the superficial soft tissues but poorly circumscribed when arising in deeper structures, such as intermuscular and intramuscular lipomas.[168] Grossly, lipomas consist of bright yellow fat separated by fine fibrous trabeculae; if the amount of fibrous tissue is appreciable, the designation of fibrolipoma may be justified. Microscopically, lipomas are composed of mature adipose tissue with no cellular atypia. Focal myxoid changes are sometimes present; if extensive, the tumor is sometimes called myxolipoma. Areas of infarction, necrosis, and calcification may occur. In contrast to subcutaneous lipomas, those located within skeletal muscle often have an infiltrative pattern of growth.[164]

Enzinger and Harney[160] have described as *spindle cell lipoma* a benign fatty tumor characteristically located in the regions of the shoulder and posterior neck of adults and composed of an admixture of mature lipocytes and uniform spindle cells set in a mucinous and fibrous background. Features that assist in the distinction with myxoid liposarcoma include the absence of lipoblasts and of a prominent plexiform vascular pattern, the presence of thick collagen bundles, and the great uniformity of the proliferating spindle cells.

Angiolipomas are well-circumscribed small tumors occurring shortly after puberty. They are often painful and multiple. They are located in the subcutis, most commonly on the trunk or extremities. The vascularity often is limited to a band of tissue on the periphery of the neoplasm. Hyaline thrombi are common. The pain correlates well with the degree of vascularity.[165]

So-called infiltrating angiolipomas are unrelated to the lesion just described; Enzinger[159] believes that they probably represent intramuscular large vessel hemangiomas in which portions of the affected muscle tissue have been replaced by fat.

Lipoblastomatosis

Vellios et al.[176] described lipoblastomatosis, which is also known as embryonal or fetal lipoma. It affects infants and young children almost exclusively; the oldest patient we have seen with this disease was a 12-year-old girl. It involves more commonly the proximal portion of the lower and upper extremities. Grossly, the lesion is soft and lobulated. It can be

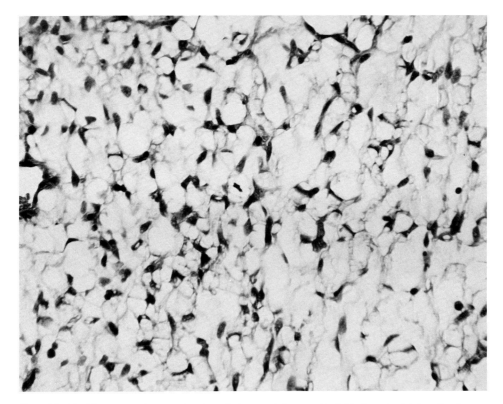

Fig. 1346 Lipoblastomatosis occurring in soft tissue of 8-year-old child. It was mistaken for liposarcoma. (×340; WU neg. 67-1169.)

well localized and superficial (sometimes designated as benign lipoblastoma) or diffusely infiltrate the deep soft tissues. Microscopically, it closely resembles fetal fat (Fig. 1346). It has often been confused with myxoid liposarcoma because of the presence of lipoblasts, a plexiform vascular pattern, and an abundant myxoid stroma. Its ultrastructural appearance is also very similar to that of myxoid liposarcoma.[155b] It is distinguished from it by the young age of the patient, distinct lobulation, and absence of giant cells or pleomorphic nuclei.[157] The clinical course is benign. In the series of Chung and Enzinger,[157] the recurrence rate was 14% and was attributed to incomplete removal of the tumor.

Liposarcoma

Liposarcoma is the most frequent soft tissue sarcoma in adults. On the other hand, its occurrence in children is exceptional.[158] The tumors are usually large and occur most frequently in the lower extremities (popliteal fossa and medial thigh), retroperitoneal, perirenal, and mesenteric region, and shoulder area.[172] Gross-

ly, they are well circumscribed, but this represents pseudoencapsulation[175] (Fig. 1347). They may have a mucoid, slimy surface suggestive of myxoma, a bright yellow appearance mimicking lipoma, or a surface resembling cerebral convolutions.

Enzinger and Winslow[161] divided these tumors into four cellular types: myxoid, round cell, well differentiated, and pleomorphic. Mixed forms occur.

The myxoid type, which is by far the commonest, has no or few mitotic figures and suggests fetal fat. As in the latter, it contains proliferating lipoblasts in different stages of differentiation, a prominent anastomosing capillary network, and a mucoid matrix rich in hyaluronidase-sensitive acid mucopolysaccharides[177] (Fig. 1348). The presence of a prominent vascular component in myxoid liposarcoma is an important feature in the differential diagnosis with myxoma. The mucoid extracellular material may accumulate in large pools, thus simulating a tumor of lymphatic vessel origin. Metaplastic cartilage is exceptionally found. Myxoid liposarcomas containing foci of pleomorphic

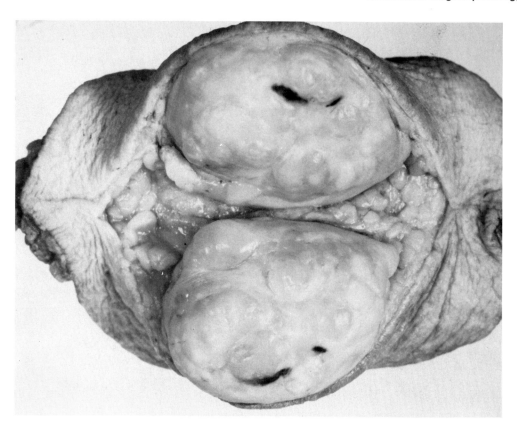

Fig. 1347 Liposarcoma of soft tissues of abdominal wall which was diagnosed by needle biopsy. Adequate excision was done. (WU neg. 66-1398.)

or round cells (designated as "poorly differentiated myxoid type" in Stout's classification or as "dedifferentiated liposarcomas" by others[161a]) are associated with a decrease in the survival rates.[167] Ultrastructurally, cells varying in appearance from primitive mesenchymal cells to typical multivacuolated and univacuolated lipoblasts are seen. The abundant capillaries are intimately related to all of these various cell types in a manner analogous to that of developing fetal adipose tissue.[155a,165a,168a]

In the round cell type, the tumor cells are small and have a distinctly acidophilic cytoplasm. The presence among them of scattered lipoblasts establishes the diagnosis. Mitoses are more common than in the myxoid form, but the vascular network is less prominent. Pseudoglandular arrangement of the tumor cells is frequent. We have seen several round cell liposarcomas misdiagnosed as hibernomas.

The well-differentiated type is often designated a lipoma, but careful examination always shows characteristic tumor cells with large, deep-staining nuclei (Fig. 1349). It is common for the malignant cells to be located within areas of dense fibrosis which are seen alternating with lipoma-like foci. Since this is nearly always a nonmetastasizing neoplasm, there is a question as to whether the designation of liposarcoma is justified for it. The term "atypical lipoma" recently has been suggested for this group of tumors.[162] Along the same line, Enzinger[159] recently has proposed the name *pleomorphic lipoma* for lipoma-like tumors containing hyperchromatic multinucleated ("floret-like") tumor cells within the fibrous septa traversing the neoplasm. As for spindle cell lipomas, the most common locations of these pleomorphic lipomas are the shoulder and posterior neck.[174a]

The pleomorphic type is highly undifferentiated, with many tumor giant cells, and is often called a rhabdomyosarcoma (Fig. 1350). On the other hand, it is likely that many tumors formerly diagnosed as pleomorphic liposarcomas actually represent malignant pleomorphic fibrous histiocytomas, as evidenced by their storiform pattern of growth.

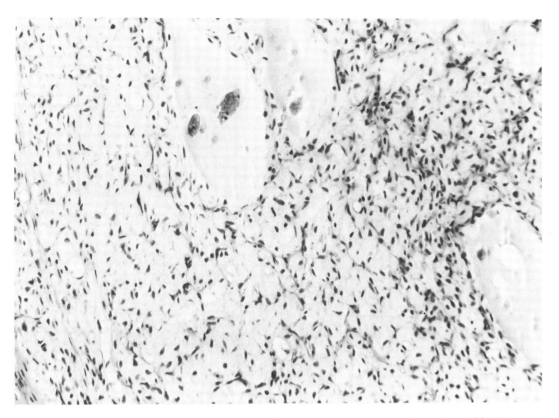

Fig. 1348 Typical myxoid liposarcoma. Note plexiform vascular pattern and abundant myxoid extracellular material, with formation of large mucoid pools.

Fat stains are of little help in the diagnosis of liposarcoma. Fat may be totally lacking in some forms of this tumor and be present in a host of soft tissue neoplasms other than liposarcoma. Benign lesions sometimes confused with liposarcoma are intramuscular myxoma, lipoblastomatosis, spindle cell lipoma, atypical (pleomorphic) lipoma, inflamed lipoma, localized lipoatrophy, and lipogranuloma (such as the one resulting from injection of liquid silicone). In general, the diagnosis of liposarcoma should be questioned for any tumor seen in the pediatric age group or any tumor that is small, superficial, or embedded within a major muscle. Although true liposarcomas can be found in the neck,[166,173] the diagnostic features of malignancy need to be assessed very critically because of the high frequency with which lesions that simulate liposarcoma occur in this location.

Both the myxoid and the well-differentiated types tend to recur locally rather than to metastasize. In contrast, the round cell and pleomorphic types often give rise to widespread metastases. In the series reported by Enzinger and Winslow,[161] the five-year survival rate of patients with myxoid and well-differentiated forms exceeded 70%, whereas in the round cell and pleomorphic varieties it amounted only to 18% (Fig. 1351). Rarely, liposarcomas have multiple foci of origin[155,163] and/or are associated with independent benign multiple lipomas in the same patient.

Hibernoma

The hibernoma is a rare benign neoplasm occurring usually in the intercapsular region and in the axilla. It forms a soft tissue mass, the cut surface of which is brown. The microscopic pattern is characteristic—an organoid arrangement of large cells that contain many vacuoles that stain for neutral fat (Fig. 1352).

This tumor received its name because it is thought to arise from brown fat similar to that seen in the hibernating glands of animals.[156] Sometimes it is seen admixed with an ordinary lipoma. This similarity is maintained at an electron microscopic level.[169,174] Malignant

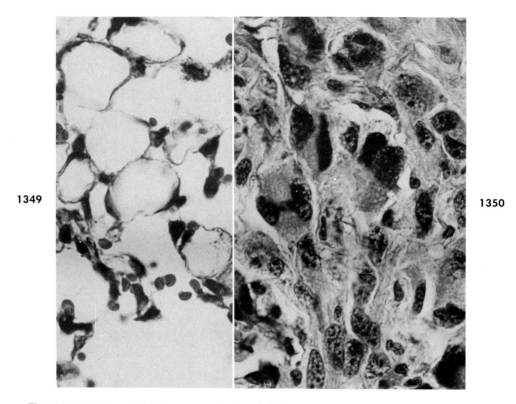

Fig. 1349 Well-differentiated liposarcoma in which individual nuclei have been compressed to crescentic shape. (×400; WU neg. 49-4502.)

Fig. 1350 Pleomorphic liposarcoma with innumerable tumor giant cells and great pleomorphism. Tumors with microscopic appearance are often incorrectly diagnosed as rhabdomyosarcomas. (×360; WU neg. 51-804.)

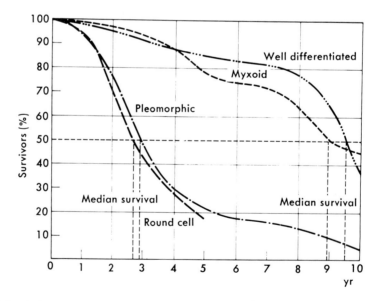

Fig. 1351 Survival rates according to histologic types in liposarcomas of retroperitoneum and lower extremity. (From Enzinger FM, Winslow DJ: Liposarcoma. A study of 103 cases. Virchows Arch [Pathol Anat] **355:**367-388, 1962; Berlin-Göttingen-Heidelberg: Springer.)

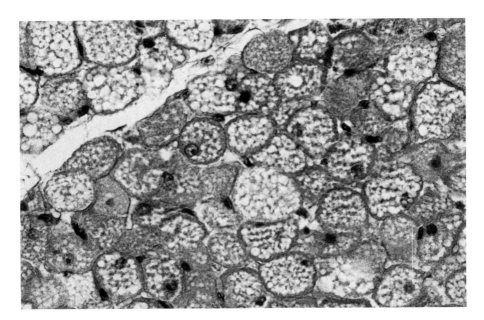

Fig. 1352 Hibernoma with large uniform cells. Vacuoles contain fat. (×40; WU neg. 49-6716.)

soft tissue tumors in which many of the tumor cells have features of brown fat have been seen; we regard them as a morphologic variant of liposarcoma.

Tumors and tumorlike conditions of blood and lymph vessels
Hemangioma

The classification of hemangiomas is unsatisfactory. In most cases, it is difficult to decide if these lesions are malformations (hamartomas) or true neoplasms. About three-fourths are present at birth, and approximately 60% occur in the head and neck area.

The *port-wine type* (nevus flammeus) occurs frequently in the skin of the face, neck, and thorax and, at times, in the skin of the extremities. It is present at birth. This lesion grows very slowly, its increase in size being proportional to the growth of the patient. In time, it becomes nodular and soft. Microscopically, this vascular lesion is of the cavernous type. It contains scattered, thin-walled, superficial telangiectatic vessels.[187] It is resistant to radiotherapy and does not regress spontaneously. This lesion may become very large and unsightly. Its treatment is often difficult.

The *strawberry type* of hemangioma is made up of cellular masses of closely packed spindle cells with spaces containing relatively little blood. Ultrastructurally, endothelial cells predominate, but perithelial cells also partici-

pate.[186a] Only rarely does this type contain a significant cavernous component. It is present at birth or appears shortly afterward and grows rapidly during the first few months of life. At this time, it is highly cellular and contains many mitotic figures (Fig. 1353). This variety is also designated as benign hemangioendothelioma. The color is an intense crimson. When the infant cries, the surface of the nodule becomes smooth. The lesion stops growing and begins to fade when the baby is about 6 months old. It becomes flaccid and pale blue and is covered with tiny wrinkles. Sections taken when the patient is 9 months of age or older show an absence of the intense cellularity and mitotic figures and the presence of increased connective tissue (Fig. 1354). Eventually it disappears completely (Fig. 1355).

In a group of ninety-three hemangiomas in seventy-seven patients studied by Lister[183] and followed from one to seven years, ninety-two out of the ninety-three lesions regressed. There is no exception to the rule that hemangiomas growing rapidly during the early months of life subsequently regress and disappear after about five years.[184] A rapid initial growth rate is not present in the port-wine type. The strawberry type must be sharply separated from the other varieties.

None of the hemangiomas becomes malignant. The so-called benign metastasizing hemangioma is a misnomer. It represents angiosarcoma. Large, deep cavernous hemangiomas may undergo thrombosis, ulceration, or infection and become lethal. Lelong et al.[181] collected fifty cases of large hemangiomas associated with thrombocytopenia. The hematologic abnormality is correctable by excision or irradiation of the hemangioma.[179,186]

We have seen hemangiomas in the soft tissues of the thigh, back, and gluteal regions. They may form poorly circumscribed, hemorrhagic masses with areas of organization and calcification. Microscopically, they contain cavernous spaces lined by normal endothelial cells. Incomplete removal may cure or be followed by recurrence. The lack of circumscription should not be construed as evidence of malignancy.

Allen and Enzinger[178] reviewed eighty-nine hemangiomas of skeletal muscle. Some of their cases were extremely cellular, with plump nuclei, mitotic figures, intraluminal papillary projections, and even infiltration of perineurial spaces. They pointed out that bona fide metastasizing angiosarcomas of skeletal muscle are exceptionally rare.

All of the aforementioned types of angiomas

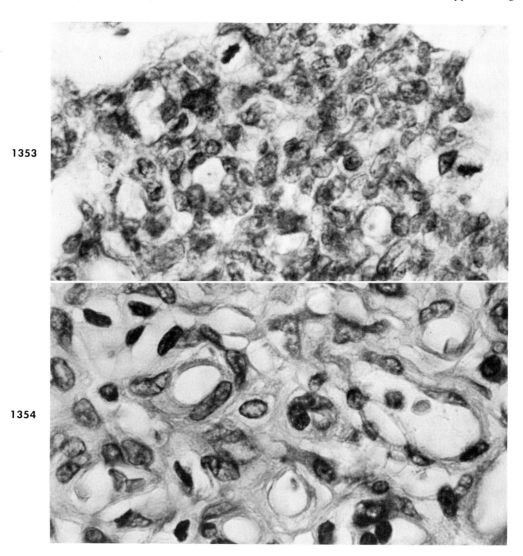

1353

1354

Fig. 1353 Highly cellular hemangioma (strawberry nevus) in 1-month-old infant. Note mitotic figures and solid masses of cells. (×480.)

Fig. 1354 Hemangioma (strawberry nevus) in 1-year-old child. Note vascular channels, decreased cellularity, and increased connective tissue. (×480.)

are composed of capillaries, either exclusively or predominantly. Rarely, hemangiomas composed of veins (venous hemangiomas) or an admixture of arteries and veins (racemose or cirsoid hemangiomas) are encountered. Thrombosis and foci of calcification are common.

The association of varicose veins, soft tissue and bone hypertrophy, and cutaneous hemangioma is known as Klippel-Trenaunay syndrome.[182]

Koblenzer and Bukowski[180] reviewed the cases of multifocal angiomatosis of skin and soft tissues associated with involvement of internal organs.

The endothelial nature of a variety of soft tissue proliferation of dubious histogenesis can now be tested by the detection in tissues of factor VIII–associated protein, a good marker for endothelial cells. This can be demonstrated in normal, hyperplastic, and well-differentiated endothelial cells by an immunoperoxidase technique[185] (Fig. 1356).

Glomus tumor

Glomus tumor, also known as glomangioma, originates in the normal neuromyoarterial glomus, an arteriovenous shunt abundantly supplied with nerve fibers and fulfilling a temperature-regulating function.[191] The classical location of the glomus tumor is the subungual region, but it can occur elsewhere in the skin and soft tissues, particularly in the flexor surface of the arms and about the knee.[188,193-195] It also has been reported in the stomach (Chapter 10), and we have seen one case in the nasal cavity and another in the trachea, below the carina. Subungual lesions are always supplied by numerous nerve fibers and are exquisitely painful, two features often absent in glomus tumors arising elsewhere. The tumor may erode the terminal phalanx or even present as an intraosseous lesion in this location.[190] Superficial lesions are well circumscribed. Glomus tumors in children tend to be multiple and of an infiltrative nature.[189] They may present clinically as varicosities of the lower extremities.

Microscopically, glomus tumors consist of blood vessels lined by normal endothelial cells and surrounded by a solid proliferation of round

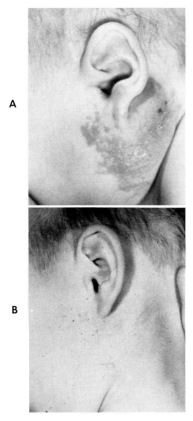

A, **B,**

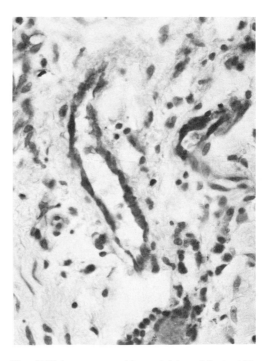

Fig. 1355 A, Extensive hemangioma (strawberry nevus) in 3-month-old infant. **B,** Same child four years later. Lesion completely disappeared without treatment.

Fig. 1356 Immunoperoxidase staining of factor VIII–associated protein. Endothelial cells of these proliferating vessels stain intensely. This can be used as cytochemical marker for endothelial cells.

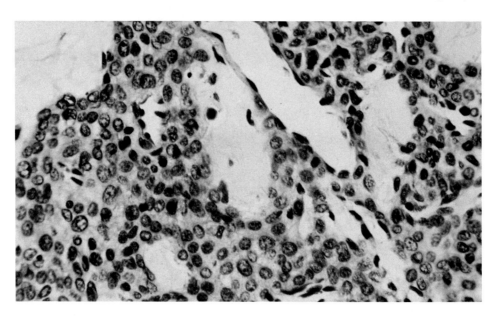

Fig. 1357 Typical glomus tumor with uniform cells and abundant vessels. It was exquisitely painful and located in subungual area. Cajal stain showed numerous neurites. (×500; WU neg. 52-3871.)

Table 70 Clinical and anatomic features of glomus tumor and hemangiopericytoma*†

	Glomus tumor	Hemangiopericytoma
Painful	Often	Rarely
Local invasion	Rare, usually in children	Frequent
Metastases	Never	Sometimes
Location	Skin, superficial soft tissues, stomach	Any tissue[203]
Multiple tumors	Sometimes	No
Histology	Organoid cells; round or oval vascular spaces, often dilated; axons are present	Diffuse elongated cells; vascular spaces often collapsed; axons are absent

*Based on the reported experience of Stout.[204,205]
†From Kuhn C III, Rosai J: Tumors arising from pericytes. Ultrastructure and organ culture of a case. Arch Pathol **88**:653-663, 1969; copyright 1969, American Medical Association.

or cuboidal "epithelioid" cells with perfectly round nucleus and acidophilic cytoplasm (Fig. 1357). By electron microscopy, the tumor cells have features of smooth muscle rather than of pericytes.[196] Three microscopic varieties were described by Masson: solid, angiomatous, and mucoid hyaline.[191,192] The solid type can be confused with sweat gland tumor or metastatic carcinoma. Often the diagnostic relationship between tumor cells and blood vessels can be clearly seen only at the very periphery of the neoplasm. Mast cells are common. Rarely, glomus tumor recurs locally; we have seen such a case in a finger that behaved in a locally malignant fashion. However, convincing cases with distant metastases have not been reported.

Hemangiopericytoma

Stout[205] regarded hemangiopericytoma as a less organoid type of glomus tumor, arising from Zimmerman's pericytes.[206] This theory was supported by the tissue culture studies of Murray and Stout.[202] The main differences with glomus tumor are summarized in Table 70. The tumor occurs principally in adults and is often deep seated.[203] In a series of 106 cases reported by Enzinger and Smith,[199] twenty-seven were in the thigh and twenty-six in the pelvic retroperitoneum. We have seen several of them in the soft tissues of the orbit. Surgical excision can be difficult because of profuse bleeding.

Grossly, hemangiopericytoma is nearly al-

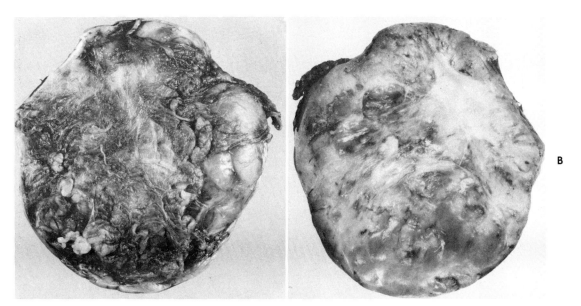

Fig. 1358 External appearance, **A**, and cross section, **B**, of hemangiopericytoma of soft tissues. Encapsulation is complete, and there are areas of cystic degeneration and fibrosis. Microscopically, mitoses were very scanty.

ways solitary and solid, with a smooth surface and a color ranging from grayish white to reddish brown; areas of hemorrhage, necrosis, and cystic degeneration are common (Fig. 1358). In about three-fourths of the cases, the tumor is well circumscribed or encapsulated. The marked vascularization of these tumors can be well demonstrated by angiographic and microangiographic studies.[197] Microscopically, the cells are spindle shaped, lack myofibrils with trichrome stains, and have a close relationship with blood vessels, being separated from the normal-appearing endothelial cells by a layer of silver-staining material composed of basement membrane material admixed with reticulin and collagen fibers (Fig. 1359). Many of the vessels are branching and exhibit a characteristic ''staghorn'' configuration. By electron microscopy, most of the tumor cells have features comparable to those of normal pericytes, whereas others appear as transitional forms with smooth muscle cells and endothelial cells.[198,200] In Stout's series,[204] 11.7% of the cases resulted in distant metastases. He was unable to predict the likelihood of malignant behavior on the basis of the microscopic appearance.

In Enzinger and Smith's series,[199] follow-up revealed local recurrence and/or metastases in nineteen of ninety-three patients with the metas-

tases more common in the lung and skeleton. The morphologic features that correlated with aggressive behavior were prominent mitotic activity, necrosis, hemorrhage, and increased cellularity. Local recurrence was an ominous sign, since it often heralded the appearance of distant metastases. These recurrences can appear five years or longer following the original excision.[201]

Although the evidence for the existence of hemangiopericytoma as a distinct entity is quite convincing, the pathologist should always keep in mind the fact that several other tumors may exhibit a pattern of growth focally indistinguishable from hemangiopericytoma. The most important are mesenchymal chondrosarcoma (distinguished by the presence elsewhere in the tumor of islands of mature cartilage), synovial sarcoma (identified by the occurrence of a biphasic pattern), fibrous histiocytoma (in which a storiform or cartwheel pattern should be apparent), and thymoma (which should have more evident epithelial foci elsewhere). Two other tumors which are perhaps histogenetically related to hemangiopericytoma but which should be kept separate from it because of their distinct natural history are angioblastic meningioma (see Chapter 27) and congenital or infantile hemangiopericytoma. The latter tends to be more superficially located than its

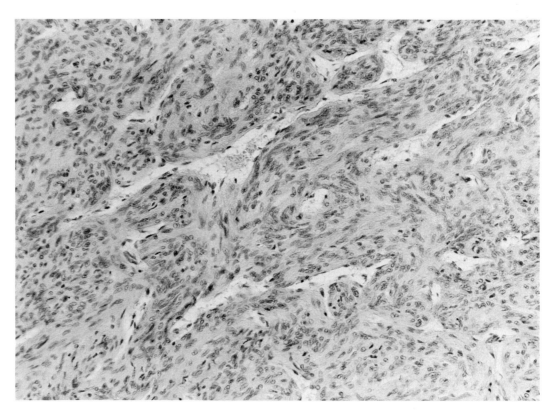

Fig. 1359 Hemangiopericytoma of soft tissue. Ramifying and somewhat collapsed vascular channels lined by flat endothelial cells show marked proliferation of spindle cells of perithelial appearance.

adult counterpart, is often multilobulated, shows increased mitotic activity, and seems also to contain a neoplastic component of endothelial cells. The latter feature, plus its invariably benign behavior despite the high mitotic activity, suggests a possible relationship with hemangioendothelioma.[199]

Angiosarcoma

The term angiosarcoma, if used without adjectives or prefixes, refers to a malignant neoplasm arising from the *endothelial cells of blood vessels*—i.e., a malignant hemangioendothelioma.[209] The lesion is highly vascular, grows in skin, muscle, or deep tissues, and occurs at any age (Fig. 1360). The soft tissue of the female breast is one of the commonest sites (Chapter 19).

The microscopic pattern of angiosarcoma is accentuated by the silver reticulin stain. The tumor cells proliferate in the vascular lumina within a reticulin sheath. They form layers and communicating channels (Fig. 1361). The latter is an important diagnostic feature. It is also seen in organizing thrombi, but practically never in hemangiomas. Lymphoid foci and clumps of hemosiderin are common. In the more solid areas, the tumor cells acquire an epithelioid nature that we have seen confused with amelanotic melanoma and metastatic carcinoma.[208] We also have seen the reciprocal error—i.e., misdiagnosing a well-vascularized liposarcoma or metastatic renal cell carcinoma as angiosarcoma.

Characteristically, angiosarcomas of the skin are multiple and involve the scalp or the face of elderly individuals. The clinical course is that of repeated local recurrences over a long period of time, followed in some cases by lymph node and pulmonary metastases.[207,208]

Lymphangioma

Most lymphangiomas represent malformations rather than true neoplasms. Three forms exist: capillary, cavernous, and cystic. The capillary form occurs in the skin, whereas the cavernous variety prefers deep soft tissues. Cystic lymphangioma is usually known as hygroma. It is a poorly defined soft tissue mass

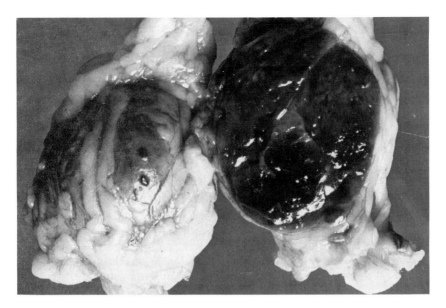

Fig. 1360 Angiosarcoma from omentum in 41-year-old woman. Tumor nodules also were present in retroperitoneum. On cross section, tumor is dark red, spongy, and of soft consistency. It proved rapidly fatal. (WU neg. 52-4780.)

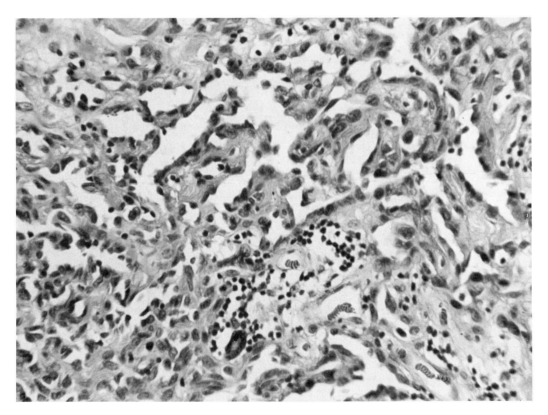

Fig. 1361 Soft tissue angiosarcoma. Freely anastomosing vascular channels are lined by atypical endothelial cells. (×350; WU neg. 73-3401.)

in the neck of children that consists of large lymphatic channels growing in loose connective tissue[214] (Fig. 1362). Large collections of lymphocytes may be present in the stroma and cause mistakes of interpretation. The lesion is usually posterior to the sternocleidomastoid muscle. It may extend into the mediastinum.

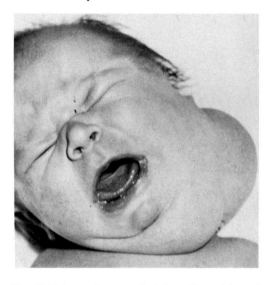

Fig. 1362 Large hygroma in infant. (From Maxwell JH: Tumors of the face and neck in infancy and childhood. South Med J **45**:292-299, 1952.)

It does not become malignant and is curable by excision.[212]

Lymphangiomyoma is the currently accepted term for a benign neoplasm originally described as lymphangiopericytoma.[211,215] It is restricted to the mediastinum and retroperitoneum, in close association with the thoracic duct and its tributaries. It occurs exclusively in females. Chylothorax and pulmonary complications are almost always present.[210] It also may result in chylous ascites and (through involvement of the wall of the ureter) in chyluria. Microscopically, a smooth muscle or pericytic component is seen in addition to the lymphatic proliferation. A relationship between lymphangioma and tuberous sclerosis was suggested by Jao et al.[213] A case of this disorder was found to be responsive to progesterone therapy.[214a]

Lymphangiosarcoma

Lymphangiosarcomas arise rarely in patients who have had long-standing massive lymphedema after radical mastectomy.[216,218] They also may develop secondary to chronic lymphedema of the lower leg.[217,219] Clinically, they present as bluish or purple elevations in the edematous skin. They are frequently multiple, although in late stages they coalesce to form a large hemorrhagic mass (Fig. 1363).

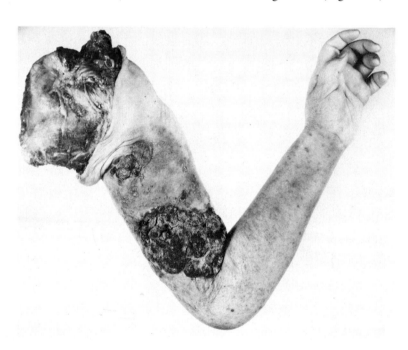

Fig. 1363 Postmastectomy lymphangiosarcoma treated by disarticulation. Large ulcerated tumor masses are present in background of lymphedema.

Microscopically, the tumors are composed of areas resembling angiosarcoma and other zones with empty endothelium-lined spaces suggesting lymphatics. The malignant cells of this lesion lie within the vascular and lymphatic lumina in contrast to Kaposi's sarcoma, in which many of the cells lie outside the vessel wall. Lymphangiosarcoma occurs at an average age of 63.9 years and an average of ten years and three months after mastectomy. Of 129 patients reviewed by Woodward et al.,[220] only eleven had survived five years or more.

Tumors of smooth muscle
Leiomyoma

Three varieties of skin and soft tissue leiomyomas exist. *Multiple leiomyomas* of the skin usually are superficial and small. They arise from the arrectores pilorum muscles. *Genital leiomyomas* are single tumors that arise from smooth muscle bundles in the superficial subcutaneous tissue of the nipple, axilla, anal region, scrotum, penis, and labia majora.[223]

Vascular leiomyomas (angioleiomyomas) arise from the wall of blood vessels. They occur most frequently in females and are usually located in the soft tissues of the lower limbs.[222] They constitute, together with traumatic neuroma, glomus tumor, eccrine spiradenoma, and angiolipoma, the classical five painful tumors of soft tissues.[221]

Grossly, these tumors are yellow or yellowish pink and fairly firm. Microscopically, those in soft tissues are made up of large numbers of vessels, usually without elastic fibers, that are mixed with smooth muscle bundles. Transitional forms with glomus tumor and hemangiopericytoma occur.

As is also the case with smooth muscle tumors of the gastrointestinal tract and uterus, soft tissue tumors may have a round cell or "epithelioid" configuration, in whole or in part. They are particularly common in the omentum and mesentery. The terms bizarre leiomyoma and leiomyoblastoma have been used for this variant. Benign and malignant forms occur. We prefer to designate these tumors as leiomyomas or leiomyosarcomas, round cell variant, classifying them as benign or malignant by using the same criteria we apply for smooth muscle tumors in general, albeit acknowledging the fact that this is not always possible.

Leiomyosarcoma

Smooth muscle tumors of soft tissue origin are relatively rare.[224,225] Most of them arise

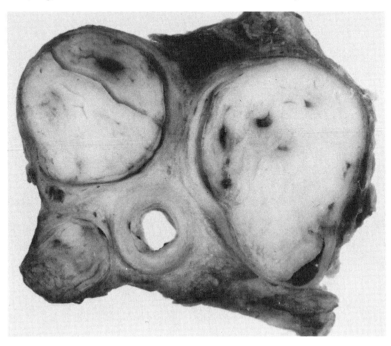

Fig. 1364 Vascular leiomyosarcoma resulting in occlusive tumor thrombi in three large veins in popliteal region. Artery is uninvolved.

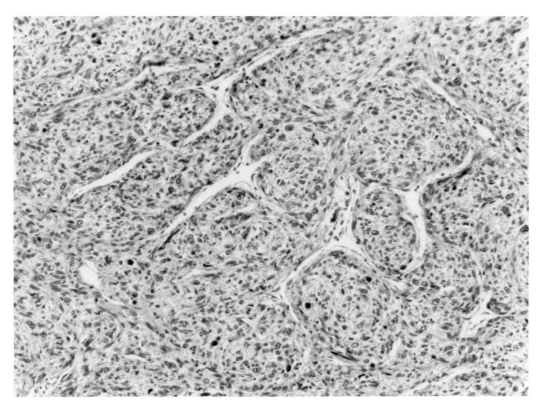

Fig. 1365 Vascular leiomyosarcoma of soft tissues. In contrast to vascular leiomyoma, mitoses are frequent and cellular atypia is present. Low-power pattern resembles hemangiopericytoma, but tumor cells contain abundant myofibrils.

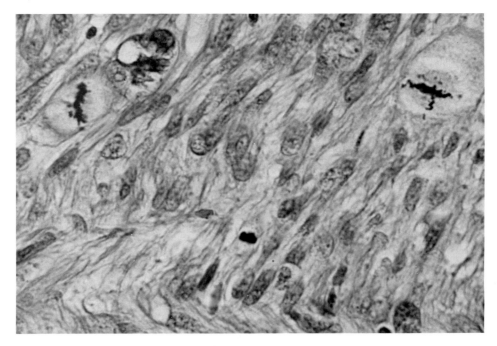

Fig. 1366 Fairly well-differentiated metastatic leiomyosarcoma. However, it showed numerous mitotic figures, both typical and atypical. (×600; WU neg. 62-8259.)

from the wall of arteries and veins of widely differing caliber, ranging from large ones (inferior vena cava, saphenous vein, femoral vein, pulmonary artery, femoral artery) to venules and arterioles[226,227,230] (Fig. 1364). Despite their grossly well-circumscribed nature, the majority eventually give rise to distant metastases, sometimes fifteen or twenty years after the excision of the primary tumor. Both the benign and malignant variants are easily enucleated. If the tumor is malignant, such enucleation results in local recurrence.[228]

Microscopically, the individual cells have elongated, blunted nuclei. Occasionally, myofibrils are demonstrated. The phosphotungstic acid–hematoxylin stain of well-differentiated tumors infrequently shows terminal myofibrils with a hooklike appearance. The reticulin extends as wavy, undulating fibers between long lines of tumor cells. Palisading of nuclei should not be a reason for calling one of these tumors neurogenous. In many of the tumors, a clearcut vascular pattern is apparent, suggesting that they represent the malignant counterpart of vascular leiomyomas (Fig. 1365). We designate these tumors as vascular leiomyosarcomas.[230a]

The gross and microscopic differentiation between the benign and malignant variant usually is not too difficult. The benign variant invariably is small, less than 2 cm in diameter, and shows practically no mitotic activity. The malignant smooth muscle tumor, which rather closely resembles a leiomyoma, invariably shows a high degree of mitotic activity[229] (Fig. 1366). Leiomyosarcomas in children are exceedingly rare.[231]

Tumor size and location are the two major prognostic factors.[230b] Mitotic activity is the morphologic feature that best correlates with biologic behavior. However, we have seen cases with all the attributes of benignancy, including an extremely low mitiotic count, which metastasized and killed the patient.

Tumors of striated muscle
Rhabdomyoma

So-called cardiac rhabdomyomas, seen in association with the tuberous sclerosis complex, are probably not true neoplasms. Bona fide benign tumors of skeletal muscle origin are exceedingly rare.[232,234] Those known as the *adult* type are found almost exclusively in the oral cavity and its vicinity. Adults are usually affected. Microscopically, the cells are well differentiated, and cross striations usually can be demonstrated. We have seen them confused with granular cell tumor and hibernoma. In contrast with the latter, the vacuolated cells of rhabdomyoma contain glycogen rather than fat. Multifocal and recurrent cases have been described.[253a]

Dehner and Enzinger[233] reported nine cases of what they reported as the *fetal* type of rhabdomyoma. Most patients were male children 3 years of age or under. The most common location was the head and neck region, particularly the posterior auricular area. Other cases have been described in the vulvovaginal region of middle-aged women.[233a] Microscopically, the lesions were very cellular, formed by immature skeletal muscle fibers (some containing cross striations) and undifferentiated mesenchymal cells. Nuclear aberrations were absent and mitoses exceedingly rare. The vulvovaginal cases tend to have a myxoid quality. Surgery was curative in every instance.

Rhabdomyosarcoma

Most childhood soft tissue sarcomas represent malignant tumors of skeletal muscle.[239] Three major categories of rhabdomyosarcoma exist, which should be kept clearly separated: pleomorphic, embryonal, and alveolar.[240]

Pleomorphic rhabdomyosarcoma, which constituted practically all the cases in the older literature,[243] is actually the least common of the three categories. It arises from myotome-derived skeletal muscle and is therefore usually located in an extremity, especially the thigh.[247,256] It occurs almost exclusively in adults. Grossly, it may be confined within fascial compartments and have the shape of the muscle from which it arises. The growth rate is often rapid. It may burst through the skin and form a fungating large mass (Fig. 1367). Microscopically, the differential diagnosis with liposarcoma and malignant pleomorphic fibrous histiocytoma is often difficult. We make the unequivocal diagnosis of pleomorphic rhabdomyosarcoma *only* if we can detect cross striations in some of the tumor cells (Fig. 1368). When defined by these criteria, pleomorphic rhabdomyosarcoma becomes a vanishingly rare and almost nonexistent neoplasm. This is a tumor in which electron microscopy can have a definite diagnostic value.[241,250] The five-year survival rate is in the range of 29%.[237,245]

Embryonal rhabdomyosarcoma arises from

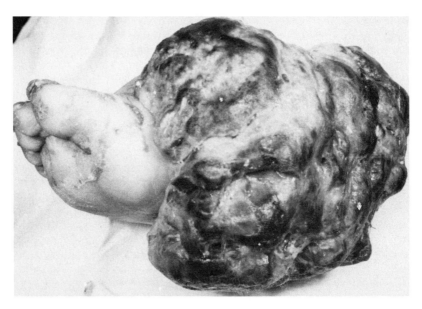

Fig. 1367 Large fungating rhabdomyosarcoma of soft tissue of ankle.

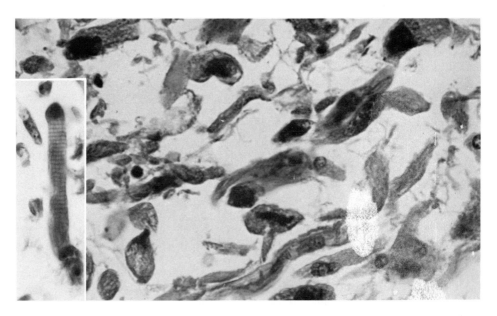

Fig. 1368 Pleomorphic rhabdomyosarcoma with tumor giant cells and tapering cytoplasmic processes. Cell in **inset** shows well-defined cross striations. (High power; WU neg. 46-1718.)

unsegmented and undifferentiated mesoderm and is more common in the head and neck region (particularly the orbit, nasopharynx, and middle ear), retroperitoneum, bile ducts, and urogenital tract.[242,246,248] Less than 5% occur in the extremities. The large majority occur in children 5 years of age or younger. Grossly, it is poorly circumscribed, white, and soft.

When growing beneath a mucosal membrane, such as vagina, urinary bladder, and nasal cavity, it frequently forms large polypoid masses resembling a bunch of grapes—hence the name sarcoma botryoides. The appearance is quite similar to that of an allergic nasal polyp.

Microscopically, the tumor cells are small and spindle shaped. Some have a deeply acido-

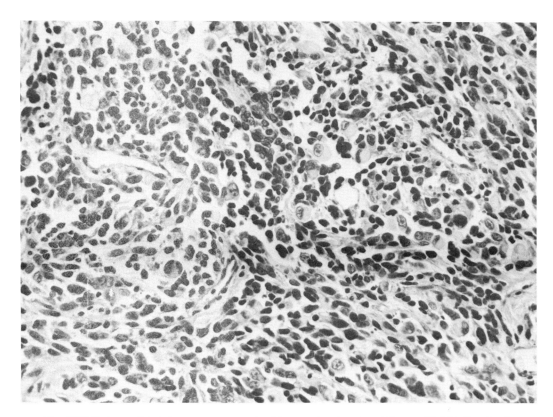

Fig. 1369 Embryonal rhabdomyosarcoma excised from perineal region of 6-year-old child. Small cells with dark nuclei alternate with larger cells with vesicular nuclei and acidophilic cytoplasm. Cross striations are not seen. (Courtesy Dr. B. Lane, New York, N. Y.)

philic cytoplasm (Fig. 1369). A feature of diagnostic value is the presence of highly cellular areas usually centered by a blood vessel, alternating with parvicellular regions with abundant mucoid intercellular material.[255] A highly characteristic feature of the polypoid ("botryoid") tumors is the presence of a dense zone of undifferentiated tumor cells immediately beneath the epithelium, a formation known as Nicholson's *cambium layer*. Skeletal muscle differentiation can be demonstrated by the presence of cross striations at a light or electron microscopic level[249a] (Fig. 1370) or by the presence of myoglobin with immunocytochemical methods[251] (Fig. 1371). Actin also can be demonstrated by the use of the latter method, but this is a less specific feature (Fig. 1372). Enzyme techniques used in muscle histochemistry and other immunohistochemical procedures[251a] also may provide evidence of muscular differentiation in otherwise poorly differentiated sarcomas.[245a,253]

The prognosis has improved markedly in recent years by the combination of surgery,

radiation therapy, and multidrug chemotherapy.[249] Approximately 80% of children may now survive when the disease is localized to the region of origin. The most common sites of metastatic involvement are lung, bone marrow, and lymph nodes. Rhabdomyosarcomas arising from genitourinary sites or extremities are particularly prone to metastasize to lymph nodes, whereas tumors originating in head and neck structures adjacent to meningeal surfaces have a high incidence of direct meningeal extension.

Occasionally, tumors in infants and children with a location and appearance otherwise characteristic of embryonal rhabdomyosarcoma are seen to contain collections of cells exhibiting neuronal, melanocytic, and/or schwannian differentiation; these have been interpreted as originating from the migratory neural crest (ectomesenchyme) and designated as *ectomesenchymoma*.[244] If this interpretation is correct, their histogenesis blends with that of some malignant tumors of peripheral nerves (see p. 1432); not much is known about their

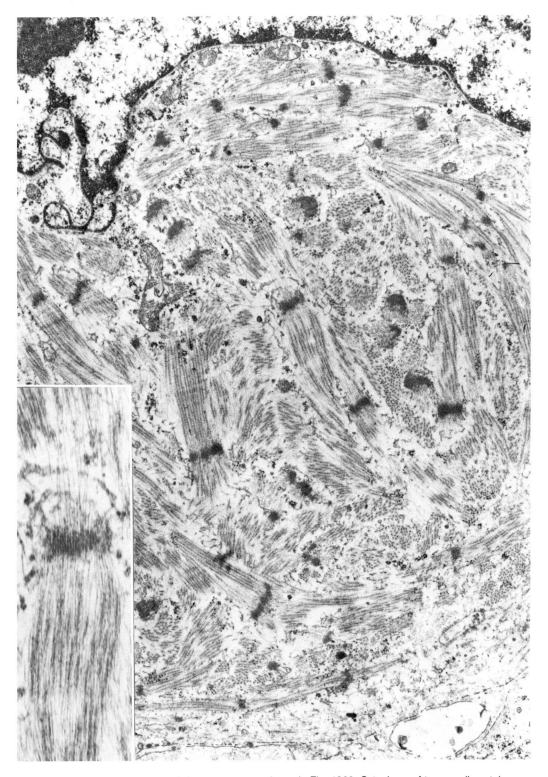

Fig. 1370 Electron micrograph from same case shown in Fig. 1369. Cytoplasm of tumor cell contains abortive cross striations, too small and haphazardly oriented to be visible with light microscope. **Inset** shows Z band and clearly visible double set of filaments. (×18,000; **inset,** ×45,000; courtesy Dr. B. Lane, New York, N. Y.)

natural history, although this does not seem to differ a great deal from that of the ordinary embryonal rhabdomyosarcoma.

Alveolar rhabdomyosarcoma was well described by Riopelle and Thériault[252] and Enterline and Horn.[236] In the past, it was usually misinterpreted as primary reticulum cell sar-

coma of soft tissues. Although clearly related to the embryonal form and occasionally coexisting with it, it should be regarded as a separate entity because of several clinical and pathologic differences with the latter. For instance, it predominates in a slightly older age group (10 to 25 years) and occurs more frequently

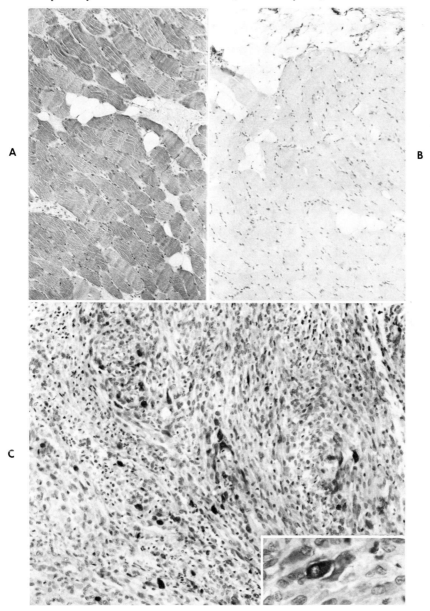

Fig. 1371 Myoglobin stain with immunoperoxidase technique. **A,** Normal skeletal muscle. Strong diffuse cytoplasmic positivity is evident. **B,** Preabsorption of antiserum with myoglobin abolishes reaction. **C,** Embryonal rhabdomyosarcoma. Cytoplasm of many tumor cells is strongly positive. This is particularly well appreciated in high-power **inset.** (**A** and **B,** From Mukai K, Rosai J, Hallaway BE: Localization of myoglobin in normal and neoplastic human skeletal muscle cells using an immunoperoxidase method. Am J Surg Pathol **3:**373-376, 1979. Copyrighted by MASSON PUBLISHING USA, Inc., New York.)

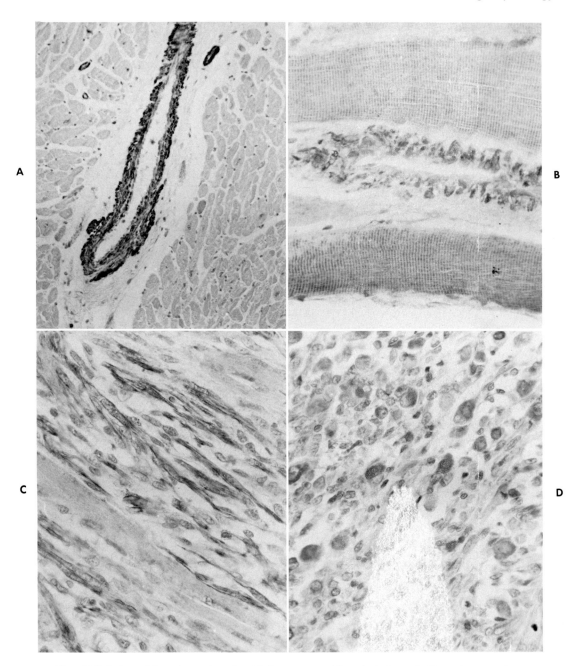

Fig. 1372 Actin staining of muscle cells with immunoperoxidase technique. **A**, Normal myocardium. Smooth muscle of vessel wall stains intensely. **B**, Normal skeletal muscle. Cross striations are dramatically demonstrated. Smooth muscle of vessel wall between two skeletal muscle fibers also stains. **C**, Fetal rhabdomyoma. There is marked cytoplasmic positivity in nearly all neoplastic cells. **D**, Embryonal rhabdomyosarcoma. Staining of variable intensity may be seen in tumor cells.

in the extremities. In a series of 110 cases reported by Enzinger,[238] the most common locations were the forearms, arms, and perirectal and perineal regions.

Microscopically, the small, round or oval tumor cells are seen separated in nests by connective tissue septa. The tumor cells in contact with these fibrous strands remain firmly attached to them, but the others tend to detach due to lack of cohesiveness, thus resulting in a typical alveolar or pseudoglandular appearance. The deep acidophilia of the cytoplasm and

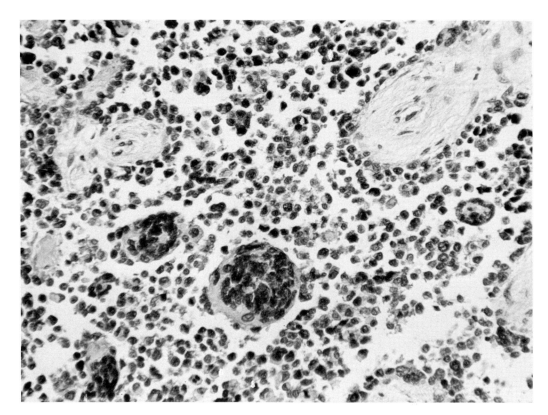

Fig. 1373 Alveolar rhabdomyosarcoma. Lack of cohesiveness of tumor cells and scattered multi-nucleated giant tumor cells are characteristic. (×300; WU neg. 73-2686.)

the presence of occasional multinucleated giant cells are important diagnostic features (Fig. 1373). Ultrastructurally, the cells have a very primitive appearance, not too dissimilar from those of Ewing's sarcoma.[235] Cross striations are rarely found in alveolar and embryonal rhabdomyosarcomas. However, the appearance of these two types is sufficiently distinctive for a definite diagnosis to be made in their absence.[254]

The prognosis of alveolar rhabdomyosarcoma remains worse than for the embryonal variety even with the most recent combined modalities of treatment. In the series reported by Enzinger,[238] 92% of the patients had died from widespread metastasis within the first four years after diagnosis. Lung and regional lymph nodes were the most common metastatic sites.

Tumors of synovial tissue
Synovial sarcoma

The synovial sarcoma is a malignant tumor arising in 80% of the cases about the knee and ankle joints in young adults[262,265] (Fig.

1374). It also occurs about the shoulder and elbow, in the region of the hip, soft tissues of the neck (particularly the retropharyngeal area)[257,267] oral cavity,[266] and anterior abdominal wall. This neoplasm grows very close to joints, tendon sheaths, and bursae, but it is rare for it to involve the synovial membrane. Grossly, this lesion forms circumscribed, firm, grayish pink tumors. Focal calcification occasionally occurs.[269a] The circumscription is false.

Microscopically, the tumor has a sarcomatous stroma and glandlike areas mimicking the arrangement of synovial membrane (Fig. 1375). Hyaluronidase-resistant mucin is often present within the glandular spaces and in the cytoplasm of the epithelial-like cells. Reticulin stains emphasize the differences between the two components. Exceptionally, squamous metaplasia is seen in the epithelial component. Hyalinization, calcification, and osseous or cartilaginous metaplasia can be present in the fibrosarcomatous component. According to Enzinger,[260] the former two features have favorable diagnostic connotations. If the fibrosarcomatous area predominates, the incorrect diag-

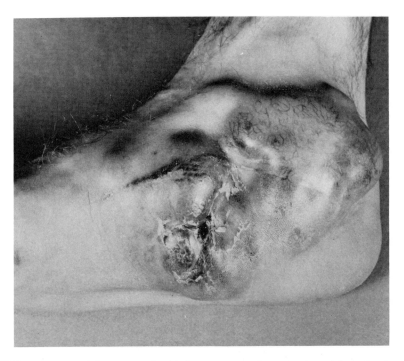

Fig. 1374 Recurrent synovial sarcoma of ankle in young man. It was inadequately excised, recurred, and distantly metastasized, causing death. (WU neg. 48-192.)

nosis may be fibrosarcoma. A careful search for an epithelial-like component should be carried out in any tumor with the appearance of fibrosarcoma located in a periarticular area. Enzinger[260] pointed out that the possibility of synovial sarcoma should be suspected in the presence of spindle cell tumors of monotonous appearance having plump-appearing nuclei, scanty mitotic activity, a focally whorled pattern, distinct lobulation, a large number of mast cells, or occasional nests of large, pale cells. It has been proposed that tumors having these features but no clear-cut epithelial foci may represent synovial sarcoma with a monophasic growth of the fibroblastic component[264a] and that clear cell sarcoma and epithelioid sarcoma are variants of synovial sarcomas with an almost monophasic growth of the epithelial component.[263] The grandlike zones of predominantly epithelial tumors may be mistaken for metastatic adenocarcinoma. By electron microscopy, these areas have features of true glandular epithelium.[264b] In all likelihood, most cases of synovial sarcoma do not arise from synovial cells but rather from mesenchymal elements with the capacity to differentiate into synovioblasts. Gabbiani et al.[261] and Dische et al.[259] have described the ultrastructural appearance of this neoplasm.

These tumors metastasize to regional lymph nodes (10%-15%). The preferable treatment of such tumors is local excision, with wide margins of normal tissue, supplemented by a high dose of radiation therapy.[268] Synovial sarcoma has been traditionally regarded as a tumor of ominous prognosis.[262] In more recent series, however, the five-year survival rate has approached 50%.[258,260,264,269] The prognosis seems to be even better for the synovial sarcomas associated with extensive calcification. Verela-Duran and Enzinger[269a] studied thirty-two of these *calcifying synovial sarcomas* and found that the five-year survival rate was 84% (Fig. 1376).

Tumors of pluripotential mesenchyme
Mesenchymoma

Stout[272] used the term *mesenchymoma* for tumors consisting of two or more mesenchymal elements in addition to fibrous tissue. Benign and malignant forms exist. The most frequent benign variant is composed of smooth muscle, fat, and blood vessels. Cartilage also can present, establishing a histogenetic link with the tumors described in the following section.[270a] It is debatable whether benign mesenchymoma is of neoplastic or hamartomatous nature.[270] The malignant variants, well described by

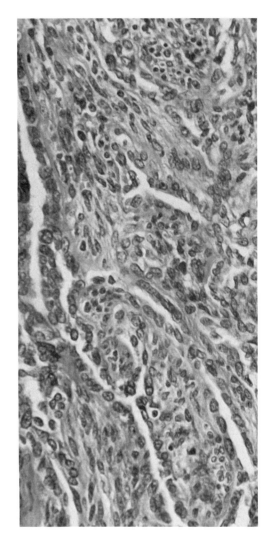

Fig. 1375 Typical synovial sarcoma with biphasic pattern composed of clefts and acinar structures lined by epithelial-like cells. These are separated by fibrosarcomatous stroma. (×350; WU neg. 72-10434.)

Stout,[272] contain multiple varieties of soft tissue sarcomas in the same neoplasm. In other words, chondrosarcoma, liposarcoma, and rhabdomyosarcoma may all be observed in a single tumor. Nash and Stout[271] reviewed forty-two cases occurring in children, nine of them present at birth.

Tumors of metaplastic mesenchyme

Soft tissue chondromas are seen most frequently in the soft tissues of the hands and feet of adults.[282] Grossly, they are lobulated, have a typical hyaline appearance, and are often calcified (Fig. 1377). Some nuclear hyperchromasia may be present and should not be interpreted as evidence of malignancy. As a matter of fact, metastasizing soft tissue cartilaginous tumors of the hands and feet are practically nonexistent.[276] The occasional presence of a cellular fibroblastic growth around the lobules may prompt confusion with juvenile aponeurotic fibroma. Histologic variants with proliferation of osteoclast-like giant cells and chondroblastic activity have been described.[274] Local recurrence is not infrequent.

Soft tissue chondrosarcomas are extremely rare.[279,284] They occur in the extremities of adult patients and exhibit a less aggressive behavior than their skeletal counterpart.[285a] Enzinger and Shiraki[277] studied thirty-four cases of a variant they designated as *extraskeletal myxoid chondrosarcoma.* Cases reported as chordoid sarcoma[283,285] probably belong to the same category. Whether the strange tumor described as parachordoma[275] is also histogenetically related to chondrosarcoma is not so clear. Well-differentiated chondrocytes were absent, and this was responsible for the difficulties in diagnosis. Glycogen was demonstrated in many of the tumor cells. Acid mucopolysaccharides were abundant in the stroma. In contrast with those present in myxoma and myxoid liposarcoma, they were partially resistant to testicular hyaluronidase treatment. Kindblom and Angervall[281] have shown that the histochemical properties of the mucosubstance formed by most chondrosarcomas (in contrast to those of benign cartilaginous tumors) are those of fetal cartilage.

Another morphologic variant of chondrosarcoma that can be found in the soft tissue is the *mesenchymal chondrosarcoma.* It has been described in the orbit, dura, trunk, retroperitoneum, and extremities.[280] Like its counterpart in the bone, it is characterized microscopically by an alternating pattern of highly cellular undifferentiated small cells (often growing in a hemangiopericytomatous fashion) and islands of well-differentiated cartilage (see Chapter 23).

Soft tissue osteosarcoma is distinguished from chondrosarcoma by applying the same criteria used for the skeletal tumors. They usually occur in the extremities of adults.[278] The prognosis is much worse than for chondrosarcoma: of the twenty-six cases reviewed by Allan and Soule,[273] twenty-one of the patients died as a result of the tumor. Extraskeletal osteosarcoma should be distinguished from

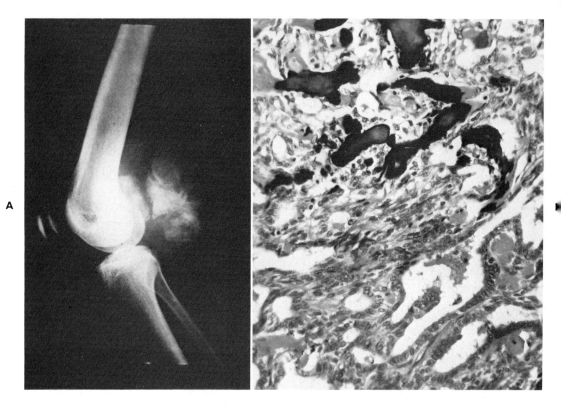

Fig. 1376 A, Roentgenogram of large calcifying synovial sarcoma located in popliteal space. **B,** Photomicrograph of same case showing biphasic component and extensive stromal calcification. (**A,** ×250; **A** and **B,** from Varela-Duran J, Enzinger FM: Calcifying synovial sarcoma. A clinicopathologic study of 32 cases. Cancer [in press].)

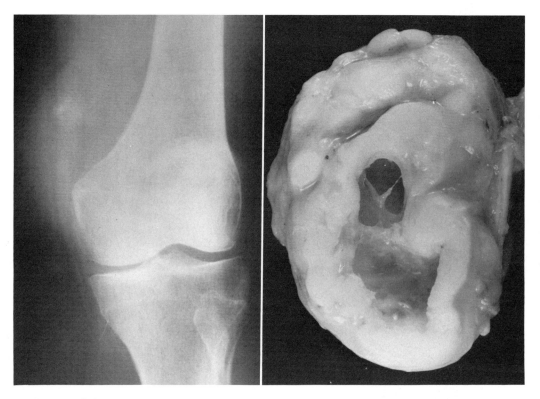

Fig. 1377 Soft tissue chondroma occurring in knee region of 71-year-old woman. As usual, tumor is partially calcified, lobulated, and focally cystic. (WU negs. 11139 and 11164.)

myositis ossificans. Nuclear atypia and lack of differentiation (''zone phenomena'') are the most important distinguishing features. It also should be differentiated from other soft tissue tumors in which metaplastic bone is formed, such as fibrosarcoma and synovial sarcoma.

Tumors of probable extragonadal germ cell origin
Teratoma

Soft tissue teratomas are uncommon.[286] They are more frequent in females and are present either at birth or in early childhood. In some cases, there is an association with twinning or malformations. The most common locations, in descending order of frequency, are retroperitoneum, mediastinum, sacrococcygeal area, base of skull, pineal region, and neck.[292] Taken

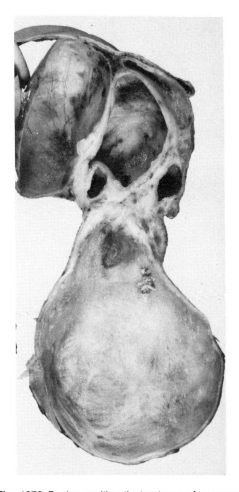

Fig. 1378 Benign multicystic teratoma of sacrococcygeal region present at birth. It was mainly composed of adult skin and neural tissue. (WU neg. 68-5325.)

as a whole, approximately three-fourths are benign. However, there are important variations in the incidence of malignancy according to location, age, and sex.[289,290] For instance, the large majority of sacrococcygeal teratomas present at birth are benign, whereas tumors in the same location discovered after the age of 2 months are often malignant.[289,291] Presence of marked bowel or bladder dysfunction indicates that the teratoma is probably malignant. Nearly all the teratomas presenting in the neck during infancy are benign, usually asymmetrical, and massive; the rare teratomas of the neck presenting in adults have a high incidence of malignancy.[288]

The terminology and diagnostic criteria used in the evaluation of these lesions is the same as for those of gonadal origin (Chapters 17 and 18). The benign form is often multicystic and contains a variety of well-differentiated tissues (Fig. 1378). The malignant types may have the appearance of teratocarcinoma, embryonal carcinoma, or yolk sac tumor. Immature neuroectodermal components are common; although they occasionally exhibit metastasizing capacity, their natural tendency is toward spontaneous maturation.[291a] Chretien et al.[287] reviewed twenty-one cases of yolk sac tumor (which they refer to as embryonal adenocarcinoma) of the sarcococcygeal region. Seven of them had other germ cell components. Local recurrence, often associated with distant metastases, resulted in the death of all twenty-one patients.

Tumors of neurogenic origin
Pigmented neuroectodermal tumor of infancy

The neurogenic origin of pigmented neuroectodermal tumor of infancy, also known as melanotic progonoma and retinal anlage tumor, is now established.[295,298] The classical location is the maxilla, but it also has been reported in the skull and mediastinum.[296,297] We also have seen it in the thigh, forearm, and epididymis. In most areas, the tumor cells are small and round, with the appearance of neuroblasts. As a matter of fact, we have seen this tumor misdiagnosed as neuroblastoma on several occasions. The diagnostic feature is the presence of pseudoglandular or alveolar formations lined by a wall of larger cells containing abundant melanin in their cytoplasm (Fig. 1379). The clinical course is almost invariably benign. Most supposedly malignant vari-

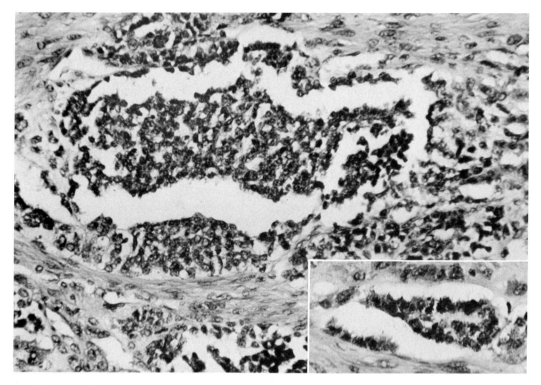

Fig. 1379 Pigmented neuroectodermal tumor of infancy. Clump of undifferentiated neuroectodermal cells has detached from peripheral portion, resulting in alveolar pattern. **Inset,** Another area of same tumor illustrating melanin-containing elements. (×300: WU neg. 73-3402; **inset,** ×350; WU neg. 73-3403.)

eties probably represent malignant teratomas with a pigmented neuroectodermal component. However, unquestionable malignant cases of pigmented neuroectodermal tumor of infancy have been seen.[296a]

Other neurogenic tumors

Exceptionally, *meningiomas* can present as a soft tissue mass at the base of the nose or scalp.[294] Anderson[293] reviewed seven benign *myxopapillary ependymomas* located in the soft tissues over the sacrococcygeal area.

Tumors of hematopoietic origin

Rarely, *malignant lymphomas* first manifest themselves by the presence of soft tissue tumor. This occurrence is more common with histiocytic and lymphocytic malignant lymphomas than with Hodgkin's disease. Most cases of *plasma cell myeloma* of soft tissue represent direct extension from underlying osseous foci. However, independent soft tissue masses also can occur. They inevitably become disseminated.

Exceptionally, nodules of *extramedullary*

hematopoiesis develop in the mediastinum or other soft tissue areas; they have been described in agnogenic myeloid metaplasia and congenital spherocytosis and in other types of anemia.[299]

Tumors of uncertain origin
Fibrous hamartoma of infancy

Enzinger[311] applied the term fibrous hamartoma of infancy to a tumorlike condition seen almost exclusively during the first two years of life and sometimes present at birth. It predominates in boys, and the most common locations are the region of the shoulder, axilla, and upper arm. It is almost always solitary. Grossly, it is poorly circumscribed and composed of whitish tissue of fibrous appearance intermixed with islands of fat.

Microscopically, the distinctive feature of this lesion is an organoid pattern, three distinct types of tissue being present: (1) well-differentiated fibrous tissue, (2) mature adipose tissue, and (3) immature, cellular areas arranged in a whorl-like pattern and resembling primitive mesenchyme. Although local recurrence may

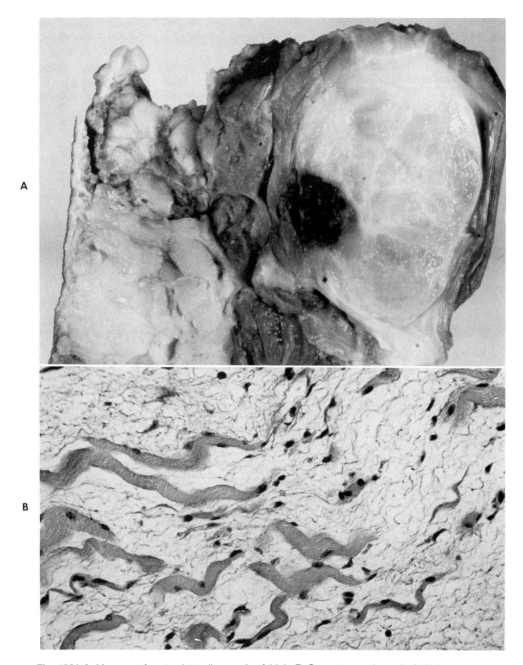

Fig. 1380 A, Myxoma of vastus lateralis muscle of thigh. **B,** Same tumor shown in **A.** Note myxomatous tissue infiltrating muscle bundles. (**A,** WU neg. 66-8361; **B,** ×300; WU neg. 67-1170.)

occur, the clinical course is basically that of a benign disease.[311]

Myxoma

Myxomas are rare neoplasms that have a mucoid, slimy gross appearance[334] (Fig. 1380, *A*). The majority are poorly circumscribed and

may infiltrate neighboring structures. They occur almost always in adults. The diagnosis of myxoma in a child should be seriously questioned. A high proportion of myxomas arise within skeletal muscle, especially those of the thigh. The prognosis is excellent. In a series of thirty-four cases reported by Enzinger,[309] there was not a single case of local recurrence. Multiple intramuscular myxomas are nearly always seen in association with fibrous dysplasia of the bones of the same extremity.[321,340]

The differential diagnosis of myxoma should be made with two groups of diseases. The first is a group of neoplasms in which myxomatous change can be a prominent secondary feature, such as liposarcoma, chondrosarcoma, smooth muscle tumors, embryonal rhabdomyosarcoma, and neurofibroma. The second is a variety of conditions resulting in focal mucinous degeneration of the skin or soft tissues, such as localized myxedema, mucous (myxoid) cyst, ganglion, follicular mucinosis (alopecia mucinosa), papular mucinosis, and cutaneous focal mucinosis.[322] It should be remembered that in myxoma the cells have a bland appearance throughout, that mitotic activity is practically absent, that lipoblasts are not identified, and, most importantly, that blood vessels are extremely scanty (Fig. 1380, *B*). The latter feature has been well demonstrated and contrasted with the high vascularity of myxoid liposarcoma in microangiographic studies.[323] Ultrastructurally, the principal cell of intramuscular myxoma resembles a fibroblast, with prominent granular endoplasmic reticulum, well-developed Golgi apparatus, and cytoplasmic filaments.[313]

Granular cell tumor

The most common location of granular cell tumor, also known as granular cell myoblastoma, is the tongue. It has been seen, however, in many other locations such as the skin, vulva, breast, larynx, bronchus, esophagus, stomach, appendix, rectum, anus, bile ducts, urinary bladder, uterus, and soft tissue.[325,338] Multiplicity of lesions can be observed, particularly in black patients.[325]

These tumors are usually small, although we have seen cases measuring up to 5 cm in diameter. They have a hard consistency and ill-defined margins. This, plus the ulceration sometimes complicating the larger cutaneous tumors, explains why they are often confused clinically and on gross inspection with a malig-

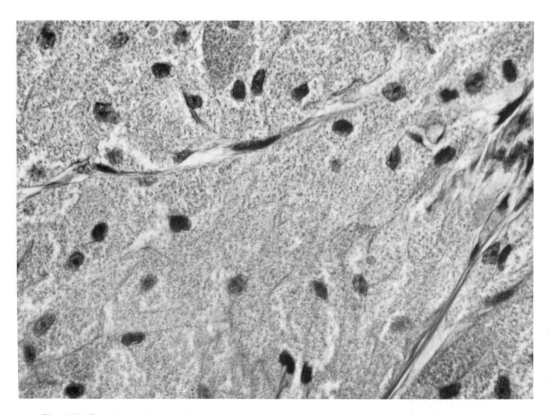

Fig. 1381 Granular cell tumor. Cells are large with finely granular cytoplasm and small dense nucleus. (×720; WU neg. 72-10437.)

nant neoplasm. The individual cells are large and their cytoplasm highly granular (Fig. 1381). Most granules are small and regular. They alternate with larger round droplets having a homogeneous eosinophilic appearance. The histochemical reactions and ultrastructural appearance of these inclusions are those of lysosomes. If the tumor grows near an epithelial surface, such as the skin, vulva, or larynx, secondary epithelial hyperplasia occurs that is often incorrectly diagnosed as carcinoma (Fig. 1382).

The large majority of the granular cell tumors pursue a benign clinical course. Most cases reported in the literature as malignant granular cell myoblastomas are in reality examples of alveolar soft part sarcoma. On the other hand, we know of a few well-documented cases of tumors with a light microscopic appearance comparable to that of granular cell tumor that resulted in distant metastases.[301,337]

The histogenesis of this lesion is still discussed, although most writers on the subject have favored a Schwann cell origin, based on histochemical and ultrastructural findings and on the occurrence of typical lesions within nerves.[307,316,318] On the other hand, changes histochemically and ultrastructurally indistinguishable from those previous discussed have been documented in neoplastic and nonneoplastic smooth muscle cells and in tumoral ameloblasts.[308,326,331] We therefore favor the view that granular cell tumor is not a specific entity but rather the expression of a degenerative change that can occur not only in Schwann's cells but also in a variety of other cell types, whether previously normal or forming part of a benign or a malignant neoplasm.

Alveolar soft part sarcoma

Alveolar soft part sarcoma, a malignant soft tissue tumor designated in the past as malignant organoid granular cell myoblastoma and malignant nonchromaffin paraganglioma, involves most often the deep soft tissues of the thigh and leg of young adults. Females are more commonly affected. We also have seen it in the oral cavity and mediastinum. Grossly, the tumors are well circumscribed, usually large, moderately firm, and gray or yellowish in color. Areas of necrosis or hemorrhage are common in the larger neoplasms.

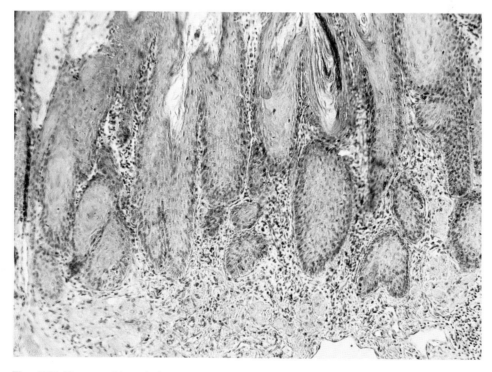

Fig. 1382 Bizarre epidermal changes overlying granular cell tumor. These changes often lead to incorrect diagnosis of cancer. (×125; WU neg. 52-3607.)

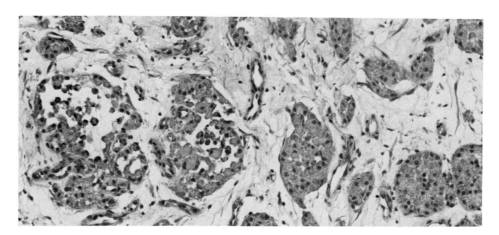

Fig. 1383 Alveolar soft part sarcoma presenting as mass in oropharyngeal region of young girl. Tumor forms well-defined lobules, some of which show central space simulating alveolus. (×150; WU neg. 72-2016A.)

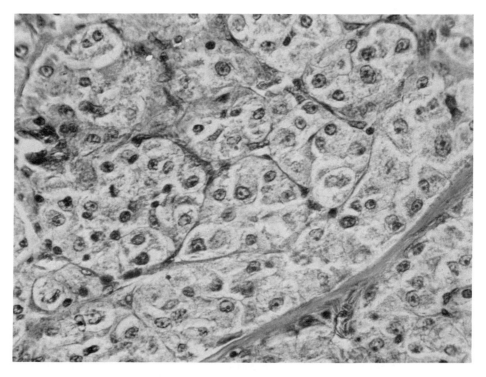

Fig. 1384 Alveolar soft part sarcoma. Note arrangement of cells, prominent nuclei and nucleoli, and abundant granular cytoplasm. (×500; WU neg. 54-4754.)

Microscopically, the tumor cells are separated by fibrous tissue into well-defined nests. Detachment of the central cells results in a typical alveolar pattern (Fig. 1383). The individual cells are large and have vesicular nuclei, *prominent nucleoli,* and a granular cytoplasm (Fig. 1384). Mitoses are exceptional. PAS stain sometimes demonstrates the presence of diastase-resistant intracytoplasmic needlelike structures. These are seen by electron microscopy as membrane-bound crystals with a periodicity of 58-100 Å, sometimes arranged in a cross-grid pattern (Fig. 1385). We have found this feature of diagnostic value in lesions of controversial nature.[330]

The tumor is highly malignant, despite its

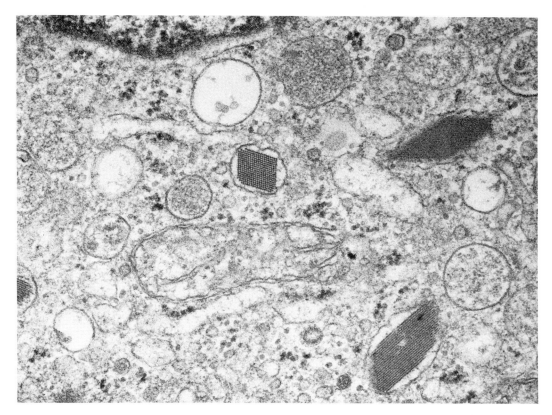

Fig. 1385 Electron microscopic appearance of alveolar soft part sarcoma. Detailed view of character-istic crystalloid inclusions that demonstrate orderly 70 Å periodicity. Both linear and cross-hatched crystalloid patterns may be noted. (×70,000; courtesy Dr. J. Sciubba, New Hyde Park, N. Y.)

deceivingly slow clinical course. Vein invasion is common. Blood-borne metastases appear in the lungs and other organs as long as fifteen years following excision of the primary tu-mor.[324]

The histogenesis of this strange neoplasm has not yet been definitely established. We be-lieve there is no convincing evidence to support the theory that this tumor represents the malig-nant counterpart of granular cell tumor or that it arises from nonchromaffin paraganglia. We agree with Fisher and Reidbard[315] that at the present time the bulk of evidence favors a myogenous derivation—i.e., that alveolar soft part sarcoma represents a distinct variant of rhabdomyosarcoma.

Clear cell sarcoma of tendons and aponeuroses

Enzinger[310] has described a malignant tumor arising chiefly from large tendons and apo-neuroses of the extremities and having a dis-tinctive microscopic appearance. The feet are

the most common site. Grossly, the tumors are firm, well circumscribed, and gray or white and cut with a gritty sensation. Microscopically, solid nests and fascicles of pale fusiform or cuboidal cells are present (Fig. 1386). The nucleoli are large and deeply basophilic. Mul-tinucleated giant cells are often seen. Abundant extracellular and intracellular iron was found in all twenty-one cases studied by Enzinger.[310]

The clinical course is characterized by slow but relentless progression with frequent local recurrences and eventual distant metasta-ses.[303,310] The histogenesis is unknown. Recent-ly, it has been found that some tumors fulfilling the morphologic criteria of clear cell sarcoma contain melanin,[304] suggesting that at least some of these tumors are, in reality, primary malignant melanomas of soft tissues. Perhaps the designation of clear cell sarcoma covers several histogenetically different neoplasms, some of melanocytic origin and others of mes-enchymal derivation, akin to synovial sar-coma.[336]

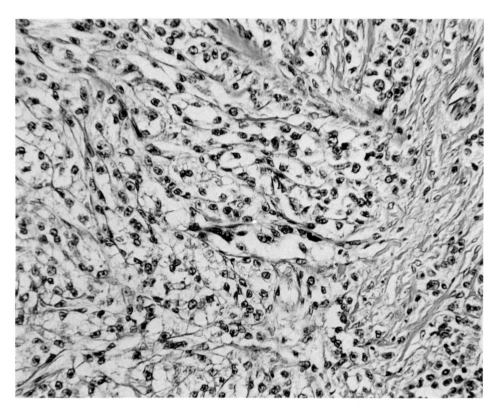

Fig. 1386 Clear cell sarcoma of soft tissue that occurred in 27-year-old woman and arose from left patellar tendon. (×300; WU neg. 66-9186; slide contributed by Dr. F. Enzinger, Washington, D. C.)

Epithelioid sarcoma

Enzinger[312] reported sixty-two cases of a malignant soft tissue tumor having a characteristic multinodular growth. The extremities are the most common location, particularly hands and fingers. The necrosis invariably seen in the center of the nodules and the epithelioid appearance of the tumor cells often results in a mistaken diagnosis of granuloma.[329] The tumors reported by Bliss and Reed[305] as ''large cell sarcomas of tendon sheath'' may be histogenetically related to epithelioid sarcoma, although several morphologic differences between the two are evident. Enzinger[312] remarked on the striking acidophilia of the tumor tissue in epithelioid sarcoma, due to the staining characteristics of the cytoplasm and the extensive desmoplasia (Fig. 1387). In his series, there was local recurrence in 85% of the patients and distant metastases in 30%. The tumor spreads to noncontiguous areas of skin, soft tissue, fascia, and bone, as well as by direct extension along fascial planes.[305a,326a] Lymph node metastases are relatively common and constitute an ominous prognostic sign.[327]

The histogenesis remains obscure. Histiocytes, fibroblasts, and synovial cells (or primitive mesenchymal cells with the capacity to differentiate into these) have all been implicated.[306,314,317,332]

Malignant giant cell tumor of soft parts

Malignant giant cell tumor of soft parts is a rare neoplasm composed of a mixture of osteoclast-like giant cells, fibroblasts, and histiocytes. The appearance is similar but not identical to that of giant cell tumor of bone.[328] Superficially located tumors are less aggressive than those situated in deeper structures. Guccion and Enzinger[320] favor a histiocytic derivation and a possible relationship with malignant fibrous histiocytoma, a concept that has been supported by a recent ultrastructural study of four cases.[300]

Extraskeletal Ewing's sarcoma

Tumors morphologically indistinguishable from Ewing's sarcoma of the bones can present as soft tissue masses. In most cases, they simply represent soft tissue extensions of tumor

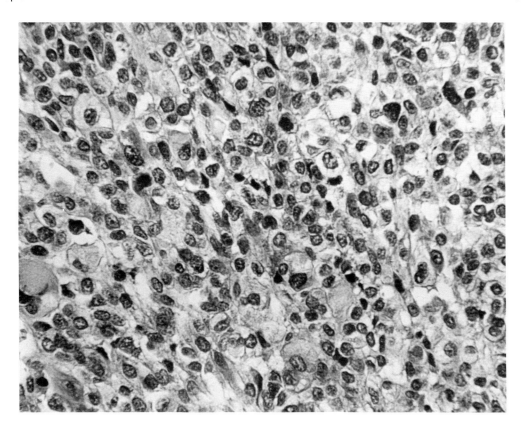

Fig. 1387 Epithelioid cell sarcoma. This rare tumor is highly cellular and at times has clear cytoplasm. (×350; WU neg. 72-10436.)

originating in the underlying bone. In some cases, however, bone involvement seems to be absent, and these are regarded as primary Ewing's sarcomas of soft tissues.[333] Angervall and Enzinger[302] reviewed thirty-nine cases affecting chiefly young adults and most commonly involving the soft tissues of the lower extremity and paravertebral region. Like their skeletal counterpart, they were composed of uniform small, round or oval cells containing cytoplasmic glycogen and sometimes arranged in a "peritheliomatous" pattern. The similarities persist at the ultrastructural level.[319,339] The course is aggressive, and distant metastases are common, particularly to lung and skeleton.

Other tumorlike conditions

In *tumoral calcinosis*, large, painless, calcified masses appear in the periarticular soft tissues, especially along extensor surfaces (Fig. 1388). The elbows and hips are the most common sites. Curiously, the knee is always spared. The serum calcium and phosphorus levels are normal. The disease may recur after excision.[344]

We prefer to designate as *Masson's hemangioma* a benign, probably nonneoplastic intravascular process that Masson first described in hemorrhoidal vessels as "vegetant intravascular hemangioendothelioma." It probably represents an exuberant organization and recanalization of a thrombus and can occur either in previously normal vessels or in varices, hemorrhoids, pyogenic granulomas and hemangiomas.[341,345] It simulates angiosarcoma because of the presence of papillary formations, anastomosing vascular channels, and plump endothelial cells. It is differentiated from it by the exclusively intravascular nature of the process, the lack of necrosis, bizarre cells, and atypical mitoses, and the characteristically fibrinous and/or hyaline appearance of the papillary stalks (Fig. 1389). Clearkin and Enzinger,[342] who refer to this process as "intravascular papillary endothelial hyperplasia," pointed out that the subcutis of the fingers, the head and neck region, and the trunk are the most common locations.

Another group of vascular proliferations that can simulate angiosarcomas microscopically is

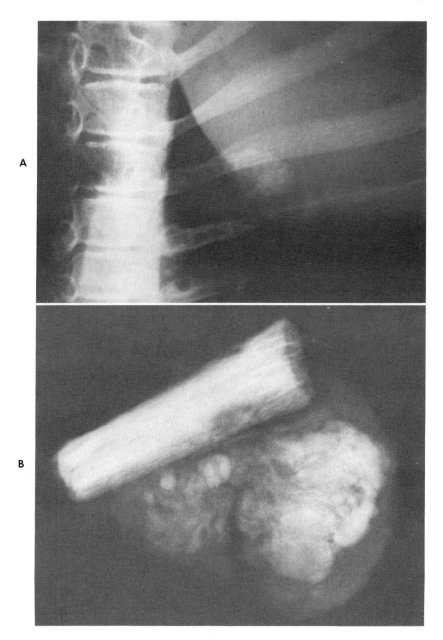

Fig. 1388 A, Roentgenogram showing area of tumoral calcinosis adjacent to posterior rib in 9-year-old child. **B,** Roentgenogram of excised specimen. Calcification is lobulated, splotchy, and independent of eighth rib.

that of the proliferative diseases of histiocytoid endothelial cells, sometimes referred to as the ''inflammatory angiomatoses.''[347,348] They are characterized by the growth of plump, acidophilic endothelial cells with indented and grooved nuclei and are often accompanied by an intense inflammatory reaction rich in eosinophils. This condition may present in the skin, soft tissue, bone, blood vessels,[346] and heart. It is more fully discussed in Chapter 3.

Bronchogenic cysts of skin and soft tissue were reported by Fraga et al.[343] The majority were discovered at or seen after birth in male infants. The most common location was the suprasternal notch and manubrium sterni.

In countries in which *hydatidosis* is en-

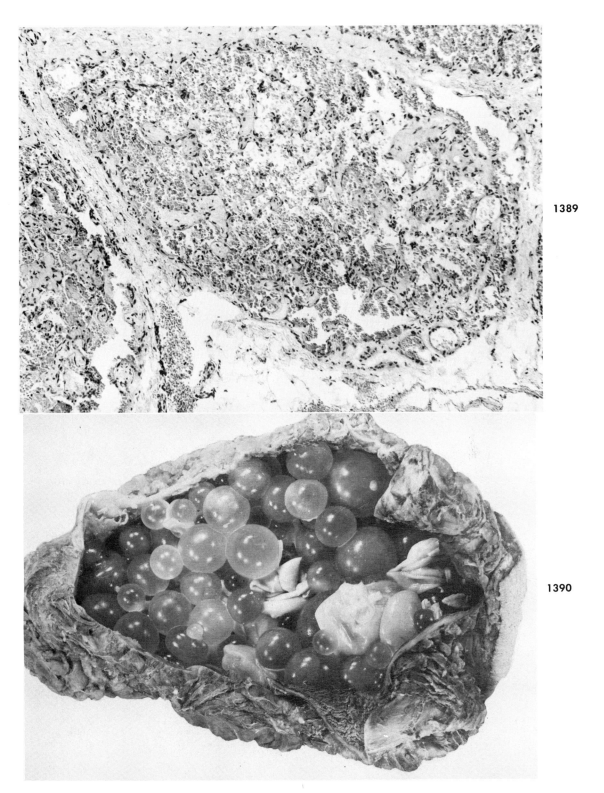

1389

1390

Fig. 1389 Masson's hemangioma. Large blood vessel shows complex papillary proliferation within lumen, covered by proliferating endothelial cells. There is no atypia or necrosis, and proliferation is confined to vessel lumen. This is not angiosarcoma but rather result of organizing and recanalizing thrombosis.

Fig. 1390 Hydatidosis presenting as soft tissue mass in gluteal region. (Courtesy Dr. E. F. Lascano, Buenos Aires, Argentina.)

demic, the disease may present as a soft tissue mass (Fig. 1390).

REFERENCES

Infection

1 Michelson E: Syndrome of trauma to the psoas muscle. Arch Surg **50:**77-81, 1945.
2 Picket WJ, Friedell MT: Large nonpulsating hematoma (false aneurysm). Surg Clin North Am **27:**153-155, 1947.

Pilonidal disease

3 Culp CE: Pilonidal disease and its treatment. Surg Clin North Am **47:**1007-1014, 1967.
4 Davage ON: The origin of sacrococcygeal pilonidal sinuses based on an analysis of four hundred sixty-three cases. Am J Pathol **30:**1191-1205, 1954.
5 Notaras MJ: A review of three popular methods of treatment of postanal (pilonidal) sinus disease. Br J Surg **57:**886-890, 1970.

Tumors

Introduction

6 Kauffman SL, Stout AP: Congenital mesenchymal tumors. Cancer **18:**460-476, 1965.
7 Soule EH, Mahour GH, Mills SD, Lynn HB: Soft-tissue sarcomas of infants and children. A clinicopathologic study of 135 cases. Mayo Clin Proc **43:**313-326, 1968.
8 Thompson DE, Frost HM, Hendrick JW, Horn RC: Soft tissue sarcomas involving the extremities and the limb girdles: A review. South Med J **64:**33-44, 1971.

Etiology

9 Hardy TJ, An T, Brown PW, Terz JJ: Postirradiation sarcoma (malignant fibrous histiocytoma) of axilla. Cancer **42:**118-124, 1978.
10 Hatfield PM, Schulz MD: Postirradiation sarcoma. Including 5 cases after x-ray therapy of breast carcinoma. Radiology **96:**593-602, 1970.
11 Monkman GR, Orwoll G, Ivins JC: Trauma and oncogenesis. Mayo Clin Proc **49:**157-163, 1974.

Diagnosis and therapy

11a Editorial: Changes in treating soft-tissue sarcomas. Br Med J **2:**562-563, 1979.
12 Lieberman Z, Ackerman LV: Principles in management of soft tissue sarcomas. Surgery **35:**350-365, 1954.
13 Rosenberg SA, Kent H, Costa J, Webber BL, Young R, Chabner B, Baker AR, Brennan MF, Chrieten PB, Cohen MH, deMoss EV, Sears HF, Seipp C, Simon R: Prospective randomized evaluation of the role of limb-sparing surgery, radiation therapy and adjuvant chemoimmunotherapy in the treatment of adult soft-tissue sarcomas. Surgery **84:**62-69, 1978.
14 Russell WO, Cohen J, Enzinger F, Hajdu SI, Heise H, Martin RG, Meissner W, Miller WT, Schmidtz RL, Suit HD: A clinical and pathological staging system for soft tissue sarcomas. Cancer **40:**1562-1570, 1977.
15 Suit HD, Russell WO, Martin RG: Sarcoma of soft tissue: clinical and histopathologic parameters and response to treatment. Cancer **35:**1478-1483, 1975.

Tumors and tumorlike conditions of fibrous tissue
Juvenile aponeurotic fibroma

16 Allen PM, Enzinger FM: Juvenile aponeurotic fibroma. Cancer **26:**857-867, 1970.
17 Goldman RL: The cartilage analogue of fibromatosis (aponeurotic fibroma). Further observations based on 7 new cases. Cancer **26:**1325-1331, 1970.
18 Keasbey LE: Juvenile aponeurotic fibroma (calcifying fibroma). Cancer **6:**338-346, 1953.
19 Lichtenstein L, Goldman RL: The cartilage analogue of fibromatosis. Cancer **17:**810-816, 1964.

Nodular and proliferative fasciitis

20 Allen PW: Nodular fasciitis. Pathology **4:**9-26, 1972.
21 Chung EB, Enzinger FM: Proliferative fasciitis. Cancer **36:**1450-1458, 1975.
22 Dahl I, Angervall L: Pseudosarcomatous proliferative lesions of soft tissue with or without bone formation. Acta Pathol Microbiol Scand [A] **85:**577-589, 1977.
23 Hutter RVP, Stewart FW, Foote FW, Jr: Fasciitis. A report of 70 cases with follow-up proving the benignity of the lesion. Cancer **15:**992-1003, 1962.
24 Kleinstiver BJ, Rodriquez HA: Nodular fasciitis. A study of 45 cases and review of the literature. J Bone Joint Surg [Am] **50:**1204-1212, 1968.
25 Konwaler BE, Keasbey L, Kaplan L: Subcutaneous pseudosarcomatous fibromatosis (fasciitis). Report of 8 cases. Am J Clin Pathol **25:**241-252, 1955.
25a Lauer DH, Enzinger FM: Cranial fasciitis of childhood. Cancer **45:**401-406, 1980.
26 Meister P, Bückmann FW, Konrad E: Extent and level of fascial involvement in 100 cases with nodular fasciitis. Virchows Arch [Pathol Anat] **380:**177-185, 1978.
26a Patchefsky AS, Enzinger FM: Intravascular fasciitis (IVF): a report of fifteen cases. Lab Invest **42:**142, 1980 (abstract).
27 Price EB, Jr, Silliphant WM, Shuman R: Nodular fasciitis: a clinicopathologic analysis of 65 cases. Am J Clin Pathol **35:**122-136, 1961.
28 Wirman JA: Nodular fasciitis, a lesion of myofibroblasts—an ultrastructural study. Cancer **38:**2378-2389, 1976.

Focal and proliferative myositis

29 Enzinger FM, Dulcey F: Proliferative myositis. Report of 33 cases. Cancer **20:**2213-2223, 1967.
29a Heffner RR Jr, Barron SA: Denervating changes in focal myositis, a benign inflammatory pseudotumor. Arch Pathol Lab Med **104:**261-264, 1980.
30 Heffner RR Jr, Armbrustmacher VW, Earle KM: Focal myositis. Cancer **40:**301-306, 1977.
31 Kern WH: Proliferative myositis. A pseudosarcomatous reaction to injury. Arch Pathol **69:**209-216, 1960.

Elastofibroma

32 Banfield WG, and Lee CK: Elastofibroma. An electron microscopic study. J Natl Cancer Inst **40:**1067-1077, 1968.
33 Järvi OH, Saxén AE, Hopsu-Havu VK, Wartiovaara JJ, Vaissalo VT: Elastofibroma. A degenerative pseudotumor. Cancer **23:**42-63, 1969.
34 Stemmermann GN, Stout AP: Elastofibroma dorsi. Am J Clin Pathol **37:**490-506, 1962.

Fibromatosis

35 Allen PW: The fibrmatoses: a clinicopathologic classi-

fication based on 140 cases. Am J Surg Pathol **1:**255-270, 305-321, 1977.

36 Allen RA, Woolner LB, Ghormley RK: Soft-tissue tumors of the sole. With special reference to plantar fibromatosis. J Bone Joint Surg [Am] **37:**14-26, 1955.

37 Battifora H, Hines JR: Recurrent digital fibromas of childhood. An electron microscope study. Cancer **27:**1530-1536, 1971.

38 Beatty EC Jr: Congenital generalized fibromatosis in infancy. Am J Dis Child **103:**620-624, 1962.

39 Bhawan J, Bacchetta C, Joris I., Majno G: A myofibroblastic tumor. Infantile digital fibroma (recurrent digital fibrous tumor of childhood). Am J Pathol **94:**19-28, 1979.

40 Bochetto JF, Raycroft JE, DeInnocentes LW: Multiple polyposis, exostosis, and soft tissue tumors. Surg Gynecol Obstet **117:**489-494, 1963.

40a Briselli MF, Soule EH, Gilchrist GS: Congenital fibromatosis. Report of 18 cases of solitary and 4 cases of multiple tumors. Mayo Clin Proc **55:**554-562, 1980.

41 Brown JB, McDowell F: Wry-neck facial distortion prevented by resection of fibrosed sternomastoid muscle in infancy and childhood. Ann Surg **131:**721-733, 1950.

42 Burry AF, Kerr JFR, Pope JH: Recurring digital fibrous tumour of childhood. An electron microscopic and virological study. Pathology **2:**287-291, 1970.

43 Conley J, Healey WV, Stout AP: Fibromatosis of the head and neck. Am J Surg **112:**609-614, 1966.

44 Coventry MB, Harris LE, Bianco AJ, Bulbulian AH: Congenital muscular torticollis (wry neck). Postgrad Med **28:**383-392, 1960.

45 Drescher E, Woyke S, Markiewicz C, Tegi S: Juvenile fibromatosis in siblings (fibromatosis hyalinica multiplex juvenilis). J Pediatr Surg **2:**427-430, 1967.

46 Editorial: The myofibroblast. Lancet **2:**1290-1291, 1978.

47 Enzinger FM: Fibrous tumors of infancy. In Tumors of bone and soft tissue. Houston, Texas, 1968, M. D. Anderson Hospital, pp. 375-396.

48 Enzinger FM: Histological typing of soft tissue tumours. International histological classification of tumours, No. 3. Geneva, 1969, World Health Organization.

49 Enzinger FM, Shiraki M: Musculo-aponeurotic fibromatosis of the shoulder girdle (extra-abdominal desmoid). Analysis of 30 cases followed up for ten or more years. Cancer **20:**1131-1140, 1967.

50 Gabbiani G, Majno G: Dupuytren's contracture. Fibroblast contraction? An ultrastructural study. Am J Pathol **66:**131-138, 1972.

51 Goslee L, Clermont V, Bernstein J, Woolley PW, Jr: Superficial connective tissue tumors in early infancy. J Pediatr **65:**377-387, 1964.

52 Hunt RT, Morgan HC, Ackerman LV: Principles in the management of extra-abdominal desmoids. Cancer **13:**825-836, 1960.

53 Ishikawa H, Mori S: Systemic hyalinosis or fibromatosis hyalinica multiplex juvenilis as a congenital syndrome. A new entity based on the inborn error of the acid mucopolysaccharide metabolism in connective tissue cells? Acta Dermatovenerol **53:**185-191, 1973.

54 Iwahara T, Ikeda A: On the ipsilateral involvement of congenital muscular torticollis and congenital dislocation of the hip. J Jap Orthop Assoc **35:**1221-1226, 1962.

55 Kim D-H, Goldsmith HS, Quan SH, Huvos AG: Intra-abdominal desmoid tumor. Cancer **27:**1041-1043, 1971.

56 Larsen RD, Posch JL: Dupuytren's contracture: with special reference to pathology. J Bone Joint Surg [Am] **40:**773-792, 1958.

57 Levine AM, Reddick R, Triche T: Intracellular collagen fibrils in human sarcomas. Lab Invest **39:**531-540, 1978.

58 Masson JK, Soule EH: Desmoid tumors of head and neck. Am J Surg **112:**615-622, 1966.

59 Pickren JW, Smith AG, Stevenson TW, Jr, Stout AP: Fibromatosis of the plantar fascia. Cancer **4:**846-856, 1951.

60 Reye RDK: Recurring digital fibrous tumors of childhood. Arch Pathol **80:**228-231, 1965.

61 Santa Cruz DJ, Reiner CB: Recurrent digital fibroma of childhood. J Cut Pathol **5:**339-346, 1978.

62 Shnitka TK, Douglas MA, Horner RH: Congenital generalized fibromatosis. Cancer **11:**627-639, 1958.

63 Skoog T: Dupuytren's contracture. Pathogenesis and surgical treatment. Surg Clin North Am **47:**433-444, 1967.

64 Staley CJ: Gardner's syndrome. Simultaneous occurrence of polyposis coli, osteomatosis and soft tissue tumors. Arch Surg **82:**420-422, 1961.

65 Stout AP: Juvenile fibromatoses. Cancer **7:**953-978, 1954.

66 Welsh RA: Intracytoplasmic collagen formations in desmoid fibromatosis. Am J Pathol **49:**515-535, 1966.

67 Woyke S, Domagala W, Olszewski W: Ultrastructure of a fibromatosis hyalinica multiplex juvenilis. Cancer **26:**1157-1168, 1970.

Fibrosarcoma

68 Chung EB, Enzinger FM: Infantile fibrosarcoma. Cancer **38:**729-739, 1976.

69 Churg AM, Kahn LB: Myofibroblasts and related cells in malignant fibrous and fibrohistiocytic tumors. Hum Pathol **8:**205-218, 1977.

70 Dehner LP, Askin FB: Tumors of fibrous tissue origin in childhood—a clinicopathologic study of cutaneous and soft tissue neoplasms in 66 children. Cancer **38:**888-900, 1976.

71 Guber S, Rudolph R: The myofibroblast. Surg Gynecol Obstet **146:**641-649, 1978.

71a Iwasaki H, Enjoji M: Infantile and adult fibrosarcomas of the soft tissues. Acta Pathol Jpn **29:**377-388, 1979.

72 Pritchard DJ, Soule EH, Taylor WF, Ivins JC: Fibrosarcoma—a clinicopathologic and statistical study of 199 tumors of the soft tissues of the extremities and trunk. Cancer **33:**888-897, 1974.

73 Soule EH, Pritchard DJ: Fibrosarcoma in infants and children—a review of 110 cases. Cancer **40:**1711-1721, 1977.

74 Stout AP: Fibrosarcoma. The malignant tumor of fibroblasts. Cancer **1:**30-63, 1948 (extensive bibliography).

75 Stout AP: Fibrosarcoma in infants and children. Cancer **15:**1028-1040, 1962.

76 van der Werf-Messing B, van Unnik JAM: Fibrosarcoma of the soft tissue. A clinicopathologic study. Cancer **18:**1113-1123, 1965.

Tumors of probable histiocytic origin

77 Alguacil-Garcia A, Unni KK, Goellner JR: Malignant fibrous histiocytoma—an ultrastructural study of six cases. Am J Clin Pathol **69:**121-129, 1978.

78 Angervall L, Kindblom L, Merck C: Myxofibrosarcoma—a study of 30 cases. Acta Pathol Microbiol
Scand [A] **85:**127-140, 1977.

79 Black WC, McGavran MH, Graham P: Nodular subepidermal fibrosis. A clinical pathologic study emphasizing the frequency of clinical misdiagnoses. Arch
Surg **98:**296-300, 1969.

80 Burkhardt BR, Soule EH, Winkelman RK, Ivins JC:
Dermatofibrosarcoma protuberans. Study of 56 cases.
Am J Surg **111:**638-644, 1966.

81 Colby TV: Malakoplakia. Two unusual cases which
presented diagnostic problems. Am J Surg Pathol **2:**
377-382, 1978.

81a Enzinger FM: Angiomatoid malignant fibrous histiocytoma. A distinct fibrohistiocytic tumor of children
and young adults simulating a vascular neoplasm.
Cancer **44:**2147-2157, 1979.

82 Feldman F, Norman D: Intra- and extraosseous malignant histiocytoma (malignant fibrous xanthoma).
Radiology **104:**497-508, 1972.

83 Fisher ER, Hellstrom HR: Dermatofibrosarcoma with
metastases simulating Hodgkin's disease and reticulum
cell sarcoma. Cancer **19:**1165-1171, 1966.

84 Fisher ER, Vuzevski VD: Cytogenesis of schwannoma
(neurilemoma), neurofibroma, dermatofibroma, and
dermatofibrosarcoma as revealed by electron microscopy. Am J Clin Pathol **49:**141-154, 1968.

85 Fretzin DF, Helwig EB: Atypical fibroxanthoma of the
skin. A clinicopathologic study of 140 cases. Cancer
31:1541-1552, 1973.

86 Fu Y, Gabbiani G, Kaye GI, Lattes R: Malignant soft
tissue tumors of probable histiocytic origin (malignant fibrous histiocytomas): general considerations and
electron microscopic and tissue culture studies. Cancer **35:**176-198, 1975.

86a Harris M: The ultrastructure of benign and malignant
fibrous histiocytomas. Histopathology **4:**29-44, 1980.

87 Hashimoto K, Brownstein MH, Jakobiec FA: Dermatofibrosarcoma protuberans—a tumor with perineural
and endoneural cell features. Arch Dermatol **110:**874-
885, 1974.

88 Hudson AW, Winkelmann RK: Atypical fibroxanthoma of the skin. A reappraisal of 19 cases in which
the original diagnosis was spindle-cell squamous carcinoma. Cancer **29:**413-422, 1972.

89 Jacoby F: Macrophages (XIV. The problem of transformation). In Willmer EN (ed): Cells and tissues
in culture. Methods, biology and physiology, vol. 2.
New York, 1965, Academic Press, Inc., pp. 63-75.

90 Kauffman SL, Stout AP: Histiocytic tumors (fibrous
xanthoma and histiocytoma) in children. Cancer **14:**
469-482, 1961.

91 Kauffman SL, Stout AP: Congenital mesenchymal
tumors. Cancer **18:**460-476, 1965.

91a Kearney MM, Soule EH, Ivins JC: Malignant fibrous
histiocytoma. A retrospective study of 167 cases.
Cancer **45:**167-178, 1980.

92 Kempson RL, Kyriakos M: Fibroxanthosarcoma of the
soft tissues. A type of malignant fibrous histiocytoma.
Cancer **29:**961-976, 1972.

93 Kempson RL, McGavran MH: Atypical fibroxanthoma
of the skin. Cancer **17:**1463-1471, 1964.

94 Kindblom L-G, Merck C, Angervall L: The ultrastructure of myxofibrosarcoma. A study of 11 cases. Virchows Arch [Pathol Anat] **381:**121-139, 1979.

95 Kroe DJ, Pitcock JA: Atypical fibroxanthoma of the
skin. Report of ten cases. Am J Clin Pathol **51:**487-
492, 1969.

96 Kyriakos M, Kempson RL: Inflammatory fibrous histiocytoma—an aggressive and lethal lesion. Cancer
37:1584-1606, 1976.

97 Lagacé R, Delage C, Seemayer TA: Myxoid variant of
malignant fibrous histiocytoma. Ultrastructural observations. Cancer **43:**526-534, 1979.

98 Meister P, Konrad E, Krauss F: Fibrous histiocytoma:
a histological and statistical analysis of 155 cases.
Path Res Pract **162:**361-379, 1978.

98a Meister P, Höhne N, Konrad E, Eder M: Fibrous
histiocytoma: an analysis of the storiform pattern.
Virchows Arch [Pathol Anat] **383:**31-41, 1979.

99 Merkow LP, Frich JC Jr, Slifkin M, Kyreages CG,
Pardo M: Ultrastructure of a fibroxanthosarcoma
(malignant fibroxanthoma). Cancer **28:**372-383, 1971.

100 Niemi KM: The benign fibrohistiocytic tumours of the
skin. Acta Derm Venereol (Stockh) **50**[suppl 63]:
1-66, 1970.

101 Oberling C: Retroperitoneal xanthogranuloma. Am J
Cancer **23:**477-489, 1935.

102 O'Brien JE, Stout AP: Malignant fibrous xanthomas.
Cancer **17:**1445-1455, 1964.

103 Ozzello L, Hamels J: The histiocytic nature of dermatofibrosarcoma protuberans—tissue culture and electron microscopic study. Am J Clin Pathol **65:**136-
148, 1976.

104 Ozzello L, Stout AP, Murray MR: Cultural characteristics of malignant histiocytomas and fibrous xanthomas. Cancer **16:**331-344, 1963.

105 Rachmaninoff N, McDonald JR, Cook JC: Sarcoma-
like tumors of the skin following irradiation. Am J
Clin Pathol **36:**427-437, 1961.

105a Santa Cruz DJ, Kyriakos M: Telangiectatic ("angiomatoid") fibrous histiocytoma of the skin. Cancer
(in press).

106 Soule EH, Enriquez P: Atypical fibrous histiocytoma,
malignant fibrous histiocytoma, malignant histiocytoma and epithelioid sarcoma. A comparative study of
65 tumors. Cancer **30:**128-143, 1972.

107 Stout AP, Lattes R: Tumors of the soft tissues. In
Atlas of tumor pathology, 2nd series, Fasc. I. Washington, D. C., 1967, Armed Forces Institute of Pathology.

108 Taxy JB, Battifora H: Malignant fibrous histiocytoma—an electron microscopic study. Cancer **40:**254-
267, 1977.

109 Taylor HB, Helwig EB: Dermatofibrosarcoma protuberans. A study of 115 cases. Cancer **15:**717-725,
1962.

110 Vernon-Roberts B: The macrophage. Cambridge,
1972, Cambridge University Press.

111 Weiss SW, Enzinger FM: Myxoid variant of malignant fibrous histiocytoma. Cancer **39:**1672-1685,
1977.

112 Weiss SW, Enzinger FM: Malignant fibrous histiocytoma—an analysis of 200 cases. Cancer **41:**2250-
2266, 1978.

113 Weiss SW, Enzinger FM, Johnson FB: Silica reaction simulating fibrous histiocytoma. Cancer **42:**2738-
2743, 1978.

Tumors and tumorlike conditions of peripheral nerves

114 Askin FB, Rosai J, Sibley RK, Dehner LP, McAlister
WH: Malignant small cell tumor of the thoracopul-
monary region in childhood: a distinctive clinicopathologic entity of uncertain histogenesis. Cancer **43:**
2438-2451, 1979.

115 Bednář B: Storiform neurofibromas of skin pigmented and nonpigmented. Cancer **10**:368-376, 1957.

116 Benedict PH, Szabó G, Fitzpatrick TB, Sinesi SJ: Melanotic macules in Albright's syndrome and in neurofibromatosis. JAMA **205**:618-626, 1968.

117 Bird CC, Willis RA: The histogenesis of pigmented neurofibromas. J Pathol **97**:631-637, 1969.

118 Bolande RP, Towler WF: A possible relationship of neuroblastoma to von Recklinghausen's disease. Cancer **26**:162-172, 1970.

118a Chen KTK, Latorraca R, Fabich D, Padgug A, Hafez GR, Gilbert EF: Malignant schwannoma. A light microscopic and ultrastructural study. Cancer **45**:1585-1593, 1980.

119 Crowe FW, Schull WJ, Neel JV: Multiple neurofibromatosis. Springfield, Ill., 1956, Charles C Thomas, Publisher.

120 D'Agostino AN, Soule EH, Miller RH: Primary malignant neoplasms of nerves (malignant neurilemonas) in patients without manifestations of multiple neurofibromatosis (von Recklinghausen's disease). Cancer **16**:1003-1013, 1963.

121 D'Agostino AN, Soule EH, Miller RH: Sarcomas of the peripheral nerves and somatic soft tissues associated with multiple neurofibromasotis (von Recklinghausen's disease). Cancer **16**:1015-1027, 1963.

122 Fisher ER, Vuzevski VD: Cytogenesis of schwannoma (neurilemoma), neurofibroma, dermatofibroma, and dermatofibrosarcoma as revealed by electron microscopy. Am J Clin Pathol **49**:141-154, 1968.

123 Ghosh BC, Ghosh L, Huvos AG, Fortner JG: Malignant schwannoma. A clinicopathologic study. Cancer **31**:184-190, 1973.

124 Gore I: Primary malignant tumors of nerve. A report of eight cases. Cancer **5**:278-296, 1952.

125 Gorlin RJ, Sedano HO, Vickers RA, Cervenka J: Multiple mucosal neuromas, pheochromocytoma and medullary carcinoma of the thyroid. A syndrome. Cancer **22**:293-299, 1968.

125a Guccion JG, Enzinger FM: Malignant schwannoma associated with von Recklinghausen's neurofibromatosis. Virchows Arch [Pathol Anat] **383**:43-57, 1979.

125b Ha'Eri GB, Fornasier VL, Schatzker J: Morton's neuroma pathogenesis and ultrastructure. Clin Orthop **141**:256-259, 1979.

126 Hill RP: Neuroma of Wagner-Meissner tactile corpuscles. Cancer **4**:879-882, 1951.

127 Hirano A, Dembitzer HM, Zimmerman HM: Fenestrated blood vessels in neurilemoma. Lab Invest **27**:305-309, 1972.

128 Holt JF; Neurofibromatosis in children. Am J Roentgenol **130**:651-639, 1978.

129 Hosoi K: Multiple neurofibromatosis (von Recklinghausen's disease), with special reference to malignant transformation. Arch Surg **22**:258-281, 1931.

130 Kamata Y: Study on the ultrastructure and acetylcholinesterase activity in von Recklinghausen's neurofibromatosis. Acta Pathol Jpn **28**:393-410, 1978.

131 Lattes R: Case A: Peripheral neuroepithelioma. Proceedings of the 39th Annual Anatomic Pathology Slide Seminar of the American Society of Clinical Pathologists. Chicago, 1975, American Society of Clinical Pathology, pp. 49-52.

132 Lazarus SS, Trombetta LD: Ultrastructural identification of a benign perineurial cell tumor. Cancer **41**:1823-1829, 1978.

133 McCarroll HR: Clinical manifestations of congenital neurofibromatosis. J Bone Joint Surg [Am] **32**:601-617, 1950.

134 Mackay B, Luna MA, Butler JJ: Adult neuroblastoma—electron microscopic observations in nine cases. Cancer **37**:1334-1351, 1976.

135 Mennemeyer RP, Hammar SP, Tytus JS, Hallman KO, Raisis JE, Bockus D: Melanotic schwannoma. Clinical and ultrastructural studies of three cases with evidence of intracellular melanin synthesis. Am J Surg Pathol **3**:3-10, 1979.

136 Oberman HA, Sullenger G: Neurogenous tumors of the head and neck. Cancer **20**:1992-2001, 1967.

137 Pineada A: Mast cells. Their presence and ultrastructural characteristics in peripheral nerve tumors. Arch Neurol **13**:372-382, 1965.

138 Raszkowski HJ, Hufner RF: Neurofibromatosis of the colon. A unique manifestation of von Recklinghausen's disease. Cancer **27**:134-142, 1971.

139 Reed RJ, Bliss BO: Morton's neuroma. Regressive and productive intermetatarsal elastofibrositis. Arch Pathol **95**:123-129, 1973.

140 Salyer WR, Salyer DC: The vascular lesions of neurofibromatosis. Angiology **25**:510-519, 1974.

141 Saxen E: Tumours of tactile end-organs. Acta Pathol Microbiology Scand **25**:66-79, 1948.

142 Schenkein I, Beuker ED, Helson L, Axelrod F, Dancis J: Increased nerve-growth-stimulating activity in disseminated neurofibromatosis. N Engl J Med **290**:613-614, 1974.

143 Scotti TM: The lesion of Morton's metatarsalgia (Morton's toe). Arch Pathol **63**:91-102, 1957.

144 Stay EJ, Vater G: The relationship between nephroblastoma and neurofibromatosis (Von Recklinghausen's disease). Cancer **39**:2550-2555, 1977.

144a Storm FK, Eilber FR, Mirra J, Morton DL: Neurofibrosarcoma. Cancer **45**:126-129, 1980.

145 Stout AP: Neurofibroma and neurilemoma. Clin Proc **5**:1-12, 1946.

146 Stout AP: Discussion of case 5. Seventeenth Seminar of the American Society of Clinical Pathologists, October, 1951.

146a Trojanowski JQ, Kleinman GM, Proppe KH: Malignant tumors of nerve sheath origin. Cancer **46**:1202-1212, 1980.

146b Tsuneyoshi M, Enjoji M: Primary malignant peripheral nerve tumors (malignant schwannomas). A clinicopathologic and electron microscopic study. Acta Pathol Jpn **29**:363-375, 1979.

147 Waggener JD: Ultrastructure of benign peripheral nerve sheath tumors. Cancer **19**:699-709, 1966.

148 Webb WR, Goodman PC: Fibrosing alveolitis in patients with neurofibromatosis. Radiology **122**:289-293, 1977.

149 White HR Jr: Survival in malignant schwannoma. An 18-year study. Cancer **27**:720-729, 1971.

150 Whitehouse D: Diagnostic value of the cafe-au-lait spots in children. Arch Dis Child **41**:316-319, 1966.

151 Williams ED, Pollock DJ: Multiple mucosal neuromata with endocrine tumors. A syndrome allied to von Recklinghausen's disease. J Pathol Bacteriol **91**:71-80, 1966.

152 Witzleben CL, Landy RA: Disseminated neuroblastoma in a child with von Recklinghausen's disease. Cancer **34**:786-790, 1974.

153 Woodruff JM: Peripheral nerve tumors showing glandular differentiation (glandular schwannomas). Cancer **37**:2399-2413, 1976.

154 Woodruff JM, Chernik NL, Smith MC, Millett WB, Foote FW: Peripheral nerve tumors with rhabdomyosarcomatous differentiation (malignant "triton" tumors). Cancer **32:**426-439, 1973.

Tumors of adipose tissue

155 Ackerman LV: Multiple primary liposarcomas. Am J Pathol **20:**789-798, 1944.

155a Battifora J, Nunez-Alonso C: Myxoid liposarcoma: study of ten cases. Ultrastruc Pathol **1:**157-169, 1980.

155b Bolen JW, Thorning D: Benign lipoblastoma and myxoid liposarcoma. A comparative light- and electron-microscopic study. Am J Surg Pathol **4:**163-174, 1980.

156 Brines OA, Johnson MH: Hibernoma, a special fatty tumor; report of a case. Am J Pathol **25:**467-479, 1949.

157 Chung EB, Enzinger FM: Benign lipoblastomatosis. An analysis of 35 cases. Cancer **32:**482-492, 1973.

158 Enterline HT, Culberson JD, Rochlin DB, Brady LW: Liposarcoma—a clinical and pathological study of 53 cases. Cancer **13:**932-950, 1960.

159 Enzinger FM: Benign lipomatous tumors simulating a sarcoma. In M. D. Anderson Tumor Institute: Management of primary bone and soft tissue tumors. Chicago, 1977, Year Book Medical Publishers, Inc., pp. 11-24.

160 Enzinger FM, Harvey DA: Spindle cell lipoma. Cancer **36:**1852-1859, 1975.

161 Enzinger FM, Winslow DJ: Liposarcoma. A study of 103 cases. Virchows Arch [Pathol Anat] **335:**367-388, 1962.

161a Evans HL: Liposarcoma. A study of 55 cases with a reassessment of its classification. Am J Surg Pathol **3:**507-523, 1979.

162 Evans HL, Soule EH, Winkelmann RK: Atypical lipoma, atypical intramuscular lipoma, and well-differentiated retroperitoneal liposarcoma. A reappraisal of 30 cases formerly classified as well differentiated liposarcomas. Cancer **43:**574-584, 1979.

163 Georgiades DE, Alcalais CB, Karabela VG: Multicentric well-differentiated liposarcomas. A case report and a brief review of the literature. Cancer **24:**1091-1097, 1969.

164 Greenberg SD, Isensee C, Gonzalez-Angulo A, Wallace SA: Infiltrating lipomas of the thigh. Am J Clin Pathol **39:**66-72, 1963.

165 Howard WR, Helwig EB: Angiolipoma. Arch Dermatol **82:**924-931, 1960.

165a Kindblom L-G, Säve-Söderbergh J: The ultrastructure of liposarcoma. A study of 10 cases. Acta Pathol Microbiol Scand [A] **87:**109-121, 1979.

166 Kindblom LG, Angervall L, Jarlstedt J: Liposarcoma of the neck. A clinicopathologic study of 4 cases. Cancer **42:**774-780, 1978.

167 Kindblom L, Angervall L, Svendsen P: Liposarcoma—a clinicopathologic, radiographic and prognostic study. Acta Pathol Microbiol Scand [Suppl] (253): 1-71, 1975.

168 Kindblom L, Angervall L, Stener B, Wickbom I: Intermuscular and intramuscular lipomas and hibernomas—a clinical, roentgenologic, histologic, and prognostic study of 46 cases. Cancer **33:**754-762, 1974.

168a Lagace R, Jacob S, Seemayer TA: Myxoid liposarcoma. An electronmicroscopic study: biological and histogenetic considerations. Virchows Arch [Pathol Anat] **384:**159-172, 1979.

169 Levine GD: Hibernoma. An electron microscopic study. Hum Pathol **3:**351-359, 1972.

170 Paarlberg D, Linscheid RL, Soule EH: Lipomas of of the hand. Including a case of lipoblastomatosis in a child. Mayo Clin Proc **47:**121-124, 1972.

171 Pack GT, Pierson JC: Liposarcoma. Surgery **36:**687-712, 1954.

172 Reszel PA, Soule EH, Coventry MB: Liposarcoma of extremities and limb girdles: study of 222 cases. J Bone Joint Surg [Am] **48:**229-244, 1966.

173 Saunders JR, Jaques DA, Casterline PF, Percarpio B, Goodloe S Jr: Liposarcomas of the head and neck. A review of the literature and addition of four cases. Cancer **43:**162-168, 1979.

174 Seemayer TA, Knaack J, Wang N, Ahmed MN: On the ultrastructure of hibernoma. Cancer **36:**1785-1793, 1975.

174a Shmookler BM, Enzinger FM: Pleomorphic lipoma: a benign tumor simulating liposarcoma. A clinicopathologic analysis of 48 cases. Cancer **47:**126-133, 1981.

175 Stout AP: Liposarcoma, the malignant tumor of lipoblasts. Ann Surg **119:**86-197, 1944.

176 Vellios F, Baez MF, Schumacher HB: Lipoblastomatosis: a tumor of fetal fat different from hibernoma. Am J Pathol **34:**1149-1155, 1958.

177 Winslow DJ, Enzinger FM: Hyaluronidase-sensitive acid mucopolysaccharides in liposarcomas. Am J Pathol **37:**497-505, 1960.

Tumors and tumorlike conditions of blood and lymph vessels
  Hemangioma

178 Allen PW, Enzinger FM: Hemangioma of skeletal muscle. An analysis of 89 cases. Cancer **29:**8-22, 1972.

179 Brizill HE, Raceuglia G: Giant hemangioma with thrombocytopenia. Blood **26:**751-756, 1965.

180 Koblenzer PJ, Bukowski MJ: Angiomatosis (hamartomatous hem-lymphangiomatosis). Report of a case with diffuse involvement. Pediatrics **28:**65-76, 1961.

181 Lelong M, Alagille D, Habib E-C, Steiner A: Memories Originaux. L'hemangiome geant du nourrisson avec thrombopenie. Arch Franc Pédiatr **21:**769-784, 1964.

182 Lindenauer SM: The Klipper-Trenaunay syndrome: varicosity, hypertrophy and hemangioma with no arteriovenous fistula. Ann Surg **162:**303-314, 1965.

183 Lister WA: The natural history of strawberry nevi. Lancet **1:**1429-1434, 1938.

184 Modlin JJ: Capillary hemangiomas of the skin. Surgery **38:**169-180, 1955.

185 Mukai K, Rosai J, Burgdorf W: Localization of factor VIII-related antigen in vascular endothelial cells using an immunoperoxidase method. Am J Surg Pathol **4:**273-276, 1980.

186 Shim WKT: Hemangiomas of infancy complicated by thrombocytopenia. Am J Surg **116:**896-906, 1968.

186a Taxy JB, Gray SR: Cellular angiomas of infancy. An ultrastructural study of two cases. Cancer **43:**2322-2331, 1979.

187 Watson WL, McCarthy WD: Blood and lymph vessel tumors. Surg Gynecol Obstet **71:**569-588, 1940.

  Glomus tumor

188 Carroll RE, Berman AT: Glomus tumors of the hand. Review of the literature and report of 28 cases. J Bone Joint Surg [Am] **54:**691-703, 1972.

189 Kohout E, Stout AR: The glomus tumor in children. Cancer **14**:555-556, 1961.

190 Lattes R, Bull DC: A case of glomus tumor with primary involvement of bone. Ann Surg **127**:187-191, 1948.

191 Masson P: Le glomus neuromyo-artériel des régions tactiles et ses tumeurs. Lyon Chir **21**:259-280, 1924.

192 Masson P: Les glomus cutanés de l'homme. Bull Soc Fr Dermatol Syphiligr **42**:1174-1245, 1935.

193 Murray MR, Stout AP: The glomus tumor. Investigations of its distribution and behavior, and the identity of its "epithelioid" cell. Am J Pathol **18**:183-203, 1942.

194 Shugart RR, Soule EH, Johnson EW: Glomus tumor. Surg Gynecol Obstet **117**:334-340, 1963.

195 Stout AP: Tumors of the neuromyoarterial glomus. Am J Cancer **24**:255-272, 1935.

196 Venkatachalam MA, Greally JG: Fine structure of glomus tumor: similarity of glomus cells to smooth muscle. Cancer **23**:1176-1184, 1969.

Hemangiopericytoma

197 Angervall L, Kindblom L-G, Nielsen JM, Stener B, Svendsen P: Hemangiopericytoma. A clinicopathologic, angiographic and microangiographic study. Cancer **42**:2412-2427, 1978.

198 Battifora H: Hemangiopericytoma: ultrastructural study of five cases. Cancer **31**:1418-1432, 1973.

199 Enzinger FM, Smith BH: Hemangiopericytoma—an analysis of 106 cases. Hum Pathol **7**:61-82, 1976.

200 Kuhn C III, Rosai J: Tumors arising from pericytes. Ultrastructure and organ culture of a case. Arch Pathol **88**:653-663, 1969.

201 McMaster MJ, Soule EH, Ivins JC: Hemangiopericytoma—a clinicopathologic study and long-term follow-up of 60 patients. Cancer **36**:2232-2244, 1975.

202 Murray MR, Stout AP: The glomus tumor. Investigation of its distribution and behavior, and the identity of its "epithelioid" cell. Am J Pathol **18**:183-203, 1942.

203 O'Brien P, Brasfield RD: Hemangiopericytoma. Cancer **14**:249-252, 1965.

204 Stout AP: Hemangiopericytoma (a study of 25 new cases). Cancer **2**:1027-1054, 1949.

205 Stout AP: Tumors featuring pericytes. Glomus tumor and hemangiopericytoma. Lab Invest **5**:217-223, 1965.

206 Zimmerman KW: Der feinere Bau der Blutcapillaren. Z Anat Entwicklungsgesch **68**:29-109, 1923.

Angiosarcoma

207 Girard C, Johnson WC, Graham JH: Cutaneous angiosarcoma. Cancer **26**:868-883, 1970.

208 Rosai J, Sumner HW, Kostianovsky M, Perez-Mesa C: Angiosarcoma of skin. A clinicopathologic and fine structural study. Hum Pathol **7**:83-109, 1976.

209 Stout AP: Hemangio-endothelioma: a tumor of blood vessels featuring vascular endothelial cells. Ann Surg **118**:445-464, 1943.

Lymphangioma

210 Cornog JL Jr, Enterline HT: Lymphangiomyoma, a benign lesion of chyliferous lymphatics synonymous with lymphangiopericytoma. Cancer **19**:1909-1930, 1966.

211 Enterline HT, Roberts D: Lymphangiopericytoma. Case report of a previously undescribed tumor type. Cancer **8**:582-587, 1955.

212 Gross RE, Hurwitt ES: Cervicomediastinal and mediastinal cystic hygromas. Surg Gynecol Obstet **87**:599-610, 1948.

213 Jao J, Gilbert S, Messer R: Lymphangiomyoma and tuberous sclerosis. Cancer **29**:1188-1192, 1972.

214 Maxwell JH: Tumros of the face and neck in infancy and childhood. South Med J **45**:292-299, 1952.

214a McCarty KS Jr, Mossler JA, McLelland R, Sieker HO: Pulmonary lymphangiomyomatosis responsive to progesterone. N Engl J Med **303**:1461-1465, 1980.

215 Wolff M: Lymphangiomyoma: clinicopathologic study and ultrastructural confirmation of its histogenesis. Cancer **31**:988-1007, 1973.

Lymphangiosarcoma

216 Eby CS, Brennan MJ, Fine G: Lymphangiosarcoma: a lethal complication of chronic lymphedema. Arch Surg **94**:223-230, 1967.

217 Herman JB: Lymphangiosarcoma of the chronically edematous extremity. Surg Gynecol Obstet **121**:1107-1115, 1965.

218 Stewart FW, Treves N: Lymphangiosarcoma in postmastectomy lymphedema. A report of six cases in elephantiasis chirurgica. Cancer **1**:64-81, 1948.

219 Whittle RJM: An angiosarcoma associated with an oedematous limb. J Fac Radiologists **10**:111-112, 1951.

220 Woodward AH, Ivins JC, Soule EH: Lymphangiosarcoma arising in chronic lymphedematous extremities. Cancer **30**:562-572, 1972.

Tumors of smooth muscle
Leiomyoma

221 Lendrum AC: Painful tumors of the skin. Ann R Coll Surg Engl **1**:62-67, 1947.

222 MacDonald DM, Sanderson KV: Angioleiomyoma of the skin. Br J Dermatol **91**:161-168, 1974.

223 Stout AP: Solitary cutaneous and subcutaneous leiomyoma. Am J Cancer **29**:435-469, 1937 (extensive bibliography).

Leiomyosarcoma

224 Bulmer JH: Smooth muscle tumors of limbs. J Bone Joint Surg [Br] **49**:52-58, 1967.

225 Dahl I, Angervall L: Cutaneous and subcutaneous leiomyosarcoma—a clinicopathologic study of 47 patients. Patho Eruop **9**:307-315, 1974.

226 Dorfman IID, Fishel ER: Leiomyosarcomas of the greater saphenous vein. Am J Clin Pathol **39**:73-78, 1963.

227 Kevorkian J, Cento DP: Leiomyosarcoma of large arteries and veins. Surgery **73**:390-400, 1973.

228 Phelan JT, Sherer W, Perez-Mesa C: Malignant smooth-muscle tumors (leiomyosarcomas) of soft-tissue origin. N Engl J Med **266**:1027-1030, 1962.

229 Stout AP, Hill WT: Leiomyosarcoma of the superficial soft tissues. Cancer **11**:844-854, 1958.

230 Thomas MA, Fine G: Leiomyosarcoma of veins. Report of 2 cases and review of the literature. Cancer **13**:96-101, 1960.

230a Varela-Duran J, Oliva H, Rosai J: Vascular leiomyosarcoma. The malignant counterpart of vascular leiomyoma. Cancer **44**:1684-1691, 1979.

230b Wile AG, Evans HL, Romsdahl MM: Leiomyosarcoma of soft tissue. A clinicopathologic study. Cancer (in press).

231 Yannopoulos K, Stout AP: Smooth muscle tumors in children. Cancer 15:958-971, 1962.

Tumors of striated muscles
Rhabdomyoma

232 Czernobilsky B, Cornog JL, Enterline HT: Rhabdomyoma. Report of case with ultrastructural and histochemical studies. Am J Clin Pathol 49:782-789, 1968.
233 Dehner LP, Enzinger FM: Fetal rhabdomyoma. An analysis of nine cases. Cancer 30:160-166, 1972.
233a di Sant'Agnese PA, Knowles DM II: Extracardiac rhabdomyoma: a clinicopathologic study and review of the literature. Cancer 46:780-789, 1980.
234 Morgan JJ, Enterline HT: Benign rhabdomyoma of the pharynx. A case report, review of the literature, and comparison with cardiac rhabdomyoma. Am J Clin Pathol 42:174-181, 1964.

Rhabdomyosarcoma

235 Churg A, Ringus J: Ultrastructural observations on the histogenesis of alveolar rhabdomyosarcoma. Cancer 41:1355-1361, 1978.
236 Enterline HT, Horn RC: Alveolar rhabdomyosarcoma. A distinctive tumor type. Am J Clin Pathol 20:356-366, 1958.
237 Enzinger FM: Recent trends in soft tissue pathology. In Tumors of bone and soft tissue. Houston, Texas, 1963, M. D. Anderson Hospital, pp. 315-332.
238 Enzinger FM: Alveolar rhabdomyosarcoma. An analysis of 110 cases. Cancer 24:18-31, 1969.
239 Gonzalez-Crussi F, Black-Schaffer S: Rhabdomyosarcoma of infancy and childhood. Problems of morphologic classification. Am J Surg Pathol 3:157-171, 1979.
240 Horn RC Jr, Enterline HT: Rhabdomyosarcoma. A clinicopathological study and classification of 39 cases. Cancer 11:181-199, 1958.
241 Horvat BI, Caines M, Fisher ER: The ultrastructure of rhabdomyosarcoma. Am J Clin Pathol 53:555-564, 1970.
242 Jaffe BF, Fox JE, Batsakis JG: Rhabdomyosarcoma of the middle ear and mastoid. Cancer 27:29-37, 1971.
243 Jönsson G: Malignant tumors of the skeletal muscles, fasciae, joint capsules, tendon sheaths and serous bursae. Acta Radiol [Suppl] (36):1-304, 1938.
244 Karcioglu Z, Someren A, Mathes SJ: Ectomesenchymoma—a malignant tumor of migratory neural crest (ectomesenchyme) remnants showing ganglionic, schwannian, melanocytic and rhabdomyoblastic differentiation. Cancer 39:2486-2496, 1977.
245 Keyhani A, Booher RJ: Pleomorphic rhabdomyosarcoma. Cancer 22:956-967, 1968.
245a Koh S-J, Johnson WW: Antimyosin and antirhabdomyoblast sera. Their use for the diagnosis of childhood rhabdomyosarcoma. Arch Pathol Lab Med 104:118-122, 1980.
246 Koop E, Tewarson IP: Rhabdomyosarcoma of head and neck in children. Ann Surg 160:95-103, 1964.
247 Linscheid RL, Soule EH, Henderson ED: Pleomorphic rhabdomyosarcomata of the extremities and limb girdles. J Bone Joint Surg [Am] 47:715-726, 1965.
248 Masson JK, Soule EH: Embryonal rhabdomyosarcoma of head and neck: report of 88 cases. Am J Surg 110:585-591, 1965.
249 Mauer HM, Moon T, Donaldson M, Fernandez C, Gehnan EA, Hammond D, Hays DM, Lawrence W, Newton W, Ragab A, Raney B, Soule EH, Sutow WW, Tefft M: The intergroup rhabdomyosarcoma study—a preliminary report. Cancer 40:2015-2026, 1977.
249a Mierau GW, Favara BE: Rhabdomyosarcoma in children: ultrastructural study of 31 cases. Cancer 46:2035-2040, 1980.
250 Morales AR, Fine G, Horn RC Jr: Rhabdomyosarcoma: an ultrastructural appraisal. Pathol Annu 7:81-106, 1972.
251 Mukai K, Rosai J, Hallaway BE: Localization of myoglobin in normal and neoplastic human skeletal muscle cells using an immunoperoxidase method. Am J Surg Pathol 3:373-376, 1979.
251a Mukai K, Schollmeyer JV, Rosai J: Immunohistochemical localization of actin: its applications in surgical pathology. Am J Surg Pathol (in press).
252 Riopelle JL, Thériault JP: Sur une forme méconnue de sarcome des parties molles; le rhabdomyosarcome alvéolaire. Ann Anat Pathol (Paris) 1:88-111, 1956.
253 Sarnat HB, de Mello DE, Siddiqui SY: Diagnostic value of histochemistry in embryonal rhabdomyosarcoma. Am J Surg Pathol 3:177-183, 1979.
253a Scrivner D, Meyer JS: Multifocal recurrent adult rhabdomyoma. Cancer 46:790-795, 1980.
254 Soule EH, Geitz M, Henderson ED: Embryonal rhabdomyosarcoma of the limbs and limb-girdles. A clinicopathologic study of 61 cases. Cancer 23:1336-1346, 1969.
255 Stobbe GD, Dargeon HW: Embryonal rhabdomyosarcoma of head and neck in children and adolescents. Cancer 3:826-836, 1950.
256 Stout AP: Rhabdomyosarcoma of the skeletal muscles. Ann Surg 123:447-472, 1946 (extensive bibliography).

Tumors of synovial tissue
Synovial sarcoma

257 Batsakis JG, Nishiyama RH, Sullinger GD: Synovial sarcomas of the neck. Arch Otolaryngol 85:327-331, 1967.
258 Crocker EW, Stout AP: Synovial sarcoma in children. Cancer 12:1123-1133, 1959.
259 Dische FE, Darby AJ, Howard ER: Malignant synovioma: electron microscopical findings in three patients and review of the literature. J Pathol 124:149-155, 1978.
260 Enzinger FM: Recent trends in soft tissue pathology. In Tumors of bone and soft tissue. Houston, Texas, 1963, M. D. Anderson Hospital, pp. 315-332.
261 Gabbiani G, Kaye GI, Lattes R, Majno G: Synovial sarcoma. Electron microscopic study of a typical case. Cancer 28:1031-1039, 1971.
262 Haagensen CD, Stout AP: Synovial sarcoma. Ann Surg 120:826-842, 1944.
263 Hajdu SI, Shiu MH, Fortner JG: Tendosynovial sarcoma—a clinicopathological study of 136 cases. Cancer 39:1201-1217, 1977.
264 Mackenzie DH: Synovial sarcoma. A review of 58 cases. Cancer 19:169-180, 1966.
264a Mackenzie DH: Monophasic synovial sarcoma—a histological entity? Histopathology 1:151-157, 1977.
264b Mickelson MR, Brown GA, Maynard JA, Cooper RR, Bonfiglio M: Synovial sarcoma. An electron microscopic study of monophasic and biphasic forms. Cancer 45:2109-2118, 1980.
265 Moberger G, Nilsonne U, Friberg S Jr: Synovial sarcoma. Histologic features and prognosis. Acta Orthop Scand [Suppl] 3:1-38, 1968.

266 Nunez-Alonso C, Gashti EN, Christ ML: Maxillo-facial synovial sarcoma. Light- and electron-microscopic study of two cases. Am J Surg Pathol **3**:23-30, 1979.

267 Roth JA, Enzinger FM, Tannenbaum M: Synovial sarcoma of the neck: a follow-up study of 24 cases. Cancer **35**:1243-1253, 1975.

268 Suit HD, Russell WO, Martin RG: Management of patients with sarcoma of soft tissue in an extremity. Cancer **31**:1247-1255, 1973.

269 van Andel JG: Synovial sarcoma. A review and analysis of treated cases. Radiol Clin Biol **41**:145-159, 1972.

269a Varela-Duran J, Enzinger FM: Calcifying synovial sarcoma. A clinicopathologic study of 32 cases. Cancer (in press).

Tumors of pluripotential mesenchyme
Mesenchymoma

270 Bures C, Barnes L: Benign mesenchymomas of the head and neck. Arch Pathol Lab Med **102**:237-241, 1978.

270a Dorfman HD, Levin S, Robbins H: Cartilage-containing benign mesenchymomas of soft tissue. Report of two cases. J Bone Joint Surg [Am] **62**:472-475, 1980.

271 Nash A, Stout AP: Malignant mesenchymomas in children. Cancer **14**:524-533, 1961.

272 Stout AP: Mesenchymoma, the mixed tumor of mesenchymal derivatives Ann Surg **127**:278-290, 1948.

Tumors of metaplastic mesenchyme

273 Allan CJ, Soule EH: Osteogenic sarcoma of the somatic soft tissues. Clinicopathologic study of 26 cases and review of literature. Cancer **27**:1121-1133, 1971.

274 Chung EB, Enzinger FM: Chondroma of soft parts. Cancer **41**:1414-1424, 1978.

275 Dabska M: Parachordoma—a new clinicopathologic entity. Cancer **40**:1586-1592, 1977.

276 Dahlin DC, Salvador AH: Cartilaginous tumors of the soft tissues of the hands and feet. Mayo Clin Proc **49**:721-726, 1974.

277 Enzinger FM, Shiraki M: Extra-skeletal myxoid chondrosarcoma. An analysis of 34 cases. Hum Pathol **3**:421-435, 1972.

278 Fine G, Stout AP: Osteogenic sarcoma of the extraskeletal soft tissues. Cancer **9**:1027-1043, 1956.

279 Goldenberg RR, Cohen P, Steinlauf P: Chondrosarcoma of extraskeletal soft tissues: report of 7 cases and review of literature. J Bone Joint Surg [Am] **49**:1487-1507, 1967.

280 Guccion JG, Font RL, Enzinger FM, Zimmerman LE: Extraskeletal mesenchymal chondrosarcoma. Arch Pathol **95**:336-340, 1973.

281 Kindblom L, Angervall L: Histochemical characterization of mucosubstances in bone and soft tissue tumors. Cancer **36**:985-994, 1975.

282 Lichtenstein L, Goldman RL: Cartilage tumors in soft tissues, particularly in the hand and foot. Cancer **17**:1203-1208, 1964.

283 Martin RF, Melnick PJ, Warner NE, Terry R, Bullock WK, Schwinn CP: Chordoid sarcoma. Am J Clin Pathol **59**:623-635, 1973.

284 Stout AP, Verner EW: Chondrosarcoma of the extraskeletal soft tissues. Cancer **6**:581-590, 1953.

285 Weiss S: Ultrastructure of the so-called "chordoid sarcoma"—evidence supporting cartilaginous differentiation. Cancer **37**:300-306, 1976.

285a Wu KK, Collon DJ, Guise ER: Extra-osseous chondrosarcoma. Report of five cases and review of the literature. J Bone Joint Surg [Am] **62**:189-194, 1980.

Tumors of probable extragonadal germ cell origin

286 Berry CL, Keelnig J, Hilton C: Teratoma in infancy and childhood: a review of 91 cases. J Pathol **98**:241-252, 1969.

287 Chretien PB, Milam JD, Foote FW, Miller TR: Embryonal adenocarcinomas (a type of malignant teratoma) of the sacrococcygeal region. Clinical and pathologic aspects of 21 cases. Cancer **26**:522-535, 1970.

288 Colton JJ, Batsakis JG, Work WP: Teratomas of the neck in adults. Arch Otolaryngol **104**:271-272, 1978.

289 Conklin J, Abell MR: Germ cell neoplasms of sarcococcygeal region. Cancer **20**:2105-2117, 1967.

290 Dehner LP: Intrarenal teratoma occurring in infancy. Report of a case with discussion of extragonadal germ cell tumors in infancy. J Pediatr Surg **8**:369-378, 1973.

291 Donnellan WA, Swenson O: Benign and malignant sacrococcygeal teratomas, Surgery **64**:834-846, 1968.

291a Gonzalez-Crussi F, Winkler RF, Mirkin DL: Sacrococcygeal teratomas in infants and children. Relationship of histology and prognosis in 40 cases. Arch Pathol Lab Med **102**:420-425, 1978.

292 Willis RA: Pathology of tumors, ed. 4, London, 1968, Butterworth & Co., Ltd.

Tumors of neurogenic origin

293 Anderson MS: Myxopapillary ependymomas presenting in the soft tissue over the sacrococcygeal region. Cancer **19**:585-590, 1966.

294 Bain GO, Shnitka TK: Cutaneous meningioma (psammoma). Arch Dermatol **74**:590-594, 1956.

295 Borello ED, Gorlin RH: Melanotic neuroectodermal tumor of infancy—a neoplasm of neural crest origin. Report of a case associated with high urinary excretion of vanilmandelic acid. Cancer **19**:196-206, 1966.

296 Clarke BE, Parsons H: An embryological tumor of retinal anlage involving the skull. Cancer **4**:78-85, 1951.

296a Dehner LP, Sibley RK, Sauk JJ Jr, Vickers RA, Nesbit ME, Leonard AS, Waite DE, Neeley JE, Ophoven J: Malignant melanotic neuroectodermal tumor of infancy. A clinical, pathologic, ultrastructural and tissue culture study. Cancer **43**:1389-1410, 1979.

297 Koudstaal J, Oldhoff J, Panders AK, Hardonk MJ: Melanotic neuroectodermal tumor of infancy. Cancer **22**:151-161, 1968.

298 Neustein HB: Fine structure of a melanotic progonoma or retinal anlage tumor of the anterior fontanel. Exp Mol Pathol **6**:131-142, 1967.

Tumors of hematopoietic origin

299 Condon WB, Safarik LR, Elzi EP: Extramedullary hematopoiesis simulating intrathoracic tumor. Arch Surg **90**:643-648, 1965.

Tumors of uncertain origin

300 Alguacil-Garcia A, Unni KK, Goellner JR: Malignant giant cell tumor of soft parts—an ultrastructural study of four cases. Cancer **40**:244-253, 1977.

301 Al-Sarraf M, Loud AV, Vaitkevicius VK: Malignant granular cell tumor histochemical and electron microscopic study. Arch Pathol **91**:550-558, 1971.

302 Angervall L, Enzinger FM: Extraskeletal neoplasm resembling Ewing's sarcoma. Cancer **36:**240-251, 1975.

303 Angervall L, Stener B: Clear-cell sarcoma of tendons. A study of 4 cases. Acta Pathol Microbiol Scand **77:**589-597, 1969.

304 Bearman RM, Noe J, Kempson RL: Clear cell sarcoma with melanin pigment. Cancer **36:**977-984, 1975.

305 Bliss BO, Reed RJ: Large cell sarcomas of tendon sheath. Malignant giant cell tumors of tendon sheath. Am J Clin Pathol **49:**776-781, 1968.

305a Bryan RS, Soule EH, Dobyns JH, Pritchard DJ, Linscheid RL: Primary epithelioid sarcoma of the hand and forearm. J Bone Joint Surg [Am] **56:**458-465, 1974.

306 Bloustein PA, Silverberg SG, Waddell WR: Epithelioid sarcoma—case report with ultrastructural review, histogenetic discussion, and chemotherapeutic data. Cancer **38:**2390-2400, 1976.

307 Budzilovich GN: Granular cell "myoblastoma" of vagus nerve. Acta Neuropathol **10:**162-169, 1968.

308 Christ ML, Ozzello L: Myogenous origin of a granular cell tumor of the urinary bladder. Am J Clin Pathol **56:**736-749, 1971.

309 Enzinger FM: Intramuscular myxoma. Am J Clin Pathol **43:**104-113, 1965.

310 Enzinger FM: Clear-cell sarcoma of tendons and aponeuroses. An analysis of 21 cases. Cancer **18:**1163-1174, 1965.

311 Enzinger FM: Fibrous hamartoma of infancy. Cancer **18:**241-248, 1965.

312 Enzinger FM: Epithelioid sarcoma. A sarcoma simulating a granuloma or a carcinoma. Cancer **26:**1029, 1041, 1970.

313 Feldman PS: A comparative study including ultrastructure of intramuscular myxoma and myxoid liposarcoma. Cancer **43:**512-525, 1979.

314 Fisher ER, Horvat B: The fibrocytic derivation of the so-called epithelioid sarcoma. Cancer **30:**1074-1081, 1970.

315 Fisher ER, Reidbord H: Electron microscopic evidence suggesting the myogenous derivation of the so-called alveolar soft part sarcoma. Cancer **27:**150-159, 1971.

316 Fisher ER, Wechsler H: Granular cell myoblastoma—a misnomer. Electron microscopic and histochemical evidence concerning its schwann cell derivation and nature (granular cell schwannoma). Cancer **15:**936-957, 1962.

317 Gabbiani G, Fu Y-S, Kaye GI, Lattes R, Majno G: Epithelioid sarcoma. A light and electron microscopic study suggesting a synovial origin. Cancer **30:**486-499, 1972.

318 Garancis JC, Komorowski RA, Kuzma JF: Granular cell myoblastoma. Cancer **25:**542-550, 1970.

319 Gillespie JJ, Roth LM, Wills ER, Einhorn LH, Willman J: Extraskeletal Ewing's sarcoma. Histologic and ultrastructural observations in three cases. Am J Surg Pathol **3:**99-108, 1979.

320 Guccion JG, Enzinger FM: Malignant giant cell tumor of soft parts. An analysis of 32 cases. Cancer **29:**1518-1529, 1972.

321 Ireland DCR, Soule EH, Ivins JC: Myxoma of somatic soft tissues—a report of 58 patients, 3 with multiple tumors and fibrous dysplasia of bone. Mayo Clin Proc **48:**401-410, 1973.

322 Johnson WC, Helwig EB: Cutaneous focal mucino-

sis. A clinicopathological and histochemical study. Arch Dermatol **93:**13-20, 1966.

323 Kindblom L, Stener B, Angervall L: Intramuscular myxoma. Cancer **34:**1737-1744, 1974.

324 Lieberman PH, Foote FW, Stewart FW, Berg JW: Alveolar soft-part sarcoma. JAMA **198:**1047-1051, 1966.

325 Moscovic EA, Azar HA: Multiple granular cell tumors ("myoblastomas"). Case report with electron microscopic observations and review of the literature. Cancer **20:**2032-2047, 1967.

326 Navarrette AR, Smith M: Ultrastructure of granular cell ameloblastoma. Cancer **27:**948-955, 1971.

326a Peimer CA, Smith RJ, Sirota RL, Cohen BE: Epithelioid sarcoma of the hand and wrist: patterns of extension. J Hand Surg **2:**275-282, 1977.

327 Prat J, Woodruff JM, Marcove RC: Epithelioid sarcoma—an analysis of 22 cases indicating the prognostic significance of vascular invasion and regional lymph node metastasis. Cancer **41:**1472-1487, 1978.

328 Salm R, Sissons HA: Giant-cell tumours of soft tissues. J Pathol **107:**27-39, 1972.

329 Santiago H, Feinerman LK, Lattes R: Epithelioid sarcoma. A clinical and pathologic study of nine cases. Hum Pathol **3:**133-147, 1972.

330 Shipkey IH, Lieberman PH, Foote FW Jr, Stewart FW: Ultrastructure of alveolar soft part sarcoma. Cancer **17:**821-830, 1964.

331 Sobel HJ, Marquet E, Schwarz R: Granular degeneration of appendiceal smooth muscle. Arch Pathol **92:**427-432, 1971.

332 Soule EH, Enriquez P: Atypical fibrous histiocytoma, malignant fibrous histiocytoma, malignant histiocytoma and epithelioid sarcoma. A comparative study of 65 tumors. Cancer **30:**128-143, 1972.

333 Soule EH, Newton W Jr, Moon TE, Tefft M: Extraskeletal Ewing's sarcoma—a preliminary review of 26 cases encountered in the intergroup rhabdomyosarcoma study. Cancer **42:**259-264, 1978.

334 Stout AP: Myxoma, the tumor of primitive mesenchyme. Ann Surg **127:**706-719, 1948.

335 Strong EW, McDivitt RW, Brasfield RD: Granular cell myoblastoma. Cancer **25:**415-422, 1970.

336 Tsuneyoshi M, Enjoji M, Kubo T: Clear cell sarcoma of tendons and aponeuroses—a comparative study of 13 cases with a provisional subgrouping into the melanotic and synovial types. Cancer **42:**243-252, 1978.

337 Usui M, Ishii S, Yamawaki S, Sasaki T, Minami A, Hizawa K: Malignant granular cell tumor of the radial nerve. Cancer **39:**1547-1555, 1977.

338 Vance SF III, Hudson RP: Granular cell myoblastoma. Clinicopathologic study of 42 patients. Am J Clin Pathol **52:**208-211, 1969.

339 Wigger HJ, Salazar GH, Blane WA: Extraskeletal Ewing sarcoma—an ultrastructural study. Arch Pathol Lab Med **101:**446-449, 1977.

340 Wirth WA, Leavitt D, Enzinger FM: Multiple intramuscular myxomas. Another extraskeletal manifestation of fibrous dysplasia. Cancer **27:**1167-1173, 1971.

Other tumorlike conditions

341 Burnett RA: A cause of erroneous diagnosis of pigmented villonodular synovitis. J Clin Pathol **29:**17-21, 1976.

342 Clearkin KP, Enzinger FM: Intravascular papillary endothelial hyperplasia. Arch Pathol Lab Med **100:**441-444, 1976.

343 Fraga S, Helwig EB, Rosen SM: Bronchogenic cysts in the skin and subcutaneous tissue. Am J Clin Pathol **56:**230-238, 1971.

344 Harkness JW, Peters HJ: Tumoral calcinosis, a report of six cases. J Bone Joint Surg [Am] **49:**721-731, 1967.

345 Kuo TT, Sayers CP, Roasi J: Masson's "vegetant intravascular hemangioendothelioma": a lesion often mistaken for angiosarcoma. Study of seventeen cases located in the skin and soft tissues. Cancer **38:**1227-1236, 1976.

346 Rosai J, Akerman LR: Intravenous atypical vascular proliferation—a cutaneous lesion simulating a malignant blood vessel tumor. Arch Dermatol **109:**714-717, 1974.

347 Rosai J, Gold J, Landy R: The histiocytoid hemangiomas. A unifying concept embracing several previously described entities of skin, soft tissue, large vessels, bone and heart. Hum Pathol **10:**707-730, 1979.

348 Wilson-Jones E: Malignant vascular tumours. Clin Exp Dermatol **1:**287-312, 1976.

25 Peritoneum, omentum, mesentery, and retroperitoneum

PERITONEUM
Inflammation

Chemical peritonitis can be caused by bile, pancreatic juice, gastric juice, and barium sulfate.[29] The peritonitis associated with the intraperitoneal extravasation of barium primarily is the result of the bacteria accompanying it. Barium peritonitis practically always follows perforation of the colon during examination of the obstructed bowel.[49]

Extravasation following injury or disease of the gallbladder, bile ducts, or duodenum causes acute or subacute peritonitis initially in the upper quadrant of the abdomen.[15] Gastric juice produces a severe peritoneal reaction because of its hydrochloric acid content, although it may be bacteriologically sterile. The release of pancreatic juice causes fat necrosis. The formation of calcium salts in large areas of fat necrosis may cause hypocalcemia.

Bacterial peritonitis may be either primary or secondary. The primary form usually is caused by streptococci or pneumococci. Aspiration of intra-abdominal fluid discloses an inflammatory exudate containing only a single type of organism. Large amounts of extracellular fluid are lost into the exudate and edema associated with generalized peritonitis. The losses may be equivalent to those of a burn covering one-half to three-fourths of the cutaneous surface.[13]

Perforation of a viscus such as a colon produces secondary peritonitis. If the fluid is aspirated, a mixture of bacterial flora rather than a single organism is found. Tuberculous and actinomycotic peritonitis may occur with few constitutional symptoms, despite extensive involvement of the peritoneum.[18,22,52] In a review of forty-seven patients with tuberculous peritonitis, Singh et al.[50] found roentgenographic evidence of pulmonary parenchymal lesions in only 6% of the cases. Search for acid-fast organisms on a direct smear of ascitic fluid is often unrewarding. The best diagnostic methods are culture of the fluid and percutaneous biopsy of the peritoneum.[33,34] Singh et al.[50] found the latter useful in 64% of their cases. Chemotherapy is the treatment of choice; surgery is reserved for those cases associated with enteritis and leading to bowel obstruction, perforation, fistula, or a mass that does not resolve with drug therapy.[49a] These specific infections are in contrast to primary streptococcal peritonitis, which produces maximal constitutional symptoms with minimal gross findings.

Pseudocysts of the peritoneal cavity may be associated with some inflammatory process such as ulcerative colitis or may follow appendectomy complicated by abscess.

Adhesions

Adhesions, with the possibility of subsequent intestinal obstruction, follow all intra-abdominal operations. They can be minimized by careful handling of tissues, reperitonealization where feasible, and removal of intraperitoneal blood clots. Ryan et al.[46] showed in an experimental model that drying of the serosa plus bleeding consistently resulted in the formation of adhesions. There is good experimental evidence to suggest that formation of peritoneal adhesions is related to a local depression of peritoneal plasminogen activator, which is the principal known peritoneal fibrin-clearing system.[4]

Innumerable agents of every description (sodium citrate, heparin, olive oil, liquid paraffin, ACTH, cortisone, pepsin, fibrinolysin, and amniotic fluid) have been used to prevent adhesions, but none has accomplished this goal. Adhesions become collagenous and strong as the cellularity of their fibrous tissue decreases with maturation. Postoperative adhesions are the most frequent cause of intestinal obstruction today.

Extensive peritoneal fibrosis ("sclerosing peritonitis") also has been described as a reaction to asbestos, in patients with the carcinoid syndrome, and following the administration of β-adrenergic-blocking drugs.[6] We have seen several cases in which no etiologic agent could be identified.[3]

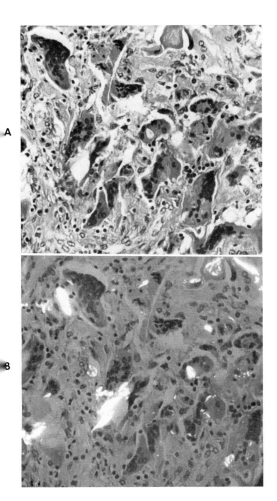

A

B

Fig. 1391 Histologic appearance of talc granuloma without, **A,** and with, **B,** polarized light. With latter, talc crystals can be seen vividly. (**A,** WU neg. 47-1049; **B,** WU neg. 47-1050.)

Reaction to foreign materials

The peritoneum reacts to all foreign substances. A great deal has been written in the past about "talc powder granuloma" of the peritoneum.[14] This followed spillage of the talc (hydrated magnesium silicate) used on surgical gloves into the peritoneal cavity at operation. Nodules formed that would be mistaken grossly for tuberculosis or metastatic cancer. Microscopically, they were shown to be formed by foreign body granulomas containing birefringent crystals. The latter are made apparent with polarizing lenses[17] or simply by lowering the condenser of the microscope (Fig. 1391).

The use of talc for surgical gloves has long been recognized as a hazard and has been replaced by other substances, such as modified starch. Although these materials elicit less reaction than talc, intraperitoneal granulomas may still develop,[21,48] usually between ten days and four weeks after a laparotomy. At reoperation, the findings are ascites, miliary peritoneal nodules, serosal inflammation, and adhesions. The appearance can closely simulate cancer, tuberculosis, and Crohn's disease. The nature of the granulomas can be identified by the presence of granules that are PAS positive and birefringent (with a Maltese cross pattern) with-

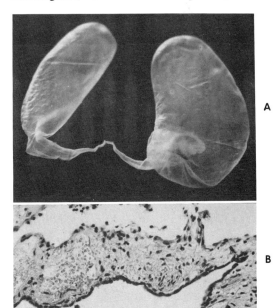

A

B

Fig. 1392 A, Thin-walled cyst containing clear fluid found free within abdominal cavity. **B,** Microscopically, it has fibrous wall and lining of flat mesothelial cells. (**A** and **B,** Courtesy Dr. E. F. Lascano, Buenos Aires, Argentina.)

in the cytoplasm of histiocytes and foreign body giant cells.[10,12] The diagnosis also may be suspected through the finding of starch granules in the aspirated peritoneal fluid. Fortunately, the disease is usually self-limited. Another source of surgical contamination is the cellulose fibers derived from disposable surgical gowns and drapes.[107a]

Mineral oil or paraffin placed in the peritoneal cavity used in the past to prevent adhesions was responsible for the formation of nodules that could be grossly mistaken for metastatic carcinoma.[37] Frozen section of these nodules is sufficient to make the diagnosis. It will show foreign body giant cells, chronic inflammation, and foamy macrophages. Similar changes follow rupture of a cystic teratoma of the ovary, in which large amounts of oily material cause a profound nodular peritoneal reaction.[2]

Cysts

Lascano et al.[32] described five cases of cysts lying loose within the abdominal cavity. They varied in diameter from 1.5-6 cm and were lined by one or several layers of mesothelial cells (Fig. 1392).

Tumors

Primary tumors

The peritoneum has a great capacity to undergo metaplasia and form papillary projections, pseudoacini, squamous nests,[11] and even cartilaginous nodules (Fig. 1393). Cirrhosis with ascites, collagen-vascular diseases (such as systemic lupus erythematosus), and viral infections are often associated with marked mesothelial proliferation (Fig. 1394).

We have observed several examples (many of them in children) of nodular mesothelial

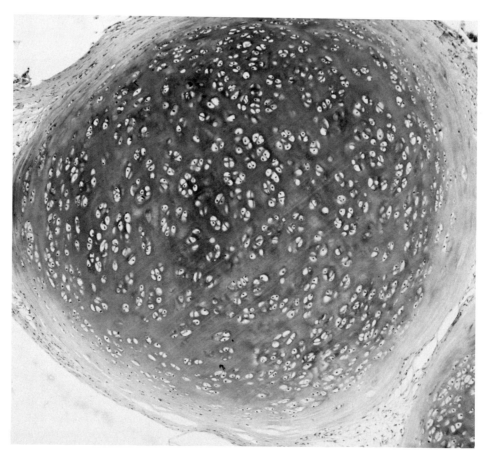

Fig. 1393 Peritoneal cartilaginous metaplasia. (Low power; WU neg. 62-90; slide contributed by Dr. J. Bauer, St. Louis, Mo.)

hyperplasia developing in hernia sacs, usually as a result of trauma or some other form of injury. This hyperplasia can simulate closely, and actually be confused with, a malignant process by virtue of the solid nature of the proliferation and the formation of papillary fronds containing psammoma bodies[45] (Fig. 1395). We have also seen foci of exuberant mesothelial hyperplasia in the serosa of an inflamed appendix (Fig. 1396) and in the fallopian tube, the latter following the rupture of an ectopic pregnancy.

In females, there is a layer of tissue sensitive to sex hormones situated underneath the peritoneal mesothelium that seems to be related to endometrial stroma.[41] It is more prominent in the pelvic parietal peritoneum and on the bladder dome. Although rather inconspicuous under normal conditions, it is probably responsible for the occurrence of ectopic decidual reaction, endometriosis, leiomyomatosis peritonealis disseminata,[31a,58a] and the exceptional cases of endometrial stromal sarcoma and mixed müllerian tumor that have been found outside the genital system (see Uterus — endometrium in Chapter 18). The pelvic mesothelium itself is closely related embryologically to the surface epithelium of the ovary and, as such, may give rise to proliferative lesions akin to those more commonly seen in the ovary. This ranges from multiple small cystic nodules seen in association with ovarian borderline serous cystomas (so-called peritoneal endosalpingiosis[7]) to the formation of malignant papillary tumors indistinguishable from ovarian serous cystadenocarcinomas[27] (Fig. 1397). Parmley and Woodruff[42] have taken the extreme view that, since tumors of the peritoneal surface and of the ovarian surface epithelium have the same basic histogenesis (i.e., all are derived from mesothelium), they should all be designated as mesotheliomas. Although conceptually this proposal is not without merit, we agree fully with Kannerstein et al.[27] that the biologic differences that exist between ovarian carcinoma or its extraovarian homologue on the one hand and peritoneal mesothelioma on the other render such a proposal impractical and potentially misleading.

Peritoneal mesotheliomas are very rare. Their very existence has been denied with the claim that they represent metastases from other neoplasms. Although it is a fact that sometimes metastatic tumors in the peritoneum, particularly those arising in the ovary, may be a source of confusion, there is no longer any question that true mesotheliomas exist. Most examples occur in patients past 35 years of age, although they may appear at any age, including childhood.[28] The frequency of mesotheli-

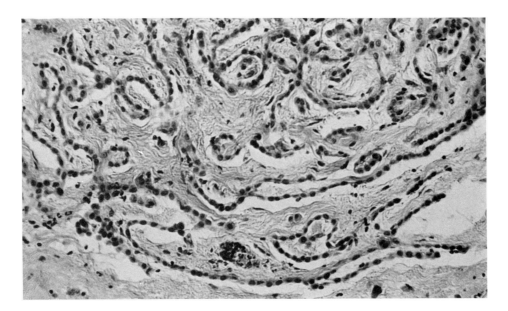

Fig. 1394 Localized area of proliferation of peritoneal mesothelium. These changes were associated with chronic inflammation. Note overproduction of fibrous tissue and pseudoacini. (×240; WU neg. 52-4549.)

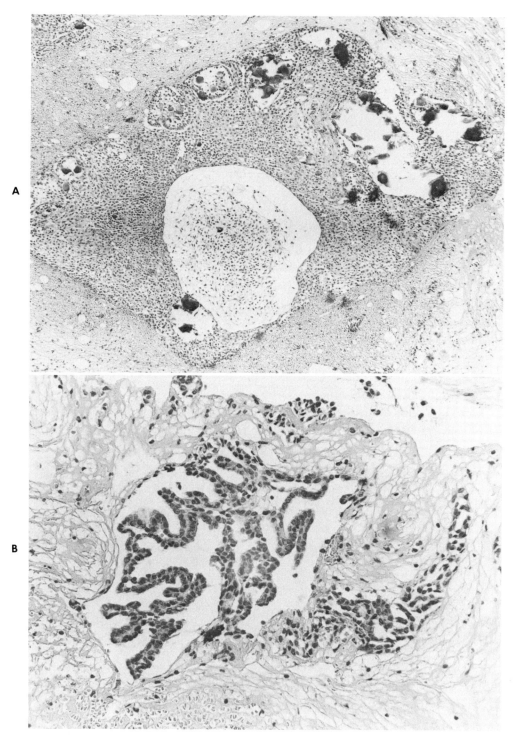

Fig. 1395 Nodular mesothelial hyperplasia in hernia sac. **A,** Predominantly solid nodule of hyperplastic mesothelial cells lines sac and obliterates lumen. Numerous psammoma bodies are present. **B,** This focus of mesothelial proliferation within sac shows papillary arrangement that may simulate mesothelioma or metastatic ovarian carcinoma. (**A,** ×63; **B,** ×290.)

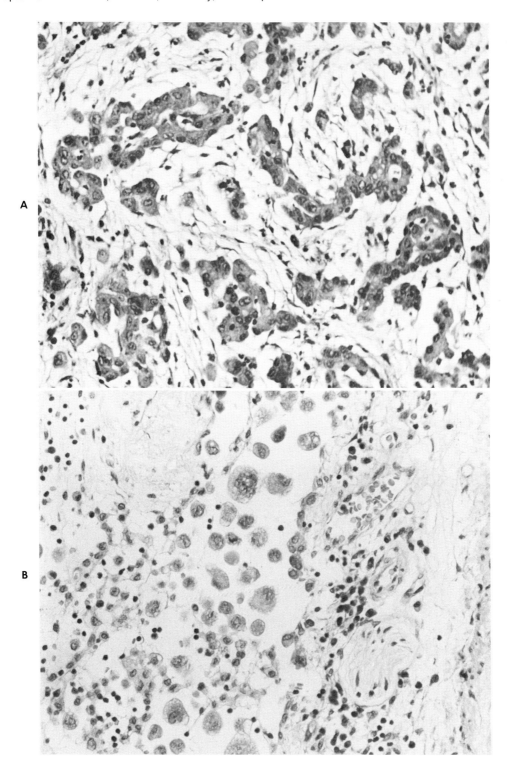

Fig. 1396 A, Intense focal mesothelial formation within tubules and extremely distorted pattern. These findings could easily be misinterpreted as metastatic adenocarcinoma. This specimen came from 49-year-old man who had appendiceal abscess. Patient is without evidence of disease over two years after operation. **B,** Mesothelial hyperplasia in lining and lumen of hernia sac. (**A,** Slide contributed by Dr. M. Ernest, Moose Jaw, Saskatchewan, Canada.)

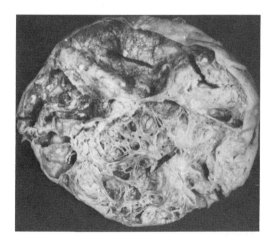

Fig. 1397 Encapsulated tumor of mesentery that measured 19 cm × 16 cm and weighed 900 gm. Cut section demonstrated its multilocular character. Microscopically it was shown to be made up of ciliated columnar cells reminiscent of the fallopian tube epithelium. It was considered that this tumor represented extraovarian serous cystadenoma. (Contributed by Major General C. C. Kapila and Major General (Retired) Sarup Narain, Poona, India.)

oma has been on the increase, presumably as a result of asbestos exposure.[40,51]

The types of mesothelioma seen in the peritoneum are similar to those of the pleura (Chapter 6), but the relative proportions vary a great deal. For example, the pure fibrous type, which is relatively common in the pleural space, constitutes only a minority of the peritoneal neoplasms.[20,54] The large majority of the peritoneal mesotheliomas are of the papillary (tubular) or mixed type, and most of them are either *solitary and benign* or *diffuse and malignant*. A diffuse benign form and a solitary malignant form have been described, but these are curiosities. Another extremely rare form of peritoneal mesothelioma is characterized by a *multicystic* configuration, simulating the appearance of cystic lymphangioma.[38a] Staining for mucosubstances and electron microscopic examination may be necessary for the differential diagnosis.

In a series of 114 peritoneal mesotheliomas reviewed by Stout,[55] there were twenty-five of the fibrous type, thirty-eight of the papillary benign solitary type, and thirty-six of the papillary diffuse malignant variety.

The fibrous type of mesothelioma presents the same bewildering microscopic picture as it does in the pleural cavity[54] (Chapter 6). The

putative evidence of mesothelial origin is based more on tissue culture studies than on the microscopic pattern, which is basically that of a fibroma.[47] The alternative explanation is that this particular type of tumor arises from submesothelial connective tissue.

The solitary benign form of papillary mesothelioma presents as a small papillary structure resembling grossly and microscopically the appearance of choroid plexus[58] (Fig. 1398). We suspect that some of these lesions are reactive rather than neoplastic. The diffuse malignant variety appears as multiple plaques or nodules scattered over the visceral and parietal peritoneum (Fig. 1399). It may be accompanied by dense intraperitoneal adhesions with shortening of the mesentery and with ascites (Fig. 1400, *A*). Complete obliteration of the peritoneal cavity may actually develop. In advanced stages, the tumor may locally invade the intestinal wall, the hilum of the spleen and liver, the gastric wall, the pancreas, and the retroperitoneum. However, distant metastases are unusual.[1,59]

The microscopic pattern is highly variable[25] (Fig. 1401). The most typical arrangement is that of papillae or tubules lined by atypical mesothelial cells, the former having vascularized fibrous cores that may contain psammoma bodies (Fig. 1400, *B*). In other instances, the mesothelial-like cells alternate with sarcomatoid spindle cells in the manner of a synovial sarcoma (Fig. 1402). The individual cells are, in general, fairly uniform, with acidophilic or vacuolated cytoplasm and large vesicular nucleus.[5] Mitoses are often difficult to find. Intracellular and extracellular mucosubstances can be present. This seems to represent acid mucopolysaccharides, since it stains with colloidal iron and Alcian blue, is removed at least partially by hyaluronidase digestion, and is PAS negative. According to Kannerstein et al.,[26] a *definitely positive* diastase-resistant PAS reaction in a poorly differentiated peritoneal malignancy rules out mesothelioma and establishes the diagnosis of carcinoma. The latter also may contain colloidal iron-positive material, but hyaluronic acid would have no effect on the reaction.

By electron microscopy, the cells of well-differentiated mesotheliomas exhibit polarity, abundant microvilli covered with fuzzy material, extracellular and intracellular neolumina formation, glycogen granules, junctional structures, tonofilaments, and basal lamina[56] (Fig.

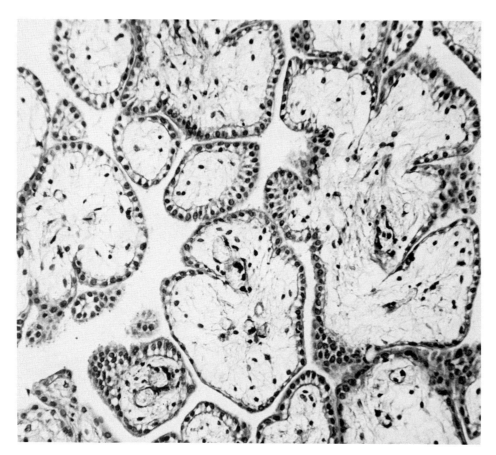

Fig. 1398 Benign papillary mesothelioma occurring in 41-year-old man. Lesion had been present for at least three years. (Low power; WU neg. 62-88; slide contributed by Dr. M. J. Zbar, Miami, Fla.)

1403). Unfortunately, the cells of less differentiated examples lack many of these distinguishing features.

Pleural and peritoneal mesotheliomas may coexist. Hypoglycemia is occasionally encountered in association with extensive mesotheliomas and is often relieved by the removal of the tumor.[36]

Metastatic tumors

All types of metastatic tumors involve the peritoneal cavity. Their gross patterns vary from single, well-defined nodules to diffuse lymphatic permeation. Variations in consistency depend upon their cellularity, amount of fibrous tissue, and mucin content. Metastatic carcinoma may simulate very closely primary malignant mesothelioma. We have observed this grossly with metastatic squamous carcinoma (Fig. 1404) and microscopically with papillary tumors of the ovary (Fig. 1405).

Pseudomyxoma peritonei is a form of peritoneal carcinomatosis in which the peritoneal cavity contains large amounts of mucinous material.[35] The primary tumor is usually a mucinous cystadenocarcinoma of the ovary, rarely of the appendix or pancreas. Microscopically, large pools of mucus are seen accompanied by hyperemic vessels and chronic inflammatory cells. *Viable epithelial glandular cells must be identified within the mucus in order to diagnose this condition.* These cells usually have a deceivingly bland appearance. Mucinous cystadenomas of the ovary and appendix can rupture and pour their content into the peritoneal cavity. The resulting condition, which is self-limited and microscopically lacks tumor cells, should not be designated as pseudomyxoma peritonei.[9,19]

Cytology

The report of a positive cytology in an effusion has great prognostic and therapeutic significance. A false positive diagnosis may

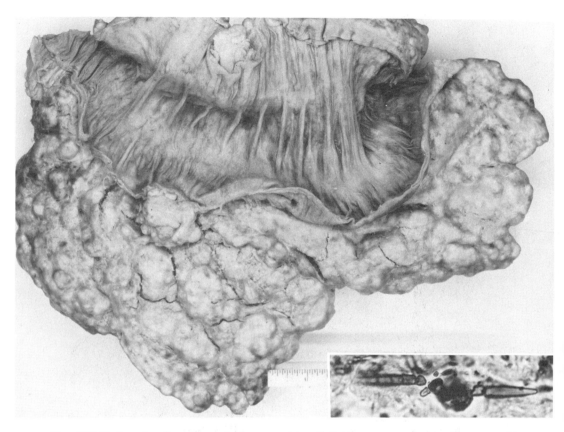

Fig. 1399 Portion of malignant mesothelioma overlying dilated transverse colon. Lesion occurred in 65-year-old male European with no history of industrial exposure to asbestos. In three sections of lower lobe, foci of asbestosis were present with asbestos bodies, fibrosis, and occasional giant cells. There were no asbestos bodies found in upper lobes. **Inset,** Classic asbestos body in lower lobe. Note chair rung appearance. (×600; WU neg. 63-2791; courtesy Dr. J. G. Thomson, Cape Town, South Africa.)

delay therapy for a potentially remedial situation. For this reason, we are conservative in our interpretation of effusions, requiring the presence of cell clusters or fragments before rendering a diagnosis of carcinoma (Figs. 1406 and 1407). Only in cases of lymphoma do we base our positive diagnoses on the findings of isolated malignant-appearing cells. When sufficient material is available, we routinely use smears from the centrifuged specimen, in addition to membrane filter preparations and cell blocks. Clinicians somehow feel insecure unless the results are based on a cell block preparation. This insecurity is unfounded. We have seen cases in which the smear preparation was positive and the cell block negative or equivocal. A smear preparation contains fewer artifacts and usually gives better nuclear detail. The finding of tumor cells in the smear preparation means the patient has a malignancy regard-

less of what the cell block shows. We have, of course, had cases in which the smear was negative and the cell block positive. Although this is unusual, we still do the cell block, but only if enough material is available.

A negative cytology report does not exclude the presence of cancer in an effusion. In 207 patients with malignant effusion, the cytology was positive in 153 (74%), whereas in 162 patients with nonmalignant effusions, there was one false positive report (0.7%).[43] Cardozo[8] was able to diagnose 67% of malignant pleural effusions and 75% of malignant ascitic effusions, with a false positive rate of 0.1%.

Patients with effusions due to lymphomas and leukemias yield positive cytology in about 55%-60% of the cases, with histiocytic lymphomas most likely to yield positive results (75%) and Hodgkin's disease least likely (25%).[38,43] At Barnes Hospital, patients with positive

Text continued on p. 1493.

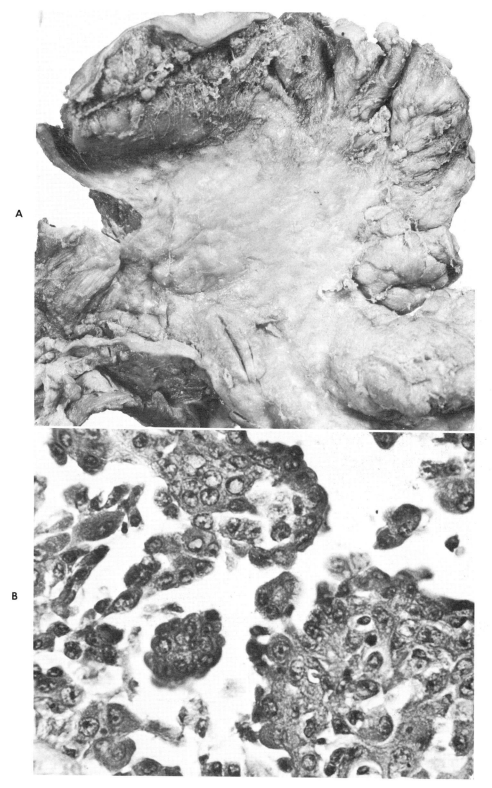

Fig. 1400 A, Malignant mesothelioma that diffusely involved peritoneal cavity. Fibrosis and shortening of mesentery are prominent. **B,** Same lesion shown in **A.** Papillary projections are prominent. (**A,** WU neg. 49-1666; **B,** ×600; WU neg. 49-1793.)

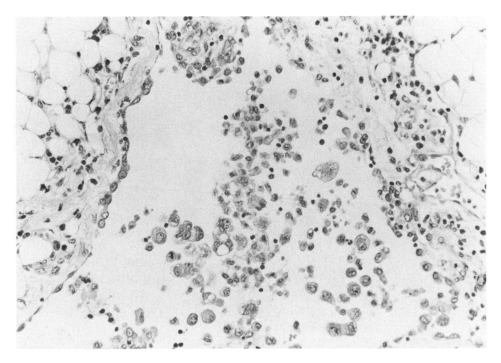

Fig. 1401 Diffuse malignant peritoneal mesothelioma. Atypical cells of mesothelial appearance line surface and detach from it in clumps. Inflammatory component is also present. (×290.)

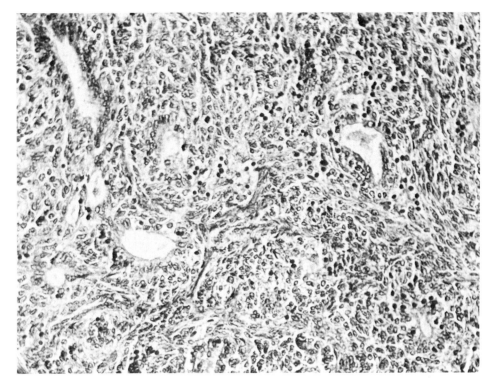

Fig. 1402 Malignant mesothelial tumor assuming pattern of synovial sarcoma. Note intimate admixture of stromal and glandular components.

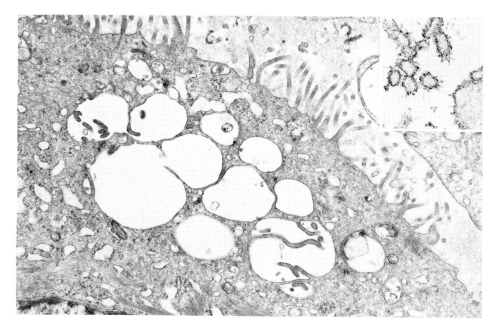

Fig. 1043 Electron microscopic appearance of cell from malignant mesothelioma demonstrating numerous micovilli in luminal surface and intracellular vacuoles also equipped with microvilli. **Inset** shows microvilli coated with acid mucopolysaccharides. (×8,000; **inset,** Hale's colloidal iron; ×45,000; from Suzuki Y, Churg J, Kannerstein M: Ultrastructure of human malignant diffuse mesothelioma. Am J Pathol **85:**241-262, 1976.)

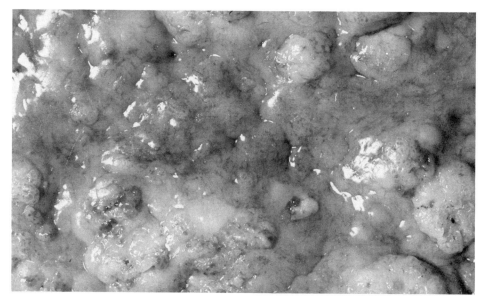

Fig. 1404 Diffuse involvement of peritoneum by metastatic squamous carcinoma simulating primary malignant peritoneal tumor. (WU neg. 52-383.)

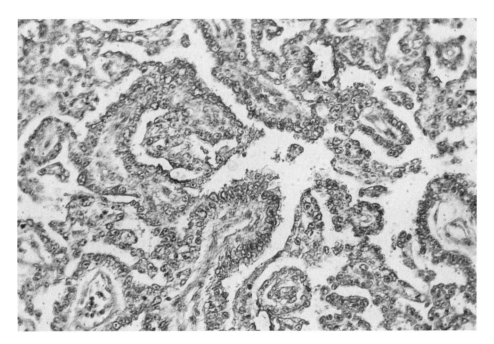

Fig. 1405 Metastatic ovarian cancer of papillary serous type closely resembling primary malignant peritoneal tumor. (×240; AFIP 314863.)

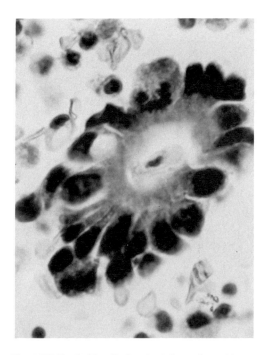

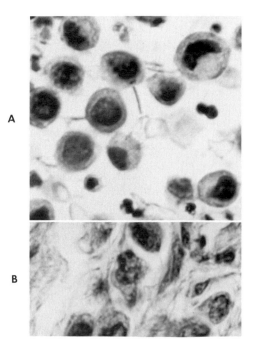

Fig. 1406 Easily identified metastatic malignant tumor. Note large, dense nuclei and atypical mitotic figure in acinus. (×900; WU neg. 52-1617.)

Fig. 1407 A, Ascitic fluid sediment with numerous tumor cells identified by their dense, large, atypical appearance. **B,** Same tumor shown in **A,** which was primary in stomach. (**A,** ×900; WU neg. 52-1621; **B,** ×900; WU neg. 52-1622.)

effusion due to carcinoma had an average survival of 3.3 months, whereas the average for those with positive effusion due to lymphoma was two months. No patient with carcinoma of the lung and positive pleural cytology survived for more than one year. All patients who survived for longer than one year had either breast or ovarian carcinoma. These patients also had the longest average survival.[31]

The most common metastatic tumors to cause pleural effusions are lung and breast carcinomas and malignant lymphomas. In ascitic fluids, carcinomas of the ovary are the most commonly encountered.[8,23,31]

False positive diagnoses have been most commonly caused by hepatic cirrhosis, congestive heart failure, tuberculosis, and pulmonary infarction.[16] Such false positive diagnoses may be made because the mesothelial cells may form pseudoacini that closely resemble adenocarcinoma[57] (Fig. 1408). Furthermore, normal mitotic figures are frequent. Mesothelial cells also may have multiple nuclei and may assume a signet-ring appearance.[24]

According to Klempman,[30] malignant mesothelioma differs from a metastatic adenocarcinoma in a cytologic preparation because true acini are not formed, binucleation and multinucleation are more common, and a combination of well-differentiated and poorly differentiated mesothelial cells is present. Arrangement in papillary clusters is common.[39,44,53]

OMENTUM

Hemorrhagic infarct of the omentum may be due to torsion or strangulation in a hernia sac. Epstein and Lempke[60] reviewed the eighty-eight reported cases of primary idiopathic segmental infarction of the greater omentum, an acute abdominal lesion usually mistaken clinically for acute appendicitis or cholecystitis. Characteristically, the infarcted segment of omentum is on the right side adherent to the cecum, ascending colon, and anterior parietal peritoneum.

Stout et al.[61] examined twenty-four solid *tumors* of the great omentum. *Leiomyomas* predominated among the benign neoplasms, and *leiomyosarcoma* was the most common malignant tumor.

MESENTERY

Mesenteric panniculitis, also called isolated lipodystrophy of the mesentery, is a rare condition grossly appearing as a diffuse, localized, or multinodular thickening of the mesentery of the small bowel. Microscopically, there is an infiltration by inflammatory cells and foamy macrophages, the latter representing a reaction to fat necrosis.[63,67] The differential diagnosis should include Weber-Christian disease and Whipple's disease. In eight of the fifty-three patients reported by Kipfer et al.,[64] a malignant lymphoma ultimately developed; other series did not show such an association.

A closely related, if not identical, condition is *retractile (sclerosing) mesenteritis*, in which the inflammation and fibrosis lead to retraction, formation of adhesions, and distortion of the intestinal loops.[68] Mesentery from both small and large bowel can be involved.[69] It is likely that at least some examples of this condition represent a variation and extension of idiopathic retroperitoneal fibrosis (see below).

Mesenteric cysts are usually incidental findings, but they may be large enough to produce symptoms. They are round and smooth, with a thin wall lined by a layer of flattened or low cuboidal cells. The content may be a serous fluid resembling plasma or a white milky fluid. In the latter instance, they are referred to as

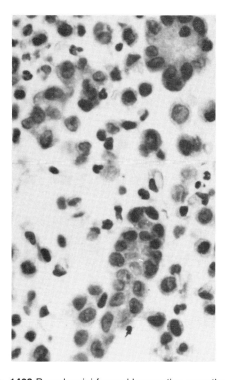

Fig. 1408 Pseudoacini formed by reactive mesothelial cells in peritoneal fluid that easily can be mistaken for metastatic carcinoma. (×600; WU neg. 48-4070.)

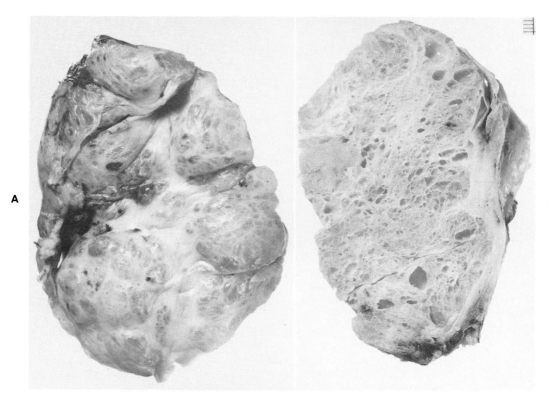

Fig. 1409 External appearance, **A**, and cross section, **B**, of benign cystic lymphangioma that was present in retroperitoneum and mesentery of 77-year-old woman who had progressive abdominal enlargement for number of years. It weighed 900 gm. Note honeycombing of specimen. Patient has now remained well for over two years. (WU neg. 61-6230.)

chylous cysts. Unlike intestinal duplications, they often can be dissected away with preservation of the adjacent intestinal segment. Most of these cysts arise from lymph vessels and are lined by endothelium, but others have a mesothelial derivation.[62]

When the cysts are extremely large, are multilocular, or have smooth muscle in the wall, we prefer to designate them as cystic lymphangiomas (Fig. 1409). As in the case of the simple cysts, the problem of differentiating them from lesions of mesothelial derivation (in this case, benign cystic mesotheliomas) arises. This may require staining for mucosubstances (often present in mesothelial lesions but invariably absent in lymphangiomas) and electron microscopy.[64a,65]

Most tumors involving the mesentery are metastatic. Yannopoulos and Stout[70] studied forty-four primary solid *tumors* of the mesentery. Two-thirds were benign. There were twelve cases of fibromatosis, seven tumors of smooth muscle origin, six tumors of adipose

tissue origin, six ''xanthogranulomas'' (which today would probably be referred to as fibrous histiocytomas), five vascular neoplasms, three neurofibromas, and five miscellaneous tumors (Fig. 1410).

In the presence of fibromatosis of the mesentery, the possibility of Gardner's syndrome should always be investigated. Giant lymph node hyperplasia (Castleman's disease) may present as a mesenteric mass associated with hematologic disturbances.[66]

RETROPERITONEUM

The retroperitoneal space is that indefinite area in the lumbar and iliac region which lies between the peritoneum and the posterior wall of the abdominal cavity. It extends from the twelfth rib and vertebra to the base of the sacrum and the iliac crest. The lateral margins correspond to the lateral borders of the quadratus lumbora muscles. The space contains the loose areolar tissue through which pass the inferior vena cava, aorta, ureters, renal vessels,

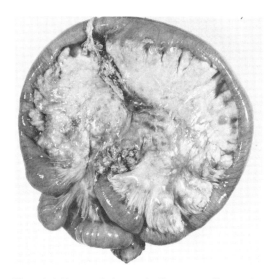

Fig. 1410 Extremely large plexiform neurofibroma involving mesentery of small bowel. It was necessary to remove 140 cm of ileum to obtain this mass, which measured 24 cm × 11 cm. Six years following operation, 22-year-old male patient was well. (From Leach WB: Giant neurofibroma of mesentery. Arch Surg **74:** 438-441, 1957; copyright 1957, American Medical Association.)

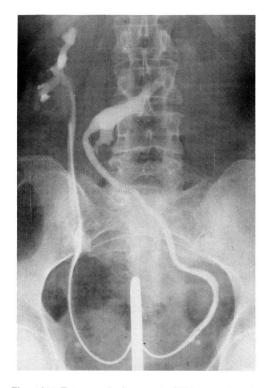

Fig. 1411 Extreme displacement of kidney and ureter in patient with large retroperitoneal tumor. (WU neg. 49-2913.)

and gonadal vessels. It contains numerous lymph nodes.

This potentially large space allows both primary and metastatic tumors to grow silently before clinical signs and symptoms appear. Symptoms are related to displacement of organs and obstructive phenomena (Fig. 1411).

Nonneoplastic conditions

Inflammatory processes from the kidney (pyelonephritis), large bowel (diverticulitis), appendix, and pancreas may result in a retroperitoneal abscess, usually due to coliform bacteria. In children, nontuberculous psoas abscesses are, in most cases, due to gram-positive cocci originating from a focus of tonsillitis, otitis media, or cutaneous furuncle. We have seen perforation of the biliary system with formation of a bile-containing cystic mass. *Infection* from a tuberculous vertebra may form a retroperitoneal cold abscess, which is often confined to the psoas muscle. *Malakoplakia* can involve the retroperitoneum and be confused with malignant fibrous histiocytoma.[106] Massive retroperitoneal *hemorrhage* in the adult is most often the result of a ruptured aortic aneurysm, trauma, hemorrhagic diathesis, or anticoagulant drug therapy.[95] Less commonly, it is of adrenal origin. Lawson et al.[94] reviewed ten cases of the latter phenomenon. In five instances the adrenal gland was the site of a pheochromocytoma, but in the other five there was no demonstrable abnormality.

We have seen a few instances of benign retroperitoneal *cysts* not connected with the adrenal gland. Their inner lining was compatible with either a mesothelial or mesonephric origin.

Idiopathic retroperitoneal fibrosis (Ormond's disease; sclerosing fibrosis) is a rare disease of obscure etiology that results in progressive renal failure by producing constriction and final obliteration of the ureters.[95b] Grossly, an ill-defined fibrous mass occupies the retroperitoneal midline, encircles the lower abdominal aorta, and displaces the ureters *medially*. The latter feature is of value to the radiologist in the differential diagnosis, since most retroperitoneal neoplasms displace the ureter laterally. More localized forms exist, in which the process is sharply circumscribed in the periureteral or renal pelvic region (Fig. 1412), around one kidney, or around the bladder.[84] Microscopically, a prominent inflammatory infiltrate composed of lymphocytes, plasma

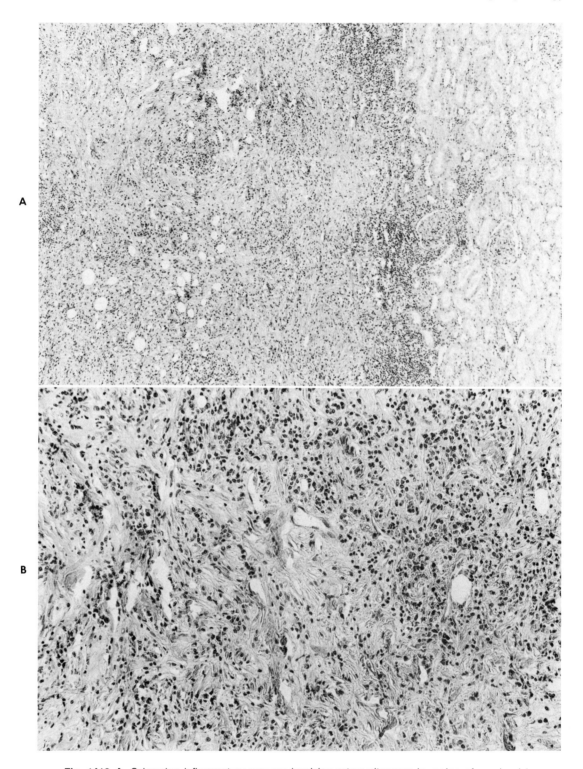

Fig. 1412 A, Sclerosing inflammatory process involving retroperitoneum in region of renal pelvis and extending into renal parenchyma. **B,** At higher magnification, fibrosing nature of process and heavy inflammatory component are evident. This should not be confused with fibromatosis or with malignant fibrous histiocytoma. (**A,** ×63; **B,** ×180.)

cells, and eosinophils, often containing germinal centers, is seen accompanied by foci of
fat necrosis, fibroblastic proliferation, and collagen deposition.[100] The fibrous tissue in the
midline tends to be more mature than that of the
periphery.[75] The wall of veins is often involved

by the inflammation.[88,99] Mitchinson[100] also
found aortic involvement in three of his cases.

Idiopathic retroperitoneal fibrosis may be
associated with a similar process in the mediastinum, sclerosing cholangitis, Riedel's thyroiditis, pseudotumor of the orbit, or generalized

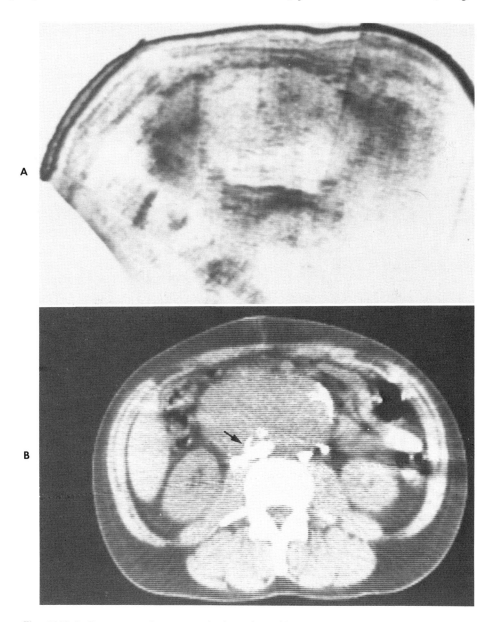

Fig. 1413 A, Transverse ultrasonography in patient with retroperitoneal metastases from testicular
germ cell tumor. Echo demonstrates massive retroperitoneal tumor lying against spine and protruding
into abdominal cavity. Complex echo pattern within tumor indicates areas of fibrosis, probably secondary to necrosis. **B,** Transverse computer tomography in same patient whose sonogram is shown
in **A.** Mass is again clearly shown. Its borders are better demarcated than in sonogram, but internal
architecture is less distinct. Darker areas at periphery of mass (arrow) represent iodide material from
previous lymphangiogram. (Courtesy Dr. S. Feinberg, Minneapolis, Minn.)

vasculitis, and this is referred to as multifocal fibrosclerosis.[76,85] Several cases have been reported secondary to the administration of methysergide and other drugs[83]; in many cases, cessation of therapy resulted in dramatic regression of the lesion. The available evidence strongly suggests that Ormond's disease represents an immunologic hypersensitivity disorder. Occasionally, the clinical and pathologic features of idiopathic retroperitoneal fibrosis can be simulated by malignant neoplasms accompanied by chronic inflammation and fibrosis, notably malignant lymphoma and signet-ring cell carcinoma of the stomach.[89,92,107]

Tumors
Primary tumors

Primary tumors of the retroperitoneal area are relatively rare. They are of many types.[80,87,96,98,103] Strictly speaking, neoplasms arising in the kidney, adrenal gland, and periaortic lymph nodes qualify in the category and are actually the commonest. However, the designation of retroperitoneal tumors has been traditionally reserved for tumors of this area arising outside these structures. Most of them have been already discussed elsewhere, particularly in Chapter 24. Here, only the peculiari-

ties of these neoplasms when they occur in this region will be described. Symptoms secondary to retroperitoneal neoplasms are vague and appear late in the course of the disease.

The classic radiologic methods for the evaluation of retroperitoneal tumors have been plain roentgenograms, barium studies of the gastrointestinal tract, and intravenous/retrograde pyelograms. These were later supplemented by selective arteriography and cavography of the inferior vena, but these techniques in turn, are being progressively replaced by computed tomography and ultrasonography[81,110] (Fig. 1413).

Liposarcoma is the most frequent retroperitoneal sarcoma. It is particularly prone to grow in the perirenal region (Fig. 1414). At the time of excision, it is usually extremely large. We have seen cases presenting as multiple independent tumor nodules in the retroperitoneum. Liposarcomas in this location have a worse prognosis than those located in the extremities (39% versus 71% in the series of Enzinger and Winslow,[78] the former figure falling to 4% at ten years). Total or near-total excision followed by radiation therapy offers the best chances of cure.[93]

Lipoma is less common than its malignant

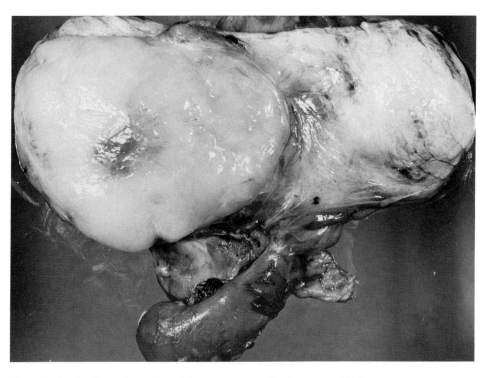

Fig. 1414 Large slimy retroperitoneal liposarcoma growing in region of kidney. (WU neg. 50-5055.)

counterpart. As the latter, it is usually very large at the time of diagnosis. It can be multiple. We have seen one such case, in which the first symptom was a mass below the inguinal ligament. Many cases reported in the literature as retroperitoneal lipomas are actually liposarcomas, particularly those in which a malignant transformation is said to have occurred.

Leiomyosarcoma is the second most common sarcoma in this area.[82] This tumor has a particular tendency to undergo massive cystic degeneration when occurring in this region.[97] Retroperitoneal smooth muscle tumors containing five or more mitoses per high-power field should be classified as leiomyosarcomas. Tumor cell necrosis or tumor size greater than 10 cm is strongly suggestive of malignancy, even in the presence of a low mitotic count. Of the thirteen cases reviewed by Kay and McNeill,[91] there was only one long-term survivor. In the series of Ranchod and Kemp-

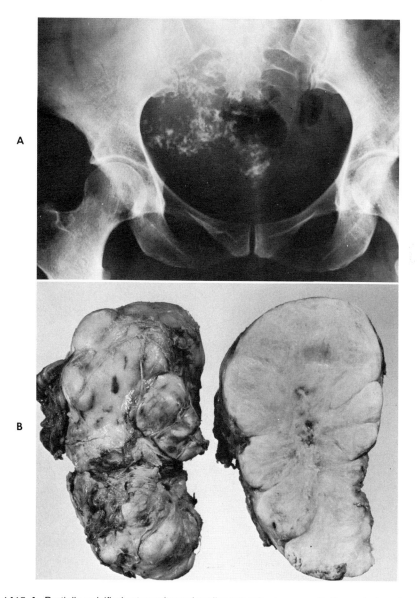

Fig. 1415 A, Partially calcified retroperitoneal malignant schwannoma. **B,** Same lesion shown in **A.** It was firm and grayish white and directly invaded vertebra, metastasized distantly, and caused death. (**A,** WU neg. 49-4366; **B,** WU neg. 49-4223.)

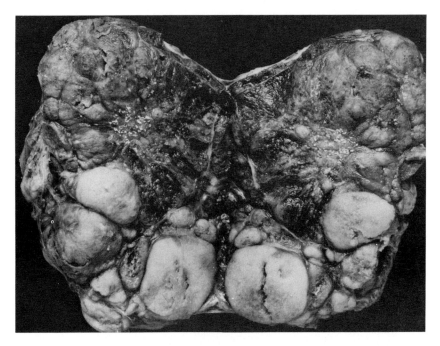

Fig. 1416 Hemorrhagic nodular ganglioneuroblastoma. (Courtesy Dr. M. Dockerty, Rochester, Minn.)

son,[104] also comprising thirteen cases, twelve of the patients died as a direct result of the neoplasm (eleven within two years of diagnosis).

Leiomyoma is exceptionally rare as a primary neoplasm, although on occasion a uterine tumor may extend into the retroperitoneal space.

Rhabdomyosarcoma is practically always of the embryonal type and limited to infants and children. The prognosis is extremely poor.

Fibromatosis may occur, sometimes in association with mediastinal involvement. In contrast to idiopathic retroperitoneal fibrosis, it lacks a prominent inflammatory component.

Fibrosarcoma is one of the rarest retroperitoneal tumors in our experience. We believe that most cases so designated in the literature are actually liposarcomas, leiomyosarcomas, or fibrous histiocytomas.[72]

Fibrous histiocytoma, on the other hand, is relatively frequent. Well-differentiated forms with large numbers of foamy macrophages and other inflammatory cells have been designated "xanthogranulomas" in the past.[101] It is inadvisable to classify these deep-seated tumors as benign no matter how bland their microscopic appearance may be in view of the fact that some of them will result in repeated recurrences and even metastases. In most cases,

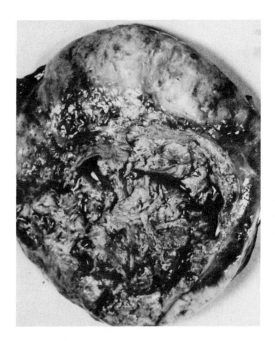

Fig. 1417 Paraganglioma arising from body of Zuckerkandl. (AFIP 270229.)

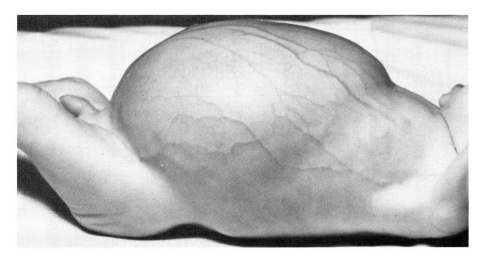

Fig. 1418 Huge benign cystic retroperitoneal teratoma in infant. Teratoma was removed successfully, and child is well. (WU neg. 52-760.)

however, atypical cytologic features (sometimes to an extreme degree) will be identified with ease.[90] We have seen a case of malakoplakia that was initially misdiagnosed as malignant fibrous histiocytoma.

Vascular tumors of several types have been described, including hemangioma, hemangiopericytoma, lymphangioma, lymphangiomyoma, and angiosarcoma.[79]

Neurogenic tumors are not nearly so common as in the mediastinum. We have seen neurilemomas, neurofibromas, and malignant schwannomas; one of the latter invaded the bone and metastasized distantly (Fig. 1415).

Tumors of sympathetic nervous tissue of the type more commonly seen in the adrenal gland also can be present in the retroperitoneum outside this gland. This includes neuroblastoma, ganglioneuroblastoma, and ganglioneuroma. These lesions often are hemorrhagic, soft, and nodular (Fig. 1416).

Paragangliomas arise outside the adrenal gland in approximately 10% of the cases. They may occur anywhere along the midline of the retroperitoneum, the best known location being Zuckerkandl's body[73,102] (Fig. 1417). Tumors arising in *heterotopic adrenal cortex* have also been reported.

Germ cell tumors are mainly represented by the *benign teratoma.*[77] This may grow large, is often cystic, and tends to occur in young children. It frequently involves the sacrococcygeal area[74] (Fig. 1418). It is often considered malignant by the surgeon because of its stubborn adherence to other structures. This

fixation is of inflammatory nature, caused by reaction to extravasated material. *Malignant teratomas*, which comprise approximately one-fourth of the cases, may have the appearance of teratocarcinoma, embryonal carcinoma, or yolk sac tumor. Exceptionally, they have been found to contain elements of Wilms' tumor.[109] *Seminomas (germinomas)* also can occur in this location. Here, even more than in the mediastinum, the possibility of a primary testicular neoplasm should be seriously investigated. Careful palpation, roentgenograms, sonography, and scrotal thermography all have been employed with varying degrees of success to detect occult testicular tumors.[95a] However, its occurrence as a primary neoplasm in the retroperitoneum has been convincingly demonstrated.[71,100a,108] In general, primary seminomas are formed by a single large mass, whereas tumors metastatic from the testis tend to involve several nodes, often on both sides of the retroperitoneum.

Tumors of ovarian type are exceptionally seen as primary retroperitoneal masses, in the pelvis or rectovaginal septum (see Chapter 18). They can be of serous, mucinous, or endometrioid type, benign or malignant. They are said to arise either from heterotopic ovarian tissue or, more likely, from invagination of the peritoneal mesothelial layer with concurrent or subsequent metaplasia.[86,105]

Metastatic tumors

Secondary neoplasms may appear in the retroperitoneal space as a result of local extension or because of lymph node involvement. The former is mainly represented by pancreatic carcinoma and primary bone neoplasms, notably sacrococcygeal chordoma.

The carcinomas most commonly giving rise to retroperitoneal lymph node metastases are those originating in testis, pancreas, uterine cervix, endometrium, and kidney.

REFERENCES

PERITONEUM

1 Ackerman LV: Tumors of the peritoneum and retroperitoneum. In Atlas of tumor pathology, Fasc. 23 and Fasc. 24. Washington, D.C., 1953, Armed Forces Institute of Pathology.

2 Auer EA, Dockerty MB, Mayo CW: Ruptured dermoid cyst of the ovary simulating abdominal carcinomatosis. Mayo Clin Proc 26:489-497, 1951.

3 Black W, Nelson D, Walker W: Multifocal subperitoneal sclerosis. Surgery 63:706-710, 1968.

4 Bockman RF, Woods M, Sargent L, Gervin AS: A unifying pathogenetic mechanism in the etiology of intraperitoneal adhesions. J Surg Res 20:1-5, 1976.

5 Bolio-Cicero A, Aguirre J, Perez-Tamayo R: Malignant peritoneal mesothelioma. Am J Clin Pathol 36:417-426, 1961.

6 Brown P, Baddeley H, Read AE, Davies JD, McGarry JMc: Sclerosing peritonitis, an unusual reaction to a β-adrenergic-blocking drug (Practolol). Lancet 2:1477-1481, 1974.

7 Burmeister RE, Fechner RE, Franklin RR: Endosalpingiosis of the peritoneum. Obst Gynecol 34:310-318, 1969.

8 Cardozo PL: A critical evaluation of 3,000 cytologic analyses of pleural fluid, ascitic fluid and pericardial fluid. Acta Cytol (Baltimore) 10:455-460, 1966.

9 Cariker M, Dockerty M: Mucinous cystadenomas and mucinous cystadenocarcinomas of the ovary. A clinical and pathological study of 355 cases. Cancer 7:302-310, 1954.

10 Coder DM, Olander GA: Granulomatous peritonitis caused by starch glove powder. Arch Surg 105:83-86, 1972.

11 Crome L: Squamous metaplasia of the peritoneum. J Pathol Bacteriol 62:61-68, 1950.

12 Davies JD, Neely J: The histopathology of peritoneal starch granulomas. J Pathol 107:265-278, 1972.

13 Davis JH: Current concepts of peritonitis. Am Surg 33:673-681, 1967.

14 Eiseman B, Seelig MG, Womack NA: Talcum powder granuloma. Frequent and serious postoperative complication. Ann Surg 126:820-832, 1947.

15 Ellis H, Adair HM: Bile peritonitis—a report of fifteen patients. Postgrad Med J 50:713-717, 1974.

16 Foot NC: The identification of neoplastic cells in serous effusions. Am J Pathol 32:961-977, 1956.

17 German WM: Dusting powder granulomas following surgery. Surg Gynecol Obstet 76:501-507, 1943.

18 Gonnella JS, Hudson EK: Clinical patterns of tuberculous peritonitis. Arch Intern Med 117:164-169, 1966.

19 Higa E, Rosai J, Pizzimbono CA, Wise L: Mucosal hyperplasia, mucinous cystadenoma and mucinous cystadenocarcinoma of appendix. A re-evaluation of appendiceal "mucocele." Cancer 32:1325-1541, 1973.

20 Hill RP: Malignant fibrous mesothelioma of the peritoneum. Cancer 6:1182-1185, 1953.

21 Holmes EC, Eggleston JC: Starch granulomatous peritonitis. Surgery 71:85-90, 1972.

22 Hughes HJ, Carr DT, Geraci JE: Tuberculous peritonitis: a review of 34 cases with emphasis on diagnostic aspects. Dis Chest 38:42-50, 1960.

23 Jarvi OH, Kunnas RJ, Laitio MT, Tyrkko JES: The accuracy and significance of cytologic cancer diagnosis of pleural effusions. Acta Cytol (Baltimore) 16:152-158, 1972.

24 Johnson WD: The cytological diagnosis of cancer in serous effusion. Acta Cytol (Baltimore) 10:161-172, 1966.

25 Kannerstein M, Churg J: Peritoneal mesothelioma. Hum Pathol 8:83-94, 1977.

26 Kannerstein M, Churg J, Magner D: Histochemistry in the diagnosis of malignant mesothelioma. Ann Clin Lab Sci 3:207-211, 1973.

27 Kannerstein M, Churg J, McCaughey WTE, Hill DP: Papillary tumors of the peritoneum in women: mesothelioma or papillary carcinoma. Am J Obstet Gynecol 127:306-314, 1977.

28 Kauffman SL, Stout AP: Mesothelioma in children. Cancer 17:539-544, 1964.

29 Kay S: Tissue reaction to barium sulfate contrast medium: histopathologic study. Arch Pathol 57:279-284, 1954.

30 Klempman S: The exfoliative cytology of diffuse pleural mesothelioma. Cancer 15:691-704, 1962.

31 Konikov N, Bleisch V, Piskie V: Prognostic significance of cytologic diagnoses of effusions. Acta Cytol (Baltimore) 10:335-339, 1966.

31a Kuo T-T, London SN, Dinh TV: Endometriosis occurring in leiomyomatosis peritonealis disseminata. Ultrastructural study and histogenetic consideration. Am J Surg Pathol 4:197-204, 1980.

32 Lascano EF, Villamayor RD, Llauró JL: Loose cysts of the peritoneal cavity. Ann Surg 152:836-844, 1960.

33 Levine H: Needle biopsy of peritoneum in exudative ascites. Arch Int Med 120:542-545, 1967.

34 Levine H: Needle biopsy diagnosis of tuberculous peritonitis. Am Rev Resp Dis 97:889-894, 1968.

35 Long RTL, Spratt JS, Dowling E: Pseudomyxoma peritonei. New concepts in management with a report of 17 patients. Am J Surg 117:162-168, 1969.

36 McPeak CJ, Papaioannou AN: Nonpancreatic tumors associated with hypoglycemia. Arch Surg 93:1019-1024, 1966.

37 Marshall SF, Forse RA: Peritoneal adhesions: report of a case of paraffinoma. Surg Clin North Am 32:903-908, 1952.

38 Melamed MR: The cytological presentation of malignant lymphomas and related diseases in effusions. Cancer 16:413-431, 1963.

38a Mennemeyer R, Smith M: Multicystic, peritoneal mesothelioma. A report with electron microscopy of a case mimicking intra-abdominal cystic hygroma (lymphangioma). Cancer 44:692-698, 1979.

39 Naylor B: The exfoliative cytology of diffuse malignant mesothelioma. J Path Bact 86:293-298, 1963.

40 Newhouse ML, Thompson H: Epidemiology of mesothelial tumors in the London area. Ann N Y Acad Sci 132:579-588, 1965.

41 Ober WB, Black MB: Neoplasms of the subcoelomic mesenchyme. Arch Pathol **59:**698-705, 1955.

42 Parmley TH, Woodruff JD: The ovarian mesothelioma. Am J Obstet Gynecol **120:**234-241, 1974.

43 Reagan JW: Exfoliative cytology of pleural, peritoneal and pericardial fluids. CA **10:**153-159, 1960.

44 Roberts HG, Campbell GM: Exfoliative cytology of diffuse mesothelioma. J Clin Pathol **23:**577-582, 1972.

45 Rosai J, Dehner LP: Nodular mesothelial hyperplasia in hernia sacs. A benign reactive condition simulating a neoplastic process. Cancer **35:**165-175, 1975.

46 Ryan GB, Grobety J, Majno G: Postoperative peritoneal adhesions. A study of the mechanisms. Am J Pathol **65:**117-140, 1971.

47 Sano ME, Weiss E, Gault ES: Pleural mesothelioma. J Thorac Surg **19:**783-788, 1950.

48 Saxen L, Saxen E: Starch granulomas as a problem in surgical pathology. Acta Pathol Microbiol Scand **64:**55-70, 1965.

49 Seaman WB, Wells J: Complications of the barium enema. Gastroenterology **48:**728-737, 1965.

49a Sherman S, Rohwedder JJ, Ravikrishnan KP, Weg JG: Tuberculous enteritis and peritonitis. Report of 36 general hospital cases. Arch Intern Med **140:**506-507, 1980.

50 Singh MM, Bhargava AN, Jain KP: Tuberculous peritonitis. An evaluation of pathogenetic mechanisms, diagnostic procedures and therapeutic measures. N Engl J Med **281:**1091-1094, 1969.

51 Smither WJ: Asbestos and mesothelioma of the pleura. Proc Roy Soc Med **59:**57-61, 1966.

52 Sochocky S: Tuberculous peritonitis. A review of 100 cases. Am Rev Respir Dis **95:**398-401, 1967.

53 Spriggs AI, Boddington MM: The cytology of effusions, ed. 2. New York, 1968, Grune & Stratton, Inc.

54 Stout AP: Solitary fibrous mesothelioma of the peritoneum. Cancer **3:**820-825, 1950.

55 Stout AP: Discussion of Case 2. Tumors of the soft tissues. Cancer Semin Penrose Cancer Hosp **2:**173-177, 1960.

56 Suzuki Y, Churg J, Kannerstein M: Ultrastructure of human malignant diffuse mesothelioma. Am J Pathol **85:**241-251, 1976.

57 Takagi F: Studies on tumor cells in serous effusion. Am J Clin Pathol **24:**663-675, 1954.

58 Wells AH: Papillomatous peritonei. Am J Pathol **11:**1011-1014, 1935.

58a Williams LJ Jr, Pavlick FJ: Leiomyomatosis peritonealis disseminata. Two case reports and a review of the medical literature. Cancer **45:**1726-1733, 1980.

59 Winslow DJ, Taylor HB: Malignant peritoneal mesotheliomas. Cancer **13:**127-136, 1960.

OMENTUM

60 Epstein LI, Lempke RE: Primary idiopathic segmental infarction of the greater omentum: case report and collective review of the literature. Ann Surg **167:**437-443, 1968.

61 Stout AP, Hendry J, Purdie FJ: Primary solid tumors of the great omentum. Cancer **16:**231-243, 1963.

MESENTERY

62 Barr WB, Yamashita T: Mesenteric cysts. Review of the literature and report of a case. Am J Gastroenterol **41:**53-57, 1964.

63 Crane JT, Aguilar MJ, Grimes OR: Isolated lipodystrophy, a form of mesenteric tumor. Am J Surg **90:**169-179, 1955.

64 Kipfer RE, Moertel CG, Dahlin DC: Mesenteric lipodystrophy. Ann Intern Med **80:**582-588, 1974.

64a Mennemeyer R, Smith M: Multicystic, peritoneal mesothelioma. A report with electron microscopy of a case mimicking intra-abdominal cystic hygroma (lymphangioma). Cancer **44:**692-698, 1979.

65 Moore JH Jr, Crum CP, Chandler JG, Feldman PS: Benign cystic mesothelioma. Cancer **45:**2395-2399, 1980.

66 Neerhout RC, Larson W, Mansur P: Mesenteric lymphoid hamartoma associated with chronic hypoferremia, anemia, growth failure and hypoglobulinemia. N Engl J Med **280:**922-925, 1969.

67 Ogden WM, Bradburn DM, Rives JD: Mesenteric panniculitis: review of 27 cases. Ann Surg **161:**864-875, 1965.

68 Reske M, Namiki H: Sclerosing mesenteritis. Report of two cases. Am J Clin Pathol **64:**661-667, 1975.

69 Tedeschi CG, Botta GC: Retractile mesenteritis. N Engl J Med **266:**1035-1040, 1962.

70 Yannopoulos K, Stout AP: Primary solid tumors of the mesentery. Cancer **16:**914-927, 1963.

RETROPERITONEUM

71 Abell MR, Fayos JV, Lampe I: Retroperitoneal germinomas (seminomas) without evidence of testicular involvement. Cancer **18:**273-290, 1965.

72 Ackerman LV: Tumors of the peritoneum and retroperitoneum. In Atlas of tumor pathology, Fasc. 23 and Fasc. 24. Washington, D.C., 1953, Armed Forces Institute of Pathology.

73 Anderson CB, Ward S, Lee J, Rosai J: Extra-adrenal retroperitoneal paraganglioma. Am Surg **40:**636-642, 1974.

74 Arnheim EE: Retroperitoneal teratomas in infancy and childhood. Pediatrics **8:**309-327, 1951 (excellent bibliography).

75 Catino D, Torack RM, Hagstrom JWC: Idiopathic retroperitoneal fibrosis. Histochemical evidence for lateral spread of the process from the midline. J Urol **98:**191-194, 1967.

76 Comings DE, Skubi KB, van Eyes J, Motulsky AG: Familial multifocal fibrosclerosis. Findings suggesting that retroperitoneal fibrosis, mediastinal fibrosis, sclerosing cholangitis, Riedel's thyroiditis, and pseudo-tumor of the orbit may be different manifestations of a single disease. Ann Intern Med **66:**884-892, 1967.

77 Engel RM, Elkins RC, Fletcher BD: Retroperitoneal teratoma. Review of the literature and presentation of an unusual case. Cancer **2:**1068-1973, 1968.

78 Enzinger FM, Winslow DJ: Liposarcoma. A study of 103 cases. Virchows Arch [Pathol Anat] **335:**367-388, 1962.

79 Gerster JCA: Retroperitoneal chyle cysts with special reference to the lymphangiomata. Ann Surg **110:**389-410, 1939 (extensive bibliography).

80 Gill W, Carter DC, Durie B: Retroperitoneal tumors. A review of 134 cases. J R Coll Surg Edinb **15:**213-221, 1970.

81 Goldberg BB, (ed): Abdominal gray scale ultrasonography. New York, 1977, John Wiley & Sons, Inc.

82 Golden T, Stout AP: Smooth muscle tumors of the

gastrointestinal tract and retroperitoneal tissues. Surg Gynecol Obstet **73:**784-810, 1941.

83 Graham JR, Suby HI, LeCompte PR, Sadowsky NL: Fibrotic disorders associated with methysergide therapy for headache. N Engl J Med **274:**359-368, 1966.

84 Harbrecht PJ: Variants of retroperitoneal fibrosis. Ann Surg **165:**388-401, 1967.

85 Hellstrom HR, Perez-Stable ED: Retroperitoneal fibrosis with disseminated vasculitis and intrahepatic sclerosing cholangitis. Am J Med **40:**184-187, 1966.

86 Hyman MP: Extraovarian endometrioid carcinoma. Review of the literature and report of two cases with unusual features. Am J Clin Pathol **68:**522-528, 1977.

87 Jacobsen S, Juul-Jorgensen S: Primary retroperitoneal tumors. A review of 26 cases. Acta Chir Scand **140:** 498-500, 1974.

88 Jones JH, Ross EJ, Matz LR, Edwards D, Davies DR: Retroperitoneal fibrosis. Am J Med **48:**203-208, 1970.

89 Jonsson G, Lindstedt E, Rubin S-O: Two cases of metastasizing scirrhous gastric carcinoma simulating idiopathic retroperitoneal fibrosis. Scand J Urol Nephrol **1:**299-302, 1967.

90 Kahn LB: Retroperitoneal xanthogranuloma and xanthosarcoma (malignant fibrous xanthoma). Cancer **31:**411-422, 1973.

91 Kay S, McNeill DD: Leiomyosarcoma of retroperitoneum. Surg Gynecol Obstet **129:**285-288, 1969.

92 Kendall AR, Lakey WH: Sclerosing Hodgkin's disease vs. idiopathic retroperitoneal fibrosis. J Urol **35:**284-291, 1961.

93 Kinne DW, Chu FCH, Huvos AG, Yagoda A, Fortner JG: Treatment of primary and recurrent retroperitoneal liposarcoma. Twenty-five-year experience at Memorial Hospital. Cancer **31:**53-64, 1973.

94 Lawson DW, Corry RJ, Patton AS, Austen WG: Massive retroperitoneal adrenal hemorrhage. Surg Gynecol Obstet **129:**989-994, 1969.

95 Leake R, Wayman TB: Retroperitoneal encysted hematomas. J Urol **68:**69-73, 1952.

95a Lee Y-TN, Gold RH: Localization of occult testicular tumor with scrotal thermography. JAMA **236:**1975-1976, 1976.

95b Lepor H, Walsh PC: Idiopathic retroperitoneal fibrosis. J Urol **122:**1-6, 1979.

96 Lofgren L: Primary retroperitoneal tumors. A histopathological, clinical and follow-up study supplemented by follow-up study of a series from the Finnish Cancer Register. Ann Acad Sci Fenn [Med] **129:**5-86, 1967.

97 Lumb G: Smooth-muscle tumours of the gastrointestinal tract and retroperitoneal tissues presenting as large cystic masses. J Pathol Bacteriol **63:**139-147, 1951.

98 Melicow MM: Primary tumors of the retroperitoneum. A clinico-pathologic analysis of 162 cases. Review of the literature and tables of classification. J Int Coll Surg **19:**401-449, 1953.

99 Meyer S, Hausman R: Occlusive phlebitis in multifocal fibrosclerosis. Am J Clin Pathol **65:**274-283, 1976.

100 Mitchinson MJ: The pathology of idiopathic retroperitoneal fibrosis. J Clin Pathol **23:**681-689, 1970.

100a Montague DK: Retroperitoneal germ cell tumors with no apparent testicular involvement. J Urol **113:**505-508, 1975.

101 Oberling C: Retroperitoneal xanthogranuloma. Am J Cancer **23:**477-489, 1935.

102 Olson JR, Abell MR: Nonfunctional nonchromaffin paragangliomas of the retroperitoneum. Cancer **23:** 1358-1367, 1969.

103 Pack GT, and Tabah EJ: Primary retroperitoneal tumors. A study of 120 cases. Surg Gynecol Obstet **90**[Suppl]:209-231, 313-341, 1954.

104 Ranchod M, Kempson RC: Smooth muscle tumors of the gastrointestinal tract and retroperitoneum. A pathologic analysis of 100 cases. Cancer **39:**255-262, 1977.

105 Roth LM, Ehrlich CE: Mucinous cystadenocarcinoma of the retroperitoneum. Obstet Gynecol **49:**486-488, 1977.

106 Terner JY, Lattes R: Malakoplakia of colon and retroperitoneum. Report of a case with a histochemical study of the Michaelis-Gutmann inclusion bodies. Am J Clin Pathol **44:**20-31, 1965.

107 Thomas MH, Chisholm GD: Retroperitoneal fibrosis associated with malignant disease. Br J Cancer **28:** 453-458, 1973.

107a Tinker MA, Burdman D, Deysine M, Teicher I, Platt N, Aufses AH Jr: Granulomatous peritonitis due to cellulose fibers from disposable surgical fabrics: laboratory investigations and clinical implications. Ann Surg **180:**831-835, 1974.

108 Veraguth P, Maillard G-F, MacGee W: Retroperitoneal seminomas without evidence of primary growth. Oncology **24:**193-209, 1970.

109 Ward SP, Dehner LP: Sacrococcygeal teratoma with nephroblastoma (Wilms' tumor): a variant of extragonadal teratoma in childhood. Cancer **33:**1355-1363, 1974.

110 Wittenberg J, Finenberg HV, Black EB, Kirkpatrick RH, Schaffer DL, Ekeda MK, Ferrucci JT Jr: Clinical efficacy of computed body tomography. Am J Roentgenol **131:**5-14, 1978 (part of a special section on the medical efficiency of computed tomography).

26 Cardiovascular system

Heart
Arteries
Veins
Lymphatics

Heart

Introduction

The heart and aorta used to be considered outside the province of the surgeon, but during the past thirty years advances in thoracic surgery have followed better understanding of the physiology of the heart and refinement of new procedures in diagnosis and treatment (cardiac catheterization, angiocardiography, hypothermia, and extracorporeal circulation). Excellent books and monographs have been written about congenital heart disease,[1,1a,2,3a] and the progress made in the field of cardiac pathology in the past few years has been reviewed.[3] Most operations for congenital cardiovascular malformations are directed toward improvement in the flow of oxygenated blood by such procedures as ligation or division of a patent ductus or the Blalock operation, the closure of interatrial and interventricular septal defects. Methods have been devised to relieve pulmonary, arotic, and mitral valvular stenosis. Coronary artery bypass graft surgery has become a widely used and effective procedure for the symptomatic treatment of ischemic heart disease. In these procedures, the surgical pathologist rarely receives tissue. If the operation fails, the cause of failure becomes the concern of the general pathologist. Therefore, the various cardiac abnormalities and their methods of treatment will not be presented in detail.

Myocardial biopsy

The performance of myocardial or endomyocardial biopsies has become an almost routine task in some hospitals.[3b] A recent report mentions that 1,300 cardiac biopsies have been taken in recent years in a single institution.[15] These biopsies can be obtained through a catheter inserted in a systemic vein through a transthoracic route or at the time of operation for a congenital or acquired heart disease.[12,16] Ideally, both light and electron miscoscopy should be carried out. This technique has been used mainly for the evaluation of the conditions discussed in the following paragraphs.

Idiopathic hypertrophic cardiomyopathy. Much information has been obtained in this disease from light and electron microscopic studies of biopsies obtained at open thoracotomy.[10] Closed chest biopsy specimens are less informative, but they will still show disarray of myofibrils and myofilaments within individual myocytes by ultrastructural examination. Unfortunately, these changes are not specific for this condition.

Idiopathic dilated cardiomyopathy. Abnormalities in the myocardial biopsy are consistently present but, again, are of a nonspecific nature.[11] A good correlation has been found between the severity of the condition clinically and the extent and degree of microscopic abnormalities,[11] although the sometimes focal nature of the changes may be misleading.

Infiltrative myocardiopathies. This is the group of cardiac disease in which endomyocardial biopsy can be particularly rewarding.

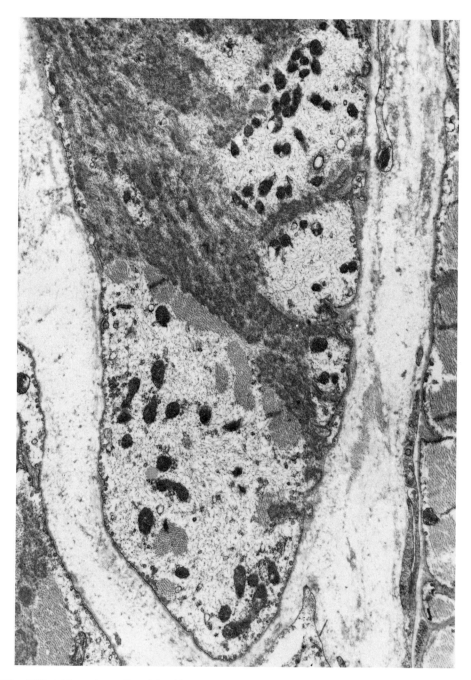

Fig. 1419 Adriamycin cardiotoxicity. Myocyte in center ("adria cell") shows extensive pale areas of loss of myofibrils and fragmentation of myofilaments. Mitochondria (dark oval structures in same areas) are not qualitatively altered. Remnants of Z bands form diagonal dense area in center. Note intact myofibril in adjacent myocyte (right edge). (Uranyl acetate–lead citrate; ×5,600; courtesy Dr. L. F. Fajardo, Stanford, Calif.)

This includes amyloidosis,[6] hemosiderosis,[5] glycogenosis, and sarcoidosis.[17] However, as Ferrans and Roberts[9] aptly pointed out, the diagnosis of most of these conditions can be made more readily by biopsy of another more readily accessible organ.

Drug-induced cardiomyopathy. The myocardial changes resulting from *adriamycin* toxicity have been well documented.[13,14] Vacuolization of cardiac myocytes, resulting from dilatation of the sarcotubular system, is the earliest change. This is followed by the appearance of the so-called "adria cell," characterized light microscopically by loss of cross striations and myofilamentous bundles, accompanied by a homogeneous basophilic staining ("myocytolysis"). Ultrastructurally, there is dissociation of sarcomers and fragmentation and loss of myofilaments. Inflammation is nil or absent, and this constitutes an important differential feature with other myocardial lesions (Figs. 1419 and 1420).

The changes are rather diffuse but seem to predominate in the subendocardial region. They are dose-dependent and are enhanced if radiation therapy also has been employed. In the latter instance, the changes just described will be in addition to those due to the radiation, mainly located in the capillaries.[4]

Cyclophosphamide may produce hemorrhagic necrosis, extensive capillary thrombosis, interstitial hemorrhage and fibrin deposition, and necrosis of myocardial fibers.[3b]

Heart transplant. The group at Stanford

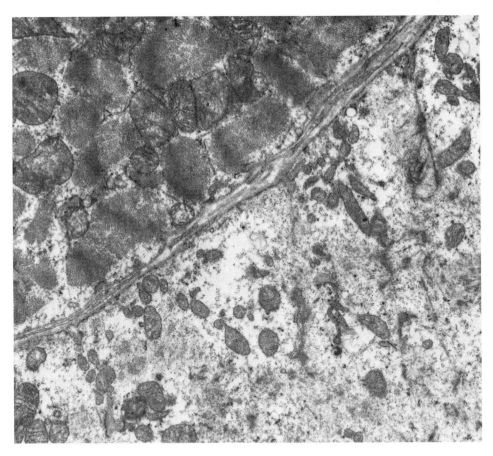

Fig. 1420 Compare transverse section of normal cardiac myocyte (upper left) with myocyte severely affected by adriamycin (lower right). There is complete disorganization of sarcomeres and extensive fragmentation of myofilaments. Mitochondria are small (compare with top). Remnants of Z bands are present near right edge. This complete loss of contractile elements in one myocyte, with preservation of adjacent cell, creates sharply defined amphophilic or basophilic areas that characterize "adria cells" in paraffin sections. (Uranyl acetate–lead citrate; ×8,200; courtesy Dr. L. F. Fajardo, Stanford, Calif.)

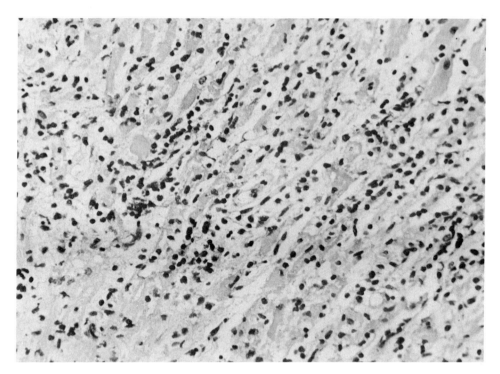

Fig. 1421 Myocardial biopsy of transplanted heart taken two weeks after operation. Signs of rejection are present in form of mononuclear cell infiltration, edema, and myocardial fiber degeneration.

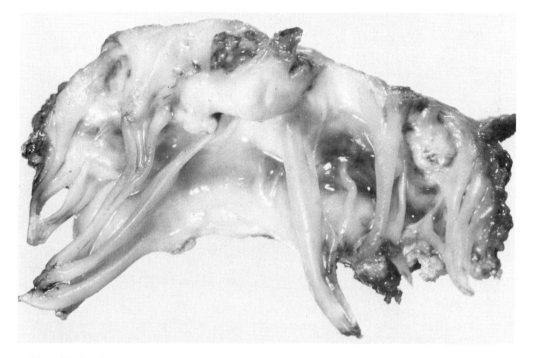

Fig. 1422 Surgical specimen of mitral valve distorted by rheumatic heart disease in 40-year-old man who had disease for over ten years. Valve was resected and replaced by prosthesis. Unfortunately, it failed. (WU neg. 62-1352.)

University has shown the usefulness of endo-myocardial biopsy for the early diagnosis and grading of transplant rejection.[3b,7,8] Signs of early rejection are interstitial edema and mono-nuclear infiltrate; these precede the clinical and electrocardiographic signs of rejection and are completely reversible if the rejection episode is successfully managed (Fig. 1421).

Cardiac valves

Operations to correct major defects of the valves by resection and prosthetic replacement are being successfully performed (Fig. 1422). Roberts and Morrow[21] emphasize that the most precise diagnosis will be made from the gross appearance of the valve and that usually the microscopic examination is of little help. Photographic and roentgenographic examination of the specimen is also well indicated. Careful examination of the gross specimen with knowledge of the clinical history often allows a distinction between a rheumatic or a congenital origin for a chronic valvulopathy to be made. Microscopically, both show fibrosis, calcification, and occasional inflammatory cells. Distinct mucinous changes were seen in twenty-one of 140 cardiac valves examined by Frable.[18] These were found to be nonspecific, inasmuch as seven of the patients suffered from congenital heart disease, four from rheumatic heart disease, and three from subacute bacterial endocarditis. In seven cases, all occurring in the aorta of adults, no specific etiology could be ascertained. There were considered examples of the "floppy valve syndrome,"[19] although the existence of such an entity is still debated.

An easy system for the identification of the many different types of artificial heart valve prostheses by the pathologist has been developed.[24] Microscopic study of these prosthetic valves has shown that, following insertion, a neoendocardium develops at the junction with the heart wall, and from there it grows centripetally over the sewing cloth toward the valve lumen. This neoformed lining can become the site of thrombus formation and bacterial or fungous infections.[20,22,23]

The pathologic changes seen in homograft valves and in heterograft (porcine) valves was summarized by Billingham.[17a]

Left atrium in mitral stenosis

Mitral valvulotomy for patients with mitral stenosis may be accompanied by biopsy of the atrial appendage. These appendages are always abnormal, showing hypertrophy of the muscle and various other alterations. About one-half of them show actual Aschoff nodules.[25] We have not been able to correlate the presence of these nodules with the postoperative course nor with clinical evidence of activity of the rheumatic process.

Coarctation of aorta

Coarctation of the aorta is usually divided into infantile and adult types, but it is probably better to call them diffuse or localized[28] (Figs. 1423 and 1424).

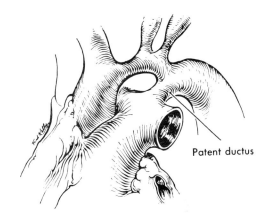

Fig. 1423 Infantile (diffuse) type of coarctation of aorta. (From Burford TH: Symposium on clinical surgery. Coarctation of aorta and its treatment. Surg Clin North Am **30**:1249-1258, 1950.)

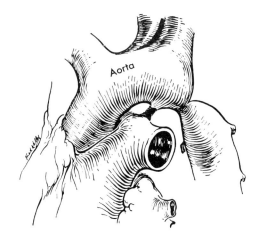

Fig. 1424 Adult (localized) type of coarctation of aorta. (From Burford TH: Symposium on clinical surgery. Coarctation of aorta and its treatment. Surg Clin North Am **30**:1249-1258, 1950.)

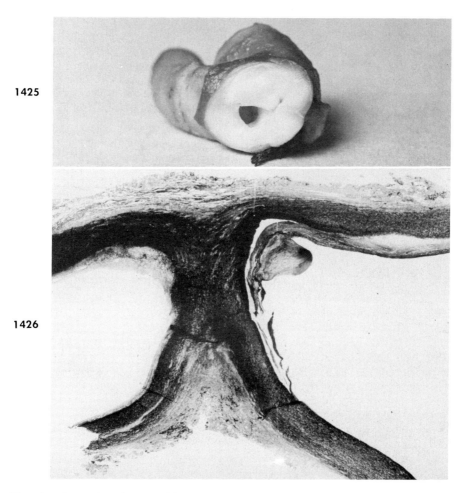

1425

1426

Fig. 1425 Coarctation of aorta, adult type, showing greatly narrowed lumen. (WU neg. 48-5295.)
Fig. 1426 Coarctation of aorta at point of constriction showing subintimal thickening and medial distortion. (Low power; WU neg. 48-6704.)

In the diffuse type, the coarctated segment lies proximal to the ductus arteriosus. This type was incompatible with life, but Gross and Hufnagel[27] used homografts to repair the defect. In the localized type, which is by far the most common, the short, narrowed segment of the aorta is at the level of the aortic insertion of the ductus or just distal to it. If resection is not done, about 60% of the patients die before 40 years of age[29] of aortic rupture, endocarditis, hypertension, or congestive failure (Fig. 1425). With present techniques, the operative risk is small and the long-term results are excellent. The operation, which consists in removal of the coarctation with end-to-end anastomosis, is best done when the patient is between 5 and 7 years of age.

Grossly, the vessel is narrowed at the point of insertion of the ligamentum arteriosum. On opening the aorta, a diaphragm-like structure lies across the lumen, through which there is an aperture usually 1 mm or less in diameter.[26] Often there is localized subintimal thickening, and beneath this the media is distorted and thickened (Fig. 1426).

Operations for coarctation of the aorta are often difficult in older patients because of advanced arteriosclerotic changes in the aorta.

Cardiac tumors

Myxomas constitute approximately 50% of primary tumors of the heart. They occur in a wide range of ages and are more common in females. A familial predisposition has been ob-

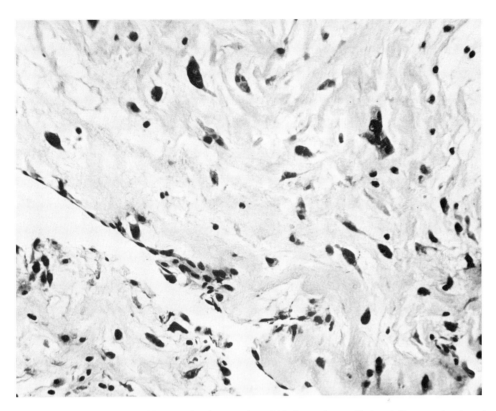

Fig. 1427 Patient (33-year-old woman), who was thought to have rheumatic heart disease, developed signs of embolism to one of large arteries of leg. Artery was opened and peculiar jellylike clot found. It was thought by surgeon to be extremely atypical. Microscopically, it showed cells with bizarre nuclei against mucoid background. This pattern was thought to be typical of myxoma, and it was predicted that patient had myxoma of left side of heart. Appropriate studies were made, and thoracic surgeon removed myxoma found in left atrium. Patient had uneventful postoperative recovery. She did not have rheumatic heart disease. (×275; WU neg. 62-7388.)

served.[45] Seventy-five per cent are located in the left atrium[41] and 25% in the right atrium. A few bilateral examples have been described.[30] They may present with signs of mitral stenosis or insufficiency, multiple emboli (Figs. 1427 and 1428), or symptoms secondary to hypergammaglobulinemia.[43,56] The diagnosis can be established by M-mode and two-dimensional echocardiography, gated radionuclide blood-pool scan, or cardiac catheterization.[47,57a] Occasionally, the diagnosis is made by histologic examination of an embolus removed at operation (Fig. 1427).

Grossly, myxomas are soft, polypoid, pale, lobulated masses often attached by a stalk to the septum near the foramen ovale. A papillary configuration may be apparent, especially if the specimen is examined under water. Calcification may occur in the tumors, and this seems to be more common in those located in the right atrium. Microscopically, round, polygonal, or stellate cells are seen surrounded by abundant loose stroma rich in acid mucopolysaccharides.[40] Although a controversy still lingers as to the reactive (exuberant thrombus) versus neoplastic nature of this process,[54] we side with the latter view.[34] The occurrence of occasional aggressive examples with invasion of the chest wall or distant metastases certainly speak in favor of this interpretation.[50,54a] The cell of origin is also in dispute. Ultrastructural examinations have suggested that myxomas arise from multipotential mesenchymal cells.[34,37] The recent demonstration of Factor VIII in the cytoplasm of the proliferating cells strongly support an endothelial (endocardial) derivation.[46b] Surgical excision of the ordinary myxoma is often curative. Several instances of local recurrence have been reported in the past; with the routine performance of partial

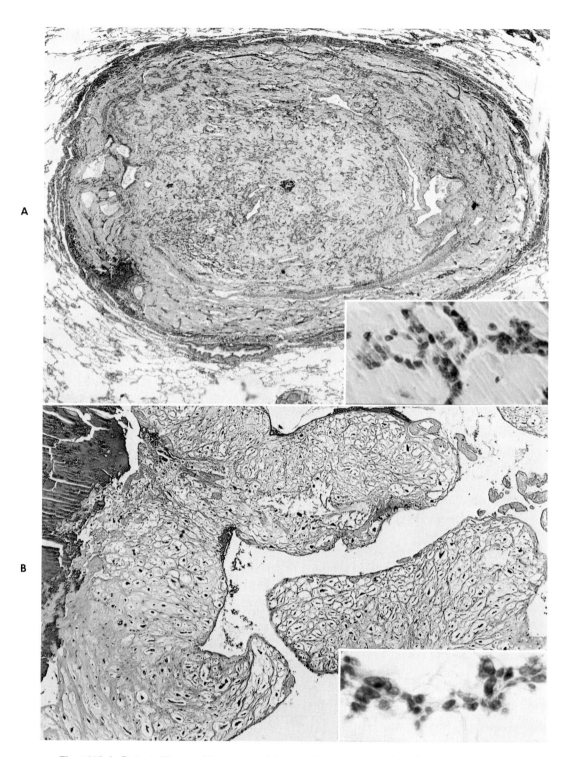

Fig. 1428 A, Patient, 28-year-old man, complained of dyspnea on exertion. Roentgenogram of chest revealed multiple small nodular densities in both lung fields. Open lung biopsy revealed tumor emboli filling branches of pulmonary artery. **Inset,** Thin rows of small regular tumor cells can be seen in abundant myxoid matrix. Pathologic diagnosis was "metastatic carcinoma, primary site undetermined." **B,** Nature of disease became obvious only nine years later, when large cardiac myxoma was removed from right atrium. Pulmonary nodules obviously represent emboli from tumor. **Inset,** Tumor cells, although larger and slightly more atypical, have same configuration and stromal background as those in lungs. (**A,** ×30; WU neg. 73-1360; **inset,** ×350; WU neg. 73-1358; **B,** ×40; WU neg. 73-1359; **inset,** ×350; WU neg. 73-1359; **A, B,** and **insets,** courtesy Dr. Y. LeGal, Strasbourg, France.)

atrial septectomy together with the excision of the tumor, they have become very rare.[50a]

Other benign primary tumors, all extremely rare, include so-called rhabdomyoma and rhabdomyomatosis, which are probably hamartomas rather than neoplasms[57]; so-called mesothelioma of the atrioventricular node,[36] which we believe to be of developmental origin and not of mesothelial nature; fibroma (fibroelastic hamartoma)[33]; granular cell tumor, frequently mistaken for rhabdomyoma[35]; hemangioma; lymphangioma; lipoma; neurilemoma[32]; and ganglioneuroma.[39,49]

Primary malignant tumors also are exceptional.[46a] They are all sarcomas, many of them undifferentiated and unclassifiable.[49] Recognizable instances of rhabdomyosarcoma, leiomyosarcoma,[31] fibrosarcoma, angiosarcoma,[53] malignant fibrous histiocytoma,[55] and primary malignant lymphoma[38] have been reported. Most patients present with intractable congestive heart failure, arrhythmias, or signs of superior vena cava obstruction. It has been pointed out that malignant tumors are more frequently found in the right side of the heart, while the benign neoplasms are more common on the left side.[31]

Involvement of the heart by metastatic carcinoma or by generalized malignant lymphoma is a commoner event but rarely seen as a surgical specimen.[42,51] In the large majority of the carcinomas metastatic to the heart, the primary tumor is in the thoracic cavity or contiguous areas and the tumor reaches the heart by metastasizing to the mediastinal lymph nodes and from there extending in a retrograde fashion to the cardiac lymphatic vessels.[44] Malignant tumors with a marked tendency to spread to the heart by the hematogenous route are malignant melanoma, renal cell carcinoma, choriocarcinoma, and childhood rhabdomyosarcoma.[48]

We have seen several cases of small nodular lesions attached to the left atrium found incidentally at the time of surgery for valvular disease. Microscopically, they were composed of solid or microcystic aggregates of cells with large vesicular nuclei (often exhibiting deep grooves) and abundant acidophilic cytoplasm, sometimes containing vacuoles. Mitoses were nearly absent. A similar process was reported as Mahaim[46] as "benign angioreticuloma of endocardium." All of our patients have remained well following excision of the mass. We believe this growth to be composed of "histiocytoid" endothelial cells, and to be of a benign nature, perhaps not even neoplastic.[52] It is important not to confuse it with metastatic carcinoma, mesothelioma, or some other malignant process.

Pericardium

Pericardial (coelomic) cysts are discussed in Chapter 7. *Pericarditis* is of importance to the surgical pathologist for several reasons. A diagnosis of tuberculous pericarditis or sarcoidosis can be made from a pericardial open biopsy.[61] Acute nonspecific pericarditis[60] and purulent pericarditis[59] are rarely biopsied, but the former may be troublesome because of the sometimes extreme degree of mesothelial hyperplasia that accompanies it and that can simulate malignancy. Chronic pericarditis often is accompanied by fibrosis and calcification, which may lead to constriction. Pathologic examination merely shows dense fibrosis with deposits of calcium and a scanty inflammatory infiltrate.

Mesotheliomas occur, but their frequency is much less than for similar tumors in the pleura or peritoneum. They may present as a single well-circumscribed mass, as multiple tumors, or as a diffuse growth encasing the heart. Sometimes, coexistence of a pleural mesothelioma is observed. Microscopically, the appearance varies from epithelial to spindle-shaped, with a frequent admixture of these elements. As in the pleura, acid mucopolysaccharides often are produced by the tumor cells. The differential diagnosis is with mesothelial hyperplasia and metastatic carcinoma. Demonstration of a continuity between the tumor and the mesothelial lining cells is a useful differential feature in regard to the latter.

Most mesotheliomas of the pericardium occur in adults and are diffuse and malignant. They may locally infiltrate the superficial myocardium and even metastasize to the mediastinal lymph nodes and lungs.[58]

Metastatic carcinoma to the pericardium usually originates in the lung, in the form of direct extension or lymphatic permeation. It may result in constrictive "pericarditis" as a result of the associated intense desmoplastic reaction.

REFERENCES
Introduction

1 Cooley DA, Hallman GL: Surgical treatment of congenital heart disease. Philadelphia, 1966, Lea & Febiger.

1a Edwards JE: Survey of operative congenital heart disease. A review. Am J Pathol **82:**408-435, 1976.

2 Keith JD, Rowe RD, Vlad P: Heart disease in infancy and childhood, ed. 2. New York, 1967, The Macmillan Co.

3 Robbins SL: Cardiac pathology—a look at the last five years. Hum Pathol **5:**9-24, 1974.

3a Taussig HB: Congenital malformations of the heart, ed. 2. Cambridge, Mass., 1960, Harvard University Press.

Myocardial biopsy

3b Billingham ME: Some recent advances in cardiac pathology. Hum Pathol **10:**367-386, 1979.

4 Billingham ME, Bristow MR, Glatstein E, Mason JW, Masek MA, Daniels JR: Adriamycin cardiotoxicity: endomyocardial biopsy evidence of enhancement by irradiation. Am J Surg Pathol **1:**17-23, 1977.

5 Buja LM, Roberts WC: Iron in the heart. Etiology and clinical significance. Am J Med **51:**209-221, 1971.

6 Buja LM, Khoi NB, Roberts WC: Clinically significant cardiac amyloidosis. Clinicopathologic findings in 15 patients. Am J Cardiol **26:**394-405, 1970.

7 Caves PK, Billingham ME, Stinson EB, Shumway NE: Serial transvenous biopsy of the transplanted human heart. Improved management of acute rejection episodes. Lancet **1:**821-826, 1974.

8 Caves PK, Stinson EB, Billingham ME, Shumway NE: Percutaneous transvenous endomyocardial biopsy in human heart recipients. Ann Thorac Surg **16:**325-336, 1973.

9 Ferrans VJ, Roberts WC: Myocardial biopsy: a useful diagnostic procedure or only a research tool? Am J Cardiol **41:**965-967, 1978.

10 Ferrans VJ, Morrow AG, Roberts WC: Myocardial ultrastructure in idiopathic hypertrophic subaortic stenosis. A study of operatively excised left ventricular outflow tract muscle in 14 patients. Circulation **45:**769-792, 1972.

11 Ferrans VJ, Massumi RA, Shugoll GL, Ali N, Roberts WC: Ultrastructural studies of myocardial biopsies in 45 patients with obstructive or congestive cardiomyopathy. In Bajusz E, Rona G, Brink AJ, Lochner A (eds): Recent advances in studies on cardiac structure and metabolism. Vol. II. The cardiomyopathies. Baltimore, 1973, University Park Press, pp. 231-272.

12 Fujita M, Neustein HB, Lurie PR: Transvascular endomyocardial biopsy in infants and small children. Myocardial findings in 10 cases of cardiomyopathy. Hum Pathol **10:**15-30, 1979.

13 Henderson IC, Frei E III: Adriamycin and the heart (editorial). N Engl J Med **300:**310-311, 1979.

14 Jaenke RS, Fajardo LF: Adriamycin-induced myocardial lesions. Report of a workshop. Am J Surg Pathol **1:**55-60, 1977.

15 Mason JW: Techniques for right and left ventricular endomyocardial biopsy. Am J Cardiol **41:**887-892, 1978.

16 Olsen EGJ: Endomyocardial biopsy. Invest Cell Pathol **1:**139-157, 1978.

17 Roberts WC, McAllister HA Jr, Ferrans VJ: Sarcoidosis of the heart. A clinicopathologic study of 35 necropsy patients (Group I) and review of 78 previously reported necropsy patients (Group II). Am J Med **63:**86-108, 1977.

Cardiac valves

17a Billingham ME: Some recent advances in cardiac pathology. Hum Pathol **10:**367-386, 1979.

18 Frable WJ: Mucinous degeneration of the cardiac valves. J Thorac Cardiovasc Surg **58:**62-70, 1969.

19 Read RC, Thal AP, Wendt VE: Symptomatic valvular myxomatous transformation (the floppy valve syndrome). A possible forme fruste of the Marfan syndrome. Circulation **32:**897-910, 1965.

20 Robboy SJ, Kaiser J: Pathogenesis of fungal infection on heart valve prostheses. Hum Pathol **6:**711-715, 1975.

21 Roberts WC, Morrow AG: Cardiac valves and the surgical pathologist. Arch Pathol **82:**309-313, 1966.

22 Silver MD: Cardiac pathology—a look at the last five years. II. The pathology of cardiovascular prostheses. Hum Pathol **5:**127-138, 1974.

23 Silver MD: Late complications of prosthetic heart valves. Arch Pathol Lab Med **102:**281-284, 1978.

24 Silver MD, Datta BN, Bowes VF: A key to identify heart valve prostheses. Arch Pathol **99:**132-138, 1975.

Left atrium in mitral stenosis

25 Clark RM, Anderson W: Rheumatic activity in auricular appendages removed at mitral valvoplasty. Am J Pathol **31:**809-819, 1955.

Coarctation of aorta

26 Edwards JE, Christensen NA, Clagett OT, McDonald JR: Pathologic considerations in coarctation of the aorta. Mayo Clin Proc **23:**324-332, 1948.

27 Gross RE, Hufnagel C: Coarctation of the aorta. N Engl J Med **233:**287-293, 1945.

28 Hanlon CR: Present status of cardiovascular surgery. JAMA **149:**1-7, 1952.

29 Reifenstein GH, Levine SA, Gross RE: Coarctation of the aorta. A review of 104 autopsied cases of the ''adult type'' 2 years of age or older. Am Heart J **33:**146-168, 1947.

Cardiac tumors

30 Anderson ST, Pitt A, Zimmet R, Kay KB, Morris KN: A case of bi-atrial myxomas with successful surgical removal. J Thorac Cardiovasc Surg **59:**768-773, 1970.

31 Bearman RM: Primary leiomyosarcoma of the heart. Report of a case and review of the literature. Arch Pathol **98:**62-65, 1974.

32 Factor S, Turi G, Biempica L: Primary cardiac neurilemmoma. Cancer **37:**883-890, 1976.

33 Feldman PS, Meyer MW: Fibroelastic hamartoma (fibroma) of the heart. Cancer **38:**314-323, 1976.

34 Feldman PS, Horvath E, Kovacs K: An ultrastructural study of seven cardiac myxomas. Cancer **40:**2216-2232, 1977.

35 Fenoglio JJ, McAllister HA: Granular cell tumors of the heart. Arch Pathol Lab Med **100:**276-278, 1976.

36 Fenoglio JJ Jr, Jacobs DW, McAllister HA Jr: Ultrastructure of the mesothelioma of the atrioventricular node. Cancer **40:**721-727, 1977.

37 Ferrans VJ, Roberts WC: Structural features of cardiac myxomas: histology, histochemistry and electron microscopy. Hum Pathol **4:**111-146, 1973.

38 Fiester RF: Reticulum cell sarcoma of the heart. Arch Pathol **99:**60-61, 1975.

39 Fine G: Primary tumors of the pericardium and heart. In Edwards JE, et al (eds): The heart. Baltimore, 1974, The Williams & Wilkins Co., pp. 189-210.

40 Fine G, Morales A, Horn RC Jr: Cardiac myxoma. A morphologic and histogenetic appraisal. Cancer **22**:1156-1162, 1968.

41 Goodwin JF: Diagnosis of left atrial myxoma. Lancet **1**:464-468, 1963.

42 Hanfling SM: Metastatic cancer to the heart. Circulation **22**:474-483, 1960.

43 Heath D: Pathology of cardiac tumors. Am J Cardiol **21**:315-327, 1968.

44 Kline IK: Cardiac lymphatic involvement by metastatic tumor. Cancer **29**:799-808, 1972.

45 Liebler GA, Magovern GJ, Park SB, Cushing WJ, Begg FR, Joyner CR: Familial myxomas in four siblings. J Thorac Cardiovasc Surg **71**:605-608, 1976.

46 Mahaim I: Les tumeurs et les polypes du coeur. Etude anatomo-clinique. Paris, 1945, Masson et Cie, pp. 321-328.

46a McAllister HA Jr, Fenoglio JJ: Tumors of the cardiovascular system. In Atlas of tumor pathology, Second Series, Fasc. 15. Washington, D. C., 1978, Armed Forces Institute of Pathology.

46b Najdi M, Gonzalez MS, Castro A, Morales AR: Factor VIII–related antigen: an endothelial cell marker. Lab Invest **42**:139, 1980 (abstract).

47 Pohost GM, Pastore JO, McKusick KA, Chiotellis PN, Kapellakis GZ, Meyers GS, Dinsmore RE, Block PC: Detection of left atrial myxoma by gated radionuclide cardiac imaging. Circulation **55**:88-92, 1977.

48 Pratt CB, Dugger DL, Johnson WW, Ainger LE: Metastatic involvement of the heart in childhood rhabdomyosarcoma. Cancer **31**:1492-1497, 1973.

49 Prichard RW: Tumors of the heart. Review of the subject and report of one hundred and fifty cases. Arch Pathol **51**:98-128, 1951.

50 Read RC, White HJ, Murphy ML, Williams D, Sun CN, Flanagan WH: The malignant potentiality of left atrial myxoma. J Thorac Cardiovasc Surg **68**:857-868, 1974.

50a Richardson JV, Brandt B III, Doty DB, Ehrenhaft JL: Surgical treatment of atrial myxomas: early and late results of 111 operations and review of the literature. Ann Thorac Surg **28**:354-358, 1979.

51 Roberts WC, Glancy DL, DeVita VT Jr: Heart in malignant lymphoma (Hodgkin's disease, lymphosarcoma, reticulum cell sarcoma and mycosis fungoides).

Study of 196 autopsy cases. Am J Cardiol **22**:85-107, 1968.

52 Rosai J, Gold J, Landy R: The histiocytoid hemangiomas. A unifying concept embracing several previously described entities of skin, soft tissue, large vessels, bone and heart. Hum Pathol **10**:707-730, 1979.

53 Rossi NP, Kioschos JM, Aschenbrener CA, Ehrenhaft JL: Primary angiosarcoma of the heart. Cancer **37**:891-894, 1976.

54 Salyer WR, Page DL, Hutchins GM: The development of cardiac myxomas and papillary endocardial lesions from mural thrombus. Am Heart J **89**:14-17, 1975.

54a Seo IS, Warner TFCS, Colyer RA, Winkler RF: Metastasizing atrial myxoma. Am J Surg Pathol **4**:391-399, 1980.

55 Shah AA, Churg A, Sbarbaro JA, Sheppard JM, Lamberti J: Malignant fibrous histiocytoma of the heart presenting as an atrial myxoma. Cancer **42**:2466-2471, 1978.

56 Silverman J, Olwin JS, Graettinger JS: Cardiac myxomas with systemic embolization. Review of the literature and report of a case. Circulation **26**:99-103, 1962.

57 Silverman JF, Kay S, McCue M, Lower RR, Brough AJ, Chang CH: Rhabdomyoma of the heart. Ultrastructural study of three cases. Lab Invest **35**:596-606, 1976.

57a Silverman NA: Primary cardiac tumors. Ann Surg **191**:127-138, 1980.

Pericardium

58 Fine G: Primary tumors of the pericardium and heart. In Edwards JE, et al (eds): The heart. Baltimore, 1974, The Williams & Wilkins Co., pp. 189-210.

59 Klacsmann PG, Bulkley BH, Hutchins GM: The changed spectrum of purulent pericarditis. An 86 year autopsy experience in 200 patients. Am J Med **63**:666-673, 1977.

60 Martin A: Acute non-specific pericarditis: a description of nineteen cases. Br Med J **2**:279-281, 1966.

61 Shiff AD, Blatt CJ, Kolp C: Recurrent pericardial effusion secondary to sarcoidosis of the pericardium: a biopsy-proved case. N Engl J Med **281**:141-143, 1967.

Arteries

Arteriosclerosis

Arteriosclerosis is a generalized progressive arterial disease associated with localized arterial occlusions and aneurysms. Its pathology has gained greater surgical significance in recent years with the development of direct operative therapy for lesions of major arteries.

The pathology of arteriosclerosis primarily consists of the following:

1 Formation of intimal *plaques,* composed of lipid deposits and proliferated spindle cells; latter seem to be of heterogenous nature, fibroblasts and smooth muscle cells predominating[38]

2 Reduplication and fragmentation of the internal elastic lamina

3 Degeneration of the media indicated by fragmentation of elastic tissue network, by hyaline, mucinoid, and collagenous degeneration of the smooth muscle, and by medial calcification

4 Adventitial fibrosis and chronic inflammatory cellular infiltration

Arteriosclerosis in an artery may present as an occlusive process when the disease attacks the intima more rapidly than the media and adventitia but may present as an aneurysm when the reverse is true. Both occlusive dis-

ease and aneurysm may exist in the same arterial system.[46]

The cause of arteriosclerosis is unknown. Factors thought important in its pathogenesis include changes in lipid metabolism, increased endothelial permeability to serum lipoprotein complexes, susceptibility of the intima to mechanical injury from flow turbulence at major bifurcations and in the presence of hypertension, elastic tissue fragmentation, and thrombosis or disruption of vasa vasorum.[6,31,34,51,61]

The areas of the arterial tree involved by arteriosclerosis that frequently are successfully treated surgically have increased rapidly so that only occlusions of the smaller peripheral arteries of the extremities remain outside the realm of operative attack.

Surgical therapy for occlusive disease of the coronary, carotid, and mesenteric arteries is being undertaken more frequently. The principal manifestations of arteriosclerosis that at present are treated surgically with some success are fusiform and saccular aneurysms of the aorta or other major arteries, dissecting aneurysm, and occlusive disease of the abdominal aorta, the iliofemoral arterial system, and, less often, the popliteal, subclavian, brachial, renal, and carotid arterial systems.[18,19,21,75]

Aneurysms
Aortic aneurysms

Aneurysms secondary to arteriosclerosis occur most frequently in the abdominal aorta. In the aorta and other arteries that become aneurysmal because of arteriosclerosis, the mechanism of development and the pathology of the arteriosclerotic aneurysms are similar.

Arterial dilatation is likely initiated by a loss of elasticity or weakening of the recoil strength in the arterial wall, which results in elongation and tortuosity as well as in dilatation. Initially, this dilatation is most often fusiform. At the same intraluminal pressure, tension developed in the arterial wall is greater the larger the diameter of the artery. The tendency for dilatation thus increases rapidly after it has begun.[23] The progressive dilatation often results in a break in the arterial well and in the development of sacculation of the aneurysm. In other words, most arteriosclerotic aneurysms proba-

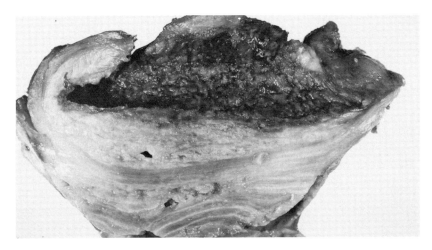

Fig. 1429 Resected abdominal aortic aneurysm that has been transected to show laminations of clot. (WU neg. 57-4850.)

bly begin as fusiform dilatations but, with the loss of structural integrity, become saccular. The sacculations nearly always are partially filled with laminated clot, which may be the source of emboli into the arteries peripheral to the aneurysm (Fig. 1429). Superimposed bacterial infection may complicate an aortic aneurysm of arteriosclerotic origin. *Salmonella* is the predominant organism, followed by *Staphylococcus*.[4]

The patient with an abdominal aneurysm may be asymptomatic and without clinical findings except for prominent abdominal aortic pulsations. The majority, however, seek treatment because of dull midabdominal or back pain associated with a pulsating, tender epigastric or retroumbilical mass that has enlarged rapidly or has been noted only recently. Painful and rapidly enlarging aneurysms will soon rupture if operative therapy is not undertaken. Retroperitoneal hemorrhages from small aneurysms may produce severe back pain with few abdominal symptoms of signs. Fistulas may develop from these aneurysms; there may be leakage into the vena cava or the duodenum or other portions of small bowel.[63] Significantly, aortoenteric fistulas also may occur as a late complication of reconstructive aortic surgery.[48a] Aneurysms of the hepatic artery may rupture into the common bile duct, those of the splenic artery into the stomach, colon, or pancreatic duct, and those of the internal iliac artery into the rectosigmoid.[2,5,30,39,58]

Patients with aneurysms of the thoracic aorta survive but a short time without surgical correction. Kampmeir[45] showed the average life expectancy after onset of symptoms to be six to eight months. The prognosis in abdominal aneurysm appears better than that in aneurysm of the thoracic aorta. Estes[28] found that one-third of patients with untreated abdominal aortic aneurysm die within one year, usually from rupture. He estimated that 90% of patients 65 years of age with untreated abdominal aortic aneurysm would be dead in eight years, whereas only 35% of persons of similar age without such an aneurysm could be expected to die.

Schatz et al.[67] reviewed 141 untreated cases of abdominal aortic aneurysms at the Mayo Clinic. The prognosis was poor when the aneurysms were accompanied by symptomatic heart disease, when they were symptomatic, and when they exceeded 7.5 cm in diameter. Only 20% of the patients with aneurysm associated with symptomatic heart disease survived five years. Of those in whom the cause of death was known, 44% died of ruptured aneurysm.

Klippel and Butcher[49] reported thirty patients with abdominal aortic aneurysms not treated operatively. Only two died of rupture. Szilagyi et al.[73] compared 223 untreated abdominal aortic aneurysms with a group of 480 treated surgically. They were able to show that modern operative mortality was significantly less than the likelihood of rupture without operation. Levy et al.[53] suggested that the presence of severe cerebral cardiovascular disease might be a contraindication to operation.

It may be concluded that once aneurysm of the aortic system is of significant size, its excision and aortic reconstitution are mandatory.[15,17,20,22]

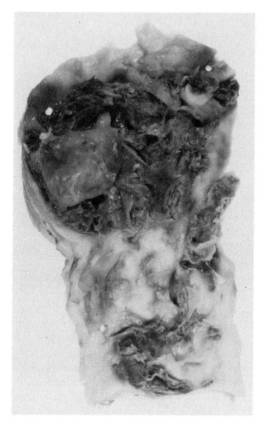

Fig. 1430 Popliteal artery aneurysm, partially thrombosed.

Popliteal artery aneurysms

Arteriosclerotic aneurysms of arteries in the extremities are rare except for the popliteal artery (Fig. 1430), although Pappas et al.[62] reported eighty-nine aneurysms of the femoral artery. The pathologic changes and the progressive enlargement of these aneurysms are similar to those in larger arteries, although the rate of progressive dilatation usually is less. Their treatment is essential to avoid acute thrombosis, embolic phenomena, or rupture as causes of severe peripheral flow deficiency and gangrene. Most patients with popliteal aneurysms are first seen because of these complications. Occasionally, such patients seek medical aid because of anterior tibial muscular necrosis. The popliteal arterial elongation associated with aneurysm formation may kink and occlude the anterior tibial artery as it passes through the interosseous membrane.[43]

Patients with popliteal aneurysms frequently have multiple aneurysms. In sixty-nine patients having 100 popliteal aneurysms, hyper-

tension and occlusive arterial disease were frequent.[32] Only three of these patients were women. Forty of the sixty-nine patinets had multiple aneurysms. Thirty-one of them had bilateral popliteal aneurysms, and the remaining had aneurysms of arteries other than the popliteal artery. The most common sites of the second aneurysm in the latter group were the abdominal aorta and the femoral artery.

Ninety-two of the aneurysms were considered purely arteriosclerotic. Syphilis, mycotic infections, and trauma entered into the diganosis of the remaining ones. In the absence of extensive gangrene, popliteal aneurysms with or without the presence of complications are best treated by excision of the aneurysm and the insertion of autologous vein grafts.

Dissecting aneurysms

Dissecting aneurysms of the aorta, if untreated, are associated with a rapidly fatal course in 75%-90% of the patients. Their etiology is related to an underlying degeneration of the elements of the media. There is an increased risk of this complication during pregnancy, although the reason for this is unclear.[9,57]

The process of dissection most commonly begins in a transverse intimal tear associated with an intimal plaque located either in the ascending aorta or in the upper descending thoracic aorta near the origin of the left subclavian artery. Once this tear develops, the intramural layers of the aorta are rapidly separated by the force of the blood entering the wall. The dissection usually involves the entire circumference of the aorta as it progresses distally. Perforation often occurs through the adventitia, resulting in early death from hemorrhage into the pericardium or pleural cavity. Lower extremity symptoms and signs of acute occlusion of the abdominal aorta may be prominent because of distal aortic or iliac luminal occlusion by the leading point of the dissection.

A subacute clinical type characteristically begins abruptly and then progresses gradually for several days before rupture and death (Fig. 1431). Finally, a chronic form occurs in a few patients who develop a reentry site from the dissected passage back into the lumen of the aorta. The occasional long-term survivor of dissecting aneurysm is encountered among these patients.

The surgical attack upon acute dissecting aneurysm of the aorta was introduced by De-

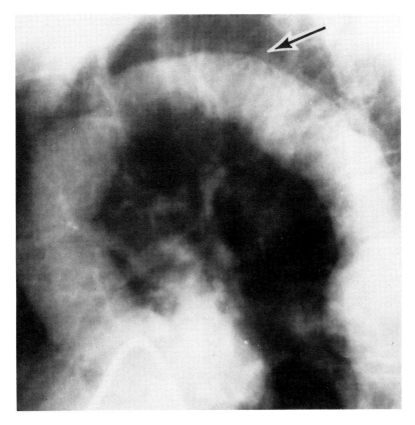

Fig. 1431 Dissecting aneurysm in 68-year-old man who died of rupture into pericardium on way to operating room. Double aortic shadow characteristic of dissecting aneurysm is indicated by arrow. (WU neg. 62-2999.)

Bakey and Cooley,[16] who succeeded in salvaging some of the patients. The fundamental principle in the surgical therapy initially introduced was the transection of the lower thoracic aorta and the establishment of a reentrance site through the intimal layer that had been dissected free by the aneurysmal process. This procedure is particularly applicable when the dissection begins in the ascending aorta. Aortic excision and graft, however, are thought to be superior if the site of beginning dissection is in the upper descending thoracic aorta. Excision is possible in most of the patients undergoing operation.[16,55]

Wheat et al.[79,80] reported the successful treatment of patients with acute dissecting aortic aneurysm by the use of antihypertensive agents. In a series of thirty-three patients so treated reported by McFarland et al.,[56] the survival rate was 52%, the mean follow-up period being more than three years. These authors emphasized the need for proper selection in deciding a surgical versus a medical therapy.

Exceptionally, dissecting aneurysms can occur in arteries other than the aorta, such as the renal, coronary, pulmonary, and carotid vessels.[81]

Diffuse arterial tortuosity and dilatation

Occasionally, a more or less generalized arterial dilatation and extreme tortuosity are seen in patients suffering from generalized arteriosclerosis. Leriche[52] reported such instances as *dolicho et mega arteria*. The mechanism of the tortuosity and generalized dilatation is thought to relate to weakening of the arterial well, but the cause for its generalized nature is not clearly understood.[68] The arteriograms of one of these are illustrated in Fig. 1432. The patient presented with a nontender pulsatile abdominal mass diagnosed initially as an abdominal aortic aneurysm. However, because of the prominence of the femoral arterial pulsation, arteriography was performed. There was marked dilatation and tortuosity of the abdominal aorta with bilateral dilatation of

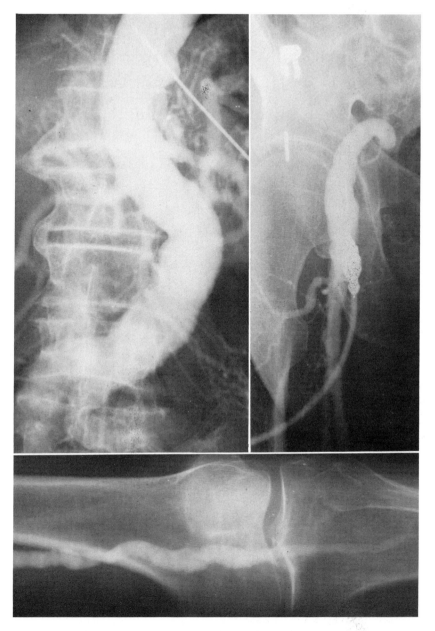

Fig. 1432 Arteriograms of abdominal aorta and femoral and popliteal arteries illustrating generalized arterial dilatation and tortuosity in patient who had pulsating intra-abdominal mass initially diagnosed as aneurysm. (WU neg. 57-4727.)

the femoral and popliteal arteries. The posterior tibial and dorsalis pedis pulses were normal bilaterally.

One need know that such arterial dilatation and tortuosity may be mistaken for intra-abdominal aneurysm since surgical attack upon such generalized tortuosity is probably not warranted in the absence of complications.

Marked enlargement and tortuosity of the femoral arterial tree in one patient were associated with lamellar deposition of thrombotic material along the wall of the tortuous and enlarged artery, with maintenance of a lumen through the thrombosis. Embolization resulted in peripheral gangrene requiring amputation. Blood flow from the center of the laminated

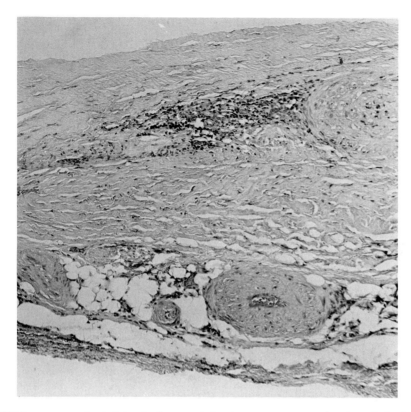

Fig. 1433 Appearance of arterial wall after amputation for gangrene secondary to embolization from mural thrombi in dilated and tortuous femoral artery. (WU neg. 57-5804.)

clot still was brisk at the time of amputation. The arterial wall showed marked loss of normal histologic structure, absence of elastic tissue, and marked fibrosis (Fig. 1433).

In another patient, marked tortuosity and enlargement of the brachial, axillary, and carotid arteries were present without localized aneurysmal formation.

Arterial substitution

Arteriosclerotic aneurysms of the abdominal aorta and the iliac arteries are best treated by excision and replacement of the involved arterial segment by synthetic cloth prostheses. Aneurysms of the popliteal arteries probably are best replaced by venous autografts. Arterial homografts are no longer used to replace diseased arterial segments because of the superiority of synthetic arterial prostheses. Degeneration of homografts resulted in an average yearly failure rate of 4.1% over ten years at the Massachusetts General Hospital.[59]

After implantation, homografts are partially replaced or encased by host collagenous tissue (Fig. 1434). In a few months they most much

of their elasticity, although fragmented elastic tissue is still demonstrable histologically over a year after implantation. The evolution of the intimal surface of both homografts and synthetic cloth prostheses after implantation consists of organization of the fibrin layer initially deposited and the development of a lining of flattened cells, which, by special staining techniques, appear nearly like normal vascular endothelium.[70] True endothelial ingrowth from the host artery occurs across the suture line for a variable distance.

Szilagyi et al.[72] reported late aneurysm formation in two of fifty-five aortic homografts and tortuous dilatation in twelve of sixty-six femoral homografts within three years after insertion. Calcification may appear in the wall of homografts after long implantation. Implantation of synthetic cloth prostheses is followed by their encasement with collagen and a decline in tensile strength of some of them. Harrison[36] showed that nylon lost 60%-90% of its strength two years after implantation in dogs. Dacron, Orlon and Teflon proved much superior in this regard.

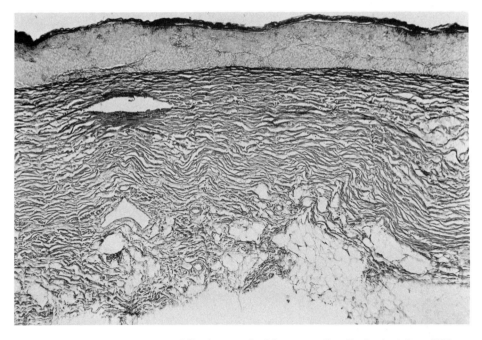

Fig. 1434 Collagenous encasement of iliac homograft eighteen months after implantation. (WU neg. 57-5807.)

Controlled experimental hypercholesterolemia in the dog[12] and rabbit[29] produced atherosclerotic changes in lyophilized homografts that were greater than those in the host arteries. Synthetic arterial substitutes have been shown to develop intimal lipid deposits in hypercholesterolemic rabbits and, after months of implantation, in man.[74] Atheromas also developed in experimentally endarterectomized arteries.[33]

Although homografts have been used extensively to replace diseased larger arteries successfully, it appears that the synthetic prostheses are superior[10,11,13] if the cloth constituting them is of the proper porosity.[37,78] Endoaneurysmorraphy and intra-aneurysmal wiring are no longer indicated in the treatment of aneurysm.

Arterial occlusive disease

Thrombotic occlusions of the major arteries often are associated with arteriosclerotic changes such as calcification, atheromatosis, and ulceration of the intima. Jørgensen[42] made a thorough review of the different factors leading to thrombosis. The occlusive process is often insidious, although final thrombotic obliteration of the lumen is occasionally quite rapid and may be clinically indistinguishable from embolization. Indeed, the differentiation of the two pathologically and at operation is quite difficult in older individuals in whom arteriosclerosis of the abdominal aorta is nearly universal. The process of occlusion probably begins in the iliac arteries near the aortic bifurcation from which thrombus formation propagates cephalad in the aorta, occasionally to the level of the renal arteries. Thrombi and emboli can become secondarily infected by fungi, particularly *Aspergillus* and *Mucor* (Fig. 1435).

The syndrome of distal aortic thrombosis (Leriche's syndrome) manifests itself with an insidious onset and gradual progression of symptoms of pain and easy fatigability in the legs, hips, and back, intermittent claudication, and sexual impotence (Fig. 1436). In this condition, arterial insufficiency in the lower extremities usually is manifested clinically by absence of pulses below the umbilicus. If the process is partial, weak pulsations may be felt or a characteristic systolic murmur heard over the abdominal aorta and the femoral arteries.

Despite the presence of intermittent claudication and the absence of pulses, many of the patients are found by arteriography to have near normal distal arteries. This patency of the peripheral arteries probably is responsible for the relative absence of muscular atrophy or of

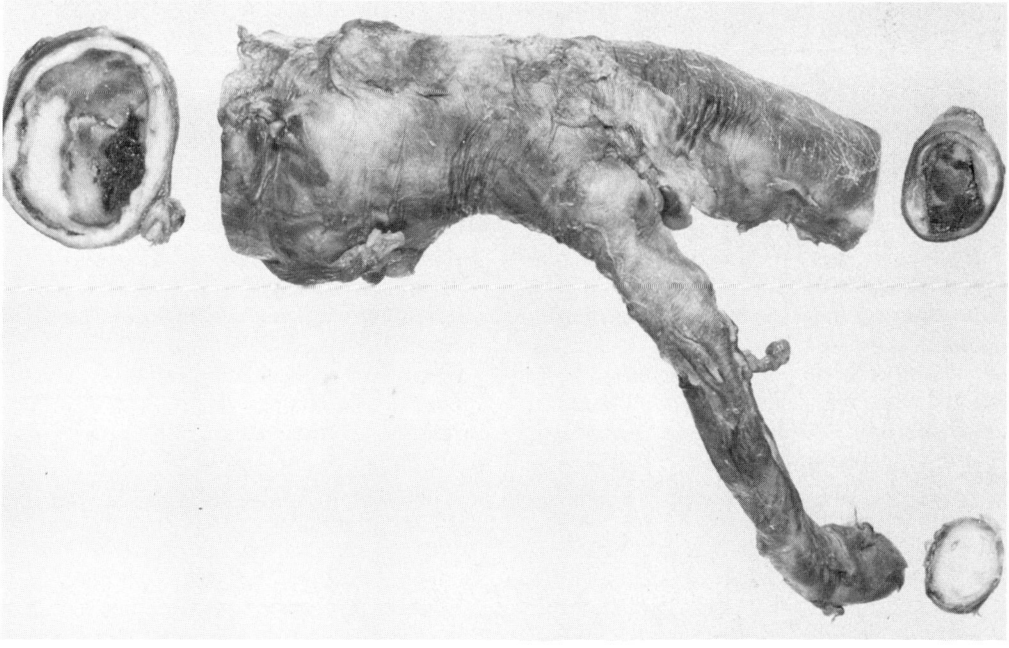

Fig. 1435 Infection of femoral artery embolus by *Aspergillus*. Hyphae are thick and septate and branch at acute angle. Patient, 59-year-old woman, had cold, pulseless lower extremity ten weeks following initial valve replacement. (Gormori's methenamine silver; ×600; WU neg. 73-55.)

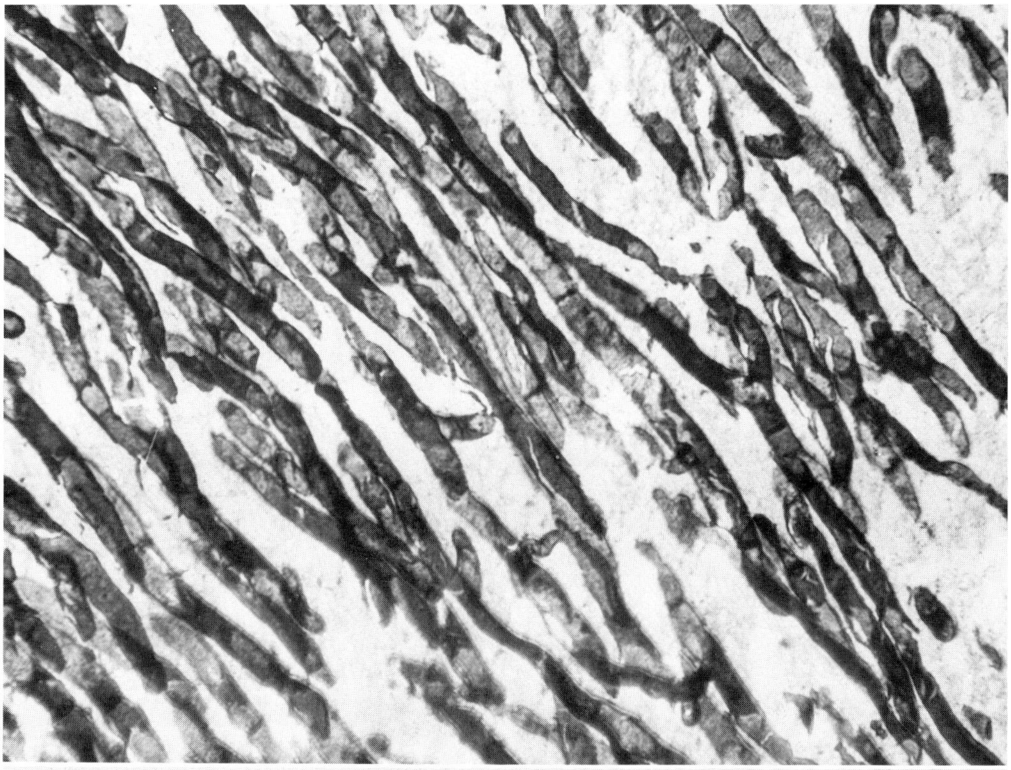

Fig. 1436 Thrombotic occlusion of distal abdominal aorta and common iliac arteries (Leriche's syndrome). (WU neg. 54-5749.)

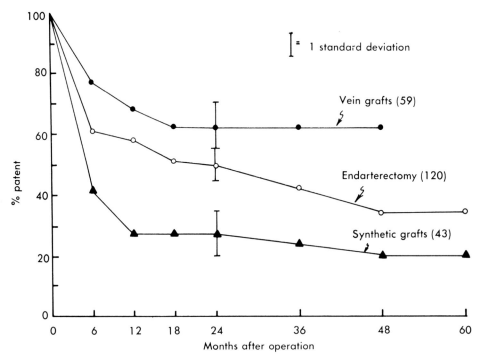

Fig. 1437 Accumulative patency rates after operations for femoral-popliteal occlusive disease. (WU neg. 66-7959.)

atrophy of skin appendages in the legs and feet of many of the patients despite their symptoms of peripheral blood flow insufficiency and lack of pulses.

Arteriosclerotic occlusive disease also frequently involves other major arterial bifurcations in the lower extremity such as those of the common iliac and common femoral arteries. In the latter instance, the intimal disease and thrombosis occur frequently in the external femoral artery just distal to the bifurcation. Other arterial segments in the lower extremity prone to early thrombotic occlusion are those associated with some degree of fascial fixation. Such areas exist (1) in the external iliac artery behind the inguinal ligament, (2) in the superficial femoral artery as it passes through the fascial ring beneath the adductor longus tendon, and (3) in the anterior tibial artery where it passes through the interosseous membrane.[26] Rodriguez-Martinez et al.[65] devised a practical, very useful dissecting technique for the pathologic evaluation of lower limbs with vascular occlusions. DeWolfe and Beven[25] described in detail the correlation between clinical and arteriographic findings.

Although arteriosclerosis is a generalized ar-

terial disease, the tendency for occlusive complications to develop early in its evolution at the sites just noted makes possible the successful treatment of patients with marked peripheral blood flow deficiency. Surgical correction of the obstructive disease, however, often only temporarily improves the peripheral blood flow because of the progressive nature of generalized arteriosclerosis.[76,77] Successful operative therapy of arterial occlusive disease relieves symptoms of ischemia but actually prevents amputation of but a few extremities.[66] However, aggressive operative therapy in properly selected patients with limited gangrene of the extremities may permit healing after amputation of only the gangrenous part.[60]

The treatment of major arterial occlusive disease is being undertaken by surgeons today using two general methods: arterial substitutes and thromboendarterectomy (intimectomy).[71]

Data from Barnes Hospital show that thromboendarterectomy is superior to arterial replacement early after treatment of arterial occlusive disease of the aorta and iliac arteries.[14] (Figs. 1437 and 1438). Autogenous venous bypass for femoral arterial occlusive disease appears to be associated with patency rates superior

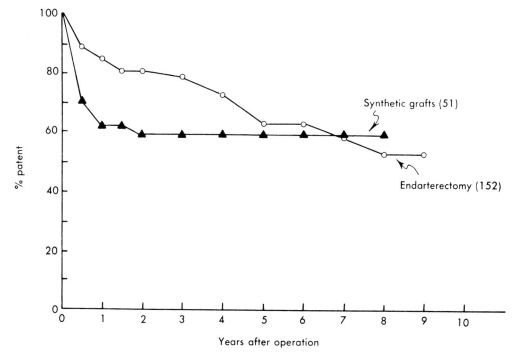

Fig. 1438 Accumulative patency rates after operations for aortic-iliac occlusive disease. (WU neg. 67-4325.)

to those following endarterectomy and synthetic bypass grafts.[24,50]

Successful results in 85%-95% of patients with occlusions of the aortic and iliac arteries have been reported by both methods of treatment.[8,44,82] Postoperative aneurysm formation and vascular thrombosis have been reported following the use of both methods. Data that will allow one to analyze the relative frequency of these complications are not available. The correction of femoral occlusive disease by endarterectomy or by the bypass arterial substitution technique has proved less beneficial than grafts in larger arteries. Approximately 70% of the patients with femoral grafts develop late thrombosis.[76]

The incidence of late failure of both endarterectomy and arterial grafting procedures will likely always be higher in the smaller femoral artery than in the aorta and iliac arteries. Results after femoral endarterectomy reported by Cannon et al.[7] indicate approximately 50% of the patients maintaining good results six months to two years after operation. Autogenous saphenous vein bypass is preferred by Linton and Darling.[54]

Thromboendarterectomy of major arteries is a technique in which the diseased intima and thrombotic material filling the lumen are dissected from the inner portion of the media in a smooth and uniform manner so that the remaining adventitia and media of the artery can continue to conduct blood (Figs. 1439 and 1440). The remaining arterial tube is lined rapidly by a fibrinoid layer that develops a pseudoendothelial surface similar to that lining an implanted arterial substitute. Likewise, early thrombosis does not occur in these segments if the transit time of the blood through them is rapid. Endarterectomized arterial segments, examined months after the operative procedure, show a fibrous type of intima with an endothelium-like covering and preservation of the remaining media and elastic tissue.[3]

Extensive medial calcification of the Mönckeberg type may occasionally be a contraindication to endarterectomy.

Studies of the elastic properties of normal human arteries and of arteriosclerotic arteries obtained at autopsy from patients of the same age have shown insignificant variations of elasticity coefficients between the two. The progressive encasement of synthetic prostheses with collagen and the similar encasement and

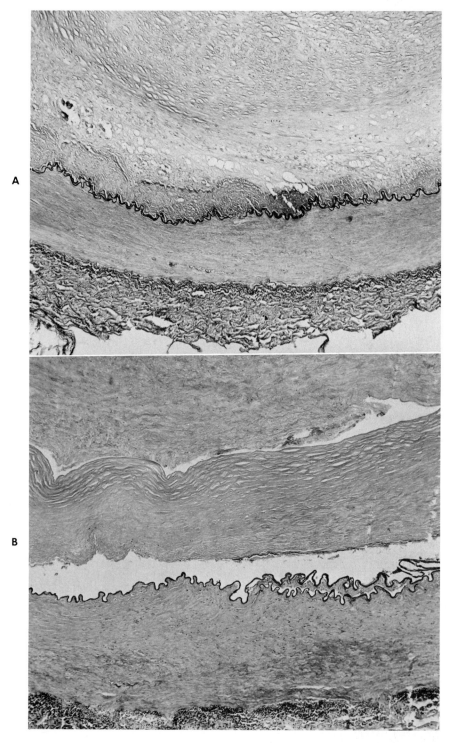

Fig. 1439 Result of endarterectomy performed upon occluded femoral artery removed at autopsy. **A,** Vessel was transected and section made from one of cut ends. **B,** Tissue section made from other cut end after simple wire loop endarterectomy. Freed intimal core was left in situ in order to demonstrate plane of cleavage developed. (**A,** WU neg. 57-5915A; **B,** WU neg. 57-5808.)

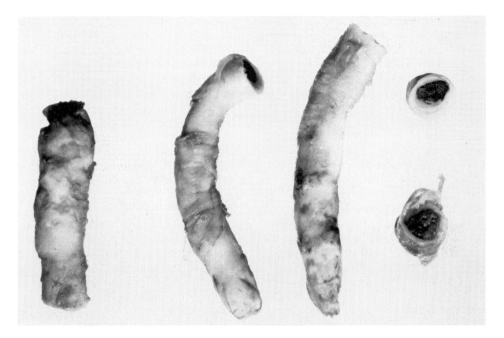

Fig. 1440 Operative specimen from femoral endarterectomy removed in cleavage plane similar to that shown in Fig. 1439. (WU neg. 61-6083.)

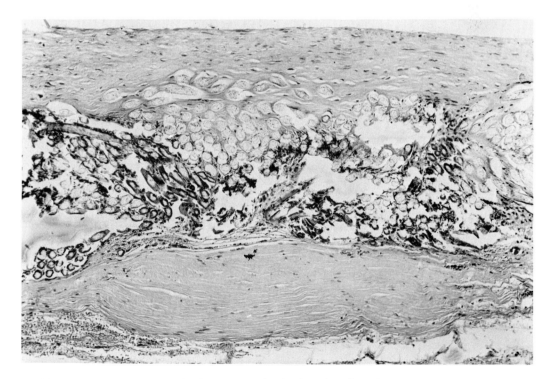

Fig. 1441 Nylon arterial prosthesis one year after implantation. Central graft material in encased in mature relatively acellular collagen, and endothelial-like lining is visible. (WU neg. 57-5805.)

invasion of fibrous tissue into the wall of homografts are associated with a reduction in the elastic properties of the implants. Their distensibility becomes much less after implantation[4] (Fig. 1441). Studies of both cloth prostheses and homografts at varying times after implantation indicate that the end result is a collagenlike tube through which the blood flows. The response of the wall of the graft to distention is no longer that of the adjacent host vessels.

In recent years, arterial embolism of atheromatous origin has become more often recognized. It may occur spontaneously or following aortic surgery or angiographic procedures.[35,69] The complications vary according to the vessels affected and include livedo reticularis and gangrene of the lower extremities, ocular symptoms, cerebral infarct, gastrointestinal bleeding, renal hypertention, and renal failure.[1,27,40,41,47,48] The frequency of atheromatous embolism correlates with the severity of ulcerative atheromatous changes in the aorta. Simultaneous embolism to various organs may lead to a mistaken clinical diagnosis of polyarteritis nodosa.[64] Random biopsies of skeletal muscle may be diagnostic in these cases.[1]

Cystic adventitial degeneration

Cystic adventitial degeneration, a rare condition almost always affecting the popliteal

artery, may cause luminal obstruction.[84] A collection of jellylike material distends the wall and bulges into the lumen (Fig. 1442). Haid et al.[85] reported a case and reviewed forty previously described. Most cases occurred in young men without a history of trauma and without general arterial changes. The microscopic structure of the involved arterial segments suggested mucinous degeneration. The cysts were lined by flattened cells. The pathogenesis is probably related to that of soft tissue ganglion.[86] Other arteries may exceptionally be affected by this condition.[83]

Fibromuscular dysplasia

Although fibromuscular dysplasia was initially regarded as a renal disease, it is now recognized that this peculiar disorder may involve a wide variety of arteries, sometimes in a multicentric fashion.[87,89,90] It usually becomes manifest during the third or fourth decades of life, although it also can be seen in children.[92] It involves large and medium-sized muscular arteries, such as the renal, carotid, axillary, and mesenteric arteries. Morphologically, it is characterized by a disorderly arrangement and proliferation of the cellular and extracellular elements of the wall, particularly the media, with the resulting distortion of the vessel lumen. The absence of necrosis, calcification, inflamma-

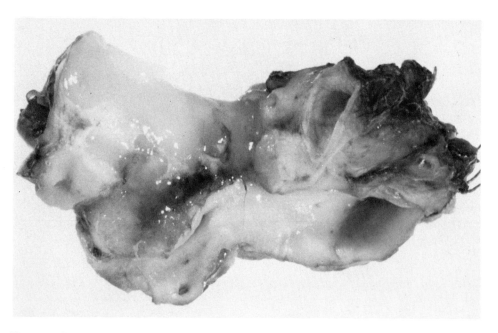

Fig. 1442 Cystic degeneration of popliteal artery. Amorphous mass of gelatinous material involves arterial wall and impinges upon lumen.

tion, and fibrinoid necrosis are important negative diagnostic features. Morphologic varieties with predominant intimal or adventitial involvement have been described.[88,91]

Mesenteric vascular occlusion

Mesenteric vascular occlusion may originate in veins or arteries. Rarely, occlusion of both occurs simultaneously. Arterial occlusion seems to be the more frequent of the two (62% of cases).[106] After the initiation of arterial or venous thrombosis, hemorrhagic infarction of the intestine and its mesentery develops if the process is rapid in onset and extensive.

Johnson and Baggenstoss[97,98] reported that venous mesenteric thrombosis often is associated with infection and cancer. This association was present in 25% of their ninety-nine patients. However, infection and cancer per se were not directly related to the mesenteric venous thrombosis. The true correlation in the 25% having infection and cancer was between portal venous and mesenteric venous obstruction.

The relative reduction in frequency of mesenteric venous occlusion has been attributed by Wilson and Block[106] to antibiotic control of many intra-abdominal infections. In the past, sepsis was thought to cause the majority of the mesenteric venous occlusions.

Occlusion of the mesenteric arterial system may be caused by emboli from thrombi in an arteriosclerotic aorta, from a fibrillating atrium, or from a mural thrombus secondary to myocardial infarction. Mesenteric arterial occlusion also may follow arteriosclerotic change in the superior mesenteric artery with local thrombosis and such rare conditions as polyarteritis or septic arteritis. Mesenteric arteries can be involved in rheumatoid disease and cause infarction.[95] Arterial and venous thrombosis, followed by ulceration and necrosis of the bowel, has been described following surgical repair of aortic coarctation.[96] The pathogenesis of this condition, which has been erroneously designated as "mesenteric arteritis," is probably related to the occurrence of hypertension during the first two postoperative days.

Infarction of the small intestine or colon, perforation, and peritonitis do not always follow mesenteric vascular occlusion, either arterial or venous. Johnson and Baggenstoss[97] reported the presence of infarction in only fifty-two of ninety-nine patinets found to have mesenteric vascular occlusions post mortem. Con-

versely, mesenteric infarct can be seen in the absence of arterial or venous occlusion.[105] This was the case in sixty-seven of 136 patients studied by Ottinger and Austen.[103] In many of these cases, the infarction was secondary to diminished cardiac output or other hypotensive states.

Infarction of the bowel depends upon the location, the extent of the occlusion, the rapidity of its onset, and the state of the collateral circulation, as well as the general physical condition of the patient. Patients with cirrhosis of the liver and portal hypertension often have episodes of cramping abdominal pain associated with low-grade fever and moderate leukocytosis that gradually recede. Several such episodes may take place before a sufficient amount of the portal venous system is occluded to cause the clinical picture of intra-abdominal catastrophe.

The clinical diagnosis of mesenteric vascular thrombosis is difficult at times because the patient does not have the classical severe abdominal pain, distention, nausea, vomiting, leukocytosis, and shock. Such a picture depends upon a massive sudden occlusion of the superior mesenteric artery or vein.

Acute occlusion of mesenteric arteries produces bowel necrosis without the early marked hypovolemic disturbances seen with extensive venous thrombosis. Of the sixty-seven patients reported by Mavor,[101] only four were in a state of peripheral vascular collapse when first examined. Bloody diarrhea is less common in arterial than in venous occlusions, although abdominal pain generally is more prominent in arterial occlusions. If the occlusion is sufficiently extensive to cause gangrene of the bowel, death from peritonitis follows if the bowel is not resected. A hypovolemic death in less than twenty-four hours, however, is often the outcome in the presence of massive venous occlusion.[93]

Of the two types of occlusion, arterial embolic occlusion is more likely to be amenable to successful treatment than is venous thrombosis. The treatment of both conditions consists primarily of early abdominal exploration and resection of nonviable bowel. The determination of viability at laparotomy may be quite difficult. The extent of small bowel resection compatible with subsequent life has been shown to be as much as three-fourths of the intestine in some patients.

To date, embolectomy has but rarely reme-

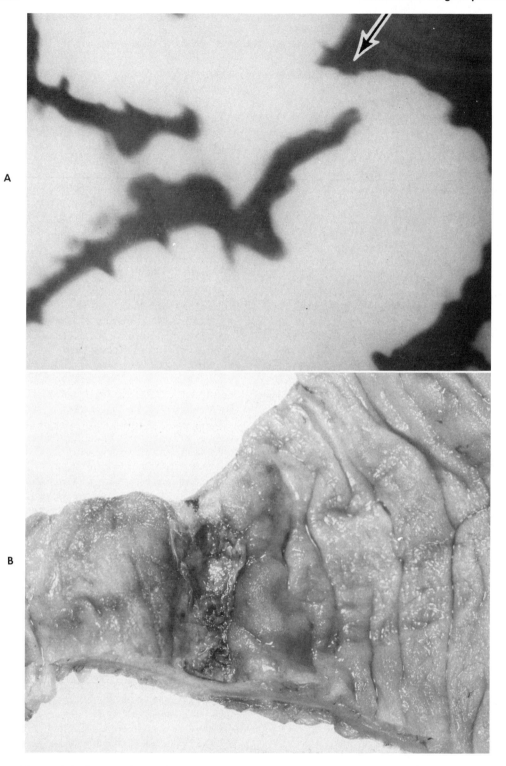

Fig. 1443 A, Segmental area of constriction (arrow) in small bowel interpreted as possible malignant neoplasm. **B,** Excised segment of lesion shown in **A** revealing well-delimited ulcer. Small segment of attached mesentery showed organized thrombi. Ulcer was on basis of vascular insufficiency. (**A,** WU neg. 64-7689; **B,** WU neg. 64-7576.)

died occlusion of the superior mesenteric artery. However, because of the serious prognosis associated with extensive small intestinal and colonic resection, this procedure probably should be attempted more often.[99]

Postoperative anticoagulant therapy and prolonged extradural anesthesia have been recommended for acute vascular occlusion in the mesentery.[100]

We have encountered three patients in whom it appears that vascular impairment of a segment of small intestine was followed by pathologic changes and clinical findings that were quite similar to those seen in Crohn's disease. One patient developed cramping abdominal pain and tenderness in the right lower quadrant approximately one month after having had a coronary thrombosis. A diagnosis of appendicitis was made, and the abdomen was explored at another hospital. The terminal ileum was described as being edematous and blue in color. It was not removed. Following the operation, the patient entered Barnes Hospital with fever, leukocytosis, and guaiac-positive stools. Roentgenograms of the small intestine were interpreted as showing Crohn's disease. Symptoms persisted for approximately six weeks, at which time the patient died of pulmonary edema. Pathologic examination showed approximately 40 cm of the terminal ileum to have submucosal thickening, mucosal ulceration, and a few giant cells. A major branch of the superior mesenteric artery contained organized thrombus. The lymph nodes contained inflammatory cells but no granulomas.[104]

Chronic intestinal ischemia produces the syndrome of abdominal angina.[102] Segmental intestinal infarction may be incident to disease of small mesenteric arteries without involvement of the proximal superior mesenteric artery. So-called nonocclusive intestinal infarction probably is related to disease in these vessels in most instances[94] (Fig. 1443).

Renal artery disease and its relationship to hypertension is discussed in Chapter 16.

Traumatic and iatrogenic injuries
Rupture

Rupture of a major vessel in the absence of an aneurysm may follow open or blunt trauma, may exceptionally occur in a spontaneous fashion through an atheromatous plaque,[119] or may be seen as a major complication of surgery or radiation therapy. Fajardo and Lee[111] reviewed eleven vascular ruptures in patients who had had previous treatment for carcinoma. The vessels involved were the aorta and the carotid and femoral arteries. Most patients were men who had been subjected to surgery and radiation therapy for epidermoid carcinomas of the oropharynx, esophagus, or genitalia. In most cases, the rupture was due to surgical rather than radiotherapeutic complications, such as necrosis of skin flaps, infections, and fistulas.

Thrombosis

Nonpenetrating trauma may result in occlusive thrombosis of a major artery such as the carotid artery following blunt trauma to the paratonsillar area.[114,118] In children, trauma and arteritis constitute the two most common causes of acquired occlusions of major arteries.[108,121] Organizing and recanalizing thrombi can exhibit a papillary pattern of anastomosing channels reminiscent of angiosarcoma[117] or else acquire a myxomatous appearance with primitive mesenchymal cells, similar to that of cardiac myxoma.[120]

Pulsating hematoma

The pulsating hematoma or false aneurysm usually results from a small perforation in the artery produced usually by a sharp instrument or a small missile. However, traumatic aneurysms occasionally follow injury to an artery by blunt trauma[107] (Fig. 1444). The defect is only a few millimeters in diameter but is sufficiently large to allow the escape of blood into the immediately surrounding tissues.

Cohen[109] emphasized the role of the adventitial layer in the development of the aneurysmal sac because of its tendency to seal off the defect in the arterial wall. Of equal importance is the nature of the surrounding tissue and the strength of its fascial structures. When strong fascial surroundings are absent, the rate of aneurysmal enlargement is quite rapid. It is slower when the area of injury is within a circumscribed fascial channel such as Hunter's canal. The blood collects about the defect in the artery until the pressure within the hematoma approaches the mean blood pressure. Enlargement of the hematoma then slows because blood returns to the arterial lumen during diastole. It is this situation that produces the characteristic to-and-fro murmur heard over the pulsating hematoma. This murmur has a rather harsh systolic component and a softer diastolic component. The murmur is not constant as is the murmur of arteriove-

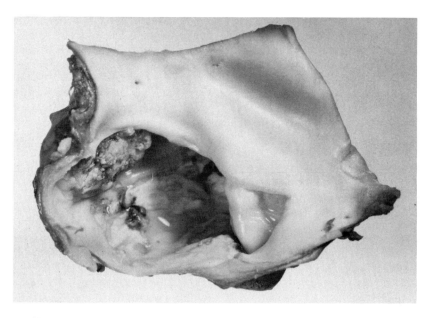

Fig. 1444 Classic traumatic aneurysm of thoracic aorta in 23-year-old man caused by automobile accident five years before operation. Note sharp line of demarcation between normal aorta and aneurysm. Aneurysm was excised and defect replaced with synthetic graft. (WU neg. 62-5338.)

nous fistula. The walls of the pulsating hematoma contain varying amounts of laminated clot, which in turn is surrounded by a rather dense fibrous tissue reaction.

The operative treatment of pulsating hematoma often is not difficult. Usually the arterial wall defect can be closed by simple suture after evacuation of the hematoma and excision of the fibrotic aneurysmal sac. Occasionally, however, arterial substitution is required.[123]

These lesions should be treated immediately upon diagnosis in order to prevent continued enlargement, pain upon compression of adjacent nerves and other structures, and ischemia of the tissues peripheral to them.[116] Since ligation of the afflicted artery, if it be a major one, is no longer the treatment of choice, waiting for collateral vessels to develop is not indicated.[115]

Acquired arteriovenous fistula

Acquired arteriovenous fistulas are seen most frequently during times of war and are produced in a manner quite similar to that of traumatic aneurysm. However, in this instance, the perforating injury involves both the artery and the adjacent vein. Such an injury usually results in a pulsating hematoma that communicates with both the arterial and the venous lumina.[112]

Following trauma, the fistula may be es-

tablished almost immediately. However, the communication between the arterial and venous systems is frequently delayed until the wound is partially organized and the thrombus in the hematoma surrounding the artery and vein is partially absorbed. Most patients present with a pulsating mass in the region of injury that can be differentiated from simple pulsating hematoma in several ways. The murmur over the pulsating region is usually continuous because of a continuous flow of arterial blood into the vein. In other words, during diastole the pressure in the pulsating hematoma about the arteriovenous communication is never sufficient to produce reversal of blood flow. In some slowly developing long-standing arteriovenous communications in the absence of a pulsating hematoma, a massive sacculation of the adjacent vein may slowly develop. This is illustrated by the following case history.

A 68-year-old black woman suffered a shotgun wound of the right thigh at the age of 38 years. A mass was first noted on the medial side of the right knee twenty-one years later. It slowly enlarged over the intervening time until it reached sufficient size to interfere with walking (Fig. 1445, *A*). The large sacculation associated with the arteriovenous fistula in this patient did not contain any laminated clots but was covered by an endothelium-like surface. The popliteal vein entered the sacculation from below

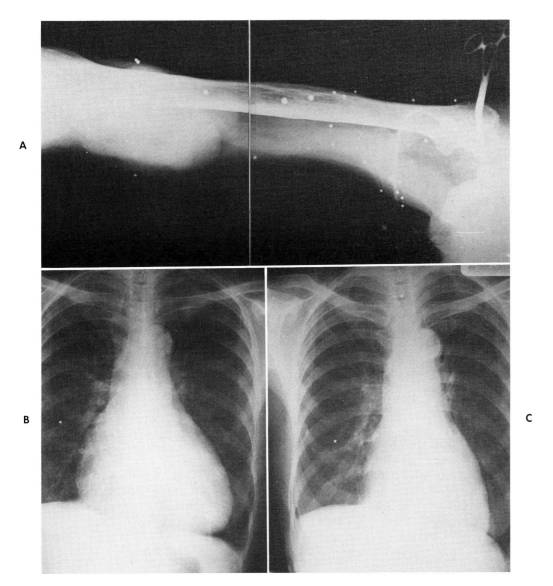

Fig. 1445 Arteriovenous fistula in 68-year-old woman. **A,** Arteriogram showing markedly enlarged femoral artery entering region of arteriovenous fistula. Pellets from original shotgun wound thirty years previously are visible. **B,** Roentgenogram before correction of arteriovenous fistula. **C,** Roentgenogram five days after operation. (**A,** WU neg. 57-980; **B** and **C,** WU neg. 57-9834.)

and the femoral vein left it above. There was a 6 mm communication between the femoral artery and the venous sac. The arteriogram showed marked femoral arterial dilatation, a characteristic finding in long-standing arteriovenous fistula. Branham's sign was positive. Occlusion of the femoral artery produced a sudden slowing of the pulse. The patient also exhibited significant cardiac enlargement but had not had difficulty with cardiac failure. Treatment consisted of ligation of the popliteal and the femoral veins near their communication with the aneurysmal sac and suture of the 6 mm arterial wall

defect. There was rapid decrease in cardiac size following the operation (Fig. 1445, *B* and *C*). The diameter of the femoral artery and the prominence of its pulsation decreased in subsequent months.

Patients with an arteriovenous fistula usually show venous dilatation about and peripheral to the fistula, as well as increased skin temperature in the area of the fistula. Despite increased temperature near the lesion, the extremity peripheral to it is usually cooler than normal since the actual peripheral blood flow is less.

When arteriovenous fistulas develop between smaller arteries and veins, the sac may be excised and the vessels ligated without difficulty. Those involving the larger arteries, such as the femoral, axillary, or popliteal artery, require the maintenance of arterial continuity. Some type of arterial substitution may be necessary occasionally in larger arteriovenous aneurysms, although transvenous closure of the defect in the arterial wall usually can be accomplished satisfactorily.[122]

The dilatation of the major artery entering an arteriovenous fistula of long standing may be marked, and the degenerative changes in the arterial wall may be extensive.[113] These changes consist of atherosclerosis, calcification, disruption of the elastic tissue network, and fibrosis. If the degeneration is sufficiently advanced, it is irreversible. In such arteries, aneurysms may develop despite the cure of the arteriovenous fistula. The dilatation of the artery entering the arteriovenous fistula is thought to result from the increased flow of blood through it.

Arteriovenous fistulas are associated with increase in cardiac output, pulse rate, and blood volume, which may lead to congestive heart failure. Such systemic results rarely, if ever, develop from a single congenital arteriovenous fistula with the exception of those that appear in the pulmonary tree. Congenital arteriovenous fistulas usually present as tumefactions containing many relatively small arteries and veins surrounded by moderately large amounts of fibrous tissue. Their treatment is primarily excisional.[110]

Thromboangiitis obliterans

Thromboangiitis obliterans is a rare thrombotic and inflammatory disease of arteries and veins of unknown etiology that has no single diagnostic, clinical, or pathologic sign. Its inflammatory component may involve entire neurovascular bundles. Although it is a generalized vascular disease, the involvement of the arteries of the lower extremities is usually most advanced, and the resultant flow deficiency is the usual reason for the patient to seek therapy. The onset of the condition occurs most often in men between 20 and 35 years of age and may be heralded by superficial migratory acute thrombophlebitis that is precipitated by undue exertion or exposure to cold.

Study of biopsies of such involved veins shows the histologic changes associated with acute intravascular thrombosis. Pathologic involvement in the arterial tree is segmental and usually is present primarily in the smaller arteries. There is a paucity of collateral flow.[125] This process has a widespread geographic distribution[129] but has been reported with increased frequency in Korea and Japan.[128]

Microscopic examination of early arterial lesions shows panarteritis, periarteritis, and thrombosis. Endothelial proliferation and periarterial fibrosis soon become prominent. The inflammatory process attacks the entire thickness of the vessel wall and perivascular tissues. Where nerves are in close proximity to the vascular tree, it involves the perineural stroma. Extension of the inflammatory process about peripheral sensory nerves may be responsible in part for the severe pain so common in afflicted extremities. In other words, neuritis as well as vascular ischemia may contribute to peripheral pain in these patients. Calcification in the arterial wall is absent. Arterial calcification on x-ray examination indicates arteriosclerosis rather than Buerger's disease.

The arterial and venous thrombosis associated with the angiitic process becomes partially recanalized. Cellularity of the organizing fibrous tissue replacing the thrombus often is prominent. Recanalization of thrombi is incomplete and is characterized by numerous small vascular channels passing through the remaining fibrous tissue (Fig. 1446).

The pathologic process ascribed to Buerger's disease may be difficult to differentiate microscopically from inflammatory and fibrotic changes that may accompany arteriosclerotic thromboses.[124,127]

The vascular process tends generally to be progressive, but in some instances the acute manifestations seem to subside, particularly in patients who cease using tobacco. Little long-term improvement is attained with or without sympathectomy as long as patients use tobacco.[131] In many of those who stop smoking, the progressive vascular occlusion appears to cease. In nearly all who continue to smoke, however, the disease progresses eventually to gangrene.

Treatment is symptomatic and includes the control of pain, the avoidance of tobacco, and cleanliness of the extremity. Late in the disease, amputations may be necessary. Sympathectomy may benefit patients with cold, tem-

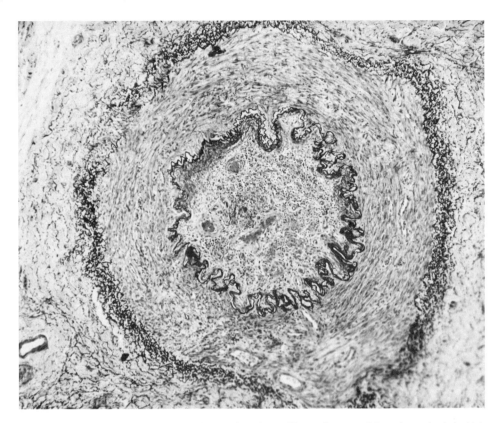

Fig. 1446 Cellular organization of occluding thrombus with small recanalizing channels thought to be compatible with Buerger's disease. Note absence of calcification. (WU neg. 58-643A.)

perature-sensitive feet or hands and those with peripheral gangrenous ulcers.

The death of persons with Buerger's disease may follow complications attending gangrene of the extremities. However, many patients with this affliction die of myocardial infarction, renal insufficiency, occlusions of mesenteric vessels and strokes. Buerger's disease should be looked upon as a rare generalized vascular disease that attacks the smaller arteries more often than the aorta and its major branches.

With the use of arteriography and careful pathologic examination, a high proportion of cases of supposed Buerger's disease have been shown actually to be arteriosclerosis. This pathologic process can be mimicked with considerable exactitude by the development of embolism and thrombosis.[132,133] This has led some investigators to postulate that Buerger's disease is not a distinct entity but rather a peculiar manifestation of arteriosclerosis. Although we agree that many cases originally diagnosed as Buerger's disease are indeed examples of arteriosclerosis, we believe that such an entity exists.[126,130,134]

Arteritis

Inflammatory diseases of the arteries have been classified on the basis of the etiologic agent involved, the caliber and location of the vessel affected, and the type of microscopic change observed. The former is obviously the most desirable but, at present, impractical, since a specific etiologic agent can be detected only for a minority of the cases, such as in syphilitic, mycotic, or tuberculous arteritis.[143,157] Gross as it seems, a division based on the vessel caliber is quite useful. Within each group, the arteritides can be further subdivided into more or less specific types on the basis of the associated condition and/or pathologic appearance.

Large vessel arteritis

There is a group of related nonsyphilitic diseases primarily affecting the aorta and its main branches and characterized by chronic inflammation and patchy destruction of the elements of the media.[136,144,151,154] They may result in aortic insufficiency, diffuse aortic tortuosity and elongation, the aortic arch syndrome, aneurysm formation, and dissection of the vessel. They are more common in adults but also have been described in children.[138] In the variety known as *Takayasu's disease*, there is chronic inflammation and fibrosis of the arterial wall, which predilects the aortic arch branches and results in absence of pulses in the upper extremities, ocular changes, and neurologic symptoms.[140,147] In later stages, superimposed changes of arteriosclerosis may obscure the diagnosis. In general, the possibility of an underlying arteritis always should be considered when arteriosclerotic changes in the aorta are seen in young or middle-aged individuals and when these changes are either segmental or occur at an unusual site. Most patients with Takayasu's disease are young, Asian, and female. In a series of sixteen autopsy cases reported from South Africa,[151a] there was segmental coronary arteritis in three

patients with the development of coronary aneurysms in two. There was coexistent tuberculosis in 37.5% of the patients, but this might well have been coincidental.

Aortic arteritis can be seen associated with rheumatoid arthritis, ankylosing spondylitis, and scleroderma.[152,156] There is a definite relationship between the type and location of a vessel and the frequency and etiology of the inflammatory diseases it may be affected by. Tuberculosis characteristically involves small vessels; rarely, it may be seen in larger vessels and result in stenosis or aneurysms.[149]

Most of the reported cases of aneurysms of the superior mesenteric artery have been either syphilitic or mycotic; the majority of the latter were associated with bacterial endocarditis.

We have encountered a single case of arteritis limited to the external iliac artery (Fig. 1447). This occurred in a 52-year-old woman whose only symptom was intermittent claudication. Arteriograms showed the aorta and peripheral arteries to be normal.

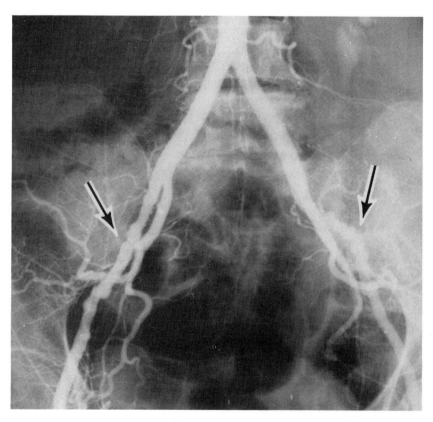

Fig. 1447 Vasculitis in 52-year-old woman showing scalloped irregularities limited to external iliac arteries. (WU neg. 62-3243.)

Medium-sized vessel arteritis

The classical example of medium-sized vessel arteritis is *polyarteritis nodosa,* formerly described at autopsy as visible nodular lesions at the points of arterial branchings. This condition should be suspected clinically if there is a history suggesting hypersensitivity, with fever, eosinophilia, and involvement of many organ systems. Infrequently, there are skin manifestations. A muscle or peripheral nerve biopsy may be diagnostic.[145] A biopsy is most rewarding in the presence of a nodule. Rarely, organs such as the gallbladder, appendix, or colon may show unsuspected lesions typical of polyarteritis. We also have seen isolated involvement of the stomach and pancreas.

In *Wegener's granulomatosis,* the arteritis is accompanied by necrosis and granulomatous reaction. Organs most commonly involved are the upper respiratory tract, lung, and kidney.

Giant cell arteritis was originally thought to be restricted to the temporal, cerebral, and retinal arteries. However, many cases with generalized arterial involvement have been described, indicating that this is a generalized disease.[135] This condition, which is most common in the older age group, is characterized by pain in the distribution of the temporal artery and localized tenderness. In other patients, central nervous system manifestations predominate.[142] Sometimes, nodulations can be palpated along the course of the artery. Microscopically, partial destruction of the wall by an inflammatory infiltrate containing multinucleated giant cells is present. Some of the multinucleated giant cells are of Langhans' type and others are of foreign body type. Many of them are intimately associated with the internal elastic lamina, and some may even contain fragments of phagocytosed elastica in their cytoplasm. It is important to emphasize that the changes are often segmental and that a negative biopsy does not rule out the diagnosis. Serial sections of the block should be always performed[141] and contralateral biopsies should be considered in selected cases.[138a] Angiography can be useful by guiding the surgeon to biopsy the diseased area.[137] Ultrastructurally, there is an accumulation of histiocytes, epithelioid cells, and giant cells at the intimal-medial junction, followed by fragmentation, degeneration, and dissolution of the internal elastic lamina.[150]

It should also be remembered that not all cases of arteritis involving the temporal artery represent examples of the entity temporal arteritis.[146,148]

The syndrome of *polymyalgia rheumatica,* characterized by muscle pain and tenderness involving mainly the muscles of the neck, shoulder, and pelvic girdle and accompanied by elevated erythrosedimentation rate, is often a manifestation of generalized giant cell arteritis.[139,153]

Degos' disease, a progressive subendothelial fibrous thickening of the wall of medium-sized arteries and arterioles, leads to vascular occlusions in many organs, particularly the skin and the digestive system, where ischemic infarcts result.[155]

Small vessel arteritis (arteriolitis)

Small vessel arteritis is the most common variety of arterial inflammation. Most examples are secondary to hypersensitivity to drugs or bacterial antigens or appear as a component of one of the "collagen" diseases. The two most important morphologic features to be determined are the nature of the inflammatory infiltrate (whether lymphocytic or neutrophilic) and the presence or absence of necrosis of the vessel wall. In the large majority of the cases, skin manifestations are prominent (Chapter 3) (Fig. 1448).

Tumors

Over twenty cases of primary malignant tumors of the aorta have been reported.[162] The majority have been labeled as fibrosarcomas or "fibromyxosarcomas"[162,165] and have been thought to arise from cells in the arterial wall. About sixty cases of sarcomas of the pulmonary trunk are on record[157a]; a few of them have been associated with abundant bone formation.[158] Cases with an appearance suggestive of endothelial origin also have been reported.[163,164] Distant metastases are common.

Tumors of smaller arteries and arterioles are discussed in Chapter 24. Malignant tumor emboli, usually originating in lung carcinomas, can lead to major arterial occlusion.[159]

Recently, we have seen several cases of a tumorlike mass involving large and medium-sized vessels (such as the femoral artery and radial vein), characterized by a solid proliferation of cells having features both of endothelial cells and histiocytes. The proliferation often occluded the lumen of the vessels and also involved its wall, sometimes extending to the adventitia. The characteristic cells, which we

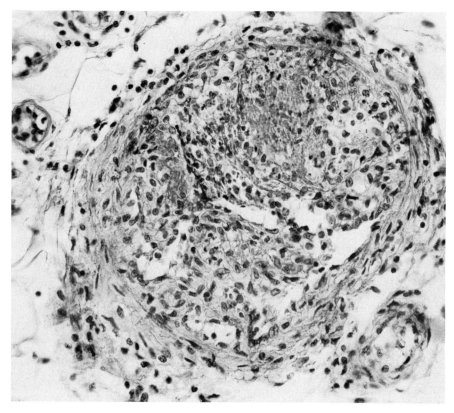

Fig. 1448 Vasculitis involving small vessel of subcutaneous tissue. Note thrombosis, inflammation, and eccentric involvement. (×340; WU neg. 51-6019.)

prefer to call *histiocytoid endothelial cells,* have large vesicular nuclei with inconspicuous nucleoli, very scanty mitoses, and prominent grooves and indentations. Their cytoplasm is abundant, acidophilic, and often vacuolated. Lymphocytes, eosinophils, and hemosiderin-laden macrophages may be seen scattered throughout the mass. Because of the solid nature of the proliferation, apparent invasion of the wall, and plump appearance of the nuclei, these lesions are often called angiosarcomas. However, their prognosis is excellent. All of the patients that we have seen are alive and well following local excision.[160] We are not sure whether this process is reactive or neoplastic but, in any event, it is obviously of indolent nature and should be treated accordingly. We believe this disease is analogous to some cases diagnosed as "angiolymphoid hyperplasia with eosinophilia" in the skin and as "low-grade hemangioendothelioma" in the skeletal system.[161]

REFERENCES
Arteriosclerosis

1 Anderson WR, Richards AM, Weiss L: Hemorrhage and necrosis of stomach and small bowel due to atheroembolism. Am J Clin Pathol **48**:30-38, 1967.
2 Ariyan S, Cahow CE, Greene FL, Stansel HC: Successful treatment of hepatic artery aneurysm with erosion into the common duct. Ann Surg **182**:169-172, 1975.
3 Barker WJ, Cannon JA, Zeldis LJ, Perry A: Anatomical results of endarterectomy. Surg Forum **6**:266-269, 1955.
4 Bennett DE, Cherry JK: Bacterial infection of aortic aneurysms. A clinicopathological study. Am J Surg **113**:321-326, 1967.
5 Bowers J, Koehler PR, Hammar SP, Nelson JA, Tolman KG: Rupture of a splenic artery aneurysm into the pancreatic duct. Gastroenterology **70**:1152-1155, 1976.
6 Butcher HR, Newton WT: Influence of age, arteriosclerosis and homotransplantation upon the elastic properties of major human arteries. Ann Surg **148**:1-20, 1958.
7 Cannon JA, Barker WF, Kawakami IG: Femoral popliteal endarterectomy in the treatment of obliterative atherosclerotic disease. Surgery **43**:76-93, 1958.

8 Cannon JA, Kawakami IG, Barker WF: The present status of aortoiliac endarterectomy for obliterative atherosclerosis. Arch Surg **82**:813-825, 1961.

9 Cavanzo FJ, Taylor HB: Effect of pregnancy on the human aorta and its relationship to dissecting aneurysms. Am J Obstet Gynecol **105**:567-568, 1969.

10 Crawford S, DeBakey ME, Cooley DA: Clinical use of synthetic arterial substitutes in three hundred seventeen patients. Arch Surg **76**:261-270, 1958.

11 Crawford ES, DeBakey ME, Morris GC, Garrett E: Evaluation of late failures after reconstructive operations for occlusive lesions of the aorta and iliac femoral and popliteal arteries. Surgery **47**:79-104, 1960.

12 Creech O Jr, Jordan GL Jr, DeBakey ME, Overton RC, Halpert B: The effect of chronic hypercholesterolemia on canine aortic transplants. Surg Gynecol Obstet **101**:607-614, 1955.

13 Creech O Jr, Deterling RA Jr, Edwards S, Julian OC, Linton RR, Shumacker H: Vascular prostheses (report of Committee for Study of Vascular Prostheses of Society for Vascular Surgery). Surgery **41**:62-80, 1957.

14 Darling RC, and Linton RR: Aortoiliofemoral endarterectomy for atherosclerotic occlusive disease. Surgery **55**:184-194, 1964.

15 Darling RC, Messina CR, Brewster DC, Ottinger LW: Autopsy study of unoperated abdominal aortic aneurysms: the case for early resection. Circulation **56**[Suppl]:161-164, 1977.

16 DeBakey ME, Cooley DA, Creech O Jr: Surgical considerations of dissecting aneurysm of the aorta. Ann Surg **142**:586-612, 1955.

17 DeBakey ME, Cooley DA, Creech O Jr: Resection of aneurysms of thoracic aorta. Surg Clin North Am **36**:969-982, 1956.

18 DeBakey ME, Crawford ES, Cooley DE, Morris GC Jr: Surgical considerations of occlusive disease of the abdominal aorta and iliac and femoral arteries: analysis of 803 cases. Ann Surg **148**:306-324, 1958.

19 DeBakey ME, Crawford ES, Cooley DA, Morris GC Jr, Garrett HE, Fields WS: Cerebral arterial insufficiency. One to 11-year results following arterial reconstructive operation. Ann Surg **161**:921-945, 1965.

20 DeBakey ME, Crawford ES, Cooley DA, Morris GC Jr, Royster TS, Abbott WP: Aneurysm of abdominal aorta—analysis of results of graft replacement therapy one to eleven years after operation. Ann Surg **160**:622-639, 1964.

21 DeBakey ME, Crawford ES, Morris GC Jr, Cooley DA: Surgical considerations of occlusive disease of the innominate carotid, subclavian, and vertebral arteries. Ann Surg **154**:698-725, 1961.

22 DeBakey ME, Creech O Jr, Morris GC Jr: Aneurysm of thoracoabdominal aorta involving the celiac, superior mesenteric, and renal arteries. Report of 4 cases treated by resection and homograft replacement. Ann Surg **144**:549-573, 1956.

23 de Takats G, Pirani CL: Aneurysms: general considerations. Angiology **5**:173-208, 1954.

24 DeWeese JA, Barner HB, Mahoney EB, Rob CG: Autogenous venous by-pass grafts and thromboendarterectomies for atherosclerotic lesions of the femoropopliteal arteries. Ann Surg **163**:205-214, 1966.

25 DeWolfe VG, Beven EG: Arteriosclerosis obliterans in the lower extremities: correlation of clinical and angiographic findings. Cardiovasc Clin **3**:65-92, 1971.

26 Dible JH: The pathology of limb ischaemia. St. Louis, 1966, Warren H. Green, Inc.

27 Eliot RS, Kanjuk VJ, Edwards JE: Atheromatous embolism. Circulation **30**:611-618, 1964.

28 Estes JE Jr: Abdominal aortic aneurysms. A study of 102 cases. Circulation **2**:258-264, 1950.

29 Fisher ER, Fisher B: The effect of induced arteriosclerosis on fresh and lyophilized aortic homografts in the rabbit. Surgery **40**:530-542, 1956.

30 Frank IN, Thompson HT, Rob C, Schwartz SI: Aneurysm of the internal iliac artery. Arch Surg **83**:956-958, 1961.

31 Getz GS, Vesselinovitch D, Wissler RW: A dynamic pathology of atherosclerosis. Am J Med **46**:657-673, 1969.

32 Gifford RW Jr, Hines EA Jr, Janes JM: An analysis and follow-up study of 100 popliteal aneurysms. Surgery **33**:284-293, 1953.

33 Gryska PF: The development of atheroma in arteries subjected to experimental thromboendarterectomy. Surgery **45**:655-660, 1959.

34 Haimovici H (ed): Atherosclerosis: recent advances. Ann N Y Acad Sci **149**:585-1068, 1968.

35 Harrington JT, Sommers SC, Kassirer JP: Atheromatous emboli with progressive renal failure: renal arteriography as the probably inciting factor. Ann Intern Med **68**:152-160, 1968.

36 Harrison JH: Synthetic materials as vascular prostheses. II. A comparative study of nylon, Dacron, Orlon, Ivalon sponge, and Teflon in large blood vessels with tensile strength studies. Am J Surg **95**:16-24, 1958.

37 Harrison JH, Davalos PA: Influence of porosity on synthetic grafts. Arch Surg **82**:8-13, 1961.

38 Haust MD, More RH, Movat HZ: The role of smooth muscle cells in the fibrogenesis of arteriosclerosis. Am J Pathol **37**:377-389, 1960.

39 Hirst AE Jr, Atteldt JE: Abdominal aortic aneurysm with rupture into the duodenum: a report of eight cases. Gastroenterology **17**:504-514, 1951.

40 Hollenhorst RW: Vascular status of patients who have cholesterol emboli in the retina. Am J Ophthalmol **61**:1159-1165, 1966.

41 Hoye SJ, Teitelbaum S, Gore I, Warren R: Atheromatous embolization: a factor in peripheral gangrene. N Engl J Med **261**:128-131, 1959.

42 Jørgensen L: Mechanisms of thrombosis. Pathobiology **2**:139-204, 1972.

43 Julian OC, Dye WS, Javid H: The use of vessel grafts in the treatment of popliteal aneurysms. Surgery **38**:970-980, 1955.

44 Julian OC, Dye WS, Olwin JH, Jordan PH: Direct surgery of arteriosclerosis. Ann Surg **136**:459-474, 1952.

45 Kampmeir RH: Saccular aneurysm of the thoracic aorta: a clinical study of 633 cases. Ann Intern Med **12**:624-651, 1938.

46 Kannel WB, Shurtleff D: The natural history of arteriosclerosis obliterans. Cardiovasc Clin **3**:37-52, 1971.

47 Kassirer JP: Atheroembolic renal disease. N Engl J Med **280**:812-818, 1969.

48 Kazmier FJ, Sheps SG, Bernatz PE, Sayre GP: Livedo reticularis and digital infarcts: a syndrome due to cholesterol emboli arising from atheromatous abdominal aneurysms. Vasc Dis **3**:12-24, 1966.

48a Kiernan PD, Pairolero PC, Hubert JP Jr, Mucha P Jr, Wallace RB: Aortic graft-enteric fistula. Mayo Clin Proc **55**:731-738, 1980.

49 Klippel AP, Butcher HR Jr: The unoperated abdominal aortic aneurysm. Am J Surg **111**:629-631, 1966.

50 Kouchoukos NT, Levy JF, Balfour JF, Butcher HR Jr: Operative therapy for femoral-popliteal arterial occlusive disease. A comparison of therapeutic methods. Circulation **35**[suppl 1]:174-182, 1967.

51 Lancet editorial: Endothelium and arteriosclerosis. Lancet **2**:1239-1241, 1967.

52 Leriche R: Physiologie, pathologique et traitement chirurgical des maladies artérielles de la vasomotricité. Paris, 1945, Masson et Cie.

53 Levy JF, Kouchoukos NT, Walker WB, Butcher HR Jr: Abdominal aortic aneurysmectomy. Arch Surg **92**:498-503, 1966.

54 Linton RR, Darling RC: Autogenous saphenous vein bypass grafts in femoropopliteal obliterative arterial disease. Surgery **51**:62-73, 1962.

55 Liotta D, Hallman GL, Milam JD, Cooley MD: Surgical treatment of acute dissecting aneurysm of the ascending aorta. Ann Thorac Surg **12**:582-592, 1971.

56 McFarland J, Willerson JT, Dinsmore RE, Austen WG, Buckley MJ, Sanders CA, DeSanctis RW: The medical treatment of dissecting aortic aneurysms. N Engl J Med **286**:115-155, 1972.

57 Mandell W, Evans EW, Walford RL: Dissecting aortic aneurysm during pregnancy. N Engl J Med **251**:1059-1061, 1954.

58 Markowitz AM, Norman JC: Aneurysm of the iliac artery. Ann Surg **154**:777-787, 1961.

59 Meade JW, Linton RR, Darling RC, Menendez CV: Arterial homografts—a long-term clinical follow-up. Arch Surg **93**:392-399, 1966.

60 Morris GC Jr, Wheeler CG, Crawford ES, Cooley DA, DeBakey ME: Restorative vascular surgery in the presence of impending and overt gangrene of the extremities. Surgery **51**:50-57, 1962.

61 National Research Council, Division of Medical Sciences: Symposium on atherosclerosis, Pub. 338. Washington, DC, 1954, National Research Council.

62 Pappas G, Janes JM, Bernatz PE, Schirger A: Femoral aneurysms—review of surgical management. JAMA **190**:489-493, 1964.

63 Reckless JPD, McColl I, Taylor GW: Aorto-enteric fistulae: an uncommon complication of abdominal aneurysms. Br J Surg **59**:458-460, 1972.

64 Richards AM, Eliot RS, Kanjuh VI, Bloemendaal RD, Edwards JE: Cholesterol embolism. A multiple system disease masquerading as polyarteritis nodosa. Am J Cardiol **15**:696-707, 1965.

65 Rodriguez-Martinez HA, Cruz-Ortiz H, Alcantara-Vazquez A, Alcorta-Anguizola B, Burgos-Mendivil J: Dissecting technique for gangrenous lower limbs with vascular occlusions. Patología (Mexico) **10**:69-78, 1972.

66 Schadt DC, Hines EA Jr, Juergens JL, Barker NW: Chronic atherosclerotic occlusion of the femoral artery. JAMA **175**:937-940, 1961.

67 Schatz IJ, Fairbairn JF II, Juergens JL: Abdominal aortic aneurysms. A reappraisal. Circulation **26**:200-205, 1962.

68 Staple TW, Friedenberg MSA, Butcher HR Jr: Arteria magna et dolicho of Leriche. Acta Radiol **4**:293-305, 1966.

69 Stout C, Hartsuck JM, Howe J, Richardson JL: Atheromatous embolism after aortofemoral bypass and aortic ligation. Arch Pathol **93**:271-275, 1972.

70 Stump MM, Jordan GL Jr, DeBakey ME, Halpert B: The endothelial lining of homografts and Dacron prostheses in the canine aorta. Am J Pathol **40**:487-491, 1962.

71 Szilagyi DE, Smith RF, Whitcomb JG: The contribution of angioplastic surgery to the therapy of peripheral occlusive arteriopathy. A critical evaluation of eight years' experience. Ann Surg **152**:660-677, 1960.

72 Szilagyi DE, McDonald RT, Smith RF, Whitcomb JG: Biologic fate of human arterial homografts. Arch Surg **75**:506-529, 1957.

73 Szilagyi DE, Smith RF, DeRusso FJ, Elliott JP, Sherrin FW: Contribution of abdominal aortic aneurysmectomy to prolongation of life. Ann Surg **164**:678-699, 1966.

74 Tarizzo RA, Alexander RW, Beattie EJ Jr, Economou SG: Atherosclerosis in synthetic vascular grafts. Arch Surg **82**:826-832, 1961.

75 Thompson JE, Kartchner MM, Austin DJ, Wheeler CG, Patman RD: Carotid endarterectomy for cerebrovascular insufficiency (stroke). Follow-up of 359 cases. Ann Surg **163**:751-763, 1966.

76 Warren R, Villavicencio JL: Iliofemoropopliteal arterial reconstructions for arteriosclerosis obliterans. N Engl J Med **260**:255-263, 1959.

77 Warren R, Gomez RL, Marston JAP, Cox JST: Femoropopliteal arteriosclerosis obliterans—arteriographic patterns and rates of progression. Surgery **55**:135-143, 1964.

78 Wesolowski SA, Fries CC, Karlson KE, DeBakey M, Sawyer PN: Porosity. Primary determinant of ultimate fate of synthetic vascular grafts. Surgery **50**:91-96, 105-106, 1961.

79 Wheat MW, Palmer RF, Bartley TD, Seelman RC: Treatment of dissecting aneurysms of the aorta without surgery. J Thorac Cardiovasc Surg **50**:364-373, 1965.

80 Wheat MW Jr, Harris PD, Malm JR, Kaiser G, Bowman FO Jr, Palmer RF: Acute dissecting aneurysms of the aorta: treatment and results in 64 patients. J Thorac Cardiovasc Surg **58**:344-351, 1969.

81 Wychulis AR, Kincaid OW, Wallace RB: Primary dissecting aneurysms of peripheral arteries. Mayo Clin Proc **44**:804-810, 1969.

82 Wylie EJ: Thromboendarterectomy for arteriosclerotic thrombosis of major arteries. Surgery **32**:275-292, 1952.

Cystic adventitial degeneration

83 Blackstrom CG, Linell F, Ostberg G: Cystic myxomatous adventitial degeneration of the radial artery with development of ganglion in the connective tissue. Acta Chir Scand **129**:447-451, 1965.

84 Flanigan DP, Burnham SJ, Goodreau JJ, Bergan JJ: Summary of cases of adventitial cystic disease of the popliteal artery. Ann Surg **189**:165-175, 1979.

85 Haid SP, Conn J Jr, Bergan JJ: Cystic adventitial disease of the popliteal artery. Arch Surg **101**:765-770, 1970.

86 Lewis GJT, Douglas DM, Reid W, Watt JK: Cystic adventitial disease of the popliteal artery. Br Med J **3**:411-415, 1967.

Fibromuscular dysplasia

87 Claiborne TS: Fibromuscular hyperplasia: report of a

case with involvement of multiple arteries. Am J Med **49:**103-105, 1970.

88 Crocker DW: Fibromuscular dysplasias of renal artery. Arch Pathol **85:**602-613, 1968.

89 Harrison EG, Hung JC, Bernatz PE: Morphology of fibromuscular dysplasia of the renal artery in renovascular hypertension. Am J Med **43:**97-112, 1967.

90 Hill LD, Anotononius JI: Arterial dysplasia: an important surgical lesion. Arch Surg **90:**585-595, 1965.

91 Hunt JC, Harrison EG Jr, Kincaid OW, Bernatz PE, Davis GP: Idiopathic fibrous and fibromuscular stenoses of the renal arteries associated with hypertension. Mayo Clin. Proc **37:**181-216, 1962.

92 Price RA, Vawter GF: Arterial fibromuscular dysplasia in infancy and childhood. Arch Pathol **93:**419-426, 1972.

Mesenteric vascular occlusion

93 Allen GJ: Mesentery, splanchnic circulation and mesenteric thrombosis. In Rhoads JE, Allen JG, Harkins HN, Moyer CA: Surgery. Principles and practice, ed. 4. Philadelphia, 1970, J. B. Lippincott Co.

94 Arosemena E, Edwards JE: Lesions of the small mesenteric arteries underlying intestinal infarction. Geriatrics **22:**122-138, 1967.

95 Bienenstock H, Minick R, Rogoff B: Mesenteric arteritis and intestinal infarction in rheumatoid disease. Arch Intern Med **119:**359-364, 1967.

96 Ho ECK, Moss AJ: The syndrome of "mesenteric arteritis" following surgical repair of aortic coarctation. Report of 9 cases and review of literature. Pediatrics **49:**40-45, 1972.

97 Johnson CC, Baggenstoss AH: Mesenteric vascular occlusion. I. Study of 99 cases of occlusion of veins. Mayo Clin Proc **24:**628-636, 1949.

98 Johnson CC, Baggenstoss AH: Mesenteric vascular occlusion. II. Study of 60 cases of occlusion of arteries and of 12 cases of occlusion of both arteries and veins. Mayo Clin Proc **24:**649-565, 1949.

99 Kleitsch WP, Connore EK, O'Neill TJ: Surgical operations on the superior mesenteric artery. Arch Surg **75:**752-755, 1957.

100 Liang H, Bernard HR, Dodd RB: The effect of epidural block upon experimental mesenteric occlusion. Arch Surg **83:**409-413, 1961.

101 Mavor GE: Superior mesenteric artery occlusion. Proc R Soc Med **54:**356-359, 1961.

102 Morris GC Jr, Crawford ES, Cooley DA, DeBakey ME: Revascularization of the celiac and superior mesenteric arteries. Arch Surg **84:**95-107, 1962.

103 Ottinger LW, Austen WG: A study of 136 patients with mesenteric infarction. Surg Gynecol Obstet **124:**251-261, 1967.

104 Pope CH, O'Neal RM: Incomplete infarction of ileum simulating regional enteritis. JAMA **161:**963-964, 1956.

105 Williams LF, Anastasia LF, Hasiotis CA, Bosniak MA, Byrne JJ: Nonocclusive mesenteric infarction. Am J Surg **114:**376-381, 1967.

106 Wilson GSM, Block J: Mesenteric vascular occlusion. Arch Surg **73:**330-345, 1956.

Traumatic and iatrogenic injuries

107 Bennett DE, Cherry JK: The natural history of traumatic aneurysms of the aorta. Surgery **61:**516-523, 1967.

108 Bickerstaff ER: Aetiology of acute hemiplegia in childhood. J Neurosurg **2:**82-87, 1964.

109 Cohen SM: Peripheral aneurysm and arteriovenous fistula. Ann R Coll Surg Engl **11:**1-30, 1952.

110 de Takats G, Pirani CL: Aneurysms: general considerations. Angiology **5:**173-208, 1954.

111 Fajardo LF, Lee A: Rupture of major vessels after radiation. Cancer **36:**904-913, 1975.

112 Gomes MMR, Bernatz PE: Arteriovenous fistulas: a review of ten-year experience at the Mayo Clinic. Mayo Clin Proc **45:**81-102, 1970.

113 Holman E: Fundamental principles governing the care of traumatic arteriovenous aneurysms. Angiology **5:**145-166, 1954.

114 Houck WS, Jackson JR, Odom GL, Young WG: Occlusion of internal carotid artery in neck secondary to closed trauma to head and neck: report of two cases. Ann Surg **159:**219-221, 1964.

115 Hughes CW, Jahnke EJ, Jr: The surgery of traumatic arteriovenous fistulas and aneurysms. A five-year follow up study of 215 lesions. Am Surg **148:**790-797, 1958.

116 Julian OC, Dye WS: Peripheral vascular surgery. In Rhoads JE, Allen JG, Harkins HN, Moyer CA: Surgery. Principles and practice, ed. 4. Philadelphia, 1970, J. B. Lippincott Co.

117 Kuo T, Sayers CP, Rosai J: Masson's "vegetant intravascular hemangioendothelioma": a lesion often mistaken for angiosarcoma. Study of seventeen cases located in the skin and soft tissues. Cancer **38:**1227-1236, 1976.

118 Pitner SE: Carotid thrombosis due to intraoral trauma. An unusual complication of a common childhood accident. N Engl J Med **274:**764-767, 1966.

119 Rodriguez HF, Rivera E: Spontaneous rupture of the thoracic aorta through an atheromatous plaque. Ann Intern Med **54:**307-313, 1961.

120 Salyer WR, Salyer DC: Myxoma-like features of organizing thrombi in arteries and veins. Arch Pathol **99:**307-311, 1975.

121 Shillito J Jr: Carotid arteritis: cause of hemiplegia in childhood. J Neurosurg **21:**540-551, 1964.

122 Shumacker HB Jr: The problem of maintaining the continuity of the artery in the surgery of aneurysms and arteriovenous fistulae. Ann Surg **127:**207-230, 1948.

123 Shumacker HB Jr, Carter KL: Arteriovenous fistulas and arterial aneurysms in military personnel. Surgery **20:**9-25, 1946.

Thromboangiitis obliterans

124 Gore I, Burrows S: A reconsideration of the pathogenesis of Buerger's disease. Am J Clin Pathol **29:**319-330, 1958.

125 Hershey FB, Pareira MD, Ahlvin RC: Quadrilateral peripheral vascular disease in the young adult. Circulation **26:**1261-1269, 1962.

126 Ishikawa K, Kawase S, Mishima Y: Occlusive arterial disease in extremities, with special reference to Buerger's disease. Angiology **13:**398-411, 1962.

127 Kelly PJ, Dahlin DJ, Janes JM: Clinicopathological study of ninety-four limbs amputated for occlusive vascular disease. J Bone Joint Surg **40:**72-78, 1958.

128 McKusick VA, Harris WS: The Buerger syndrome in the Orient. Bull Johns Hopkins Hosp **109:**241-291, 1961.

129 McKusick VA, Harris WS, Ottesen OE, Goodman RM: The Buerger syndrome in the United States. Bull Johns Hopkins Hosp **110:**145-176, 1962.

130 McKusick VA, Harris WS, Ottesen OE, Shelley WM,

Bloodwell DB: Buerger's disease: a distinct clinical and pathologic entity. JAMA **181:**93-100, 1962.

131 Selbert S: Etiology of thromboangiitis obliterans. JAMA **129:**5-9, 1954.

132 Theis FV: Thromboangiitis obliterans: a 30-year study. J Am Geriatr Soc **6:**106-117, 1958.

133 Wessler S, Ming S-C, Gurewich V, Greiman DG: A critical evaluation of thromboangiitis obliterans. The case against Buerger's disease. N Engl J Med **262:** 1149-1160, 1960.

134 Williams G: Recent views on Buerger's disease. J Clin Pathol **22:**573-577, 1969.

Arteritis

135 Cardell BS, Hanley T: A fatal case of giant cell or temporal arteritis. J Pathol Bacteriol **63:**587-597, 1951.

136 Domingo RT, Maramba MD, Torres LF, Wesolowski SA: Acquired aortoarteritis. A worldwide vascular entity. Arch Surg **95:**780-790, 1967.

137 Elliott PD, Baker HL Jr, Brown AL Jr: The superficial temporal artery angiogram. Radiology **102:**635-638, 1972.

138 Gonzalez-Cerna JL, Villavicencio L, Molina B, Bessudo L: Nonspecific obliterative aortitis in children. Ann Thorac Surg **4:**193-204, 1967.

138a Goodman BW Jr: Temporal arteritis. Am J Med **67:** 839-852, 1979.

139 Hamilton CR Jr, Shelley WM, Tumulty PA: Giant cell arteritis: including temporal arteritis and polymyalgia rheumatica. Medicine (Baltimore) **50:**1-27, 1971.

140 Judge RD, Currier RD, Gracie WA, Figley MM: Takayasu arteritis and the aortic arch syndrome. Am J Med **32:**379-392, 1962.

141 Klein RG, Campbell RJ, Hunder GG, Carney JA: Skip lesions in temporal arteritis. Mayo Clin Proc **51:**504-510, 1976.

142 Kolodny EH, Rebeiz JJ, Caviness VS, Richardson EP: Granulomatous angiitis of the central nervous system. Arch Neurol **19:**510-524, 1968.

143 Manion WC: Infectious angiitis. In Orbison JL, Smith DE, (eds): The peripheral blood vessels. Baltimore, 1963, The Williams & Wilkins Co., pp. 221-231.

144 Marquis Y, Richardson JP, Ritchie AC, Wigle ED: Idiopathic medial aortopathy and arteriopathy. Am J Med **44:**939-954, 1968.

145 Maxeiner SR, McDonald JR, Kirklin JW: Muscle biopsy in the diagnosis of periarteritis nodosa. Surg Clin North Am **32:**1225-1233, 1952.

146 Morgan GJ Jr, and Harris ED Jr: Non-giant cell temporal arteritis. Arthritis Rheum **21:**362-366, 1978.

147 Nasu T: Pathology of pulseless disease: a systematic study and critical review of 21 autopsy cases reported in Japan. Angiology **14:**225-242, 1963.

148 O'Brien JP: A concept of diffuse actinic arteritis. Br J Dermatol **98:**1-13, 1978.

149 O'Leary M, Nollet DJ, Blomberg DJ: Rupture of a tuberculous pseudoaneurysm of the innominate artery into the trachea and esophagus: report of a case and review of the literature. Hum Pathol **8:**458-467, 1977.

150 Parker F, Healey LA, Wilske KR, Odland GF: Light and electron microscopic studies on human temporal arteries with special reference to alterations related to senescence, atherosclerosis and giant cell arteritis. Am J Pathol **79:**57-80, 1975.

151 Restrepo C, Tejeda C, Correa P: Nonsyphilitic aortitis. Arch Pathol **87:**1-12, 1969.

151a Rose AG, Sinclair-Smith CC: Takayasu's arteritis. A study of 16 autopsy cases. Arch Pathol Lab Med **104:** 231-237, 1980.

152 Roth LM, Kissane JM: Panaortitis and aortic valvulitis in progressive systemic sclerosis (scleroderma). Report of case with perforation of an aortic cusp. Am J Clin Pathol **41:**287-296, 1964.

153 Royster TS, DiRe JJ: Polymyalgia rheumatica and giant cell arteritis with bilateral axillary artery occlusion. Am Surg **37:**421-426, 1971.

154 Schrire V, Asherson RA: Arteritis of the aorta and its major branches. Q J Med **33:**439-463, 1964.

155 Strole WE Jr, Clark WH, Isselbacher KJ: Progressive arterial occlusive disease (Kohlmeier-Degos). A frequently fatal cutaneosystemic disorder. N Engl J Med **276:**195-201, 1967.

156 Valaitis J, Pilz CG, Montgomery MM: Aortitis with aortic valve insufficiency in rheumatoid arthritis. Arch Pathol **63:**207-212, 1957.

157 Whelan TJ Jr, Baugh JH: Nonatherosclerotic arterial lesions and their management. I. Trauma. II. Inflammatory lesions of arteries. Curr Probl Surg, pp. 3-76, Feb., 1967.

Tumors

157a Bleisch VR, Kraus FT: Polypoid sarcoma of the pulmonary trunk: analysis of the literature and report of a case with leptomeric organelles and ultrastructural features of rhabdomyosarcoma. Cancer **46:**314-324, 1980.

158 Murthy MSN, Meckstroth CV, Merkle BH, Huston JT, Cattaneo SM: Primary intimal sarcoma of pulmonary valve and trunk with osteogenic sarcomatous elements. Report of a case considered to be pulmonary embolus. Arch Pathol Lab Med **100:**649-651, 1976.

159 Prioleau PG, Katzenstein AA: Major peripheral arterial occlusion due to malignant tumor embolism. Cancer **42:**2009-2014, 1978.

160 Rosai J, Akerman LR: Intravenous atypical vascular proliferation. A cutaneous lesion simulating a malignant blood vessel tumor. Arch Dermatol **109:**714-717, 1974.

161 Rosai J, Gold J, Landy R: The histiocytoid hemangiomas. A unifying concept embracing several previously described entities of skin, soft tissue, large vessels, bone and heart. Hum Pathol **10:**707-730, 1979.

162 Salm R: Primary fibrosarcoma of aorta. Cancer **29:** 73-83, 1972.

163 Sladden RA: Neoplasia of aortic intima. J Clin Pathol **17:**602-607, 1964.

164 Steffelaar JW, van der Heul RO, Blackstone E, Vos A: Primary sarcoma of the aorta. Arch Pathol **99:**139-142, 1975.

165 Stevenson JE, Burkhead H, Trueheart RE, McLaren J: Primary malignant tumor of the aorta. Am J Med **51:** 553-559, 1971.

Veins

Thrombophlebitis—thromboembolism
Stasis ulcers
Varicose veins

Thrombophlebitis—thromboembolism

Thrombophlebitis is a thrombotic disease of veins accompanied by varying degrees of inflammation. The venous wall is edematous, the intima irregularly ulcerated, and the media infiltrated with chronic inflammatory cells (Fig. 1449). As the acute inflammatory phase of the disease subsides, varying amounts of fibrous tissue and collagen are deposited in the adventitia and in the media. During the acute phase, the thrombus becomes attached more or less firmly to the denuded intima.

The process of thrombophlebitis is associated with edema of the part, which may be minimal or marked. When there is but little edema and few or no clinical signs of acute inflammation in the extremity, the venous thrombosis has been termed phlebothrombosis or bland noninflammatory venous thrombosis.[15] The noninflammatory type of thrombophlebitis probably is more frequently associated with pulmonary emboli than is thrombophlebitis with more marked signs of inflammation. However, the rigid separation of phlebothrombosis from thrombophlebitis is not possible pathologically or practical clinically. These conditions are merely different degrees of the same process.

Thrombophlebitis may involve only the superficial veins such as the saphenous vein. The vein is acutely inflamed and tender, and the overlying skin is usually red. When such thrombosis of the superficial veins occurs, there is usually little edema. However, thrombophlebitic edema may develop with marked rapidity and be of great volume if the process extends into the deep venous system. Rapid shifts of extracellular fluid into the leg may be sufficiently massive to cause shock.[12] In such instances,

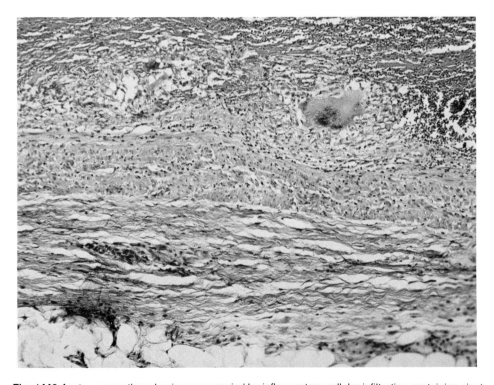

Fig. 1449 Acute venous thrombosis accompanied by inflammatory cellular infiltration containing giant cells. (WU neg. 58-6275.)

the extremity may become so swollen that cutaneous blebs develop, followed by cutaneous necrosis (phlegmasia cerulea dolens).[20] Thrombophlebitis of this severity, however, is rare. The usual postoperative or posttraumatic acute thrombophlebitis causes initially a painful, tender, swollen, cool, and mottled or grayish white extremity.

Purulent or septic thrombophlebitis occasionally is seen in association with abscess or other infection usually occurring in the peritoneal cavity or pelvis. Stein and Pruitt[21] found this complication in 4.6% of 521 burned patients who had been treated by venous catheterization. Purulent thrombophlebitis at any location is associated with marked chills and high temperature because of the bacteremia arising from the infected intravascular thrombus.

Pulmonary embolism is often thought to be primarily a complication of some surgical procedure or trauma such as fracture, particularly of the lower extremity, but the incidence of this complication is as high on medical as on surgical services.[10] Some of the factors thought to favor intravenous thrombosis and subsequent pulmonary embolism are neoplasms, cardiac disease, venous stasis from any cause, infection in the immediate area of veins, trauma, spasm of vessels, intimal injury, increased ability of the blood to coagulate, and immobilization of the limbs.[5] The use of oral contraceptives is causally related to the presence of thromboembolic phenomena.[7,19] Vessey and Doll[22] estimated that the risk of venous thromboembolism is approximately nine times greater in women taking contraceptives than in those who do not. Irey et al.[8] described distinctive vascular lesions in association with thrombosis in arteries and veins of twenty young women receiving oral contraceptives. However, the basic etiology or initiating mechanisms of thrombosis are not known. The importance of endothelial surface injury and defects has been emphasized by Samuels and Webster,[18] using the technique devised by O'Neill.[16]

Pulmonary embolism is seen in all forms of thrombophlebitis. Sudden massive pulmonary emboli frequently occur in patients without antecedent symptoms or signs of peripheral thrombophlebitis.

The greatest percentage of thrombi resulting in pulmonary embolization are thought to originate in the veins of the lower extremity. Rössle[17] found that 27% of patients over 20 years of age harbored thrombi in the veins of

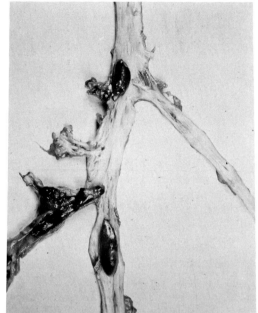

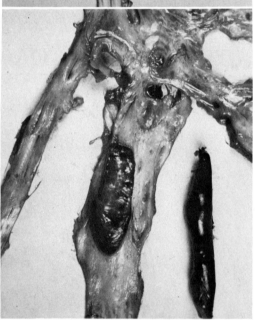

Fig. 1450 A, Multiple venous thrombi. Lower thrombus is lying in valve pocket at upper end of superficial femoral vein. Middle one on left is lying in proximal end of profunda femoris vein, while upper thrombus is lying in common femoral vein at junction of long saphenous vein. **B,** Thrombus arising in valve pocket at upper end of superficial femoral vein. Lines of Zahn can be clearly seen. Postmortem clot is shown for comparison. (**A** and **B,** From McLachlin J, Paterson JC: Some basic observations on venous thrombosis and pulmonary embolism. Surg Gynecol Obstet **93:** 1-8, 1951; by permission of Surgery, Gynecology & Obstetrics.)

the calf at autopsy. The study of Hunter et al.[6] confirmed these observations and indicated that the thrombosis occurred in over 50% of middle-aged or older persons confined to bed.

McLachlin and Paterson[11] stressed the finding of intravascular thromboses arising in relationship to the valve pockets. In 100 complete dissections of the veins of the pelvis and lower extremities, they showed gross venous thrombi in 34%, and in over one-half of these there were pulmonary emboli (Fig. 1450). In their series, the thrombi found in thirty-four patients totaled seventy-six—six in the pelvic veins, forty-nine in the thigh veins, and twenty-one in the leg veins. In other words, they found that 75% of the venous thrombi arose in the veins of the thigh and pelvis and 25% in the smaller veins of the calf and feet, with 92% arising in the lower extremities. Similar findings were reported by Beckering and Titus.[2]

Crane[4] concluded that the evaluation of all data available concerning the origin of fatal pulmonary emboli indicates that approximately 85% of them arise in the legs. This figure may well be 90% in postsurgical patients and 80% in cardiac or medical patients.

Stasis ulcers

The chief immediate complication of thrombophlebitis is pulmonary embolus, and the principal long-term complication is stasis ulceration.

The treatment of acute thrombophlebitis attempts to limit the extension of the process and to prevent pulmonary embolization. Elevation, rest with the maintenance of good hydration, elastic support, and possibly anticoagulant therapy are the initial measures. The effectiveness of anticoagulant therapy as usually administered for thromboembolic disease has been questioned.[3] Ligation of the venous system above the area of intravascular clotting is occasionally indicated when lesser measures fail to prevent pulmonary embolus.

As the acute phase of the disease subsides, measures must be taken to avoid later stasis disease in the lower extremity. The use of elastic supports to help control any dependent edema in the extremity is imperative and may be required for many months or years. With the passage of time, collateral venous channels may develop and communicate with the superficial venous systems, resulting in secondary superficial varicosities. Recanalization of the major deep veins usually is associated with this process. Any significant varicosities in the postphlebitic extremity should be removed.

For reasons not clearly understood, the prevention and control of stasis ulceration are quite difficult in the presence of subcutaneous varicosities. The preventive measures directed toward control of dependent edema often are not carried out by patients suffering from thrombophlebitis, so that after several years cutaneous pigmentation, brawny edema, dermal and subcutaneous fibrosis, extensive secondary varicosities, and ulceration of the skin in the lower one-third of the leg develop. Although stasis ulcers are seen in patients who have a history of past thrombophlebitis, such a history commonly is absent (only 50% of the patients seen in the Washington University Clinics have such a history). Even in patients having thrombophlebitis, the exact pathogenesis of the process leading to ulceration is unknown.

The diagnosis of stasis disease is usually not difficult. Only occasionally are ulceration, pigmentation, and surrounding fibrosis confused with other forms of ulceration. Before extensive treatment of a patient with advanced chronic leg ulcer, careful evaluation of the arterial blood supply should be made. Any significant arterial flow deficiency will likely result in failure of surgical therapy for ulceration. Correction of major arterial occlusion should be made when possible before treatment of the stasis ulcer in those patients in whom both are present. Obviously, the other rare causes

Table 71 Chronic stasis ulcer (time of recurrence of ulcer after operative therapy)*

Years after operation	At risk	Number of patients developing recurrent stasis ulcer in interval	Healed	Accumulative % of patients without ulcer
0-1	107	8	99	92
1-2	90	8	81	84
2-3	69	4	65	79
3-4	55	0	55	79
4-5	53	1	52	77
5-6	45	0	45	77
6-7	40	2	38	74
7-8	29	3	26	66
8+	16	0	16	66

*Three of five patients whose ulcer recurred after five postoperative years had had arterial occlusive disease develop.

of ulceration such as specific infections and neoplasms must be excluded. All ulcers should be cultured and any unusual-appearing ones biopsied before excisional therapy is undertaken.

If ulceration has not yet appeared or is not extensive or chronic in nature, the total removal of the varicose veins with ligation of perforating veins may control the process. If stasis ulceration is extensive, chronic, and long standing, it is best treated by excision and stripping of all superficial varicosities of the extremity after high ligation and division of the saphena magna and its tributaries at the saphenal-femoral junction. The ulcer and its base should be excised down to normal tissue with removal of all the inelastic thickened skin and fascia about it. The cutaneous-fascial defect should then be

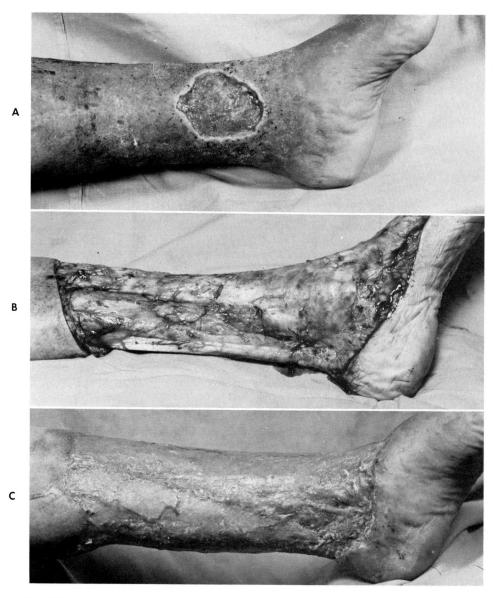

Fig. 1451 A, Long-standing chronic stasis ulcer refractory to nonoperative therapy. **B,** Fibrotic skin, subcutaneous tissue, and fascia have been widely excised. Periosteum and peritendineum were not removed. **C,** Extremity two years after operation. (**A,** WU neg. 57-5074; **B,** WU neg. 55-4561; **C,** WU neg. 57-5549.)

covered with a partial thickness cutaneous autograft.[13] The results of this form of therapy at Barnes Hospital are shown in Table 71.

The extent of excision often required for advanced stasis ulceration is shown in Fig. 1451. In most instances, the depth of the excision should include the fascia overlying the muscle, for in the presence of long-standing stasis ulcers, the fascial fibrosis and thickening are quite extensive. This also facilitates ligation of the perforating veins that are invariably present beneath the area of stasis fibrosis.

Varicose veins

Varicose veins occur more frequently in women than in men. Their incidence is much higher in obese women, particularly those who have had several pregnancies. Varicosities developing in women after pregnancy may be secondary to deep venous thrombosis.

Larson and Smith[9] reported that 213 of 491 patients (43%) had a definite family history of varicose veins, indicating some hereditary disposition. The superficial veins of the leg become dilated and tortuous and lose valvular function. Microscopically, there is fibrosis beneath the endothelium and in the wall, with secondary elastosis and loss of muscle. Calcification may occur.

Primary or simple varicosities often develop in the second and third decades of life and may be present for many years without causing symptoms or complications. The likelihood of thrombosis with propagation into the deep venous system and the likelihood of the development of the postphlebitic syndrome are sufficiently great to warrant the removal of varicose veins. The use of sclerosing agents is contraindicated because of the danger of deep venous thrombosis as well as the temporary nature of the superficial venous occlusion obtained. The operative removal of varicosities is best performed by venous stripping techniques and excisions.[1,14]

REFERENCES

1 Agrifoglio G, Edwards EA: Results of surgical treatment of varicose veins. JAMA **178**:906-911, 1961.
2 Beckering RE Jr, Titus JL: Femoral-popliteal venous thrombosis and pulmonary embolism. Am J Clin Pathol **52**:530-537, 1969.
3 Butcher HR Jr: Anticoagulant drug therapy for thrombophlebitis in the lower extremities—an evaluation. Arch Surg **80**:864-875, 1960.
4 Crane C: Deep venous thrombosis and pulmonary embolism. N Engl J Med **257**:147-157, 1957.
5 DeBakey ME: Collective review: critical evaluation of problem of thromboembolism. Int Abstr Surg **98**:1-27, 1954.
6 Hunter WC, Krygier JJ, Kennedy JC, Sneedend VD: Etiology and prevention of thrombosis of the deep leg veins. Surgery **17**:178-190, 1945.
7 Inman WHW, Vessey MP: Investigation of deaths from pulmonary coronary and cerebral thrombosis and embolism in women in childbearing age. Br Med J **2**:193-199, 1968.
8 Irey NS, Manion WC, Taylor HB: Vascular lesions in women taking oral contraceptives. Arch Pathol **89**:1-8, 1970.
9 Larson RA, Smith FS: Varicose veins: evaluation of observations in 491 cases. Mayo Clin Proc **18**:400-408, 1943.
10 McCartney JS: Postoperative pulmonary embolism. N Engl J Med **257**:147-157, 1957.
11 McLachlin J, Paterson JC: Some basic observations on venous thrombosis and pulmonary embolism. Surg Gynecol Obstet **93**:1-8, 1951.
12 Moyer CA: Nonoperative surgical care. In Rhoads JE, Allen JG, Harkins HN, Moyer CA: Surgery. Principles and practice, ed. 4, Philadelphia, 1970, J. B. Lippincott Co.
13 Moyer CA, Butcher HR: Stasis ulcers: an evaluation of the effectiveness of three methods of therapy and the implication of obliterative cutaneous lymphangitis as a credible etiologic factor. Ann Surg **141**:577-587, 1955.
14 Myers TT: Results of the stripping operation in the treatment of varicose veins. Mayo Clin Proc **29**:583-590, 1954.
15 Ochsner A, DeBakey ME, DeCamp PT: Venous thrombosis, analysis of 580 cases. Surgery **29**:1-20, 1951.
16 O'Neill JF: The effects of venous endothelium of alterations in blood flow through the vessels in vein walls and the possible relation to thrombosis. Ann Surg **126**:270-288, 1947.
17 Rössle R: Ueber die Bedeutung und die Entstehung der Wadenvenenthrombosen. Virshows Arch [Pathol Anat]**300**:180-189, 1937.
18 Samuels PB, Webster DR: The role of venous endothelium in the inception of thrombosis. Ann Surg **136**:422-438, 1952.
19 Sartwell PE, Masi AT, Arthes FG, Greene GR, Smith HE: Thromboembolism and oral contraceptives: an epidemiological case-control study. Am J Epidemiol **90**:365-380, 1969.
20 Stallworth JM, Bradham GB, Kletke RR, Price RG Jr: Phlegmasia cerulea dolens: a 10-year review. Ann Surg **161**:802-811, 1965.
21 Stein JM, Pruitt BA Jr: Suppurative thrombophlebitis: a lethal iatrogenic disease. N Engl J Med **282**:1452-1455, 1970.
22 Vessey MP, Doll R: Investigation of relation between use of oral contraceptives and thromboembolic disease. A further report. Br Med J **2**:651-657, 1969.

Lymphatic vessels

Introduction

With the exception of certain rare tumors related to lymph vessels, such as diffuse lymphangioma and lymphangiosarcoma (Chapter 24), the primary lymphatic disease encountered clinically is lymphedema. Of course, chylothorax and chyloascites occur, but in nearly all instances these processes are secondary to trauma, neoplastic disease, or some infectious process.

Lymphedema

Lymphedema may be classified as postinfectious, posttraumatic, obstructive, and idiopathic. Obstructive lymphedema is most often seen following the obstruction of regional lymph nodes by neoplastic invasion or following their removal, as in radical mastectomy or in radical groin dissection. The development of lymphedema of the arm after radical mastectomy is thought more likely to follow in those patients in whom postoperative infection has produced fibrosis in the axilla or in those patients having persistent cancer in the axilla. However, lymphedema is seen in patients who give a history of as little trauma as a severely sprained ankle or following such infections as a furuncle.

Many patients give no history of trauma or infection associated with the onset of their lymphedema. In such instances, the lymphedema usually is termed idiopathic or lymphedema praecox. Congenital lymphedema is usually considered in this category and is differentiated from lymphedema praecox only in that the patient has had some degree of swelling of the extremity since infancy. Idiopathic lymphedema may develop in persons up to the age of 40 years.[10]

Pathology

The obstructive nature of neoplastic involvement of regional lymph nodes is obvious. Improved injection techniques combined with magnification roentgenography may serve to delineate accurately normal fine lymphatic channels as well as tumor involvement[7,8,12] (Fig. 1452).

The swelling of lymphedema is usually slowly progressive. There is dilatation of the dermal lymphatics as well as the deeper fascial lymphatics[2] (Fig. 1453). When the degree of swelling is advanced, there is a depression of hair follicles and gross dermal edema. In such cases, the cutaneous lymphatics may be sufficiently dilated to be associated with lymphorrhea following minor cutaneous abrasions or needle punctures (Fig. 1454). Tissue sections of such skin usually show markedly dilated dermal lymphatics.

All forms of lymphedema probably are in some way associated with inadequate lymphatic drainage.[5] Drinker and Yaffey[3] postulated that the increased protein content of the lymph present in chronic lymphatic stasis stimulates the deposition of fibrous tissue in the skin, subcutaneous tissue, and fascia. Such fibrosis aggravates the degree of inadequate lymphatic drainage and makes the disease slowly progressive.

Whatever the mechanism is, the slowly progressive nature of lymphedema in many patients is associated with dermal thickening and collagenous deposition in the subcutaneous tissues and fascia. Bouts of superficial cellulitis and lymphangitis often become superimposed upon the lymphedema in an extremity. In some patients, recurrent bouts of such infections are completely incapacitating. The presence of recurrent infection in such an extremity appears to hasten the deposition of collagen and may result in such a large amount of fibrotic replacement of subcutaneous fat and normal dermal structures as to make demonstration of dermal lymphatics impossible.

Kinmonth et al.[6] reported the presence of dilated, valveless, deep lymphatic channels in idiopathic lymphedema. These were visualized at operation after the injection of patent blue dye and by roentgenologic lymphangiography. Although many varicose-like lymphatic trunks were found in their patients, in none was a definite proximal site of lymphatic channel obstruction discovered.

In a few patients with idiopathic lymphedema having no clinical evidence or history of lym-

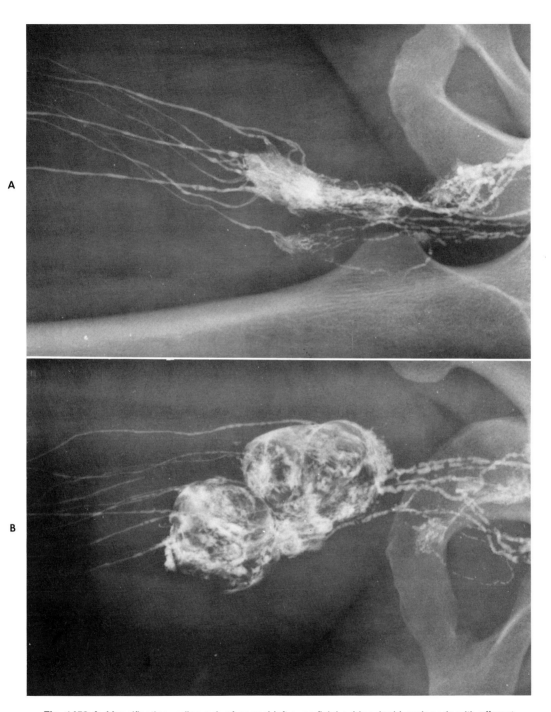

Fig. 1452 A, Magnification radiograph of normal left superficial subinguinal lymph node with afferent and efferent lymphatic channels in 40-year-old woman. **B,** Magnification radiograph of enlarged right superficial subinguinal lymph node with malignant infiltration secondary to primary melanoma of skin of heel. Same patient as shown in **A.** (**A** and **B,** From Isard HJ, Ostrum BJ, Cullinan JE: Magnification roentgenography. A "spot-film" technic. Med Radiogr Photogr **38:**92-109, 1962.)

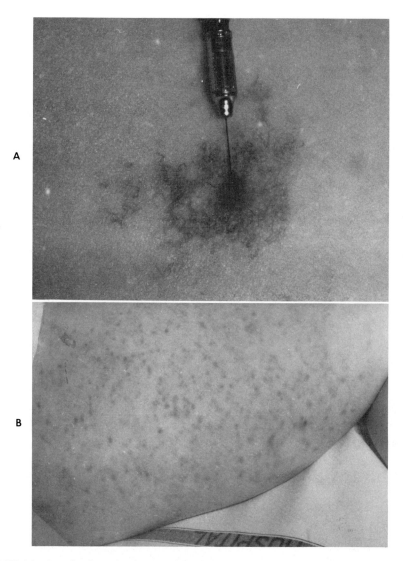

Fig. 1453 Injection of enlarged cutaneous lymphatics with 4% sky blue dye. Patient had obstructive lymphedema in inguinal region caused by Hodgkin's disease. **A,** Initial injection was made on lateral aspect of thigh. **B,** Four hours after injection, extensive retrograde filling of cutaneous lymphatics on skin of medial thigh had occurred. (**A** and **B,** From Butcher HR Jr, Hoover AL: Abnormalities of human superficial cutaneous lymphatic cannulation. Ann Surg **142:**633-653, 1955.)

phangitis or cellulitis in the extremity, enlarged regional lymph nodes have been removed. Microscopically, they contain a mild chronic inflammatory response, sinusoidal fibrosis, and markedly dilated lymphatic channels (Fig. 1455). Despite such findings, the pathogenesis responsible for the inadequate lymph drainage in most cases of lymphedema remains unknown.[1] Direct communication between lymph nodes and veins has been demonstrated by Pressman and Simon.[9]

Treatment

Treatment of lymphedema consists primarily of elevation of the extremity, compression, and massage, which must be maintained during many years of supervision. Recurrent bouts of streptococcal lymphangitis may be prevented by daily administration of penicillin orally. Such conservative measures will control the lymphedema sufficiently to avoid operation in many patients. Operative therapy is indicated only when the extent of subcutaneous fibrosis,

A 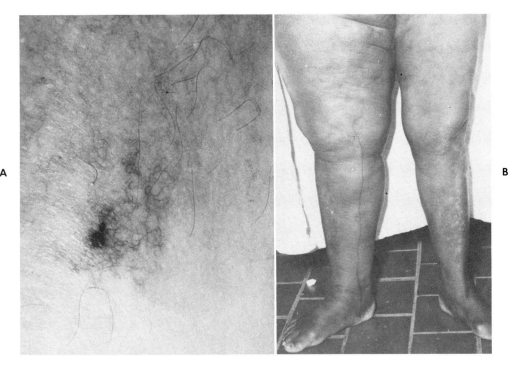 B

Fig. 1454 Dye-filled skin lymphatics in leg of patient with obstructive lymphedema. **B,** Following cutaneous puncture for injection of lymphatics, dye-containing lymph flowed from site. (**A** and **B,** From Butcher HR Jr, Hoover AL: Abnormalities of human superficial cutaneous lymphatic cannulation. Ann Surg **142:**633-653, 1955.)

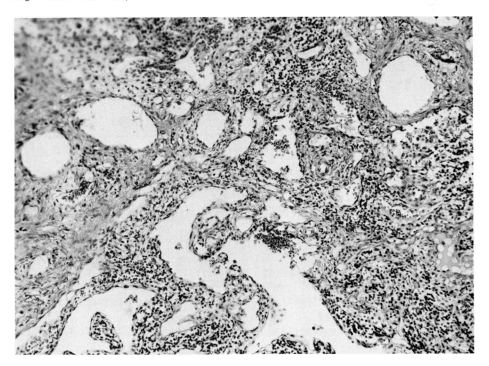

Fig. 1455 Markedly dilated lymph channels in enlarged lymph node removed from groin of patient with idiopathic lymphedema of obstructive type.

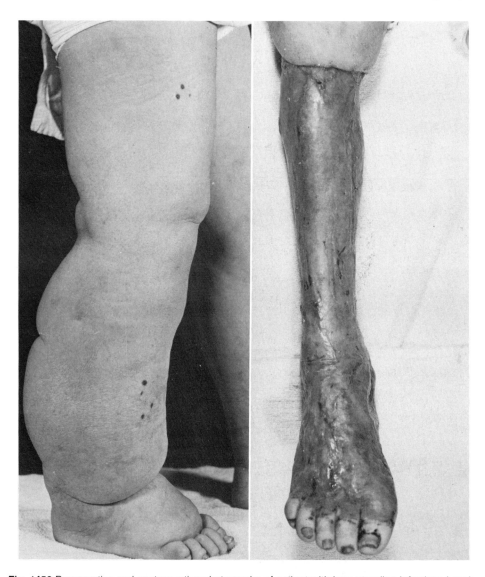

Fig. 1456 Preoperative and postoperative photographs of patient with long-standing infectious lymphedema. All fibrotic skin, subcutaneous tissue, and fascia were removed and defect was covered with split-thickness cutaneous autografts. (WU negs. 54-2266 and 54-2881; from Butcher HR Jr, Hoover AL: Abnormalities of human superficial cutaneous lymphatic cannulation. Ann Surg **142:**633-653, 1955.)

infection, and massive swelling is sufficient to handicap the patient markedly.[10,11]

The operation most useful is the excision of the thickened fibrotic skin, the edematous subcutaneous tissue, and the thickened fascia overlying the muscles, followed by the immediate application of split-thickness cutaneous autografts (Fig. 1456). The Sistrunk modification of the Kondoleon operation is no longer considered of value. The use of hyaluronidase and long, nonabsorbable subcutaneous sutures extending from the lymphedematous areas into the normal subcutaneous tissue have not proved of value.[4]

In patients with sufficiently severe lymphedema to require excision of the skin, subcutaneous tissue, and fascia of the extremity, gross examination of the excised portions shows dense fibrotic bands and sheets extending through the markedly swollen subcutaneous tissue. Pockets of fluid may be found in the intervening tissue spaces at operation. The skin over the fibrotic dermis may be atrophic in some areas and hyperplastic and keratotic in

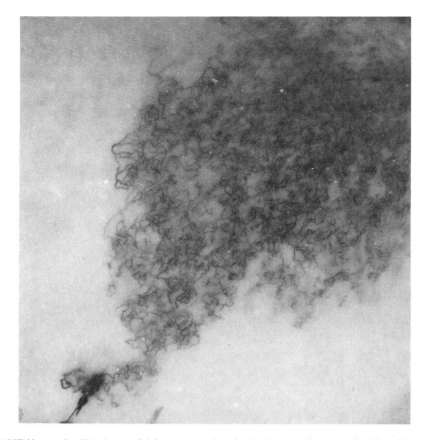

Fig. 1457 Unusually dilated superficial cutaneous lymphatics in skin of patient with idiopathic lymph-edema. (From Butcher HR Jr, Hoover AL: Abnormalities of human superficial cutaneous lymphatic cannulation. Ann Surg **142:**633-653, 1955.)

others. The collagenous thickening of the dermis is usually extreme. Lymphatic channels as such are often not seen histologically in such skin and subcutaneous tissue. This is particularly true if the process has been associated with multiple episodes of dermal infection. Dilated dermal lymphatics may be demonstrated histologically and by dye injection techniques in the skin of a lymphedematous extremity unassociated with long-standing episodes of infection (Fig. 1457).

The dermal and subcutaneous fibrosis similar to that seen in advanced forms of lymphedema also occurs about long-standing chronic stasis ulcers. The obliteration of dermal lymphatics, however, cannot be related primarily to the etiology of stasis ulcers since similar obliteration occurs in the fibrotic skin of long-standing lymphedema, a condition rarely associated with chronic ulceration of the lower extremity.

REFERENCES

1 Blocker TG Jr, Smith JR, Dunton EF, Protas JM, Cooley RM, Lewis SR, Kirby EJ: Studies of ulceration and edema of the lower extremity by lymphatic cannulation. Surgery **149:**884-896, 1959.
2 Butcher HR Jr, Hoover AL: Abnormalities of human superficial cutaneous lymphatics associated with stasis ulcers, lymphedema, scars and cutaneous autographs. Ann Surg **142:**633-653, 1955.
3 Drinker CK, Yaffey JM: Lymphatics, lymph and lymphoid tissue. Their physiological and clinical significance. Cambridge, Mass., 1941, Harvard University Press.
4 Foley WT: The treatment of lymphedema. Surg Gynecol Obstet **101:**25-34, 1955.
5 Kinmonth JB, Taylor GW: The lymphatic circulation in lymphedema. Ann Surg **139:**129-136, 1954.
6 Kinmonth JB, Taylor GW, Tracy GD, Marsh JD: Primary lymphoedema. Clinical and lymphangiographic studies of a series of 107 patients in which the lower limbs were affected. Br J Surg **95:**1-10, 1957.
7 McPeak CJ, Constantinides SG: Lymphangiography in malignant melanoma. A comparison of clinicopathologic and lymphangiographic findings in 21 cases. Cancer **17:**1586-1594, 1964.

8 Pomerantz M, Ketcham AS: Lymphangiography and its surgical applications. Surgery **53**:589-597, 1963.

9 Pressman JJ, Simon MB: Experimental evidence of direct communications between lymph nodes and veins. Surgery **113**:537-541, 1961.

10 Schirger A, Harrison EG Jr, Janes JM: Idiopathic lymphedema. JAMA **182**:124-132, 1962.

11 Thompson N: Surgical treatment of chronic lymphedema of extremities. Surg Clin North Am **47**:445-503, 1967.

12 Wallace S: Dynamics of normal and abnormal lymphatic systems as studied with contrast media. Cancer Chemother Rep **52**:31-58, 1968.

27 Neuromuscular system

Central nervous system and
  peripheral nerves
Skeletal muscle

Central nervous system and peripheral nerves

CENTRAL NERVOUS SYSTEM
Congenital diseases

Most congenital malformations of the central nervous system that are amenable to surgical correction are associated with defects of the overlying bony structures. A less common group is represented by defects in the cerebrospinal fluid pathways.

Ectopia

Nodular collections of mature neural tissue, predominantly formed by astrocytic elements but occasionally also containing neurons and meningothelial cells, are sometimes found adjacent to the structures of the central nervous system. Nasal glioma (nasal glial heterotopia), the most common variety, is discussed in Chapter 6. Goldring et al.[1] found ectopic neural

1555

tissue in the occipital bone of an adult. We have seen a well-circumscribed soft nodule in the soft tissues of the buttock composed of mature glial cells and ganglion cells, partially surrounded by a cleft lined by hyperplastic meningothelial cells, apparently not connected with the spinal canal. It is likely that all these lesions represent peculiar variants of the encephaloceles and meningomyeloceles described below.

Spina bifida

The group of malformations called spina bifida represent failures in the closure of midline structures over the neural tube. They range from a completely open neural tube (craniorachischisis) to the unperceptible lesions of occult spina bifida. The most common site of these defects is the lumbosacral region of the spine, accounting for over 70% of cases.[2] The second most common site is the cervical or occipitocervical region, whereas occasional defects can be found at all points along the cerebrospinal axis. Fisher et al.[2] reported the association of these lesions with other congenital defects in over one-fourth of the patients. Hydrocephalus is the most common, usually due to the Arnold-Chiari malformation that is invariably present.[4]

The lesions are designated as meningocele, meningomyelocele, syringomyelocele, myelocele, and encephalocele according to the nature of the wall and content of the sac (Fig. 1458). Meningomyeloceles and syringomyeloceles are about three times as common as simple meningoceles and are more serious lesions because of the greater deficit resulting from them.

Motor disability and sensory disturbance are the most common defects that result from these lesions, some degree of the former being detectable in 91% of the patients. Involvement

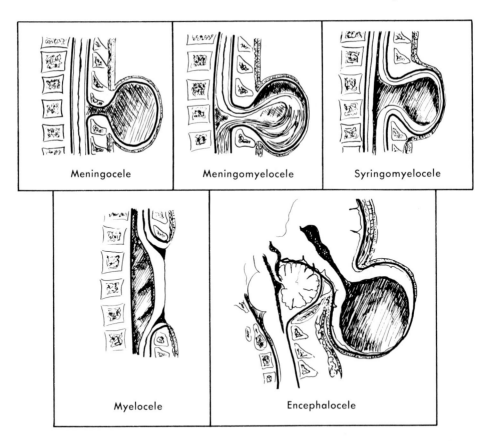

Fig. 1458 Schematic drawing of main varieties of malformations of central nervous system that require surgical intervention. (Adapted, with permission, from THE CIBA COLLECTION OF MEDICAL ILLUSTRATION by Frank H. Netter, M.D. © Copyright 1953, 1972 CIBA Pharmaceutical Company, Division of CIBA-GEIGY Corporation. All rights reserved.)

of the urinary and anal sphincters occur in about two-thirds and one-half of the patients, respectively, and is responsible for the most serious threat to the patient's life other than the accidental rupture or erosion of the sac with consequent meningitis. Nevertheless, Mawsdley et al.[3] report that about 35% of all patients survive and that about 40% of survivors have no or minor handicaps.

The sac of a meningocele is composed of a more or less complete outer layer of skin over an irregular layer of dense collagenous tissue mixed with various amounts of fat and representing tissue derived probably from the dermis, subcutaneous tissue, and dura mater. The inner lining is a thin, smooth layer of flattened cells. In the more common meningomyeloceles, syringomyeloceles, and encephaloceles, varying types and amounts of nerve tissue are found in or attached to the walls. Normally developed myelinated nerves or nerve roots are most commonly found, but pieces of choroid plexus or islands of isolated neuroglial tissue are often present. The latter can be discovered at considerable distances from the main cavity or mass of central nervous tissue.

If the lesions are not too large, operative repair may be successful in obliterating the sac. The progression of hydrocephalus, when present, may be halted, but neurologic deficit is never improved. Fisher et al.[2] reported that when neither hydrocephalus nor neurologic disability is present, they rarely appear after operation. Operative mortality and postoperative deficit are much greater in patients with spinal lesions than in those with cranial lesions, the majority of the latter being normal after operation.

Epidermoid, dermoid, and other congenital cysts

Epidermoid cysts of the central nervous system usually are classified as tumors, yet they are not neoplasms. These are rare lesions that comprise less than 1% of all tumors of the central nervous system. The transition examples mentioned in the preceding paragraphs indicate their kinship to congenital deformities, and their usual sites of occurrence confirm the impression.

They are found, for the most part, in the spinal cord, in the suprasellar region (where they are a variety of the craniopharyngioma and have a similar embryonic basis), in the pineal region (which in the early embryo, is at the apex of the cephalic flexure and consequently in a position immediately beneath the ectoderm), and at various positions over the convexities of the cerebral hemispheres (where they are associated with defects in the diploë, so that the mass may be predominantly beneath the dura or within the skull or beneath the scalp with perplexing unpredictability). According to Manno et al.,[8] 40% of the epidermoid cysts of the spinal cord (as distinguished from dermoid sinuses and teratomas) arise from implantation of epidermis by lumbar puncture or trauma.

Other examples are found in the cerebellopontine angle, sylvian fissure, temporal lobe, or petrous portion of the temporal bone, where their embryologic origins are less clear but are probably associated with the formation of the pharynx, middle ear, and base of the skull.[6] These lesions should not be confused with the so-called cholesteatomas of the middle ear that are associated with chronic inflammation and may erode through the temporal bone to extradural positions.

The cysts of the central nervous system are largely within the leptomeninges and only rarely are located within or seem to arise within the brain substance.[11] Like similar lesions in other organs, they have a central mass of desquamated squamous cells, the iridescence of which has resulted in the names of pearly tumors and cholesteatomas. About this central mass there is a layer of squamous epithelium that is essentially epidermis and then a layer of fibrous tissue continuous usually with the leptomeninges and equivalent to the corium. In some tumors, skin appendages such as sweat or sebaceous glands and hair follicles are present in this outer layer, so that the terminologies of *dermoid cyst* in contradistinction to epidermoid cyst have been applied (Fig. 1459). No detectable differences in the biology of the two groups are apparent.[7]

Depending upon whether there has been an escape of the contents of the cyst, the surrounding fibrous tissue may contain evidence of a foreign body reaction and chronic inflammation. The adjacent brain substance shows only the effects of pressure that may lead to a loss of neurons with diffuse hypertrophy and hyperplasia of astrocytes.

The symptomatology of these lesions is that of very slowly expanding tumors, unless there is a rupture, whereupon the signs of acute meningeal irritation supervene.[9] Most of the lesions

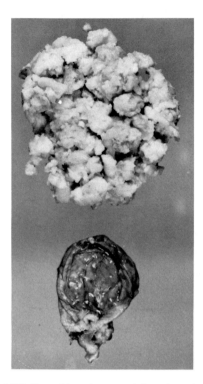

Fig. 1459 Dermoid cyst removed from frontal region of 15-year-old girl. Content of cyst (top) is white, granular, friable material representing keratin. Cyst wall (bottom) is thin and translucent and has smooth inner surface. Microscopically, it was composed of mature squamous epithelium with skin appendages. (WU neg. 66-3615.)

become manifest in early adult life. Apparently, the lesion expands at about the same rate as its surrounding encasement until after puberty. It then either continues to increase in size, while the other tissues cease to grow, or there is accelerated accumulation of the contents of the sac. Sizable lesions sometimes cause such severe displacement and deformity of the structures of the central nervous system as to cause amazement at the degree of anatomic deformity that this delicate organ can tolerate with apparent complete physiologic compensation. The very slow enlargement of the lesion is probably the explanation for such unusual cases. Exceptionally, squamous cell carcinomas will develop from these cysts.[12]

Enterogenous cysts lined by intestinal epithelium can occur within the spinal canal.[10] They are also known as enteric cysts, neuroenteric cysts, and gastrocystomas. They are thought to arise from persistence of a portion of the neurenteric canal, a minute tubelike structure joining the gut and the neuroectoderm during embryogenesis. Most cases are found in a ventral position, often near the cervicothoracic junction of young patients.

Ependymal cysts are extremely rare. Most examples are found intracranially in the subarachnoid space, usually on top of the cerebral hemispheres but sometimes within the brain. In contrast to epidermoid and dermoid cysts, most ependymal cysts are found in adults. Microscopically, the lining is made up of ciliated cuboidal cells.[5]

Colloid (neuroepithelial) cysts are discussed on p. 1585.

Hydrocephalus

Hydrocephalus may be secondary to congenital defects of the nervous system or its coverings, or it may follow other lesions such as tumors, inflammations, or hemorrhages. The first type is sometimes misnamed primary hydrocephalus, whereas the problems of the second group are largely those of the underlying disease.

When hydrocephalus is secondary to congenital defects, the deformity is apparent at birth or develops soon thereafter. It is probably always associated with a block in the pathways of the flow of cerebrospinal fluid, although it is undeniable that such a block is difficult to demonstrate in all patients. Hyperactivity of the choroid plexuses might be a contributing factor in some instances, such as those of a choroid papilloma. A common site of the block is at the aqueduct of Sylvius, which may be obliterated or narrowed by congenital malformation so that it is a group of small branching channels.[13] It may also be narrowed by a tumor or a vascular malformation in the mesencephalon, or a severe ependymitis may result in obliteration of the canal.

The outflow paths of the fourth ventricle, the foramina of Luschka and Magendie, are other sites of possible obstruction. The drainage from the cisterna magna may be impaired by adhesions at its margin or by the pressure of the edge of the foramen magnum in patients with the Arnold-Chiari malformation. The flow and final absorption of fluid can be affected by adhesions or obliteration of the subarachnoid space over the base of the brain or the convexities. Absence or destruction of the arachnoidal villi is a final possibility.

Cases are classified as communicating or noncommunicating hydrocephalus, depending upon whether or not a communication between the lumbar sac and the lateral ventricles can be demonstrated. This classification is of greater aid in eliminating the possibility of obstruction at certain sites (such as in congenital aqueductal stenosis) than it is in establishing the location of the obstruction at any particular site.

The pathologic histology of hydrocephalus is usually disappointing and often obscure.[14] Surgical treatment is aimed at the palliative removal of the excess fluid from some point above the block by any of several ingenious routes—catheters from the lateral ventricles into the cervical subarachnoid space, the cervical subcutaneous tissues, the pleural or peritoneal cavities, a ureter, or the middle ear. In some patients, the process spontaneously resolves itself for unknown reasons, and it is sometimes surprising how little neurologic or mental deficit may result from really tremendous deformity.

Obstructive hydrocephalus is almost entirely internal hydrocephalus (i.e., it is characterized by dilated ventricles). External hydrocephalus is almost always due to extensive cortical malformation or destruction, porencephaly, or meningeal lesions such as subdural hematomas or hygromas.

Arnold-Chiari deformity and platybasia

The Arnold-Chiari deformity and basilar depression are two lesions that result in malarrangements between the central nervous system and its bony encasement. Surgical revision of the bones at the foramen magnum may be effective in decompressing the brainstem and spinal cord and relieving symptoms that have arisen on that basis.

The Arnold-Chiari malformation is primarily one of the hindbrain. The pons, medulla, and cervical cord are elongated and sometimes acutely flexed. The cerebellar tonsils are deformed and extend as a cuff ventrally and caudally around the medulla. This results in the medulla lying in the foramen magnum and in the foramina of Luschka and Magendie lying below the level of the atlanto-occipital articulation. The upper spinal roots consequently take an upward course instead of running directly lateral. The deformity is usually, but not always, associated with a lumbar meningomyelocele and caudal fixation of the lower spinal cord.[16] Because the openings of the fourth ventricle are below the foramen magnum, which is

wedged full of medulla and cerebellum, spinal fluid cannot rise over the cerebral hemispheres to its usual site of maximal absorption, and a communicating hydrocephalus develops.

The deformity of basilar depression is primarily of the pars basilaris of the occipital bone with consequent flattening of the angle of decline of the clivus and impingement of the rim of the foramen magnum on the medulla.

Various other malformations of the skull have restrictive effects upon the growth and function of the brain. These conditions have been referred to as craniostenosis.[15] The bone or other surrounding tissue removed at surgical revision of these relationships is, of course, of normal histologic appearance.

Congenital cerebral diseases and brain biopsy

Cortical biopsy is occasionally employed for specific diagnosis, particularly in children.[21] This procedure should be carefully planned so that maximal utilization may be made of the valuable material obtained.[23] The best sites for biopsy should be chosen in conference among the clinician, surgeon, and pathologist and preparations made for the utilization of appropriate procedures of staining, electron microscopy, histochemistry, and analytic chemistry.

Despite such planning and the rather dire circumstances necessary to justify a biopsy, only about one-third yield a specific diagnosis, another third show abnormalities that are not diagnostic, and the remainder may yield normal tissue. Svennerholm[22] points out that most of the conditions specifically diagnosed can be easier diagnosed by other procedures and suggests that biopsy is really of more value for research than for diagnosis. As medical science is more successful in prolonging life, biopsy may be the only opportunity to learn more about the early phases of some diseases before late, nonspecific and secondary changes obliterate more essential features.[17]

Cellular inclusions in herpes, cytomegalic, and Dawson's encephalitis are examples of fairly specific morphologic landmarks, as are globoid cells in Krabbe's leukodystrophy and the brown granular bodies of metachromatic leukodystrophy.[18,19] Fairly specific structural features in neurons in amaurotic familial idiocy, Alzheimer's disease, and Pick's disease may be demonstrated. Landing and Rubinstein[20] describe the features of many of these disorders in great detail and also point out other sites of biopsy that may yield helpful information, such as the liver in metachromatic leukodystrophy.[24]

Vascular diseases
Saccular aneurysms

Saccular aneurysms of the cerebral arteries comprise most of the acquired abnormalities of vessels that can be relieved by surgical treatment.[26] They have been called congenital and berry aneurysms, but the fact that very few have ever been found in children and infants indicates that they are usually not present at birth, although certain important factors of formation may be congenital.

These lesions are the single most common cause of massive subarachnoid hemorrhage and occur most frequently in patients past the fourth decade and in those with hypertension. It has even been observed that patients with coarctation of the aorta and consequently hypertension in the carotid and brachial circulations have an apparently increased incidence of saccular aneurysms. About 80% of the lesions occur in that part of the circle of Willis derived from the carotid arteries, rostral to the posterior communicating arteries, with a great majority occurring within 3 cm of the terminations of the carotid arteries. The middle cerebral artery is most frequently involved, followed by the internal carotid and anterior cerebral arteries.

Multiple lesions may be found at postmortem examinations in perhaps one-fourth of the patients,[32] but it is unusual for more than one lesion to give symptoms. The problem of multiple lesions is important because the refinement of cerebral angiography has made the preoperative localization of these lesions much easier and has occasionally succeeded in demonstrating aneurysms that were not the site of the bleeding or symptoms. The coincidence of aneurysms and angiomas has been commented upon by Boyd-Wilson.[25]

The pathology of the saccular aneurysm is not of diagnostic importance, for the lesion is

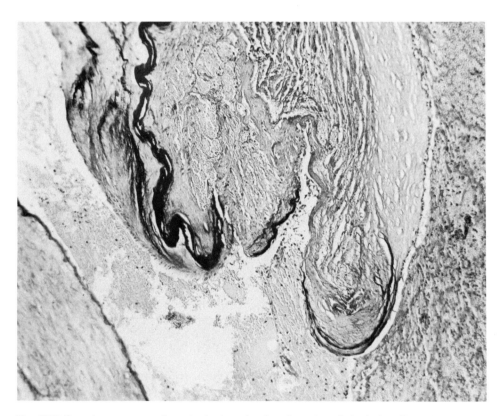

Fig. 1460 Saccular aneurysm of cerebral artery showing disruption of elastic lamella and muscularis at lip of mouth of aneurysm. Lumen of artery is to left and that of aneurysmal sac to right. (Verhoeff-van Gieson; ×125; WU neg. 52-4241.)

rarely examined before death. Nearly all occur in or very near the acute angles of bifurcations of the cerebral arteries, but when the sac is 1 cm or more in diameter, it is difficult, if not impossible, to define the site of its opening. This occurrence at the bifurcations has been explained by Forbus[29] as due to the maximum impact of the bloodstream at these points plus the presence of folds or defects in the muscle of the media in these sites.

Interpretation of the role of these medial defects has caused much controversy and misunderstanding.[27,30] They occur in as many as one-third of the bifurcations of sizable cerebral arteries, even in newborn infants.[34,36] It is therefore certain that they are not the sole factor in the formation of aneurysms, and probably they are more important in their localization than in their development. As Forbus[29] pointed out, the necessary prerequisite for initiation of the aneurysm is probably a defect or weakening of the strongest layer of the wall—the elastic lamella (Fig. 1460). This would obviously be accelerated by increased intraluminal pressure and would most likely occur at the point of maximum impact, especially if that point overlies a discontinuity of the muscular media.

Other authors, particularly Dandy,[28] took exception to this view and maintained that most aneurysms occur on the straight parts of vessels at the sites of incomplete absorption of embryonic branches. They support this contention with the observation that anomalies in the vessels of the circle of Willis in patients with aneurysms are more than usually frequent.

Regardless of the primeval nature of the origins of the aneurysms, the walls of the sacs are composed principally of fibrous connective tissue, and the elastic membrane and muscular media disappear at the edges of the mouth in ordinary microscopic sections. By electron microscopy,[31] smooth muscle cells, fine elastic fibers, and altered basement membranes can be observed and present appearances reminiscent of similar changes in the inner layers of arteries that are developing arteriosclerosis.

There are usually arteriosclerotic plaques in the wall of the sac or in the vessel about its mouth. Walker and Allegra[37] suggested that the fortuitous severity of such plaques may be the initiating factor that accomplishes the destruction of the elastic lamella and weakens the wall of the vessel. However, the correlation of aneurysms with general arteriosclerosis of the cerebral vessels is poor. Factors in the rupture of the lesions are not known other than the suggestion of overdistention of the fibrous sac.

After rupture, the effects on the surrounding brain vary with the site and direction of the rupture. The bleeding may occur simply into the subarachnoid space, or if the stream of blood under arterial pressure points toward cerebral substance, the effect may be much like that of a hose playing on sand with extensive dissection and destruction of tissue. Aneurysms of the anterior cerebral arteries sometimes dissect the opposite frontal lobe if the rupture is properly oriented, giving rise to evidence of hemorrhage and enlargement on the side of the normal artery. Rupture of the hemorrhage into the ventricles is not uncommon in fatal cases and usually occurs by dissection through the inferior and medial frontal lobe at the anterior extremity of the lateral ventricle.

Richardson and Hyland[33] reported that approximately 50% of patients with ruptured aneurysms recover with no therapy other than bed rest, and Slosberg[35] obtained successful results in twelve of fifteen patients treated only with induced hypotension. Repeated hemorrhages occur in one of every seven patients.

Arteriovenous fistulas

Other than the communications between arteries and veins that arise in angiomas, intracranial arteriovenous fistulas develop principally between the internal carotid artery and the cavernous sinus because that is the only intracranial site where there is juxtaposition of a sizable artery and vein. Many are said to be of traumatic origin secondary to basilar skull fractures, but others develop from ruptured aneurysms of the internal carotid artery.

Symptoms include bruit, pulsating exophthalmos on the affected side, and evidence of disturbances of function of the third, fourth, and sixth nerves. Little can be said for the pathology of the lesions other than the gross observation of the communication between the artery and the vein, some surrounding fibrous reaction, and occasionally sclerotic plaques in the artery, fistula, or even the vein.

Temporal (giant cell) arteritis

Among the intrinsic diseases of the blood vessels of the head, temporal or granulomatous (giant cell) arteritis is most likely to come to the attention of the neurosurgeon. It is a febrile, self-limited disease of variable duration and unknown etiology. The greatest incidence is in women and in the seventh decade of life.

Prominent local signs are headache and pain in various structures of the head, but systemic symptoms such as malaise, anorexia, and weakness may be present. Involvement of the eye, with complete or partial loss of vision, may occur in as many as one-third of the patients. Cerebral symptoms may suggest focal ischemic damage or an encephalitis.[38]

A tender nodule is usually palpable along the course of the temporal artery. The disease may involve other cranial arteries and has been reported to occur concomitantly with similar lesions in arteries elsewhere.

Histologically, temporal arteritis is a fibrosis of the intima with focal necrosis and granulomas of the media characterized by the presence of a few giant cells and an infiltrate of round cells but very few or no eosinophils. Kimmelstiel et al.[39] described the giant cells in association with the disrupted internal elastic membrane and considered the presence of fragments of that tissue in the cytoplasm of the giant cells as pathognomonic of this entity. Otherwise, the changes are similar to those of polyarteritis nodosa.

Another variety of giant cell granulomatous angiitis confined to the central nervous system has been distinguished from temporal arteritis.[40] This is a diffuse involvement of small arteries and veins. The histologic appearance, and probably the pathogenesis, are similar to those of temporal arteritis. Therapy with steroids apparently has some beneficial effect. Earlier reports probably have not separated cases of this type from other examples of arteritis involving cranial arteries.

Effects of vascular insufficiency

The effects on the brain of vascular insufficiency are responsible for a great deal of morbidity but are usually common general pathologic processes of no special interest to the surgical pathologist. Two conditions, however, can give rise to a difficult symptomatology of acute intracranial pressure and may be recognized only on exploration and biopsy: acute encephalomalacia and pseudotumor cerebri.

Acute encephalomalacia

Acute encephalomalacia or ischemic infarction, in its early stages, may be accompanied by tremendous edema and swelling of the af-fected tissue and ventricular displacement suggestive of a tumor. The surgeon has no difficulty in recognizing the tissue as abnormal, and rarely is there an opportunity to demonstrate the actual causative lesion in the deeply buried blood vessel serving the involved region.

Although the arterial circulation of the brain is endarterial in pattern, there are innumerable communications at the capillary and precapillary levels between the distributions of the various major arteries. It is apparently by means of these connections that fluid enters the damaged tissue to cause the remarkable swelling. Pathologically, this tissue is usually seen only in the acute phase when its gross characteristics are principally its softness and moistness.

Microscopically, the elements of the tissue are irregularly separated, and perivascular and pericellular spaces are widened but empty. There may be small foci of diapedesis of erythrocytes. The most frequent definite histologic change is a leukostasis in the capillaries and small vessels with occasional small fibrin thrombi and migration of leukocytes through the vascular walls. Neurons may retain an essentially normal appearance for several days after the onset of symptoms. There is no evidence of proliferative glial reaction. The lack of lymphocytic cellular infiltrate about larger vessels and the lack of the evidence of damage or death of individual neurons distinguish this picture from that of an encephalitis. Not until three to five days after the onset do macrophages, peripheral vascular proliferation, and other better-recognized reactions to an infarct appear.

Pseudotumor cerebri

Pseudotumor cerebri consists of the rather sudden appearance of the signs of increased intracranial pressure without other signs or symptoms suggestive of etiologic factors.[41,42] Almost one-half the cases occur in persons in the third decade of life. The ventricular system is normal on ventriculography, and the cerebrospinal fluid is normal to examination and analysis. Zuidema and Cohen[43] determined by follow-up of a large series that there were three etiologic groups into which such cases could be eventually assigned:

1 Early and otherwise undetectable brain tumors
2 Dural sinus thrombosis that is usually a sequela of upper respiratory infection
3 A large idiopathic group in which the prognosis for recovery is very good

If the brain is biopsied, the tissue is usually remarkably normal, but occasionally it may present the histologic picture of acute encephalomalacia.

Traumatic diseases

Patients with acute traumatic lesions of the central nervous system comprise a high percentage of those treated by the neurosurgeon. Wounds create difficult and perplexing problems in diagnosis and therapy but supply very little material of pathologic interest. The physics of the distribution of forces about the skull and the physiology of acute cranial and spinal injuries are fields of study in themselves.[45]

Acute concussion leaves no recognizable morphologic equivalent. Contusion of the brain results only in physical disruption of its substance and acute hemorrhages. Material from more chronic lesions of traumatic origin, however, is more likely to come to the attention of the pathologist during the operative relief of posttraumatic epilepsy.[44]

Dural-cortical cicatrix

The dural-cortical cicatrix as the lesion responsible for much posttraumatic epilepsy has been ably investigated and explained by Penfield and Jasper.[46] A fibrous scar and adhesions develop between the dura matter and other extra-arachnoidal fibrous tissue and the brain substance.

Penetrating wounds of the brain and its coverings are most likely to be responsible for the development of this lesion, although it can follow skull fractures, hemorrhages, or abscesses.[47] It is less commonly a postoperative complication because its development is dependent upon the introduction of extraneous fibrous tissue into the brain wound rather than upon the amount of cerebral substance destroyed or removed. This connective tissue stimulates the proliferation of astrocytes that bind it to the surrounding viable brain. Capillaries grow out from the implant of fibrous tissue into the substance of the central nervous system and anastomose with the normal vascular bed in that site. This supplies a direct union of the external and internal carotid circulations.

Because the external carotid circulation is subject to much greater variation in flow due to greater vasomotor activity, the amount of blood in this newly formed abnormal bed is subject to considerable variation. This unstable vascular bed inevitably has at least an indirect effect on the blood supply of the surrounding cortex, and it is postulated that its variations are the trigger mechanism for the convulsions.

Surgical therapy of this condition consists of accurate delimitation of the electrically abnormal cortex by means of electrocorticograms and its excision along with the overlying fibrous adhesions. The pathologic specimen is an irregular mixture of fibrous and glial tissue that is usually characterized by distinct astrocytic gliosis. There may be macrophages, hemosiderin, or other evidences of the process of the acute injury depending upon its nature and the length of time since its occurrence.

Cortical excisions for jacksonian epilepsy are sometimes performed in the absence of cortical meningeal adhesions or scars. Such specimens are usually remarkably normal in appearance but deserve full examination since they occasionally contain evidence of an otherwise silent tumor.

Epidural hematoma

Hemorrhage in the epidural space is most often arterial and posttraumatic and is due to the rupture of an artery such as the middle meningeal incidental to a fracture involving the foramen by which the artery enters the skull.[48] These lesions are acute surgical emergencies. A much more rare epidural hemorrhage may be of venous origin following trauma and of chronic duration.[49]

Subdural hematoma

Subdural hematomas are of two varieties, occurring most commonly at the two extremes of life, infancy and old age.

The type seen in infants is the result of intracranial hemorrhage that usually has occurred at the time of birth. The infant's skull is deformed and distorted by the pressure and process of birth. This places a tension and shearing force on certain structures such as the tentorium, vein of Galen, and other bridging veins. If a major vessel ruptures, the infant dies during or soon after birth, but if bleeding is slow and slight, there may be only the symptoms of lethargy that later deepen into coma. Enlargement of the head may be one of the first noticeable signs. Because of the lack of full myelination in infancy, paralytic and motor phenomena that might be expected are often lacking.

The diagnosis and even the therapy can often be performed by aspiration through the fontanel. However, fluid tends to reaccumulate in the sacs. On exploration, a thin gray membrane is found forming a sac in the subdural space.

It is filled with blood, bloody fluid, or sometimes yellow or clear fluid. The membrane itself may have yellow foci, especially on its inner surface. It is usually loosely adherent to the dura but not to the arachnoid.

Microscopically, these subdural hematomas are usually thin membranes composed of fibroblasts and relatively few blood vessels. The inner surface is often covered by a rather thick single layer of flattened cells that are probably fibroblasts. In the interstices of the tissue there are relatively few lymphocytes and histiocytes and, occasionally, foci of hemosiderin. The appearance is rarely as similar to granulation tissue as is often seen in subdural hematomas in adults. Once the blood has been removed, these membranes are apparently completely resorbed into the dura unless there is a bleeding point or a tear in the arachnoid that allows fluid to return. On rare occasions, the membranes may calcify.[52]

Essentially the same lesion sometimes develops in response to cerebrospinal fluid that has escaped into the subdural space, where it cannot be resorbed. Such lesions are called subdural hygromas. Their formation is apparently dependent upon the lack of absorptive abilities on the part of the subdural space. The fluid is supplied through the tear in the arachnoid that presumably has something of a valvular action. The membrane about the pocket of fluid is not essential to its formation or retention and may consist of little more than adhesions between the dura and the arachnoid.

Subdural hematomas in adults are considerably different lesions. Trauma to the head is almost always responsible for their formation, although there may be other factors such as a bleeding tendency or the widened subarachnoid spaces of arteriosclerotic cerebral atrophy that makes it possible for this trauma to be so slight as to pass unnoticed.

The initial lesion must be a rupture of a small bridging vein in the subdural space, although some authors have suggested that bleeding from arteries or capillaries might also be responsible. This rupture often occurs in the contrecoup position because these veins are stretched by the displacement of the skull in the line of the blow and at the same time are subjected to the convergence of the transmitted forces that pass around the vault of the skull. The initial blow may cause a period of unconsciousness due to concussion or even contusion

of the brain. In the latter instance, the patient's course is usually stormy from the very start, but it is also just as characteristic for the patient to recover consciousness and be essentially free of symptoms for a period of several weeks. There then appear, often rather suddenly, the signs and symptoms of increased intracranial pressure that may be accompanied by motor and paralytic phenomena, for these lesions are often near the motor cortex.

Pathologically, the well-developed lesion is a discoid sac filled with dark, partially laked blood (Fig. 1461). The gray membrane of the sac may be several millimeters thick. It is grossly similar on all sides of the hemorrhage but is attached to the dura on the outer side. It is smooth and unattached to the arachnoid on the inner side.

Microscopically, the membrane is composed of large fibroblasts, capillaries with thick endothelial walls, newly formed vessels and endothelial buds, and an infiltrate of histiocytes and lymphocytes (Fig. 1462). Many of the histiocytes contain hemosiderin, and hematoidin may be present to supply a grossly visible golden color. The histologic picture is quite similar to that of granulation tissue except for the absence of prominent numbers of granular leukocytes.

The mechanisms of the development of the complete symptom-producing lesion have been well investigated. Leary[51] showed that there were four recognizable anatomic stages which could supply a basis for an estimate of the time from the onset of hemorrhage.

1 For the first eighteen hours, the subdural blood remained fluid or formed soft, nonadherent clots.

2 During the second and third days, the clots were recognizably firmer and adherent to the dura.

3 From the fourth day through the second week, the blood was very dark, clotted, and sometimes separated from a yellow fluid. Evidence of organization was visible on the dural surface, but there was no inner covering or neomembrane.

4 The last stage consisted of formation of the neomembrane, which was observed in one of his patients to be completely formed thirty-nine days after injury. After the complete double membrane is formed, it may persist for months or even years with no reliable anatomic changes to represent its age.

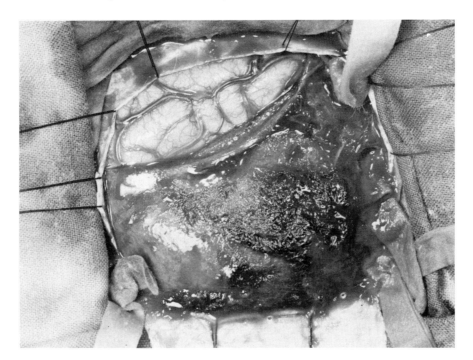

Fig. 1461 Subdural hematoma. Dura has been reflected downward, exposing neomembrane and hematoma in situ, and normal underlying pia-arachnoid and brain are exposed in upper part of field. (WU neg. 52-5356; courtesy Dr. H. G. Schwartz, St. Louis, Mo.)

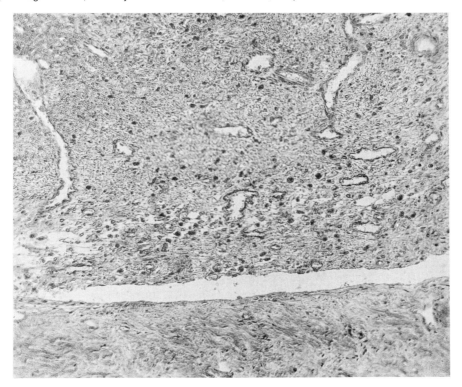

Fig. 1462 Subdural hematoma. Cleft demarcates coarse collagenous tissue of dura from overlying organized membrane of hematoma. (Masson trichrome; ×125; WU neg. 52-4240.)

The mechanism of the production of symptoms of a space-occupying lesion by an old subdural hematoma is obscure because of contradictory results form the study of different cases. A most attractive thesis, although it has apparently never been demonstrated in experimental animals, is that the hematoma begins to behave as an osmometer. With completion of the enclosing membrane, the hemorrhage becomes a volume of fluid that contains cells, proteins, and salts. Zollinger and Gross[55] demonstrated that the surrounding sac had the properties of a semipermeable membrane when removed intact and connected to an osmometer. Furthermore, the protein content of the fluid in old subdural hematomas is one-third or less than that of whole blood due to disintegration of the proteins and imbibition of fluid by means of osmotic forces. The source of this new fluid is probably the plasma of the capillaries in the surrounding membrane, and its method of accumulation accounts for the late onset of symptoms. The hemorrhage does not have a space-occupying effect until the sac is closed and its volume increased. However, there are also other phenomena that may help explain the clinical course.

Hemorrhages of various ages recognizable by the stage of preservation of erythrocytes are often seen within the membrane, so some of the increase of volume (particularly in hematomas that have been evacuated) may be due to fresh hemorrhages from the thin capillaries in the membrane. There is also a controversy as to the role of intradural hemorrhage in the formation of this lesion, but, to say the least, that theory has not gained general acceptance and would apparently apply more often to the lesions of vascular disease or hemorrhagic dyscrasias than to those of trauma.

It recently has been postulated on the basis of electron microscopic studies that (1) there is not a subdural space in the normal human brain but rather a complex, tight layer of cells—the interface layer—composed of the innermost portion of the dura (the dural border cells) and the outermost portion of the arachnoid; (2) subdural lesions form within a sheet of torn dural border cells and not within a preexistent tissue compartment; (3) the neomembrane is the result of proliferation and thickening of the layer of dural border cells.[50,53]

Therapy consists of evacuation of the hemorrhage. The membranes often have been removed against the possibility of their refilling, but experience has shown this is not always necessary or advisable.[54] The success of treatment apparently depends more upon the condition of the underlying brain than upon the operative procedure itself. Since many persons with these lesions are elderly, their brains are atrophied by the effects of arteriosclerosis and arteriolosclerosis. With removal of the hematoma, the displaced and compressed cerebral tissue does not expand and return to its normal position, and functional improvement is equally unsatisfactory. Histologic examination of the underlying cortex will show principally thickening of the small vessels and loss of neurons with a slight hypertrophy and hyperplasia of astrocytes.

Chronic arachnoiditis and arachnoidal cyst

Chronic arachnoiditis may follow the introduction of foreign substances into the subarachnoid space. This is most likely to occur in the region of the lumbar sac and to be characterized by involvement of the spinal roots of the cauda equina, but occasionally a similar etiology is blamed for the formation of pockets of fluid in the subarachnoid space that are called arachnoidal cysts. The lesion may be a sequela of accidents during spinal anesthesia, and its crippling effects may be as severe as a paraplegia.[58]

The pathologic findings are usually more obvious in situ than they are in a histologic section. A distinct thickness, grayness, and opacity of the membrane can be observed at operation. Microscopically, the most that can usually be seen is a bland fibrous membrane that is several times thicker than the normal pia-arachnoid but that contains no evidence of inflammation beyond a few lymphocytes. Only very rarely are foreign substances, macrophages, and giant cells of a foreign body reaction identifiable.

Not all arachnoidal cysts are clearly of this origin. Some are undoubtedly congenital, but all are characterized by the nonspecific histologic character of their walls.

There are also other rare cystic lesions such as epidural cerebrospinal cysts that are due to herniation of a sac of pia-arachnoid through a congenital or acquired defect of the dura. These can occur in the spinal vertebral canal and give the signs and symptoms of cord compression like a tumor.[57] Miller and Elder[56] reported ten cases of paraspinal cysts occurring as a complication of laminectomy, probably the result of a tear in the dura-arachnoid layer. The cysts communicated with the arachnoid space and were lined by flattened connective tissue cells.

Cysts also occur at the intervertebral foramina, particularly of the sacrum, where they may compress the spinal nerves. These are often filled with a rather glairy fluid and are thought to be isolated diverticula of pia-arachnoid.

Ruptured intervertebral discs

Ruptured intervertebral discs are lesions of possibly traumatic origin and are of importance principally for the effects they produce on the central nervous system.[59] The great majority of these lesions occur between the lumbar vertebrae and produce signs of irritation and destruction of fibers in the roots of the cauda equina. They also occur at higher sites, where they cause pressure upon the spinal cord itself. In these instances, the root pain characteristic of the lower lesions is not prominent. Instead, there result confusing syndromes suggestive of such degenerative diseases as amyotrophic lateral sclerosis.

The material removed at operation is only fibroelastic cartilage that may show slight degenerative changes such as fibrillar stroma and focal calcification. The essential pathologic changes are probably in the outer layers of the intervertebral disc, which are weakened and destroyed and allow the central portions to herniate. As such, they are not observed or available for study.

Inflammatory diseases

Inflammatory diseases of the central nervous system that are subject to surgical treatment are of two types. In one, the process is focal and behaves as a space-occupying lesion (abscesses, granulomas). In the second, inflammatory changes in the meninges create the necessity of decompressing the underlying nerve tissue or of relieving the obstruction in the flow of cerebrospinal fluid (hydrocephalus following meningitis and an obscure condition that can be termed a chronic pachymeningitis).

Chronic pachymeningitis

Chronic pachymeningitis has been customarily ascribed to syphilis. The typical lesion is said to be a gummatous inflammation of the dura mater in the cervical region that forms a collar about the spinal cord and compresses

it. There are, however, other cases in which there is great thickening of the dura mater in relatively wide expanses of the skull as well as in the vertebral canal. The membrane may reach a thickness of 1 cm and have the consistency of a tendon.

The symptomatology varies with the site of maximum involvement and is likely to include signs of pressure on various cranial nerves, the brainstem, or the spinal cord. Fever is sometimes present.[60]

Grossly, the tissue is a tough grayish yellow membrane several millimeters in thickness. Microscopically, it is composed of fibroblasts, collagenous fibers, and a light infiltrate of lymphocytes, plasma cells, and a few leukocytes and eosinophils. The cellular infiltrate is often concentrated in perivascular foci, and there may be small areas of necrosis. The blood vessels may be thickened and contain a few inflammatory cells in their walls.

The occurrence of fever in this disease and the localization of the lesion in the dura over the base of the skull have suggested that it may be related to chronic infection and inflammation of sinuses or retropharyngeal tissues. There is no evidence of syphilis in most patients. The course is apparently mildly progressive, and surgical removal of the thickened membrane can give worthwhile relief by decompression of involved structures.

Brain and spinal abscess

Experience with *brain abscess* has changed greatly in the years since the introduction of modern chemotherapeutic agents.[63,66] Although acute and chronic mastoiditis, which formerly anteceded a majority of brain abscesses, have declined markedly, the incidence of brain abscess appears to be about the same as it was previously.

This lesion occurs predominantly in the earlier decades of life. The symptoms are essentially those of an acute intracranial tumefaction. Headache, fever, and vomiting are the most common symptoms, and nausea, seizures, hemiplegia, and other neurologic symptoms may be observed. It is sometimes remarked that bradycardia is more common with abscesses than with tumors, presumably because of the more acute development of elevated intracranial pressure.

Two-thirds or more of the abscesses formerly were associated with local suppurative disease in the adjacent ear or nasal sinuses and one-fourth with suppurative pulmonary disease or bacterial endocarditis. The remainder followed trauma or incidental conditions or were of idiopathic origin. In the series reported by Kerr et al.,[65] one-half arose from direct extension from the ear, sinuses, or skull, and one-third were of hematogenous origin. These groupings also indicate the principal methods by which the infection reaches the brain:

1 By contiguous spread, utilizing infected thrombi in veins
2 By emboli in the arterial bloodstream or possibly distant venous embolization by way of the vertebral veins
3 By direct inoculation or unknown methods

The abscesses of the first group are associated with infection of the middle ear or sinuses about equally, although formerly they arose from the mastoid from four to nine times as frequently as from the sinuses. Lesions arising by contiguous spread and localizing in the frontal lobe or anterior fossa are characteristically associated with frontal sinusitis and subsequent osteomyelitis. Those of the middle fossa follow chronic middle ear infection. The cerebellar abscesses are associated with infected thrombosis of the lateral sinus or chronic labyrinthitis which, in turn, follows infection of the middle ear or mastoid. The abscess is not always immediately adjacent to the focus of chronic infection, however, for the inoculum can apparently be carried as an infected embolus in cerebral or diploic veins for considerable distances. In general, the proportion of temporal lobe to cerebellar involvement in abscesses following ear disease is approximately two to one, but only one-eighth of all abscesses occur in the posterior fossa.

Lesions that arise by hematogenous spread are distributed to the various parts of the brain according to their volumes. Many of the particularly unfavorable cases of multiple abscesses develop lesions by this mechanism.

The initial focus of involvement in an abscess is apparently immediately beneath the cortex which, with its high content of astrocytes, retains the developing lesion and prevents its outward rupture, although extension toward and into the ventricles is not so opposed.[61,64] Judging by our knowledge of the development of abscesses elsewhere, there must be an early stage of diffuse pyogenic inflammation followed by liquefaction of tissue and then formation of a pyogenic membrane. In the brain, this membrane is much like that of abscesses in other tissues. There is an inner zone of necrotic tissue and fibrin heavily infiltrated with leukocytes and a middle zone of proliferated capillaries and fibroblasts, which respond unusually extensively for lesions of the central nervous tissue. These zones are infiltrated with leukocytes and histiocytes which phagocytize the lipids of the destroyed brain. Beyond this, there is a zone of astrocytic glial proliferation that is naturally characteristic of abscesses in this tissue. A plane of cleavage often exists in this region so that well-encapsulated abscesses can be enucleated with removal of very little adherent surrounding brain. The pyogenic membrane about an abscess of the brain requires at least two weeks for complete development, but its first traces in wounds can be seen grossly is as few as four or five days.

The bacterial etiology of brain abscesses may be staphylococci, streptococci, pneumococci, or various other organisms, especially gram-negative rods. Pneumococci and beta hemolytic streptococci are much less frequent causative organisms than formerly, while anaerobic streptococci and enterococci are of increased importance. Many abscesses today are sterile by culture at the time of operation.

Many different methods of surgical treatment of abscesses have been used. The single most important contribution to their effective therapy has been the modern antibiotics. It has been long recognized that operation upon a well-encapsulated lesion may give the most favorable result, but many patients become desperately ill before complete encapsulation takes place. Mortality rates of greater than 40% were the rule before the spread of infection could be so well controlled by drugs, but a rate of less than 20% may now be expected if the abscesses are not multiple. Excision and treatment of early abscesses in the stages before encapsulation may be even more effective.[67] It is significant that in one series of cerebellar abscesses, only two of nine patients survived before the advent of penicillin, whereas eight of nine survived when penicillin was used. Chemotherapy is not the whole answer, however, and there remains the necessity of surgical drainage or removal of loculated suppuration.

Spinal abscess usually is located in the epidural space. *Staphylococcus areus* is the most common etiologic agent. In one series, osteomyelitis was the source of infection in 38% of the cases and bacteremia in 26%; 16% of the cases were due to postoperative infection.[62]

Granulomatous diseases

Granulomas of the central nervous system may be caused by tuberculosis, syphilis, or various fungous diseases, such as cryptococcosis, actinomycosis, or mucormycosis. Because of their space-occupying properties, these lesions present a clinical picture essentially that of a tumor. They make up 2%-3% of a group of lesions diagnosed at first as tumors. The infectious inoculum of these lesions is borne by the blood to the central nervous system, and its localization there is consequently dependent upon the relative size and vascularity of the various areas. Being a disease of adults, granulomas are, therefore, relatively more common in the posterior fossa than are primary glial tumors.

The histology of these lesions is comparable to that of the same diseases as they occur elsewhere with perhaps a relatively less prominent fibroblastic component in their composition. Tuberculous infections can be accompanied by multiple cerebral infarcts due to tuberculous arteritis. Fungous lesions vary from those that are more properly described as abscesses to others that are quite solid and like tuberculomas or gummas.[68,69,70] The specific diagnosis rests upon the recognition of the causative organisms either in tissues or by culture.

Other inflammatory diseases

Parasitic infestation of the central nervous system by *Cysticercus, Amoeba,* or *Echinococcus* is rare in this country. Depending upon the number and size of the lesions, they can present the symptoms of either space-occupying masses or a more diffuse process suggestive of an encephalitis. Rayport et al.[72] have reported an interesting case in which hydatids of *Echinococcus* in the vertebra resulted in a compression myelopathy.

A case of *plasma cell granuloma* (inflammatory pseudotumor) that involved the spinal cord meninges and led to symptoms of spinal cord compression has been reported.[71]

Tumors
Introduction

Neoplasms of the central nervous system have several unique features, some as the result of the very specialized tissue from which they originate and others from the anatomic peculiarities of this region.[75a] This should not detract from the fact that, by and large, their morphologic patterns and biologic behavior can be adequately studied by applying the same principles and techniques as those employed for tumors elsewhere in the body. Knowledge of the age of the patient, exact location of the tumor, and its gross appearance at operation are essential pieces of information that the pathologist should possess in order to properly evaluate a microscopic slide. Examination by frozen section at the time of operation is as accurate for neural neoplasms as it is for tumors in general.[73,74]

Much has been argued about the value of silver and gold impregnation techniques (principally those of Golgi, Cajal, and del Rio Hortega) in the identification of central nervous system neoplasms. Some pathologists believe they are essential for the proper classification of these tumors and advocate their use as a routine procedure.[76] Others seriously doubt their diagnostic utility. It seems obvious that they have greatly contributed to our understanding of this family of neoplasms and that the researcher in the field might still profit from them, as he might profit from electron microscopic examination, tissue culture studies, or histochemical techniques. But we must agree with Willis,[78] Kernohan and Sayre,[75] Rubinstein,[77] and many others that, in the overwhelming majority of the cases, examination of sections from formalin-fixed, paraffin-embedded material stained with hematoxylin-eosin (sometimes supplemented by PTAH, reticulin, or other stains) is perfectly adequate for the classification and prognostic evaluation of tumors of the central nervous system.

Tumors of neuroglial cells
Astrocytoma

Tumors originated from adult astrocytes are the most common type of glioma and, for that matter, the most common primary neoplasms of the central nervous system. All ages are affected. It is very useful to divide astrocytomas into clinicopathologic varieties on the basis of their different age incidence, location, and biologic behavior.

Cerebral astrocytomas are generally tumors of adults. Their gross boundaries are very difficult to define. They are solid, whitish or gray, and may infiltrate the cortex, white matter, or basal ganglia. The microscopic diagnosis is often difficult, since the cells are mature

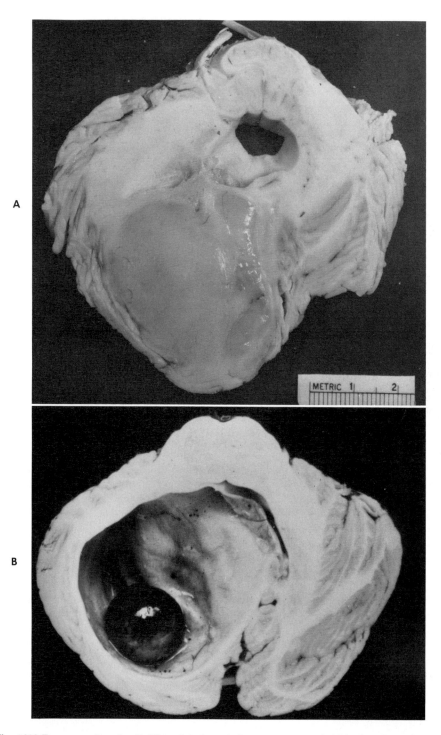

Fig. 1463 Two examples of well-differentiated cerebellar astrocytoma of children, illustrating two most common forms of gross presentation. **A,** Predominantly solid neoplasm of gray color and firm consistency. **B,** Cystic tumor with sharply circumscribed, hemorrhagic mural nodule. (**A,** UVa neg. 11,148; **B,** WU neg. 72-5924; from Rubinstein LJ: Seminario de Neuropatología, Mérida, Yucatán. Bol Asoc Mex Patol AC **7:**13-59, 1969; courtesy Dr. J. E. Olvera-Rabiela, Mexico City, Mexico.)

and widely scattered between normal structures. The only clue to the diagnosis in a biopsy may be slight nuclear enlargement and hyperchromasia, with accumulation of cells beneath the pia, around neurons or surrounding the Virchow-Robin spaces.[101] The cytologic appearance seen in a small biopsy may not be representative of the whole neoplasm. We have seen many cases in which extremely well-differentiated astrocytes in the superficial portion of the tumor coexisted with highly atypical cells in deeper areas. Grading of these tumors is, therefore, of little prognostic value.

Cerebellar astrocytomas are predominantly tumors of children.[86] They may occupy the cerebellar hemispheres or the vermis or even extend within the cavity of the fourth ventricle. Grossly, they may appear solid, of a homogeneous gray color, firm consistency, and ill-defined borders, or as a cystic mass with a mural, frequently hemorrhagic nodule (Fig. 1463). Microscopically, cellular areas composed of mature fibrillary astrocytes are present, often surrounding microcystic formations containing an eosinophilic amorphous material (Fig. 1464). Multinucleated astrocytes may be seen, but mitoses are exceptional. Rosenthal's fibers, representing amorphous aggregates of unknown composition in the glial cell process, often can be identified.[88] Ultrastructurally, numerous filaments and microtubules are seen (Fig. 1465). Cerebellar astrocytomas are among the most benign tumors of the brain. Their successful removal will result in a complete and permanent cure.[80]

Astrocytomas of the third ventricle are sometimes called pilocytic (hairlike), because of the marked elongation of the tumor cells which has been responsible in the past for the erroneous designation of this tumor as polar spongioblastoma. Specific silver stains, growth in tissue culture, and electron microscopic studies have clearly demonstrated their astrocytic nature.[91,100] Rosenthal's fibers and microcystic areas often are encountered.

Astrocytomas of the pons and medulla are generally tumors of children. Grossly, they are solid, gray or whitish and result in a symmetri-

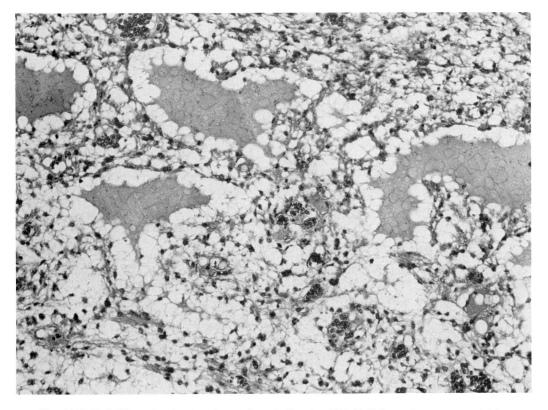

Fig. 1464 Well-differentiated astrocytoma of cerebellum in child. Multiple cystic spaces containing proteinaceous material are characteristic. (×175; WU neg. 73-2665.)

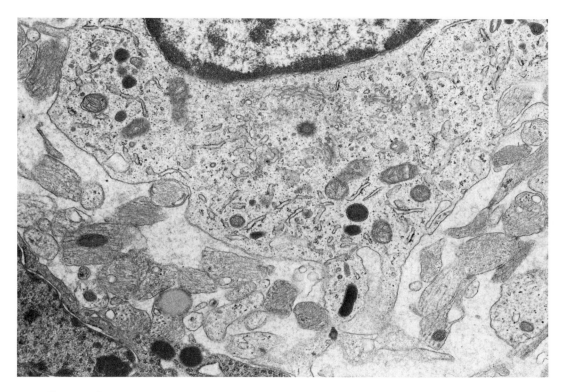

Fig. 1465 Grade II astrocytoma of fourth ventricle characterized by intercellular processes containing numerous thick microfilaments, occasional microtubules and small numbers of mitochondria, endoplasmic reticulum, and ribosomes. (×16,850.)

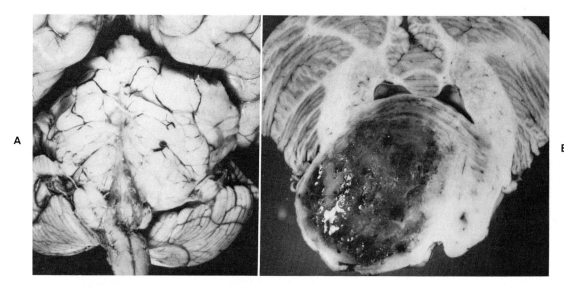

Fig. 1466 A, External appearance of astrocytoma of pons, illustrating symmetrical enlargement of structure often seen in this tumor. **B,** Cross section of astrocytoma of pons, showing hemorrhagic tumor of ill-defined margins partially obliterating fourth ventricle. (**A,** WU neg. 72-5923; **B,** WU neg. 72-5926; courtesy Dr. J. E. Olvera-Rabiela, Mexico City, Mexico.)

cal enlargement of the pons and medulla (Fig. 1466). Microscopically, a whole spectrum of cytologic atypia can be found, even within the same neoplasm. A significant portion of the cells has pilocytic configuration.

Astrocytomas of the spinal cord are more common in the thoracic and cervical segments. They are solid, of firm consistency, and often elongated. They are characteristically intramedullary in location; however, a few primary extramedullary tumors have been observed, presumably arising from the heterotopic glial tissue that is occasionally found in the subarachnoid space.[81] Microscopically, they display no specific characteristics. Like those of the brainstem and third ventricle, they may contain pilocytic elements.

Astrocytomas of the optic nerve constitute the majority of the tumors collectively named "optic nerve glioma," the remaining being oligodendrogliomas. The distinction is difficult and often requires silver impregnation techniques. In children, optic nerve astrocytomas are slow growing and usually behave as benign neoplasms. In adults, this tumor is often highly aggressive and fatal.[92]

In *diffuse astrocytoma (gliomatosis cerebri)*, neoplastic astrocytes are seen occupying extensive areas of the cerebrum, cerebellum, and brainstem without producing a grossly evident tumor mass.[83] Most cells are microscopically mature but, as in other astrocytomas, anaplastic foci are occasionally detected.

It is obvious that age, location, and gross features, in conjunction with the microscopic appearance, play an important role in the characterization of the varieties of astrocytomas already mentioned. In addition, there are histologic features that need to be recognized and evaluated independently of the foregoing. The occurrence of *pilocytic astrocytomas* has already been alluded to. It probably represents a secondary feature dictated by the disposition of the preexisting nerve fibers and has no particular prognostic significance. Although the pilocytic cells are almost always well differentiated, this does not preclude the existence of anaplastic elements in other portions of the tumor. *Gemistocytic astrocytomas*, in which the tumor astrocytes are characterized by an abundant, brightly acidophilic cytoplasm, can be seen as a pure form (particularly in the cerebellum or, in patients with tuberous sclerosis, in the wall of the lateral ventricles) or, most commonly, intermingled with areas of ordinary astrocytoma. Their presence has no prognostic significance but for the fact that they appear most commonly in well-differentiated neoplasms.

Astrocytic tumors formed by compact small cells that arrange themselves around blood vessels were designated as *astroblastomas* by Bailey and Bucy.[79] Only rarely are they present as a pure form. In most instances, this pattern of growth is seen focally as an otherwise typical astrocytoma or in an undifferentiated glioma.

Kepes et al.[95a] have identified what they regard as another distinctive form of supratentorial astrocytoma, which they designate as *pleomorphic xanthoastrocytoma*. This tumor occurs in young patients, involves the leptomeninges extensively, and has a relatively favorable prognosis. Microscopically, there is marked pleomorphism, including bizarre giant cells and mitotic figures, but no necrosis. Many of the tumor cells contain cytoplasmic fat and are surrounded by reticulin fibers, thus simulating a mesenchymal tumor and specifically a fibrous histiocytoma (fibrous xanthoma).[95a] However, the astrocytic lineage was demonstrated by the presence of glial fibrillary acidic protein.[95b]

The most important feature to evaluate in the microscopic examination of an astrocytoma is the presence of atypia of the tumor astrocytes, evidenced by nuclear enlargement, nucleolar prominence, and mitotic activity, often accompanied by vascular proliferation and areas of necrosis. The occurrence of these alterations can be regarded as a reliable sign forecasting aggressive clinical behavior, which may be manifest by local invasion of the surrounding parenchyma and meninges, spread through the cerebrospinal fluid pathways, and, exceptionally, by metastatic involvement of distant organs. On the other hand, the absence of these atypical features in a biopsy specimen should not be used as conclusive evidence that the tumor lacks these properties. Astrocytomas are well known for their marked variations in degrees of maturity from area to area. This variability, although rare in cerebellar tumors, is quite common in neoplasms of the cerebral hemispheres.

The astrocytic lineage of many cytologically malignant glial neoplasms is evident with the use of special stains or, in hematoxylin-eosin sections, by the common intermingling of well-differentiated elements. The identification of glial fibrillary acidic protein by immunohisto-

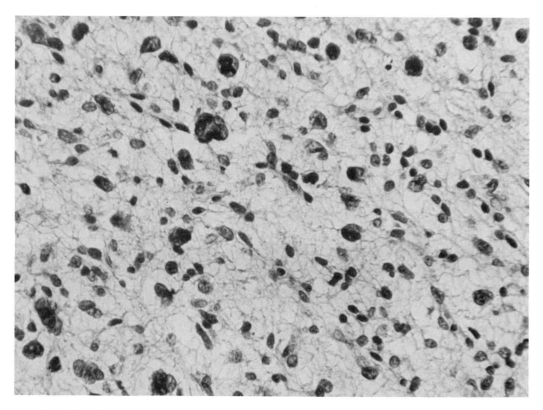

Fig. 1467 Malignant astrocytoma of cerebral hemisphere. Despite marked cytologic atypia, astrocytic nature of tumor is evident even in routinely stained sections. (×300; WU neg. 73-2689.)

chemical techniques is particularly useful in this regard, this protein being absent in cells of the oligodendroglial, neuronal, and meningothelial series.[81a, 85a,104a] The term *malignant astrocytoma* is properly applied to this tumor type (Fig. 1467). In other cases, however, the dedifferentiation is so great that an astrocytic origin cannot be established. The designation of *glioblastoma multiforme* has traditionally been given to this variety.[94] This term is unsatisfactory on several grounds. First, it implies an origin from (or at least a relationship with) the embryonal glioblast that has not been proved. Second, it conveys the impression of a specific tumor type when it simply represents the undifferentiated form of all types of gliomas. Admittedly, the large majority of tumors called glioblastoma multiforme are of astrocytic origin, as demonstrated by special stains, immunohistochemistry for glial fibrillary acidic protein,[85a,104a] tissue culture, and electron microscopy,[98] but oligodendrogliomas and ependymomas may result in an identical microscopic appearance. Therefore, it seems more logical to simply call these tumors *undifferentiated gliomas.* The majority occur in the cerebral hemispheres (particularly frontal lobes) of adults, but they also can present in childhood.[82] Grossly, they often have a sharper border than their better differentiated counterparts. Areas of necrosis are almost always encountered. Cystic degeneration and hemorrhage may be present (Figs. 1468 and 1469). Invasion of the meninges and ventricular cavities is a common event. Multiple foci are sometimes found.[104]

Microscopically, highly cellular areas, which are always present, alternate with large necrotic foci. In many cases, the tumor cells show a wide diversity of sizes and shapes—hence the designation of "multiforme." Round, polygonal, oval, and markedly elongated elements can all be present. Intranuclear "inclusion bodies" are frequent.[99] They represent cytoplasmic invaginations lying within nuclear folds.[97] It is not uncommon to find multinucleated tumor giant cells with abundant acidophilic cytoplasm (Fig. 1470). Tumors in which

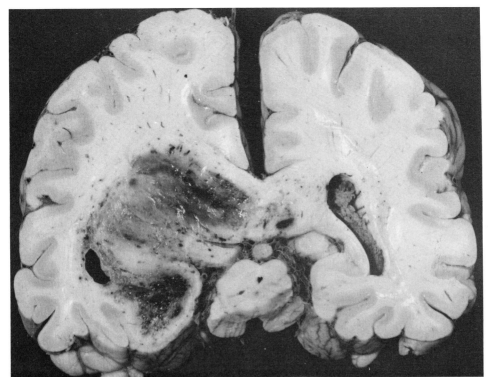

1468

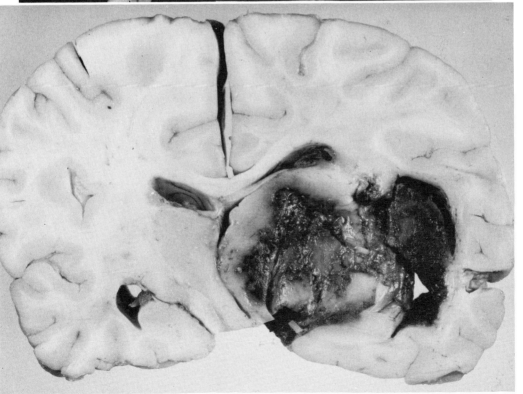

1469

Fig. 1468 Undifferentiated glioma of left parietal and temporal lobes with extension into corpus callosum. Variegated surface and foci of hemorrhage are characteristic. (UVa neg. 11,026.)

Fig. 1469 Massive hemorrhage within substance of undifferentiated glioma. This complication is often the first clinical manifestation of disease. Note marked displacement of midline structures. (WU neg. 72-2479.)

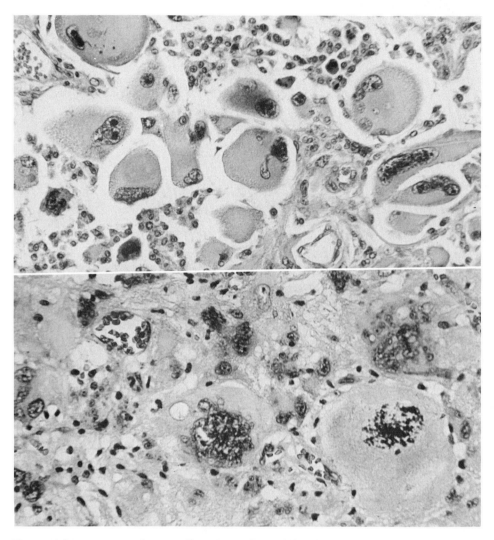

Fig. 1470 Bizarre tumor cells in undifferentiated glioma. Although tumors containing such elements have been interpreted by some as sarcomas, special staining techniques and electron microscopy have clearly evidenced their glial derivation. (×300; WU negs. 73-2683 and 73-2688.)

these cells represent the predominant type have been regarded in the past as sarcomas, but there is now convincing ultrastructural evidence for their glial derivation.[89,96] Paradoxically, gliomas with these features seem to be associated with a slightly better prognosis.[80a]

It is characteristic for the tumor cells of undifferentiated glioma to concentrate around foci of the necrosis, resulting in a palisading effect (Fig. 1471, A). This is an important differential feature with metastatic carcinoma, since in the latter the necrosis tends to spare perivascular collections of tumor cells, leading to the so-called ''perithelial'' effect. Another constant microscopic feature of undifferentiated gliomas

is represented by the vascular changes. The most common abnormality is a marked proliferation of the endothelium (and perhaps also the perithelium) of the capillaries, resulting in the formation of highly cellular nests with a narrow central lumen (Fig. 1471, B). It should be remarked that this change also can be seen, although less commonly, in oligodendrogliomas, well-differentiated astrocytomas, and even metastatic carcinomas. Other vascular changes of undifferentiated gliomas include perivascular fibrosis, marked dilatation of the lumen, and thrombosis. Ultrastructurally, the vascular changes include fenestration, widened intercellular junctions, increase in pinocytotic

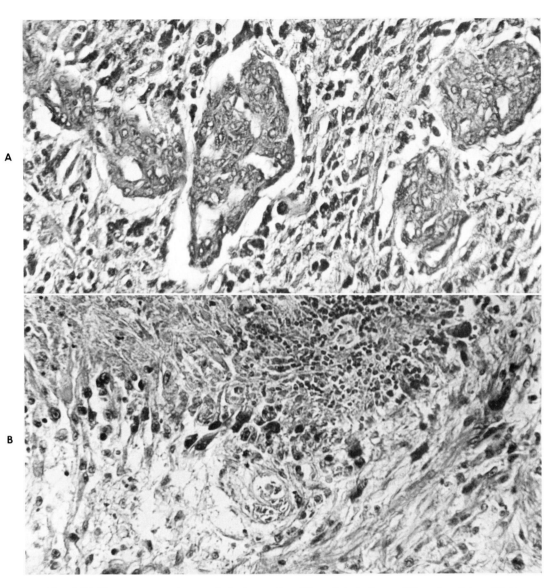

Fig. 1471 Two common microscopic features of undifferentiated glioma. Although not completely specific, they are of considerable diagnostic value. **A,** Marked proliferation of blood vessels within tumor mass. Both endothelial and perithelial cells participate. **B,** Palisading of tumor cells around foci of necrosis. Note fact that necrosis shows no particular relationship to blood vessels. (**A,** ×300; WU neg. 73-2687; **B,** ×300; WU neg. 73-2684.)

vesicles, and infolding of the luminal surface.[90] Cases have been described in which glioblastoma multiforme was interpreted as coexisting with sarcoma, the latter presumably arising from the proliferating endothelial cells or fibroblasts of the stroma.[85,87] An increased incidence of extracranial metastases has been observed in this particular variety.[103] An alternative explanation for these lesions is that they represent glioblastomas with focal sarcomatoid transfor-

mation, analogous to the more common spindle cell metaplasia and desmoplastic reaction that is sometimes seen in these tumors, especially in areas of meningeal invasion.

Undifferentiated gliomas infiltrate the central nervous system locally and often extend to the overlying subarachnoid space, from which location they can spread away from the primary site. Spinal subarachnoidal seeding from a primary intracranial tumor has been thought to be uncommon, but Erlich and Davis[84] found it in five of twenty patients. Of all primary tumors of the central nervous system, undifferentiated gliomas are the ones most commonly associated with the production of extracranial metastases. The most important factor in the development of this complication is direct access of the glioma to the extrameningeal tissues.[95c] This is preceded in most cases by a surgical intervention,[102] but it may be seen in its absence.[93] The most common sites are the lungs and cervical lymph nodes. Undifferentiated gliomas are among the most malignant tumors of the human body.[105] The two-year mortality following operation approaches 90%. Jelsma and Bucy[95] showed that two favorable prognostic signs, relatively speaking, are gross circumscription of the tumor and young age of the patient. Radiation therapy in high doses can induce a retardation in tumor growth but almost never a total sterilization; furthermore, "late delayed" radiation necrosis of the adjacent white matter and other forms of injury can occur.[80b]

Oligodendroglioma

A rare form of glioma, oligodendroglioma presents most often as a slow-growing neoplasm in adults,[106a,114] although there is also a small peak in childhood. Grossly, it is well circumscribed, soft, and sometimes of a gelatinous appearance. Cystic changes are very common. Foci of calcification are present in 70% of the cases and are sufficiently numerous in 40% to be detectable roentgenographically. Microscopically, the most common and best known pattern is that of a uniformly cellular neoplasm composed of round cells with a small darkly staining nucleus, clear cytoplasm, and clearly defined cell membrane (Fig. 1472). This type is most commonly seen in the cerebral hemispheres, although the cerebellum and spinal cord also may be affected. In the second variety, most frequently seen in the optic nerve and chiasma and in the corpus callosum, the tumor cells are elongated. Transitions often occur. At the periphery of the neoplasm, it is not uncommon for the tumor cells to surround neurons in a fashion similar to that of reactive glial cells.[111] Morphologic variations that may result in diagnostic difficulties include separation into well-defined nests by connective tissue septa, accumulation of a PAS-positive cytoplasmic mucosubstance, formation of signet-ring cells,[110] and aggregates of large cells rich in eosinophilic granular cytoplasm, somewhat similar to reactive astrocytes. Takei et al.[113] confirmed the oligodendroglial nature of

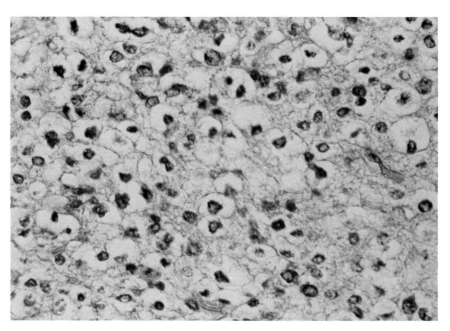

Fig. 1472 Oligodendroglioma with typical perinuclear clear zones of unstained cytoplasm. (×750; WU neg. 52-4237.)

the latter by electron microscopy and showed that the granules correspond to cytoplasmic bodies of autophagic-vacuole type. In most cases, other glial elements (particularly astrocytes) are present in addition to the oligodendrocytes. If these two cell types are present in approximately equal amounts, the designation of *mixed glioma* is justified. Ultrastructurally, a striking concentric arrangement of cytoplasmic processes of the tumor cells was described by Robertson and Vogel.[109]

The behavior of this tumor is quite erratic. Presence of marked cytologic atypia can be correlated with a biologically aggressive tumor, but the reverse is not necessarily true. Local recurrence is to be expected in approximately

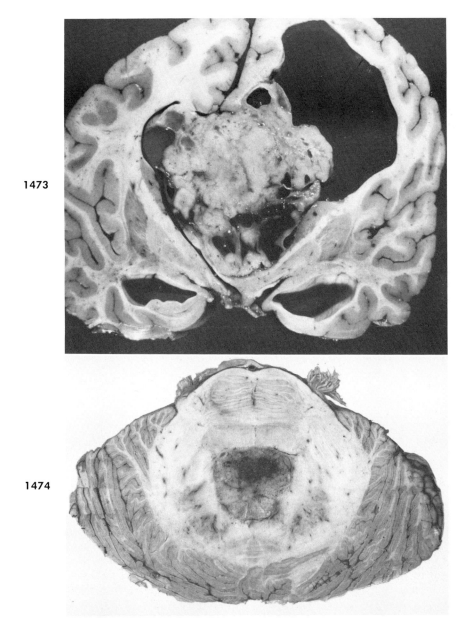

1473

1474

Fig. 1473 Large septal ependymoma, with secondary hyrocephalus. (WU neg. 72-5943; courtesy Dr. J. E. Olvera-Rabiela, Mexico City, Mexico.)
Fig. 1474 Ependymoma of fourth ventricle. This tumor should be distinguished from choroid plexus papilloma. (Courtesy Dr. E. Lascano, Buenos Aires, Argentina.)

50% of the cases.[108] Clinical malignancy is manifested by dissemination through the cerebrospinal pathways and, exceptionally, by the appearance of distant metastases.[106,112] A case has been described of an oligodendroglioma associated with a sarcoma-like component, a phenomenon analogous to that previously mentioned in connection with astrocytomas.[107]

Ependymoma

Ependymoma constitues only 5% of all intracranial gliomas in adults and 8%-9% in children.[118] On the other hand, it represents the most common intramedullary glioma. It may be seen in all ages. The most common locations are the ventricles (particularly the fourth), the lumbosacral portion of the spinal cord, and the filum terminale (Figs. 1473 and 1474). The majority of the intracranial tumors occur in children, while the large majority of the intraspinal tumors are seen in adults.[123] In a significant proportion of cases, anatomic connection of the tumor with the ventricular cavity cannot be demonstrated.[119] We have seen extraneural ependymomas appearing in the soft tissues of the sacrococcygeal region.[115] The tumor is almost always solitary, except in the variant known as supependymoma and in patients with Recklinghausen's disease.

Grossly, the most common appearance of ependymoma is that of a well-circumscribed, granular, friable gray mass. When located in the filum terminale, it typically presents as a fusiform enlargement of this structure (Fig. 1475).

Microscopically, the most important distinguishing feature (although not always demonstrable in biopsy material) is the presence of ependymal rosettes. These are ductlike structures with a round or elongated central lumen around which columnar tumor cells are arranged concentrically. The nuclei lie in a basal position. Cilia and blepharoplasts often can be demonstrated. These rosettes, which in this location are diagnostic of ependymomas, should be clearly differentiated from Wright's rosettes of neuroblastomas and medulloblastomas. The latter are an expression of neuroblastic differentiation and are therefore never present in ependymomas. Formation of perivascular pseudorosettes is another feature of ependymoma and often the only clue to the diagnosis. In routinely stained sections, these structures appear quite similar to those of astroblastoma, although specific silver impregna-

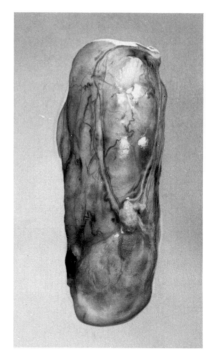

Fig. 1475 Ependymoma of spinal cord. Elongated shape and encapsulation are characteristic. (WU neg. 51-3014.)

tions differentiate them easily.[125] Foci of calcification can be identified in 15% of the cases. Occasionally, foci of metaplastic bone and cartilage are encountered.[122] It is not uncommon for ependymomas to be admixed with an astrocytic component, thus constituting a form of mixed glioma. Malignant histologic variants, which are rare, are recognized by the usual features of malignancy, such as invasive properties, cytologic atypia, and large foci of necrosis. These tumors can be properly called malignant ependymomas, and an aggressive clinical behavior can be predicted.[128] This implies seeding of the subarachnoid space and, exceptionally, extraneural metastases. On the other hand, a "benign" microscopic appearance does not guarantee a benign clinical evolution, although this will be the case in the majority of the instances. Ultrastructurally, tumor ependymal cells retain many of the features of the normal parent cells, particularly their specialized connections, cilia, ciliary rootlets (blepharoplasts), and microvilli.[120] Location of the tumor is a very good prognostic indicator; this is partially dependent on the microscopic type of the tumor[123] (Fig. 1476).

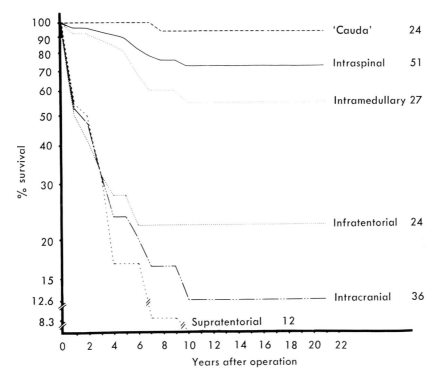

Fig. 1476 Cumulative survival rates for ependymoma depending on its location. (From Mørk SJ, Løken AC: Ependymoma. A follow-up study of 101 cases. Cancer **40**:907-915, 1977.)

There are two types of ependymomas that deserve to be treated separately because of their distinctive clinicopathologic features: myxopapillary ependymoma and subependymoma.

Myxopapillary ependymoma occurs exclusively in the region of the conus medullaris and filum terminale. It constitutes the majority of tumors of this region.[116,121] Grossly, it presents as a fusiform enlargement of the filum terminale sometimes attached to the meninges. Microscopically, the distinctive feature is the presence of papillae centered by dilated blood vessels, surrounded by an abundant mucinous stroma and covered by one or more layers of regular cuboidal tumor cells (Fig. 1477). Fusion of adjacent papillae results in a complicated reticular pattern. A very common mistake is to confuse these tumors with chordomas. Rawlinson et al.[124] have described the fine structural appearance of this neoplasm. The prognosis is generally good, although exceptional cases with distant metastases have been reported.[126]

Subependymomas most often represent an incidental necropsy finding in the cerebral ventricles, where they present as multiple small nodules protruding into the cavity. Microscopically, they seem to be composed of an admixture of ependymal cells and subependymal astrocytes.[117] Rarely, they are symptomatic.[127]

Mixed glioma

It is not generally recognized that a relatively large proportion of glial tumors of the central nervous system have a composite cell population composed of varying mixtures of oligodendroglioma, astrocytoma and ependymoma.[129] The different cell types may be separated in clumps or be closely intermingled. The two most common combinations are oligodendroglioma-astrocytoma and ependymoma-astrocytoma. Probably the term should be restricted to those tumors in which there is roughly an equivalent amount of two or more cell types. The others are better designated on the basis of the predominant population. Mixed gliomas can be graded using the same criteria as applied to astrocytomas; this grading correlates well with prognosis.[129]

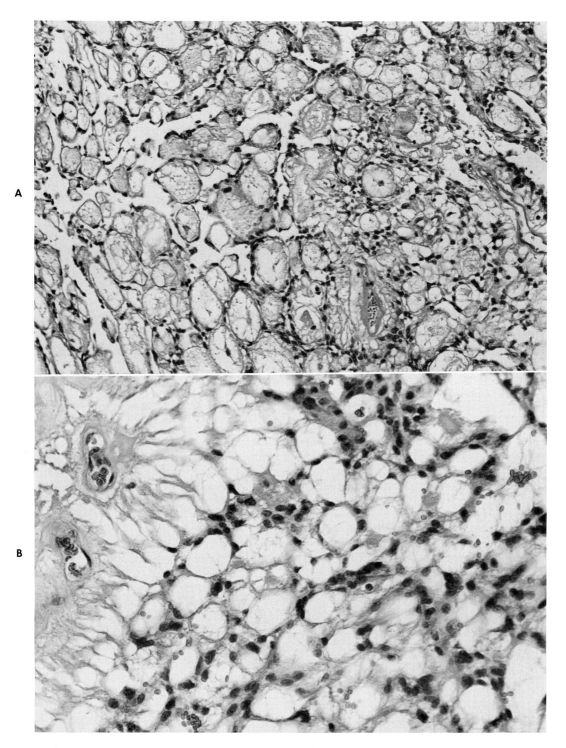

Fig. 1477 Myxopapillary ependymoma of cauda equina. **A,** Small cuboidal ependymal cells line papillae containing large amount of myxoid intercellular material. **B,** Reticulated appearance of tumor can result in mistaken diagnosis of chordoma. Note relationship with blood vessel wall. (**A,** ×150; WU neg. 73-2662; **B,** ×300; WU neg. 73-2953.)

Tumors and tumorlike conditions of choroid plexus

Although tumors of the choroid plexus can be regarded as variants of ependymoma, their highly specialized nature and distinctive appearance justify a separation from the latter.

Choroid papilloma is by far the commonest variety. Young male children are most commonly affected. The cavity and lateral recesses of the fourth ventricle are the commonest sites of involvement. The appearance of a large tumor mass in the cerebellopontine angle is a frequent form of presentation. In younger children, the tumor prefers the lateral ventricles, where it may reach a large size. The internal hydrocephalus frequently encountered may be due to secretory activity by the tumor.[137] The primarily intraventricular growth is responsible for the paucity of symptoms in the early stages of the disease.

Grossly, choroid plexus papilloma appears as an intraventricular mass of obvious papillary configuration (Fig. 1478). Microscopically, the tumor duplicates the structure of the normal choroid plexus, with its formation of fibrovascular fronds lined by a single layer of uniform cuboidal or columnar cells of almost epithelial appearance[132] (Fig. 1479). The similarities with benign papillary mesothelioma are striking. Exceptionally, mucus-producing columnar cells are present. Excision is curative. A few instances of microscopically benign choroid plexus papillomas that have seeded throughout the neuraxis have been documented.[138]

Choroid carcinomas are extremely rare.[136] Although they retain some of the papillary configuration of the papillomas, they differ from them because of invasion of the adjacent brain and the presence of malignant cytologic features (Fig. 1480). Most of the cases have occurred in children and have shown a marked

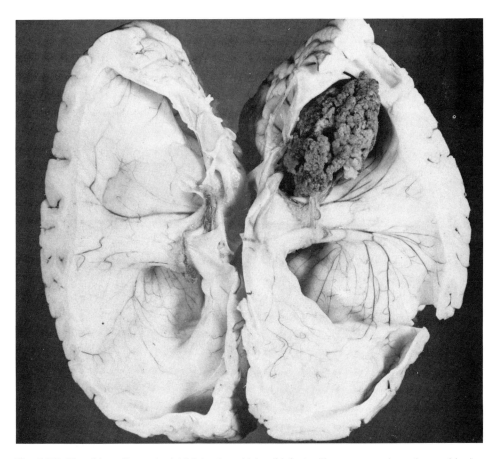

Fig. 1478 Choroid papilloma in right lateral ventricle of infant with accompanying advanced hydrocephalus. (WU neg. 50-3245.)

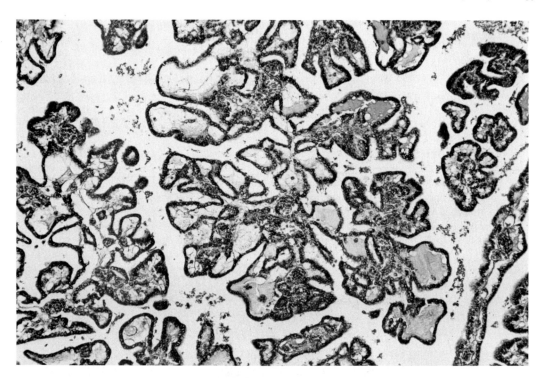

Fig. 1479 Choroid plexus papilloma removed from right lateral ventricle of 8-month-old male infant. Tumor is made of innumerable papillary fronds lined by cuboidal epithelium and supported by delicate fibrovascular cores. (×150; WU neg. 73-2661.)

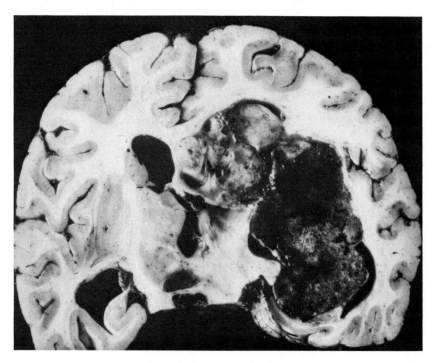

Fig. 1480 Carcinoma of choroid plexus filling lateral ventricle and invading brain substance. (Courtesy Dr. J. E. Olvera-Rabiela, Mexico City, Mexico.)

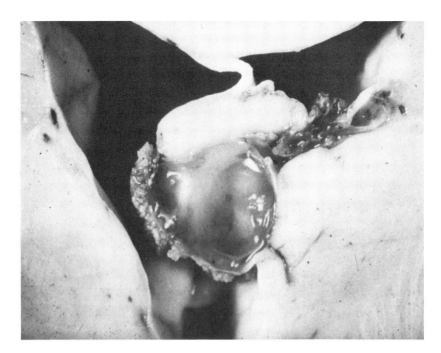

Fig. 1481 Typical gross appearance of colloid cyst of third ventricle. It is easy to imagine how this formation may result in acute hydrocephalus. (Courtesy Dr. J. E. Olvera-Rabiela, Mexico City, Mexico.)

propensity for spread throughout the ventricular and subarachnoid spaces. Great caution should be exercised in the diagnosis of choroid carcinomas, especially in adults. *The large majority of papillary and/or glandular malignant tumors involving the ventricles represent metastatic carcinoma.*

Not infrequently, collections of foamy macrophages are found incidentally in the choroid plexus, resulting in the formation of a yellowish plaque or nodule. Although they have been sometimes dignified with the designation of *xanthogranuloma*, they do not represent true neoplasms and are of no clinical significance.[131]

Colloid (neuroepithelial) cysts occur most commonly in the anterior part of the third ventricle, but they can develop in any part of the cerebral ventricular system.[135] Whether they arise from the paraphysis, ependymal pouches from the diencephalon, or the choroid plexus epithelium is still unsettled.[130,134] The cyst is usually unilocular and contains a fluid which may appear clear or milky (Fig. 1481). The wall is quite thin, made of fibrous tissue, and lined by one layer of low cuboidal epithelium, sometimes ciliated.[133] It may reach a diameter of 3 or 4 cm. Cysts measuring 1 cm or less

are usually asymptomatic. The cases that become clinically manifest frequently do so during the third or fourth decade. Acute hydrocephalus, sometimes fatal, may develop as a result of blockage of the foramen of Monro. Operative removal of the cyst results in relief of almost all symptoms, except those due to permanent damage of neighboring structures.

Tumors of primitive neuroepithelial cells

Rubinstein[162] has lucidly discussed the cytogenesis, morphology, and possible relationships of embryonal tumors of the central nervous system—i.e., tumors which arise during embryonal, fetal, or early postnatal development from tissues that are still immature. Although in an individual case the distinction may not be easy, this group of neoplasms should be clearly separated from those previously discussed, which are presumed to arise from adult differentiated cells. As is usually the case with embryonal tumors in general, those originating in the central nervous system almost always affect infants or children. They may arise at any stage of the differentiation process and thereby acquire a wide spectrum of morphologic patterns.[143,148] The best defined varieties are given specific names, as indicated in Table 72, but it should be realized that mixed and intermediate forms are not infrequently encountered.

Medulloepithelioma

Medulloepithelioma is the most undifferentiated member of the group, in the sense that it recapitulates the structure of the primitive medullary epithelium and shows minimal or no signs of neuroblastic, spongioblastic, or ependymal differentiation.[151] All of the few reported cases have occurred in infants or children.[166,167] The cerebral hemispheres have been the preferred location, either in or near the ventricular system. Microscopically, the tumor is made up of tubules and papillae lined by columnar or cuboidal cells, often pseudostratified and with high mitotic activity. Since malignant teratomas may contain neural elements with an identical appearance, this possibility should always be eliminated by generous sampling of the tumor. The differential diagnosis should also include malignant ependymoma, choroid plexus carcinoma, and metastatic carcinoma. The former is identified by the presence of rosettes, blepharoplasts, and/or ependymal rosettes. Ultrastructurally, the appearance of this tumor is similar to that of the fetal neural tube.[158] The behavior of medulloepithelioma is that of a highly malignant tumor, prone to local recurrence, leptomeningeal spread, and distant metastases.

Medulloblastoma

Medulloblastoma is the commonest and most controversial of all the embryonal neuroectodermal tumors. Despite all the arguments and uncertainties regarding its cytogenesis and the justified criticisms that have been voiced to the term medulloblastoma, there is little doubt that it constitutes a definite clinicopathologic entity.

More than one-half of the cases occur in the first decade of life.[146] Medulloblastoma accounts of over 25% of all intracranial tumors in children. *It occurs exclusively in the cerebellum.* The classical presentation is that of a midline tumor involving the vermis and often extending into the fourth ventricle. Rarely, it is found in one of the cerebellar hemispheres.

Grossly, it is soft, friable, and well circumscribed. Its color varies from gray to pinkish (Fig. 1482). Microscopically, it is a highly cellular neoplasm. The nuclei are closely packed, hyperchromatic, relatively uniform, and round, oval, or carrot-shaped. In the absence of previous radiation therapy, the presence of giant or bizarre cells makes the diagnosis of medulloblastoma very unlikely. The cytoplasm is scanty, and the cytoplasmic margins are indistinct.[145] Rosettes centered by neurofibrillary material are encountered in approximately one-third of the cases. These should not be confused with areas of perivascular arrangement of the tumor cells, which may also occur. Matakas et al.[153] found no evidence of differentiation toward neuronal or glial structures in the nine cases they examined ultrastructurally.

Spread of medulloblastoma takes place through several routes. Subpial permeation is particularly common, as are also infiltration of the subarachnoid space and spread through the cerebrospinal fluid. Extraneural metastases also occur, particularly to bone and cervical lymph nodes.[147,156] Osseous metastases may be osteoblastic, osteolytic, or mixed[141] (Fig. 1483). The treatment consists of surgical removal of as much tumor as possible, followed by radiation therapy to the entire cerebrospinal axis. In a series of eighty-two cases reviewed by Bloom et al.,[142] 40% of the patients completing treatment survived five years and 30% ten

Table 72 Correlation between normal cytogenesis of central nervous system and embryonal neuroepithelial tumors

Stage of cytogenesis	Normal cell	Tumor
First	Neuroepithelial (matrix) cell	Medulloepithelioma
Second	Neuroblast	Medulloblastoma Neuroblastoma
Third	Spongioblast	Polar spongioblastoma
	Ependymoblast	Ependymoblastoma

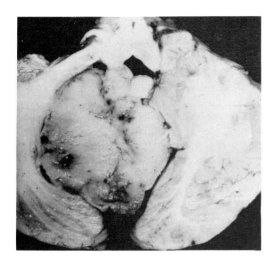

Fig. 1482 Cerebellar medulloblastoma in child. Tumor involves vermis and extends into fourth ventricle. (Courtesy Dr. J. E. Olvera-Rabiela, Mexico City, Mexico.)

years. The major cause of treatment failure is local recurrence in the posterior fossa.[152]

A well-defined variant of medulloblastoma (designated as "desmoplastic" by Rubinstein and Northfield[164]) has been described in an older age group, involving the cerebellar hemispheres, extending into the leptomeninges, and accompanied by abundant reticulin formation. Although originally regarded as a malignant mesenchymal tumor and designated "circumscribed arachnoidal cerebellar sarcoma," several authors have convincingly shown its link with the "classic" medulloblastoma.[164] Its prognosis is somewhat better than that of the latter.[145] Transitional and mixed forms have been described.[165] Another variant of medulloblastoma is characterized by the presence of embryonal skeletal muscle fibers in an otherwise typical neoplasm.[144,155]

The cytogenesis of this tumor has been a subject of heated discussions for decades. It is now more or less agreed that it arises from

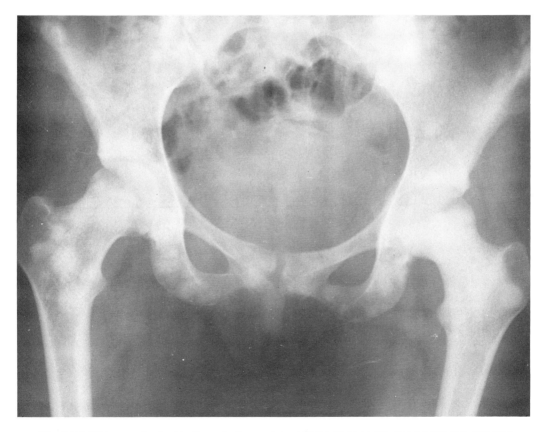

Fig. 1483 Widespread osteoblastic metastases of medulloblastoma in 12-year-old girl who also had local recurrence in posterior fossa of tumor treated by surgery and irradiation five years previously. (WU neg. 71-6738.)

the primitive cells that originate in the neuro-epithelial roof of the fourth ventricle to migrate upward and laterally to form the external granular layer of the cerebellar cortex.[149] Although cases with spongioblastic, astrocytic, and even oligodendroglial differentiation have been observed,[163] the differentiation, if present at all, is almost always in the direction of neuroblasts.[150] In this respect, medulloblastoma can be regarded in most instances as a peculiar clinicopathologic variant of neuroblastoma.[157,159]

Other embryonal tumors

Rare embryonal tumors of controversial cytogenesis include cerebral neuroblastoma, polar spongioblastoma, and ependymoblastoma.

Cerebral neuroblastoma closely resembles adrenal neuroblastoma on the one hand and cerebellar medulloblastoma on the other. Like them, it probably represents a malignant tumor of neuroblastic derivation.[154,164] In some cases, beginning differentiation toward neurons has been observed.[139]

Polar spongioblastoma faithfully recapitulates the architectural pattern of normal migrating polar spongioblasts.[160] Microscopically, uniform elongated cells are seen growing in a parallel fashion with a striking palisading effect.

Rubinstein[161] suggested the designation of *ependymoblastoma* (in a quite different sense from that previously used by Bailey and Cushing[140]) for a highly malignant embryonal tumor in which differentiation toward ependymal cells can be demonstrated. Whether it is justified to regard this as a specific tumor type distinct from medulloepithelioma and malignant ependymoma remains to be determined.

Tumors of neuronal cells

Whereas tumors containing adult neurons are not uncommon in the autonomic nervous system, their occurrence in the central nervous system is exceptional. It is likely that, here too, they form as a result of maturation of tumors originally composed of primitive neuroblastic cells. In a few reported examples, mature neurons make the bulk of the tumor, which is then designated as *ganglioneuroma*. In the majority of the cases, however, there is in addition a conspicuous astrocytic component (analogous to the schwannian element of peripheral tumors)—hence the term *ganglioglioma*.[168] Most cases have occurred in children and young adults, and the preferred locations have been the floor of the third ventricle, the hypothalamus, and the temporal lobe.[169] Occasionally, multiple foci are encountered.[170]

Microscopically, the abnormal neurons and astrocytes are characteristically surrounded by a prominent fibrovascular stroma, which we have seen confused with hemangioma. Ordinary astrocytomas can simulate gangliogliomas by entrapment of normal neurons. Also, some astrocytomas contain tumor glial cells with abundant acidophilic cytoplasm of polygonal shape and large vesicular nucleus, thus simulating the appearance of a neuron.

If all the elements present in a ganglioneuroma or ganglioglioma appear microscopically mature, a benign clinical behavior will follow in the large majority of the cases.

Tumors of meningothelial cells

Tumors of several different origins may arise from, or be connected with, the anatomic struc-

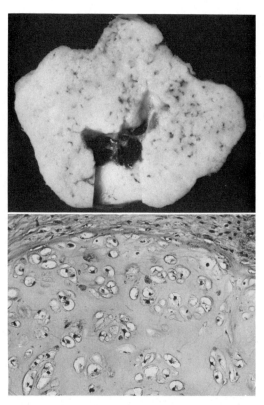

Fig. 1484 Chondroma of cerebral meninges. **A,** Gross appearance is that of well-circumscribed, lobulated mass of glistening white cut surface. **B,** Microscopic appearance of same tumor. Lobule of mature cartilage is partially surrounded by dense fibrous tissue. (**A,** WU neg. 66-7871; **B,** ×150; WU neg. 73-2682.)

tures composing the dura mater and lepto-meninges.[174] It is unfortunate that the designation of meningioma has often been indiscriminately applied to such tumors regardless of their histogenesis. Following this nomenclature, a lipoma becomes a lipoblastic meningioma, a chondroma is designated a chondromatous meningioma, etc. (Fig. 1484). It is probably better to restrict the term meningioma to the specific neoplasm arising from, and composed of, meningothelial (arachnoid) cells.

Most examples occur in adults, and there is a definite predilection for females. These tumors may be encountered in many sites, including the parasagittal region, lateral cerebral convexity, falx cerebri (Fig. 1485), base of the brain (particularly the sphenoid ridge), olfactory grooves, pontocerebellar angles, petrous ridge of the temporal bone, spinal canal (especially the thoracic segments), and inside the cerebral ventricles (most often on the left side).[174,181] We also have seen them in the orbit, nasal cavity, paranasal sinuses, bones of the skull, and soft tissues of the glabella.[180,193]

Lopez et al.[183] studied twenty-five cases of cutaneous meningiomas and divided them into three categories: Type I occurs in the scalp, face, or paravertebral region of children and young adults and is usually present at the time of birth; Type II presents around sensory organs of the head and along the course of cranial and spinal nerves of adults; Type III represents a cutaneous extension of a central nervous system meningioma through the skull. The prognosis is better for Type I than for the other two types. They also convincingly showed that a continuum exists between meningocele, meningeal hamartomas, and Type I cutaneous meningiomas, all of them arising from arachnoidal cap cells displaced during embryogenesis.

The gross appearance of the meningioma is that of a well-circumscribed, often lobulated

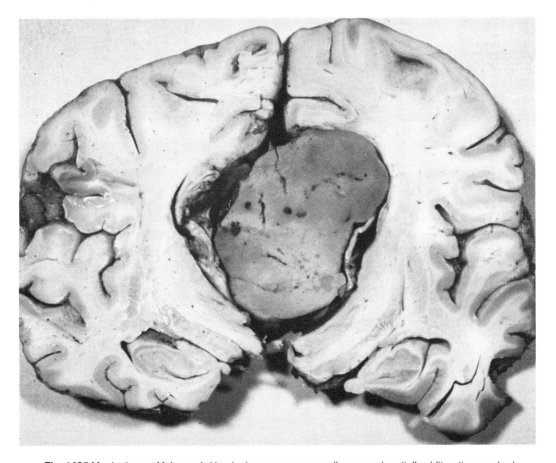

Fig. 1485 Meningioma of falx cerebri impinging upon corpus callosum and partially obliterating cerebral ventricles. There were no localizing symptoms, and clinical diagnosis was viral encephalitis. (WU neg. 73-2735.)

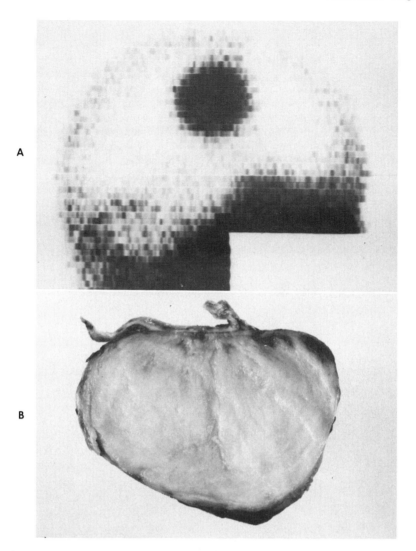

Fig. 1486 Parasagittal meningioma in 51-year-old man. **A,** Tc99m scan showing round hot area in frontoparietal region. **B,** Same tumor. It is well circumscribed, gray, homogeneous, and of firm consistency. Portion of dura attached to neoplasm may be seen at upper edge. (**A,** WU neg. 72-2786; **B,** WU neg. 72-2866.)

solid tumor of gray color and firm consistency (Fig. 1486). Calcification is common and often can be recognized roentgenographically and on gross inspection. The cut section exhibits a whorling configuration not unlike that of uterine leiomyomas. Most meningiomas have a round or oval shape, but some (known as *meningiomas en plaque*) grow in a diffuse sheetlike manner over the convexity of the brain. Hyperostosis of the neighboring bone is a common finding and an important roentgenographic sign (Fig. 1487).

Microscopically, the tumoral meningothelial cells may appear round, polygonal, oval, or spindle shaped (Fig. 1488). Their nuclei are regular, round or oval, and leptochromatic. The cytoplasm has a pale eosinophilic hue, and the cytoplasmic borders are indistinct. Rarely, round eosinophilic inclusions which are PAS positive and diastase resistant are seen in the cytoplasm.[174a] Mitoses are exceptional. Ultrastructurally, the most distinctive features are the pronounced interdigitations of the plasma membrane, the abundance of cytoplasmic microfilaments, and the presence of several types of cell junc-

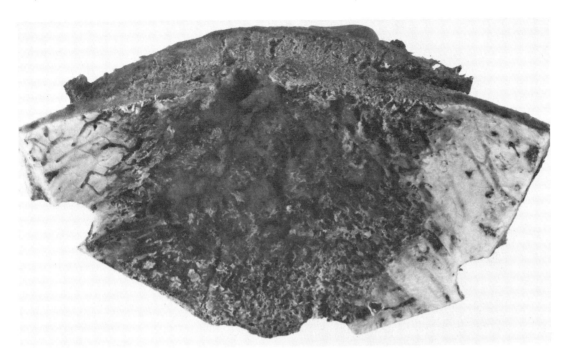

Fig. 1487 Marked hyperostosis in bone overlying meningioma *en plaque.*

tions, including hemidesmosome-like formations[172,173,186] (Fig. 1489). The tumor cells often are arranged in nests and concentric whorls,
the latter sometimes containing psammoma
bodies in their centers.[177] Blood vessels with
thick hyaline walls are very prominent in some
examples, to the point that a mistaken diagnosis
of hemangioma can be made. Meningiomas
also can be confused microscopically with
metastatic carcinoma, astrocytoma, and neurilemoma. Features supporting the diagnosis of
meningiomas in these instances are the presence
of laminated whorls (never seen in neurilemomas), indistinct cell borders resulting in a syncytial appearance, and short and plump nuclei
with a sharply delineated membrane.[179] Cellular whorls are a very important distinguishing
feature of meningiomas, especially in frozen
sections. However, they are far from pathognomonic; Kepes and Kernohan[178] have described them in various types of metastatic
carcinoma (including melanoma), medulloblastoma, and giant cell glioblastoma. Collections
of foamy macrophages and foci of metaplastic
bone are well recognized secondary features.
Occasionally, a heavy infiltration by lymphocytes and plasma cells is seen around the neoplastic cells.[176] Focally, the tumor cells may
be stellate, with slender processes surrounding

microcystic spaces.[180a] The subdivision of
meningiomas into microscopic types, such as
syncytial, psammomatous, meningothelioma-
tous, etc. is probably unwarranted in view of
their similar biologic behavior.[192]

The large majority of meningiomas follow
a benign clinical course and are permanently
cured by surgical excision. Local recurrence
supervenes in about 10% of the cases.[191] Extension into the dura mater, major sinuses, and
skull is a feature inherent to this neoplasm and
not a sign of malignancy. On the other hand,
well-documented cases of bona fide *malignant
meningiomas* exist. According to Rubinstein,[188] features in a meningioma which when
present should raise the possibility of malignancy include invasion of the adjacent brain,
papillary configuration, and presence of numerous mitotic figures. Distant metastases have
been observed along the cerebrospinal fluid
pathways as well as extracranially.[190] Ludwin
et al.[184] studied seventeen cases of *papillary
meningioma* and found that this pattern was
invariably associated with other histologic features of malignancy. Several of these tumors
occurred in children, and there was a high rate
of local recurrence and/or distant metastases.
They believe that this tumor is a distinct clinicopathologic variant of meningioma.

The tumor that Bailey et al.[171] designated as *angioblastic meningioma* needs to be clearly separated from those just described. Microscopically, it is a highly vascular neoplasm, the blood vessels being separated by closely packed cells with ill-defined cytoplasm (sometimes containing neutral fat) and oval or fusiform nuclei. Some examples show a striking similarity to hemangiopericytoma of soft tissues. The appearance is strikingly similar to that of hemangiopericytoma of soft tissues (Fig. 1490), and it seems likely that it repre-

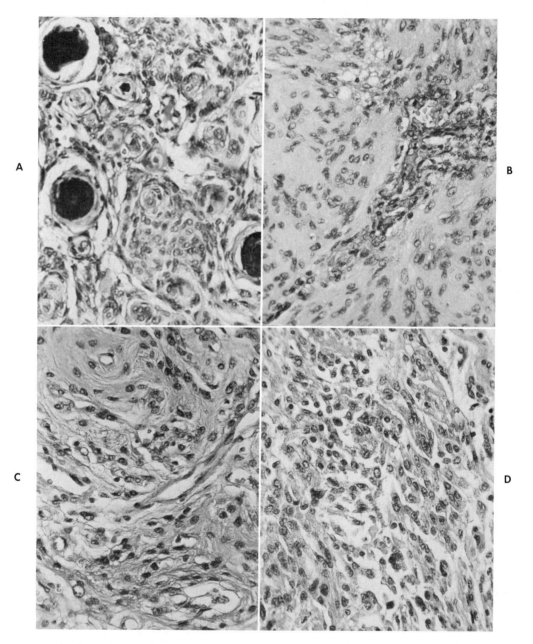

Fig. 1488 Four histologic appearances of meningioma. **A,** Small, well-defined whorls and psammoma bodies. **B,** Tumor cells with abundant fibrillary cytoplasm arranged in indistinct whorls. **C,** Tumor with marked vascularity and focal hyaline changes. **D,** Invasive meningioma, with atypical cytologic features. (**A-D,** ×280; **A,** WU neg. 49-3364; **B,** WU neg. 52-4262; **C,** WU neg. 52-4263; **D,** WU neg. 52-4264.)

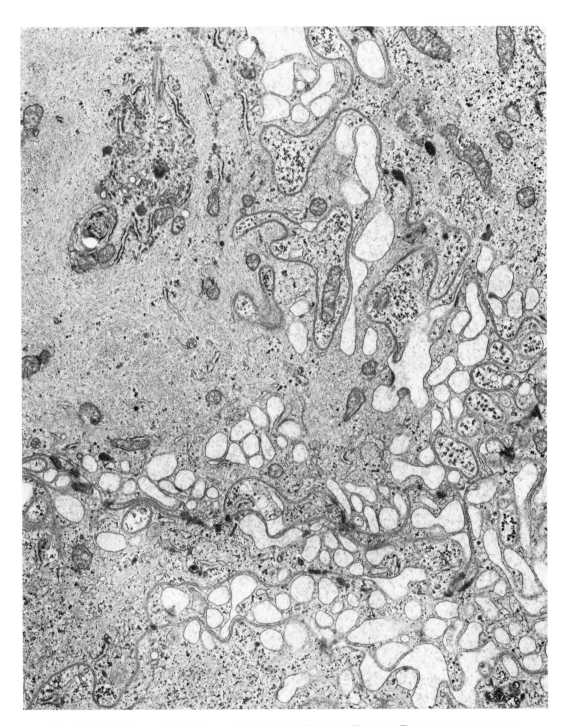

Fig. 1489 Meningioma. Cell bodies contain abundant thick microfilaments. There are numerous cytoplasmic interdigitating processes between cells, which are attached by desmosomes. (×11,200.)

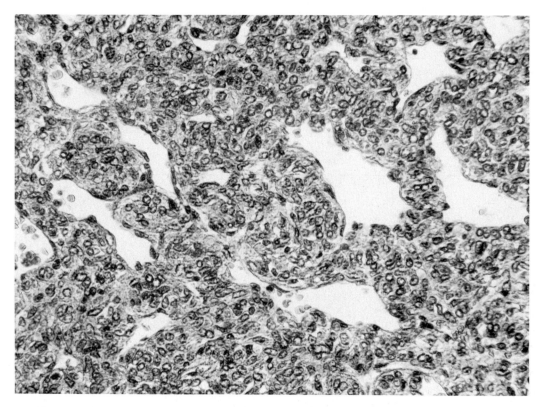

Fig. 1490 "Angioblastic meningioma." Morphologic similarities with hemangiopericytoma of soft tissue are evident. (×350; WU neg. 73-2668.)

sents the central nervous system counterpart of this tumor. When thus defined, angioblastic meningioma exhibits a different angiographic pattern[185] and a more aggressive behavior than the usual meningioma. Local recurrence is common, and extracranial metastases are not rare.[182,187] In a series of twenty-six cases from the Mayo Clinic, there was recurrence in 80% of the patients and metastases in 23%.[175]

Angioblastic meningioma should be distinguished from well-vascularized meningioma, which also can resemble cerebellar hemangioblastoma.[189] In one such case that we examined ultrastructurally, the tumor cells had unmistakable meningothelial features (Fig. 1491).

Exceptionally, meningiomas are found harboring metastases of carcinoma. The most common "donor" cancers have been from the breast and lung.[172a]

Tumors of melanocytes

The melanocytes normally present in the pia mater may give rise to a variety of disorders, most of which can be classified into one of two categories: neurocutaneous melanosis and primary meningeal melanoma.

In *neurocutaneous melanosis*, a disease of infants and children, diffuse pigmentation of the meninges resulting from proliferation of mature autochthonous melanocytes is associated with giant cutaneous nevi and occasionally with peripheral neurofibromas.[198] Internal hydrocephalus is the main complication of the central nervous system component of the disease.

Primary meningeal melanoma, which may occur as a complication of neurocutaneous melanosis, presents as a more or less circumscribed tumor mass or as a diffuse leptomeningeal process.[195,197] The latter form is differentiated from neurocutaneous melanosis by the atypia of the tumor cells, which is, however, less marked than that usually exhibited by cutaneous melanomas. Young adults are more commonly affected. The prognosis is poor. Metastasis from a cutaneous melanoma should be carefully ruled out before accepting any case as being of primary meningeal origin (Fig.

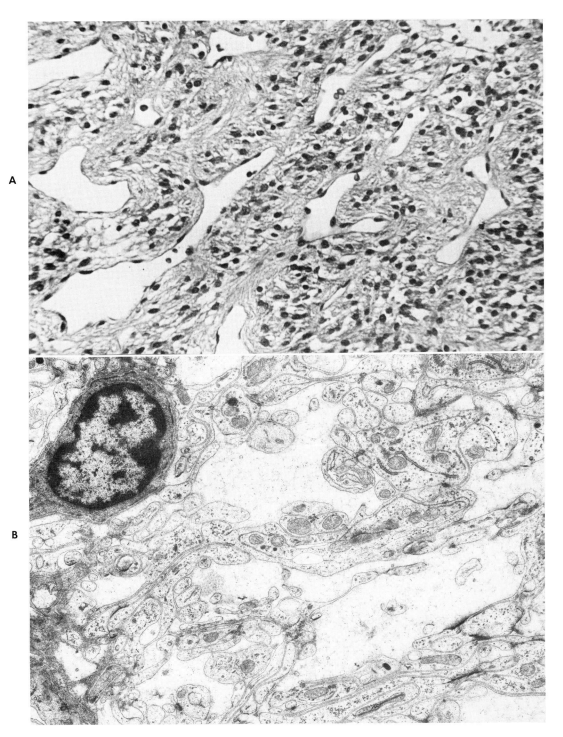

Fig. 1491 "Angioblastic meningioma" attached to dura of frontoparietal region in 44-year-old woman. **A,** Microscopic appearance of tumor. Resemblance to cerebellar hemangioblastoma is striking. **B,** Electron microscopic appearance of same tumor. There are complicated evaginations of plasmalemma, connected by desmosomes and partially surrounded by basal lamina. (**A,** ×300; WU neg. 73-2952; **B,** uranyl acetate–lead citrate; ×500; courtesy Dr. J. Bilbao, Toronto, Ontario, Canada.)

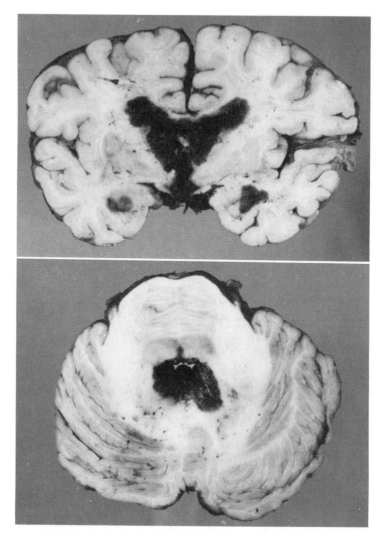

Fig. 1492 Leptomeningeal and ventricular spread of metastatic malignant melanoma. Primary tumor had been excised eighteen months previously from skin of back. (WU negs. 67-5089 and 67-5091.)

1492). Cases of primary malignant melanomas of the central nervous system with extraneural metastases have been described,[196] but it is difficult, if not impossible, in most of them to rule out the alternative possibility that the central nervous system tumor is yet another metastasis of undetected (? spontaneously disappearing) primary lesion.

It also should be pointed out that melanin can be observed in a variety of central nervous system tumors other than those strictly composed of cells with the morphologic features of melanocytes. These include craniopharyngioma, intracranial teratoma, melanotic medulloblastoma, melanotic progonoma, and a tumor that was interpreted as melanotic cerebral ependymoma.[194]

Tumors and malformations of blood vessels

Arteriovenous malformations also are known as arteriovenous angiomas, but the former designation is preferable since they are not true neoplasms.[201] Although congenital, they usually become manifest in late childhood and adolescence. A common complication is the production of repeated subarachnoid or intracerebral hemorrhages.[208] Most examples are found along the course of the middle cerebral artery. The cerebral choroid plex-

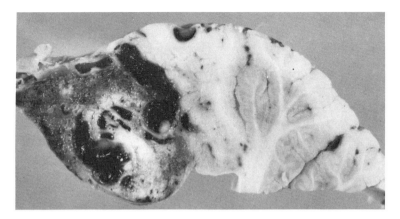

Fig. 1493 Hemangioblastoma of cerebellum. Tumor is well circumscribed, granular, and markedly vascular. (WU neg. 72-5929; courtesy Dr. J. E. Olvera-Rabiela, Mexico City, Mexico.)

us, cerebellum, and spinal cord are less often affected.[203] Usually, the lesion is quite superficial in character—i.e., restricted to the leptomeninges and the immediate cortical areas.

Grossly, large tortuous blood vessels are seen traversing thickened and hemorrhagic meninges and penetrating between atrophic cortical convolutions. Microscopically, some vessels can be identified as arteries and others as veins, but the majority represent hybrids difficult to classify. Secondary changes such as hyaline thickening, arteriosclerosis, calcification, and thrombosis are common.

Pure *venous malformations* are most commonly seen in the spinal cord and its meninges in adults.[212] The thoracic and cervical portions are the sites of predilection.[200,202,219] A well-known variant of venous malformation is Sturge-Weber disease, in which extensive venocapillary malformations of a cerebral hemisphere are associated with a cutaneous "port-wine hemangioma" in the region of the trigeminal nerve.[199,218] Arteriovenous malformations of the spinal cord also can be associated with segmentally related cutaneous hemangiomas.[207]

Cavernous hemangiomas have a structure quite reminiscent of the similarly called cutaneous lesions. Markedly dilated capillaries are seen side by side with little intervening parenchyma. The subcortical region of the cerebral hemisphere is the preferred location. As with hemangiomas elsewhere, multiplicity and multicentric involvement of other organs are not infrequent.

Hemangioblastoma is the most enigmatic member of the group. Its classical location is the cerebellar hemispheres, but it also can occur in the vermis, spinal cord, medulla, and, exceptionally, the cerebral hemispheres.[209,215] It usually becomes clinically manifest during the third or fourth decade of life. It may be the only abnormality present or represent a component of *von Hippel–Lindau disease* in association with angiomatosis of the retina, renal and pancreatic cysts, and, occasionally, papillary cystadenoma of the epididymis[214] and renal cell carcinoma.[210] It also has been reported in association with syringomyelia,[213] pheochromocytoma,[211] and erythrocythemia,[206] the latter as the result of the secretion of an erythropoietin-like substance by the tumor.[217]

Grossly, hemangioblastoma is well circumscribed, soft, yellowish or brown, and often cystic (Fig. 1493). Microscopically, an anastomosing network of capillary vessels is invariably seen. This feature is responsible for the tumor name, its typical angiographic presentation, and the general belief that it represents a primary vascular neoplasm (Fig. 1494). We favor the alternative theory that the true tumor cells of this well-vascularized lesion are those located between the blood vessels and often designated as "stromal cells." They are large, round, or polygonal and have a pale cytoplasm that often contains abundant neutral fat (Fig. 1495). The nuclei are usually small and uniform. In some instances, however, bizarre hyperchromatic forms are observed. They are of no particular prognostic significance. The nature of these cells is obscure. In some instances, they contain glial fibrillary acidic protein, which identifies them as astrocytes, but

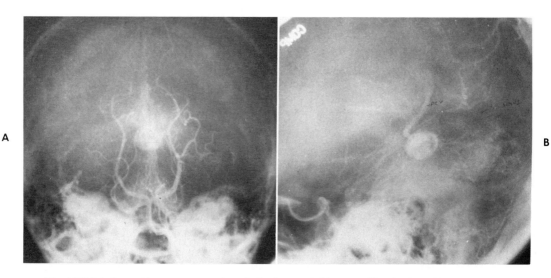

Fig. 1494 Arteriographic appearance of cerebellar hemangioblastoma. Vertebral arteriogram illustrated in **A** shows early in arterial phase a round dense homogeneous blush in midline of culmen of cerebellum. **B** corresponds to venous phase. (**A**, WU neg. 73-3127; **B**, WU neg. 73-3128.)

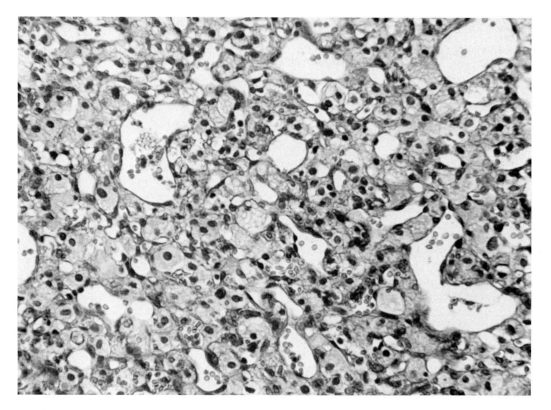

Fig. 1495 Hemangioblastoma of cerebellum. Tumor cells grow among intricate network of capillaries. They contain central normochromatic nuclei and abundant acidophilic (frequently foamy) cytoplasm. (×350; WU neg. 73-2667.)

in others this protein is totally absent.[209a] Ultrastructurally, their most prominent feature is an abundant electron-lucent cytoplasm, with a complex arrangement of branching and intercommunicating vesicular and tubular profiles of smooth and rough endoplasmic reticulum (Fig. 1496). Numerous mitochondria, annulate lamellae, and lipid droplets also are noticeable. The electron microscopic appearance does not resemble that of glial, meningothelial, endothelial, or perithelial cells or, for that matter, that of any normal cell known to occur in this area.[204] It has been suggested that all these cells arise from primitive vasoformative elements and that the "stromal" cells are histogenetically related to the endothelial cells and pericytes[205,216]; we find this hypothesis unconvincing.

The treatment is surgical, and the prognosis is good. The main hazard is local recurrence,

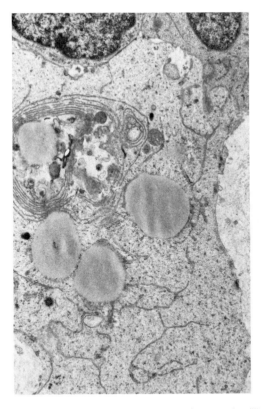

Fig. 1496 Ultrastructural appearance of "stromal cell" of cerebellar hemangioblastoma. Most conspicuous feature is presence of complex anastomosing membranous system in cytoplasm, sometimes arranged in concentric circles. Fat globules also are evident. (Uranyl acetate–lead citrate; ×8,400.)

either as a result of incomplete removal or because of multicentricity.

Tumors of lymphoreticular system

Secondary involvement of the central nervous system, particularly of the meninges, epidural space, and nerve roots, is a common event in malignant lymphoma and leukemia during the late stages of their evolution.[227,240,242] Among the acute leukemias, it is seen more commonly in the lymphocytic and undifferentiated forms than in the myelocytic leukemia or the acute blastic crisis of chronic myelocytic leukemia.[250] Among the malignant lymphomas, central nervous system involvement is seen more commonly with the non-Hodgkin's lymphomas than in Hodgkin's disease. The highest incidence is found in patients with diffuse lymphomas (especially of histiocytic and lymphoblastic types) and those with nodular histiocytic lymphomas. Patients who develop central nervous system lymphoma usually had extranodal disease at initial staging.[230] Some of the lymphocytic lymphomas exhibit plasmacytoid differentiation and may be associated with dysproteinemia.[226] Central nervous system involvement also can be seen, although exceptionally, in mycosis fungoides and plasma cell myeloma.[224,238,244] In patients with acute myelocytic leukemia, the development of an intracranial mass ("granulocytic sarcoma") can be the first manifestation of relapse.[235] In other instances, neurologic involvement represents the initial manifestation of a lymphoma or leukemia in which physical or roentgenographic examination shows to be in other organs as well. We are concerned here with the rarer instances in which a careful clinical study of the patient fails to uncover extraneural foci.

Malignant lymphoma of histiocytic type (reticulum cell sarcoma) is sometimes referred to as microglioma or microgliomatosis.[233,241,245] It seems increasingly evident that these terms, when applied to large cell lymphomas of the central nervous system, are all inaccurate. This is because the majority of these neoplasms are not made up of histiocytes, microglial cells, or reticulum cells but rather of lymphocytes belonging to the B cell series.[232] This neoplasm is probably not so rare as the paucity of reported cases might suggest. Review of reference cases has convinced us that many cases go unrecognized because of the common tendency to label all poorly differentiated primary tumors of the central nervous system as malignant glioma or glioblastoma multiforme.[223] Some have been observed in patients with congenital immune deficiencies,[221] following immunosuppression,[247] or as a complication of lymphomatoid granulomatosis.[243] Most patients are either young children or elderly adults.[220,246] Any region of the central nervous system can be affected, although the cerebral hemispheres are the most common site. In the series of Henry et al.,[229] the localization was as follows: cerebrum, 70; brainstem, 21; cerebellum, 14; spinal cord, 4. Multicentric foci are frequent.

Malignant lymphoma of the histiocytic type most commonly presents as an ill-defined gray, granular mass. Microscopically, the appearance is that of a large cell lymphoma similar to that seen outside the central nervous system, both by light and electron microscopic criteria.[231] Approximately one-half of the cases have the features of immunoblastic sarcoma. Taylor et al.[248] studied twenty-four cases of primary central nervous system lymphoma with an immunoperoxidase technique and demonstrated definite cytoplasmic immunoglobulin staining in thirteen, usually (but not always) monoclonal. Most of the positive cases exhibited some degree of plasmacytoid differentiation. In a few instances, the presence of a serum paraprotein has been documented in the absence of extraneural disease.[236] A striking perivascular distribution, accompanied by the deposition of concentric rings of reticulin fibers, is an important distinguishing feature.[229] Leptomeningeal spread is frequent. Extraneural foci eventually develop in a minority of cases. The clinical course is usually rapidly fatal,[237,246] although radiation therapy has resulted in prolonged survival in several instances.[234]

Malignant lymphoma of lymphocytic type primarily involving the central nervous system is almost always found in one of two sites: the meninges and the spinal epidural space, particularly in the thoracic portion.[222,228] *Plasmacytoma* of the central nervous system is exceptional; it presents as a meningeal or intracerebral mass in the absence of systemic myeloma.[239]

Although Hodgkin's disease can involve the central nervous system secondarily, we have never seen a case of primary central nervous system involvement. This has been the experience of most other authors,[225] with the outstanding exception of the series of Henry et al.[229]; 17% of their cases of primary lymphomas

of the central nervous system were diagnosed as Hodgkin's disease, an amazing figure especially in view of the fact that they were all regarded as belonging to the lymphocyte predominance type.

A case of primary intracranial *Burkitt's lymphoma* occurring in an infant has been recently reported.[249]

Lymphomatoid granulomatosis, a lymphoreticular proliferative process with angiocentric features, may involve the central nervous system, usually in association with lung disease but exceptionally as an isolated finding.[234a]

Tumors of nerve roots

The morphologic appearance of tumors of the nerve roots, their biologic behavior, and the problems of histogenetic interpretation they present are those of the most common types occurring outside the cranial cavity and spinal canal, which are discussed in Chapter 24. *Neurilemomas* (schwannomas) are by far the commonest. Most cases are seen in adults,[253] but pediatric cases also have been reported.[251] They have a strong predilection for two sites: the cerebellopontine angle and the spinal extramedullary space. The former arise practically always in the acoustic nerve, especially its vestibular branch (Fig. 1497). Enlargement of the internal auditory canal is an early finding and an important roentgenographic sign. *The presence of bilateral acoustic neurilemomas should be regarded as a probable indication of Recklinghausen's disease.* Spinal neurilemomas have a predilection for the posterior (sensory) roots of the lumbar region.[257] Not infrequently, the tumor extends outside the spinal canal through an intervertebral foramen to form a large soft tissue mass ("dumbbell tumor").

Microscopically, the main source of difficulty lies in the differential diagnosis with meningioma. The presence of foci of microcystic degeneration (Antoni B areas), vascular changes, and collections of foamy macrophages should lead to the correct diagnosis. Some neurilemomas contain melanin. Most, but not all, of these pigmented tumors have behaved in an aggressive fashion.[253a] The electron microscopic appearance of neurilemomas is distinctive.[252] The treatment is surgical. The outcome of the operation is directly related to the size of the neoplasm. The larger the tumor, the higher the operative mortality rate and the possibilities of permanent residual

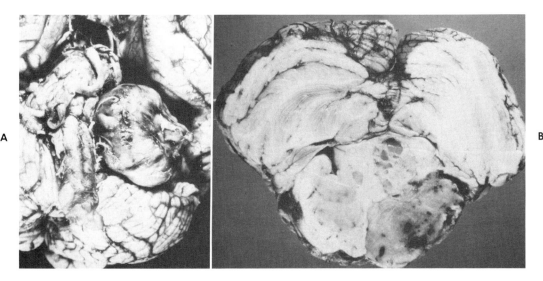

Fig. 1497 A, External appearance of neurilemoma of cerebellopontine angle. Tapered end of acoustic nerve on one side and compression of pons and medulla on other are well appreciated. **B,** Cross section of acoustic neurilemoma. Tumor compression has resulted in focal degenerative change of pons. (**A,** WU neg. 72-5942; **B,** WU neg. 72-5934; **A** and **B,** courtesy Dr. J. E. Olvera-Rabiela, Mexico City, Mexico.)

damage.[254] If the excision is only partial, recurrence of symptoms is common. Interruption of vital arterial supply to the tegmentum of the pons is the main hazard of the operation.[254]

Neurofibromas of the central nervous system are always multiple and an expression of Recklinghausen's disease. Both cranial and spinal nerve roots may be involved. In addition to neurofibromas, patients with Recklinghausen's disease may present with a bewildering variety of neural tumors and hamartomas. These include neurilemomas (particularly bilateral acoustic tumors), meningiomas, ependymomas, astrocytomas, and optic nerve gliomas.[256] Syringomyelia is another frequently associated abnormality.[255]

Tumors of germ cell origin

Tumors presumably arising from misplaced germ cell elements can occur within the cranial cavity and, much less commonly, in the spinal cord.[266] Like extragonadal germ cell tumors in general, they are located almost exclusively in midline structures, particularly within the pineal gland, in the parapineal area, and in a suprasellar or even intrasellar position.[260,262] Their common relationship with the pineal gland, plus a vague similarity with the embryonic structure of this organ, has resulted in many of these tumors being mistakenly re-

garded as pinealomas,[263] a misconception still held in some circles in spite of convincing arguments to the contrary.[270-272]

All varieties of germ cell tumors have been described, including germinoma (a term proposed by Friedman[261] for neoplasms having the morphologic features of seminoma or dysgerminoma, regardless of site of origin), embryonal carcinoma, adult teratoma, choriocarcinoma, and yolk sac tumor.[258,264,267] Alphafetoprotein and human chorionic gonadotropin secretion can be encountered with the nonseminomatous types and can be detected in the tumor cell cytoplasm by immunocytochemical techniques.[265] Combinations of these tumor types commonly occur. Their gross and microscopic features are identical to the homologous gonadal tumors.

Grossly, germinomas are soft, grayish, friable, and granular. Infiltration beneath the ependyma of the wall of the third ventricle is common. Two or more independent foci may be present. Microscopically, they consist of tumor cells with large, vesicular nuclei and pale, glycogen-containing cytoplasm that are irregularly divided in groups by thin fibrous strands infiltrated by inflammatory cells (Fig. 1498). The lymphocytic and sometimes granulomatous reaction accompanying these neoplasms is sometimes so intense that the true nature of the

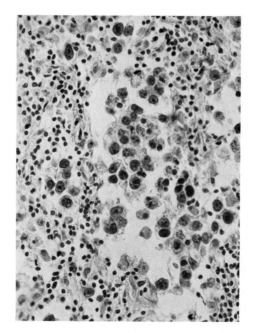

Fig. 1498 Germinoma of pineal region. Poorly cohesive nests of large tumor cells are surrounded by fibrous strands heavily infiltrated by lymphocytes. (×280; WU neg. 52-4267.)

lesion may be missed in a small biopsy.[272] The ultrastructural appearance is identical to that of the corresponding gonadal neoplasm.[269]

The majority of the patients with germ cell neoplasms are young adult males.[259] Symptoms derive from pressure effects upon the regions of the rear of the third ventricle and over the mesencephalon. Oculomotor and visual disturbances are common. Diabetes insipidus, emaciation, and precocious puberty occur less frequently.[268] Local extension within the third ventricle is common. Occasionally, it spreads to other ventricles and even into the meningeal space.[259] The surgical approach is understandably difficult. Excision, whether partial or apparently complete, should be followed by radiation therapy. Germinomas are extremely radiosensitive neoplasms. Of seven patients with suprasellar germinoma who survived the operation and were treated with radiation therapy, five were alive and well from three to eighteen years later.[272] Serial cytologic examination of the cerebrospinal fluid has been recommended to detect early recurrences, which would justify additional therapy to the spinal cord. Adult teratomas, although radioresistant, can be cured by total removal. Conversely, embryonal carcinomas, choriocarcinomas, yolk sac tumors, and their combinations are almost invariably fatal.[272a]

Tumors of pineal gland

Once germ cell tumors are excluded from the category of tumors of the pineal gland, true neoplasms of the pineal gland become a curiosity. They supposedly arise from the pineal parenchymal cells and are classified into pineocytomas and pineoblastomas according to their degree of differentiation.

Pineocytomas present as solid, well-circumscribed tumors replacing the pineal body. Microscopically, the tumor cells are small and uniform, with round nucleus and eosinophilic cytoplasm, separated in nests by delicate connective tissue strands. The overall microscopic appearance and the argyrophilia that the tumor cells often exhibit have suggested to some a link with paraganglioma.[273,276] However, the few electron microscopic studies that have been performed have failed to demonstrate dense-core neurosecretory granules; instead, differentiation toward neuronal and astrocytic lines was described.[274] The relationship of the tumor cells with blood vessels may cause confusion with ependymoma and astroblastoma. Actually, even a normal pineal gland may suggest ependymoma to the uninitiated. The majority of pineocytomas have behaved in a benign fashion, but the number of reported cases is too small to make any generalizations about their natural history.

The name *pineoblastoma* has been given to an extremely rare, highly malignant neoplasm occurring in young people and histologically resembling tumors of the medulloblastoma-neuroblastoma group.[275] It is an infiltrating neoplasm that commonly spreads via the cerebrospinal fluid.[272b] Electron microscopic studies have shown features reminiscent of photoreceptor cells in the pineal gland of lower vertebrates and human fetal pineal glands.[273a]

Tumors of other mesenchymal cells

Lipomas of the central nervous system often are found attached to the meninges (hence their previous designation of lipomatous meningiomas). Those located in the spine predominate in the thoracic region and often have an intramedullary component.[277] *Chondromas* appear as bosselated masses of glistening appearance, usually attached to the inner side of the dura mater (Fig. 1484).

Primary sarcomas are extremely rare tumors, most frequently found in infants and children.[282] The majority arise from the dura, but leptomeningeal and parenchymal cases also have been observed. In some instances, the previous use of radiation therapy has been incrimated in their causation.[290,292] A rare variant characterized by diffuse meningeal involvement has been designated *meningeal meningiomatosis*.[279] Sometimes a definite diagnosis of tumor type can be made, such as fibrosarcoma, rhabdomyosarcoma, chondrosarcoma, or mesenchymal chondrosarcoma.[278,280,282,284,288,291] In many cases, however, the specific cell type involved remains elusive despite the most exhaustive morphologic study. Lately, a number of benign and malignant *fibrous histiocytomas* of the brain and meninges have been reported.[280,286] Their microscopic appearance is similar to that of the analogous extraneural tumors. A storiform pattern of growth is usually present, as well as Touton-like multinucleated tumor cells.

Before making such a diagnosis, alternative possibilities of meningioma or astrocytoma with desmoplastic reaction and spindle cell metaplasia (including the recently described pleomorphic xanthoastrocytoma[281]) should be ruled out by a thorough sampling of the tumor.

Most primary *rhabdomyosarcomas* of the central nervous system have been found in the brainstem of children.[287] They are probably related to medulloblastomas with skeletal muscle differentiation (so-called medullomyoblastomas), just as rhabdomyosarcomas of the kidney are probably related to Wilms' tumor with skeletal muscle foci. Other rhabdomyosarcomas of the central nervous system have been reported in the cerebrum of adults; these have been thought to arise from multipotential mesenchymal tissues in the leptomeninges.[285]

The *mesenchymal chondrosarcoma* presents as a cranial or spinal meningeal tumor and has a morphologic appearance identical to that of its osseous counterpart (see Chapter 23) and characterized by the admixture of primitive undifferentiated mesenchymal cells and well-defined islands of hyaline cartilage. In a series of twelve cases reviewed by Scheithauer and Rubenstein,[289] five led to local recurrence and one to lung metastases.

Excluded from this group are the following "entities": circumscribed arachnoidal cerebellar sarcoma, monstruocellular sarcoma, and giant cell fibrosarcoma. The reasons we do not regard them as authentic sarcomas have

been given elsewhere in this chapter. Occasionally, a malignant tumor is seen that seems to contain both a glial and a sarcomatous component. Two morphologic varieties are described. In one, known as *gliosarcoma*, it is thought that the glioma is primary and that the sarcoma arises from the highly hyperplastic vessels that accompany the tumor. In the other, designated as *sarcoglioma*, the sarcomatous element, which is centrally located, is supposed to be the primary event; the glial malignant component is postulated to arise on the basis of the reactive glial proliferation that is frequently seen around the sarcoma.[283] These proposals are highly imaginative and backed by considerable authority. Yet, it seems to us that the alternative explanation (i.e., that these tumors represent gliomas with an undifferentiated, sarcomatoid component) is just as likely. Naturally, these considerations do not apply to collision tumors, in which two separate and distinct primary neoplasms, such as meningioma and glioma, are found close to each other or even sharing a common side.

Tumors of pituitary gland

Pituitary neoplasms constitute approximately 10% of the intracranial tumors. The large majority arise from the endocrine cells of the adenohypophysis and are designated as *pituitary adenomas.* Naturally, most examples are found within the confines of the sella turcica. However, since aberrant adenohypophyseal cells are known to occur in the pituitary infundibulum, pituitary stalk, floor of the third ventricle, and in the sphenoid bone between the nasopharynx and the pituitary fossa, the appearance of pituitary adenomas in one of these locations is not unexpected, even if exceptional.[301] Grossly, pituitary adenomas are usually solid and soft. Their color varies from gray to red according to the degree of vascularity. Cystic and hemorrhagic changes may occur in the larger tumors. A characteristic gross appearance is that of a tumor occupying both the intrasellar and suprasellar areas, with a central constriction produced by the diaphragm and the circle of Willis.

The microscopic pattern in hematoxylin-eosin sections varies from case to case, the differences being based on the relative degrees of cellularity and vascularity (Figs. 1499 and 1500). Kernohan and Sayre[326] classified their cases into a *diffuse* type, highly cellular, with scanty stroma and blood vessels; a *sinusoidal*

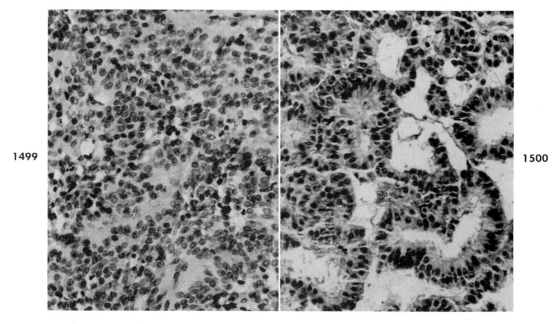

Fig. 1499 Pituitary adenoma of diffuse type. (×280; WU neg. 52-4265.)
Fig. 1500 Pituitary adenoma with glandular arrangement of tumor cells. This pattern is uncommon in our experience. (×280; WU neg. 49-3365.)

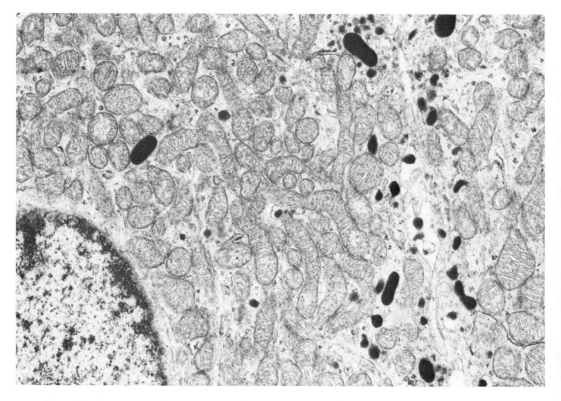

Fig. 1501 Oncocytoma of pituitary gland. Cytoplasm is packed with mitochondria and also contains secretory granules in peripheral cytoplasm.

type, having an architecture which recapitulates that of the normal gland; and a *papillary* type, in which pseudopapillae centered by a blood vessel and covered by tumor cells are noted. Transitional and mixed forms often occur. There is apparently no relation between these microscopic types and prognosis. The tumor cells are similar in all three varieties. They are generally round or polygonal and have a round or oval nucleus and a variable amount of cytoplasm, which may be basophilic, amphophilic, acidophilic, or clear. Mitoses are scanty or absent. Occasional bizarre hyperchromatic nuclei may occur including giant and ring forms with prominent nucleoli. It has been suggested that this nuclear configuration is indicative of endocrine hyperfunction.[336] Rarely, the tumor cells have the morphologic appearance of oncocytes[298,329] (Fig. 1501); one such case has been reported in association with Cushing's disease.[309] Calcification occurs in about 7% of pituitary adenomas and seems to

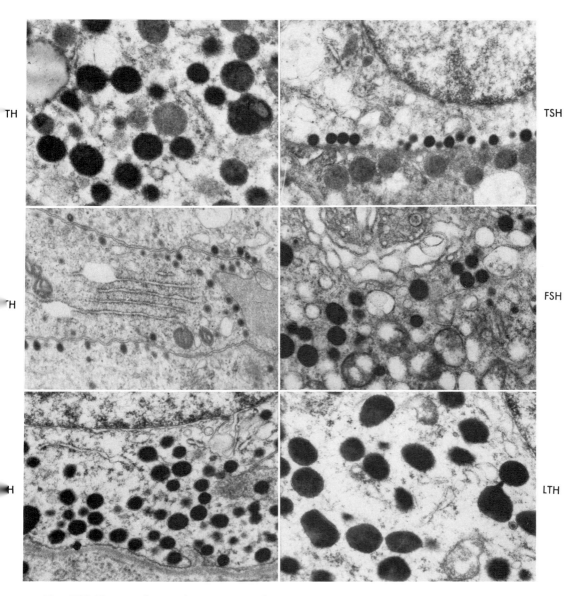

TH   TSH

ᵀH   FSH

ᴴ   LTH

Fig. 1502 Electron microscopic appearance of secretory granules of six major cell types of human anterior pituitary gland. (Uranyl acetate–lead citrate; ×21,000; courtesy Dr. I. von Lawzewitsch, Buenos Aires, Argentina.)

Table 73 Histochemical and ultrastructural features of normal pituitary cells and of the corresponding tumors

Hormone	Normal cell					Tumor	
	Chemical composition and molecular weight	Hematoxylin-eosin	Special stains	Granules (E.M.) in rat	Granules (E.M.) in human (tentative)	Usual appearance on H & E sections	Diameter of most granules (E.M.)
Growth hormone (STH or GH)	Protein ~21,000	Acidophil (alpha cell)	PAS, -; orange G, +; erythrosin, -	300-350 mμ; abundant; throughout cytoplasm	350-400 mμ	Acidophil or "chromophobe"	350-450 mμ (densely granulated tumors) 100-250 mμ (sparsely granulated tumors)
Adrenocorticotropic hormone (ACTH)*	Protein ~4,500	? Basophil and chromophobe (beta, R, or zeta cell)	PAS, +; orange G, -; erythrosin, -	200-300 mμ; more numerous in peripheral cytoplasm	200-300 mμ	Basophil or "chromophobe"	250-450 mμ
Thyrotropic hormone (TSH)	Glycoprotein ~28,000	Basophil (beta cell)	PAS, +; orange G, -; erythrosin, -	150-200 mμ; more numerous in peripheral cytoplasm	80-150 mμ	Basophil or "chromophobe"	100-150 mμ
Prolactin (LTH)	Protein ~25,000	Acidophil (eta cell)	PAS, -; orange G, -; erythrosin, +	600-900 mμ; scanty or irregular shape	100-200 mμ in width; 600-900 mμ in length	Acidophil or "chromophobe"	500-600 mμ (densely granulated tumors) 200-300 mμ (sparsely granulated tumors)
Luteinizing hormone (LH or ICSH)	Glycoprotein ~26,000	Basophil (delta₁ cell)	PAS, +; orange G, -; erythrosin, -	200-250 mμ; throughout cytoplasm or concentrated in periphery	100-250 mμ or ICSH)	?	?
Follicle-stimulating hormone (FSH)	Glycoprotein ~50,000	Basophil (delta₂ cell)	PAS, +; orange G, -; erythrosin, -	200-250 mμ; throughout cytoplasm or concentrated in periphery	150-300 mμ	?	?

*Melanocyte stimulating hormone (β-MSH) seems to be present in the same cell that manufactures ACTH, probably in the same secretory granules.

be more common in prolactin-secreting neo-plasms.[333] The deposition of an amyloid-like substance also has been documented in some of these tumors.[300]

We have seen pituitary adenomas composed of uniform tumor cells of clear cytoplasm confused with oligodendrogliomas. We also have seen adenomas made up of oval cells with oval acidophilic cytoplasm and eccentric nucleus mistaken for plasma cell myeloma. The most common error, however, is the misinterpretation of a papillary type of pituitary adenoma as an ependymoma.

The traditional classification of pituitary adenomas into chromophobe, acidophil, and basophil varieties correlates so poorly with the specific cell types and the corresponding patterns of hormone secretion that there is little use in maintaining it.[304,358] It has become evident that most normal "chromophobe" cells simply represent specific cells of one kind or another in which the number of granules is not large enough to be obvious at a light microscopic level.[316] The same seems to be true of the so-called chromophobe adenomas.[338] Acidophilic pituitary tumors also have been shown to be highly heterogenous. In an immunohistochemical study of twenty-eight such cases by Halmi and Duello,[313] 8 showed no

immunostaining, 11 stained only for prolactin, 3 stained only for growth hormone, 5 contained mostly growth hormone cells and some prolactin cells, and 1 contained predominantly prolactin cells but also numerous growth hormone cells.

There is now general agreement that each of the major hormones of the adenohypophysis is secreted by a single cell type. The identification of these cells and the correlation with a given hormone have been achieved in some animals (particularly the rat) by careful histochemical and electron microscopic studies under normal and abnormal conditions and, most of all, by immunocytochemical methods.[295,296,318,343,344] (Table 73). Understandably, the corresponding information on the normal human pituitary gland is not nearly so complete. However, correlation with the animal models and studies in several disease processes has permitted at least a tentative classification of cell types[294,299,347,350,370] (Fig. 1502). The same approach should be followed in the case of the neoplasms. Hematoxylin-eosin stains should be routinely supplemented by PAS–hematoxylin–light green–orange G,[338] and, if possible by immunohistochemical and electron microscopic examination.[330,332,346] (Fig. 1503). Biochemical and immunochemical procedures

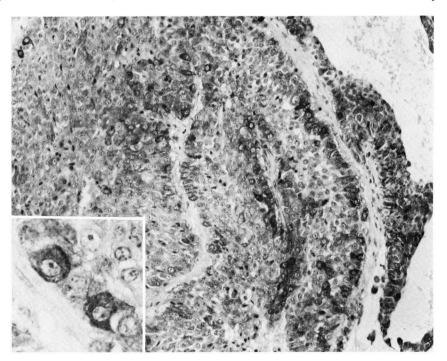

Fig. 1503 ACTH-producing pituitary adenoma stained for ACTH with immunoperoxidase technique. **Inset** shows two strongly positive cells.

in tumor extracts and in tumors grown in tissue culture also can be very informative but require highly specialized techniques.[328]

The types of pituitary adenomas already identified include STH, ACTH, TSH, and LTH cell types. A certain proportion of these tumors secrete more than one hormone.[317]

Adenomas of the STH cell type may result in gigantism or acromegaly if functioning at a clinical level or, more commonly, be unaccompanied by signs of hyperfunction. If the series reported by McCormick and Halmi,[338] only 3% of the acidophilic adenomas produced typical acromegaly. The few tumors composed of highly granulated cells appear acidophilic in hematoxylin-eosin sections. The others, which constitute the majority, have the appearance of "chromophobe adenomas."[372] Growth hormone can be demonstrated by immunohistochemical techniques[307a]; some correlation exists between the serum levels and the staining of this hormone in tissues. By electron microscopy, secretory granules measuring 300-400 mμ can be identified in every case.[335] The endoplasmic reticulum is disposed in concentric arrays. Bundles of cytoplasmic microfilaments are sometimes encountered.[362] Presence of fibrous bodies and multiple centrioles are said to be highly suggestive of the sparsely granulated variant of this tumor type.[320]

The functioning examples of *adenomas of the ACTH cell type*, which constitute approximately 7% of the cases,[338] result in the production of Cushing's syndrome. Female pa-

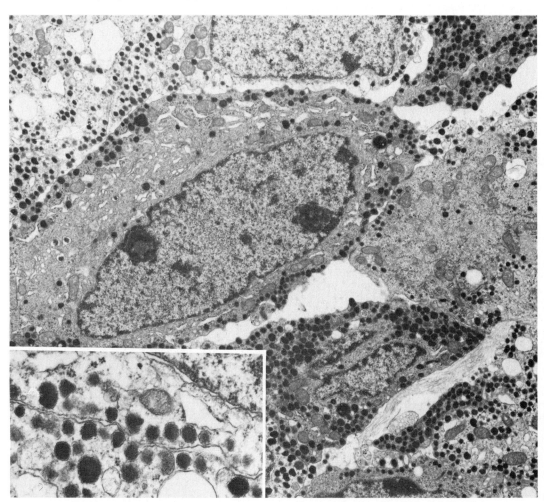

Fig. 1504 Ultrastructural appearance of ACTH cell pituitary adenoma. Secretory granules arrange themselves in parallel rows along cell membranes. **Inset,** Higher magnification of secretory granules. (×7,450; **inset,** ×16,850.)

tients predominante. Approximately 10% of all cases of Cushing's syndrome are accompanied by an overt pituitary adenoma.[357,360] Some workers maintain that the incidence of pituitary adenomas in Cushing's disease is actually much higher (over 80% of the cases) and advocate their removal by selective transsphenoidal resection.[359] Tyrrell et al.[369] performed this operation in twenty patients and found seventeen tumors. The size of the neoplasms ranged from 3-10 mm. Most of them were located within the body of the anterior lobe of the pituitary gland either centrally or in the lateral lobes. The diagnosis of pituitary adenoma was confirmed histologically in fourteen. The very small size and fragmentation of the sample may render the diagnosis difficult or even impossible. Immunohistochemical staining for ACTH may be very helpful in this regard by demonstrating that in one or more of the fragments all of the cells are positive for this hormone. Removal of the hyperplastic adrenal glands

in these patients may result in rapid enlargement or even massive hemorrhagic infarct of the pituitary neoplasm. Nelson et al.[345] have estimated that about 10% of patients with Cushing's disease and adrenal cortical hyperplasia who undergo total adrenalectomy later develop clinical signs of a pituitary neoplasm. The condition is known as Nelson's syndrome.[331] By light microscopy, the tumor cells may appear basophil, amphophil, acidophil or, more commonly, "chromophobe." Ultrastructurally, the secretory granules may concentrate along the cell membrane or be found scattered throughout the cytoplasm. Their diameter show considerable variations, ranging in one series from 200-700 mμ (Fig. 1504). Perinuclear microfilaments, 70 Å in diameter, are usually present and constitute an important diagnostic feature of ACTH-producing tumors[354] (Fig. 1505); they are probably equivalent to the Crooke's change seen in nonneoplastic ACTH cells in cases of Cushing's disease; their appearance is

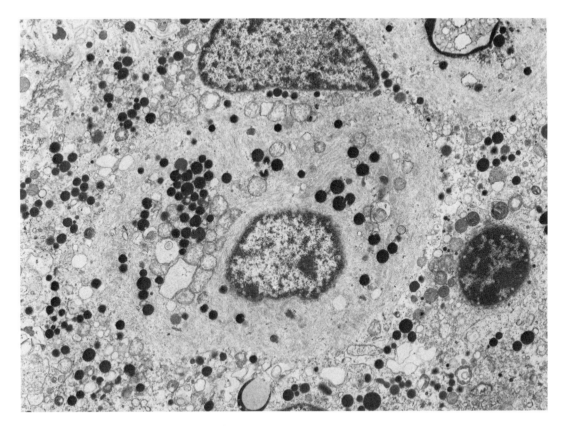

Fig. 1505 Pituitary adenoma in 25-year-old woman with Cushing's disease. Immunoperoxidase staining revealed presence of ACTH. Ultrastructurally, cells contained large dense-core secretory granules; in addition, occasional cells had large numbers of microfilaments representing Crooke's hyaline change. (×7,450.)

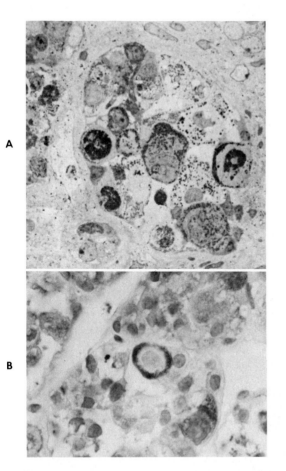

Fig. 1506 Crooke's change in pituitary cells in patient with Cushing's disease. **A,** Toluidine blue stain of epoxy-embedded section. **B,** ACTH stain (immuno-peroxidase).

probably dependent upon the level of circulating corticosteroids[331] (Fig. 1506).

Occasional basophil, densely granulated adenomas of ACTH type are endocrinologically silent, the reason for this lack of function not being apparent.[319a]

The presence of *adenomas of THS cell type* had been suggested by the reports of pituitary adenomas associated with hyperthyroidism[322] and confirmed by Hamilton et al.[315] by the finding of elevated serum TSH levels on radio-immunoassay. The ultrastructural features of this tumor type have been described by Samaan et al.[361] Capella et al.[302] made the interesting observation that most of these tumors are argyrophilic.

The situation in regard to *adenomas of the LTH (prolactin) cell type* is somewhat similar. Their existence had been long suspected by

the reported cases of pituitary adenomas associated with galactorrhea and amenorrhea (Forbes-Albright syndrome)[306,307] and finally documented by the thoroughly investigated case of Peake et al.[348] The incidence of this tumor, or at least its recognition, is on the rise.[352,356,364] An analysis of 235 patients with galactorrhea (5.5% of whom were males) showed that 20% of all patients, and 34% of the women with associated amenorrhea, had roentgenologically evident pituitary tumors; these patients had the highest serum prolactin concentrations.[327] Immunohistochemical techniques with Sternberger's method using specific antibodies against prolactin have been well described[314]; the granules often are concentrated along one nuclear pole.[314]

The light microscopic appearance of this tumor is similar to that of *STH cell adenoma*, but ultrastructurally it differs by the larger size of its secretory granules (500-600 mμ). The tumor cells are elongated or polyhedral and show complex interdigitations. The secretory granules are characteristically sparse and show no particular predilection for any region of the cytoplasm.[353] Some of these granules are found in the extracellular space between two cells, a phenomenon described as "misplaced exocytosis."[319]

Horvath et al.[320] have described under the term "acidophilic stem adenoma" four neoplasms that share ultrastructural and immunocytochemical features of growth hormone-secreting and prolactin-secreting cells.

As far as we know, the *FSH* and *LH* cells are the only ones for which no corresponding tumor in human beings has yet been conclusively demonstrated, although its occurrence in experimental animals is well known.[312] However, Kohler et al.[328] have found production of LH in several human pituitary adenomas grown in tissue culture. Tumors composed of more than one cell type, and therefore secreting two or more hormones, also occur.

Pituitary adenomas as a group are more frequent in adults and show a slight predilection for males. In a small percentage of patients, the pituitary tumor is one of the components of the multiple endocrine adenomatosis syndrome Type I.[297,369a] They may become clinically evident as a result of the increased secretion of a specific hormone by the tumor cell as previously outlined, by signs of hypopituitarism secondary to destruction of the normal gland, and/or by symptoms or signs resulting from the compression of adjacent structures. Enlargement and erosion of the floor of the sella turcica is a very common finding and an important roentgenologic sign. Suprasellar extension, present in 10%-20% of the cases, results in visual symptoms as a result of compression of the optic chiasm. Extraocular tumor palsies occur in 5%-10% of the patients. In 5%-10% of all pituitary tumors, actual invasion of neighboring structures is encountered, such as the anterior, middle, or posterior fossa, cavernous sinus, optic nerves, chiasm, nasopharynx, or nasal cavity.[325,341] We prefer to designate these tumors as "invasive adenomas" rather than as carcinomas. Exceptionally, pituitary neoplasms are found to implant along the subarachnoid space and even to metastasize distantly, particularly to the liver.[305,339] This phenomenon has been reported with nonfunctioning tumors as well as with neoplasms associated with Cushing's syndrome.[351,357] As in most other endocrine tumors, the correlation between microscopic appearance and biologic behavior is poor. Some of the invasive or metastasizing neoplasms have an obviously malignant cytologic appearance, but the majority do not appreciably differ from the ordinary pituitary adenoma. "Pituitary apoplexy" is a rare complication of adenomas. It represents a massive hemorrhagic infarct within the tumor and is most often seen in adenomas associated with acromegaly or Cushing's syndrome.[357]

The therapeutic approach to pituitary adenomas varies in different clinics. Both surgical excision and radiation therapy can be employed, the results being largely comparable. The choice of therapy sometimes depends on the clinical circumstances but most often on local preference.[303,334,341,365] A few cases of sarcoma developing as a possible late complication of radiation therapy for pituitary adenoma have been reported.[293,310,371] The average latent period is ten years, and the average tissue dose of irradiation is over 7,000 R.[311]

Craniopharyngioma is not a tumor of pituitary origin but is included in this discussion because of its invariable close correlation with the pituitary gland. Children and adults are equally affected. Its location is usually suprasellar, although it may occupy the sella as well (Fig. 1507, *A*). Cystic degeneration is an extremely common finding, the content of the cyst being a straw-colored or brown fluid rich in cholesterol crystals. Focal calcification is al-

most invariably present. In about 75% of the cases, it is prominent enough to be detectable roentgenographically. The microscopic appearance is very similar to that of ameloblastoma of the jaws. Anastomosing epithelial islands with a palisaded layer of cells and a center of stellate cells are characteristic (Fig. 1507, *B*). Foci of squamous metaplasia, microcystic degeneration, calcification, and reactive gliosis are often found. Small epithelial strands trapped in the peripheral reactive glial tissue may result in a mistaken diagnosis of carcinoma. Cystic adamantinomas also should be differentiated from epidermoid and other cysts occurring in this region although this may prove difficult or even impossible in some cases.[349] The most important features that favor a diagnosis of carniopharyngioma are the basal palisading and the stellate reticulum. The electron microscopic appearance of craniopharyngioma has been well described by Ghatak et al.[308]

Although minor microscopic differences exist between craniopharyngioma and ameloblastoma of the jaws, comparative morphologic and histochemical studies and the finding in several cases of craniopharyngioma of undeniable tooth structures is conclusive evidence of a related embryologic origin, the intracranial tumor probably arising from a buccal equivalent of the embryonic enamel organ present in Rathke's pouch.[323,363,368]

Symptoms are dominated by those of hydrocephalus, especially in the younger patients, and of pressure upon the chiasm and optic tracts. Signs of hypothalamic involvement such as diabetes insipidus are common. Total surgical excision is the treatment of choice. In one series, most postoperative morbidity and all postoperative mortality occurred after second and third operations for recurrent tumor.[342]

Granular cell tumors arising from the stalk or posterior lobe of the pituitary gland usually represent an incidental autopsy finding,[337] but in a few cases they have attained enough size to produce symptoms and require surgical intervention.[366] Their morphologic appearance and histochemical reactions are similar to those of their more common peripheral counterpart. Granular cell tumors also can occur in the cerebral hemispheres.[340]

Metastatic carcinoma to the pituitary gland and sella trucica is a common finding in autopsy material, particularly in cases of breast and lung carcinoma.[355] Microscopic examination of pitu-

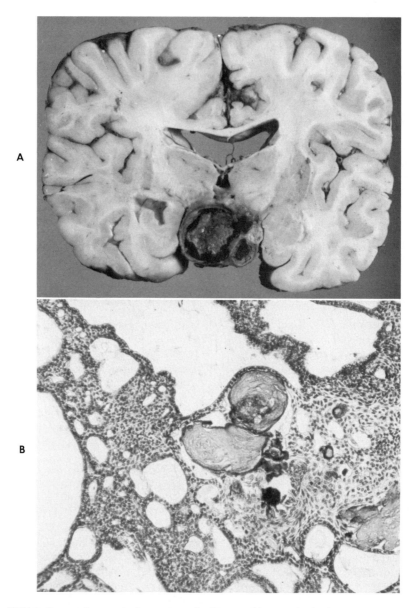

Fig. 1507 A, Suprasellar craniopharyngioma in 47-year-old man who had surgery fifteen years previously, but tumor could not be excised because of its size. Despite subsequent radiation therapy, progressive tumor growth led to compression of optic chiasm, pituitary gland, and cerebral peduncles. Note good circumscription of tumor and its variegated appearance. **B,** Microscopic appearance of craniopharyngioma of suprasellar region. Solid epithelial nests with calcification, collections of "shadow cells," and peripheral palisading alternate with cystic areas. (**A,** WU neg. 62-5191; **B,** ×90; WU neg. 73-2681.)

itary glands surgically removed as part of the treatment of breast carcinoma reveals a strikingly high incidence of unsuspected metastatic involvement.[324] This is always the expression of generalized disease and of little clinical significance, although on occasion it results in diabetes insipidus.[321] In most cases, the metas-

tases are localized either in the posterior lobe alone or in the posterior and anterior lobes together.[367]

Other primary tumors

Paraganglioma can involve the central nervous system in several ways. Glomus jugulare tumors may invade it directly. Carotid tumors and other paragangliomas can metastasize there by the hematogenous route. The possibilities that pineocytoma and cerebellar hemangioblastoma may be related to paraganglioma have been advanced but never substantiated. Two cases of convincing primary *paragangliomas* in the cauda equina have been reported.[373] They can be confused with ependymoma; actually, one of the cases was reported as such.[374] Electron microscopy reveals numerous dense-core neurosecretory granules, as in paraganglioma elsewhere.

Tumors of metastatic origin

Tumors of diverse origins can secondarily involve the central nervous system, either by direct extension or in the form of hematogenous metastases. They are important because they can mimic the features of primary neoplasms both clinically and pathologically. They also can present with the clinical picture of subdural hematoma.[375] The excision of a solitary brain metastasis may precede the detection of a primary visceral neoplasm by several years. Furthermore, the neurologic manifestations may be so prominent that its removal permits an appreciably comfortable life.[380] Local extension is common in *pituitary adenomas*, as previously indicated. *Glomus jugulare tumors* often extend into the posterior fossa and present as pontocerebellar angle tumors (Chapter 15). *Carcinomas* of nasopharynx, paranasal sinuses, and ear may spread into the meninges and nerve roots of the base of the brain. This is also the case with *embryonal rhabdomyosarcomas* of the nasopharynx and ear. We have seen a *basal cell carcinoma* of the scalp penetrate into the skull and invade the cerebral meninges. *Sacrococcygeal chordomas* often produce symptoms of nerve root compression as a result of extension around the cauda equina. *Spheno-occipital chordomas* have a special propensity for penetrating the sella turcica, thus simulating a pituitary neoplasm.

Blood-borne metastatic tumors comprise approximately 4% of the intracranial tumors in surgical series and as many as 27% in some large autopsy series. Carcinomas predominate greatly over the sarcomas. The primary sites, in approximate order of frequency, are lung (65%), breast (30%), malignant melanoma (10%), kidney, colon, pancreas, prostate, stomach, and testis. Malignant melanomas have a particularly great tendency to metastasize to the central nervous system. In a series of 122

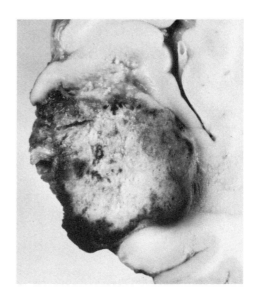

Fig. 1508 Metastatic carcinoma of temporal lobe. Primary tumor was in lung. Note sharp circumscription of tumor and surrounding edema. (WU neg. 72-1778.)

patients with clinically advanced malignant melanoma of the skin, the incidence of metastases to the central nervous system diagnosed clinically was 46% and at autopsy 75%.[376] The metastatic foci may appear as well-circumscribed nodules in the dura and neural parenchyma or as a diffuse meningeal and ventricular carcinomatosis (Fig. 1492). Gonzalez-Vitale and Garcia-Bunuel[379] have suggested that in the latter instance the malignant cells reach the cerebrospinal leptomeninges via perineural, endoneural, and perivascular lymphatics and sheaths through the intervertebral and possibly cranial foramina. In general, metastatic nodules are better delimited than primary tumors and are surrounded by more pronounced edema (Fig. 1508). Vascular endothelial proliferation of the type most commonly seen with glial tumors is occasionally present. Any site of the brain can be affected, but the posterior portion of the sylvian fissure is a favorite location because of the dominance of the middle cerebral artery as a continuation of the internal carotid artery. In a series from the Lahey Clinic, the localization was as follows: frontal region, 60; parietal region, 52; temporal region, 41; cerebellum, 35; occipital region, 23; calvarium, 15; brainstem, 8; meninges, 4.[381] Metastatic tumors involving the spine have a strong preference for the thoracic segment of the epidural space, although intramedullary deposits also may occur.[377,378]

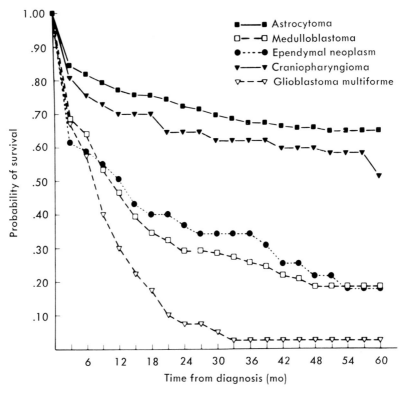

Fig. 1509 Probability of survival with each of five most common central nervous system neoplasms in children. (From Farwell JR, Dohrmann GJ, Flannery JT: Central nervous system tumors in children. Cancer **40**:3123-3132, 1977.)

Clinicopathologic correlation

Tumors of the central nervous system exhibit a rather close correlation between their microscopic types and certain clinical and anatomic parameters. Thus, knowledge of the age of the patient and exact location of the tumor frequently allows for a fairly accurate prediction of the tumor type to be expected, a piece of information that can prove quite useful to the pathologist when examining a small biopsy of a central nervous system neoplasm, particularly at the time of frozen section. The accompanying list, compiled from the surgical cases seen at Barnes Hospital and from several published series,[382-392] summarizes this information. Each major anatomic heading contains the main tumor types to be expected, listed according to their relative frequency. The probability of survival in the five most common central nervous systems neoplasms in children is shown in Fig. 1509.[385]

Cerebral meninges

Meningioma
Metastatic carcinoma

Direct extension from glial tumors
Direct extension from skull tumors
Malignant lymphoma
Primary sarcoma
Melanosis and malignant melanoma

Cerebral hemispheres—adults

Astrocytoma
Undifferentiated glioma
Metastatic carcinoma
Oligodendroglioma
Ependymoma
Arteriovenous malformation
Malignant lymphoma

Cerebral hemispheres—children

Astrocytoma
Ependymoma
Undifferentiated glioma
Sarcoma
Oligodendroglioma

Thalamus and basal ganglia

Undifferentiated glioma
Astrocytoma
Metastatic carcinoma

Corpus callosum and septum pellucidum

Undifferentiated glioma
Astrocytoma
Oligodendroglioma
Metastatic carcinoma

Third ventricle

Colloid cyst
Epidermoid cyst
Craniopharyngioma
Astrocytoma (pilocytic)
Ependymoma
Meningioma
Choroid plexus papilloma
Pituitary adenoma

Lateral ventricles

Ependymoma
Meningioma
Choroid plexus papilloma
Metastatic carcinoma

Pineal region

Germ cell tumors
Astrocytoma
Pinealoma

Region of sella turcica and chiasm—adults

Pituitary adenoma
Meningioma
Craniopharyngioma
Germ cell tumors
Malignant lymphoma
Chordoma

Region of sella turcica and chiasm—children

Craniopharyngioma
Germ cell tumors
Meningioma
Pituitary adenoma

Foramen magnum

Meningioma
Neurilemoma

Brainstem

Astrocytoma
Ependymoma
Undifferentiated glioma
Metastatic carcinoma

Fourth ventricle—adults

Ependymoma
Undifferentiated glioma
Astrocytoma
Choroid plexus papilloma
Metastatic carcinoma

Fourth ventricle—children

Ependymoma
Medulloblastoma

Choroid plexus papilloma
Astrocytoma

Cerebellar vermis—children

Medulloblastoma
Astrocytoma

Cerebellar hemispheres—adults

Astrocytoma
Metastatic carcinoma
Hemangioblastoma
Medulloblastoma

Cerebellar hemispheres—children

Astrocytoma
Medulloblastoma
Hemangioblastoma

Cerebellopontine angle

Neurilemoma
Meningioma
Cholesteatoma
Choroid plexus papilloma
Paraganglioma
Astrocytoma

Spinal cord—intramedullary

Ependymoma
Astrocytoma

Spinal cord—extramedullary

Neurilemoma
Meningioma
Metastatic carcinoma
Malignant lymphoma

Cauda equina—adults

Myxopapillary ependymoma
Metastatic undifferentiated glioma
Metastatic carcinoma
Malignant lymphoma
Chordoma

Cauda equina—children

Metastatic medulloblastoma
Invasion by sacrococcygeal germ cell tumors
Myxopapillary ependymoma

Local and regional effects of intracranial tumors

The most common general signs of intracranial neoplasms are headache, papilledema, vomiting, giddiness, convulsions, abducens palsy, disturbances of mentation, and, less commonly, bradycardia and respiratory dysrhythmias. The plain roentgenogram supplies certain other signs of increased intracranial pressure or space-occupying lesions such as evidence of atrophy about the sella turcica and on the inner table of the skull and detectable shift in the position of a calcified pineal body, whereas special roentgenographic techniques such as ventriculography and arteriography can indicate specifically the location of a lesion. Echoencephalography with ultrasound may be helpful in detecting a shift of midline structures and even the position of parts of tumors or other lesions without subjecting the patient to an operative procedure.[393]

Examples of specific or focal signs are the uncinate fits that accompany involvement of the temporal lobe in the neighborhood of the hippocampus, field defects resulting from interruption of the optic tracts or projection fields, recognizable disturbance of cerebellar functions from involvement of the cerebellum, and, less frequently, recognizable deficit in extrapyramidal activity characteristic of the corpus striatum or sensory disturbance of a nature that can be recognized as thalamic in origin. Lesions in the brainstem and spinal cord often can be almost pinpointed by careful consideration of the disturbances of particular functions known to be associated with tracts or nuclei that are of constant location.

None of these signs, either general or focal,

gives any but inferential evidence, however, of the nature of the underlying lesion.

In addition to the diagnostic import of the phenomenon underlying the signs and symptoms of increased intracranial pressure, certain pathologic conditions are created by this pressure and account for important complications that constantly lurk as unpleasant possibilities in the background of most neurosurgical cases. Principal among these are the herniations that occur at the foramen magnum and through the incisura tentorii. These are most likely to accompany supratentorial space-taking lesions The compression of the medulla as a consequence of its being wedged between the cerebellar tonsils and the rim of the foramen magnum is rarely a lethal mechanism but has been blamed for death due to respiratory or cardiac arrest. This accounts for the general reluctance of neurosurgeons to consent to diagnostic lumbar punctures in patients suspected of having space-occupying cerebral lesions. Such events are fortunately rare, and careful examinations of the entire medical histories of a very high percentage of patients with brain tumors will reveal that a lumbar puncture was per-

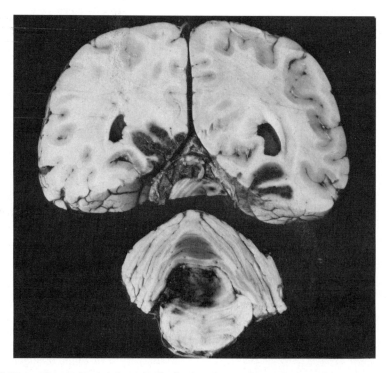

Fig. 1510 Bilateral hemorrhagic infarcts in distribution of posterior cerebral arteries and venous hemorrhages in tegmentum of pons that resulted from incisural and foramen magnum herniations in untreated astrocytoma of frontal lobe. (WU neg. 50-1272.)

formed at some time after the onset of symptoms and before operation with no appreciable untoward effects.

Hemorrhages into the mesencephalon and pons are more commonly proved complications of increased intracranial pressure with herniations at the incisura and the foramen magnum (Fig. 1510). Poppen et al.[396] observed an incidence of 14% in 258 fatal cases of supratentorial lesions. The lesions are particularly prone to occur shortly after operations but may occur spontaneously. It is impossible to estimate how often they may develop without a fatal outcome, but their occurrence in patients who survive is occasionally suggested by the signs of increased disturbance of oculomotor and pyramidal tract function with depression of consciousness or coma. The demonstration of old hemorrhages in these sites at autopsy, however, is very uncommon.

These hemorrhages appear to be of venous or capillary origin because of their infiltrative nature. Were they arterial, a lesion of more destructive and dissecting character would be expected. A satisfactory explanation of their pathogenesis is founded upon the fact that a large portion of the venous drainage of the brainstem flows upward to join Rosenthal's vein and finally Galen's vein. The herniation of tissue into the incisura tentorii compresses this path of venous outflow and is followed by congestion and rupture of vessels in the venous bed. On the other hand, there is interesting evidence that the hemorrhages are related rather specifically to the dynamics of the blood pressure and the increased intracranial pressure[395] and might arise from focal arterial necrosis.[394]

Infarction of the medial and inferior temporal and occipital cortices also occurs as a complication of transtentorial herniation. In this event, the posterior cerebral arteries are compressed in their course around the mesencephalon, and the resulting lesions are usually symmetrical hemorrhagic infarcts. The lesions obviously involve the visual cortex, but the comatose condition of the patient generally prevents recognition of the resulting defects.

Cytology

The use of spinal fluid cytology as a diagnostic method has, in the past, been impeded by the need for a simple and reliable concentration procedure for recovery of the limited number of cells found in spinal fluid specimens. The introduction of special membrane filters permits about 100% cellular recovery and a simplified approach to the problem. The method recommended by Rich[401] is used in most laboratories and is quite satisfactory.

Spinal fluid cytology is of value in patients in whom an intracranial tumor is suspected but other diagnostic procedures have been unrewarding.[398,399] The recovery of tumor cells depends upon whether the tumor has made contact with the subarachnoid space and its ability to exfoliate cells.[402] Meningiomas, although having access to the subarachnoid space, infrequently shed cells, whereas medulloblastomas do so quite readily. Metastatic tumors are more frequently identified than are primary intracranial neoplasms. Tumor cells have been diagnosed cytologically in 40%-50% of patients with cranial metastases, whereas they are detected on an average of 30%-40% in patients with primary lesions. Low-grade gliomas have yielded positive cytology in about 20% of cases studied, while the higher grade tumors have been positive in 40% of cases. Patients with acute lymphoblastic or myeloblastic leukemia have been shown to have immature leukocytes in the spinal fluid at some time during the course of their disease in over 60% of cases.[397,400] Due to the scanty cellular material, the finding of even a few cells that are not consistent with cells normally found in a normal spinal fluid makes the diagnosis of tumor usually a simple task. False positives are rare.[401]

PERIPHERAL NERVES

Routinely processed biopsies of peripheral nerves can provide diagnostic information in a few selected diseases, such as periarteritis nodosa, amyloidosis, sarcoidosis, leprosy, and metachromatic leukodystrophy. On the other hand, they are of little use in the evaluation of the much more common primary degenerative conditions. Proper evaluation of a nerve biopsy in these cases includes a battery of special stains for neurites, myelin, and various enzymes, quantitative estimations, examination of teased fiber preparations, conduction velocity studies in vitro, and electron microscopic examination.[409,413] The sural nerve is particularly suited for biopsy because of its common involvement in peripheral nerve diseases, its superficiality, and its primarily sensory nature. Dyck and Lofgren[408] have described a technique for fascicular biopsy of this nerve that results in only minimal sensorial deficit.

Pathologically, degenerative peripheral neuropathies can be divided in two broad categories. In *axonal (wallerian) degeneration*, the central axon is the primary site of the disease, eventually leading to collapse of the myelin sheath. In *segmental demyelination*, the myelin sheath (and therefore Schwann's cell) is the site of degeneration. The disease begins near the nodes of Ranvier, eventually leading to disappearance of the myelin sheath of an entire internode.[411]

Many are the causes of peripheral neuropathy.[407,414] Some are genetically determined, such as peroneal muscular atrophy (Charcot-Marie-Tooth disease) and hereditary hypertrophic interstitial neuropathy (Dejerine-Sottas disease). A large percentage arise on the basis of a metabolic derangement, such as nutritional deficiency, diabetes, chronic liver disease, uremia, or porphyria.[403,410,415] A form of neuropathy of special interest is that associated with malignant tumors. It is seen more commonly with carcinoma, particularly of the bronchogenic type,[405] but it also has been observed with malignant lymphoma and myeloma.[405,406,416] It may present as a purely sensorial neuropathy with paresthesias due to degeneration of dorsal root ganglion cells or as a symmetrical distal mixed neuropathy secondary to segmental demyelination.[405] The rare occurrence of direct metastatic involvement of the nerve by carcinoma and lymphoma has been reported by Barron et al.[404] In a large percentage of polyneuropathies, the cause remains undetermined.[412]

REFERENCES
CENTRAL NERVOUS SYSTEM
Congenital diseases
Ectopia

1 Goldring S, Hodges FH Jr, Luse SA: Ectopic neural tissue of occipital bone. J Neurosurg **21**:479-484,1964.

Spina bifida

2 Fisher RG, Uihlein A, Keith HM: Spina bifida and cranium bifidum. Study of 530 cases. Mayo Clin Proc **27**:33-38, 1952.

3 Mawdsley T, Rickham PP, Roberts JR: Long term results of early operation of open myelomeningoceles and encephaloceles. Br Med J **1**:663-666, 1967.

4 Russell DS: Observations on the pathology of hydrocephalus. Medical Research Council Special Report Series, No. 265, London, 1949, His Majesty's Stationery Office.

Epidermoid, dermoid, and other congenital cysts

5 Leech RW, Olafson RA: Epithelial cysts of the neuraxis. Presentation of three cases and a review of the origins and classification. Arch Pathol Lab Med **101**:196-202, 1977.

6 Leidler F, Smith DE, Woolsey RD: Intracranial epidermoid cyst. Am J Clin Pathol **21**:852-857, 1951.

7 MacCarty CS, Leavens ME, Love JG, Kernohan JW: Dermoid and epidermoid tumors in the central nervous systems of adults. Surg Gynecol Obstet **108**:191-198, 1959.

8 Manno NJ, Uihlein A, Kernohan JW: Intraspinal epidermoids. J Neurosurg **19**:754-765, 1962.

9 Mount LA: Congenital dermal sinuses as a cause of meningitis, intraspinal abscess and intracranial abscess. JAMA **139**:1263-1268, 1949.

10 Scoville WB, Manlapaz JS, Otis RD, Cabieses F: Intraspinal enterogenous cyst. J Neurosurg **20**:704-706, 1963.

11 Ulrich J: Intracranial epidermoids. A study of their distribution and spread. J Neurosurg **21**:1054-1058, 1964.

12 Wong SW, Ducker TB, Powers JM: Fulminating parapontine epidermoid carcinoma in a four-year-old boy. Cancer **37**:1525-1531, 1976.

Hydrocephalus

13 Beckett RS, Netsky MG, Zimmerman HM: Developmental stenosis of the aqueduct of Sylvius. Am J Pathol **26**:755-787, 1950.

14 Russell DS: Observations on the pathology of hydrocephalus. Medical Research Council Special Report Series, No. 265. London, 1949, His Majesty's Stationery Office.

Arnold-Chiari deformity and platybasia

15 Fairman D, Horrax G: Classification of craniostenosis. J Neurosurg **6**:307-313, 388-395, 1949.

16 List CF: Neurologic syndromes accompanying developmental anomalies of occipital bone, atlas and axis. Arch Neurol Psychiatry **45**:577-616, 1941.

Congenital cerebral diseases and brain biopsy

17 Borberg A: Clinical and genetic investigations into tuberous sclerosis and Recklinghausen's neurofibromatosis. Contribution to elucidation of interrelationship and eugenics of syndromes. Acta Psychiatr Neurol Suppl 71, pp. 3-239, 1951.

18 Davidson C, Jacobson SA: Generalized lipoidosis in a case of amaurotic familial idiocy. Am J Dis Child **52**:345-360, 1936.

19 Hain RF, LaVeck GD: Metachromatic leuko-encephalopathy. Pediatrics **22**:1064-1073, 1958.

20 Landing BH, Rubinstein JH: Biopsy diagnosis of neurologic diseases in children, with emphasis on the lipidoses. In Aronson SM, Volk BW (eds): Cerebral sphingolipidoses. A symposium on Tay-Sach's disease and allied disorders. New York, 1962, Academic Press, Inc. (this volume has other relative papers).

21 McMenemey WH: Cerebral biopsy and special methods for study of cerebrospinal fluid. In Bailey OT, Smith DE (eds): The central nervous system. Baltimore, 1968, The Williams & Wilkins Co.

22 Svennerholm L: Chemical examination of neural biopsy material. General aspects. Acta Neurol Scand **41**[Suppl 13]:281-284, 1965.

23 Wagner JA, Wisotzkey H: Cerebral cortical biopsy: a new vista for the pathologist. South Med J **56**:415-418, 1963.

24 Wolfe HJ, Pietra GG: The visceral lesions of metachromatic leukodystrophy. Am J Pathol **44**:921-930, 1964.

Vascular diseases
Saccular aneurysms

25 Boyd-Wilson JS: The association of cerebral angiomas with intracranial aneurysms. J Neurol Neurosurg Psychiatr **22**:218-223, 1959.

26 Burger PC, Vogel FS: Cerebrovascular disease. Teaching monograph. Am J Pathol **92**:257-314, 1978.

27 Crompton MR: The pathogenesis of cerebral aneurysms. Brain **89**:797-814, 1966.

28 Dandy WE: Intracranial arterial aneurysms. New York, 1969, Hafner Publishing Co.

29 Forbus WD: On the origin of miliary aneurysms of the superficial cerebral arteries. Bull Hopkins Hosp **47**:239-284, 1930.

30 Glynn LE: Medial defects in the circle of Willis and their relation to aneurysm formation. J Pathol Bacteriol **51**:213-222, 1940.

31 Lang ER, Kidd M: Electron microscopy of human cerebral aneurysms. J Neurosurg **22**:554-562, 1965.

32 McCormick WF, Nofzinger JD: Saccular intracranial aneurysms. An autopsy study. J Neurosurg **22**:155-159, 1965.

33 Richardson JC, Hyland HH: Intracranial aneurysms. Medicine (Baltimore) **20**:1-83, 1941.

34 Sahs AL: Observations on the pathology of saccular aneurysms. J Neurosurg **24**:792-806, 1966.

35 Slosberg PS: Medical treatment of intracranial aneurysm. Neurology **10**:1085-1089, 1960.

36 Smith DE, Windsor RB: Embryologic and pathogenic aspects of the development of cerebral saccular aneurysms. In Fields WS (ed): Pathogenesis and treatment of cerebrovascular disease. Springfield, Ill., 1961, Charles C Thomas, Publisher, pp. 367-386.

37 Walker AE, Allegra GW: The pathology and pathogenesis of cerebral aneurysms. J Neuropathol Exp Neurol **13**:248-259, 1954.

Temporal (giant cell) arteritis

38 Hollenhorst RW, Brown JR, Wagener HP, Shick RM: Neurologic aspects of temporal arteritis. Neurology **10**:490-498, 1960.

39 Kimmelstiel P, Gilmour MT, Hodges HH: Degeneration of elastic fibers in granulomatous giant cell arteritis (temporal arteritis) Arch Pathol **54**:157-168, 1952.

40 Kolodny EH, Rebiez JJ, Caviness VS Jr, Richardson EP Jr: Granulomatous angiitis of the central nervous system. J Neuropathol Exp Neurol **27**:125-126, 1968.

Effects of vascular insufficiency
Pseudotumor cerebri

41 Conn HO, Dunn JB, Newman HA, Belkin GA: Pulmonary emphysema simulating brain tumor. Am J Med **22**:524-533, 1957.

42 Foley J: Benign forms of intracranial hypertension—"toxic" and "otitic" hydrocephalus. Brain **78**:1-41, 1955.

43 Zuidema GD, Cohen SJ: Pseudotumor cerebri. J Neurosurg **11**:433-441, 1954.

Traumatic diseases

44 Penfield W, Flanigin H: Surgical therapy of temporal lobe seizures. Arch Neurol Psychiatry **64**:491-500, 1950.

45 Tedeschi CG: Cerebral injury by blunt mechanical trauma. Review of literature. Medicine (Baltimore) **24**:339-357, 1945.

Dural-cortical cicatrix

46 Penfield W, Jasper H: Epilepsy and the functional anatomy of the human brain. Boston, 1954, Little, Brown and Co.

47 Walker AE: Posttraumatic epilepsy. Springfield, Ill., 1949, Charles C Thomas, Publisher.

Epidural hematoma

48 Gallagher JP, Browder EJ: Extradural hematoma. Experience with 167 patients. J Neurosurg **29**:1-12, 1968.

49 Stevenson GC, Brown HA, Hoyt WF: Chronic venous epidural hematoma at the vertex. J Neurosurg **21**:887-891, 1964.

Subdural hematoma

50 Friede RL, Schachenmayr W: The origin of subdural neomembranes. II. Fine structure of neomembranes. Am J Pathol **92**:69-84, 1978.

51 Leary T: Subdural hemorrhages. JAMA **103**:897-903, 1934.

52 McLaurin RL, McLaurin KS: Calcified subdural hematomas in childhood. J Neurosurg **24**:648-655, 1966.

53 Schachenmayr W, Friede RL: The origin of subdural neomembranes. I. Fine structure of the dura-arachnoid interface in man. Am J Pathol **92**:53-68, 1978.

54 Svien HJ, Gelety JE: On the surgical management of encapsulated subdural hematomas. A comparison of the results of membranectomy and simple evacuation. J Neurosurg **21**:172-177, 1964.

55 Zollinger R, Gross RE: Traumatic subdural hematoma. An explanation of the late onset of pressure symptoms. JAMA **103**:245-249, 1934.

Chronic arachnoiditis and arachnoidal cyst

56 Miller PR, Elder FW Jr: Meningeal pseudocysts (meningocele spurius) following laminectomy. Report of ten cases. J Bone Joint Surg [Am] **50**:268-276, 1968.

57 Nugent GR, Odom GL, Woodhall B: Spinal extradural cysts. Neurology **9**:397-405, 1959.

58 Rosenbaum HE, Long F, Hinchey T, Trufant SA: Paralysis following saddle-block anesthesia. Arch Neurol Psychiatry **68**:783-790, 1952.

Ruptured intervertebral discs

59 Strully KJ, Gross SW, Schwartzmann J, von Storch TJC: Progressive spinal cord disease. Syndromes associated with herniation of cervical intervertebral discs. JAMA **146**:10-12, 1951.

Inflammatory diseases
Chronic pachymeningitis

60 Hassin GB: Circumscribed suppurative (nontuberculous) peripachymeningitis. Arch Neurol Psychiatry **20**:110-129, 1928.

Brain and spinal abscess

61 Atkinson EM: Abscess of the brain: its pathology, diagnosis and treatment. London, 1934, Medical Publications, Ltd.

62 Baker AS, Ojemann RG, Swartz MN, Richardson

EP Jr: Spinal epidural abscess. New Engl J Med **293:**463-468, 1975.

63 Carey ME, Chow SN, French LA: Experience with brain abscesses. J Neurosurg **36:**1-9, 1972.

64 Carmichael FA, Kernohan JW, Adson AW: Histopathogenesis of cerebral abscess. Arch Neurol Psychiatry **42:**1001-1029, 1939.

65 Kerr FWL, King RB, Meagher JN: Brain abscess — a study of forty-seven consecutive cases. JAMA **168:**868-872, 1958.

66 Samson DS, Clark R: Current review of brain abscesses. Am J Med **54:**201-210, 1973.

67 Wright RL, Ballantine HT Jr: Management of brain abscesses in children and adolescents. Am J Dis Child **114:**113-122, 1967.

Granulomatous diseases

68 Canton CA, Mount LA: Neurosurgical aspect of cryptococcosis. J Neurosurg **8:**143-156, 1951.

69 Kreuger EG, Norsa L, Kenney M, Price PA: Nocardiosis of the central nervous system. J Neurosurg **11:**226-233, 1954.

70 Schneider RC, Rand RW: Actinomycotin brain abscess. J Neurosurg **6:**255-259, 1949.

Other inflammatory diseases

71 Eimoto T, Yanaka M, Kurosawa M, Ikeya F: Plasma cell granuloma (inflammatory pseudotumor) of the spinal cord meninges. Report of a case. Cancer **4:**1929-1936, 1978.

72 Rayport M, Wisoff HS, Zaiman H: Vertebral echinococcosis. Report of case of surgical and biological therapy with review of the literature. J Neurosurg **21:**647-659, 1964.

Tumors
Introduction

73 Burger, PC, Vogel FS: Frozen section interpretation in surgical neuropathology. I. Intracranial lesions. Am J Surg Pathol **1:**323-347, 1977.

74 Burger PC, Vogel FS: Frozen section interpretation in surgical neuropathology. II. Intraspinal lesions. Am J Surg Pathol **2:**81-95, 1978.

75 Kernohan JW, Sayre GP: Tumors of the central nervous system, In Atlas of tumor pathology, Fasc. 35, Washington, D. C., 1952, Armed Forces Institute of Pathology.

75a Leestma JE: Brain tumors. Am J Pathol **100:**243-316, 1980.

76 Polak M: Blastomas del sistema nervioso central y periférico. Patología y ordenación histogenética. Buenos Aires, 1967, Lopez Libreros Ed.

77 Rubinstein LJ: Tumors of the central nervous system. In Atlas of tumor pathology, Second Series, Fasc. 6, Washington, DC, 1972, Armed Forces Institute of Pathology.

78 Willis RA: Pathology of tumours, ed. 4, London, 1967, Butterworth & Co.

Tumors of neuroglial cells
Astrocytoma

79 Bailey P, Bucy PC: Astroblastomas of the brain. Acta Psychiatr Neurol **5:**439-461, 1960.

80 Bucy PC, Thieman PW: Astrocytomas of the cerebellum. A study of a series of patients operated upon over 28 years ago. Arch Neurol **18:**14-19, 1968.

80a Burger PC, Vollmer RT: Histologic factors of prog-

nostic significance in the glioblastoma multiforme. Cancer **46:**1179-1186, 1980.

80b Burger PC, Mahaley S Jr, Dudka L, Vogel FS: The morphologic effects of radiation administered therapeutically for intracranial gliomas. A postmortem study of 25 cases. Cancer **44:**1256-1272, 1979.

81 Cooper IS, Craig WM, Kernohan JW: Tumors of the spinal cord: primary extramedullary gliomas. Surg Gynecol Obstet **92:**183-190, 1951.

81a De Armond SJ, Eng LF, Rubinstein LJ: The application of glial fibrillary acidic (GFA) protein immunohistochemistry in neuro-oncology. A progress report. Path Res Pract **168:**374-394, 1980.

82 Dohrmann GJ, Farwell JR, Flannery JT: Glioblastoma multiforme in children. J Neurosurg **44:**442-448, 1976.

83 Dunn J Jr, Kernohan JW: Gliomatosis cerebri. Arch Pathol **64:**82-91, 1957.

84 Erlich SS, Davis RL: Spinal subarachnoid metastasis from primary intracranial glioblastoma multiforme. Cancer **42:**2854-2864, 1978.

85 Feigin IH, Gross SW: Sarcoma arising in glioblastoma of the brain. Am J Pathol **31:**633-653, 1955.

85a Gambetti P, Roessmann U, Velasco ME: Immunofluorescence technique for rapid diagnosis of glial tumors. Am J Surg Pathol **4:**277-280, 1980.

86 Gjerris F, Klinken L: Long-term prognosis in children with benign cerebellar astrocytoma. J Neurosurg **49:** 179-184, 1978.

87 Goldman RL: Gliomyosarcoma of the cerebrum. Report of a unique case. Am J Clin Pathol **52:**741-744, 1969.

88 Grcevic N, Yates PO: Rosenthal fibres in tumours of the central nervous system. J Pathol Bacteriol **73:** 467-472, 1957.

89 Hadfield MG, Silverberg SF: Light and electron microscopy of giant-cell glioblastoma. Cancer **30:** 989-996, 1972.

90 Hirano A, Matsui T: Vascular structures in brain tumors. Hum Pathol **6:**611-621, 1975.

91 Hossman KA, Wechsler W: Zur Feinstruktur menschlicher spongioblastome. Dtsch Z Nervenheilk **197:** 327-351, 1965.

92 Hoyt WF, Meshel LG, Lessell S, Schatz NJ, Suckling RD: Malignant optic glioma of adulthood. Brain **96:** 121-132, 1973.

93 Hulbanni S, Goodman PA: Glioblastoma multiforme with extraneural metastases in the absence of previous surgery. Cancer **37:**1577-1583, 1976.

94 Jellinger K: Glioblastoma multiforme: morphology and biology. Acta Neurochir **42:**5-32, 1978.

95 Jelsma R, Bucy PC: The treatment of glioblastoma multiforme of the brain. J Neurosurg **27:**388-400, 1967.

95a Kepes JJ: "Xanthomatous" lesions of the central nervous system: definition, classification and some recent observations. Neuropathology **4:**179-213, 1979.

95b Kepes JJ, Rubinstein LJ, Eng LF: Pleomorphic xanthoastrocytoma: a distinctive meningocerebral glioma of young subjects with relatively favorable prognosis. A study of 12 cases. Cancer **44:**1839-1852, 1979.

95c Liwnicz BH, Rubinstein LJ: The pathways of extraneural spread in metastasizing gliomas. A report of three cases and critical review of the literature. Hum Pathol **10:**453-467, 1979.

96 Lynn JA, Panopio IT, Martin JH, Shaw ML, Race GJ,

Ultrastructural evidence for astroglial histogenesis of the monstruocellular astrocytoma (so-called monstruocellular sarcoma of brain). Cancer **22:**356-366, 1968.

97 Robertson DM, MacLean JD: Nuclear inclusions in malignant gliomas. Arch Neurol **13:**287-296, 1965.

98 Rubinstein LJ, Herman MM, Foley VL: In vitro characteristics of human glioblastomas maintained in organ culture systems. Light microscopic observations. Am J Pathol **71:**61-76, 1973.

99 Russell DS: The occurrence and distribution of intranuclear "inclusion bodies" in gliomas. J Pathol Bacteriol **35:**625-634, 1932.

100 Russell DS, Bland JOW: Further notes on the tissue culture of gliomas with special reference to Bailey's spongioblastoma. J Pathol Bacteriol **39:**375-380, 1934.

101 Scherer HJ: Structural development in gliomas. Am J Cancer **34:**333-351, 1938.

102 Smith DR, Hardman JM, Earle KM: Metastasizing neuroectodermal tumors of the central nervous system. J. Neurosurg **31:**50-58, 1969.

103 Smith DR, Hardman JM, Earle KM: Contiguous glioblastoma multiforme and fibrosarcoma with extracranial metastasis. Cancer **24:**270-276, 1969.

104 Solomon A, Perret GE, McCormick WF: Multicentric gliomas of the cerebral and cerebellar hemispheres. Case report. J Neurosurg **31:**87-93, 1969.

104a Velasco ME, Dahl D, Roessmann U, Gambetti P: Immunohistochemical localization of glial fibrillary acidic protein in human glial neoplasms. Cancer **45:**484-494, 1980.

105 Weir B: The relative significance of factors affecting postoperative survival in astrocytomas, grade 3 and 4. J Neurosurg **38:**448-452, 1973.

Oligodendroglioma

106 Best PV: Intracranial oligodendromatosis. J Neurol Neurosurg Psychiatry **26:**249-256, 1963.

106a Chin HW, Hazel JJ, Kim TH, Webster JH: Oligodendrogliomas. I. A clinical study of cerebral oligodendrogliomas. Cancer **45:**1458-1466, 1980.

107 Pasquier B, Couderc P, Pasquier D, Panh MH, N'Golet A: Sarcoma arising in oligodendroglioma of the brain. A case with intramedullary and subarachnoid spinal metastases. Cancer **42:**2753-2758, 1978.

108 Roberts M, German WJ: A long term study of patients with oligodendrogliomas. Follow-up of 50 cases, including Dr. Harvey Cushing's series. J Neurosurg **24:**697-700, 1966.

109 Robertson DM, Vogel FS: Concentric lamination of glial processes in oligodendrogliomas. J Cell Biol **15:**313-334, 1962.

110 Rubinstein LJ: Tumors of the central nervous system. In Atlas of tumor pathology, Second Series, Fasc. 6. Washington, DC, 1972, Armed Forces Institute of Pathology.

111 Scharenberg K: Blastomatous oligodendroglia as satellites of nerve cells. A study with silver carbonate. Am J Pathol **30:**957-967, 1954.

112 Spataro J, Sacks O: Oligodendroglioma with remote metastases. Case report. J. Neurosurg **28:**373-379, 1968.

113 Takei Y, Mirra SS, Miles ML: Eosinophilic granular cells in oligodendrogliomas. An ultrastructural study. Cancer **38:**1968-1976, 1976.

114 Weir B, Elvidge AR: Oligodendrogliomas. An analysis of 63 cases. J Neurosurg **29:**500-525, 1968.

Ependymoma

115 Anderson MS: Myxopapillary ependymomas presenting in the soft tissue over the sacrococcygeal region. Cancer **19:**585-590, 1966.

116 Ayres WW: Ependymoma of the cauda equina. A report of the clinicopathologic aspects and follow-up studies of eighteen cases. Milit Med **122:**10-35, 1958.

117 Chason JL: Subependymal mixed gliomas. J Neuropathol Exp Neurol **15:**461-470, 1956.

118 Dohrmann GJ, Farwell JR, Flannery JT: Ependymomas and ependymoblastomas in children. J Neurosurg **45:**273-283, 1976.

119 Fokes EC Jr, Earle KM: Ependymomas: clinical and pathological aspects. J Neurosurg **30:**585-594, 1969.

120 Goebel HH, Cravioto H: Ultrastructure of human and experimental ependymomas. A comparative study. J Neuropathol Exp Neurol **31:**54-71, 1972.

121 Kernohan JW, Fletcher-Kernohan E: Ependymomas. A study of 109 cases. Assoc Res Nerv Ment Dis Proc **16:**182-209, 1937.

122 Mathews T, Moossy J: Gliomas containing bone and cartilage. J Neuropathol Exp Neurol **33:**456-471, 1974.

123 Mørk SJ, Løken AC: Ependymoma. A follow-up study of 101 cases. Cancer **40:**907-915, 1977.

124 Rawlinson DG, Herman MM, Rubinstein LJ: The fine structure of a myxopapillary ependymoma of the filum terminale. Acta Neuropathol **25:**1-13, 1973.

125 Rubinstein LJ: Tumors of the central nervous system. In Atlas of tumor pathology, Second Series, Fasc. 6. Washington, D.C., 1972, Armed Forces Institute of Pathology.

126 Rubinstein LJ, Logan WJ: Extraneural metastases in ependymoma of the cauda equina. J Neurol Neurosurg Psychiatry **33:**763-770, 1970.

127 Scheithauer BW: Symptomatic subependymoma. J Neurosurg **49:**689-696, 1978.

128 Wolff M, Santiago H, Duby MM: Delayed distant metastasis from a subcutaneous sacrococcygeal ependymoma; case report with tissue culture, ultrastructural observations and review of the literature. Cancer **30:**1046-1067, 1972.

Mixed glioma

129 Hart MN, Petito CK, Earle KM: Mixed gliomas. Cancer **33:**134-140, 1974.

Tumors and tumorlike conditions of choroid plexus

130 Ariëns-Kappers JA: The development of the paraphysis cerebri in man with comments on its relationship to the intercolumnar tubercle and its significance for the origin of cystic tumors in the third ventricle. J Comp Neurol **102:**425-509, 1955.

131 Ayres WW, Haymaker W: Xanthoma and cholesterol granuloma of the choroid plexus; report of the pathologic aspects in 29 cases. J Neuropathol Exp Neurol **23:**431-445, 1964.

132 Carter LP, Beggs J, and Waggener JD: Ultrastructure of three choroid plexus papillomas. Cancer **30:**1130-1136, 1972.

133 Coxe WS, Luse SA: Colloid cyst of third ventricle. An electron microscopic study. J Neuropathol Exp Neurol **23:**431-445, 1964.

134 Shuangshoti S, Netsky MG: Neuroepithelial (colloid) cysts of nervous system: further observations on pathogenesis, location, incidence and histochemistry. Neurology **16:**887-903, 1966.

135 Shuangshoti S, Roberts MP, Netsky MG: Neuroepithelial (colloid) cysts. Arch Pathol **80**:214-224, 1965.

136 Shuangshoti S, Tangchai P, Netsky MG: Primary adenocarcinoma of the choroid plexus. Arch Pathol **91**:101-106, 1971.

137 Smith JF: Hydrocephalus associated with choroid plexus papillomas. J Neuropathol Exp Neurol **14**:442-449, 1955.

138 Wolfson WL, Brown WJ: Disseminated choroid plexus papilloma. An ultrastructural study. Arch Pathol Lab Med **101**:366-368, 1977.

Tumors of primitive neuroepithelial cells

139 Ahdevaara P, Kalimo H, Torma T, Haltia M: Differentiating intracerebral neuroblastoma. Cancer **40**:784-788, 1977.

140 Bailey P, Cushing H: A classification of the tumors of the glioma group on a histogenetic basis with a correlated study of prognosis. Philadelphia, 1966, J. B. Lippincott Co.

141 Banna M, Lassman LP, Pearce GW: Radiological study of skeletal metastases from cerebellar medulloblastoma. Br J Radiol **43**:173-179, 1970.

142 Bloom HJG, Wallace ENK, Henz JM: Treatment and prognosis of medulloblastoma in children: study of 82 verified cases. Am J Roentgenol Radium Ther Nucl Med **105**:43-62, 1969.

143 Boesel CP, Suhan JP, Bradel EJ: Ultrastructure of primitive neuroectodermal neoplasms of the central nervous system. Cancer **42**:194-201, 1978.

144 Bofin PJ, Ebels E: A case of medullomyoblastoma. Acta Neuropathol (Berl) **2**:309-311, 1963.

145 Chatty EM, Earle KM: Medulloblastoma. A report of 201 cases with emphasis on the relationship of histologic variants to survival. Cancer **28**:977-983, 1971.

146 Crue BL Jr: Medulloblastoma. Springfield, Ill., 1958 Charles C Thomas, Publisher.

147 Drachman DA, Winter TS III, Karon M: Medulloblastoma with extracranial metastases. Arch Neurol **9**:518-530, 1963.

148 Feigin I, Budzilovich GN: Tumors of neurons and their precursors. J Neuropathol Exp Neurol **33**:483-506, 1974.

149 Kadin ME, Rubinstein LJ, Nelson JS: Neonatal cerebellar medulloblastoma originating from the fetal external granular layer. J Neuropathol Exp Neurol **29**:583-600, 1970.

150 Kane W, Aronson SM: Gangliogliomatous maturation in cerebellar medulloblastoma. Acta Neuropathol (Berl) **9**:273-279, 1967.

151 Karch SB, Urich H: Medulloepithelioma: definition of an entity. J Neuropathol Exp Neurol **31**:27-53, 1972.

152 McFarland DR, Horwitz H, Saenger EL, Bahr GK: Medulloblastoma. Review of prognosis and survival. Br J Radiol **42**:198-214, 1969.

153 Matakas F, Cervós-Navarro J, Gullotta F: The ultrastructure of medulloblastomas. Acta Neuropathol (Berl) **16**:271-284, 1970.

154 Miller AA, Ramsden F: A cerebral neuroblastoma with unusual fibrous tissue reaction. J Neuropathol Exp Neurol **25**:328-340, 1966.

155 Misugi K, Liss L: Medulloblastoma with cross-striated muscle: a fine structural study. Cancer **25**:1279-1285, 1970.

156 Oberman HA, Hewitt WC Jr, Kalivoda AJ: Medulloblastomas with distant metastases. Am J Pathol **39**:148-160, 1963.

157 Polak M: On the true nature of the so-called medulloblastoma. Acta Neuropathol (Berl) **8**:84-95, 1967.

158 Pollak A, Friede RL: Fine structure of medulloepithelioma. J Neuropathol Exp Neurol **36**:712-725, 1977.

159 Rio Hortega P del: Nomenclatura y clasificación de los tumores del sistema nervioso. Buenos Aires, 1945, Lopez & Etchegoyen.

160 Rubinstein LJ: Discussion on polar spongioblastomas. Acta Neurochir (Wien) [suppl] **10**:126-132, 1964.

161 Rubinstein LJ: The definition of the ependymoblastoma. Arch Pathol **90**:35-45, 1970.

162 Rubinstein LJ: Cytogenesis and differentiation of primitive central neuroepithelial tumors. J Neuropathol Exp Neurol **31**:7-26, 1972.

163 Rubinstein LJ: Tumors of the central nervous system. In Atlas of tumor pathology, Second Series, Fasc. 6. Washington, DC, 1972, Armed Forces Institute of Pathology.

164 Rubinstein LJ, Northfield DWC: Medulloblastoma and so-called "arachnoidal cerebellar sarcoma": critical re-examination of a nosologic problem. Brain **87**:379-412, 1964.

165 Schenk EA: Medulloblastoma. Relationship to meningeal sarcoma. Arch Pathol **82**:363-368, 1966.

166 Treip CS: A congenital medulloepithelioma of the midbrain. J Pathol Bacteriol **74**:357-363, 1957.

167 von Epps RR, Samuelson DR, McCormick WF: Cerebral medulloepithelioma. Case report. J Neurosurg **27**:568-573, 1967.

Tumors of neuronal cells

168 Courville CB: Ganglioglioma, tumor of the central nervous system. Review of the literature and report of two cases. Arch Neurol Psychiatry **24**:439-491, 1930.

169 Steegmann AT, Winer B: Temporal lobe epilepsy resulting from ganglioglioma. Report of an unusual case in an adolescent boy. Neurology **11**:406-412, 1961.

170 Wahl RW, Dillard SH Jr: Multiple ganglioneuromas of the central nervous system. Arch Pathol **94**:158-164, 1972.

Tumors of meningothelial cells

171 Bailey P, Cushing H, Eisenhardt L: Angioblastic meningiomas. Arch Pathol **6**:953-990, 1928.

172 Cervós-Navarro J, Vazquez JJ: An electron microscopic study of meningiomas. Acta Neuropathol (Berl) **13**:301-323, 1969.

172a Chambers PW, Davis RL, Blanding JD Jr, Buck FS: Metastases to primary intracranial meningiomas and neurilemomas. Arch Pathol Lab Med **104**:350-354, 1980.

173 Copeland DD, Bell SW, Shelburne JD: Hemidesmosome-like intercellular specializations in human meningiomas. Cancer **41**:2242-2249, 1978.

174 Cushing HW, Eisenhardt L: Meningiomas: their classification, regional behavior, life history and surgical end results. Springfield, Ill., 1938, Charles C Thomas, Publishers.

174a Font RL, Croxatto JO: Intracellular inclusions in meningothelial meningioma. A histochemical and ultrastructural study. J Neuropathol Exper Neurol **39**:575-583, 1980.

175 Goellner JR, Laws ER Jr, Soule EH, Okazaki H: Hemangiopericytoma of the meninges. Mayo Clinic experience. Am J Clin Pathol **70**:375-380, 1978.

176 Horten BC, Urich H, Stefoski D: Meningiomas with conspicuous plasma cell-lymphocytic components. A

report of five cases. Cancer **43**:258-264, 1979.

177 Kepes J: Observations of the formation of psammoma bodies in meningiomas. J Neuropathol Exp Neurol **20**: 255-262, 1961.

178 Kepes JJ: Cellular whorls in brain tumors other than meningiomas. Cancer **37**:2232-2237, 1976.

179 Kepes J, Kernohan JW: Meningiomas: Problems of histological differential diagnosis. Cancer **12**:364-370, 1959.

180 Kjeldsberg CR, Minckler J: Meningiomas presenting as nasal polyps. Cancer **29**:153-156, 1972.

180a Kleinman GM, Liszczak T, Tarlov E, Richardson EP Jr: Microcystic variant of meningioma. A light-microscopic and ultrastructural study. Am J Surg Pathol **4**:383-389, 1980.

181 Kobahashi S, Okazaki H, MacCarthy CS: Intraventricular meningiomas. Mayo Clin Proc **46**:735-741, 1971.

182 Kruse F Jr: Hemangiopericytoma of the meninges (angioblastic meningioma of Cushing and Eisenhardt). Clinicopathologic aspects and follow-up studies in 8 cases. Neurology **11**:771-777, 1961.

183 Lopez DA, Silvers DN, Helwig EB: Cutaneous meningiomas—a clinicopathologic study. Cancer **34**:728-744, 1974.

184 Ludwin SK, Rubinstein LJ, Russell DS: Papillary meningioma: a malignant variant of meningioma. Cancer **36**:1363-1373, 1975.

185 Marc JA, Takei Y, Schechter MM, Hoffman JC: Intracranial hemangiopericytomas. Angiography, pathology and differential diagnosis. Am J Roentgenol Radium Ther Nucl Med **125**:823-832, 1975.

186 Napolitano L, Kyle R, Fisher ER: Ultrastructure of meningiomas and the derivation and nature of their cellular components. Cancer **17**:233-241, 1964.

187 Pitkethly DT, Hardman JM, Kempe LG, Earle KM: Angioblastic meningiomas. Clinicopathologic study of 81 cases. J Neurosurg **32**:539-544, 1970.

188 Rubinstein LJ: Tumors of the central nervous system. In Atlas of tumor pathology, Second Series, Fasc. 6. Washington, D.C., 1972, Armed Forces Institute of Pathology.

189 Russell DS, Rubinstein LJ: Pathology of tumors of the nervous system, ed. 4. Baltimore, 1977, The Williams & Wilkins, Co.

190 Shuangshoti S, Hongsaprabhas C, Netsky MG: Metastasizing meningioma. Cancer **26**:832-841, 1970.

191 Simpson D: The recurrence of intracranial meningiomas after surgical treatment. J Neurol Neurosurg Psychiatry **20**:22-39, 1957.

192 Skullerud K, Löken AC: The prognosis in meningiomas. Acta Neuropath (Berl) **29**:337-344, 1974.

193 Suzuki H, Gilbert EF, Zimmerman B: Primary extracranial meningioma. Arch Pathol **84**:202-206, 1967.

Tumors of melanocytes

194 McCloskey JJ, Parker JC Jr, Brooks WH, Blacker HM: Melanin as a component of cerebral gliomas. The melanotic cerebral ependymoma. Cancer **37**: 2373-2379, 1976.

195 Pappenheim E, Bhattacharji SK: Primary melanoma of the central nervous system. Arch Neurol **7**:101-113, 1962.

196 Pasquier B, Couderc P, Pasquier D, Panh MH, Arnould JP: Primary malignant melanoma of the cerebellum. A case with metastases outside the nervous system. Cancer **41**:344-351, 1978.

197 Silbert SW, Smith KR, Jr, Horenstein S: Primary leptomeningeal melanoma. An ultrastructural study. Cancer **41**:519-527, 1978.

198 Slaughter JC, Hardman JM, Kempe LG, Earle KM: Neurocutaneous melanosis and leptomeningeal melanomatosis in children. Arch Pathol **88**:298-304, 1969.

Tumors and malformations of blood vessels

199 Alexander GL, Norman RM: The Sturge-Weber syndrome. Bristol, 1960, John Wright & Sons, Ltd.

200 Bailey WL, Sperl MP: Angiomas of the cervical spinal cord. J Neurosurg **30**:560-568, 1969.

201 Brihaye J, Blackwoord W: Arteriovenous aneurysm of the cerebral hemispheres. J Pathol Bacteriol **73**:25-31, 1957.

202 Brion S, Netsky MG, Zimmerman HM: Vascular malformations of the spinal cord. Arch Neurol Psychiatry **68**:339-361, 1952.

203 Carleton CC, Cauthen JC: Vascular (''arteriovenous'') malformations of the choroid plexus. Arch Pathol **99**: 286-288, 1975.

204 Castaigne P, David M, Pertviset B, Escourolle R, Poirier J: L'ultrastructure des hémangioblastomes du système nerveux central. Rev Neurol **118**:5-26, 1968.

205 Chaudhry AP, Montes M, Cohn GA: Ultrastructure of cerebellar hemangioblastoma. Cancer **42**:1834-1850, 1978.

206 Cramer F, Kimsey W: Cerebellar hemangioblastomas. Review of 53 cases, with special reference to cerebellar cysts and the association of polycythemia. Arch Neurol Psychiatry **67**:237-252, 1952.

207 Doppman JL, Wirth FP Jr, Di Chiro G, Ommaya AK: Value of cutaneous angiomas in the arteriographic localization of spinal-cord arteriovenous malformations. N Engl J Med **281**:1440-1444, 1969.

208 Henderson WR, Gomez R de RL: Natural history of cerebral angiomas. Br Med J **4**:571-574, 1967.

209 Hoff JT, Ray BS: Cerebral hemangioblastoma occurring in a patient with von Hippel-Lindau disease. Case report. J Neurosurg **28**:365-368, 1968.

209a Kepes JJ, Rengachary SS, Lee SH: Astrocytes in hemangioblastomas of the central nervous system and their relationship to stromal cells. Acta Neuropathol (Berl) **47**:99-104, 1979.

210 Melmon KL, Rosen SW: Lindau's disease. Review of the literature and study of a large kindred. Am J Med **36**:595-617, 1964.

211 Nibbelink DW, Peters BH, McCormick WF: On the association of pheochromocytoma and cerebellar hemangioblastoma. Neurology **19**:455-460, 1969.

212 Pia HW: Diagnosis and treatment of spinal angiomas. Acta Neurochir **28**:1-12, 1973.

213 Poser CM: The relationship between syringomyelia and neoplasm. Springfield, Ill., 1956. Charles C Thomas, Publisher.

214 Price EB Jr: Papillary cystadenoma of the epididymis: a clinicopathologic analysis of 20 cases. Arch Pathol **90**:456-470, 1971.

215 Silver ML, Hennigar G: Cerebellar hemangioma (hemangioblastoma). A clinicopathological review of 40 cases. J Neurosurg **9**:484-494, 1952.

216 Spence AM, Rubinstein LJ: Cerebellar capillary hemangioblastoma: its histogenesis studied by organ culture and electron microscopy. Cancer **35**:326-341, 1975.

217 Waldmann TA, Levin EH, Baldwin M: The association of polycythemia with a cerebellar hemangioblastoma. The production of an erythropoiesis stimulating factor by the tumor. Am J Med **31**:318-324, 1961.

218 Wohlwill FJ, Yakovlev PI: Histopathology of meningofacial angiomatosis (Sturge-Weber's disease). Report of four cases. J Neuropathol Exp Neurol **16:** 341-364, 1957.

219 Wyburn-Mason R: The vascular abnormalities and tumours of the spinal cord and its membrane. London, 1943, Henry Kimpton.

Tumors of lymphoreticular system

220 Adams JH, Jackson JM: Intracerebral tumours of reticular tissue: the problem of microgliomatosis and reticulo-endothelial sarcomas of the brain. J Pathol Bacteriol **91:**369-381, 1966.

221 Brand MM, Marinkovich VA: Primary malignant reticulosis of the brain in Wiskott-Aldrich syndrome. Arch Dis Child **44:**536-542, 1969.

222 Bucy PC, Jerva MJ: Primary epidural spinal lymphosarcoma. J Neurosurg **19:**142-152, 1962.

223 Burstein SD, Kernohan JW, Uihlein A: Neoplasms of the reticuloendothelial system of the brain. Cancer **16:** 289-305, 1963.

224 Clarke E: Cranial and intracranial myelomas, Brain **77:**61-81, 1954.

225 Cuttner J, Meyer R, Huang YP: Intracerebral involvement in Hodgkin's disease. Cancer **43:**1497-1506, 1979.

226 Edgar R, Dutcher TF: Histopathology of the Bing-Neel syndrome. Neurology **11:**239-245, 1961.

227 Griffin JW, Thompson RW, Mitchinson MJ, de Kiewiet JC, Wellard FH: Lymphomatous meningitis. Am J Med **51:**200-208, 1971.

228 Haddad P, Thaell JF, Kiely JM, Harrison EG, Miller RH: Lymphoma of the spinal extradural space. Cancer **38:**1862-1866, 1976.

229 Henry JM, Heffner RR Jr, Dillard SH, Earle KM, Davis RL: Primary malignant lymphomas of the central nervous system. Cancer **34:**1293-1302, 1974.

230 Herman TS, Hammond N, Jones SE, Butler JJ, Byrne GE Jr, McKelvey EM: Involvement of the central nervous system by non-Hodgkin's lymphoma. The Southwest Oncology Group experience. Cancer **43:** 390-397, 1979.

231 Horvat B, Pena C, Fisher ER: Primary reticulum cell sarcoma (microglioma) of brain. Arch Pathol **87:** 609-616, 1969.

232 Houthoff HJ, Poppema S, Ebels EJ, Elema JD: Intracranial malignant lymphomas. Acta Neuropathol (Berl) **44:**203-210, 1978.

233 Jellinger K, Radaskiewicz TH, Slowik F: Primary malignant lymphoma of the central nervous system in man. Acta Neuropathol [Suppl] (Berl) **6:**95-102, 1975.

234 Kernohan JW, Uihlein A: Sarcomas of the brain. Springfield, Ill., 1962, Charles C Thomas, Publisher.

234a Kokmen E, Billman JK Jr, Abell MR: Lymphomatoid granulomatosis clinically confined to the CNS. A case report. Arch Neurol **34:**782-784, 1977.

235 Krishnamurthy M, Nusbacher N, Elguezabal A, Seligman BR: Granulocytic sarcoma of the brain. Cancer **39:**1542-1546, 1977.

236 Lambert CD, Trewby PN: Microglioma with paraproteinaemia. J Neurol Neurosurg Psychiatry **37:**835-840, 1974.

237 Littman P, Wang CC: Reticulum cell sarcoma of the brain. A review of the literature and a study of 19 cases. Cancer **35:**1412-1420, 1975.

238 Lundberg WB, Cadman EC, Skeel RT: Leptomeningeal mycosis fungoides. Cancer **38:**2149-2153, 1976.

239 Mancilla-Jimenez R, Tavassoli FA: Solitary meningeal plasmacytoma. Report of a case with electron microscopic and immunohistologic observations. Cancer **38:** 798-806, 1976.

240 Marshall G, Roessmann U, van der Noort S: Invasive Hodgkin's disease of brain. Report of two new cases and review of American and European literature with clinical-pathologic correlations. Cancer **22:**621-630, 1968.

241 Miller AA, Ramsden F: Primary reticulosis of the central nervous system. "Microgliomatosis." Acta Neurochir **11:**439-478, 1963.

242 Moore EW, Thomas LB, Shaw RK, Freireich EJ: The central nervous system in acute leukemia. A postmortem study of 117 consecutive cases, with particular reference to hemorrhages, leukemia infiltrations, and the syndrome of meningeal leukemia. Arch Intern Med **105:**451-468, 1960.

243 Reddick RL, Fauci AS, Valsamis MP, Mann RB: Immunoblastic sarcoma of the central nervous system in a patient with lymphomatoid granulomatosis. Cancer **42:**652-659, 1978.

244 Rosai J, Spiro J: Central nervous system involvement by mycosis fungoides. Acta Derm Venereol (Stockh) **48:**482-488, 1968.

245 Russell DS, Marshall AHE, Smith FB: Microgliomatosis. A form of reticulosis affecting the brain. Brain **71:**1-15, 1948.

246 Samuelsson S-M, Werner L, Poutén J, Nathorst-Windahl G, Thorell J: Reticuloendothelial (perivascular) sarcoma of the brain. Acta Neurol Scand **42:**567-580, 1966.

247 Schneck SA, Penn I: De-novo brain tumors in renal transplant recipients. Lancet **1:**983-986, 1971.

248 Taylor CR, Russell R, Lukes RJ, Davis RL: An immunohistological study of immunoglobulin content of primary central nervous system lymphomas. Cancer **41:**2197-2205, 1978.

249 Valsamis MP, Levine PH, Rapin I, Santorineou M, Shulman K: Primary intracranial Burkitt's lymphoma in an infant. Cancer **37:**1500-1507, 1976.

250 Wolk RW, Masse SR, Conklin R, Freireich EJ: The incidence of central nervous system leukemia in adults with acute leukemia. Cancer **33:**863-869, 1974.

Tumors of nerve roots

251 Anderson MS, Bentinck BR: Intracranial schwannoma in a child. Cancer **29:**231-234, 1972.

252 Cravioto H: The ultrastructure of acoustic nerve tumors. Acta Neuropathol **12:**116-140, 1969.

253 Erickson LS, Sorenson GD, McGavran MH: A review of 140 acoustic neurinomas (neurilemmoma). Laryngoscope **75:**601-627, 1965.

253a Lowman RM, Livolsi VA: Pigmented (melanotic) schwannomas of the spinal canal. Cancer **46:**391-397, 1980.

254 Olivecrona H: Acoustic tumors. J Neurosurg **26:**6-13, 1967.

255 Rodriguez HA, Berthrong M: Multiple primary intracranial tumors in von Recklinghausen's neurofibromatosis. Arch Neurol **14:**467-475, 1966.

256 Rubinstein LJ: Tumors of the central nervous system. In Atlas of tumor pathology, Second Series, Fasc. 6. Washington, D.C., 1972, Armed Forces Institute of Pathology.

257 Sloof JL, Kernohan JW, MacCarthy CS: Primary intramedullary tumors of the spinal cord and filum terminale. Philadelphia, 1964, W. B. Saunders Co.

Tumors of germ cell origin

258 Bestle J: Extragonadal endodermal sinus tumours originating in the region of the pineal gland. Acta Pathol Microbiol Scand **74**:214-222, 1968.

259 Dayan AD, Marshall AHE, Miller AA, Pick FJ, Rankin NE: Atypical teratomas of the pineal and hypothalamus. J Pathol Bacteriol **92**:1-28, 1966.

260 DeGirolami U, Schmidek H: Clinicopathological study of 53 tumors of the pineal region. J Neurosurg **39**:455-462, 1973.

261 Friedman NB: Germinoma of the pineal; its identity with germinoma (''seminoma'') of the testis. Cancer Res **7**:363-368, 1947.

262 Ghatak NR, Hirano A, Zimmerman HM: Intrasellar germinomas: a form of ectopic pinealoma. J Neurosurg **31**:670-675, 1969.

263 Globus JH, Silbert S: Pinealomas. Arch Neurol **25**:937-984, 1931.

264 Nishiyama RH, Batsakis JG, Weaver DK, Simrall JH: Germinal neoplasms of the central nervous system. Arch Surg **93**:342-347, 1966.

265 Norgaard-Pedersen B, Lindholm J, Albrechtsen R, Arends J, Diemer NH, Rushede J: Alpha-fetoprotein and human chorionic gonadotropin in a patient with a primary intracranial germ cell tumor. Cancer **41**:2315-2320, 1978.

266 Pickens JM, Wilson J, Myers GG, Grunnet ML: Teratoma of the spinal cord. Report of a case and review of the literature. Arch Pathol **99**:446-448, 1975.

267 Prioleau G, Wilson CB: Endodermal sinus tumor of the pineal region. Case report. Cancer **38**:2489-2493, 1976.

268 Puschett JB, Goldberg M: Endocrinopathy associated with pineal tumor. Ann Intern Med **69**:203-219, 1968.

269 Ramsey HJ: Ultrastructure of a pineal tumor. Cancer **18**:1014-1025, 1965.

270 Russell DS: The pinealoma: its relationship to teratoma. J Pathol Bacteriol **56**:145-150, 1944.

271 Russell DS: ''Ectopic pinealoma'': its kinship to atypical teratoma of the pineal gland. Report of a case. J Pathol Bacteriol **68**:125-129, 1954.

272 Simson LR, Lampe I, Abell MR: Suprasellar germinomas. Cancer **22**:533-544, 1968.

272a Tavcar D, Robboy SJ, Chapman P: Endodermal sinus tumor of the pineal region. Cancer **45**:2646-2651, 1980.

Tumors of pineal gland

272b Borit A, Blackwood W, Mair WGP: The separation of pineocytoma from pineoblastoma. Cancer **45**:1408-1418, 1980.

273 Costero I, Earle KM: Pinealoma: a variety of argentaffinoma? Nature (Lond) **199**:190, 1963.

273a Kline KT, Damjanov I, Katz SM, Schmidek H: Pineoblastoma: an electron microscopic study. Cancer **44**:1692-1699, 1979.

274 Nielsen SL, Wilson CB: Ultrastructure of a ''pineocytoma.'' J Neuropathol Exp Neurol **34**:148-158, 1975.

275 Rubinstein LJ: Tumors of the central nervous system. In Atlas of tumor pathology, Second Series, Fasc. 6. Washington, D.C., 1972, Armed Forces Institute of Pathology.

276 Smith WT, Hughes B, Ermocilla R: Chemodectoma of the pineal region, with observations on the pineal body and chemoreceptor tissue. J Pathol Bacteriol **92**:69-76, 1966.

Tumors of other mesenchymal cells

277 Ammerman BJ, Henry JM, Girolami UD, Earle KM: Intradural lipomas of the spinal cord. A clinicopathological correlation. J Neurosurg **44**:331-336, 1976.

278 Bailey OT, Ingraham FD: Intracranial fibrosarcomas of the dura mater in childhood: pathological characteristics and surgical management. J Neurosurg **2**:1-15, 1945.

279 Black BK, Kernohan JW: Primary diffuse tumors of the meninges (so-called meningeal meningiomatosis). Cancer **3**:805-819, 1950.

280 Kepes JJ, Kepes M, Slowik F: Fibrous xanthomas and xanthosarcomas of the meninges and the brain. Acta Neuropathol (Berl) **23**:187-199, 1973.

281 Kepes JJ, Rubinstein LJ, Eng LF: Pleomorphic xanthoastrocytoma: a distinctive meningocerebral glioma of young subjects with relatively favorable prognosis. A study of 12 cases. Cancer **44**:1839-1852, 1979.

282 Kernohan JW, Vihlein A: Sarcomas of the brain. Springfield, Ill., 1962, Charles C Thomas, Publisher.

283 Lalitha VS, Rubinstein LJ: Reactive glioma in intracranial sarcoma: a form of mixed sarcoma and glioma (''sarcoglioma''). Report of eight cases. Cancer **43**:246-257, 1979.

284 Mena H, Garcia JH: Primary brain sarcomas. Light and electron microscopic features. Cancer **42**:1298-1307, 1978.

285 Min K-W, Gyorkey F, Halpert B: Primary rhabdomyosarcoma of the cerebrum. Cancer **35**:1405-1411, 1975.

286 Ming-Yan Lam R, Colah SA: Atypical fibrous histiocytoma with myxoid stroma. A rare lesion arising from dura mater of the brain. Cancer **43**:237-245, 1979.

287 Pasquier B, Coudarc P, Pasquier D, Hong PM, Pellat J: Primary rhabdomyosarcoma of the central nervous system. Acta Neurpathol (Berl) **33**:333 342, 1975.

288 Raskind R, Grant S: Primary mesenchymal chondrosarcoma of the cerebrum. Report of a case. J Neurosurg **24**:676-678, 1966.

289 Scheithauer BW, Rubinstein LJ: Meningeal mesenchymal chondrosarcoma. Report of 8 cases with review of the literature. Cancer **42**:2744-2752, 1978.

290 Schrantz JL, Araoz CA: Radiation induced meningeal fibrosarcoma. Arch Pathol **93**:26-31, 1972.

291 Shuangshoti S, Piyaratn P, Viriyapanich PL: Primary rhabdomyosarcoma of cerebellum: necropsy report. Cancer **22**:367-371, 1968.

292 Waltz TA, Brownell B: Sarcoma: a possible late result of effective radiation therapy for pituitary adenoma. Report of two cases. J Neurosurg **24**:901-907, 1966.

Tumors of pituitary gland

293 Ahmad K, Fayos JV: Pituitary fibrosarcoma secondary to radiation therapy. Cancer **42**:107-110, 1978.

294 Bain J, Ezrin C: Immunofluorescent localization of the LH cell of the human adenohypophysis. J Clin Endocrinol Metab **30**:181-184, 1970.

295 Baker BL: Studies on hormone localization with emphasis on the hypophysis. J Histochem Cytochem **18**:1-40, 1970.

296 Baker BL, Yu Y-Y: The thyrotropic cell of the rat hypophysis as studied with peroxidase-labelled antibody. Am J Anat **131**:55-71, 1971.

297 Ballard HS, Frame B, Hartsock RJ: Familial multiple

endocrine adenoma-peptic ulcer complex. Medicine (Baltimore) **43:**481-516, 1964.

298 Bauserman SC, Hardman JM, Schochet SS Jr, Earle RM: Pituitary oncocytoma. Indispensable role of electron microscopy in its identification. Arch Pathol Lab Med **102:**456-459, 1978.

299 Bergland RM, Torack RM: An ultrastructural study of follicular cells in the human anterior pituitary. Am J Pathol **57:**273-297, 1969.

300 Bilbao JM II, Horvath E, Hudson AR, Kovacs K: Pituitary adenoma producing amyloid-like substance. Arch Pathol **99:**411-415, 1975.

301 Borit A, Blanshard TP: Sphenoidal pituitary adenoma. Hum Pathol **10:**93-96, 1979.

302 Capella C, Usellini L, Frigerio B, Buffa R, Fontana P, Solcia E: Argyrophil pituitary tumors showing TSH cells or small granule cells. Virchows Arch [Pathol Anat] **381:**295-312, 1979.

303 Chang CH, Pool L: The radiotherapy of pituitary chromophobe adenomas: an evaluation of indication, technic and result. Radiology **89:**1005-1016, 1967.

304 Doniach I: Cytology of pituitary adenomas. J R Coll Physicians Lond **6:**299-307, 1972.

305 Epstein JA, Epstein BS, Molho L, Zimmerman HM: Carcinoma of the pituitary gland with metastasis to the spinal cord and roots of the canda equina. J Neurosurg **21:**846-853, 1964.

306 Finn JW, Mount LA: Galactorrhea in males with tumors in the region of the pituitary gland. J Neurosurg **35:**723-727, 1971.

307 Forbes AP, Henneman PH, Griswold GC, Albright F: Syndrome characterized by galactorrhea, amenorrhea and low urinary FSH: comparison with acromegaly and normal lactation. J Clin Endocrinol Metab **14:**265-271, 1954.

307a Fukaya T, Kageyama N, Kuwayama A, Takanohashi M, Okada C, Yoshida J, Osamura Y: Morphofunctional study of pituitary adenomas with acromegaly by immunoperoxidase technique and electron microscopy. Cancer **45:**1598-1603, 1980.

308 Ghatak NR, Hirano A, Zimmerman HM: Ultrastructure of a craniopharyngioma. Cancer **27:**1465-1475, 1971.

309 Gjerris A, Lindholm J, Riishede J: Pituitary oncocytic tumor with Cushing's disease. Cancer **42:**1818-1822, 1978.

310 Gonzalez-Vitale JC, Slavin RE, McQueen JD: Radiation-induced intracranial malignant fibrous histiocytoma. Cancer **37:**2960-2963, 1976.

311 Greenhouse AH: Pituitary sarcoma. JAMA **190:**269-273, 1964.

312 Griesbach WE, Purves HD: Basophil adenomata in the rat. Hypophysis after gonadectomy. Br J Cancer **14:**49-59, 1960.

313 Halmi NS, Duello T: 'Acidophilic' pituitary tumors. A reappraisal with differential staining and immunocytochemical techniques. Arch Pathol Lab Med **100:**346-351, 1976.

314 Halmi NS, Parsons JA, Erlandsen SL, Duello T: Prolactin and growth hormone cells in the human hypophysis: a study with immunoenzyme histochemistry and differential staining. Cell Tiss Res **158:**497-507, 1975.

315 Hamilton CR Jr, Adams LC, and Maloof F: Hyperthyroidism due to thyrotropin-producing pituitary chromophobe adenoma. N Engl J Med **283:**1077-1080, 1970.

316 Harris GW, Donovan BT (eds): The pituitary gland. Berkeley, 1966, University of California Press.

317 Heitz PU: Multihormonal pituitary adenomas. Hormone Res **10:**1-13, 1979.

318 Herlant M: The cells of the adenohypophysis and their functional significance. Int Rev Cytol **17:**299-382, 1964.

319 Horvath E, Kovacs K: Misplaced exocytosis: distinct ultrastructural feature in some pituitary adenomas. Arch Pathol **97:**221-224, 1974.

319a Horvath E, Kovacs K, Killinger DW, Smyth HS, Platts ME, Singer W: Silent corticotropic adenomas of the human pituitary gland. A histologic, immunocytologic, and ultrastructural study. Am J Pathol **98:**617-638, 1980.

320 Horvath E, Kovacs K, Singer W, Ezrin C, Kerenyi NA: Acidophil stem cell adenoma of the human pituitary. Arch Pathol Lab Med **101:**594-599, 1977.

321 Houck WA, Olson KB, Horton J: Clinical features of tumor metastasis to the pituitary. Cancer **26:**656-659, 1970.

322 Jackson IMD: Hyperthyroidism in a patient with a pituitary chromophobe adenoma. J Clin Endocrinol Metab **25:**491-494, 1965.

323 Kalnins V: Calcification and amelogenesis in craniopharyngiomas. Oral Surg **31:**366-379, 1971.

324 Kaufman B, Lapham LW, Shealy CN, Pearson OH: Transphenoidal yttrium 90 pituitary ablation. Acta Radiol **5:**17-25, 1966.

325 Kay S, Lees JK, Stout AP: Pituitary chromophobe tumors of the nasal cavity. Cancer **3:**695-704, 1950.

326 Kernohan JW, Sayre GP: Tumors of the pituitary gland and infundibulum. In Atlas of tumor pathology. Sect. X, Fasc. 36. Washington, D.C., 1956, Armed Forces Institute of Pathology.

327 Kleinberg DL, Noel GL, Frantz AG: Galactorrhea: a study of 235 cases, including 48 with pituitary tumors. N Engl J Med **296:**589-600, 1977.

328 Kohler PO, Bridson WE, Rayford PL, Kohler SE: Hormone production by human pituitary adenomas in culture. Metabolism **18:**782-788, 1969.

329 Kovacs K, Horvath H: Pituitary "chromophobe" adenoma composed of oncocytes. Arch Pathol **95:**235-239, 1973.

330 Kovacs K, Horvath E, Exrin C: Pituitary adenomas. Pathol Annu **12:**341-382, 1977.

331 Kovacs K, Horvath E, Kerenyi NA, Sheppard RH: Light and electron microscopic features of a pituitary adenoma in Nelson's syndrome. Am J Clin Pathol **65:**337-343, 1976.

332 Landolt AM: Ultrastructure of human sella tumors. Acta Neurochir [Suppl] **22:**1-167, 1975.

333 Landolt AM, Rothenbuhler V: Pituitary adenoma calcification. Arch Pathol Lab Med **101:**22-27, 1977.

334 Levene MB: Pituitary radiotherapy. Radiol Clin North Am **5:**333-348, 1967.

335 Lewis PD, Van Noorden S: Pituitary abnormalities in acromegaly. Arch Pathol **94:**119-126, 1972.

336 Lewis PD, Van Noorden S: "Nonfunctioning" pituitary tumors. A light and electron microscopical study. Arch Pathol **97:**178-182, 1974.

337 Luse SA, Kernohan JW: Granular cell tumors of the stalk and posterior lobe of the pituitary gland. Cancer **8:**616-622, 1955.

338 McCormick WF, Halmi NS: Absence of chromophobe adenomas from a large series of pituitary tumors. Arch Pathol **92:**231-238, 1971.

339 Madonick MJ, Rubinstein LJ, Dacso MR, Ribner, H: Chromophobe adenoma of pituitary gland with subarachnoid metastasis. Neurology **13:**836-840, 1963.

340 Markesbery WR, Duffy PE, Cowen D: Granular cell tumors of the central nervous system. J Neuropathol Exp Neurol **32:**92-109, 1973.

341 Martins AN, Hayes GJ, Kempe LG: Invasive pituitary adenomas. J Neurosurg **22:**268-276, 1965.

342 Matson DD, Crigler JF Jr: Management of craniopharyngioma in childhood. J Neurosurg **30:**377-390, 1969.

343 Mikami S: Light and electron microscopic investigations of six types of glandular cells of the bovine adenohypophysis. Z Zellforsch Mikrosk Anat **105:** 457-482, 1970.

344 Nakane PK: Classifications of anterior pituitary cell types with immunoenzyme histochemistry. J Histochem Cytochem **18:**9-20, 1970.

345 Nelson DH, Meakin JW, Thorn GW: ACTH-producing pituitary tumors following adrenalectomy for Cushing's syndrome. Ann Intern Med **52:**560-569, 1960.

346 Olivier L, Vila-Porcile E, Racadot O, Peillon F, Racadot J: Ultrastructure of pituitary tumor cells: a critical study. In Tixier-Vidal A, Farquhar MG (eds): Ultrastructure in biological systems. Vol. 7. The anterior pituitary. New York, 1975, Academic Press, Inc.

347 Paiz C, Hennigar GR: Electron microscopy and histochemical correlation of human anterior pituitary cells. Am J Pathol **59:**43-73, 1970.

348 Peake GT, McKeel DW, Jarett L, Daughaday WH: Ultrastructural, histologic and hormonal characterization of a prolactinrich human pituitary tumor. J Clin Endocrinol Metab **29:**1383-1393, 1969.

349 Petito CK, DeGirolami U, Earle KM: Craniopharyngiomas. A clinical and pathological review. Cancer **37:**1944-1952, 1976.

350 Phifer RF, Spicer SS, Orth DN: Specific demonstration of the human hypophyseal cells which produce adrenocorticotropic hormone. J Clin Endocrinol Metab **31:**347-361, 1970.

351 de S. Queiroz L, Facure NO, Facure JJ, Modesto NP, Faria LD: Pituitary carcinoma with liver metastases and Cushing's syndrome. Report of a case. Arch Pathol **99:**32-35, 1975.

352 Reichlin S: The prolactinoma problem [editorial]. N Engl J Med **300:**313-315, 1979.

353 Robert F, Hardy J: Prolactin-secreting adenomas. A light and electron microscopical study. Arch Pathol **99:**625-633, 1975.

354 Robert F, Pelletier G, Hardy J: Pituitary adenomas in Cushing's disease. A histologic, ultrastructural, and immunocytochemical study. Arch Pathol Lab Med **102:**448-455, 1978.

355 Roessmann U, Kaufman B, Friede RL: Metastatic lesions in the sella turcica and pituitary gland. Cancer **25:**478-480, 1970.

356 Rogol AD, Eastman RC: Prolactin and pituitary tumors [editorial]. Am J Med **66:**547-548, 1979.

357 Rovit RL, Duane TD: Cushing's syndrome and pituitary tumors. Pathophysiology and ocular manifestations of ACTH-secreting pituitary adenomas. Am J Med **46:**416-427, 1969.

358 Russfield AB: Human pituitary tumors. In Sommers SC (ed): Pathology annual, vol. 2. New York, 1967, Appleton-Century-Crofts, pp. 332-350.

359 Salassa RM, Laws ER Jr, Carpenter PC, Northcutt RC: Transsphenoidal removal of pituitary microadenoma in Cushing's disease. Mayo Clin Proc **53:**24-28, 1978.

360 Salassa RM, Kearns TP, Kernohan JW, Sprague RG, MacCarthy CS: Pituitary tumors in patients with Cushing's syndrome. J Clin Endocrinol Metab **19:** 1523-1539, 1959.

361 Samaan NA, Osborne BM, Mackay B, Leavens ME, Duello TM, Halmi NS: Endocrine and morphologic studies of pituitary adenomas secondary to primary hypothyroidism. J Clin Endocrinol Metab **45:**903-911, 1977.

362 Schochet SS Jr, McCormick WF, Halmi NS: Acidophil adenomas with intracytoplasmic filamentous aggregates. A light and electron microscopic study. Arch Pathol **94:**16-22, 1972.

363 Seemayer TA, Blundell JS, Wiglesworth FW: Pituitary craniopharyngioma with tooth formation. Cancer **29:**423-430, 1972.

364 Sherman BM, Schlechte J, Halmi NS, Chapler FK, Harris CE, Duello TM, VanGilder J, Granner DK: Pathogenesis of prolactin-secreting pituitary adenomas. Lancet **2:**1019-1021, 1978.

365 Svien HJ, Colby MY Jr, Kearns TP: Comparison of results after surgery and after irradiation in pituitary chromophobe adenomas. Acta Radiol [Ther] (Stockh) **5:**53-66, 1966.

366 Symon L, Ganz JC, Burston J: Granular cell myoblastoma of the neurohypophysis. Report of two cases. J Neurosurg **35:**82-89, 1971.

367 Teears RJ, Silverman EM: Clinicopathologic review of 88 cases of carcinoma metastatic to the pituitary gland. Cancer **36:**216-220, 1975.

368 Timperley WR: Histochemistry of Rathke pouch tumours. J Neurol Neurosurg Psychiatry **31:**589-595, 1968.

369 Tyrrell JB, Brooks RM, Fitzgerald PA, Cofoid PB, Forshaw PH, Wilson CB: Cushing's disease. Selective trans-sphenoidal resection of pituitary microadenomas. N Engl J Med **298:**753-758, 1978.

369a Veldhuis JD, Green JE III, Kovacs E, Worgul TJ, Murray FT, Hammond JM: Prolactin-secreting pituitary adenomas. Association with multiple endocrine neoplasia, Type I. Am J Med **67:**830-837, 1979.

370 von Lawzewitsch I, Dickmann GH, Amezúa L, Pardal C: Cytological and ultrastructural characterization of the human pituitary. Acta Anat (Basel) **81:**286-316, 1972.

371 Waltz TA, Brownell B: Sarcoma: possible late result of effective radiation therapy for pituitary adenoma. Report of two cases. J Neurosurg **24:**901-907, 1966.

372 Young DG, Bahn RC, Randall RV: Pituitary tumors associated with acromegaly. J Clin Endocrinol Metab **25:**249-259, 1965.

Other primary tumors

373 Horoupian DS, Kerson LA, Saiontz H, Valsamis M: Paraganglioma of cauda equina. Clinicopathologic and ultrastructural studies of an unusual case. Cancer **33:**1337-1348, 1974.

374 Miller CA, Rorack RM: Secretory ependymoma of the filum terminale. Acta Neuropathol (Berl) **15:**240-250, 1970.

Tumors of metastatic origin

375 Ambiavagar P-C, Sher J: Subdural hematoma sec-

ondary to metastatic neoplasm. Report of two cases and a review of the literature. Cancer **42:**2015-2018, 1978.

376 Amer MH, Al-Sarraf M, Baker LH, Vaitkevicius VK: Malignant melanoma and central nervous system metastases. Incidence, diagnosis, treatment and survival. Cancer **42:**660-668, 1978.

377 Auld AW, Buerman A: Metastatic spinal epidural tumors. An analysis of 50 cases. Arch Neurol **15:**100-108, 1966.

378 Edelson RN, Deck MDF, Posner JB: Intramedullary spinal cord metastases. Clinical and radiographic findings in nine cases. Neurology **22:**1222-1231, 1972.

379 Gonzalez-Vitale JC, Garcia-Bunuel R: Meningeal carcinomatosis. Cancer **37:**2906-2911, 1976.

380 Haar F, Patterson RH Jr: Surgery for metastatic intracranial neoplasm. Cancer **30:**1241-1245, 1972.

381 Lang EF, Slater J: Metastatic brain tumors: results of surgical and nonsurgical treatment. Surg Clin North Am **44:**865-872, 1964.

Clinicopathologic correlation

382 Bodian M, Lawson D: The intracranial neoplastic diseases of childhood. A description of their natural history based on a clinicopathological study of 129 cases. Br J Surg **40:**368-392, 1953.

383 Cheek WR, Taveras JM: Thalamic tumors. J Nuerosurg **24:**503-513, 1966.

384 Dastur DK, Lalitha VS: Pathological analysis of intracranial space-occupying lesions in 1000 cases including children. Part 2. Incidence, types and unusual cases of glioma. J Neurol Sci **8:**143-170, 1968.

385 Farwell JR, Dohrmann GJ, Flannery JT: Central nervous system tumors in children. Cancer **40:**3123-3132, 1977.

386 Kernohan JW: Tumors of the spinal cord; a review. Arch Pathol **32:**843-883, 1941.

387 Koos WT, Miller MH: Intracranial tumors of infants and children. St. Louis, 1971, The C. V. Mosby Co.

388 Low NL, Correll JW, Hammill JF: Tumors of cerebral hemispheres in children. Arch Neurol **13:**547-554, 1965.

389 Marsden HB, Steward JK: Gliomas and other intracranial tumors. In Tumors in children. Recent results in cancer research, vol. 13. New York, 1968, Springer-Verlag New York, Inc., pp. 86-130.

390 Pecker J, Ferrand B, Javalet A: Tumors of third ventricle. Neurochirurgie **12:**7-136, 1966.

391 Yasuoka S, Okazaki H, Daube JR, MacCarty CS: Foramen magnum tumors. J Neurosurg **49:**828-838, 1978.

392 Zülch KJ: Brian tumors. Their biology and pathology, ed. 2. New York, 1965, Springer Publishing co.

Local and regional effects of intracranial tumors

393 Dreese MJ, Netsky MG: Studies of lateral reflections in the echo-encephalogram. Neurology **14:**521-528, 1964.

394 Friede RL, Roessmann U: The pathogenesis of secondary midbrain hemorrhages. Neurology **16:**1210-1216, 1966.

395 Klintworth GK: The pathogenesis of secondary brain-stem hemorrhages as studied in a experimental model. Am J Pathol **47:**525-536, 1965.

396 Poppen JL, Kendrick JF, Hicks SF: Brain stem hemorrhages secondary to supratentorial space-taking lesions. J Neuropathol Exp Neurol **11:**267-279, 1952.

Cytology

397 Aaronson AG, Hajdu SI, Melamed MR: Spinal fluid cytology during chemotherapy of leukemia of the central nervous system in children. Am J Clin Pathol **63:**528-537, 1975.

398 Gondos B, King EB: Cerebrospinal fluid cytology: diagnostic accuracy and comparison of different techniques. Acta Cytol **20:**542-547, 1976.

399 Kline TS: Cytological examination of the cerebrospinal fluid. Cancer **15:**591-597, 1962.

400 Nies BS, Malmgren RA, Chu EW, Del Vecchio PR, Thomas LB, Freireich EJ: Cerebrospinal fluid cytology in patients with acute leukemia. Cancer **18:**1385-1391, 1965.

401 Rich JR: A survey of cerebrospinal fluid cytology. Bull Los Angeles Neurol Soc **34:**115-131, 1969.

402 Wertlake PT, Markovits BA, Stellar S: Cytologic evaluation of cerebrospinal fluid with clinical and histologic correlation. Acta Cytol **16:**224-239, 1972.

PERIPHERAL NERVES

403 Appenzeller O, Kornfeld M, MacGee J: Neuropathy in chronic renal disease. A microscopic, ultrastructural, and biochemical study of several nerve biopsies. Arch Neurol **24:**449-461, 1971.

404 Barron KD, Rowland LP, Zimmerman HM: Neuropathy with malignant tumor metastases. J Nerv Ment Dis **131:**10-31, 1960.

405 Brain WR, Adams RD: In Brain WR, Norris FH (eds): The remote effects of cancer on the nervous system. New York, 1965, Grume & Stratton, Inc., p. 216.

406 Dayan AD, Gardner-Thorpe C: Peripheral neuropathy and myeloma. J Neurol Sci **14:**21-35, 1971.

407 Dyck PJ: Peripheral neuropathy. Changing concepts, differential diagnosis and classification. Med Clin North Am **52:**895-908, 1968.

408 Dyck PJ, Lofgren EP: Nerve biopsy. Choice of nerves, method, symptoms, and usefulness. Med Clin North Am **52:**885-893, 1968.

409 Dyck PJ, Thomas PK, Lambert EH (eds): Peripheral neuropathy. Philadelphia, 1979, W. B. Saunders Co.

410 Knill-Jones RP, Goodwill CJ, Dayan AD, and Williams R: Peripheral neuropathy in chronic liver disease: clinical, electrodiagnostic, and nerve biopsy findings. J Neurol Neurosurg Psychiatry **35:**22-30, 1972.

411 Locke S: Axons, Schwann cells and diabetic neuropathy. Bull N Y Acad Med **43:**784-791, 1967.

412 Prineas J: Polyneuropathies of undetermined cause. Acta Neurol Scand [Suppl] **44:**1-72, 1970.

413 Schlaepfer WW: Axonal degeneration in the sural nerves of cancer patients. Cancer **34:**371-381, 1974.

414 Thomas PK: Peripheral neuropathy, Br Med J **1:**349-351, 1970.

415 Thomas PK, Hollinrake K, Lascelles RG, O'Sullivan DJ, Baillod RA, Moorhead JF, Mackenzie JC: The polyneuropathy of chronic renal failure. Brain **94:**761-780, 1971.

416 Walsh JC: The neuropathy of multiple myeloma. An electrophysiological and histological study. Arch Neurol **25:**404-414, 1971.

Skeletal muscle

Nonneoplastic diseases of the skeletal muscle system can be divided into six major categories:

1 *Neurogenic atrophy,* secondary to partial or total denervation of the muscle segment; the term *amyotrophy,* which simply means ''muscle atrophy,'' sometimes used as synonym for neurogenic atrophy

2 *Muscular dystrophies,* thought to represent genetically determined primary degenerative diseases of the muscle fibers

3 *Myositis,* either infectious or immunologically induced

4 *Myopathies,* a term which in a generic sense embraces all muscle diseases but which usually is restricted to primary degenerative conditions that are noninflammatory, nondystrophic, and not caused by denervation

5 *Traumatic and circulatory disturbances*

6 *Disorders of function* not accompanied by significant structural changes by the usual microscopic examination; includes some disorders of neuromuscular transmission and of supraspinal tonal regulation

An internationally agreed comprehensive classification of the neuromuscular disorders has been published by the Research Group on Neuromuscular Diseases.[1]

Techniques of pathologic examination

The adequate study of muscle biopsies is a highly specialized endeavor, requiring a careful evaluation of the patient, a rigorous biopsy technique, and the performance of a battery of sophisticated techniques on the processed material.[9a,12,15] When properly done, it often allows the disease to be classified into one of the five major categories previously noted and sometimes provides enough information for the diagnosis of a specific condition.[6] In selected cases, muscle biopsy should be combined with biopsy of the skin or of a peripheral nerve. The most

common and successful application of muscle biopsy is in the differential diagnosis of progressive muscle wasting.[8] When the morphologic abnormalities seen in the muscle biopsy are correlated with the results of other tests, such as enzyme determinations, electromyography, determination of motor and sensory nerve conduction times, and repetitive motor nerve stimulation, it is usually possible to determine whether the primary disease is in the spinal cord, peripheral nerves, or neuromuscular function or in the muscle fiber itself.[13,14] To attempt to make a specific diagnosis with a single muscle biopsy without knowledge of the clinical and laboratory findings is simply to invite disaster. Many of the morphologic changes seen are nonspecific. There is often a marked discrepancy between the severity of the symptoms and the degree

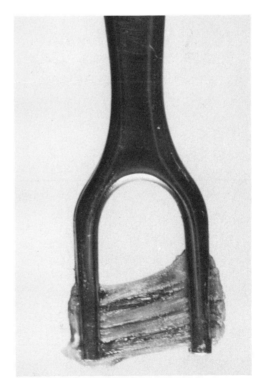

Fig. 1511 Clamp used for skeletal muscle biopsy. Specimen is maintained in this position throughout fixation step, thus minimizing retraction and distortion of muscle fibers. (WU neg. 71-10454.)

1629

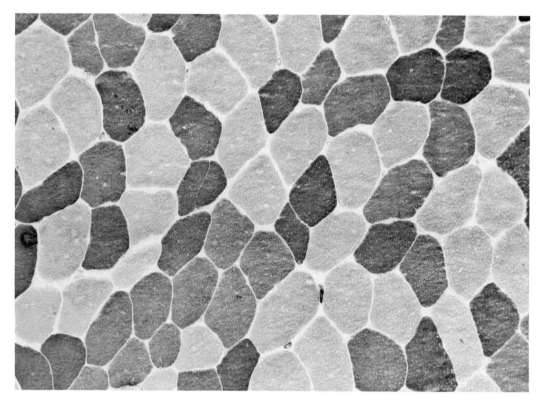

Fig. 1512 ATPase stain in normal skeletal muscle. Type I (light) and Type II fibers can be easily distinguished. (×150; WU neg. 73-3540.)

of pathologic abnormalities. Furthermore, minor microscopic alterations in muscle are often seen in the absence of any specific muscle disease, as demonstrated by Pearson[11] and by Clawson et al.[2] in careful autopsy studies.

The muscle chosen for biopsy should be one *moderately* affected by the disease. Muscles with minimal changes or with total atrophy usually fail to provide diagnostic information. Pain to palpation and electromyographic changes may be of help in this selection. Care should be taken to avoid the muscle area needled at electromyography as the biopsy site, since marked degenerative and inflammatory changes always follow the procedure.[9] In some conditions, it is important to examine a piece of muscle that includes the terminal innervation, the latter having been located by surface electric stimulation. Care is needed to obtain good fixation with a minimum of contraction of the muscle fragment. This is best accomplished by removing the sample of muscle in a special clamp that can hold the specimen throughout fixation (Fig. 1511). Ideally, at least two sections should be made to show muscle

fibers in cross section as well as longitudinal section. In the selected cases, particularly in those of a metabolic nature, the performance of a needle biopsy is a safe and cost-effective technique.[2a] Masson's trichrome and Mallory's phosphotungstic acid–hematoxylin are useful additions to the routine hematoxylin-eosin in the evaluation of formalin-fixed, paraffin-embedded material. Whenever possible, this should be supplemented by enzymatic histochemical techniques performed on fresh frozen sections. This allows a sharp separation of the muscle fibers into two distinct categories: *Type I fibers,* characterized by high mitochondrial oxidative enzyme activity, and *Type II fibers,* rich in myofibrillar enzymes.[5] (Fig. 1512). We employ the DPNH dehydrogenase reaction for the identification of the first type and ATPase for the second. The distinction is important because these two fiber types show selective susceptibility to several diseases.[4] Direct immunofluorescence staining for immunoglobulins and complement will often show deposition of these substances in the vessel wall, sarcolemma basement membrane,

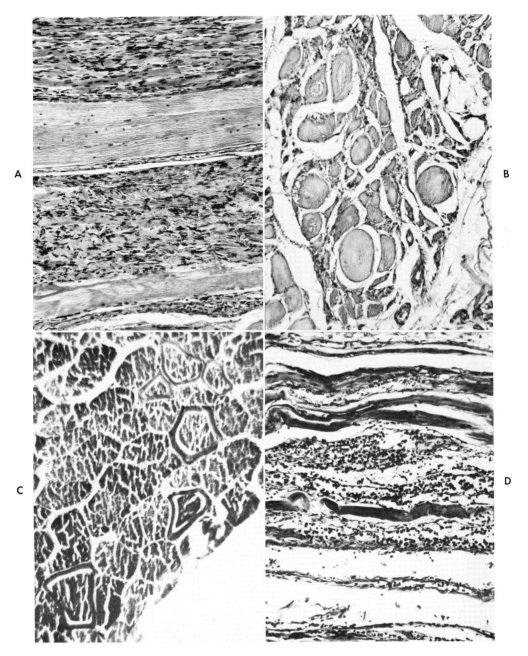

Fig. 1513 Four patterns of reaction in primary diseases of muscle. **A,** Fascicular atrophy in amyotrophic lateral sclerosis. **B,** Dystrophy with irregular, large, hyalinized fibers. **C,** Ringed fibers as occur in myotonic states, especially myotonic dystrophy. **D,** Polymyositis with disrupted fibers and heavy cellular infiltration. (**A,** ×125; UVa neg. 6308; **B,** ×125; UVa neg. 6308; **C,** Masson; ×260; UVa neg. 6308; courtesy Dr. A. G. Smith, Memphis, Tenn.; **D,** ×125; UVa neg. 6308; courtesy Dr. C. E. Wheeler, Chapel Hill, N. C.)

and/or fibers in most cases of collagen-vascular diseases.[10] Finally, electron microscopic examination has proved of great value in the evaluation of the several types of myopathy.[3,7]

Neurogenic atrophy (amyotrophy)

The normal size of muscle fibers varies in different muscles as well as with the age and physical development of the individual. Most muscles of the extremities have fibers that average about 50μ in diameter, whereas external ocular muscles regularly contain uniformly small fibers of 20μ-25μ in diameter.[18]

Skeletal muscle fibers hypertrophy with exercise and decrease in diameter and volume with disuse. Such atrophic changes are particularly pronounced if a fiber is denervated and loses its tonic stimuli.

The muscles in diseases characterized by neurogenic atrophy contain fibers that are reduced to 20μ or less in diameter, yet they retain normal structural features such as cross striations. The sarcolemmal nuclei may increase slightly in size, and their nucleoli become more prominent. Combined with the decreased fiber size, this results in a considerable apparent increase in the number of nuclei, although it is not certain whether an absolute increase actually takes place.

The most characteristic feature of biopsies from patients with neurogenic atrophy consists of large groups of small atrophic fibers with persisting islands of smaller groups of normal or hypertrophied fibers (Fig. 1513, *A*). This group is considered to be due to the atrophy of fibers by motor units as their anterior horn cells or major nerve fibers are destroyed. "Group lesions" often occur in neurogenic atrophy, but they are not pathognomonic of this condition. They also have been described in muscular dystrophy, malnutrition, and disuse atrophy.[22] In the early stages of neurogenic muscle disease, the atrophy may be represented only by scattered small angular fibers wedged between normal fibers. Histochemical staining often reveals "type grouping" instead of the normal mosaic pattern of Type I and Type II fibers.[17] "Target fibers" often appear. These are best demonstrated with the myofibrillary ATPase reaction and are regarded as characteristic of denervation atrophy.[21,22] Intravital or supravital staining of motor nerve filaments and end-plates reveals a characteristic pattern of branching of subterminal intramuscular nerve fibers, with collateral reinnervation and degeneration of end-plates.[20]

Occasionally, focal degenerative changes simulating myopathy may appear during the late stages of neurogenic atrophy, perhaps due to reinnervation by neighboring motor neurons.[16,19] It is not until late in these diseases that structural changes in the atrophied fibers and interstitial tissue occur. Sarcoplasm and myofibrils may disappear, sometimes with persistence of rows of sarcolemmal nuclei,

and finally fibers are completely destroyed. Interstitial connective tissue increases slowly in amount, and there may be moderate infiltration of fat cells into the fascicles. It takes about eleven months for significant fibrosis to appear following denervation. Cellular infiltrations in the interstitial tissues and regenerative proliferation of fragments of muscle fibers form no part of the histologic pattern in these muscles.

Neurogenic atrophy can be secondary to diseases of the spinal cord, motor nerve roots, or peripheral nerves. Types of spinal muscular atrophies include the genetically determined infantile (Werdnig-Hoffmann) and juvenile spinal muscular atrophies, the amyotrophies due to congenital, infectious, and traumatic diseases of the spinal cord, and a large group of diseases of unknown etiology, such as motor neuron (Aran-Duchenne) disease.

Muscular dystrophies

The muscular dystrophies are an inherited group of conditions that has been classically regarded as a primary degenerative condition of the muscle, although the possibilities of an abnormal microvascular supply of muscle[31a] or an aberration of the normal controlling influence of the nervous system on muscle also have been considered.[26] Recently, evidence has been presented that these diseases are the result of an alteration in fluidity of the cell membrane of the skeletal muscle fibers.[30]

Muscular dystrophies are classified into different types on the basis of age of onset, regional distribution of the muscle involvement, and pattern of genetic transmission. The commonest varieties are *Duchenne's (pseudohypertrophic) type,* a severe generalized disease affecting children and inherited by either a sex-linked or a recessive gene, and the *facioscapulohumeral (Landouzy-Dejerine) type,* a disease of adults with a dominant pattern of inheritance and first involving the muscles of the face and shoulder girdle. Other recognized varieties of muscular dystrophy are the limb-girdle type, distal myopathy, ocular myopathy, and oculopharyngeal muscular type.[31] Also included in this category are the myotonic disorders, of which dystrophia myotonica is the commonest.

The microscopic appearance of the muscle is quite similar in all these clinical varieties of dystrophy and is mainly dependent on the stage of the disease at the time of biopsy. There is random variation in size of the muscle fibers (without the grouping of neurogenic atrophy),

atrophy and disappearance of the muscle fibers with progressive replacement by fat and fibrous tissue, and degenerative changes, characterized by increased eosinophilia, loss of cross striations, disorganization of myofibrils, and granular, hyaline, or vacuolated appearance of the sarcoplasm (Fig. 1513, *B*). The sarcolemmal nuclei are enlarged, increased in number, and sometimes arranged in chains along the center of the muscle fiber.[24,27] This latter change, as well as ringed fibers, is particularly prominent in dystrophia myotonica.[33] (Fig. 1513, *C*). Inflammatory reaction, phagocytosis, and regeneration (as indicated by the presence of basophilic muscle fibers), although frequently present, rarely reach the severity seen in polymyositis.[29]

Histochemically, muscular dystrophies exhibit preservation of myofibrillary ATPase activity and focal loss of mitochondrial enzymatic activity.[25] Ultrastructurally, mitochondrial abnormalities and disruption and loss of myofilaments are constant findings.[23,28] Muscular dystrophy carriers exhibit changes qualitatively similar but of lesser severity.[28] According to Schroder and Adams,[32] the most characteristic fine structural feature of dystrophia myotonica is the presence of large sarcoplasmic aggregates of disordered myofilaments and other organelles.

Myositis

Inflammatory diseases of muscle can be divided into two groups: those of recognized infectious etiology (viral, bacterial, fungous, or parasitic) and those probably mediated by immunologic mechanisms. The better known forms of infectious myositis are due to trichinosis, superimposed bacterial infection in a muscle of an ischemic extremity, and gas gangrene. The infrequent granulomatous myositis due to tuberculosis, atypical mycobacteriosis, sarcoidosis, or syphilis also belongs to this category.[39] Immunologically mediated myositis is characterized by generalized involvement—hence the term polymyositis. The disease may be restricted to the skeletal muscle system or, more commonly, be a manifestation of a systemic "collagen disease," such as dermatomyositis, lupus erythematosus, rheumatic fever, rheumatoid arthritis, scleroderma, polyarteritis nodosa, or Sjogren's syndrome.[35,36] Polymyositis developing after the age of 40 years is associated with visceral carcinoma in a high percentage of patients.

Polymyositis primarily affects the girdle muscles. It can closely simulate various types of muscular dystrophy on clinical grounds,[38,40] but the two diseases are easily distinguished by examination of a muscle biopsy. Microscopically, the acute form is expressed by a combination of inflammatory, degenerative, and regenerative changes, such as granular and floccular degeneration, fragmentation and phagocytosis of muscle fibers, and interstitial infiltrations of lymphocytes, plasma cells, macrophages, and occasional neutrophils and eosinophils (Fig. 1513, *D*). Evidence of regeneration consists of buds or separate masses of basophilic sarcoplasm in which there are central large or multiple nuclei. This disease may be overwhelming and fatal, but many patients recover.

Chronic polymyositis, on the other hand, is a more relentlessly progressive disease. The histologic appearance of the muscles may be that of intense inflammation even late in the course of the disease in some patients, but in many the changes consist of a greater interstitial fibrosis with less inflammatory cellular infiltration and evidence of regenerative reaction by the muscle fibers. Adams et al.[34] emphasized the particular atrophy, vacuolation, and destruction of fibers at the periphery of muscle fascicles in this condition. It may progress to complete destruction of the muscle, fibrous contracture, and even metaplastic bone formation.

Histochemically, the affected muscle fibers show extensive loss of myosin ATPase as a result of destruction of myofibrils. On the other hand, mitochondrial oxidative enzymatic activity usually is preserved. Ultrastructurally, the most significant finding in polymyositis is the frequent occurrence of filamentous or tubular structures resembling paramyxovirus nucleocapsid.[37] Whether they indeed represent viral structures or a peculiar cytoplasmic reaction to injury, their almost constant occurrence in cases of dermatomyositis is of diagnostic significance. Other changes include disorganization and loss of myofilaments, mitochondial alterations, and dilation of endoplasmic reticulum[41]

Myopathies

The nondystrophic, noninflammatory primary degenerative muscle diseases can be divided into two distinct categories. The first is comprised of a large group of acquired myopathies secondary to or at least associated with a variety of endocrine, metabolic, neoplastic, and immunologically mediated disorders or with the administration of drugs or toxins. We are referring to the myopathies seen in association with hyperthyroidism,[69] myxedema, hypopituitarism, acromegaly, Cushing's disease, Addison's disease, primary aldosteronism, hyperparathyroidism, osteomalacia, glycogen storage disease, nutritional deficiency, carcinomatosis,[42,45,46] and myasthenia gravis, as well as those appearing after the administration of chloroquine,[70] emetine,[47] plasmocid,[67] vincristine,[76] tri-ortho-cresyl-phosphate (TOCP),[68] steroid, ACTH, and alcohol.[60,62,66]

The microscopic appearance is nonspecific. In some cases, no morphologic alterations are present. In the majority, however, scattered degenerative changes of the muscle fibers are present, sometimes accompanied by an inflammatory infiltrate. The differential diagnosis with muscular dystrophy and polymyositis may be impossible on morphologic grounds. This is also the case at an electron microscopic level.[71]

Most types of glycogenosis involve skeletal muscle, their common morphologic denominator being the accumulation of glycogen in the sarcoplasm.[56] The tinctorial and ultrastructural appearance of the glycogen granules and their location within the sarcoplasm vary according to the types of glycogenosis.[58]

The second group of myopathies, sometimes referred to as "benign congenital myopathies," become symptomatic in infancy or childhood, the usual way of presentation being proximal or diffuse muscle weakness ("floppy infants"). They are unaccompanied by elevation of serum enzyme levels, run an essentially nonprogressive clinical course, and have a definite familial incidence.[65] Among this group, an ever-increasing number of more or less distinct varieties have been singled out in recent years, principally on the basis of some supposedly specific fine structural feature.

In *nemaline myopathy*, threadlike or rodlike structures appear within an otherwise normal sarcoplasm.[75] These structures stain with Mallory's PTAH and Masson's trichrome. Ultrastructurally, the nemaline structures have a tetragonal filamentous structure with a perpendicular periodicity of 125Å-200Å, thus closely resembling hypertrophic Z bands.[48,52] This condition is a possible cause of rapidly fatal infantile hypotonia.[51] *Central core disease* is characterized by the presence of "cores" in the central areas of the sarcoplasm that are PAS-positive and fail to rotate polar-

ized light.[73] Ultrastructural study of the "core" shows focal decrease of mitochondria, myofibrillar degeneration, and decrease of glycogen and sarcotubular profiles.[54] *Multicore disease* shows qualitatively similar changes but differs from the former by virtue of the pleomorphism of the cores, their smaller size, and their greater number per unit area in the affected fibers.[50] In *centronuclear (myotubular) myopathy*, most of the myofibers contain central nuclei, the appearance thus resembling that of embryonal myotubules.[55,63,77] *"Mitochondrial" myopathies* are so named because of the striking mitochondrial abnormalities seen on electron microscopic examination. These consist of enlargement, abnormal shapes, and presence of inclusions.[74] Other "entities" that have been described are cystalline intranuclear inclusion myopathy,[59] reducing body myopathy,[43] and fingerprint body myopathy.[49]

It is becoming evident that many of these ultrastructural features are not specific for their respective entities. The sampling error inherent in any electron microscopic study and the limited present knowledge on the ultrastructural variations of normalcy or of physiologic reaction in human muscle call for caution in the interpretation of these findings. Rodlike structures and "cores" have been produced by tenotomy.[61] Mitochondrial abnormalities similar to those described by Shy et al.[74] have been found in hypothyroid myopathy,[57,64] neuropathy,[53] myositis,[44] and muscular atrophy.[72]

Traumatic and circulatory disturbances

Several types of reaction may arise in muscle as the result of hemorrhage or ischemia. *Myositis ossificans* has been discussed in Chapter 23. *Volkmann's contracture* represents a complication of too tightly applied casts and bandages and is probably the result of ischemia due principally to interruption of the venous drainage. Microscopically, large amounts of cellular fibrous tissue are seen replacing a destroyed muscle, of which only a few fibers may eventually persist.

Violent contraction or hard exercise in the untrained individual may lead to rupture of muscle sheaths, with herniation or hemorrhages in the muscle. A particularly interesting form is the "anterior tibial compartment syndrome" in which initial edema or hemorrhage increases the volume of a rather rigidly confined muscle and results in progressive destruction of the remainder of the muscle apparently by ischemia.[78] The connective tissue in these muscles reacts rapidly with the formation of considerable fibrosis.

REFERENCES

1 Research Group on Neuromuscular Diseases: Classification of the neuromuscular disorders: appendix A. Minutes of the Meeting of the Research Group on Neuromuscular Diseases, Sept. 21, 1967. J Neurol Sci **6:**165-177, 1968.

Techniques of pathologic examination

2 Clawson BJ, Noble JF, Lufkin NH: Nodular inflammatory and degenerative lesions of muscles from 450 autopsies. Arch Pathol **43:**579-589, 1947.

2a Edwards R, Young A, Wiles M: Needle biopsy of skeletal muscle in the diagnosis of myopathy and the clinical study of muscle function and repair. N Engl J Med **302:**261-271, 1980.

3 Engel AG: Ultrastructural reactions in muscle disease. Med Clin North Am **52:**909-931, 1968.

4 Engel WK: Selective and nonselective susceptibility of muscle fiber types. Arch Neurol **22:**97-117, 1970.

5 Engel WK: The essentiality of histo- and cytochemical studies of skeletal muscle in the investigation of neuromuscular disease. Neurology **12:**778-794, 1962.

6 Engel WK, Brooke MH: Muscle biopsy as a clinical diagnostic aid. In Fields WS (ed): Neurological diagnostic techniques. Springfield, Ill., 1966, Charles C Thomas, Publisher, pp. 90-146.

7 Hudgson P: The value of electron microscopy in muscle biopsies. Proc R Soc Med **63:**14-18, 1970.

8 Hughes J: Pathology of muscle. In Bennington JL (ed): Major problems in pathology, vol. IV. Philadelphia, 1974, W. B. Saunders Co.

9 Hughes JT, Brownell B: Muscle biopsy in the diagnosis of neurological and muscle disease. In Dyke SC (ed): Recent advances in clinical pathology, ser. 5. London, 1968, J. & A. Churchill, Ltd., chap. 20.

9a Manz HJ: Pathology of skeletal muscle: principles of reaction patterns and histochemistry and experience with 195 biopsies. Virchows Arch [Pathol Anat] **386:**1-19, 1980.

10 Oxenhandler R, Adelstein EH, Hart MN: Immunopathology of skeletal muscle. The value of direct immunofluorescence in the diagnosis of connective tissue disease. Hum Pathol **8:**321-328, 1977.

11 Pearson CM: Incidence and type of pathologic alterations observed in muscle in a routine autopsy survey. Neurology **9:**757-766, 1959.

12 Pearson CM, Mostofi FK (eds): The striated muscle. Baltimore, 1973, The Williams & Wilkins Co.

13 Samaha FJ: Electrodiagnostic studies in neuromuscular disease. N Engl J Med **282:**1244-1247, 1971.

14 Vasella F, Richterich R, Rossi E: The diagnostic value of serum creatine kinase in neuromuscular and muscular disease. Pediatrics **35:**322-330, 1965.

15 Walton JN (ed): Disorders of voluntary muscle, ed. 2. Boston, 1969, Little, Brown and Co.

Neurogenic atrophy (amyotrophy)

16 Emery AEH: The nosology of the spinal muscular atrophies. J Med Genet **8:**481-495, 1971.

17 Engel WK, Brooke MH: Muscle biopsy as a clinical diagnostic aid. In Fields WS (ed): Neurological diagnostic techniques. Springfield, Ill., 1966, Charles C Thomas, Publisher, pp. 90-146.

18 Greenfield JG, Shy GM, Alvord EC, Berg L: An Atlas of muscle pathology in neuromuscular diseases. Edinburgh, 1957, E. & S. Livingstone, Ltd.

19 Hasse GR, and Shy GM: Pathological changes in muscle biopsies from patients with peroneal muscular atrophy. Brain **83:**631-637, 1960.

20 Pearce J, Harriman DGF: Chronic spinal muscular atrophy. J Neurosurg Psychiatry **29:**509-520, 1966.

21 Schotland DL: An electron microscopic study of target fibers, target-like fibers and related abnormalities in human muscle. J Neuropathol Exp Neurol **28:**214-228, 1969.

22 Zacks SI: Recent contributions to the diagnosis of muscle disease. Hum Pathol **1:**465-498, 1970.

Muscular dystrophies

23 Aleu FP, and Afifi AK: Ultrastructure of muscle in myotonic dystrophy. Am J Pathol **45:**221-232, 1964.

24 Bell CD, Conen PE: Histopathological changes in Duchenne muscular dystrophy. J Neurol Sci **7:**529-544, 1968.

25 Brooke MH, Engel WK: The histologic diagnoses of neuromuscular diseases: a review of 79 biopsies. Arch Phys Med Rehabil **47:**99-121, 1966.

26 Dubowitz V: Muscular dystrophy—where is the lesion? Dev Med Child Neurol **13:**238-240, 1971.

27 Engel WK, Brooke MH: Muscle biopsy as a clinical diagnostic aid. In Fields WS, (ed): Neurological diagnostic techniques. Springfield, Ill., 1966, Charles C Thomas, Publisher, pp. 90-146.

28 Fisher ER, Cohn RE, Denowski TS: Ultrastructural observations of skeletal muscle in myopathy and neuropathy with special reference to muscular dystrophy. Lab Invest **15:**778-793, 1966.

29 Pearce GW, Walton JN: Progressive muscular dystrophy. The histopathological changes in skeletal muscle obtained by biopsy. J Pathol Bacteriol **83:**535-550, 1962.

30 Pickard NA, Gruemer H-D, Verrill HL, Issacs ER, Robinow M, Nance WE, Myers EC, Goldsmith B: Systemic membrane defect in the proximal muscular dystrophies. N Engl J Med **299:**841-846, 1978.

31 Research Group on Neuromuscular Diseases: Classification of the neuromuscular disorders: Appendix A. Minutes of the Meeting of the Research Group on Neuromuscular Diseases, Sept. 21, 1967. J Neurol Sci **6:**165-177, 1968.

31a Rowland LP: Pathogenesis of muscular dystrophies. Arch Neurol **33:**315-321, 1976.

32 Schroder JM, Adams RD: The ultrastructural morphology of the muscle fiber in myotonic dystrophy. Acta Neuropathol **10:**218-241, 1968.

33 Wohlfart G: Dystrophia myotonica and myotonia congenita. Histopathologic studies with special reference to changes in the muscle. J Neuropathol Exp Neurol **10:**109-124, 1951.

Myositis

34 Adams RD: Diseases of muscle. A study in pathology, ed. 3. Hagerstown, Md., 1975, Harper & Row, Publishers, Inc.

35 Bohan A, Peter JB: Polymyositis and dermatomyositis. N Engl J Med **292:**344-347, 403-407, 1975.

36 Brooke MH, Engel WK: The histologic diagnosis of neuromuscular diseases: a review of 79 biopsies. Arch Phys Med Rehabil **47:**99-121, 1966.

37 Chou S-M: Myxovirus-like structures and accompany-

ing nuclear changes in chronic polymyositis. Arch Pathol **86:**649-658, 1968.

38 Dowben RM, Vawter GF, Bradfonbrenner A, Sniderman P, Kaegy RD: Polymyositis and other diseases resembling muscular dystrophy. Arch Intern Med **115:** 584-594, 1965.

39 Gardner-Thorpe C: Muscle weakness due to sarcoid myopathy. Six case reports and an evaluation of steroid therapy. Neurology **22:**917-928, 1972.

40 Munsat TL, Piper D, Cancilla P, Mednick J: Inflammatory myopathy with facioscapulohumeral distribution. Neurology **22:**335-347, 1972.

41 Rose AL, Walton JN, Pearce GW: Polymyositis: an ultramicroscopic study of muscle biopsy material, J Neurol Sci **5:**457-472, 1967.

Myopathies

42 Azzopardi JG: Systemic effects of neoplasia: neuromyopathies. In Harrison CV (ed): Recent advances in pathology, ed. 8. Boston, 1966, Little, Brown and Co.

43 Brooke MH, Neville HE: Reducing body myopathy, a new disease. Neurology **21:**412-413, 1971.

44 Cape CA, Johnson WW, and Pitner SE: Nemaline structures in polymyositis. A nonspecific pathological reaction of skeletal muscles. Neurology **20:**494-502, 1970.

45 Croft PB, Wilkinson M: Carcinomatous neuromyopathy. Its influence in patients with carcinoma of the lung and carcinoma of the breast. Lancet **1:**184-188, 1963.

46 Croft PB, Wilkinson M: The incidence of carcinomatous neuromyopathy in patients with various types of carcinoma. Brain **88:**427-434, 1965.

47 Duane DD, Engel AG: Emetine myopathy. Neurology **18:**274, 1968.

48 Engel AG, Gomez MR: Nemaline (Z disk) myopathy: observations on the origin, structure, and solubility properties of the nemaline structures. J Neuropathol Exp Neurol **26:**601-619, 1967.

49 Engel AG, Angelini C, Gomez MR: Fingerprint body myopathy. A newly recognized congenital muscle disease. Mayo Clin Proc **47:**377-388, 1972.

50 Engel AG, Gomez MR, Groover RV: Multicore disease. A recently recognized congenital myopathy associated with multifocal degeneration of muscle fibers. Mayo Clin Proc **46:**666-681, 1971.

51 Gillies C, Raye J, Vasan U, Hart WE, Goldblatt PJ: Nemaline (rod) myopathy. A possible cause of rapidly fatal infantile hypotonia. Arch Pathol Lab Med **103:** 1-5, 1979.

52 Gonatas NK, Shy GM, Godfrey EH: Nemaline myopathy. The origin of nemaline structures. N Engl J Med **274:**535-539, 1966.

53 Gonatas N, Evangelista I, Martin J: A generalized disorder of nervous system, skeletal muscle, and heart resembling Refsum's disease and Hurler's syndrome. II. Ultrastructure. Am J Med **42:**169-178, 1967.

54 Gonatas NK, Perez MC, Shy GM, Evangelista I: Central core disease of skeletal muscle. Ultrastructural and cytochemical observations in 2 cases. Am J Pathol **47:** 503-524, 1965.

55 Headington JT, McNamara JO, Brownell AK: Centronuclear myopathy: histochemistry and electron microscopy. Report of two cases. Arch Pathol **99:**16-24, 1975.

56 Hers HG: Glycogen storage disease. Adv Metab Disord **1:**1-44, 1964.

57 Hudgson P, Brodley WG, Jenkison M: Familial "mitochondrial" myopathy. A myopathy associated with dis-

ordered oxidative metabolism in muscle fibers. J Neurol Sci **16:**343-370, 1972.

58 Hug G, Garancis JC, Schubert WK, and Kaplan S: Glycogen storage disease, Types II, III, VIII, and IX. Am J Dis Child **111:**457-474, 1966.

59 Jenis EH, Lingquist RR, Lister RC: New congenital myopathy with crystalline intranuclear inclusions. Arch Neurol **20:**281-287, 1969.

60 Kahn LB, Meyer JS: Acute myopathy in chronic alcoholism: a study of 22 autopsy cases, with ultrastructural observations. Am J Clin Pathol **53:**516-530, 1970.

61 Karpati G, Carpenter S, Eisen AA: Experimental corelike lesions and membrane rods; a correlative morphological and physiological study. Arch Neurol **27:**237-251, 1972.

62 Klinkerfuss G, Bleisch V, Dioso MM, Perkoff GT: A spectrum of myopathy associated with alcoholism. II. Light and electron microscopic observations. Ann Intern Med **67:**493-510, 1967.

63 Munsat TL, Thompson LR, Coleman RS: Centronuclear ("myotubular") myopathy. Arch Neurol **20:** 120-131, 1969.

64 Norris FH, and Panner BJ: Hypothyroid myopathy. Arch Neurol **14:**574-589, 1966.

65 Pearson CM, Coleman RF, Fowlder WM, Jr, Mommaerts W, Munsat TL, Peter JB: Skeletal muscle. Ann Intern Med **63:**614-650, 1967.

66 Perkoff GT, Dioso MM, Bleisch V, Klinkerfuss G: A spectrum of myopathy associated with alcoholism. I. Clinical and laboratory features. Ann Intern Med **67:** 481-492, 1967.

67 Price HM, Pease DC, Pearson CM: Selective actin filament and Z-band degeneration induced by plasmocid. An electron microscopic study. Lab Invest **11:**549-562, 1962.

68 Prineas J: Tri-ortho-cresyl-phosphate (TOCP) myopathy. Arch Neurol **21:**150-156, 1969.

69 Ramsay ID: Muscle dysfunction in hyperthyroidism. Lancet **2:**931-934, 1966.

70 Rewcastle NB, Humphrey JG: Vacuolar myopathy. Clinical histochemical and microscopic study. Arch Neurol **12:**570-582, 1965.

71 Santa T: Fine structure of the human skeletal muscle in myopathy. Arch Neurol **20:**479-489, 1969.

72 Shafiq SA, Milhorat AT, Gorycki MA: Giant mitochondria in human muscle with inclusions. Arch Neurol **17:**666-671, 1967.

73 Shy GM, Magee AR: A new congenital non-progressive myopathy. Brain **79:**610-621, 1956.

74 Shy GM, Gonatas NK, Perez M: Two childhood myopathies with abnormal mitochondria. I. Megaconial myopathy. II. Pleoconial myopathy. Brain **89:**133-158, 1966.

75 Shy GM, Engel WK, Somers JE, Wanko T: Nemaline myopathy: a new congenital myopathy. Brain **86:**793-810, 1963.

76 Slotweiner P, Song SK, Anderson PJ: Spheromembranous degeneration of muscle induced by vincristine. Arch Neurol **15:**172-176, 1966.

77 Spiro AJ, Shy GM, Gonatas NK: Myotubular myopathy: persistence of fetal muscle in an adolescent boy. Arch Neurol **14:**1-14, 1966.

Traumatic and circulatory disturbances

78 Leach RE, Hammond G, Stryker WS: Anterior tibial compartment syndrome. J Bone Joint Surg [Am] **49:**451-462, 1967.

28 Eyes and ocular adnexa

Morton E. Smith, M.D.*

*Director of Ophthalmic Pathology and Professor, Departments of Ophthalmology and Pathology, Washington University School of Medicine, St. Louis, Mo.

This chapter will cover primarily those entities that come to the attention of the surgical pathologist; therefore, entities seen most often at postmortem examination will be excluded. In order for the surgical pathologist to develop the proper orientation to the pathology of the eyes and ocular adnexa, he should have some idea of the relative frequency of lesions coming

1637

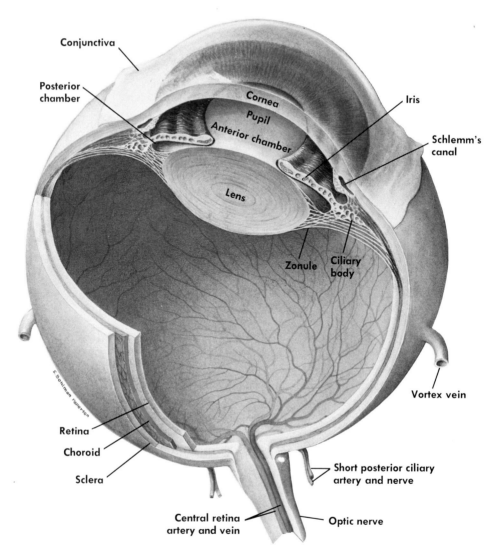

Conjunctiva

Posterior
chamber

Cornea

Pupil

Anterior chamber

Iris

Schlemm's
canal

Lens

Zonule

Ciliary
body

Retina

Choroid

Sclera

Vortex vein

Short posterior ciliary
artery and nerve

Central retina
artery and vein

Optic nerve

Fig. 1514 Human eye. (From Newell FW: Ophthalmology: principles and concepts, ed. 4. St. Louis, 1978, The C. V. Mosby Co.)

to the laboratory. For example, in a year's time, the surgical pathology resident and the ophthalmology resident at the Washington University Medical Center in St. Louis* are responsible for the pathologic diagnosis on approximately 200 enucleated globes (excluding autopsy globes), 200 corneal "buttons" from corneal transplant patients, 15 orbital biopsies, 35 conjunctival biopsies, 70 lid biopsies, 40 temporal artery

biopsies, and 6 iris and ciliary body biopsies. Throughout this chapter, mention will be made of the most common lesions in each of these categories.

As with all surgical specimens, a complete description of the lesion and a meaningful clinical history are invaluable. Clinical photographs are especially helpful in ophthalmic pathology.

EYELIDS

Most of the pathologic processes that involve the eyelids are those that involve the skin in general and are considered in detail in Chapter

---

*All tissue removed by an ophthalmic surgeon at our institution is reviewed and officially diagnosed by both the surgical pathology resident and the ophthalmology resident under the supervision of a faculty member trained in ophthalmic pathology.

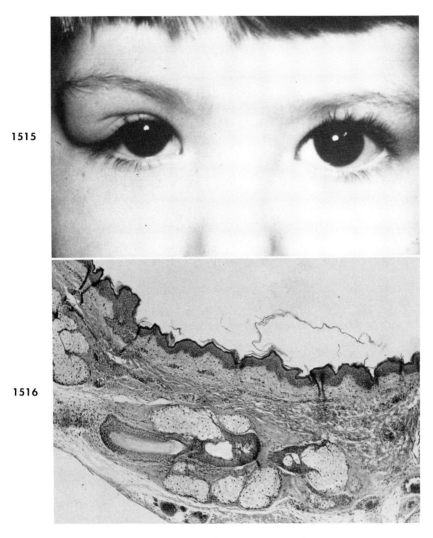

Fig. 1515 Dermoid cyst of right upper eyelid. (WU neg. 67-3508.)
Fig. 1516 Dermoid cyst of eyelid and brow. Cyst lumen is located in upper right corner. (×55; AFIP 722706.)

3. Some consideration, however, is given here to those lesions that are either peculiar to the lids or present particular problems in this location.

Developmental anomalies

Dermoid cysts typically involve the upper eyelid along the brow margin and may represent forward extension of a mass primarily intra-orbital (Fig. 1515). These lesions rest on, and often are firmly attached to, the periosteum of the bony orbital rim. They are soft, nontender, oval or round, and usually about 1 cm in diameter.

Microscopically, the cysts are lined by well-differentiated epidermal and dermal tissues containing all of the usual skin appendages (Fig. 1516). The lumen is filled with keratinous debris, sebum, and hairs. In places where these contents have been extruded into the surrounding tissues, a severe foreign body inflammatory reaction may be observed.

Nevi dating from birth may be observed in either the cutaneous or the conjunctival surface of the eyelids. The lid margin is a common site for benign nevi (Fig. 1517). They tend to be of the junctional or compound type and, like those in other areas, may give rise to malignant melanoma. Fortunately, this is a very rare event.

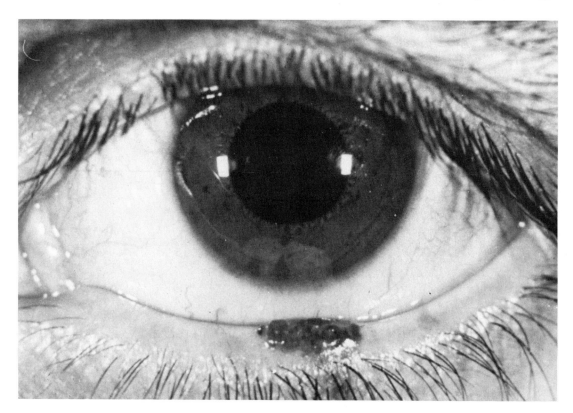

Fig. 1517 Nevus of margin of lower eyelid. (WU neg. 79-1627.)

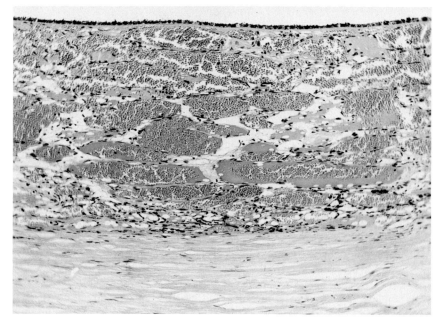

Fig. 1518 Hemangioma of choroid in eye enucleated from 42-year-old white woman who had had a port-wine facial hemangioma since birth and ipsilateral glaucoma since early childhood. (×115; AFIP 759801.)

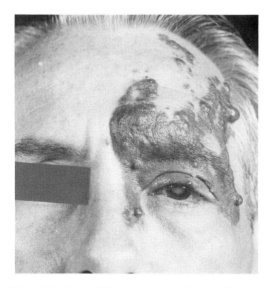

Fig. 1519 Sturge-Weber syndrome. Patient, 42-year-old white man, had had facial hemangioma all his life and was blind in ipsilateral eye because of retinal degeneration, glaucoma, and cataract. Choroidal hemangioma was found in enucleated eye, but clinical study failed to disclose evidence of intracranial lesion. (AFIP 761707; courtesy Veterans Administration Hospital, Hines, Ill.)

A more diffuse and deeply situated melanotic lesion of the lids is the nevus of Ota (congenital oculodermal melanosis). This is a form of extrasacral mongolian spot involving the face in areas supplied by the first and second branches of the trigeminal nerve. Associated conjunctival, scleral, and orbital pigmentation is present in many of the cases. This type of nevus occurs more frequently in Orientals and Blacks than in Caucasians. Caucasians with this condition seem to have a greater than normal predilection for ocular or orbital malignant melanomas.[20]

Angiomas may be small lesions confined to the eyelid or may extend deep into the orbit. Hemangiomas are more common than lymphangiomas. The histopathologic characteristics have been described elsewhere (Chapter 3).

The so-called port-wine stain (nevus flammeus) is of special interest not only because of its great cosmetic effect, but also because it may be associated with malformations in other tissues (Fig. 1518). In the Sturge-Weber syndrome, the facial hemangioma may be associated with a choroidal hemangioma, glaucoma, and a meningeal hemangioma, all on the ipsilateral side (Fig. 1519).

Neurofibromas and plexiform neuromas may be isolated developmental lesions of the eyelid, or they may be merely a part of Reck-

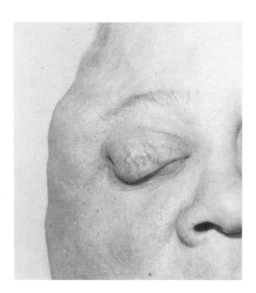

Fig. 1520 Severe unilateral deformity of face in patient with Recklinghausen's neurofibromatosis. (AFIP 55-17512; courtesy Dr. L. L. Calkins, Kansas City, Kan.)

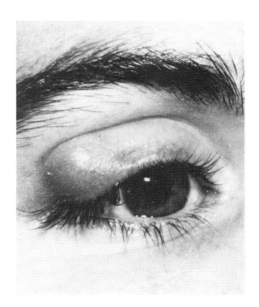

Fig. 1521 Chalazion of right upper eyelid. (WU neg. 79-1631.)

linghausen's neurofibromatosis. Although believed to be present from birth, these tumors frequently show accelerated growth during childhood or later. When associated with Reck-

linghausen's disease, there may be marked asymmetry of the face due to diffuse hypertrophy and pendulousness of all of the facial tissues on one side (Fig. 1520).

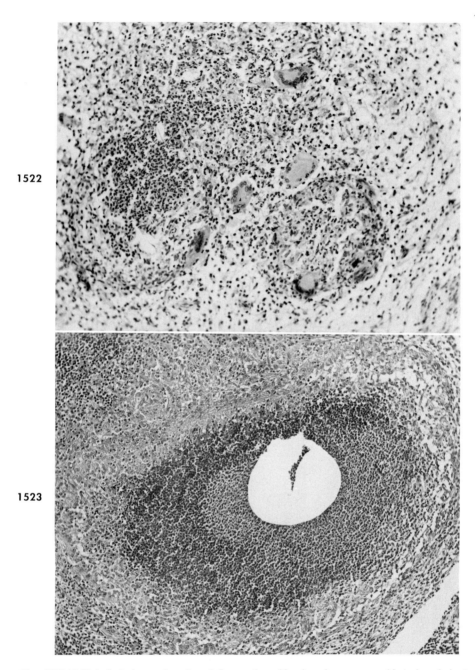

1522

1523

Fig. 1522 Multiple foci of granulomatous inflammation with microabscesses and Langhans' giant cells in chalazion. (×137; AFIP 91218.)
Fig. 1523 Presence of pools of fat in center of many of granulomas is characteristic of chalazia. (×115; AFIP 732397.)

Inflammation

Inflammation of the eyelids may be the result of viral, rickettsial, bacterial, mycotic, or parasitic infections, of chemical or physical irritants, of hypersensitivity states, or of systemic dermatologic disorders. These inflammatory processes are rarely biopsied and are of relatively little practical significance to pathologists.

Chalazion

Chalazion is an extremely common lesion. It represents a lipogranuloma that develops in and about a meibomian gland, presumably as a consequence of the combined effects of obstruction and nonspecific infection of the excretory passages of the gland. The sebaceous material, discharged into the tarsus as a result of the meibomitis, provokes an intense granulomatous inflammatory reaction (Fig. 1521).

Although it begins as a deep-seated process, the chalazion not infrequently erupts through the conjunctival surface of the eyelid. Ordinarily, this lesion is readily recognized and treated, but if, after curettage, one or more recurrences develop, the clinician should be alert to the possibility of a meibomian gland tumor that has previously escaped recognition. In such cases, excision and histopathologic study are indicated.

Microscopically, the typical chalazion reveals multiple foci of granulomatous inflammation (Fig. 1522). In the center of many of the focal granulomas there is a small globule of fat, which in paraffin sections presents simply as an empty round to ovoid space (Fig. 1523).

Metabolic disorders

Xanthelasmas are slightly elevated yellow plaques located on the medial aspect of the upper and lower eyelids (Fig. 1524). They are rarely indicative of any serious systemic disturbance and usually are removed for cosmetic reasons. Most of the patients are in the fifth or sixth decade of life. Patients with familial hypercholesterolemia may develop these lesions at a younger age.

Microscopically, these lesions show large pale-staining fat-laden histiocytes throughout the subepithelial tissues.

Localized *amyloidosis* can occur in the eyelids and conjunctiva. It presents as a chronic painless tumefaction usually not associated with any systemic disease.[22]

Cysts

Benign cysts of the skin of the eyelids and along the lid margins are relatively common, comprising about one-third of lesions removed from the lids. The most common of these are the keratinous cysts discussed in Chapter 3. Another relatively frequent cyst is the cyst of Moll's glands, often referred to as sudoriferous cysts or simply ductal cysts. These present as

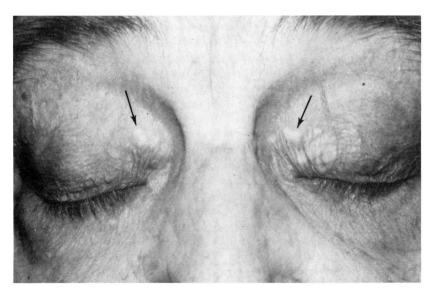

Fig. 1524 Xanthelasma of upper eyelids in patient who had no other systemic findings. (WU neg. 67-4281.)

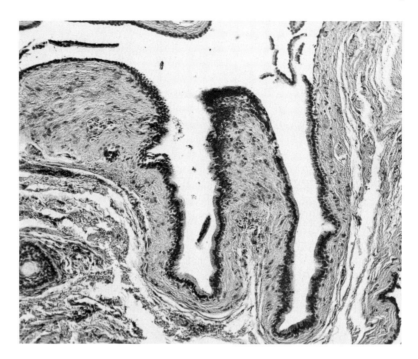

Fig. 1525 Simple cyst of eyelid margin believed to be secondary to obstruction of duct of Moll's gland (sudoriferous cyst). (×110; AFIP 750918.)

thin-walled transparent vesicles at the lid margin. Microscopically, they are simple cysts lined by atrophic cuboidal or flattened epithelial cells with an empty lumen (Fig. 1525).

Tumors and tumorlike lesions
Tumors of surface epithelium

Basal cell carcinomas are by far the most frequent of all true neoplasms arising in any of the palpebral tissues.[15,16] The overwhelming majority are easily excised without sequelae. On rare occasion, they may invade the orbit or nose or both, and exenteration of the orbit may become necessary. Microscopic examination of the margins by frozen section at the time of operation is a useful technique for ensuring that total removal of the tumor has been achieved.[19a]

Basal cell carcinomas arise from the cutaneous surface of the eyelids and rarely, if ever, from the conjunctiva. This point is of some diagnostic significance, for *papillomas* of the palpebral conjunctiva may resemble basal cell carcinoma. When such a lesion is excised and sectioned in such a way that its topographic orientation in relation to the conjunctival surface of the lid is not apparent and if the pathologist is not informed of the clinical appearance of the tumor, an erroneous diagnosis of basal cell carcinoma can be made (Fig. 1526).

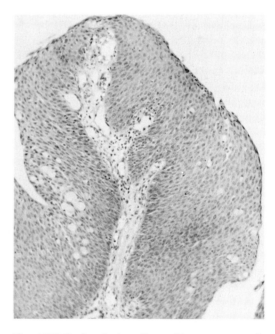

Fig. 1526 Conjunctival papilloma. Many mucous cells are scattered about in acanthotic nonkeratinized epithelium. (×125; AFIP 230075; from Friedenwald JS, Wilder HC, Maumenee AE, Sanders TE, Keyes JEL, Hogan MJ, Owens WC, Owens EU: Ophthalmic pathology: an atlas and textbook. Philadelphia, 1952, W. B. Saunders Co.)

Squamous cell carcinomas often have been cited as responsible for about 10%-20% of all malignant epithelial tumors of the eyelid. Experience, however, indicates that squamous cell carcinoma is much less frequent than that, accounting for less than 3% of malignant tumors of the eyelids.[21]

Nonneoplastic keratotic lesions

Nonneoplastic keratotic lesions may resemble squamous cell carcinomas so closely that even experienced clinicians and pathologists have much difficulty in differential diagnosis.

The lesions include such entities as papilloma, pseudoepitheliomatous hyperplasia, keratoacanthoma, inverted follicular keratosis, seborrheic keratosis, senile keratosis, and cutaneous horns.[17,18] The histopathologic features of these lesions are described in Chapter 3.

Melanotic tumors

Nevi have already been mentioned (p. 1639) since they are generally considered to be congenital or developmental tumors, even though their presence may not be recognized until growth or pigmentation takes place during adolescence or later.

Acquired melanosis is a condition that may involve either or both surfaces of the eyelid in association with the conjunctiva and is described under conjunctiva and cornea (p. 1662).

Malignant melanoma of the eyelid is rare. It may originate from a nevus that has been present for many years, from an acquired melanosis or variable duration, or from what is be-lieved to have been previously normal skin or conjunctiva.

In general, malignant melanomas of the lid carry a very grave prognosis, for they tend to metastasize early by lymphatics and the bloodstream. This is in decided contrast with malignant melanomas of the bulbar conjunctiva (p. 1661) and of the uvea (p. 1685), which have a much more favorable prognosis.

Glandular and other adnexal tumors

Sebaceous gland adenomas and adenocarcinomas may arise from the cutaneous sebaceous glands, the glands of Zeis, or the meibomian gland.

Solitary adenomas of the meibomian and Zeis glands are rarely seen in the laboratory, although they may be more common than is generally believed. The meibomian gland tumors, for example, may simulate a chalazion and be removed by curettage. Such curettings are rarely submitted for microscopic examination. Hence, one does not know how often such tumors are missed. In the case of malignant tumors, however, recurrence is likely. It is for this reason that recurrent chalazia are often excised and sent to the pathology laboratory. In reviewing the histories of patients with meibomian gland carcinomas, it is impressive that the usual story is one of repeated curettages for chalazia before a neoplasm is suspected and a biopsy obtained.

In the series of seventy-eight sebaceous carcinomas of the eyelid recorded by Boniuk and Zimmerman,[19] thirty presented clinically as a

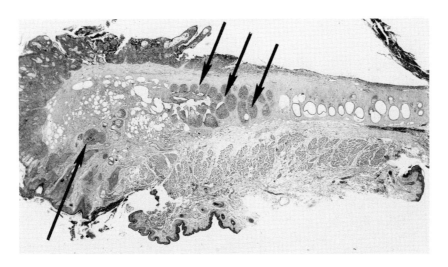

Fig. 1527 Full-thickness section of eyelid showing sebaceous gland carcinoma arising from meibomian glands (arrows) as well as pagetoid invasion of skin. (×5; WU neg. 72-6065.)

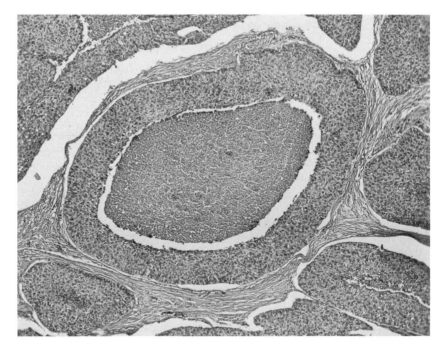

Fig. 1528 Adenocarcinoma of meibomian gland. Plugs of completely necrotic tumor fill central portions of ductlike tubular masses of neoplastic tissue. (×65; AFIP 541358.)

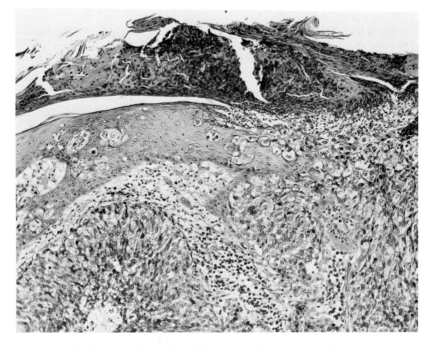

Fig. 1529 Pagetoid involvement of skin of eyelid in patient with carcinoma of meibomian gland. (×115; AFIP 804889.)

chalazion. In twelve patients, the clinical picture was that of a chornic blepharoconjunctivitis, but seven tumors were mistaken for basal cell carcinoma. Following early complete excisonal surgery, the prognosis is good. In Boniuk and Zimmerman's series,[19] however, orbital invasion occurred in 17%, lymph node metastasis developed in 28%, and the tumors proved fatal in 14% of the patients.

Malignant meibomian gland tumors show considerable histologic and cytologic variation, merging with adenomas on the one hand and with very anaplastic epithelial tumors of uncertain histogenesis on the other. The former are easily recognized, first by their position within the tarsus and their obvious anatomic relation to the meibomian gland and second by their cytologic characteristics. In such tumors, the cells continue to exhibit sebaceous differentiation (Fig. 1527), which is very dramatically brought out by frozen sections stained for fat. More rapidly growing tumors may be characterized by extensive necrosis of the central areas of neoplastic lobules, giving rise to a comedocarcinoma pattern (Fig. 1528). Pagetoid involvement of the overlying skin can occur[21a] (Fig. 1529).

Trichilemmoma, a benign adnexal tumor believed to originate from the outer hair sheath (trichilemma) and mostly composed of glycogen-rich clear cells, can involve the eyelid and eyebrow.[20a]

Wright and Font[22a] have described twenty-one cases of a *mucinous sweat gland adenocarcinoma* of the eyelid, homologous to the adenocystic carcinoma of the skin seen in other cutaneous locations (see Chapter 3). Local recurrent was common, but distant metastases occurred in only one case.

LACRIMAL PASSAGES

Diseases of the lacrimal passages that are of importance to the surgical pathologist are characterized by epiphora, the imperfect drainage of tears so that they flow over the lid margin onto the cheek, and by varying degrees of swelling, induration, and inflammation of the lower eyelid at its nasal end. While inflammatory obstructions of these passages are common, neoplastic lesions are rare.

Canaliculitis and dacryocystitis

Canaliculitis and dacryocystitis may be the result of direct spread of inflammatory processes in such neighboring structures as the conjunctiva or nose, but more often their pathogenesis is obscure. Acute and chronic types are recognized, and the inflammatory reaction may be suppurative, granulomatous, or necrotizing, with the formation of fistulous tracts to the skin surface below the eyelid near the base of the nose.

The lacrimal passages become filled with purulent exudate in the acute suppurative types, whereas in the chronic forms the passages are narrowed by the inflammatory thickening of the walls of the lacrimal canal or sac. Frequently, there are also hyperplasia of the lining epithelium and hypersecretion of mucus. At times, the degree of papillomatous or adenomatous hyperplasia of the sac may give rise to difficulties in differential diagnosis.

Mucocele

Lacrimal mucocele is another complication of chronic inflammation of the lacrimal sac. A low-grade obstructive lesion with a relatively intact and possibly hypersecreting mucosa may lead to great distention of the sac by accumulated secretions.

The contents of the cyst may be clear or milky, fluid or gelatinous, fibrinous or flocculent, sterile or infected. Microscopically, the cyst wall reveals varying degrees of atrophy, degeneration, hyperplasia, and hypersecretion of the mucosa and chronic inflammation of the subepithelial tissues.

Dacryolithiasis

Dacryolithiasis and concretions in the lacrimal canaliculus are of uncertain pathogenesis, but they generally are believed to be the result of low-grade inflammatory process. Mycotic infections are believed by some authorities to account for most "tear stones." If such concretions are crushed and examined microscopically, they will be seen to contain myriad mycelial elements embedded in a relatively acellular matrix. Others, however, are laminated, mineralized stones without recognizable fungous or bacterial forms.

Tumors

Neoplasms of the lacrimal passages are rare. Papillomas similar to those arising in the conjunctival surface of the eyelid (p. 1644), may form in the punctum, within the canaliculus, or in the sac. Inflammatory pseudoepitheliomatous hyperplasia, however, is seen more often.

From the clinical point of view, it is usually

not possible to differentiate malignant tumors of the lacrimal passages from benign neoplasms and pseudotumors. Dacryocystography has become an important part of the clinical evaluation of lacrimal sac tumors.

All malignant tumors of the lacrimal passages except carcinoma are exceedingly rare, and even carcinoma is distinctly uncommon. These tumors are usually moderately well-differentiated squamous carcinomas, similar in appearance to those arising from the mucosa of the nose or in the conjunctiva. They tend to form papillary projections into the lumen and spread along natural surfaces, but they also infiltrate directly into adjacent tissues.[23]

LACRIMAL GLAND

Lacrimal gland lesions are divided into nonepithelial and epithelial. The nonepithelial lesions, which make up about 65% of lacrimal gland lesions, include inflammatory pseudotumor, lymphoid hyperplasia, nonspecific dacryoadenitis, Sjogren's syndrome, sarcoid, lymphoma, and leukemia. Of the epithelial tumors, benign mixed cell tumor (pleomorphic adenoma) is the most common.

Dacryoadenitis

When chronic dacryoadenitis is associated with enlargement of the parotid or other salivary glands, it has been referred to as *Mikulicz's syndrome*. This may be the result of a variety of specific diseases, including sarcoidosis, tuberculosis, syphilis, mumps, Graves' disease, malignant lymphoma, and leukemia.

The term *Mikulicz's disease* is being used less and less, for no one knows exactly what Mikulicz's patients had, and it is doubtful whether there is a specific disease of the lacrimal and salivary glands, other than that responsible for Sjögren's syndrome, that is sufficiently distinctive in its clinical and/or histopathologic picture to justify this eponymic designation.[27]

The benign lymphoepithelial lesion of the salivary glands described by Godwin[26] has been equated with Mikulicz's disease, but the patients usually present clinical evidence of Sjögren's syndrome. The occurrence of the benign lymphoepithelial lesion in the lacrimal glands and its relationship to Sjögren's syndrome have been discussed by Font et al.[24] The typical lesion is shown in Fig. 586 (p. 573).

The lacrimal gland also may be involved in a unilateral chronic nongranulomatous inflammatory process with no associated involvement of salivary glands, no systemic manifestations, and no features of Sjögren's syndrome. As a matter of fact, this is the type of dacryoadenitis the surgical pathologist sees most frequently. Bilateral lacrimal gland enlargement with a histologic picture of chronic dacryoadenitis has been reported in a patient with diffuse elevation of IgG and IgA fractions.[29]

Atrophy; Sjögren's syndrome

Sjögren's syndrome is characterized by a failure of lacrimal and conjunctival secretions and consequent keratoconjunctivitis sicca, usually in postmenopausal women. Typically, there is evidence of a systemic disorder affecting mucous membranes and their associated glands. It is believed that degeneration of the secretory portions of the lacrimal and salivary glands is the essential feature of the pathologic anatomy in Sjögren's syndrome, although such secondary changes as lymphocytic infiltration, fibrosis, and hyalinization are commonly present.

The benign lymphoepithelial lesion (Fig. 586, p. 573), while not pathognomonic of Sjögren's syndrome, is often associated with it that it carries more diagnostic significance than any other histopathologic finding.[24]

Tumors

Most neoplasms of the lacrimal gland arise in the orbital lobe where the gland is firmly attached to the orbital rim about the lacrimal fossa. The bone tends to restrict growth in its direction. Hence, the enlarging tumor characteristically displaces the eye downward and nasally (Fig. 1530).

The histopathologic characteristics of lacrimal gland tumors are similar to those of the

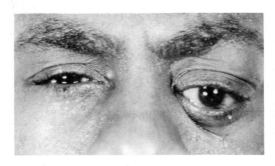

Fig. 1530 Pleomorphic adenoma of left lacrimal gland in 38-year-old black man. Proptosis was accompanied by severe visual loss. (AFIP 62-931; courtesy Veterans Administration Hospital, Jefferson Barracks, Mo.)

salivary glands (Chapter 11). Whereas pleo-morphic adenomas are by far the most com-mon, they do not predominate to the degree that some writers have suggested (90%). Pleo-morphic adenomas account for about 50%-60%, carcinomas in pleomorphic adenomas for 5%-10%, adenoid cystic carcinomas for 20%-30%, and other carcinomas for 5%-10%.[26a,27a]

Because so many of these lacrimal gland tumors have not been completely and adequate-ly removed at the initial operation, there has been an excessively high recurrence rate.[28] It is even more difficult to treat the recurrences, for these are often multiple. The carcinomas have a very poor prognosis.[25,30]

In addition to the epithelial tumors of the lacrimal gland, malignant lymphomas, lym-phoid pseudotumors, and chronic inflammatory processes are important causes of enlargement of the gland. In a patient who is in good general health and who presents no evidence of a sys-temic disease, the discovery of a lymphomatous tumor in the lacrimal fossa rarely heralds the development of malignant lymphoma or leu-kemia. In fact, in the majority of cases there is a polymorphism suggestive of a reactive inflammatory process, although in other cases the rather pure proliferation of lymphocytes makes it quite impossible to rule out a lym-phocytic lymphoma or leukemia. The lacrimal glands may, of course, become involved along with other tissues in a leukemia or malignant lymphoma.

ORBIT

The hallmark of disease of the orbit is ex-ophthalmos. This may not necessarily be caused by a true neoplasm, and therefore the surgical pathologist may never see any speci-men from many patients who present with this finding. For example, the most common cause for exophthalmos is dysthyroid ophthalmopathy and rarely is a biopsy taken in these cases.

As for the relative frequency of lesions that cause exophthalmos, many of the statistics that have been reported merely reflect the bias of the specialist involved. For example, to the radiolo-gist one of the most common orbital lesions producing displacement of the eye is a muco-cele arising from a paranasal sinus. The oph-thalmologist, however, would place mucocele far below such entities as dysthyroid ophthal-mopathy, hemangioma, and inflammatory pseudotumor.

Congenital and developmental conditions
Angioma

Angiomas are relatively common orbital tu-mors, with hemangiomas occurring much more commonly than lymphangiomas.

In the infant, these soft, blue, compressible tumors are diffuse throughout the orbit and often

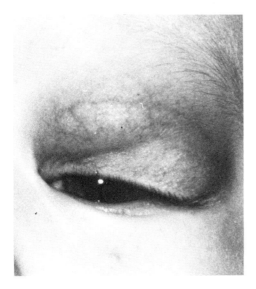

Fig. 1531 Capillary hemangioma of left orbit and eye-lid. (WU neg. 79-1630.)

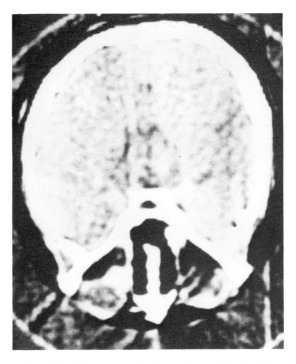

Fig. 1532 CT scan showing hemangioma of right orbit. (WU neg. 79-1636.)

extend forward into the eyelids (Fig. 1531). Surgical removal is difficult; fortunately, however, most of these lesions spontaneously regress by 4 years of age. If the tumor is so large that the visual axis of the eye is covered and the eye is at risk for the development of deprivation amblyopia, such lesions often can be reduced in size following a short course of systemic steroids or small doses of radiotherapy.

In the adult, these tumors are usually encapsulated, are situated close to the back of the eye, and can be surgically "shelled" out. The CT scan reveals a discrete round mass that is enhanced by contrast dye (Fig. 1532).

These tumors rarely present difficulties in histopathologic diagnosis, for they are not significantly dissimilar from angiomas elsewhere. In the infant the lesion is usually the capillary type and in the adult the cavernous type.

Peripheral nerve tumors

Peripheral nerve tumors are also basically hamartomatous lesions, but they are much less common in the orbit than are the vascular tumors. These orbital tumors may be merely one of a number of manifestations of Recklinghausen's disease, but on occasion they are also encountered as isolated lesions.

There may be a gross deformity of the orbit and eyelids (Fig. 1520) and upon palpation of the lid has been referred to as "a bag of worms."

Systemic diseases
Dysthyroid ophthalmopathy

The most common cause of orbital disease and of exophthalmos is dysthyroid ophthalmopathy, in which there is some dysfunction between the pituitary-thyroid axis. When seen with the ocular problems, the patient may be hyperthyroid, hypothyroid, or euthyroid. Often there is a history of hyperthyroidism or some form of treatment in the past.

Unilateral orbital involvement occurs with sufficient frequency in both forms of dysthyroid ophthalmopathy to warrant this condition always being considered in the differential diagnosis of orbital tumors (Fig. 1533).

Histopathologic changes observed in the severe cases which are most likely to come to the attention of surgical pathologists include widespread edema and chronic inflammation of all the orbital tissues. The most striking gross alterations are observed in the extraocular

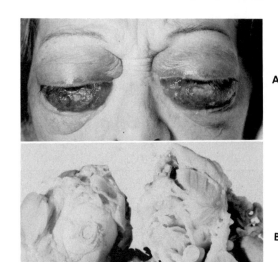

Fig. 1533 A, Malignant exophthalmos of about ten months' duration in 65-year-old white woman who finally died of congestive heart failure. **B,** At autopsy, extraocular muscles were found to be massively thickened. (**A** and **B**, AFIP 692463.)

muscles, which may be massively enlarged (Fig. 1533). Muscle fibers degenerate and become hyalinized. A great increase in the interstitial connective tissue, including both cellular elements and ground substance, is observed particularly in the muscles but also in the other orbital tissues.

Histiocytoses and juvenile xanthogranuloma

Exophthalmos may rarely be caused by orbital involvement by Hand-Schüller-Christian disease, Letterer-Siwe disease, eosinophilic granuloma, or juvenile xanthogranuloma.

Inflammatory processes

The orbit may become secondarily inflamed by lesions arising in the face, eyes, nose, sinuses, orbital bones, blood vessels, brain, and meninges. Generally, it is only when such inflammations simulate neoplasms that orbital exploration is undertaken and tissue is obtained for histopathologic diagnosis.

Specific granulomas, including those of tuberculosis and sarcoidosis, are rare.

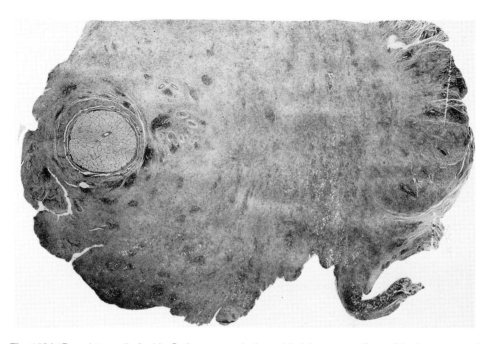

Fig. 1534 "Pseudotumor" of orbit. Optic nerve and other orbital tissues are "frozen" in dense mass of nonspecific chronic inflammatory tissue. (×5½; AFIP 35691.)

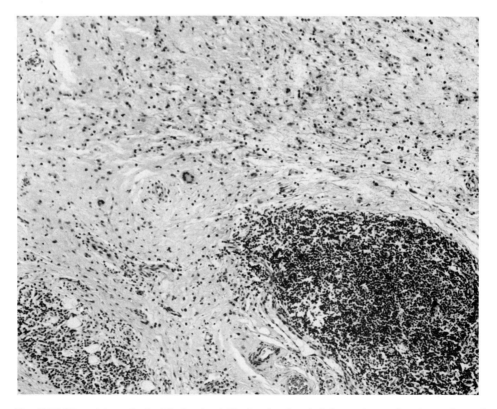

Fig. 1535 "Pseudotumor" of orbit showing infiltration by chronic inflammatory cells, giant cells, and generalized fibrosis. (×90; WU neg. 67-4223.)

Nonspecific chronic inflammations ("pseudotumors" of orbit) are very much more frequent than are the specific infectious granulomas.

Undoubtedly, these pseudotumors represent an etiologically and pathogenetically heterogeneous group. The pathologic features they share include the following:

1 The formation of an indurated orbital mass often surrounding the optic nerve and incorporating one or more of the extraocular muscles (Fig. 1534)

2 A tissue reaction that includes exudation of fluid, excessive production of ground substance, the mobilization of chronic inflammatory cells, vascular proliferation, and hyperplasia of connective tissue (Fig. 1535)

3 The absence of demonstrable etiologic agents or of otherwise diagnostic histopathologic alterations indicative of such specific disease entities as Hodgkin's disease, temporal arteritis, etc.

This is not to say, however, that the microscopic features are uniform from case to case. In some instances, the proliferation of blood vessels and ground substance resembles that of exuberant granulation tissue. At times, the lymphoid hyperplasia with follicle formation is of such intensity that the picture resembles that which is characteristic of orbital malignant lymphomas (p. 1653). Other cases with prominent involvement of extraocular muscles suggest the possibility of dysthyroid ophthalmopathy.

A well-developed granulomatous reaction about small pools of fat is observed in certain cases. Such lesions may suggest traumatic fat necrosis. Others containing large numbers of cholesterol clefts and many foamy macrophages and giant cells suggest an area of old suppuration or hemorrhage. Periphlebitis is prominent in certain cases, and some of these may present a significant eosinophilia suggesting the possibility of a hypersensitivity angiitis. Rarely, the picture merges with that of sclerosing hemangioma or fasciitis.[34]

Patients with pseudotumors are usually in the third to fifth decade and in good health. The exophthalmos is of relatively sudden onset and in at least one-half of the patients is associated with moderate to severe orbital pain and with lid and conjunctival edema. Diplopia is often present, secondary to limitation of ocular motility in one or more fields of gaze, but visual acuity is usually unimpaired.

The lesion often can be palpated through the eyelids; if so, the surgeon may be able to reach it easily for a biopsy. Deeper lesions are not so readily accessible for biopsy and, if the clinical signs and symptoms are characteristic for inflammatory pseudotumor, steroids are often given without a biopsy, especially since systemic steroids often produce dramatic alleviation of signs and symptoms. The CT scan can be helpful in localizing the lesion.

Primary tumors
Connective tissue tumors

Connective tissue tumors of the orbit, both benign and malignant, are extremely rare. Only the *rhabdomyosarcoma* is encountered with any degree of regularity, and this is the most frequently observed tumor in the orbit in children.[36]

This neoplasm characteristically occurs between the ages of 5 and 15 years with a rather sudden onset and a rapidly progressive course. Although the tumor can occur anywhere in the orbit, there is a slightly higher incidence of an upper nasal location, displacing the eye downward and outward (Fig. 1536). Microscopically, it resembles the rhabdomyosarcomas of childhood seen in other anatomic locations (Chapter 24).

Lipomas, fibrous histiocytomas, hemangiopericytomas, chondromas, osteomas, and their malignant counterparts have all been reported,

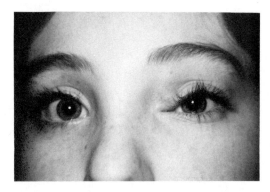

Fig. 1536 Rhabdomyosarcoma presenting as palpable mass in upper medial quadrant of left orbit with only minimal downward and lateral displacement of eye. (WU neg. 67-3507; from Smith ME: The differential diagnosis of unilateral exophthalmos. In Gay AJ, Burde RM (eds): Clinical concepts in neuro-ophthalmology. International Ophthalmology Clinics, vol. 7, no. 4, Boston, 1967, Little, Brown and Co.)

but they are extremely rare. One possible exception to this statement concerns the occurrence of osteosarcomas and other sarcomas arising in the orbital tissues as a late complication of extensive radiation therapy.[33] Many of the hemangiopericytomas have behaved in an aggressive fashion.[34a]

Reactive fibroblastic proliferations such as nodular fasciitis may be mistaken for sarcomas.[32]

Lymphoid tumors

Lymphoid tumors of the orbit present great difficulties in histopathologic diagnoses. Such lesions may develop in the course of a previously recognized malignant lymphoma or leukemia, but much more often the lymphoid tumor of the orbit, lacrimal gland, or conjunctiva is not accompanied by any clinical or hematologic evidence of a systemic disease.[30a]

Microscopically, lymphoid tumors of the orbit fall into three main groups. The smallest but most important contains those lesions that are quite obviously malignant neoplasms, usually non-Hodgkin's lymphomas of poorly differentiated lymphocytic or ''histiocytic'' types.[36b] The two largest groups include the following:

1 Those lesions that are fairly obvious examples of severe reactive hyperplasia
2 Those lesions that are characterized by a rather uniform but widespread proliferation of lymphocytes

In the former, one frequently observes considerable polymorphism, a variety of cell types participating, vascular proliferation, and prominent follicles with reactive centers. It is the latter group, characterized by a monotonous lymphocytic proliferation, frequently with apparent infiltration of orbital fat, blood vessels, and nerves, that presents most of the exceedingly difficult problems in differential diagnosis.[36a] Careful evaluation of the cytologic features in well-made preparations remains as the most important criterion for their separation into benign and malignant varieties, which is not always possible.[35a] At present, we believe that most of these lesions are benign, for they generally respond to very small doses of radiation, are not associated with other evidence of systemic disease, and do not recur or metastasize following therapy. It is possible, however, that much longer periods of follow-up will be required to ascertain the behavior of these lesions properly.

Glioma of optic nerve

Gliomas of the optic nerve are relatively rare slow-growing tumors that usually arise within the orbital segment of the nerve.[37]

Considerable cytologic variation is observed among the gliomas, not only from case to case but also in different portions of a given tumor. Varying degrees of cellularity are observed, but generally these neoplasms are characterized by a low order of anaplasia. This is especially true about the margins of the tumor, where it is often impossible to be certain where reactive gliosis ends and neoplasia begins. Typically, there are areas of intense mucinous degeneration within the tumor. Frequently in such areas the tumor cells appear to be virtually lost in the abundant hyaluronidase-sensitive mucoid accumulations.

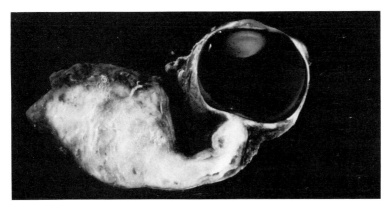

Fig. 1537 Glioma that has produced massive enlargement of orbital segment of optic nerve. Tumor has completely effaced characteristic architectural features of nerve and its meninges. (AFIP 842777.)

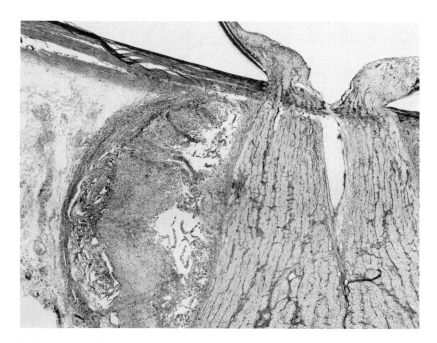

Fig. 1538 Section through optic nerve just anterior to main mass of this glioma reveals minimal alteration of parenchyma of nerve but greatly thickened meninges. Combination of infiltrating tumor and arachnoidal proliferation is responsible for this meningeal thickening. (×20; AFIP 65035.)

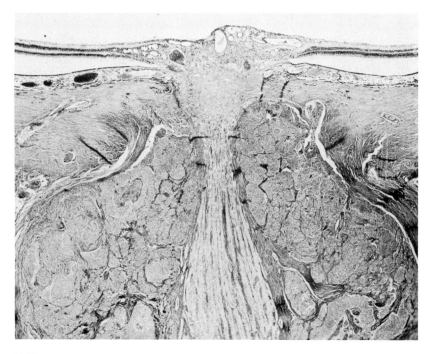

Fig. 1539 Meningioma of optic nerve. Meninges are greatly thickened, and optic nerve reveals severe compression atrophy. (×21; AFIP 55939.)

Small tumors limited to the optic nerve can be adequately managed by resection alone; for the more extensive lesions, biopsy followed by irradiation is recommended.[31a]

As these gliomas increase in size, they tend to form a bulbous enlargement of the nerve (Fig. 1537). They also extend along the nerve peripherally toward the eye and centrally toward the brain. In so doing, they often produce great enlargement of the optic canal, an important diagnostic sign for the radiologist. In such cases, the optic nerve fibers are likely to be completely destroyed, and the optic disc typically presents the ophthalmoscopic characteristics of primary optic atrophy.

Another growth pattern exhibited by a majority of optic nerve gliomas is for infiltration to take place through the pia. This leads to great thickening of the arachnoid (Fig. 1538). This is partly the result of more exuberant growth of the tumor cells once they have reached the arachnoid, but equally important is the reactive proliferation of arachnoidal cells. At times, this has created difficulties in differential diagnosis between glioma and meningioma.

Gliomas of the optic nerve typically make their presence known during the first decade of life with minimal exophthalmos, optic nerve atrophy, or papilledema and a characteristic thickening of the nerve on CT scan. There is a distinct association of these tumors and Recklinghausen's disease. There is recent evidence that the overwhelming majority of optic nerve gliomas are so slow growing that surgical intervention is seldom warranted.

Meningioma

Meningiomas of the orbit may arise from the meninges of the optic nerve (Fig. 1539) and are felt to be more aggressive tumors than the meningiomas of the sphenoidal ridge.[35] However, some authors feel that meningiomas of the orbit need not be operated on until severe proptosis or proof of posterior extension occurs.

Those tumors arising from the orbital meninges generally produce some visual loss, optic atrophy, and exophthalmos. Those arising from the inner portion of the sphenoidal ridge produce more severe compression of the optic nerve within the optic canal, resulting in papilledema or optic atrophy before proptosis. The CT scan, of course, has facilitated the diagnosis and localization of these tumors (Fig. 1540).

The microscopic diagnosis is usually not a problem for the pathologist. Perioptic meningiomas are almost always the meningothelial type.

Secondary tumors

Direct spread from adjacent structures can occur with primary intraocular tumors such as retinoblastoma or uveal malignant melanomas. Carcinomas of the paranasal sinuses also may fail to produce diagnostic symptoms until orbital extension has occurred.

Chronic disease of the frontal or ethmoid sinuses may produce a *mucocele* that erodes through the wall of the sinus to produce an inferolateral displacement of the globe. The

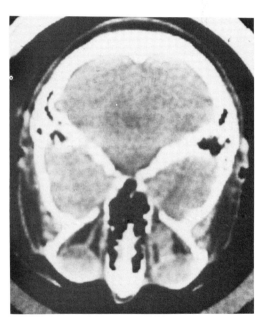

Fig. 1540 CT scan showing perioptic meningioma of left orbit. (WU neg. 79-1635.)

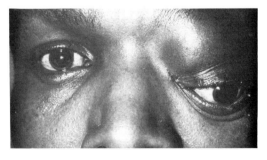

Fig. 1541 Mucocele producing downward and lateral displacement of left eye. (WU neg. 69-7637; from del Regato JA, Spjut HJ: Ackerman and del Regato's Cancer, ed. 5. St. Louis, 1977, The C. V. Mosby Co.)

onset is usually insidious, and the enlargement is symptomless and slow (Fig. 1541).

Histopathologically, this cystic mass is lined by mucus-secreting sinus mucosa with variable degrees of inflammation and scarring.

Hematogenous metastases to the orbit may be seen, on occasion, with many different tumors, but rarely are these initial manifestations of a carcinoma. Even the neuroblastoma, which has a notorious reputation for its orbital metastases, rarely does so before other diagnostic signs appear.

Most important in this regard is the distinct possibility that a primary embryonal rhabdomyosarcoma might be misinterpreted as a metastatic tumor. Another important possibility to be considered when an undifferentiated "round cell sarcoma" is found in a child's orbital tissues is acute leukemia. Such orbital lesions may make their appearance before peripheral blood studies are diagnostic, but bone marrow aspirates will usually furnish a conclusive answer. In the case of adults, an orbital metastasis may, on rare occasions, be the initial manifestation of carcinoma of the breast, bronchus, or kidney.

CONJUNCTIVA

Lesions of the conjunctiva are thin and tend to fold into distorted patterns when placed into fixative. To prepare the tissue so that the pathologist can orient it properly, the surgeon should spread the lesion onto a small piece of filter paper and allow it to dry onto the filter paper for a few seconds before gently placing the filter paper with the adherent specimen into the jar of fixation. Specimens should never be put onto sponges of any kind since these will expand when placed into the fixative, thus distorting the specimen.

Congenital and developmental lesions
Dermoid tumors

Dermoid tumors of the bulbar conjunctiva are firm, localized, elevated opaque masses that typically occur at the limbus, often encroaching upon the cornea (Fig. 1542). These are solid choristomatous masses, not to be confused with dermoid cysts of the orbit.

Over the lesion, the surface epithelium and the subepithelial connective tissue present the histologic features characteristic of epidermis and dermis, respectively. Typically, a few hairs project from the tumor. The bulk of the mass is composed of thick bundles of collagen. In some lesions, skin appendages are few, and adipose tissue is abundant. These are known as dermolipomas, and they usually are situated in the upper outer fornix. Ocular dermoids may be part of Goldenhar's syndrome, in which there are extra-auricular appendages and vertebral abnormalities.

Nevi

Nevi of the bulbar conjunctiva, like those of the skin, may be observed from birth, or they

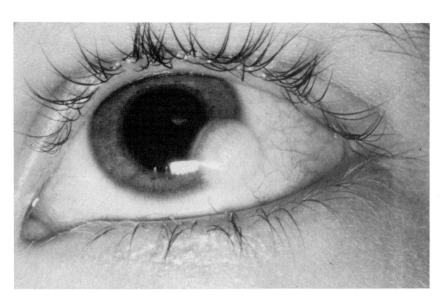

Fig. 1542 Limbal dermoid in child. (WU neg. 67-4282.)

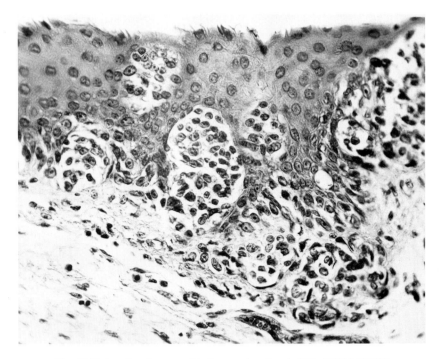

Fig. 1543 Junctional nevus of bulbar conjunctiva (×305; AFIP 819328.)

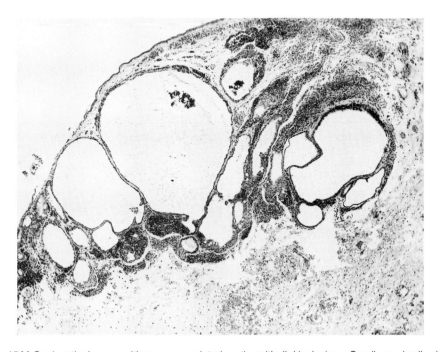

Fig. 1544 Conjunctival nevus with many associated cystic epithelial inclusions. Small round cells about large cysts are not inflammatory cells but nevus cells. This epibulbar lesion may be analogous to hairy dermal nevi of skin. (×48; AFIP 713602.)

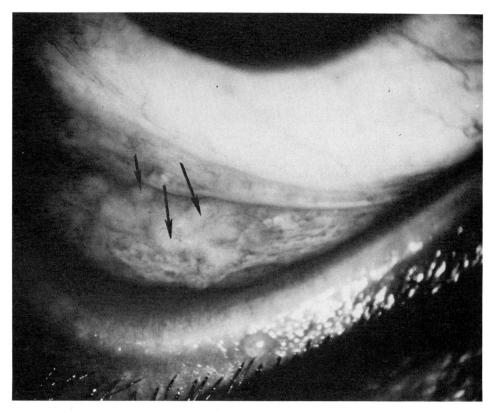

Fig. 1545 Conjunctival granulomas in sarcoidosis. (WU neg. 79-1632.)

may become noticeable at any time during childhood, adolescence, or later. At times, a nevus known to have been present since infancy appears to become much larger and more pigmented at puberty (Fig. 1552).

Characteristically, conjunctival nevi are discrete, flat, or slightly elevated lesions located on the globe in the interpalpebral zone near the limbus, but they vary greatly in size, shape, and position. They also exhibit much variation in degree of pigmentation, about one-third being essentially amelanotic.

Microscopically, conjunctival nevi are almost always of the junctional (Fig. 1543) or compound varieties. Counterparts of the common dermal nevus of the skin are rarely observed. Frequently, there are numerous solid and cystic inclusions of conjunctival epithelium intimately incorporated into the subepithelial component of these nevi. At times, the epithelial inclusions may so dominate the clinical and histopathologic picture (Fig. 1544) that the nevoid nature of the lesion is overlooked. The presence of the epithelial inclusions is

supportive evidence for benignity since they are rare in melanomas.

Inflammation

Inflammatory lesions of the conjunctiva do not often give rise to the type of diagnostic or therapeutic problem that requires excision and histopathologic study. One lesion that deserves mention is the *chronic granuloma* characteristic of sarcoidosis (Fig. 1545). A noncaseating granulomatous tubercle can be found in about one-fourth of patients with sarcoidosis.[39] Ligneous conjunctivitis is a peculiar form of chronic pseudomembranous conjunctivitis that presents as a woody induration of the eyelids plus the formation of a pseudomembrane on the tarsal conjunctiva. The cardinal feature histologically is the presence of large hyaline masses.[40]

Degeneration

Pinguecula is a very common degenerative process affecting primarily the subepithelial connective tissues of the bulbar conjunctiva in

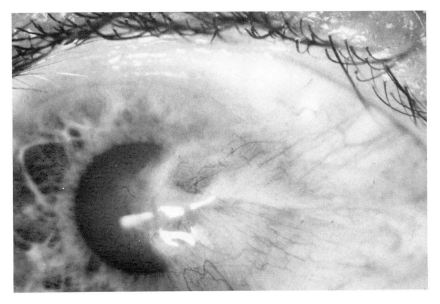

Fig. 1546 Pterygium that has grown over pupillary axis and has interfered with vision. (WU neg. 67-4284.)

the interpalpebral region. This gives rise to an elevated yellowish lesion over which the epithelium may become atrophic or thickened. Since these lesions are not progressive, they are seldom excised.

Histologically, the most characteristic feature is senile elastosis affecting a band-like zone beneath the epithelium. Secondary hyalinization and calcareous degeneration also may be observed. Typically, the epithelium over pingueculae becomes atrophic, but at times it becomes so acanthotic and dyskeratotic that the erroneous diagnosis of carcinoma may be made.

Pterygium extends into the cornea and is therefore a more important lesion than the pinguecula (Fig. 1546).

Microscopically, there is usually some senile elastosis but also a variable amount of acute and chronic inflammation and congestion of blood vessels.

Tumors and related lesions
Papilloma

Papillomas are relatively common lesions of the conjunctiva with a tendency for recurrence after apparent complete excision. In children, the papillomas are often multiple. The lesions have a typical papillomatous or "mulberry" surface appearance with small vessels coming up to the surface (Fig. 1547).

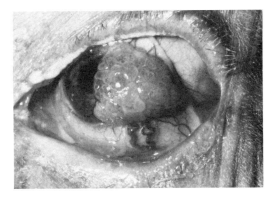

Fig. 1547 Extensive papilloma of bulbar conjunctiva. (WU neg. 72-6272.)

Microscopically, the typical papilloma reveals pronounced acanthosis and varying degrees of keratinization, dyskeratosis, and nonspecific inflammation (Fig. 1526).

Carcinoma in situ

Carcinoma in situ, also known as intraepithelial epithelioma, is often erroneously referred to as "Bowen's disease" by the ophthalmic surgeon. Bowen's disease, however, is a lesion of the skin and not of mucous membranes.

Carcinoma in situ of the bulbar conjunctiva varies considerably in its clinical appearance. It may present as an area of leukoplakia, as a papilloma, or as a complication of pterygium or pinguecula (Fig. 1548).

The histopathologic characteristics of carcinoma in situ of the conjunctiva and cornea are similar to those observed elsewhere in the mucous membranes (Fig. 1549), or the lesion may mimic Bowen's disease of the skin.[41]

There are many lesions removed from the conjunctiva that do not fall clearly into either of the categories of papilloma or carcinoma in situ. They are often not quite so benign to be called papilloma, yet there are not enough changes to warrant a classification of carcinoma in situ. These are referred to as dysplastic lesions of the conjunctiva.

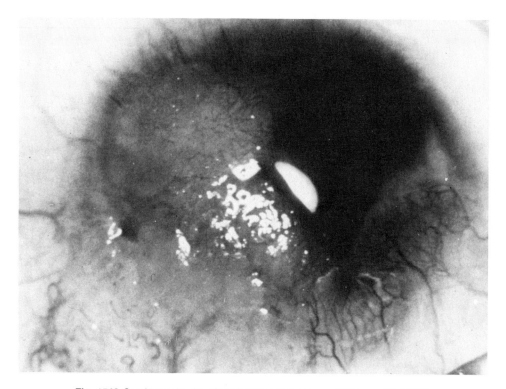

Fig. 1548 Carcinoma in situ of conjunctiva and cornea. (WU neg. 79-1633.)

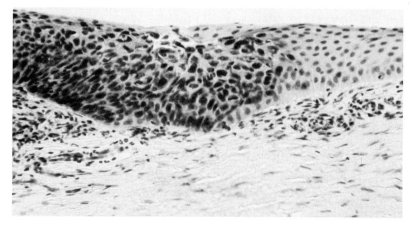

Fig. 1549 Carcinoma in situ in which there is abrupt transition from essentially normal conjunctival epithelium to intraepithelial neoplasm. (×160; WU neg. 67-5356.)

Squamous cell carcinoma

Invasive squamous cell carcinoma of the conjunctiva is rare but is seen at least more often than basal cell carcinoma of the conjunctiva.[38]

Clinically, significant infiltrative carcinoma (Fig. 1550) is seldom observed in the United States, probably because it is a common prac-

tice to excise early "precancerous" or "in situ cancerous" lesions long before they become infiltrative. Such lesions, as well as the majority of early invasive carcinomas of the limbal area, can be adequately controlled by excisional therapy. Rarely in the United States is it necessary to resort to radical surgery for these tumors[41] (Fig. 1551).

Malignant melanoma

Malignant melanoma of the conjunctiva is quite rare; it may arise without an apparent precursor lesion, or it may be a sequela of a nevus or of acquired melanosis[42] (Figs. 1552 and 1553).

Nevus origin

Nevi of the conjunctiva rarely become malignant; yet it has been reported that about one-third of melanomas of the conjunctiva arise from preexisting nevi (Fig. 1554).

Histologically, these tumors also have shown evidence of the occurrence of malignant change in previously benign compound nevi. Subsequent behavior of these histologically malignant melanomas has been difficult to predict. Many, particularly the pedunculated limbal lesions, have neither recurred or metastasized even though removed by simple excision. Others have produced multiple recurrences or have metastasized.

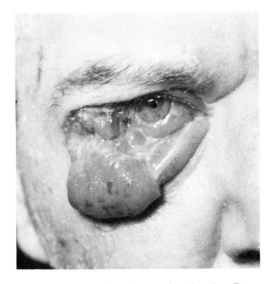

Fig. 1550 Epidermal carcinoma of conjunctiva. Tumor grew rapidly over four-month period. (WU neg. 64-3837.)

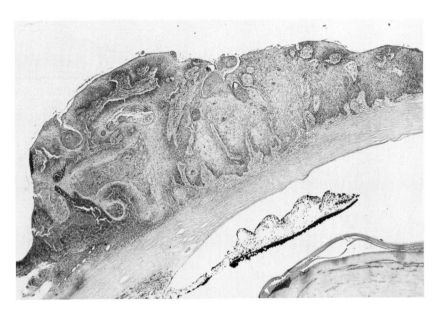

Fig. 1551 Carcinoma of limbus. Exophytic growth pattern with formation of papillomatous mass is typical of more advanced limbal carcinomas. Even in such large tumors, corneoscleral stroma tends to prevent neoplasm from invading intraocular tissues. (×18; AFIP 785865.)

Acquired melanosis—benign and malignant

Acquired melanosis is also referred to as precancerous and cancerous melanosis.[44] The condition is characterized clinically by the insidious development (typically in the fifth decade) of a diffuse nonelevated granular pigmentation of the conjunctiva. it has a poor prognosis due to the frequency with which it gives rise to metastasizing malignant melanoma (Figs. 1553 and 1555).

Usually, a period of two to ten years elapses between the onset of benign acquired melanosis and the development of malignant melanoma. During this interval, the extent of the lesion and the degree of pigmentation may fluctuate spon-

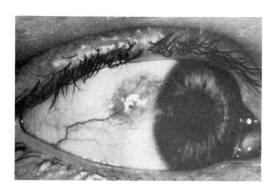

Fig. 1552 Pigmented lesion at limbus that proved to be benign nevus. (WU neg. 69-2209; from del Regato JA, Spjut HJ: Ackerman and del Regato's Cancer, ed. 5. St. Louis, 1977, The C. V. Mosby Co.; courtesy Registry of Ophthalmic Pathology, Armed Forces Institute of Pathology.)

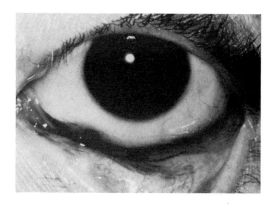

Fig. 1553 Malignant melanoma of conjunctiva in lower cul-de-sac arising from lesion of acquired melanosis. (WU neg. 69-2211; from Zimmerman LE: Discussion of Pigmented tumors of the conjunctiva. In Boniuk M (ed): Ocular and adenexal tumors, St. Louis, 1964, The C. V. Mosby Co.; courtesy Registry of Ophthalmic Pathology, Armed Forces Institute of Pathology; AFIP 56-9886.)

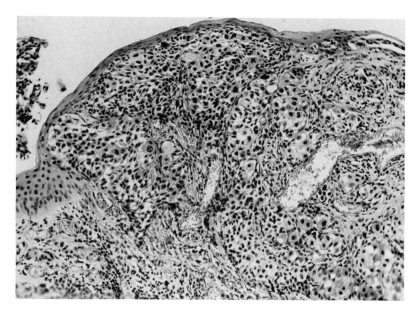

Fig. 1554 Malignant melanoma arising in nevus known to have been present since childhood. Patient, 59-year-old white woman, stated that lesion suddenly became quite large several months before it was excised. (×135; AFIP 643700.)

taneously. The disease affects the bulbar conjunctiva most commonly, but associated lesions
of the cornea, palpebral conjunctiva, and skin
of the eyelids are not uncommon.

Because the term precancerous melanosis has
led to the unwarranted assumption that the lesion will inevitably give rise to a malignant
melanoma despite the fact that fewer than one
in five cases actually progress to cancerous
melanosis, we believe this term should be
dropped. We recommend Zimmerman's classification[45] which is based on the histopathologic
appearance of the lesions.

Stage I—Benign acquired melanosis

A *With minimal junctional activity* —In some cases,
the tissue shows only hyperpigmentation of the
epithelium, while in others a few clusters of nevus
cells (atypical melanocytes) also may be seen in
the affected epithelium.

B *With marked junctional activity* —In addition to
hyperpigmentation, there are many nests of nevus
cells, some of which appear rather disturbing,
and there are engorged vessels and inflammatory
cells in the substantia propria.

Stage II—Cancerous acquired melanosis

A *With minimal invasion* —This would correspond
to the early malignant melanomas that other pathologists have variously designated as "super-

ficial malignant melanoma" or "incipient malignant melanoma." In addition to changes indicated previously, there are focal areas in which
the full thickness of the affected epithelium is
replaced by extremely disturbing, very atypical
melanocytes, often with mitotic activity in evidence. Often foci of invasion of the superficial
substantia propria can be demonstrated.

B *With marked invasion* —A fully developed, frankly invasive malignant melanoma is present in
addition to the other changes listed in Stage I and
Stage IIA.

The transition from the benign to the cancerous state may not be apparent clinically,
although usually there are areas that become
elevated, nodular, ulcerated, and/or more
deeply pigmented.

No therapy is recommended for most patients
with benign acquired melanosis (Stage IA),
and orbital exenteration has been recommended
for frank malignant melanoma arising in an extensive area of acquired melanosis (Stage IIB).
Between these extremes lie the real therapeutic
problems. We recommended careful follow-up
plus antiinflammatory measures for Stage IB
and wide excisional surgery for Stage IIA with
preservation of the eye and eyelids when feasible. Cryotherapy and radiation are presently
being evaluated.

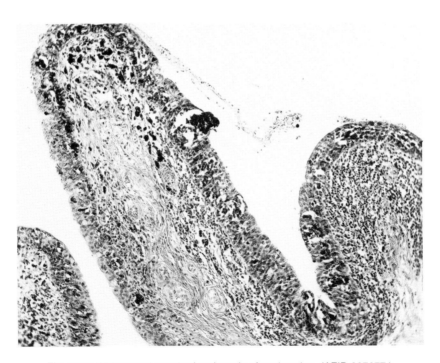

Fig. 1555 Widespread acquired melanosis of conjunctiva. (AFIP 897677.)

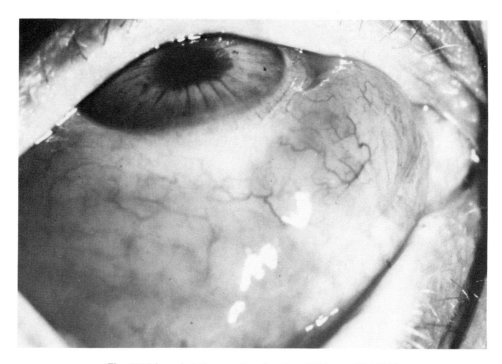

Fig. 1556 Lymphoid tumor of conjunctiva. (WU neg. 79-1634.)

Lymphoid tumors

Lymphomatous tumors analogous to those of the eyelid and the orbit (p. 1653) may present as salmon-colored smooth masses in the conjunctiva (Fig. 1556). As with the lid and orbital lesions, they may range from obvious cancer to benign lymphoid hyperplasias.[43]

Cysts

Benign epithelial-lined inclusion cysts of the conjunctiva usually arise after accidental or surgical trauma or, rarely, de novo.

CORNEA

A major source of knowledge about corneal pathology comes from the study of corneal "buttons" submitted to the laboratory after corneal transplantation (keratoplasty). The most common diseases that account for keratoplasties are primary and secondary endothelial decompensation, fibrosis and vascularization (such as herpes simplex keratitis), keratoconus, and failed previous grafts.

Endothelial decompensation

When the endothelium of the cornea decompensates, it leads to chronic edema of the stroma and epithelium. Bullae of the epithelium break down, causing severe pain, and eventually there is diffuse scarring with reduced vision. When the process is primary (i.e., with no apparent antecedent factors), it is referred to as Fuch's dystrophy and occurs most frequently in females past 50 years of age. It is a bilateral process, although often asymmetrical.

When the endothelial decompensation occurs some time after intraocular surgery, especially after cataract extraction, it often is referred to clinically as "aphakic bullous keratopathy." The clinical appearance and the histopathologic appearance of these buttons is similar in both situations.

The histopathology is characterized by a paucity of endothelial cells, thickening of Descemet's membrane, and the formation of excrescences of Descemet's membrane, clinically referred to as guttata (Fig. 1557). If the process has been severe, changes in the epithelium occur, including edema of the basal cells, bullae formation, and pannus formation. A pannus is a fibrovascular ingrowth between the epithelium and Bowman's membrane.[47]

Fibrosis and vascularization

Many buttons from keratoplasty procedures will show a diffuse, nonspecific fibrosis and vascularization throughout the corneal stroma.

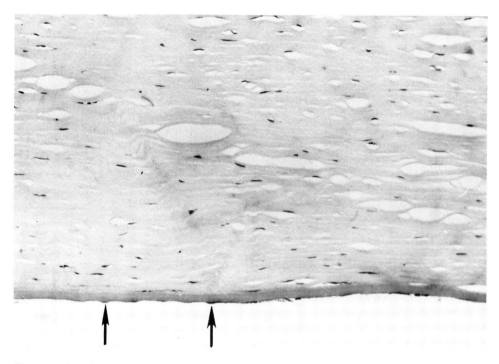

Fig. 1557 Endothelial decompensation. There is paucity of endothelial cells. Descemet's membrane is thickened, and there are excrescences along its posterior edge (arrows).

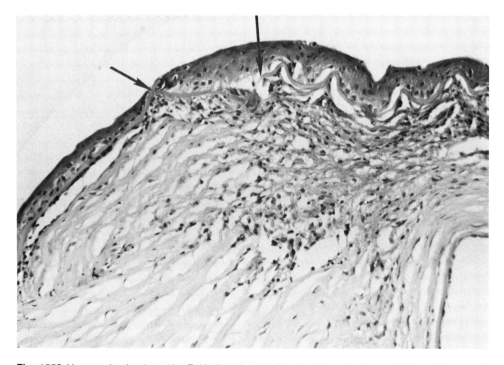

Fig. 1558 Herpes simplex keratitis. Epithelium is irregular, and there is fragmentation of Bowman's membrane (arrows). Chronic inflammatory cells infiltrate anterior stroma.

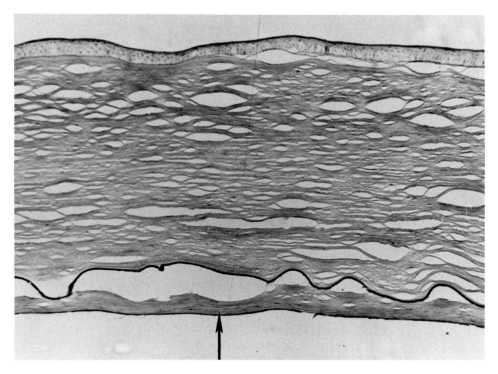

Fig. 1559 Regraft of corneal button. Note fibrous retrocorneal membrane posterior to Descemet's membrane (arrow).

Such a histopathologic picture would be seen with traumatic scars, chemical burns, or healed ulcerative keratitis secondary to infections. One particular infection that is common is herpes simplex keratitis, in which the histopathology is characterized by irregularity of the epithelium, patchy loss of Bowman's membrane, infiltration of the anterior stroma by lymphocytes and plasma cells, and diffuse fibrosis and vascularization of the stroma (Fig. 1558). In several cases, there is often a granulomatous reaction surrounding Descemet's membrane.[46] Inclusion bodies are only occasionally seen.

Keratoconus

Keratoconus is a congenital ectasia of the central cornea usually becoming manifest in the first decade of life. It tends to progress until fibrosis decreases the vision and necessitates corneal transplantation. Histopathologically, there are central thinning and fibrosis. Often the "button" will appear wrinkled on the slide, and this artifact is an instant clue to the pathologist that this is a case of keratoconus.

Failed previous grafts

For a variety of reasons, corneal grafts may become opaque and a second graft is done. The button from the second procedure will often show nonspecific changes such as fibrosis, vascularization, and inflammatory cell infiltration throughout the stroma. At the peripheral edges of the button, there are the full-thickness scars of the previous procedure. A fibrous retrocorneal membrane is present in about half the cases (Fig. 1559).

Other entities for which keratoplasties done

Other rarer entities for which keratoplasties are done include interstitial keratitis and the various hereditary dystrophies.

INTRAOCULAR TISSUES

Surgical pathology of the eye itself differs from most of the rest of surgical pathology for several important reasons.

In the first place, biopsies of intraocular tissues are rarely feasible. The important exceptions are the iris and the ciliary body. Lesions of the iris and/or ciliary body can be removed by iridectomy or iridocyclectomy. This is especially true for melanomas confined to these structures.

In the second place, most of the eyes reaching the surgical pathology laboratory are obtained as a result of enucleation. Usually the globe is intact but free of such accessory tissues as the extraocular muscles and orbital fat. Much less often, the eye is eviscerated, and only fragments of the intraocular tissues are submitted for microscopic study. In such cases, it is rarely possible to arrive at a satisfactory diagnosis and clinicopathologic correlation. Eyes that are enucleated or eviscerated usually have been diseased for a long period of time and have become blind. Severe pain and unsightliness are the common immediate reasons for removing the eye. In these cases it is the responsibility of the pathologist not merely to arrive at a definitive diagnosis but also to reconstruct the sequence of events that took place from the onset of ocular disease to the final stages that led to enucleation.

This brings us to another distinctive characteristic of ophthalmic pathology. Frequently, the initial pathologic process becomes completely obscured by the subsequent series of events. For example, the patient may first complain of visual disturbance produced by a cataract. The lens opacification progresses, and cataract extraction is performed. Defective wound healing follows, and surface epithelium grows down into the anterior chamber. This leads to secondary glaucoma for which one or more additional surgical procedures are performed. These, in turn, may be complicated by hemorrhage, infection, or retinal detachment. Finally, the eye may become shrunken (phthisical) and disfiguring. A period of several years to a decade or more usually is required for such a series of events to take place.

Intraocular neoplasms represent an exception to the generalization just given. Since only in the case of iris and small ciliary body tumors is it ordinarily possible to excise the neoplasm, the procedure usually followed is to recommend enucleation for other uveal and retinal neoplasms. The aim here is to arrive at a correct clinical diagnosis early, long before such secondary pathologic processes as cataract formation, massive retinal detachment, glaucoma, uveitis, or phthisis complicate the picture. Therefore, the pathologist often observes a much less confusing array of pathologic changes and has less difficulty making a diagnosis in eyes removed because of intraocular neoplasms than in other enucleated eyes. This, however, is not invariably the case, for if the tumor has been present and growing for a long period of time, it, too, may lead to a wide assortment of secondary processes that sometimes confuse the pathologist as well as the clinician.

Congenital and developmental malformations

Many congenital and developmental malformations of the eye are rarely seen by the surgical pathologist but are seen only at postmortem examination.[58] Congenital abnormalities typify the point made earlier—i.e., the initial pathologic process becomes completely obscured by the subsequent series of events occurring in that eye.

Congenital glaucoma

Congenital glaucoma is characterized by an elevation in the intraocular pressure due to a malformation of the tissues in the region of the anterior chamber angle. The precise nature of this malformation is still not clear, but there seems to be either an incomplete separation of the iris root from the trabeculae or the retention of an embryonic membrane, or both.

The increased intraocular pressure leads to retinal and optic nerve degeneration, corneal edema and scarring, and global enlargement (buphthalmos). Unilateral congenital glaucoma may occur in Recklinghausen's disease or in the Sturge-Weber syndrome.

When there is a more obvious architectural distortion of the iris and angle of the anterior chamber, it is referred to as the anterior chamber cleavage syndrome[56] or iridogoniodysgenesis. Depending upon the degree of angle malformation, other various designations are used (e.g., Rieger's syndrome and Axenfeld's syndrome). This group of malformations is also often associated with a developmental glaucoma.

Retrolental fibroplasia

Retrolental fibroplasia, also called the retinopathy of prematurity, is an acquired form of developmental disorder resulting from the unique sensitivity of retinal blood vessels of the premature retina to oxygen.[55]

Much of the retinal periphery of a baby born after only six or seven months of gestation is completely avascular. If such a premature in-

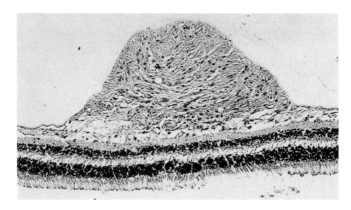

Fig. 1560 Tuberous sclerosis showing glial nodule or hamartoma projecting against vitreous body from nerve fiber layer of retina. (×90; AFIP 511046.)

fant is given high concentrations of oxygen, normal vascularization of the retinal periphery may be inhibited. Vasoconstriction and actual obliteration of the terminal vessels may follow prolonged oxygen therapy. Later, upon withdrawal of oxygen, pathologic neovascularization occurs. These newly formed vessels frequently invade the vitreous, leak serum or blood, and eventually lead to organization of the vitreous, retinal detachment, and blindness.

Phakoma

Phakomas are hamartomatous malformations often associated with extraocular lesions as a part of well-defined clinicopathologic syndromes.[50] These include Bourneville's syndrome (tuberous sclerosis), Recklinghausen's disease (neurofibromatosis), the Sturge-Weber syndrome (encephalotrigeminal angiomatosis), Lindau–von Hippel disease (angiogliomatosis), ataxia-telangiectasia, and Wyburn-Mason syndrome.

In tuberous sclerosis, the most characteristic intraocular lesions are glial plaques and nodules in the nerve fiber layer of the retina which clinically may simulate a retinoblastoma (Fig. 1560). Neurofibromas and plexiform neuromas in the eyelid and orbit and gliomas of the optic nerve are the usual lesions observed in neurofibromatosis.

Hemangioma of the choroid (Fig. 1518) is the most common intraocular lesion of the Sturge-Weber syndrome. Ipsilateral glaucoma is often associated with the Sturge-Weber syndrome or Recklinghausen's disease. Abnormally large tortuous arteries and veins leading to a retinal nodule composed of vascular, endothelial, and glial tissues are characteristic of Lindau–von Hippel disease. Vitreous disturbance and retinal detachment are common complications. In ataxia-telangiectasia there are telangiectatic conjunctival vessels, and in the Wyburn-Mason syndrome there are arteriovenous shunts of the retinal vessels.

Persistent hyperplastic primary vitreous

A congenital condition, persistent hyperplastic primary vitreous refers to the persistence and hyperplasia of the fibrovascular tunic of the lens and part of the hyaloid vascular system.[53] It is usually unilateral and occurs in a microphthalmic eye. Clinically, this anomaly is manifested by a white reflex behind the pupil (leukokoria). Varying degrees of fibrous tissue are seen behind the lens, and often there is a cataract. Differentiation from retinoblastoma is not so great a problem as in the past, but occasionally these eyes are enculeated because retinoblastoma cannot be ruled out.

Histologically, there is a dense fibrovascular retrolental mass, and the elongated ciliary processes are enmeshed in this tissue. Remnants of the hyaloid artery system are present, and the retina may appear normal or show evidence of retinal dysplasia (Figs. 1561 and 1562).

Retinal dysplasia

A congenital anomaly, retinal dysplasia may occur as part of the 13-15 trisomy syndrome or merely in a unilateral malformed eye not associated with other systemic anomalies.[49,52] An example of the latter situation would be in the case of persistent hyperplastic primary vitreous, as previously mentioned.

Dysplastic retina is characterized histologi-

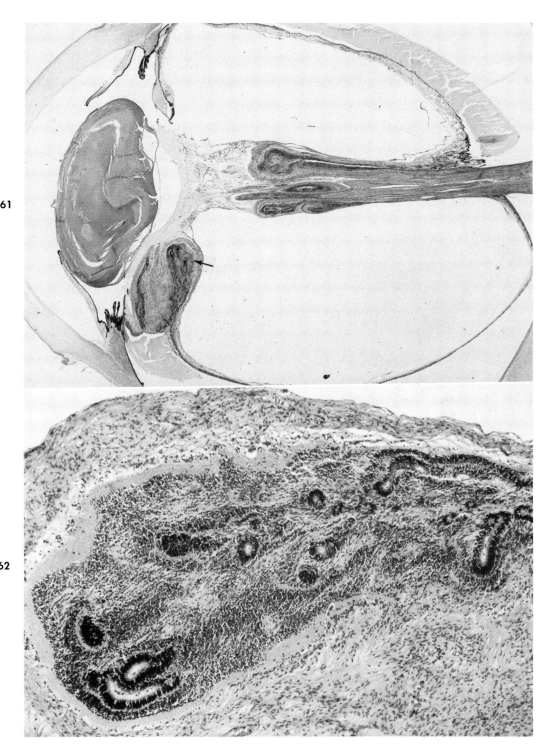

Fig. 1561 Persistent hyperplastic primary vitreous. Behind lens lies fibrovascular mass to which remnant of hyaloid system attaches. In some cases of persistent hyperplastic primary vitreous, there may be areas of retinal dysplasia (arrow). (×12; WU neg. 67-4230.)
Fig. 1562 Retinal dysplasia. Within retina are branching tubes composed of abortive elements of rod and cone layer. (×90; WU neg. 67-4229.)

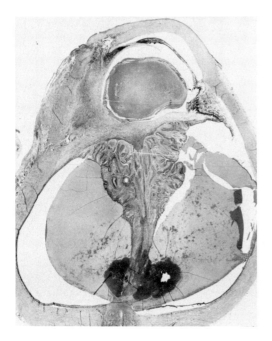

Fig. 1563 Penetrating wound of eye and multiple minute intraocular foreign bodies (palm splinters) led to formation of dense mass of inflammatory tissue in anterior segment on one side. Organization of vitreous has been complicated by retinal detachment. Blood clots are attached to stalk of detached retina near optic disc. (×4; AFIP 737587.)

cally by a series of straight branching tubes composed of abortive elements of the rod and cone layers (Fig. 1562), and it is believed that this represents disturbed differentiation of neural ectoderm.

Other congenital entities

Other congenital entities that are only rarely seen by the surgical pathologist include the rubella syndrome,[48,57] Lowe's syndrome, Fabry's syndrome,[51] and aniridia, in which the nonfamilial case may be associated with Wilms' tumor.[54]

Trauma

Trauma to the globe can be accidental or surgical. The complications that may ensue after severe trauma may eventually lead to blindness and pain, necessitating enucleation. In fact, ocular trauma is the most common reason for eyes reaching the ophthalmic pathology laboratory of a general hospital. Often there are instances in which the surgical pathologist will be expected to identify tissue that has been removed from an eye that is being sutured

following a severe laceration. What the ophthalmic surgeon wants to know is whether any retina is extruded through the wound. If so, this information may influence further management of the case.

Although some eyes are so extensively damaged that immediate removal is necessary, most of the injured eyes are removed at varying intervals because of secondary changes such as organization of hemorrhage, glaucoma, retinal detachment, infections, inflammation, or complete atrophy (phthisis bulbi) (Fig. 1563).

Histopathologic diagnosis is usually not a problem, but a search should be made for retained intraocular foreign bodies such as metal, vegetation, and cilia. Retained intraocular iron and copper may produce siderosis and chalcosis, respectively.

Besides the aforementioned secondary changes (e.g., diffuse fibrosis, secondary glaucoma, inflammation, etc.), certain specific complications associated with trauma include sympathetic ophthalmia, phacoanaphylactic endophthalmitis, postcontusion angle deformity, fibrous downgrowth, and epithelial downgrowth. These will be considered subsequently under other headings.

Inflammation

Inflammation of the eye, as elsewhere, may be either acute or chronic, granulomatous or nongranulomatous.

Acute inflammation

Acute intraocular inflammation is often infectious in origin. The causative organism is usually a bacterium or fungus and is generally introduced through a perforating wound (Fig. 1564). Occasionally, however, the infection is hematogenous. There have been reports of endogenous fungous endophthalmitis,[60,62] and metastatic endophthalmitis also has been reported after injection of addictive drugs.[64]

Initially, there is a massive purulent reaction in the anterior and vitreous chambers, and the process is called endophthalmitis. As the infection spreads, other intraocular tissues, such as the retina, uvea, and eventually the cornea and sclera, may become involved. At this stage, the term panophthalmitis is applicable. Before the advent of antibiotic therapy, eyes affected by severe panophthalmitis were frequently eviscerated or enucleated early. Today the infection often can be controlled, but subsequent organization of the exudate leads to

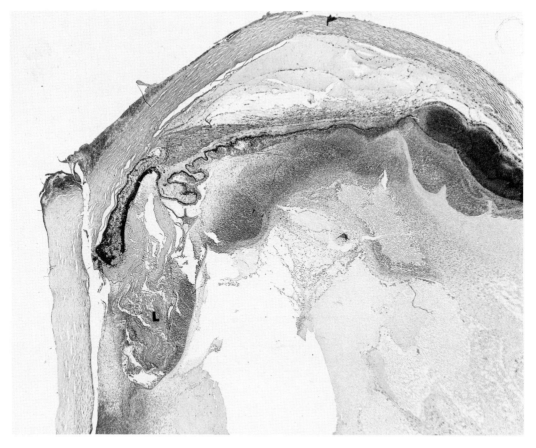

Fig. 1564 Endophthalmitis showing infiltration of all intraocular structures by acute inflammatory cells. Lens, **L,** is necrotic. Organism presumably gained entrance through corneal wound. (×15; WU neg. 67-4233.)

phthisis bulbi (p. 1676). A cause of noninfectious endophthalmitis or panophthalmitis that is not unusual is massive necrosis of a uveal malignant melanoma or a metastatic carcinoma.[61]

Chronic nongranulomatous inflammation

In chronic nongranulomatous inflammation of the eye, the uveal tract is primarily involved. In anterior uveitis (iridocyclitis), the tissues are typically infiltrated by plasma cells in a rather diffuse fashion (Fig. 1565), but occasionally we see nodular lymphocytic infiltrates. In posterior uveitis (choroiditis) the round cell infiltration also may be diffuse, but frequently it is focal or scattered as multiple discrete lesions. In choroiditis the overlying retina is usually involved by spread of the inflammatory reaction—hence the term chorioretinitis. In choroiditis, even if prolonged, enucleation is

not often necessary, for the eyes do not become painful. However, with recurrent iridocyclitis, the inflammatory reaction often produces adhesions between the iris and the cornea (anterior synechiae) (Fig. 1566) or between the iris and the lens (posterior synechiae) (Fig. 1567), and secondary glaucoma results. If this condition is intractable, enucleation is almost inevitable. Often, the process is of such a long-term nature that when the eye is enucleated, all that is recognized is the massive scarring that is found in phthisis bulbi due to any cause.

The etiology and pathogenesis of nongranulomatous uveitis can rarely be ascertained clinically or pathologically. Occasionally, an entity presents a characteristic picture such as is seen in herpes zoster ophthalmicus in which there is a chronic inflammatory cell infiltration around the posterior ciliary nerves and vessels.[63] Behçet's disease produces an obliterative vasculitis of the retinal vessels.

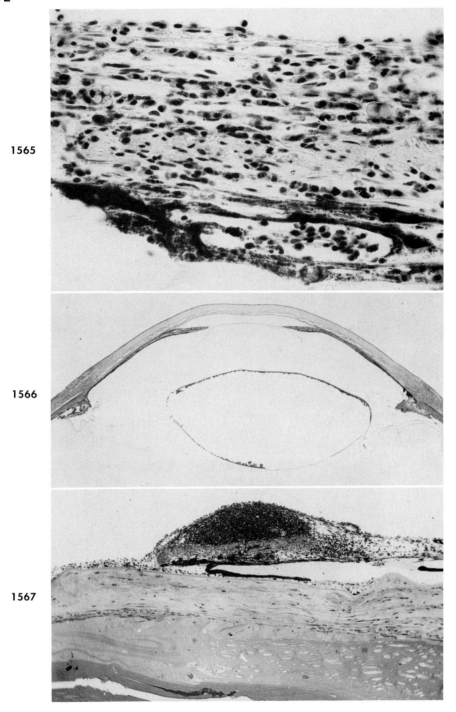

Fig. 1565 Nongranulomatous iritis in which atrophic iris is diffusely infiltrated by plasma cells and several Russell bodies are present. Irregular degenerative and proliferative changes may be observed in pigment epithelium. (×360; AFIP 698722.)

Fig. 1566 Same lesion illustrated in Fig. 1565 showing chronically inflamed iris almost completely adherent to cornea and anterior chamber virtually obliterated. (×8).

Fig. 1567 Nongranulomatous iritis with posterior synechiae. Iris is firmly attached to lens, which reveals widespread degeneration of its cortex and fibrous metaplasia of its subcapsular epithelium. (×25; AFIP 184111.)

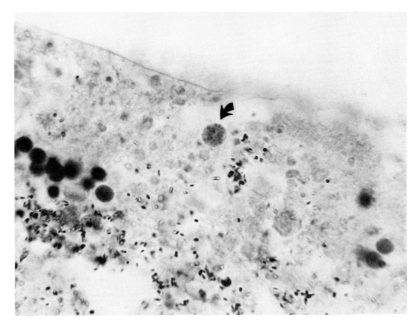

Fig. 1568 Encysting proliferative forms (arrow) of *Toxoplasma gondii* found in necrotic retina. Small particles are pigment granules from necrotic retinal pigment epithelium, whereas larger round structures represent pyknotic retinal nuclei. (×1000; AFIP 754058.)

Granulomatous inflammation

Granulomatous inflammation may be the result of a specific infection such as toxoplasmosis, tuberculosis, syphilis, nematodiasis, and cytomegalic inclusion disease. Also associated with granulomatous reactions are such entities as sarcoidosis and the collagen diseases. It should be kept in mind, however, that as with the nongranulomatous cases, the etiology often cannot be ascertained.

The inflammatory process in granulomatous uveitis may be diffuse, or there is a more localized area of destruction in which the causative agent or otherwise diagnostic lesion will be found.

The term granulomatous uveitis is misleading, for often the most diagnostic lesions are not found in the iris, ciliary body, or choroid but rather in the retina, vitreous, or sclera. The diagnostic lesions of toxoplasmosis are found in the retina, those of nematodiasis in the vitreous or retina, and those of the rheumatoid group in the sclera between the limbus and the equator.

Toxoplasmosis

Although ocular toxoplasmosis is an important entity, it actually is quite rare to receive such globes in the pathology laboratory. The histopathology is characterized by a focal area of coagulative necrosis of the retina surrounded by a granulomatous inflammation in the adjacent choroid and sclera. Within the area of necrotic retina, cysts of *Toxoplasma gondii* can be found[66] (Fig. 1568).

Nematodiasis

Nematodiasis is a broad term encompassing a variety of parasitic diseases. The one form of ocular nematodiasis that has been found with considerable frequency in the United States and Great Britain is a type of visceral larva migrans, probably produced in most cases by wandering larvae of *Toxocara canis*. This is principally an infection of children between the ages of 3 and 14 years.[67]

Almost without exception, those children who have had ocular infection have not had clinical evidence of systemic visceral larva migrans, and those who have had the systemic form have not had ocular lesions. Typically, a single migrating larva finds its way, hematogenously, into the eye and comes to rest in the vitreous or on the inner surface of the retina (Fig. 1569).

A pronounced infiltration by acute and chronic inflammatory cells, often with intense eosinophilia, is observed in these tissues.

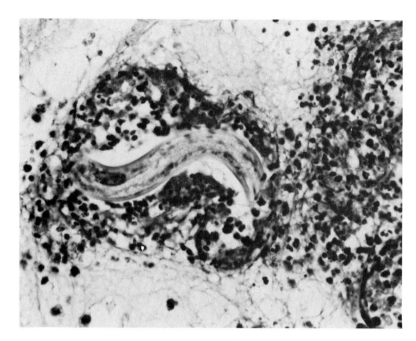

Fig. 1569 Nematode larva, probably *Toxocara canis,* surrounded by inflammatory cells in vitreous body. (×220; AFIP 298563.)

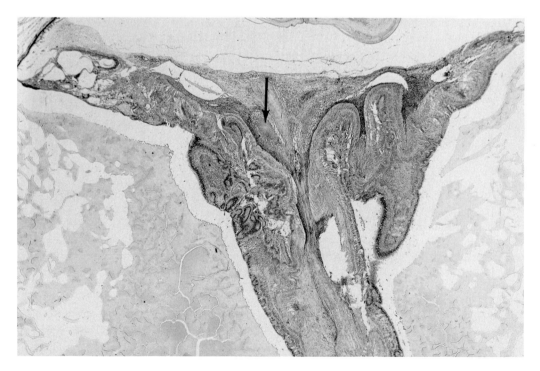

Fig. 1570 Nematode endophthalmitis in which inflammatory reaction in vitreous has led to retinal detachment. Parasite was found in area of necrosis (arrow). (×15; WU neg. 67-4234.)

Eventually, the inflammatory reaction in the vitreous leads to organization and contracture of this structure with consequent detachment of the retina (Fig. 1570). This leads to leukokoria, and the eye is enucleated because retinoblastoma cannot be ruled out.

As the nematode larvae die, they often stimulate the formation of a typical granulomatous inflammatory reaction about them. It is usually necessary to make serial sections to find these minute granulomas. The typical inflammatory reaction with intense eosinophilia observed in the vitreous is presumptive evidence of nematodiasis.[65]

Posttraumatic uveitis

Following penetrating injury of the eye, the development of a granulomatous uveitis always causes great concern because of the possibility of sympathetic uveitis, a dreaded disease in which injury to one eye gives rise to severe inflammation that sometimes progresses to blindness in the uninjured eye as well as in the injured eye. Fortunately, sympathetic uveitis is extremely rare today. Other causes of posttraumatic granulomatous inflammation are lens-induced endophthalmitis (phacoanaphylaxis), foreign bodies, and blood in the vitreous.

Sympathetic uveitis

Sympathetic uveitis is probably the best example of a pure granulomatous uveitis, for the significant lesion in this disease is confined to the uveal tissues. Typically, the process involves the entire uveal tract. There may, of course, be associated inflammatory lesions in other tissues due to the original trauma, the presence of foreign bodies, etc., but the reaction of sympathetic uveitis itself is purely uveal.

There is a dense, diffuse infiltration of the choroid by lymphocytes (Fig. 1571), and often the ciliary body and iris are similarly involved. Superimposed upon this lymphocytic infiltrate are small, irregular, patchy accumulations of large, pale-staining epithelioid cells which, upon high magnification, will often be found to contain finely dispersed melanin granules (Fig. 1572). Polymorphonuclear leukocytes are characteristically lacking, plasma cells are rare, but eosinophils are often included in moderate numbers.

The reaction involves the outer and middle coats of the choroid, extending into the scleral canals along ciliary vessels and nerves, sometimes to the episcleral surface. The choriocapillaris, on the other hand, is typically uninvolved. Clusters of epithelioid cells between Bruch's

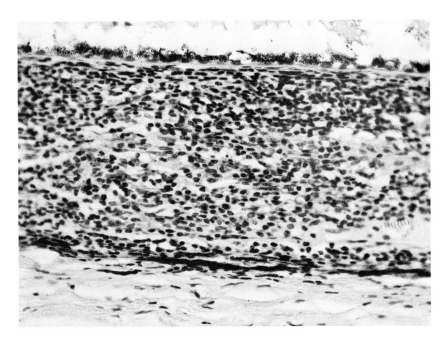

Fig. 1571 Sympathetic uveitis. Uveal tissues are diffusely infiltrated by lymphocytes, and there are small, irregular collections of pale-staining epithelioid cells. (×300; AFIP 731769.)

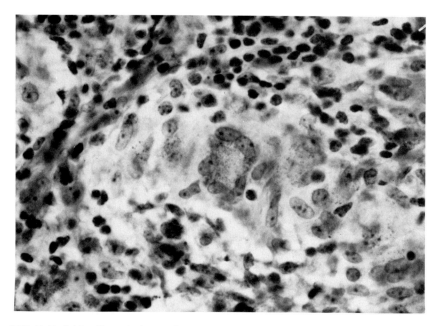

Fig. 1572 Epithelioid cells and giant cells containing finely dispersed uveal pigment granules that are characteristically present in sympathetic uveitis. (×655; AFIP 37381; from Friedenwald JS, Wilder HC, Maumenee AE, Sanders TE, Keyes JEL, Hogan MJ, Owens WC, Owens EU: Ophthalmic pathology: an atlas and textbook. Philadelphia, 1952, W. B. Saunders Co.)

membrane and the retinal pigment epithelium, referred to as Dalen-Fuchs nodules, are often seen.

Phacoanaphylaxis

Phacoanaphylactic endophthalmitis usually follows penetrating injury to the lens, but a few cases have been observed following spontaneous rupture of a swollen cataractous lens. It is characterized by a granulomatous inflammatory reaction centered about an area of lens perforation. The process is believed to be the result of acquired hypersensitivity to lens protein.[69]

A typical zonal pattern of inflammatory reaction is observed in most cases (Fig. 1573, A). In the area in which the lens capsule is broken, there is a massive invasion of the lens by inflammatory cells. Centrally and immediately surrounding individual lens fibers are polymorphonuclear leukocytes. Peripheral to this is a wall of epithelioid and giant cells about which is a broader, more diffuse zone of granulation tissue and round cell infiltration (Fig. 1573, B). The iris reveals a variable degree of plasma cell infiltration, and posterior synechiae are commonly formed.

Ordinarily, the posterior uveal tract is not inflamed, but characteristically there is a perivasculitis of the retinal vessels. In a considerable number of cases, however, phacoanaphylactic endophthalmitis and sympathetic uveitis are coexistent.[68]

Degeneration

Degenerative changes are usually the result of other primary processes such as trauma or inflammation. The most advanced stage of ocular degeneration in which all tissues are involved is called phthisis bulbi.

Phthisis bulbi

Phthisis bulbi represents the final stage of ocular degeneration in which the production of aqueous humor is so markedly reduced that the intraocular pressure falls (hypotony) and the globe shrinks (Fig. 1574).

The causes of phthisis bulbi are myriad, but most phthisical eyes reaching the surgical pathology laboratory have been injured, either accidentally or as a result of surgical procedures.

Phthisical eyes are enucleated for several reasons. Many are enucleated because they are disfiguring and others because they become irritable because of periodic hemorrhages or bouts

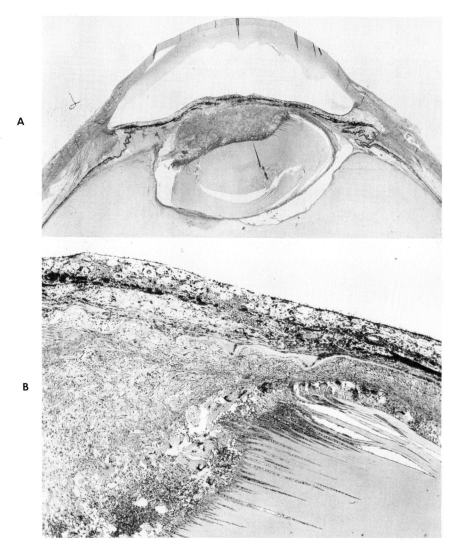

Fig. 1573 A, Phacoanaphylactic endophthalmitis resulting from penetrating wound that ruptured capsule of anterior lens. Dense infiltrate of acute and chronic inflammatory cells is present in area of lens damage. **B,** Higher magnification of lesion illustrated in **A.** Polymorphonuclear leukocytes are present in and about disintegrating lens fibers. Peripheral to them is wall of macrophages, epithelioid cells, and giant cells, and about entire lesion there is broad zone of granulation tissue. (**A,** ×10; AFIP 339621; **B,** ×53.)

of uveitis. Some are enucleated for prophylactic reasons—the fear of sympathetic uveitis or of malignant melanoma, either of which may develop long after the eye has become blind and phthisical.

All tissues are affected to varying degrees in phthisis bulbi, and the degree of shrinkage is also variable. The eye may be soft and spongy or stony hard due to calcification and ossification. Typically, the media are opaque. Corneal scars, exudates in the anterior and

posterior chambers, and advanced cataract formation prevent visualization of the inner eye. The vitreous is usually destroyed, and the retina is completely detached. Extensive areas of osseous metaplasia frequently are observed along the inner surface of the choroid posteriorly. The uvea is often edematous, and pools of serous exudate may separate it from the wrinkled sclera.

In phthisis bulbi that has followed extensive endophthalmitis or panophthalmitis, the

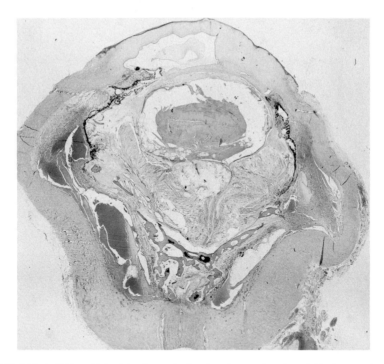

Fig. 1574 Phthisis bulbi in which globe is markedly shrunken, sclera is wrinkled, and all intraocular tissues reveal severe degenerative changes, including foci of ossification. (×7½; AFIP 276925.)

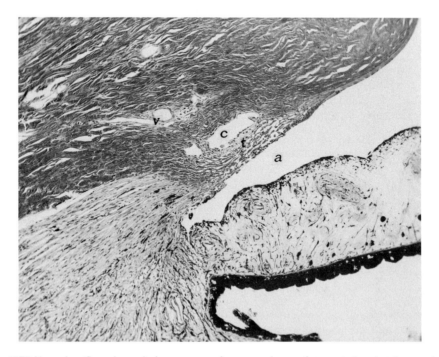

Fig. 1575 Normal outflow channels for passage of aqueous humor from anterior chamber angle, **a,** include corneoscleral trabecula, **t,** Schlemm's canal, **c,** and intrascleral plexus of veins, **v.** (Verhoeff–van Gieson; ×70; AFIP 630832.)

various intraocular tissues often are so necrotic and replaced by scar tissue that most of the internal architecture of the eye is effaced.

Glaucoma

Glaucoma is conveniently placed here, since it represents another condition of diverse etiology characterized by widespread degeneration of ocular tissues. The essential feature of the glaucomas is an unphysiologic state of increased intraocular pressure, due in almost all cases to impaired outflow of aqueous humor. Aqueous humor is produced by the ciliary processes and discharged into the posterior chamber. It flows forward between the lens and the iris, through the pupil, into the anterior chamber. Aqueous humor leaves the anterior chamber via the trabecular meshwork, which is present in the deep layers of the peripheral cornea, just in front of the anterior chamber angle (Fig. 1575). After passing through the trabecula, aqueous humor enters Schlemm's canal and leaves the eye via the plexus of intrascleral and episcleral veins along the corneoscleral limbus. When the impaired aqueous drainage follows some known or suspected antecedent disease, we speak of secondary glaucoma. Here the surgical pathologist may play an important role in determining the antecedent disease.

Primary glaucoma

The primary glaucomas are not associated with antecedent disease but are either the "chronic simple" type or the "angle-closure" type. In the former, there are certain degenerative changes in the trabecular meshwork and the connective tissues about Schlemm's canal. The exact nature of these changes remain obscure. These eyes seldom reach the pathology laboratory since the process is usually insidious and often does not cause enough pain to necessitate enucleation.

Acute and chronic angle-closure glaucoma is due to anatomic and physiologic peculiarities of the tissues and the spaces of the anterior chamber that predispose to blockage of the outflow channels by the iris root. Chronic attacks of angle-closure glaucoma may lead to extensive adhesions of the iris root to the tra-

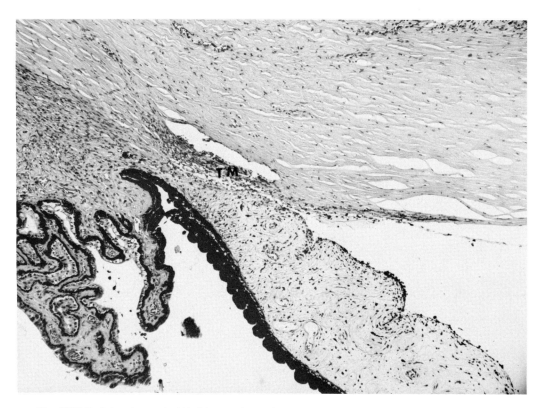

Fig. 1576 Peripheral aspect of iris lying against trabecular meshwork, **TM,** producing peripheral anterior synechia and blocking outflow of aqueous. (×90; WU neg. 67-4224.)

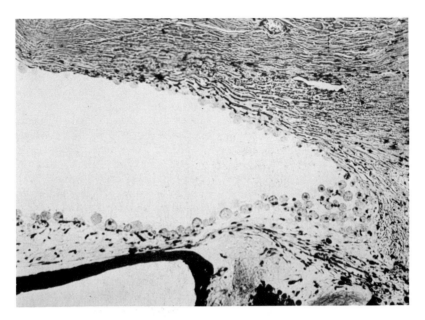

Fig. 1577 Outflow channels blocked by macrophages in anterior chamber in phacolytic glaucoma (glaucoma secondary to lysis and escape of lens protein into aqueous humor). (×75; AFIP 609920; from Flocks M, Littwin CS, Zimmerman LE: Phacolytic glaucoma. Clinicopathologic study of 138 cases of glaucoma associated with hypermature cataract. Arch Ophthalmol **54:**37-45, 1955; copyright 1955, American Medical Association.)

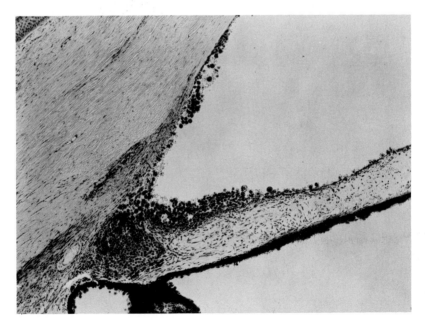

Fig. 1578 Anterior chamber angle and outflow channels filled with deeply pigmented cells dispersed into aqueous humor from malignant melanoma of iris. (×50; AFIP 176188.)

becular meshwork (peripheral anterior synechia, Fig. 1576), and if this glaucoma becomes intractable, it may necessitate enucleation because of pain.[72]

Secondary glaucoma

Secondary glaucoma may be a complication of numerous primary processes, including trauma, inflammation, neoplasia, and malformation. The sites of obstruction to the outflow of aqueous humor are numerous, but the most vulnerable areas are the pupil and the angle of the anterior chamber. Formation of pupillary membranes as a result of organization of hemorrhages and exudates or the development of extensive adhesions between the iris and the lens (posterior synechiae) as a consequence of iritis (Fig. 1567) are the usual mechanisms leading to pupillary obstruction.

The outflow channels in the anterior chamber angle may become obstructed by particulate matter or by the formation of extensive adhesions between the root of the iris and the peripheral cornea (peripheral anterior synechiae) (Fig. 1576). Particulate matter clogging the passages between the anterior chamber and Schlemm's canal is usually cellular—red blood cells after massive hemorrhage into the anterior chamber,[70] leukocytes in certain types of uveitis[71] (Fig. 1577), tumor cells, particularly with diffuse melanomas of the iris (Fig. 1578). Following accidental trauma or surgery, conjunctival and/or corneal epithelium may grow between the wound edges and eventually line the anterior chamber and iris, thus blocking the outflow of aqueous (clinically referred to as "epithelial downgrowth") (Fig. 1579). Fibrous downgrowth is the extension of dense fibrous tissue from the cornea into the anterior chamber through a gap in the posterior aspect of a corneal wound.

One of the common causes of secondary glaucoma encountered by the ophthalmic pathologist is the development of a neovascular membrane on the surface of the iris. This membrane, known as rubeosis iridis, is eventually associated with some degree of peripheral anterior synechia, thus causing blockage of the outflow channels (Fig. 1580).

Rubeosis iridis can occur following several different conditions. It occurs most commonly in diabetes or following occlusion of the central retinal artery or vein. Other conditions associated with rubeosis include carotid artery occlusion, long-standing retinal detachment, chronic uveitis, and intraocular neoplasms.

Damage to the outflow channels may occur as a result of blunt trauma to the eye and give

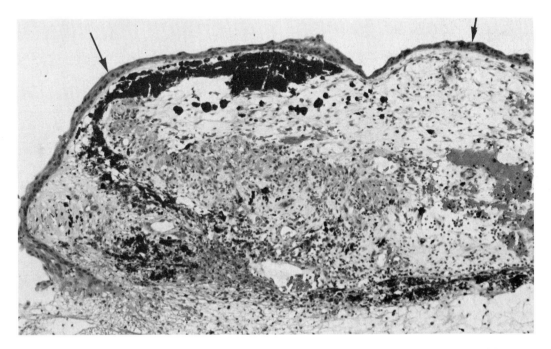

Fig. 1579 In this case of postcataract extraction, layer of epithelium has grown down wound into anterior chamber to lie on surface of iris (arrows). (×100; WU neg. 72-3172.)

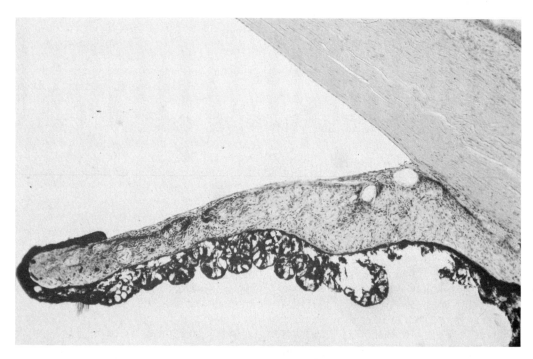

Fig. 1580 Rubeosis iridis in diabetes. Angle of anterior chamber is occluded by peripheral anterior synechia, and fibrovascular membrane (rubeosis iridis) covers anterior surface of iris. Contraction of this membrane has pulled pigment epithelium anteriorly to produce "ectropion uvea." There is marked diabetic vacuolization of pigment epithelial cells. (×90; WU neg. 67-4225.)

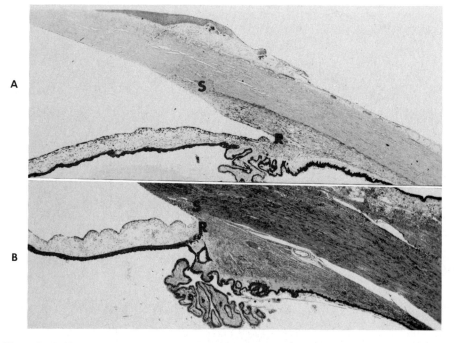

Fig. 1581 A, Recession of angle of anterior chamber. **B,** Normal angle. In **A,** iris root, **R,** is retrodisplaced with reference to scleral spur, **S,** and contour of atrophic ciliary body is fusiform instead of normal wedge shape. (**A** and **B,** ×21; AFIP 58-7578.)

rise to a chronic glaucoma. This situation is often associated with a recession of the anterior chamber angle. Histologically, the iris root insertion appears retrodisplaced, and there is atrophy of the ciliary body (Fig. 1581).

Regardless of the type and cause of glau-coma, certain degenerative changes are typi-cally produced after periods of variable dura-tion. When glaucoma begins in childhood, the tissues tend to stretch, and the globe may be-come greatly enlarged (buphthalmos). When its onset is in adult life, however, the tissues tend

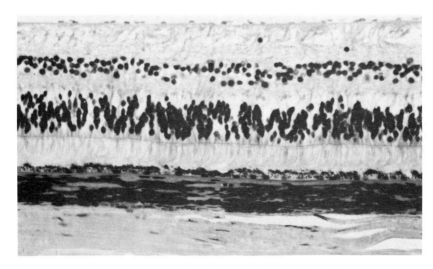

Fig. 1582 Retina in chronic glaucoma revealing widespread loss of ganglion cells and nerve fibers and reduction of cells in inner nuclear layer but relatively well-preserved visual cells. (×230; AFIP 49729; from Friedenwald JS, Wilder HC, Maumenee AE, Sanders TE, Keyes JEL, Hogan MJ, Owens WC, Owens EU: Ophthalmic pathology: an atlas and textbook. Philadelphia, 1952, W. B. Saunders Co.)

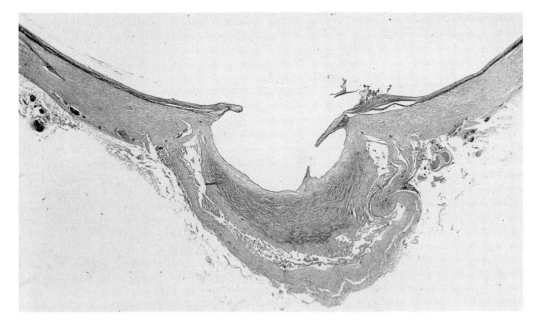

Fig. 1583 Deep excavation (cupping) of optic disc and severe atrophy of optic nerve, which are im-portant complications of chronic glaucoma. (×12; WU neg. 67-4235.)

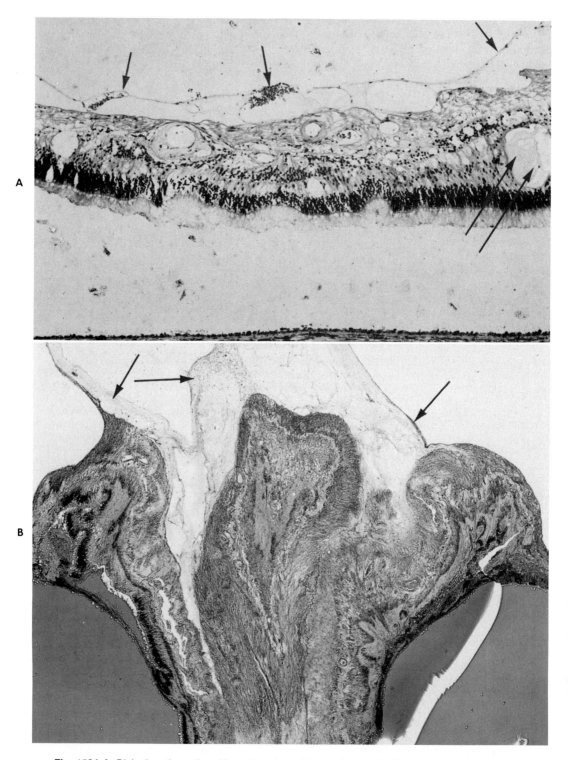

Fig. 1584 A, Diabetic retinopathy with scattered exudates in deep retinal layers (double arrows) and early neovascularization extending from inner surface of retina into vitreous (single arrows). **B,** Diabetic proliferative retinopathy (arrows) has caused complete retinal detachment. (**A,** ×90; WU neg. 72-3170; **B,** ×34; WU neg. 72-3171.)

to resist stretching, and normal ocular dimensions are maintained.

The elevated intraocular pressure typically affects the inner retinal layers to a much more pronounced degree than it does the outer layers. A common observation is the presence of rather well-preserved rods and cones and an intact outer nuclear layer when virtually all ganglion cells have disappeared and the nerve fiber and inner nuclear layers have become reduced to one-half or one-third their normal thickness (Fig. 1582).

Degeneration of nerve fibers is especially noteworthy in the region of the optic disc. This leads to excavation or cupping of the nerve head, posterior bowing of the lamina cribrosa, and severe atrophy of the optic nerve (Fig. 1583). Often, discrete areas of scleral ectasia are observed, particularly in the equatorial regions. These are lined by uveal tissue and therefore have a bluish color—hence the name staphyloma (grapelike swelling).

Diabetes

Ocular diabetes is rapidly becoming one of the most common causes of blindness in western society. Diabetes can cause a variety of pathologic conditions within the eye. These conditions may lead to complete blindness and, if associated with pain, the eyes often do reach the pathology laboratory.[74]

The retina often shows scattered hemorrhages and exudates, and there may be the development of neovascular tissue that grows from the inner surface of the retina into the vitreous (Fig. 1584, *A*). This condition, known as proliferative retinopathy, can cause a retinal detachment that usually does not respond well to surgical treatment (Fig. 1584, *B*).

As previously mentioned, secondary glaucoma may result from the development of diabetic rubeosis iridis with peripheral anterior synechia (Fig. 1580). Many eyes from diabetic patients will also manifest vacuolization of the iris pigment epithelium. These vacuoles have been demonstrated to contain glycogen (Fig. 1580) and are related to the level of the blood sugar at the time of enucleation similar to Armanni-Ebstein nephropathy.[73]

Tumors and pseudotumors

Tumors of the intraocular tissues are neither numerous in type nor frequent in occurrence. From a practical standpoint, discussion may be limited to malignant melanomas, conditions confused with malignant melanomas of the uvea, retinoblastomas, conditions confused with retinoblastoma, and metastatic carcinomas.

Malignant melanoma

Melanomas arising from the pigmented or potentially pigment-producing cells of the uvea are the most frequent primary intraocular neoplasms in adults. The tumor arises from any point in the uveal tract, with the choroid and ciliary body being more frequent than the iris. Melanoma of the iris presents as an elevated mass with varying degrees of pigmentation and often with distortion of the pupil and the pres-

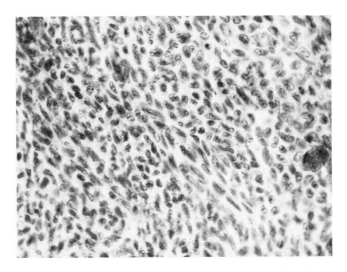

Fig. 1585 Spindle A type of melanoma cells. (×510; AFIP 49801.)

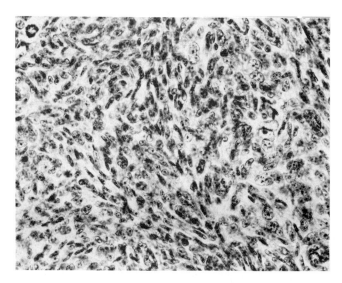

Fig. 1586 Spindle B type of melanoma cells that are larger and more pleomorphic than spindle A cells. Most of nuclei contain prominent nucleoli. (×305; AFIP 232296.)

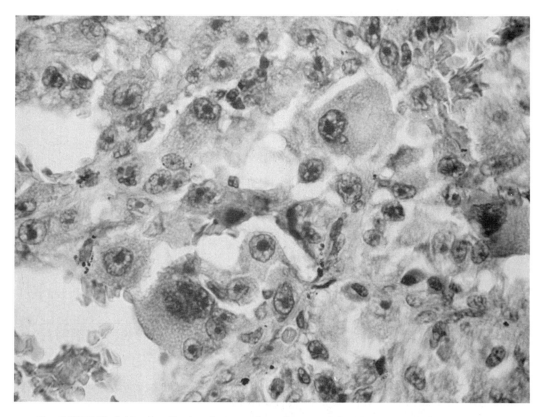

Fig. 1587 Epithelioid cells with abundant cytoplasm, large nuclei, and extremely prominent nucleoli. (×600; WU neg. 69-7517; from del Regato JA, Spjut HJ: Ackerman and del Regato's Cancer, ed. 5. St. Louis, 1977, The C. V. Mosby Co.)

ence of prominent vessels on the tumor (Fig. 1595). The choroidal melanoma also may vary in pigmentation but characteristically is an irregular, slate-gray, solid, subretinal tumor producing an overlying retinal detachment and decreased vision.

An extensive study of ocular melanomas and nevi has shown that most malignant melanomas of the uveal tract probably develop from pre-existing nevi.[92-94] The Callender classification[76,88] based on the cytologic characteristics of these tumors was used for many years to determine prognostic significance. Recently, that classification has been slightly modified.[86] Three main cell types are recognized: spindle A, spindle B, and epithelioid. From their combinations and patterns, various tumor types are defined.

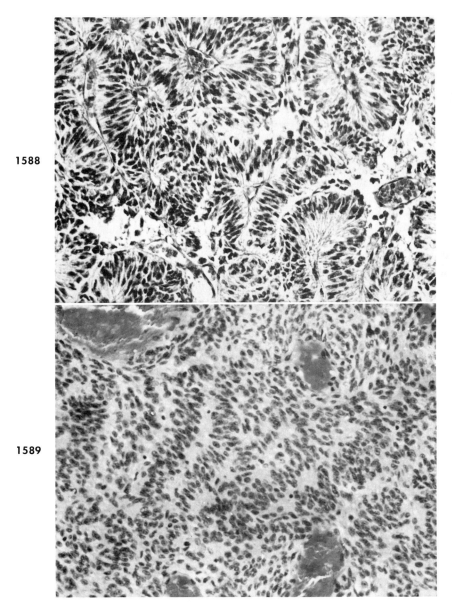

Fig. 1588 Fascicular type of melanoma composed of spindle cells arranged about dilated capillaries. (×250; AFIP 231963.)

Fig. 1589 Fascicular type of melanoma in which spindle-shaped cells are arranged with their nuclei in parallel rows. (×230; AFIP 48427.)

Spindle A cells are rather slender, very benign-appearing spindle-shaped cells that have relatively small fusiform nuclei and no nucleoli (Fig. 1585). Frequently, the chromatin is arranged in a linear fashion along the central axis of the nucleus.

Spindle B cells are larger and more pleomorphic, merging on the one hand with spindle A cells and on the other with epithelioid cells.

Typically, they possess large ovoid nuclei containing prominent nucleoli (Fig. 1586). Mitotic activity may be more marked. Spindle cells (A and B) tend to be quite cohesive.

Epithelioid cells are still larger and more irregular (Fig. 1587). They have an abundance of cytoplasm and may be truly gigantic. Multinucleated forms are not unusual. The nuclei are large, and their nucleoli often are striking-

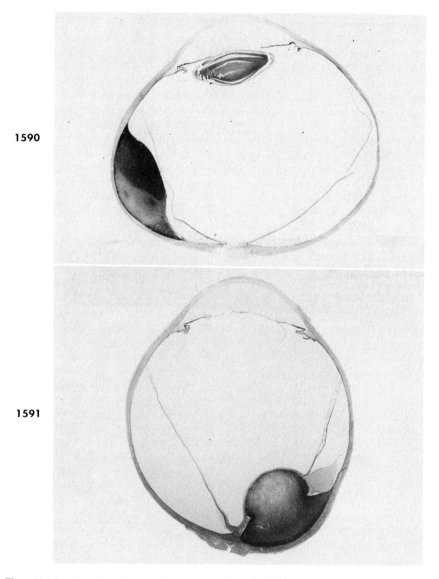

1590

1591

Fig. 1590 Malignant melanoma of choroid that has not broken through Bruch's membrane but has elevated retina. Most of retinal separation observed in this section is artifactitious. (×3; AFIP 79372; from Friedenwald JS, Wilder HC, Maumenee AE, Sanders TE, Keyes JEL, Hogan MJ, Owens WC, Owens EU: Ophthalmic pathology: an atlas and textbook. Philadelphia, 1952, W. B. Saunders Co.)
Fig. 1591 Malignant melanoma of choroid which, by erupting through Bruch's membrane, has formed mushroom-shaped subretinal mass. (×3; AFIP 289600.)

ly prominent. In some tumors, many bizarre nuclei may be seen. Epithelioid cells are characteristically less cohesive than the spindle cells.

As might be anticipated from the cytologic characteristics of these different types of melanomatous tumors, the spindle A type is essentially a benign neoplasm, whereas the epithelioid tumors are much more prone to metastasize. In fact, recent retrospective evidence has shown there were no deaths associated with pure spindle A tumors, and this should now be considered a nevus.[86]

It is rather unusual for these tumors to be composed of a single cell type. A mixture of spindle A and B cells or a mixture of spindle and epithelioid cells is very common. Certain of the spindle cell tumors present a fascicular pattern due to the palisading of nuclei (Figs. 1588 and 1589). The cell type is still one of the most important criteria for prognosis, and, in general, predictions concerning prognosis can be remembered as follows: Roughly two-thirds to three-fourths of patients with spindle cell melanomas (i.e., spindle A and spindle B or pure spindle B) will still be alive in five years, whereas roughly two-thirds to three-fourths of patients with pure epithelioid melanomas will be dead of their tumor in five years. A patient with a mixed cell melanoma (i.e., spindle plus epithelioid) has roughly a fifty-fifty chance of surviving five years.

Besides cell type, the other most important

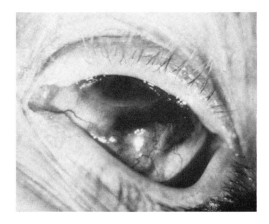

Fig. 1592 Malignant melanoma of choroid breaking through sclera and presenting under conjunctiva. (WU neg. 69-2213; from del Regato JA, Spjut HJ: Ackerman and del Regato's Cancer, ed. 5. St. Louis, 1977, The C. V. Mosby Co.; courtesy Registry of Ophthalmic Pathology, Armed Forces Institute of Pathology.)

criterion for predicting prognosis is size of the tumor, with larger tumors naturally having a worse prognosis than smaller ones.[80] Furthermore, the larger ones tend to be epithelioid.

Other criteria that worsen the prognosis include necrosis of the tumor and extraocular extension. In the past, the amount of pigmentation of the tumor and the amount of reticulum were thought to influence prognosis, but these latter criteria are no longer believed to be as reliable as cell type, size, and extraocular extension.

Another extremely important fact concerning the prognosis of uveal tumors is the very benign behavior of almost all neoplasms of the iris. This is especially true of those iris tumors that are sufficiently small and localized to be excisable by iridectomy or iridocyclectomy.[75,82,95]

Choroidal melanomas, regardless of their cytologic characteristics, tend to grow inward as discoid, globular, or mushroom-shaped masses, first elevating and then detaching the retina (Figs. 1590 and 1591). Less commonly, they spread diffusely and extend out along scleral canals into the orbit[81] (Figs. 1592 to 1594). Visual disturbance due to retinal detachment is therefore a much more frequent presenting complaint than is the formation of an orbital tumor. Not infrequently the patient remains asymptomatic until the tumor has grown sufficiently to become necrotic and produce such complications as endophthalmitis, massive intraocular hemorrhage, and/or secondary glaucoma.

At times, malignant melanomas of the posterior uvea are not discovered until the enucleated eye is examined in the laboratory. Iris tumors are much more often recognized early, for they can be seen by the patient and his family long before other symptoms appear (Figs. 1595 and 1596).

It should be remembered that all the aforementioned data is based on globes that have been enucleated. A recent reappraisal of survival data on patients with uveal melanomas has led to the impression that the mortality rate before enucleation is low, estimated at 1% per year, and this mortality rate rises abruptly following enucleation, reaching a peak of 8% during the second year after enucleation.

The provocative point, therefore, that has been raised is that enucleation as performed in the past may have for some patients an adverse rather than a beneficial effect with respect

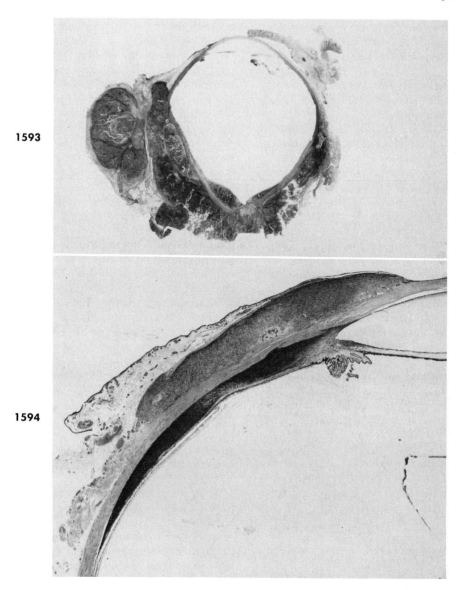

Fig. 1593 Massive orbital extension from small choroidal melanoma that has occurred as result of diffuse spread along natural passages through sclera and optic nerve. (×2; AFIP 159090; from Friedenwald JS, Wilder HC, Maumenee AE, Sanders TE, Keyes JEL, Hogan MJ, Owens WC, Owens EU: Ophthalmic pathology: an atlas and textbook. Philadelphia, 1952, W. B. Saunders Co.)

Fig. 1594 Diffuse malignant melanoma of ciliary body and choroid that extended forward through scleral canals to form large subconjunctival mass that encroached upon cornea. (×9; AFIP 824055.)

to the development of metastatic disease from malignant melanoma of the choroid and ciliary body.[96,96a] A statistical study recently concluded did not support this contention,[91a] but long-term prospective studies of untreated patients with melanoma is indicated. In fact, many ophthalmologists are not resorting to immediate enucleation of eyes with clinically small melanomas that remain relatively stationary in growth.

Conditions confused with malignant melanoma of uvea

Clinically, there are many lesions that simulate malignant melanoma,[83] but histopathologic problems in differential diagnosis are infre-

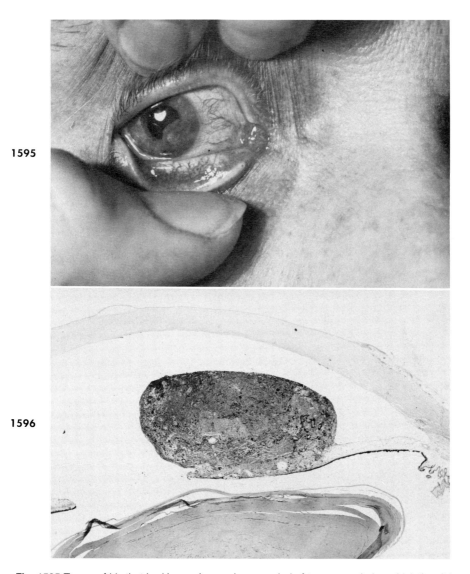

1595

1596

Fig. 1595 Tumor of iris that had been observed over period of ten years, during which time it became progressively larger and encroached upon pupil. Iridectomy revealed it to be of spindle A cell type. Tumor recurred and necessitated enucleation for secondary glaucoma fifteen years after iridectomy. (AFIP 749919; courtesy Dr. M. E. Nugent, Bismarck, N. D.)
Fig. 1596 Melanomas of iris frequently are clearly visible through cornea. Hence their duration and rate of growth often are known by patient or his family long before other subjective or objective manifestations appear. (×13; AFIP 272658.)

quent.[78,79] The latter consist primarily of differentiating nevi from spindle cell melanomas (especially in the case of iris tumors removed by iridectomy). Rarely, the problem concerns the differentiation of amelanotic epithelioid melanomas from metastatic carcinoma or distinguishing certain amelanotic spindle cell melanomas with a fascicular pattern from

neurofibromas, neurilemomas, or leiomyomas (especially in the ciliary body, where smooth muscle is so abundant).

Conditions that often present confusing clinical problems in differential diagnosis include metastatic carcinoma, localized hemorrhage beneath the retina or between the pigment epithelium and choroid (Fig. 1597), focal

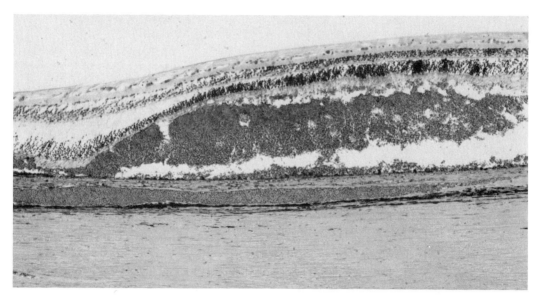

Fig. 1597 Focal hemorrhage under retina was mistaken clinically for melanoma. (×90; WU neg. 72-3167.)

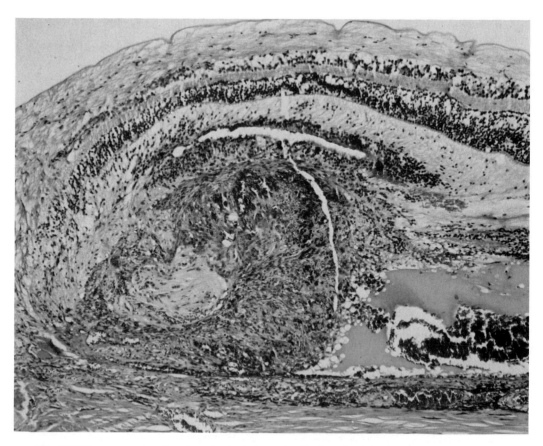

Fig. 1598 Focal area of proliferation of retinal pigment epithelium that has elevated retina to simulate melanoma. (×90; WU neg. 72-3169.)

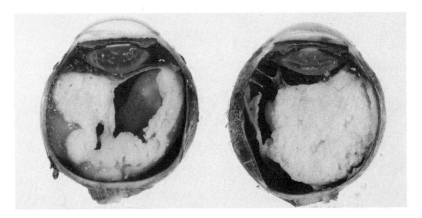

Fig. 1599 Bilateral retinoblastoma showing presence of white mass consisting of detached retina and neoplastic tissue immediately behind lens in each eye. (AFIP 635460.)

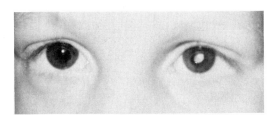

Fig. 1600 Prominent white reflex present in dilated pupil of left eye due to retinoblastoma.

areas of proliferation of the retinal pigment epithelium (Figs. 1598), posterior scleritis, and benign tumors such as nevi and hemangiomas. Melanocytomas are congenital benign pigmented tumors occurring in the disc or in the uveal tract that may be mistaken for melanomas.[85,96]

In recent years, the clinician has been aided by such techniques as fluorescein angiography,[84] radioactive phosphorus uptake, and ultrasonography.[87,90]

Retinoblastoma

Retinoblastomas are the most common intraocular neoplasm of children. Generally believed to be congenital and derived from the incompletely differentiated retinal cells, they nevertheless are seldom recognized until considerable growth has taken place. They are usually diagnosed between the ages of 16 months and 2 years. Although most cases arise sporadically, the influence of heredity has been well shown in many. Bilaterality is present in 30% of all cases and in over 90% of the familial cases (Fig. 1599).

These tumors characteristically present as a leukocoria (white pupillary reflex) (Fig. 1600) or less often as a stabismus when the tumor is in the macula. Rarely, extraocular extension with the formation of an orbital mass is the presenting manifestation.

Retinoblastomas may be flat and diffuse or elevated and may show multicentric foci of origin, especially in the hereditary type. They made protrude into the vitreous (endophytic type) (Fig. 1601), often with vitreous seeding, or they may grow between the retina and the pigment epithelium (exophytic type). Since the tumors tend to outgrow their blood supply, necrosis is often extensive, and many minute foci of calcification are often present in these areas of necrosis (Fig. 1602). In fact, these areas of calcification may be appreciated by x-ray examination prior to enucleation.

Cytologically, the tumors are composed of dense masses of small round cells with hyperchromatic nuclei and scanty cytoplasm (Fig. 1603). In the more differentiated tumors, the cells are often arranged in rosettes (Fig. 1604) and fleurettes. Light and electron microscopic studies have confirmed that these tumors are neuronal neoplasms rather than gliomas as was suspected by many in years past.[102,103]

A most important practical consideration for the surgical pathologist concerns examination of the optic nerve in order to determine the extent of invasion by the tumor (Fig. 1605). Ordinarily, the ophthalmic surgeon who suspects a retinoblastoma will try to obtain a long segment of optic nerve attached to the globe. Transverse sections of the nerve should be examined microscopically at the level of surgical transection and at various levels along the

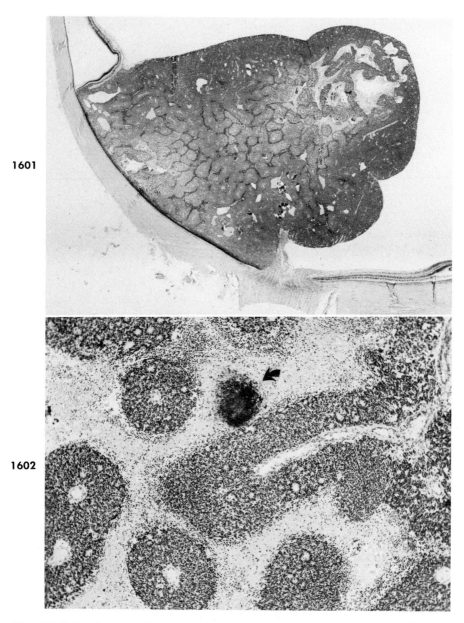

Fig. 1601 Retinoblastoma, highly cellular neoplasm with scanty stroma. Tumor tends to outgrow its blood supply, and irregular areas of necrosis are commonly observed. (×12; AFIP 747443.)
Fig. 1602 Retinoblastoma showing typical pattern of collar of viable cells about nutrient vessels. Foci of calcification (arrow) occur within areas of coagulation necrosis. (×80; AFIP 147292.)

nerve. The prognosis is poor in tumors that have invaded the nerve and extended to the plane of transection or into the meninges. These tumors are very likely to extend along the nerve to the brain or be carried there by the subarachnoid fluid. Another histopathologic finding that carries a grave prognosis is massive invasion of the uveal tract.

In most unilateral cases, the tumor is so large that the eye is no longer salvageable, and enucleation should be performed immediately. If tumor has extended to the surgically cut end of the nerve, radiation to the orbit and systemic chemotherapy should then be carried out. In patients with bilateral retinoblastoma, the less affected eye is treated with radiother-

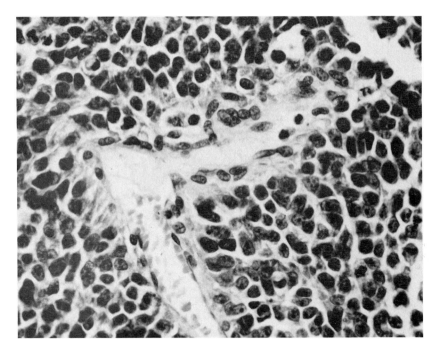

Fig. 1603 Undifferentiated retinoblastomas composed of relatively large anaplastic cells have less favorable prognosis than those that contain highly differentiated rosettes. (×400; AFIP 190088; from Friedenwald JS, Wilder HC, Maumenee AE, Sanders TE, Keyes JEL, Hogan MJ, Owens WC, Owens EU: Ophthalmic pathology: an atlas and textbook. Philadelphia, 1952, W. B. Saunders Co.)

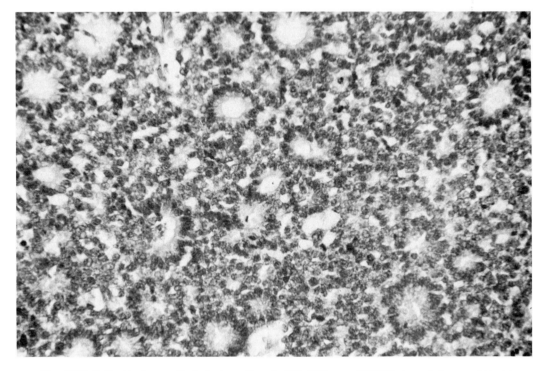

Fig. 1604 Retinoblastoma with typical rosettes. (×600; WU neg. 69-7513; from Ackerman LV, del Regato JA: Cancer, ed. 4. St. Louis, 1970, The C. V. Mosby Co.)

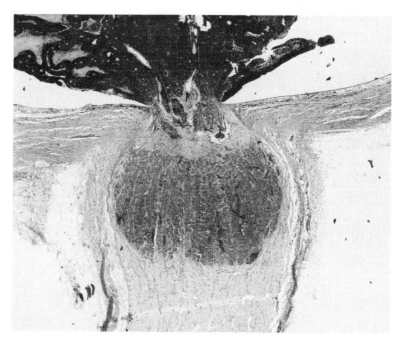

Fig. 1605 Retinoblastomas exhibit definite tendency to spread out of globe by way of optic nerve. It is therefore of utmost importance for surgical pathologist to determine whether such optic nerve extension has occurred and, if it has, to what extent. (×14; AFIP 57-344.)

apy and at times in combination with chemotherapy. The success rate for life of the patient and for preservation of vision is quite good. Tumor recurrences are then treated with photocoagulation, cryotherapy, and cobalt disks.

Conditions confused with retinoblastoma

Any disease process (congenital malformations, developmental disorders, inflammatory processes, trauma, etc.) that leads to retinal detachment or a retrolental mass in a child under 6 years of age must be suspected as a possible retinoblastoma.[100,101]

Lesions in this category include traumatic or idiopathic retinal detachments, retrolental fibroplasia, persistent hyperplastic primary vitreous, massive retinal gliosis, Coats' disease, nematodiasis, astrocytomas of tuberous sclerosis, and medulloepitheliomas.

Persistent hyperplastic primary vitreous and nematodiasis have already been discussed (pp. 1668 and 1673). Massive retinal gliosis is a relatively uncommon condition in which a large elevated scar develops near the disc and posterior pole following hemorrahge (e.g., in newborn infants) or inflammation. Coats' disease is an exudative retinopathy associated with retinal detachment and foci of telangiectatic retinal vessels. It is usually unilateral and occurs in young children, more often in males. Medulloepitheliomas are rare tumors that resemble histologically the embryonic retina.

Metastatic carcinoma

Although metastatic sarcomas to the eye are rare, metastatic carcinomas are actually common intraocular tumors in adults. In fact, if one were to routinely do serial sections on all autopsy eyes, cases of metastatic carcinoma would outnumber primary melanoma. The difference, of course, is that most of the patients were asymptomatic for ocular symptoms while alive. The most common primary lesions involved are the breast in the female and the lung in the male, with the gastrointestinal tract next in frequency.[104-106] Occasionally, the ocular metastasis may be the initial manifestation of the disease, and the primary lesion is discovered only after the eye has been enucleated.

The posterior choroid is most often affected by metastatic carcinoma (Fig. 1606). Anterior uveal involvement is much less common, and retinal metastases are rare. Although diffuse thickening of the choroid along both sides of the optic nerve is most characteristic, large,

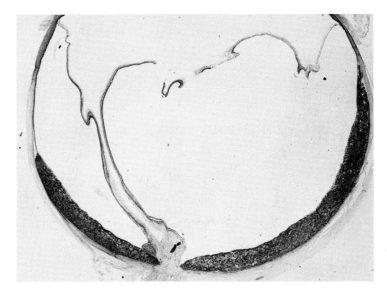

Fig. 1606 Metastatic carcinoma from breast producing diffuse thickening of choroid posteriorly. (×6; AFIP 638509.)

bulky tumor masses resembling malignant melanomas also may be observed.

Leukemia and malignant lymphoma

The eye is often involved in leukemic and lymphomatous processes, and the intraocular structures are no exception. In fact, ocular involvement is present in at least 50% of all patients who die of leukemia or allied disorders.[107] The histologic findings consist largely of leukemic infiltrations and hemorrhages, particularly in the vascular structures of the eye—i.e., the choroid and retina.[107,109]

There is often confusion concerning these lesions as to whether they are true neoplasms of the reticuloendothelial system or merely benign lymphoid hyperplasias. It has been shown by Ryan et al.[108] that this unusual form of intraocular pseudotumor probably occurs more often than had been appreciated in the past.

Other tumors

Rare tumors include *leiomyomas* of the ciliary body and iris, pigmented and nonpigmented *neuroepitheliomas* of the iris, ciliary body, and retinal pigment epithelium, and hemartomatous lesions—e.g., hemangiomas, neurofibromas, and astrocytomas.

Juvenile xanthogranuloma can occur in the iris and can cause a spontaneous hyphema and/or secondary glaucoma. It occurs almost exclusively in young children and is associated with the same lesions of the skin from which a biopsy diagnosis can be made.[110]

Cytology

In certain cases, the pathologist may be called upon to examine material that has been aspirated from either the aqueous or the vitreous and has been passed through a millipore filter. Cases in which this has proved beneficial include histiocytic lymphoma,[111] retinoblastoma,[113] and phacolytic glaucoma.[112]

TECHNIQUE FOR EXAMINATION AND OPENING OF ENUCLEATED EYES

It is very important that the eye be fixed well, oriented properly, examined with the aid of a dissecting microscope, and transilluminated before it is opened.

Good fixation is obtained by placing the intact surgical specimen in a pint of 10% aqueous formalin. It is not necessary to open the eye, to cut windows into the sclera, or to inject formalin into the vitreous in order to obtain good fixation for routine histopathologic techniques. After twenty-four hours in formalin, the globe should be washed in running tap water for several hours and then placed in 60% ethyl alcohol. Formalin is the fixative of choice because it penetrates readily, does not discolor and opacify the ocular tissues, and is generally very satisfactory for most staining procedures.

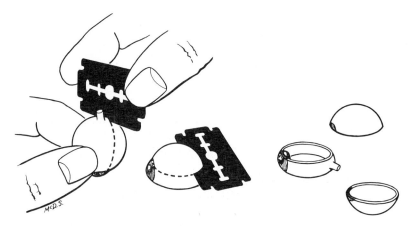

Fig. 1607 Steps used in opening whole eyes. See text for description.

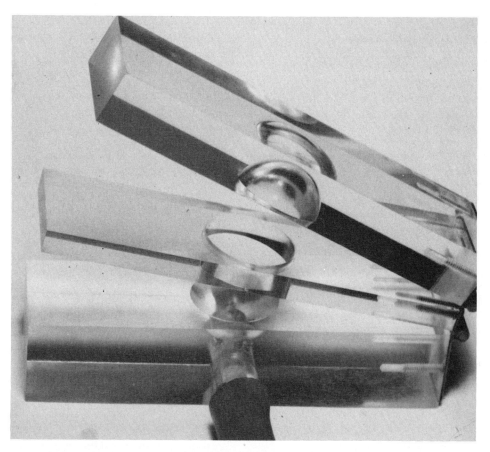

Fig. 1608 "Ophthalmotome" that can be used for cutting eyes. Model shown is fashioned after original instrument constructed by Herreman, de Buen, and Cortez. (WU neg. 67-4484.)

There is some evidence that glutaraldehyde may have some advantages over formalin for routine fixation.[116]

At the time of gross examination, it is imperative that the pathologist have a good summary of the clinical history and the results of ophthalmologic examination. If there have been accidental or surgical injuries to the globe, their sites should be determined before the eye is opened. Likewise, any particular lesion of interest observed in the fundus must be known so that the globe may be advantageously positioned when it is being opened.

Every effort should be made to open the eye in such a way that the plane of section will include the cornea, pupil, lens, and optic nerve, along with the lesion of principal clinical interest. If there is no focal lesion that requires a particular plane of section, the horizontal plane is used in order to obtain the macula in the block.

Many minute lesions of interest that would ordinarily be overlooked with the naked eye can be detected if the ×7 objective of a binocular dissecting microscope is used. Likewise, transillumination of the globe before it is opened will frequently reveal discrete shadows or areas of increased translucency. A substage microscope lamp in a darkened room is very satisfactory for this purpose. Rotation of the globe over the light source will often reveal in sharp outline the presence of intraocular tumors. Such shadows should then be delineated on the sclera with an indelible pencil.

When the presence of intraocular foreign bodies is suspected, it is good practice to examine the globe roentgenologically before it is opened.

The eye is opened with the aid of a double-edged razor blade. During sectioning, a right-handed individual holds the eye with the left hand, cornea down against the cutting block (Fig. 1607). The razor blade is held between the thumb and middle finger of the right hand. With a sawing motion, the eye is opened from back to front. The plane of section begins adjacent to the optic nerve and ends through the periphery of the cornea. After the interior of the globe is examined, a second plane of section, parallel to the first, is made, again passing from back to front. During this step, the eye is placed flat on its cut surface (Fig. 1607).

An alternate method of opening the globe is with the use of a plastic apparatus known as an "ophthalmotome" that was developed by Herreman, de Buen, and Cortez and later revised by Smith.[114,115] This device holds the eye within a compartment while the razor is passed through the different sections of the plastic block (Fig. 1608).

As a result of the two-step procedure, either with the "ophthalmotome" or by hand, a disc-shaped slab about 8 mm in thickness containing the cornea, pupil, lens, and optic nerve is obtained. This slab may be carried through the automatic tissue processor along with other surgical specimens that are to be embedded in paraffin. With experience, excellent paraffin sections may be cut on the rotary microtome, although it is technically easier to obtain good histologic preparations with celloidin embedding and use of a sliding microtome.

REFERENCES
GENERAL REFERENCES

1 Apple D, Rabb M: Clinicopathologic correlation of ocular disease. A text and stereoscopic atlas ed 2. St. Louis, 1978, The C. V. Mosby Co.
2 Beck K, Jensen OA: External ocular tumors. Textbook and atlas. W. B. Saunders Co., 1978, Philadelphia.
3 Duane T: Clinical ophthalmology. New York, 1976, Harper & Row, Publishers, Inc.
4 Ferry AP (ed): Ocular and adnexal tumors. Int Ophthalmol Clin **12:**1-269, 1972.
5 Fine B, Yanoff M: Ocular histology. A text and atlas. New York, 1972, Harper & Row, Publishers, Inc.
6 Henderson JW: Orbital tumors. Philadelphia, 1973, W. B. Saunders Co.
7 Hogan MJ, Zimmerman LE: Ophthalmic pathology. An atlas and textbook, ed. 2. Philadelphia. 1962, W. B. Saunders Co.
8 Hogan MJ, Alvarado JA, Weddell JE: Histology of the human eye. Philadelphia, 1971, W. B. Saunders Co.
9 Jakobiec FA: Ocular and adnexal tumors. Birmingham, Ala., 1978, Aesculapius Publishing Co.
10 Peyman, G, Apple D, Sanders D: Intraocular tumors. New York, 1977, Appleton-Century-Crofts.
11 Reese AB: Tumors of the eye, ed. 2. New York, 1976, Harper & Row, Publishers, Inc.
12 Yanoff M, Fine B: Ocular pathology. A text and atlas, New York, 1975, Harper & Row, Publishers, Inc.
13 Zimmerman LE: Changing concepts concerning the malignancy of ocular tumors. Arch Ophthalmol **78:** 166-173, 1967.
14 Zimmerman LE, Font R, Ts'o M: Application of electron microscopy to histopathologic diagnosis. Trans Am Acad Ophthalmol Otolaryngol **76:**101-107, 1972.

EYELIDS

15 Aurora AL, Blodi FC: Lesions of the eyelids: a clinicopathologic study. Surv Ophthalmol **15:**94-104, 1970.
16 Boniuk M: Tumors of the eyelids. Int Ophthalmol Clin **2:**239-317, 1962.
17 Boniuk M, Zimmerman LE: Eyelid tumors with reference to lesions confused with squamous cell car-

cinoma. II. Inverted follicular keratosis. Arch Ophthalmol **69:**698-707, 1963.

18 Boniuk M, Zimmerman LE: Eyelid tumors with reference to lesions confused with squamous cell carcinoma. III. Keratoacanthoma. Arch Ophthalmol **77:** 29-40, 1967.

19 Boniuk M, Zimmerman LE: Sebaceous carcinomas of the eyelid, eyebrow, caruncle, and orbit. Trans Am Acad Ophthalmol Orolaryngol **72:**619-642, 1068.

19a Chaflin J, Putterman AM: Frozen section control in the surgery of basal cell carcinoma of the eyelid. Am J Ophthalmol **87:**802-809, 1979.

20 Henkind P, Friedman A: External ocular pigmentation. Int Ophthalmol Clin **11:**87-111, 1971.

20a Hidayal AA, Font RL: Trichilemmoma of eyelid and eyebrow. A clinicopathologic study of 31 cases. Arch Ophthalmol **98:**844-847, 1980.

21 Kwitko ML, Boniuk M, Zimmerman LE: Eyelid tumors with reference to lesions confused with squamous cell carcinoma. I. Incidence and errors in diagnosis. Arch Ophthalmol **69:**693-697, 1963.

21a Russel WG, Page DL, Hough AJ, Rogers LW: Sebaceous carcinoma of meibomian gland origin. The diagnostic importance of pagetoid spread of neoplastic cells. Am J Clin Pathol **73:**504-511, 1980.

22 Smith ME, Zimmerman LE: Amyloidosis of the eyelid and conjunctiva. Arch Ophthalmol **75:**42-56, 1966.

22a Wright JD, Font RL: Mucinous sweat gland adenocarcinoma of eyelid. A clinicopathologic study of 21 cases with histochemical and electron microscopic observations. Cancer **44:**1757-1768, 1979.

LACRIMAL PASSAGES

23 Ryan SJ, Font RL: Primary epithelial neoplasms of the lacrimal sac. Am J Ophthalmol **76:**73-88, 1973.

LACRIMAL GLAND

24 Font RL, Yanoff M, Zimmerman LE: Benign lymphoepithelial lesion of the lacrimal gland and its relationship to Sjögren's syndrome. Am J Clin Pathol **48:**365-376, 1967.

25 Forrest AW: Pathologic criteria for effective management of epithelial lacrimal gland tumors. Am J Ophthalmol **71:**178-192, 1971.

26 Godwin JT: Benign lymphoepithelial lesion of the parotid gland (adenolymphoma, chronic inflammation, lymphoepithelioma, lymphocytic tumor, Mikulicz's disease). Cancer **5:**1089-1103, 1952.

26a Ludwig ME, LiVolsi VA, McMahon RT: Malignant mixed tumor of the lacrimal gland. Am J Surg Pathol **3:**457-462, 1979.

27 Meyer D, Yanoff M, Hanno H: Differential diagnosis in Mikulicz syndrome, Mikulicz's disease, and similar disease entities. Am J Ophthalmol **70:**516-524, 1971.

27a Perzin KH, Jakobiec FA, LiVolsi VA, Desjardins L: Lacrimal gland malignant mixed tumors (carcinomas arising in benign mixed tumors): a clinico-pathologic study. Cancer **45:**2593-2606, 1980.

28 Sanders TE, Ackerman LV, Zimmerman LE: Epithelial tumors of the lacrimal gland. A comparison of the pathologic and clinical behavior with those of the salivary glands. Am J Surg **104:**657-665, 1962.

29 Yanoff M, Nix R, Swan D: Bilateral lacrimal gland enlargement associated with a diffuse gamma globulin elevation. Ophthalmol Res **1:**245-253, 1970.

30 Zimmerman LE, Sanders TE, Ackerman LV: Epithelial tumors of the lacrimal gland: prognostic and therapeutic significance of histologic types. Int Ophthalmol Clin **2:**337-367, 1962.

ORBIT

30a Astarita RW, Minckler D, Taylor CR, Levine A, Lukes RJ: Orbital and adnexal lymphomas. A multiparameter approach. Am J Clin Pathol **73:**615-621, 1980.

31 Blodi F, Gass D: Inflammatory pseudotumor of the orbit. Trans Am Acad Ophthalmol Otolaryngol **71:** 303-323, 1967.

31a Dosoretz DE, Blitzer PH, Wang CC, Linggood RM: Management of glioma of the optic nerve and/or chiasm. An analysis of 20 cases. Cancer **45:**1467-1471, 1980.

32 Font R, Zimmerman LE: Nodular fasciitis of the eye and adnexa: a report of ten cases. Arch Ophthalmol **75:**475-481, 1966.

33 Forrest AW: Tumors following radiation about the eye. Int Ophthalmol Clin **2:**543-553, 1962.

34 Garner A: Pathology of "pseudotumors" of the orbit: a review. J Clin Pathol **26:**639-648, 1973.

34a Henderson JW, Farrow GM: Primary orbital hemangiopericytoma. An aggressive and potentially malignant neoplasm. Arch Ophthalmol **96:**666-673, 1978.

35 Karp L, Zimmerman L, Borit A, Spencer W: Primary intraorbital meningiomas. Arch Ophthalmol **91:**24-28, 1974.

35a Knowles DM II, Jakobiec FA: Orbital lymphoid neoplasms. A clinicopathologic study of 60 patients. Cancer **46:**576-589, 1980.

36 Knowles D, Jakobiec F, Potter G, Jones IS: Ophthalmic striated muscle neoplasms. Surv Ophthalmol **21:** 219-261, 1976.

36a Morgan G, Harry J: Lymphocytic tumours of indeterminate nature: a 5-year follow-up of 98 conjunctival and orbital lesions. Br J Ophthalmol **62:**381-383, 1978.

36b Tewfik HH, Platz CE, Corder MP, Panther SK, Blodi FC: A clinicopathologic study of orbital and adnexal non-Hodgkin's lymphomas. Cancer **44:**1022-1028, 1979.

37 Verhoeff FA: Tumors of optic nerve. In Penfield WC: Cytology and cellular pathology of the nervous system, vol. 3. New York, 1932, Hoeber Medical Division, Harper & Row, Publishers, pp. 1029-1039.

CONJUNCTIVA

38 Blodi FC: Squamous cell carcinoma of the conjunctiva. Doc Ophthalmol **34:**93-108, 1973.

39 Bornstein J, Frank M, Radnec D: Conjunctival biopsy in the diagnosis of sarcoidosis. N Engl J Med **267:**60-64, 1962.

40 Chambers J, Blodi F, Golden B, McKee A: Ligneous conjunctivitis. Trans Am Acad Ophthalmol Otolaryngol **73:**996-1004, 1969.

41 Irvine AR Jr: Epibulbar squamous cell carcinoma and related lesions. In Ferry AP (ed): Ocular and adnexal tumors. Int. Ophthalmol Clin **12:**71-83, 1972.

42 Jay B: Naevi and melanomata of the conjunctiva. Br J Ophthalmol **49:**169-204, 1965.

43 Morgan G: Lymphocytic tumours of the conjunctiva. J Clin Pathol **24:**585-595, 1971.

44 Reese AB: Precancerous and cancerous melanosis. Am J Ophthalmol **61:**1272-1277, 1966.

45 Zimmerman LE: Criteria for management of melanosis [correspondence]. Arch Ophthalmol **76:**307-308, 1966.

CORNEA

46 Green WR, Zimmerman LE: Granulomatous reaction to Descemet's membrane. Am J Ophthalmol **64:**555-558, 1967.

47 Waring G, Rodrigues M, Laibson P: Corneal dystrophies II. Endothelial dystrophies. Surv Ophthalmol **23:**147-168, 1978.

INTRAOCULAR TISSUES
Congenital and developmental malformations

48 Boniuk M, Zimmerman LE: Ocular pathology in the rubella syndrome Arch Ophthalmol **77:**455-473, 1967.

49 Cogan DG, Kuwabara T: Ocular pathology of the 13-15 trisomy syndrome. Arch Ophthalmol **72:**246-247, 1964.

50 Font R, Ferry AP: The phakomatoses. In Ferry AP (ed): Ocular and adnexal tumors. Int Ophthalmol Clin **12:**1-50, 1972.

51 Font RL, Fine BS: Ocular pathology in Fabry's disease. Histochemical and electron microscopic observations. Am J Ophthalmol **73:**419-430, 1972.

52 Hunter WS, Zimmerman LE: Unilateral retinal dysplasia. Arch Ophthalmol **74:**23-30, 1965.

53 Jensen OA: Persistent hyperplastic primary vitreous. Acta Ophthalmol **46:**418-429, 1968.

54 Miller RW, Fraumeni JF, Jr, Manning MD: Association of Wilms' tumor with aniridia, hemihypertrophy, and other congenital malformations. N Engl J Med **270:**922-927, 1964.

55 Reese AB (moderator): Symposium on retrolental fibroplasia. Trans Am Acad Ophthalmol Otolaryngol **59:**7-41, 1955.

56 Reese AB, Ellsworth RM: The anterior chamber cleavage syndrome. Arch Ophthalmol **75:**307-318, 1968.

57 Zimmerman LE: The histopathologic basis for ocular manifestations of the congenital rubella syndrome. Am J Ophthalmol **65:**837-862, 1968.

58 Zimmerman LE, Font RL: Some recent advances in the pathogenesis and histopathology of congenital malformations of the eye. JAMA **196:**684-696, 1966.

Inflammation
Acute inflammation/Chronic nongranulomatous inflammation/Granulomatous inflammation

59 Beaver PC: Larva migrans. Exp Parasit **5:**587-621, 1956.

60 Fishman LS, Griffin JR, Sapico FL, Hecht R: Hematogenous Candida endophthalmitis. N Engl J Med **286:**675-681, 1972.

61 Levine R, Williamson DE: Metastatic carcinoma simulating a postoperative endophthalmitis. Arch Ophthalmol **83:**59-60, 1970.

62 Michelson PE, Stark W, Reeser F, and Green WR: Endogenous Candida endophthalmitis. Report of 13 cases and 16 from the literature. Int Ophthalmol Clin **11:**125-147, 1971.

63 Naumann G, Gass D, Font R: Histopathology of herpes zoster ophthalmicus. Am J Ophthalmol **65:** 533-541, 1968.

64 Sugar S, Mandell G, Shaler J: Metastatic endophthalmitis associated with injection of addictive drugs. Am J Ophthalmol **71:**1055-1058, 1971.

65 Wilder HC: Nematode endophthalmitis. Trans Am Acad Ophthalmol Otolaryngol **54:**99-109, 1950.

66 Wilder HC: Toxoplasma chorioretinitis in adults. Arch Ophthalmol **48:**127-136, 1952.

67 Wilkinson C, Welch R: Intraocular Toxocara. Am J Ophthalmol **71:**921-930, 1971.

Posttraumatic uveitis

68 Easom H, Zimmerman LE: Sympathetic ophthalmia and bilateral phacoanaphylaxis. Arch Ophthalmol **72:** 9-15, 1964.

69 Verhoeff FH, Lemoine AN: Endophthalmitis phacoanaphylactica. Transactions of the International Congress of Ophthalmology, Washington, D.C., April 25, 1922.

Degeneration
Glaucoma

70 Fenton R, Zimmerman L: Hemolytic glaucoma. Arch Ophthalmol **70:**236-239, 1963.

71 Flocks M, Littwin CS, Zimmerman LE: Phacolytic glaucoma. Arch Ophthalmol **54:**37-45, 1955.

72 Kolker AE, Hetherington J Jr: Becker-Shaffer's Diagnosis and therapy of the glaucomas, ed. 4. St. Louis, 1976, The C. V. Mosby Co.

Diabetes

73 Smith ME, Glickman P: Diabetic vacuolation of the iris pigment epithelium. Am J Ophthalmol **79:**875-877, 1975.

74 Yanoff M: Ocular pathology in diabetes mellitus. Am J Ophthalmol **67:**21-38, 1969.

Tumors and pseudotumors
Malignant melanoma

75 Ashton N, Wybar K: Primary tumours of the iris. Ophthalmologica **151:**97-113, 1966.

76 Callender GR: Malignant melanotic tumors of the eye: a study of histologic types in 111 cases. Trans Am Acad Ophthalmol Otolaryngol **36:**131-142, 1931.

77 Char DH: The management of small choroidal melanomas. Surv Ophthalmol **22:**377-386, 1978.

78 Ferry AP: Lesions mistaken for malignant melanoma of posterior uvea. Arch Ophthalmol **72:**463-469, 1964.

79 Ferry AP: Lesions mistaken for malignant melanoma of iris. Arch Ophthalmol **74:**9-18, 1965.

80 Flocks M, Gerende JH, Zimmerman LE: The size and shape of malignant melanomas of the choroid and ciliary body in relation to prognosis and histologic characteristics—a statistical study of 210 tumors. Trans Am Acad Ophthalmol Otolaryngol **59:**740-758, 1955.

81 Font R, Spaulding A, Zimmerman LE: Diffuse malignant melanoma of the uveal tract: a clinicopathologic report of 54 cases. Trans Am Acad Ophthalmol Otolaryngol **72:**877-895, 1968.

82 Forrest A, Keeper R, Spencer W: Iridocyclectomy for melanomas of the ciliary body: a follow-up study of pathology and surgical morbidity. Am J Ophthalmol **85:**1237-1249, 1978.

83 Gass JMD: Differential diagnosis of intraocular tumors. St. Louis, 1974, The C. V. Mosby Co.

84 Gass JMD: Fluorescein angiography. An aid in the differential diagnosis of intraocular tumors. In Ferry AP (ed): Ocular and adnexal tumors. Int. Ophthalmol Clin **12:**85-120, 1972.

85 Howard GM, Forrest AW: Incidence and location of melanocytomas. Arch Ophthalmol **77:**61-66, 1967.

86 McLean I, Zimmerman LE, Evans R: Reappraisal of Callender's spindle A type of malignant melanoma of choroid and ciliary body. Am J Ophthalmol **86:** 557-564, 1978.

87 Ossoinig KC: Preoperative differential diagnosis of

tumors with echography. In Blodi FC (ed): Current concepts of ophthalmology, vol 4, St. Louis, 1974, The C. V. Mosby Co., pp. 264-343.

88 Paul EV, Parnell BL, Fraker M: Prognosis of malignant melanomas of the choroid and ciliary body. Int. Ophthalmol Clin 2:387-402, 1962.

89 Reese AB: Tumors of the eye, ed. 2. New York, 1963, Hoeber Medical Division, Harper & Row, Publishers.

90 Shields JA: Current approaches to the diagnosis and management of choroidal melanomas. Surv Ophthalmol 21:443-463, 1977.

91 Shields JA, Hagler WS, Federman JL, Jarrett WH III, Carmichael PL: The significance of the P_{32} uptake test in the diagnosis of posterior uveal melanomas. Trans Amer Acad Ophthalmol Otolaryngol 79:297-306, 1975.

91a Seigel D, Myers M, Ferris F III, Steinhorn SC: Survival rates after enucleation of eyes with malignant melanoma. Am J Ophthalmol 87:761-765, 1979.

92 Yanoff M, Zimmerman LE: Histogenesis of malignant melanomas of the uvea. I. Nevi of choroid and ciliary body. Arch Ophthalmol 76:784-796, 1966.

93 Yanoff M, Zimmerman LE: Histogenesis of malignant melanomas of the uvea. II. The relationship of uveal nevi to malignant melanomas. Cancer 20:493-507, 1967.

94 Yanoff M, Zimmerman LE: Histogenesis of malignant melanomas of the uvea. III. The relationship of congenital ocular melanocytosis and neurofibromatosis to uveal melanomas. Arch Ophthalmol 77:331-336, 1967.

95 Zimmerman LE: Clinical pathology of iris tumors. Am J Clin Pathol 39:214-228, 1963.

96 Zimmerman LE: Melanocytes, melanocytic nevi, and melanocytomas. Invest Ophthalmol 4:11-41, 1965.

96a Zimmerman LE, McLean IW: An evaluation of enucleation in the management of uveal melanomas. Am J Ophthalmol 87:741-760, 1979.

97 Zimmerman LE, McLean I, Foster W: Does enucleation of the eye containing a malignant melanoma prevent or accelerate the dissemination of tumor cells? Br J Ophthalmol 62:420-425, 1978.

Retinoblastoma

98 Abramson D, Ellsworth R, Zimmerman L: Nonocular cancer in retinoblastoma survivors. Trans Amer Acad Ophthalmol Otolaryngol 81:454-457, 1976.

99 Bishop J, Madson E: Retinoblastoma. Review of the current status. Surv Ophthalmol 19:342-366, 1975.

100 Howard GM, Ellsworth RM: Differential diagnosis of retinoblastoma. A statistical survey of 500 children. Am J Ophthalmol 60:610-612, 1965.

101 Kogan L, Boniuk M: Causes for enucleation in childhood with special reference to pseudogliomas and retinoblastomas. Int Ophthalmol Clin 2:507-524, 1962.

102 Ts'o MO, Fine BS, Zimmerman LE: The nature of retinoblastoma. II Photoreceptor differentiation: an electron microscopic study. Am J Ophthalmol 69:350-359, 1970.

103 Ts'o MO, Zimmerman LE, Fine BS: The nature of retinoblastoma. I. Photoreceptor differentiation: a clinical and histopathologic study. Am J Ophthalmol 69:339-349, 1970.

Metastatic carcinoma

104 Albert DM, Rubenstein R, Scheie H: Tumor metastasis to the eye. Part I. Incidence in 213 adult patients with generalized malignancy. Am J Ophthalmol 63:724-726, 1967.

105 Ferry AP: Metastatic carcinoma of the eye and ocular adnexa. Int Ophthalmol Clin 7:615-658, 1967.

106 Ferry A, Font R: Carcinoma metastatic to the eye and orbit. Arch Ophthalmol 92:276-286, 1974.

Leukemia and malignant lymphoma

107 Allen R, Straatsma B: Ocular involvement in leukemia and allied disorders. Arch Ophthalmol 66:490-508, 1961.

108 Ryan S, Zimmerman LE, King FM: Reactive lymphoid hyperplasia. An unusual form of intraocular pseudotumor. Trans Am Acad Ophthalmol Otolaryngol 76:652-671, 1972.

109 Vogel M, Font R, Zimmerman LE, Levine R: Reticulum cell sarcoma of the retina and uvea. Am J Ophthalmol 66:205-215, 1968.

Other tumors

110 Zimmerman LE: Ocular lesions of juvenile xanthogranuloma: nevoxanthoendothelioma. Trans Am Acad Ophthalmol Otolaryngol 69:412-442, 1965.

Cytology

111 Barr CC, Green WR, Payne JW, Knox DL, Jensen AD, Thompson RL: Intraocular reticulum-cell sarcoma: clinicopathologic study of four cases and review of the literature. Surv Ophthalmol 19:224-239, 1975.

112 Goldberg MF: Cytological diagnosis of phacolytic glaucoma utilizing millepor filtration of the aqueous. Br J Ophthalmol 51:847-853, 1967.

113 Wolter JR, Naylor B: A membrane filter method: used to diagnose intraocular tumor. J Pediatr Ophthalmol 5:36-38, 1968.

TECHNIQUE FOR EXAMINATION AND OPENING OF ENUCLEATED EYES

114 Herreman R, De Buen S, Cortés T: Oftalmótomo: un nuevo aparato para secionar los ojos en el laboratorio de anatomía patológica. Rev Fac Med (Mexico) 7:157-167, 1965.

115 Smith ME: A method for immediate gross sectioning of enucleated globes. Am J Ophthalmol 77:413-414, 1974.

116 Yanoff M, Fine BS: Glutaraldehyde fixation of routine surgical eye tissue. Am J Ophthalmol 63:137-140, 1967.

appendix

Guidelines for handling of most common and important surgical specimens

Some general guidelines for the procedure, description, and sampling of the most common and important surgical specimens received in the laboratory are set forth in the following pages. They are mainly derived from personal experience in our institutions, although the *Gross room manual* used for years in the Surgical Pathology Laboratory at Barnes Hospital in St. Louis, and considerably expanded by the surgical pathologists at Stanford University, was freely used as a model for many of the procedures. These instructions can be used in the form of a manual or be copied on microfiche cards to facilitate their reading by the prosector.

Naturally, not all types of specimens or eventualities could be covered. The guidelines presented herewith will be useful only if they are taken as *general recommendations* for a typical specimen showing a typical lesion. All kinds of modifications need to be made according to the specific circumstances of the case. Each specimen is unique and presents special problems of dissection and description that will be missed or mishandled if the prosector rigidly follows these general guidelines. Also it should be pointed out that the guidelines reflect only one way of working up a specimen. There are probably no two laboratories in the country that process and describe tissues in exactly the same fashion. What we are describing here is a series of procedures that we have found useful and reliable over the years, fully realizing that they are not the only ones or even necessarily the best.

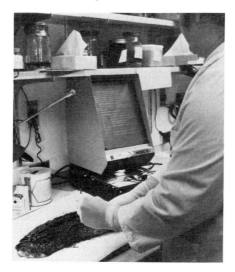

APPENDIX—APPENDECTOMY

Procedure

1 Measure organ (length and greatest diameter).
2 Divide into halves by cutting a cross section 2 cm from tip.
3 Cut cross sections of proximal fragment at 5 mm intervals.
4 Divide distal fragment in two by a longitudinal cut.

Description

1 Length and greatest diameter
2 External surface: fibrin? pus? hemorrhage? hyperemia? perforation? condition of mesentery
3 Wall: any localized lesions?
4 Lumen: obliterated? dilated? content: fecaliths? stones?

Sections for histology

1 Proximal one-third, close to surgical margin: one cross section
If tumor is present in the specimen, paint the surgical margin with India ink and take an additional section from it.
2 Mid one-third: one cross section
3 Distal one-third: one longitudinal section

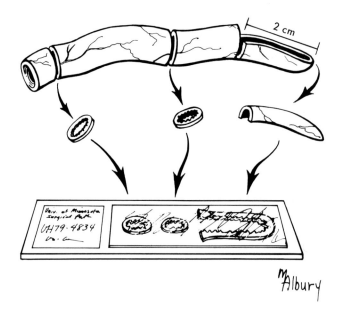

BLADDER—CYSTECTOMY

Procedure

1 Two options are available depending on the type of lesion present and the status of the organ when received in the laboratory (see accompanying drawings):

   a Open with scissors in a Y shape through the anterior wall, pin on a corkboard, and fix overnight in formalin.

   b Fill with formalin; fix overnight and divide into anterior and posterior halves by first cutting the lateral bladder walls with scissors and then sectioning the prostate with a sharp knife, beginning at the bladder neck and being careful to make the cut through the urethra. See instructions for Injection of specimens — General guidelines. The injection can be performed through the urethra with a Foley catheter, with a 50 ml syringe with large-bore needle inserted through the bladder dome after the urethra has been clamped or tied, or by filling the bladder with formalin-soaked cotton.

2 Take two Polaroid photographs and identify in one of them the site of the sections to be taken.

Description

1 Size of bladder; length of ureters; other organs present
2 Tumor characteristics: size (including thickness), location, extent of invasion, shape (papillary, ulcerated)
3 Appearance of nonneoplastic mucosa; thickness of bladder wall away from tumor

Sections for histology

1 Tumor: at least three sections, through bladder wall
2 Bladder neck: one section
3 Trigone: two sections
4 Anterior wall: two sections
5 Posterior wall: two sections
6 Dome: two sections
7 Any abnormal-looking area in bladder mucosa if not included in previous sections
8 Ureters: three cross sections of each
9 In males: prostate and seminal vesicles
10 Other organs present
11 Perivesical lymph nodes if any

Continued

BLADDER—CYSTECTOMY cont'd

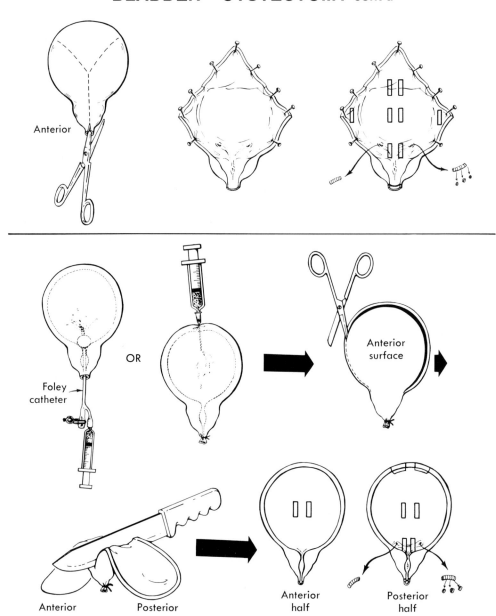

Anterior

Foley catheter

OR

Anterior surface

Anterior   Posterior

Anterior half

Posterior half

BONE—FEMORAL HEAD EXCISION

Procedure

1 Examine articular and cut surfaces.
2 Measure diameter and thickness.
3 Take photographs if indicated.
4 Hold the specimen with a specially devised clamp (a meatball maker works quite well) or in a vise and cut through the center of the articular surface (fovea) with a band saw (see accompanying drawing).
5 Make a parallel cut about 3 mm from the first cut while holding the specimen in the same position.
6 Examine a cut section of the slice; take a photograph and roentgenogram. Make parallel cuts through remaining pieces if indicated.

Description

1 Type of excision; side if known
2 Diameter and thickness
3 Articular surface: smooth or irregular?
4 Synovial membrane at edges: hypertrophic? papillary?
5 Cut surface: thickness of articular cartilage; bone exposed? subchondral eburnation? cysts? (if so, size and content) areas of necrosis? (if so, size and appearance)

Sections for histology

1 Take two sections from the most abnormal areas, at least one including the articular surface (see accompanying drawing).
2 Two options are available for obtaining these sections. The first is more expeditious and quite adequate and is the one to be used in most instances. The second is more time-consuming and requires extra care but provides slightly better results.
   a Cut the sections from the fresh slice with a fine band saw or strong knife, depending upon the amount and hardness of the bone; fix thoroughly in formalin and decalcify.
   b Fix a whole slice in formalin for several hours or overnight; decalcify thoroughly; cut desired sections with a scalpel or submit material in its entirety if facilities are available.

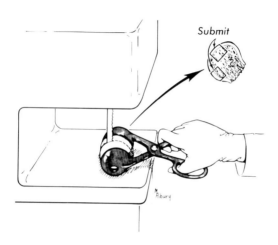

Submit

BONE MARROW—FRAGMENTS FROM ASPIRATE

Procedure

1 The material is obtained by aspiration and usually allowed to clot before fixation.
2 Alternatively, the marrow particles can be concentrated "by ejecting the aspirate, before it clots, onto a slanted slide and into a [fixative] solution. The latter is rapidly filtered and the residue is processed by usual histologic technics."*

Description

1 Approximate amount of material
2 Appearance and relative amount of marrow particles in relation to blood clots

Sections for histology

1 Submit the material in its entirety unless blood clots are excessive.
2 If clots are excessive, select areas with largest concentration of marrow particles.
3 Decalcification is generally not needed for this material.

---

*From Rywlin AM, Marvan P, Robinson MJ: A simple technic for the preparation of bone marrow smears and sections. Am J Clin Pathol **53**:389-393, 1970; reproduced with permission.

BONE MARROW—NEEDLE BIOPSY

Procedure

The needle biopsy should be fixed immediately after it is obtained. Zenker's fixative is preferable.

Description

1 Number, length, and diameter of fragments
2 Color and consistency; homogeneous?

Sections for histology

1 Submit the material in its entirety.
2 If bilateral biopsies were performed, submit them separately.
3 Decalcify only after the tissue is properly fixed and washed and for the shortest time that will allow proper sectioning.

BONE MARROW—RIB FROM THORACOTOMY

Procedure

Sometimes a rib is submitted together with a specimen of pneumonectomy or lobectomy. Gross examination alone is adequate if no gross abnormalities are detected. However, an opportunity to study the status of the patient's bone marrow should not be overlooked. Proceed as follows:

1 Measure the length and diameter of the rib.
2 With a saw cut a piece about 2 cm long from the fresh specimen, having bone marrow at both ends.
3 Place between pliers longitudinally and squeeze until bone marrow is expressed from both ends (see accompanying drawing). Let the marrow fall in a container with fixative or scrape it out with a blade.
4 Fix and submit for microscopic examination; decalcification is not necessary.
5 Cut the remainder of the rib longitudinally along its entire length and examine cut sections.

Description

1 Identification of side and number of rib if information is provided
2 Length and greatest diameter
3 Appearance of bone marrow on cut section: color, amount; any irregularities?

Sections for histology

1 If no abnormalities are observed, submit only bone marrow preparation as described under Procedure (without decalcifying).
2 If gross abnormalities are present, cut blocks, fix, decalcify, and submit for histology.

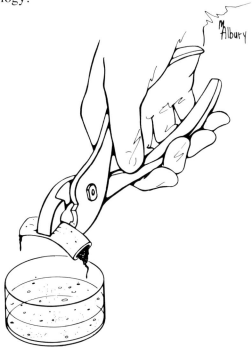

BREAST—BIOPSY AND LOCAL EXCISION

Procedure

1 Measure the specimen prior to cutting. Weigh if amount of material is substantial (over 50 gm).
2 If indicated, take a roentgenogram of the specimen.
3 If indicated, take a sample for hormone receptor studies (see instructions for Hormone receptor assays — Sampling).
4 Fix for a few hours or overnight before sectioning.
5 Cut parallel slices 3-4 mm thick.

Description

1 Dimensions and consistency of specimen
2 Appearance of cut sections: fibrosis, cysts (size, number, content), calcification, tumor masses (size, color, borders, consistency, necrosis)

Sections for histology

1 Small specimens: Submit in their entirety (up to five cassettes).
2 Larger specimens: Thorough sampling. At least two-thirds of the breast tissue (exclusive of adipose tissue) should be processed.
3 If a roentgenogram of the specimen has been taken, all positive or suspicious areas should be submitted, labeled so that the presence of calcification in the section can be correlated with the roentgenographic appearance.

BREAST—MASTECTOMY

(Adapted and quoted in part from National Cancer Institute: Standardized management of breast specimens recommended by Pathology Working Group, Breast Cancer Task Force. Am J Clin Pathol **60**:789-798, 1973; reproduced with permission.)

Procedure
First day

1 Weigh the specimen.
2 Orient the specimen. In radical mastectomy cases, use the axillary fat as a marker for the lateral side and the surgical section of the muscle as a marker for the upper side. Place the specimen on the cutting board, posterior side up, with its most inferior point toward the dissector. The specimen is oriented as if the dissector were standing behind it. Note that at the junction of the upper and middle thirds of the pectoralis major the muscle fibers run in a nearly horizontal direction.
3 Dissect lymph nodes groups as follows:
Radical mastectomy:
   a Arrange the pectoral muscles and axillary contents in their anatomic positions, using the cut attachments of the pectoral muscle fibers as guides. The axillary contents, which are sometimes partially detached from the muscle during operation, when properly arranged will form a broadly linear fatty mass extending upward and laterally, crossing the posterior surface of the pectoralis minor muscle.
   b Using the pectoralis minor muscle as a guide, divide the axilla into three segments:
   • Level I (low): inferior to lower border of muscle
   • Level II (middle): between upper and lower borders of muscle
   • Level III (high): superior to upper border of muscle
   Remove each separately and fix overnight; Carnoy's solution is preferred because, besides fixing, it clears the fat somewhat.
   c Remove the pectoralis minor muscle and search for the interpectoral (Rotter's) nodes; these usually are found near the lateral edge of the posterior surface of the pectoralis major. If no nodes are apparent, submit the adipose tissue from this site.
   d Remove the pectoralis major muscle and look for evidence of tumor invasion.
Modified mastectomy:
   a Separate the axillary tissue from the breast.
   b Since the landmarks used in radical mastectomy specimens are not present, divide the axillary tissue into a higher and a lower half and fix overnight in separate containers.
4 Turn the specimen around, with the skin side up and the 6 o'clock position nearest the dissector—i.e., as if the dissector were facing the patient.
5 Evaluate features of the external appearance and measure. Palpate the specimen for masses or nodularity. With a water-resistant marker, draw a vertical line passing through the nipple and another perpendicular to it, also passing through the nipple. This will divide the breast specimen into four quadrants: upper outer, lower outer, lower inner, and upper inner.

Continued

6 Remove the nipple and areola, using scalpel, forceps, and scissors, and fix the specimen thus obtained overnight.

7 With a long sharp knife, cut the entire breast longitudinally into slices about 2 cm thick. One of the cuts should be exactly through the level of the nipple, using as a guide the vertical line previously made in the skin; this will allow a precise separation of slices belonging to the inner and outer halves of the breast. Lay out the slices in order on a flat surface, maintaining orientation. Examine each slice carefully; take photographs and roentgenograms if indicated. Take a sample for hormone receptor studies if indicated (see instructions for Hormone receptor assays—Sampling). Fix all the slices overnight, keeping their orientation by either laying them flat sequentially in a long pan (preferable) or by stringing them together.

Second day

1 Lymph node specimens (radical or modified mastectomies): Shred the axillary tissue and dissect out all lymph nodes, which stand out as white nodules. A minimum of twenty lymph nodes should be found in the usual radical mastectomy.

2 Nipple specimen: If following fixation the nipple is erect, cut as indicated in the accompanying drawing. If it is retracted or inverted, cut several parallel sections, about 2-3 mm apart, perpendicular to the skin surface through the nipple and areola.

3 Breast specimen: reexamine the slices, make additional cuts if necessary, and take sections for histology according to instructions below.

Description

It is preferable to make short notes at the time the specimen is examined the first day and to dictate the whole case the second day.

1 Side (right or left) and type of mastectomy: superradical, radical, modified, simple, subcutaneous

2 List of structures included in specimen: skin, nipple, breast, major and minor pectoralis muscles, fascia, axillary tissue, chest wall structures

3 Weight and dimensions (greatest length of skin and length perpendicular to it)

4 Features of external appearance:
   a Shape and color of skin
   b Location and extent of skin changes (scars, recent surgical incisions, erythema, edema, flattening, retraction, ulceration)
   c Appearance of nipple and areola (erosions, ulceration, retraction, inversion)
   d Location of lesions and other features, which can be designated by stating their distance from nipple and quadrant or their direction in clock face numerals
   e Description of abnormalities on palpation if any

5 Features of cross sections:
   a Relative amounts of fat and parenchyma

b Cysts and dilated ducts: size, number, location, content

c Masses: quadrant and distance from nipple, depth beneath skin, size, shape, consistency, color; necrosis? hemorrhage? calcification? relation or attachment to skin, muscle, fascia, or nipple

d Lymph nodes if present: number of nodes in each group, size of largest node in each group, and size and locations of nodes containing grossly evident tumor

Sections for histology

1 Breast: Take three sections of tumor; sample all lesions noted grossly or roentgenographically; take at least one section from each quadrant (using as guidelines the previously made marks made on the skin) in the following order:

- Upper outer quadrant (UOQ)
- Lower outer quadrant (LOQ)
- Lower inner quadrant (LIQ)
- Upper inner quadrant (UIQ)

2 Nipple: See under Procedure.

3 Pectoralis major muscle (in radical mastectomies): Take one section from any grossly abnormal area or, if none is found, from the area closest to the tumor.

4 Lymph nodes: All identified nodes should be processed for histology. Small nodes are submitted entirely; nodes over 0.5 cm in diameter are sliced. If the axillary fat is grossly involved, a representative section should be taken. Label in the following order:

Radical mastectomy:

- Low axillary (Level I)
- Mid axillary (Level II)
- High axillary (Level III)
- Interpectoral (Rotter's) or, if none found, adipose tissue from this site

Modified mastectomy:

- Lower half
- Upper half

(For this operation it is better not to use the terms low, mid, and high as are used for radical mastectomies.)

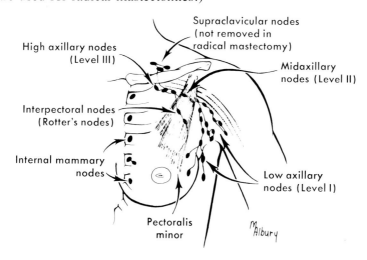

BREAST—MASTECTOMY cont'd

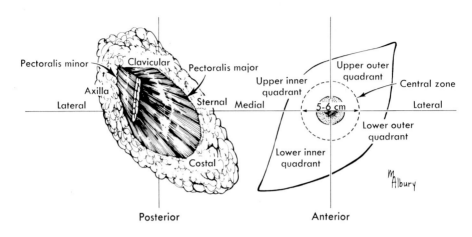

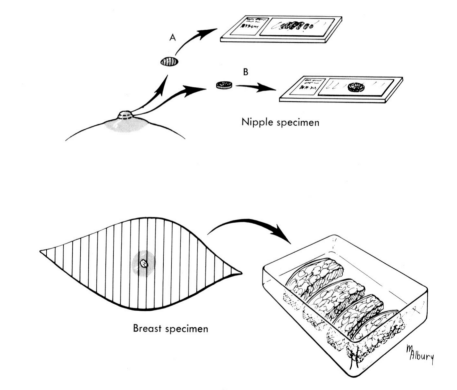

Upper and middle drawings redrawn after National Cancer Institute: Standardized management of breast specimens recommended by Pathology Working Group, Breast Cancer Task Force. Am J Clin Pathol **60**:789-798, 1973; reproduced with permission.

CELL SURFACE MARKERS—SAMPLING

This has become an important and established technique for the evaluation of lymphoreticular proliferations. It may help in identifying a given proliferation as lymphoreticular, in separating a reactive from a neoplastic process, and in specifically identifying the cellular type of proliferation (B lymphocyte, T lymphocyte, histiocyte).

If facilities for the performance of this test are available, it should be used in:

- All specimens from lymph nodes, spleen, or thymus in which the possibility of a proliferative lymphoreticular process is considered
- All tumors with clinical or gross features suggestive of malignant lymphoma
- All tissues in patients with known malignant lymphoma or leukemia in which the possibility of involvement by the disease exists.

The specimen should be received fresh. Ideally, a $2 \times 2 \times 1$ cm piece should be taken for this purpose, placed in a Petri dish having in its bottom a layer of filter paper wet (not overly soaked) with saline solution and submitted to the laboratory immediately. If the specimen is not large enough for a $2 \times 2 \times 1$ cm piece to be taken, sample a fragment as large as feasible.

Note: If cell surface marker studies are to be done in combination with chromosomal or tissue culture studies, in which a piece of tissue needs to be put in culture medium under sterile conditions, it is not necessary to follow the foregoing procedure. Rather, a piece from the sample in the culture medium can be used for this purpose.

CHROMOSOMAL ANALYSIS—SAMPLING

Chromosomal analysis of surgically excised tissues (using direct and indirect techniques) can be useful in the differential diagnosis between reactive and neoplastic processes, and it can demonstrate a specific chromosomal defect associated with a particular type of tumor.

Cut a piece of viable tissue in the fresh state as soon as possible after excision under sterile conditions, drop in a bottle containing culture medium, and submit to the genetics laboratory. The piece should be about 0.5-1 cm in diameter or as large a sample as allowable. If immediate transportation to the laboratory is not feasible, store temporarily in the refrigerator at 4° C.

CULTURES—BACTERIAL, FUNGAL, AND VIRAL

Whenever a fresh specimen is received in the laboratory and there is some indication (clinical, gross appearance, frozen section, etc.) that it may be involved by an infectious process, cultures should be taken, unless this has already been done in the operating room.

Large specimens

Several techniques can be used for large operative specimens (lung, spleen, etc.) received intact in the fresh state:
1. a Burn the surface close to the area to be cultured with a red-hot spatula.
    b Make a deep cut through this sterilized surface with a sterile blade.
    c Cut a portion of tissue from the inside, using sterile forceps and scalpel or scissors. A size of 1 × 1 × 1 cm is recommended.
    d Put the specimen in a sterile container. This method is generally preferable to the one that follows.
2. a Burn the surface as noted in **1 a** and make a deep cut through it with a sterile blade.
    b Introduce a sterile swab stick (such as Culturette) through the opening, push beyond the cut into the tissue, remove, and place in appropriate transport medium.
3. For cystic processes that need to be cultured for anaerobic organisms: Aspirate with a sterile syringe and needle (about 1-4 ml), expel air bubble from the syringe, and inject the sample into an anaerobic vial. If a vial is not available, put a rubber cork on the end of the needle.

Small specimens

1. If the specimen is submitted fresh in a sterile container with the request for bacteriologic studies to be carried out:
    Open the container, cut a portion of tissue with sterile instruments, and transfer to a sterile container.
2. If the need for culture becomes evident after the fresh specimen has been handled in a nonsterile fashion, proceed as follows:
    a Cut a piece of the tissue (approximately 1 × 1 × 1 cm) with a sterile blade.
    b Sterilize a pair of clean forceps by dipping them in ethanol and flaming.
    c Holding the specimen with the sterilized forceps, wash thoroughly with sterile saline solution.
    d Lay specimen down in a sterile container. Sterilize the forceps again and pick up the specimen in a different portion.
    e Repeat the washing with sterile solution.
    f Put the specimen in a sterile container.

All specimens

1. Send specimens to the microbiology laboratory as soon as possible after they have been obtained, properly identified with patient's name and surgical pathology number. If a specimen cannot be sent immediately, place it in the refrigerator at 4° C.

CULTURES—BACTERIAL, FUNGAL, AND VIRAL cont'd

2 Specify the cultures desired and organisms suspected. The usual requests are the following:
- Routine (includes aerobic and the less fastidious anaerobic)
- Anaerobic
- Acid-fast organisms
- Fungi
- Viruses

3 After a sample has been taken for cultures, it is advisable to make a smear from an adjacent area, fix it in alcohol, and stain for the microorganisms suspected (Gram's Ziehl-Neelsen, etc.).

ELECTRON MICROSCOPY—SAMPLING

Fixative

Several fixatives are available for electron microscopy. The most commonly used is 2.5% glutaraldehyde in Millonig's buffer, in amounts of 3-4 ml per vial, which is kept refrigerated at 4° C. The working solution can be stored for up to one month.

Sampling from fresh tissue

Fresh tissue is highly preferable to routinely fixed material. It is imperative for tissue to be handled *immediately* after excision.

1 Put the specimen on a clear cutting board (such as a heavy plastic card) and cut 1 mm thick slices with a sharp razor blade.

2 Place several drops of electron microscopy fixative in another area of the cutting board, place the tissue slice on top, and cover with a few drops of fixative.

3 Chop the slide into 1 mm cubes with a sharp razor blade and immerse them in cold (4° C) fixative. Five to fifteen fragments of tissue are adequate. If the specimen has grossly different areas, submit for electron microscopy in separate containers.

4 Submit to electron microscopy laboratory for processing; the tissue can remain in the electron microscopy fixative for several days at 4° C.

Sampling from routinely fixed tissue

In routinely fixed tissue, there is usually extensive fixation artifact, but at times recognizable diagnostic electron microscopy features are retained (such as desmosomes, neurosecretory granules, melanosomes, etc).

1 Cut a 1 mm slice from an *edge* of the specimen that was in direct contact with the fixative.

2 Proceed as for fresh tissues.

ESOPHAGUS—ESOPHAGECTOMY

Procedure

Two options are available:

1 a Dissect the specimen in the fresh state; open longitudinally from one end to the other, trying to cut on the side opposite the tumor (see accompanying drawing **A**). If a portion of stomach is included, open along the greater curvature in continuity with the esophageal cut (see accompanying drawing **B**).

b Dissect the periesophageal fat and look for lymph nodes. Divide into three portions: adjacent, proximal, and distal to the tumor (the latter might include the cardioesophageal nodes).

c Pin the specimen in a corkboard, mucosal side up, and float in a large formalin container with the specimen on the underside; fix overnight.

d Take two Polaroid photographs and identify in one of them the sites of the sections to be taken.

e Paint the surgical specimens with India ink after the specimens are fixed; this includes both mucosal ends and the soft tissue around the tumor.

2 Fill the lumen with gauze or cotton impregnated with formalin; fix overnight; cut with scissors longitudinally on the side opposite the tumor; complete the division by cutting with a long knife on the opposite side.

Description

1 Length and diameter or circumference of specimen; proximal stomach included? (if so, its length along lesser and greater curvature?)

2 Tumor: size, appearance (fungating? rolled edges? ulcerated?); involve entire organ circumferentially? depth of invasion; extension into stomach and adjacent organs; distance from both lines of resection.

3 Mucosa: appearance of nonneoplastic mucosa; recognizable esophageal mucosa *distal* to tumor? lumen dilated proximal to tumor?

4 Wall: thickened? varices?

5 Stomach if present: features of cardioesophageal junction and of gastric mucosa

6 Lymph nodes: nunber found, size of largest; appear grossly involved by tumor?

Continued

Sections for histology

1 Tumor: four longitudinal sections, one including a portion of nonneoplastic mucosa proximal to tumor and another a portion distal to tumor
2 Nonneoplastic mucosa: two to three transverse sections, at different distances from tumor edge, proximally and/or distally, depending on location of tumor
3 Stomach if present: two sections, one including gastroesophageal junction
4 Proximal line of resection
5 Distal line of resection
6 Lymph nodes:
    a Adjacent to tumor
    b Proximal to tumor
    c Distal to tumor

A

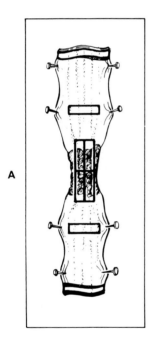

B

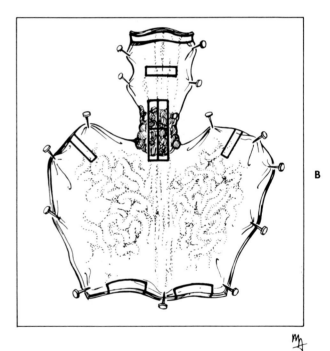

EXTREMITIES—AMPUTATION FOR GANGRENE

(Quoted [with minor changes] from Rodriguez-Martinez HA, Cruz-Ortiz H, Alcantara-Vazquez A, Alcorta-Anguizola B, Burgos-Mendivil J: Dissecting technique for gangrenous lower limbs with vascular occlusions. Pathología **10**:69-78, 1972; reproduced with permission.)

Procedure

1 Removal of femoral, popliteal, and posterior tibial neurovascular bundles and peroneal vessels:

   a Place the extremity on a dissecting board with the posterior surface upward. The dissection will be completed more rapidly if an assistant holds the specimen and helps to retract flaps.

   b Incise longitudinally the skin over the midline of the popliteal region, and the upper two-thirds of the posterior tibial region [see accompanying diagram].

   c Incise obliquely the skin from the lower end of the first incision to 2 cm below the posterior border of the medial malleolus [see accompanying diagram].

   d With a scalpel or knife, cut through the subcutaneous tissue and superficial fascia of the entire incision.

   e In the posterior femoral and popliteal regions separate, with blunt and sharp dissection, the semitendinous, semimembranous, and medial head of the gastrocnemius muscles from the biceps femoris and lateral head of the gastrocnemius. This maneuver will expose the sciatic and posterior tibial nerves and the femoral and popliteal vessels.

   f Deepen the incisions made in steps **b** and **c** in the posterior tibial region, cutting through the gastrocnemius and soleus muscles and the tendo calcaneus. This will show, underneath the intermuscular fascial septum, the posterior tibial neurovascular bundle and the peroneal vessels.

   g Beginning at their upper end, dissect and excise the sciatic and posterior tibial nerves down to the place where the latter nerve joins the popliteal vessels.

   h Beginning at their upper end, dissect and excise the femoral and popliteal vessels down to the place where the latter vessels join the posterior tibial nerve.

   i Excise en bloc the popliteal vessels and the posterior tibial nerve.

   j Continue with the removal of the entire posterior tibial neurovascular bundle, down to the lowest portion of the skin incision, and transect it there. The bundle should be excised together with neighboring portions of muscle and fascia.

   k Lastly, remove the peroneal vessels together with contiguous muscle fibers. These vessels are chiefly located behind the fibula and the interosseous membrane and within the muscle fibers of the flexor hallucis longus.

2 Removal of the anterior tibial neurovascular bundle:

   a Place the extremity with its anterior surface upward.

   b Incise longitudinally the skin, from a point located between the head

Continued

A21

of the fibula and the tibial tuberosity to a joint equidistant between both malleoli [see accompanying diagram].

c With a scalpel or knife, cut through the subcutaneous tissue and superficial fascia of the whole incision.

d In the middle portion of the incision, with scissors or knife, cut through the fibers of the tibialis anterior muscle down to the interosseous membrane. This will uncover part of the anterior tibial neurovascular bundle.

e With sharp or blunt dissection, separate partially the regional muscular masses in the upper portion and the tendons in the lower portion, so as to expose lengthwise the anterior tibial neurovascular bundle.

f Cut across the lowest portion of the anterior tibial neurovascular bundle. Pull the bundle downwards and excise it together with portions of adjacent muscles and interosseous membrane. The upper end of the bundle becomes loose just exerting traction downward.

3 Removal of the tissue block with the dorsalis pedis vessels:

a Trace a 3-4 cm wide rectangle over the dorsum of the foot, extending from the lowest part of the anterior tibial incision to the proximal portion of the first interosseous space.

b Following the sides of the rectangle, cut through the skin, subcutaneous tissue, superficial fascia, regional muscles and tendons, and deep fascia. Actually, cut down to the very dorsal surface of the regional bones.

c With a scalpel or knife, excise the whole tissue block, clearing away all the soft tissues from the underlying bones. The vessels lie very deep in this region.

4 Removal of the tissue blocks with the medial and lateral plantar vessels:

a Place the extremity with the posterior surface upward.

b Trace a rectangle on the sole with the following anatomic landmarks: posterior border of the medial malleolus, medial side of the foot, base of the metatarsal bones, and lateral side of the foot. The transverse limits can also be determined, approximately, dividing the sole in fifths.

c Following the sides of the rectangle, cut through the skin, subcutaneous tissue, plantar aponeurosis and fascia, and regional muscles and tendons. In fact, cut down to the very plantar surfaces of the regional bones.

d With sharp dissection, remove the entire tissue block so as to leave fully exposed the regional bones and ligaments.

e Bisect longitudinally the tissue block. The medial half represents the tissue block of the medial plantar vessels, while the lateral half represents the tissue block of the lateral plantar vessels.

5 Takes samples of skin and soft tissues from areas of ulceration, necrosis, or infection and from bone if indicated. Now the extremity can be disposed of.

6 Fix all the excised tissues overnight in formalin. The neurovascular bundles should be pinned down on corkboard.

7 Once neurovascular bundles are well fixed, cut transversely every 4-5 mm and examine carefully the wall and lumen of vessels.

Description

1 Type of amputation; side of extremity
2 Length and circumference
3 Appearance of skin: ulcers (size, extent), hemorrhage, stasis dermatitis
4 Subcutaneous tissue; muscle; bone and joints
5 Appearance of major arteries and veins: atherosclerosis (degree), thrombosis

Sections for histology

1 Skin
2 Major arteries, veins, and nerves according to accompanying diagram or an abbreviated version of it
3 Skeletal muscle
4 Bone and joint (when pertinent)

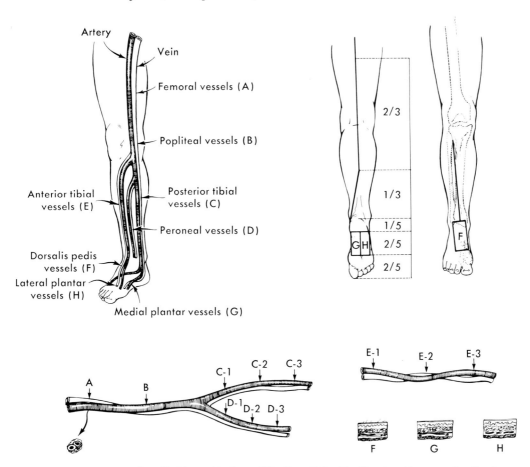

Diagrams redrawn after Rodriguez-Martinez HA, Cruz-Ortiz H, Alcantara-Vazquez A, Alcorta-Anguizola B, Burgos-Mendivil J: Dissecting technique for gangrenous lower limbs with vascular occlusions. Patología **10**:69-78, 1972; reproduced with permission.

EXTREMITIES—AMPUTATION FOR OSSEOUS TUMOR

Procedure

1 Measure the length and circumference (including a measure of the circumference at the level of the tumor if this is apparent or known).

2 Determine the presence, position, and dimensions of biopsy sites.

3 Search for the major lymph node groups, identify, and place in separate containers.

4 Cut a cross section of the proximal bone margin with a band saw.

5 Dissect out all the soft tissues (down to the periosteum) around the involved bone with a scalpel, forceps, and scissors. Review the clinical and roentgenographic findings before proceeding. If there is any indication (from the roentgenograms or at the time of dissection) of soft tissue extension by the tumor, dissect *around* this area and keep it in continuity with the bone. If, from the roentgenograms, the tumor does not seem to involve the joint, cut through it; if it does, leave the joint intact and make a cross section with the band saw through the adjacent noninvolved bone, approximately 5-10 cm from the joint. If a previous incision site is present, take a sample for histology at this time, along the entire course of the incision.

6 Cut longitudinally the bone specimen thus obtained with a band saw. In most cases, a section dividing the specimen into an anterior and a posterior half is preferable; in others, sagittal, lateralized, or even oblique cuts are to be recommended. The type of bone involved and the location of the tumor as seen roentgenographically will determine which plane of section will give the most information.

7 Examine the cut section and take regular and two sets of Polaroid photographs; identify in one set of the latter the site of the sections to be taken.

8 Examine under Wood's light if tetracycline had been administered before amputation (to detect satellite foci).

9 Cut a parallel section with the band saw, producing a slice about 5 mm thick. Use a saw guide for this purpose. Take a roentgenogram of the slice. Make additional cuts of the remaining bone pieces if indicated. It might be desirable to take additional photographs (regular and Polaroid) at this time.

10 Quickly dissect the soft tissues that had been peeled off the involved bone; cut sagitally with the band saw all major bones that were left in this portion of the specimen, and examine carefully for other foci of tumor or other lesions. Open the major joints and examine them.

Description

1 Type of amputation; side of extremity

2 Length and circumference of extremity, including circumference at level of tumor

3 Presence, position, and dimensions of biopsy sites

4 Tumor characteristics:

   a Location: bone involved; diaphysis, metaphysis, or epiphysis? medulla, cortex, or periosteum? epiphyseal line apparent? (if so, tumor crossing it?) tumor involve articular cartilage and joint cavity? tumor extend into soft tissue? periosteum elevated by tumor? (if so, to what extent?) invaded by tumor? if previous incision present, evidence of tumor extension along it?

   b Features of tumor: size, shape, color, borders, consistency; appear to be bone-forming, cartilaginous, fibrous, or myxoid? cystic changes, hemorrhage, or necrosis?

   c Distance of tumor to osseous margin of resection

5 Appearance of bone away from tumor; satellite lesions? any fluorescent foci seen if examined under Wood's light?

6 Appearance of remaining extremity, if abnormal; if not, so state; skin, subcutaneous fat, muscles, major vessels and nerves, other bones, joints

7 Appearance and approximate number of lymph nodes found

Sections for histology

1 Tumor: four sections or more depending on case
All grossly dissimilar areas should be sampled. Whenever possible, sections should be taken to include the periphery of the tumor *and* adjacent cortex, medulla, epiphyseal line, articular cartilage, periosteum, and soft tissues.

2 Previous incision site (if present) taken all along its course

3 Section from grossly noninvolved bone, midway between tumor and margin of resection
If the tumor involves upper end of a bone, take this section from midportion of proximally located bone.

4 Osseous margin of resection

5 Any abnormal-looking areas elsewhere in bone, soft tissues, or skin

6 Lymph nodes: if grossly normal, only representative ones; if grossly abnormal or there is clinical suspicion of metastases, all of them

EXTREMITIES—AMPUTATION FOR SOFT TISSUE TUMOR

Procedure

1 Measure the length and circumference (including a measure of the circumference at the level of the tumor).

2 Determine the presence, position, and dimensions of biopsy sites.

3 Search for the major lymph node groups, identify, and place in separate containers.

4 Cut through the skin and carefully dissect the subcutaneous fat, muscles, and major arteries, veins, and nerves *around* the tumor, avoiding cutting through the latter. Use an anatomy atlas as a guide if necessary. Try to determine as accurately as possible the relationship of the tumor with the following structures: skin, subcutaneous fat, specific muscles, arteries, veins, and nerves, periosteum, and bone. Mark some of the major anatomic landmarks with tags if indicated.

5 As soon as all the margins of the tumor have been determined, remove the entire area with a good margin of normal tissues using a scalpel and scissors.

6 Two options are available for studying the specimen thus obtained as outlined below. The first is used in most instances, but the second is preferable in selected cases. In either case, if a previous incision site it present, take a sample for histology at this time along the entire course of the incision.

   a Divide the tumor into slices with a large, sharp knife. Continue the dissection with the forceps, scissors, and scalpel to determine the tumor relationship with the structures previously mentioned. Place several pieces from different areas in formalin, fix for several hours or overnight, and trim to place in cassettes.

   b Place the entire specimen in a large pan containing formalin, cover with a towel, leave in the refrigerator at 4° C overnight, and cut parallel slices with a large, sharp knife. Take roentgenograms if pertinent. Take two Polaroid photographs and identify in one of them the site of the sections to be taken.

7 Quickly dissect the soft tissues from the rest of the extremity, looking for other foci of tumor or other lesions.

8 Cut the major bones of the extremities longitudinally with a band saw. Make one of the sections through the area of bone closest to the soft tissue tumor. Examine for tumor extension or other lesions.

9 Open the major joints and examine them.

Description

1 Type of amputation; side of extremity

2 Length and circumference of extremity, including circumference at level of tumor

3 Presence, position, and dimensions of biopsy sites

4 Tumor characteristics:
  a Primary location: subcutaneous fat; muscle compartment(s) (specify which); fascial planes.
  b Tumor extension into and relation with skin, subcutaneous fat, deep fascia, muscle, periosteum, bone, joint vessels, and nerves (specify which); presence of obvious vascular or neural involvement by tumor
  c If previous incision present, evidence of tumor extension along it?
  d Size (three dimensions), shape, color, borders (encapsulated? pushing? infiltrating?), consistency, secondary changes (cysts, necrosis? hemorrhage?)
  e Presence of myxoid changes, foci of calcification, cartilage, or bone
  f Shortest distance of tumor from margin of resection
5 Appearance of remaining extremity if abnormal (if not, so state); skin, subcutaneous fat, muscles, major vessels and nerves, bone (tumor invasion? osteoporosis? bone marrow?), joints (osteoarthritis?)
6 Appearance and approximate number of lymph nodes found

Sections for histology

1 Tumor: four sections or more depending on case
  All grossly dissimilar areas should be sampled. Whenever possible, sections should be taken to include the periphery of the tumor *and* adjacent fat, muscle, skin, periosteum, vessels, and/or more nerves.
2 Previous incision site (if present) taken all along its course
3 Lymph nodes: if grossly normal, only representative ones; if grossly abnormal or if clinical suspicion of metastases, all of them
4 Proximal margins of resection: subcutaneous fat and muscle (plus skin and/or bone if indicated)

EYES—ENUCLEATION

Procedure

1 Fix the intact ocular globe in formalin for twenty-four hours before sectioning; it is not advisable to open the eye, to cut windows into the sclera, or to inject fixative into the vitreous.

2 Wash in running tap water for one or more hours and, optionally, place in 60% ethyl alcohol for a few more hours.

3 Review the summary of the clinical history and the results of the ophthalmologic examination prior to sectioning.

4 Measure anteroposterior, horizontal, and vertical dimensions of the globe, length of the optic nerve, and horizontal dimensions of the cornea.

5 Look for sites of accidental or surgical injuries.

6 Transilluminate the globe before opening it. A substage microscope lamp in a darkened room is satisfactory. Rotate the globe over the light source; if abnormal shadows are detected, mark them on the sclera with an indelible pencil.

7 Examination of the globe with a ×7 objective of a dissecting microscope can be carried out to detect minute lesions.

8 If intraocular foreign bodies or retinoblastoma is suspected, take a roentgenogram of the globe before it is opened.

9 If choroidal malignant melanoma is suspected, sample at least one of the vortex veins from each of the four quadrants (see accompanying drawing).

10 Open the eye with a sharp razor blade by holding the globe with the left hand, cornea down against the cutting block, and holding the blade between the thumb and middle finger of the right hand. Open the eye with a sawing motion from back to front. The plane of section should begin adjacent to the optic nerve and end through the periphery of the cornea. The plane of section is dependent on whether a lesion has been detected in the previous steps. If it has not, cut the globe along a horizontal plane, using as surface landmarks the superior and inferior oblique insertions and the long postciliary vein (see accompanying drawing). If a lesion has been found, modify the plane of section so that the lesion will be included in the slab.

11 Examine the interior of the globe.

12 Place the eye flat on its cut surface and make a second plane of section, parallel to the first, again passing from back to front.

13 Examine carefully the ~8 mm disk-shaped slab thus obtained, which should contain the cornea, pupils, lens, and optic nerve. Take regular and Polaroid photographs if indicated.

Description
Intact eye

1 Side of the globe (see accompanying drawing); anteroposterior, horizontal, and vertical dimensions

2 Length of optic nerve

3 Horizontal and vertical dimensions of cornea

4 Anterior segment: surgical incisions? corneal opacification? iris abnormalities? lens present?

5 Transillumination findings

Slab

1 Corneal thickness; anterior chamber depth; configuration of anterior chamber angle

2 Condition of iris, ciliary body, and lens

3 Condition of choroid, retina, vitreous body, and optic disk

4 If tumor present: location, size, color, edges, consistency, presence of hemorrhage or necrosis, ocular structures involved, extension into optic nerve

Sections for histology

1 Entire eye slab

2 Any (other) abnormal areas

3 In tumors, particularly retinoblastoma: cross section of surgical margin of optic nerve

4 In suspected malignant melanoma: sample from at least one of vortex veins from each of four quadrants

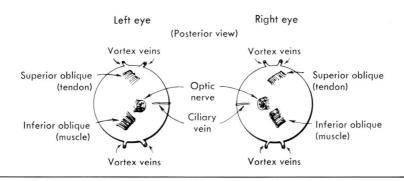

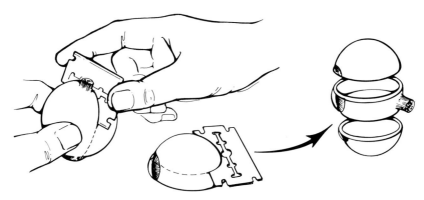

FALLOPIAN TUBES—LIGATION

Procedure

1 Keep specimens from right and left tubes separate.
2 Measure the length and diameter of each.

Description

1 Length and diameter of each specimen.
2 Do they appear to be a complete segment of each tube? lumen present?

Sections for histology

1 All tissue received, identified as to right and left tube
2 Very important that tissue be sectioned on end; instructions to histotechnician or embedding in agar may be necessary.

FALLOPIAN TUBES—SALPINGECTOMY

Procedure

1 Fix the specimen before sectioning. If the tubes are attached to the uterus, they should be fixed in that position.
2 Measure the length and greatest diameter.
3 If the tube is relatively normal in size, serially section at 5 mm intervals and examine. Make the cuts incomplete so that the pieces remain attached by the serosa.
4 If the tube is obviously enlarged, make one complete longitudinal section, followed by parallel sections if necessary.

Description

1 Length and greatest diameter
2 Serosa: fibrin? hemorrhage? fibrous adhesions to ovary or other organs?
3 Wall: abnormally thick? ruptured?
4 Mucosa: atrophic? hyperplastic? appearance of fimbriated end; inverted?
5 Lumen: patent? dilated? content; diameter if abnormally large
6 Masses: size, appearance, invasion
7 Cysts in paraovarian region: diameter, thickness of wall, content; sessile or pedunculated?
8 In cases of suspected ectopic pregnancy: embryo or placenta identified? amount of hemorrhage; rupture?

Sections for histology

1 For incidental tubes without gross abnormalities: three cross sections of each tube, taken from the proximal, mid, and distal portions, submitted in the same cassette (see accompanying drawing).

2 For tubes with suspected ectopic pregnancy: submit any tissue with gross appearance of products of conception. If none is grossly identified, submit several sections from the wall in the area of hemorrhage as well as several from the *intraluminal clot*. If products of conception are not identified microscopically, submit additional sections.

3 For tubes with other lesions: as many as needed to adequately examine any abnormal areas. If tumor is present, at least three sections must be taken to include grossly uninvolved mucosa.

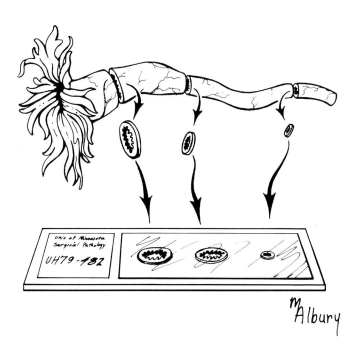

FETUS—ABORTION

Procedure

Depending on size, keep intact, cut sagitally, or dissect.

Description

1 Crown-rump or crown-heel length (see accompanying drawings), sex and weight
2 Approximate length of gestation (see accompanying table)
3 General condition: well preserved? macerated?
4 Anomalies and other changes
5 Umbilical cord: appearance

Sections for histology

1 Small embryos: submit whole embryo or one-half, depending on size.
2 Large fetuses: Submit sections only if grossly abnormal areas are found.

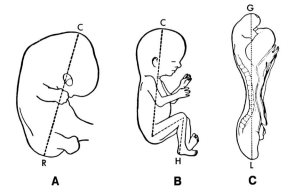

Measurement of embryos. **A,** Crown-rump length. **B,** Crown-heel length. **C,** Greatest length. (From Arey LB: Developmental anatomy, ed. 7. Philadelphia, 1974, W. B. Saunders Co.)

Relations of age, size, and weight in the human embryo*

Age of embryo	Crown-heel length (mm)	Crown-heel length (mm)‡	External diameter of chorionic sac (mm)	Weight in grams	Amount of increase each month when value at start of month equals unity	
					CR length	Weight
One week	0.1†	. . . .	0.2			
Two weeks	0.2†	. . . .	3			
Three weeks	2.0	. . . .	10			
Four weeks	5.0	. . . .	20	.02	49.0	40000.00
Five weeks	8.0	. . . .	25			
Six weeks	12.0	. . . .	30			
Seven weeks	17.0	19.0	40			
Two lunar months	25.0	30.0	50	1	3.6	49.00
Three lunar months	56.0	73.0	. . . .	14	1.4	13.00
Four lunar months	112.0	157.0	. . . .	105	1.0	6.50
Five lunar months	160.0	239.0	. . . .	310	0.43	1.95
Six lunar months	203.0	296.0	. . . .	640	0.26	1.07
Seven lunar months	242.0	355.0	. . . .	1080	0.14	0.69
Eight lunar months	277.0	409.0	. . . .	1670	0.14	0.55
Nine lunar months	313.0	458.0	. . . .	2400	0.13	0.43
Full term (38 weeks)	350.0	500.0	. . . .	3300	0.12	0.38

*From Arey LB: Developmental anatomy, ed 7. Philadelphia, 1974, W. B. Saunders Co.
†Total length of embryonic disc.
‡Recent study (Iffy L, Shepard TH, Jakobovits A, Lemire RJ, Kerner P: The rate of growth in young human embryos of Streeter's horizons XIII to XXIII. Acta Anat 66:178-186, 1967): 7 wk = 23 mm; 8 wk = 32 mm.

GALLBLADDER—CHOLECYSTECTOMY

Procedure

1 Open the entire organ longitudinally as soon as feasible after excision; otherwise the mucosa will quickly undergo autolytic changes.
2 If stones are present, wash them, estimate the number and the size of the largest, and cut one or several of them with a scalpel.
3 Search for lymph nodes along the bladder neck.
4 In cases of carcinoma, the organ also can be studied by extracting the bile with a syringe, filling the lumen with formalin, fixing overnight at 4° C, and cutting the specimen with scissors and a scalpel.

Description

1 Length and greatest diameter of gallbladder
2 Serosa: thickened? fibrous adhesions? fibrin?
3 Wall: thickened? if so, focally or diffusely? hemorrhage?
4 Mucosa: color, appearance, ulcerated? hyperplastic? cholesterosis?
5 Cystic duct: dilated? impacted with stones? lymph nodes present? size and appearance
6 Approximate volume, color, and consistency of bile
7 Stones: approximate number, shape, and size range; color and appearance on cross section; type of stone (see accompanying table)

Sections for histology

1 Two sections from mucosa to serosa taken through areas that appear grossly more abnormal
2 Cystic duct and lymph nodes if they appear grossly abnormal

Types of gallstones*

Type of stone	Incidence	Composition	Appearance
Pure	10%	Cholesterol	Solitary; crystalline surface
		Calcium bilirubinate	Multiple; jet black; crystalline or amorphous
		Calcium carbonate	Grayish white; amorphous

Mixed	80%	Cholesterol and calcium bilirubinate	Multiple, faceted or lobulated, laminated, and crystalline on cut surfaces
			Hue:
			  Yellow—cholesterol
			  Black—calcium bilirubinate
			  White—calcium carbonate

		Cholesterol and calcium carbonate	
		Calcium bilirubinate and calcium carbonate	
		Cholesterol, calcium bilirubinate, and calcium carbonate	
Combined	10%	Pure gallstone nucleus with mixed gallstone shell	Largest of gallstones when single Hue depends on composition of shell
		Mixed gallstone nucleus with pure gallstone shell	

*Slightly modified from Halpert B: Gallbladder and biliary ducts. In Anderson WAD, Kissane JM (eds): Pathology, ed. 7. St. Louis, 1977, The C. V. Mosby Co.

HEART—VALVE REPLACEMENT

(Adapted from Roberts WC, Morrow AG: Cardiac valves and the surgical pathologist. Arch Pathol **82:**309-313, 1966. Copyright 1966, American Medical Association.)

Procedure

1 Fix the specimen before sectioning
2 Take Polaroid photographs and a roentgenogram in every case. For atrioventricular valves, photograph from both atrial and ventricular aspects. For aortic valves, photograph from both aortic and ventricular aspects.

Description
Atrioventricular valve

1 Leaflets fibrotic, calcified, or normal?
2 Fibrosis or calcification focal or diffuse?
3 Fibrosis or calcification distributed on leaflets? (only at margins? on one surface? on both?)
4 Leaflets immobile, shortened, stretched, or normal?
5 Commissures fused? (if so, to what extent?)
6 Chordae tendineae intact, ruptured, shortened, elongated, fused, or normal?
7 Papillary muscles normal in number, scarred, hypertrophied, or elongated?
8 Valve incompetent, stenotic, or both?
9 If incompetent, due to scanty valvular tissue, dilated annulus, or ruptured chordae or to ruptured, scarred, or shortened papillary muscle?

Semilunar valves

1 Same as for atrioventricular valve in most respects plus:
2 Number of cusps present
3 Cusps of equal or unequal size?

Sections for histology

Several sections, including free edge; decalcify if necessary

HORMONE RECEPTOR ASSAYS—SAMPLING

(Adapted from Keffer JH: Hormone-receptor assays and cancer of the breast. The pathologist's role [editorial]. Am J Clin Pathol **70**:719-720, 1978; reproduced with permission.)

Biochemical determination of receptors for different steroids hormones (estrogens, progesterone, androgens) has become an established technique for the evaluation of several surgically excised tissues, particularly breast carcinoma. It correlates with clinical response to hormone therapy and, according to some, also with clinical response to chemotherapeutic agents. In some cases of metastatic cancer, it may provide some indication of the site of origin of the primary lesion. Sampling should be taken of recurrent or metastatic carcinoma even if the original tumor had been previously assayed in order to establish the continued presence or absence of the receptor.

1 Examine tissue in the fresh state, immediately after excision; select a sample carefully, avoiding areas of necrosis, adipose tissue, and other nonsuitable areas.

2 Cut a sample measuring approximately 1 cm in greatest diameter (or as large as allowable). The instruments should be clean but not necessarily sterile.

3 Freeze quickly in liquid nitrogen, in isopentane, or with freon spray.

4 Store in the deep freezer until the sample is ready to be delivered (in the frozen state) to the appropriate laboratory.

5 Submit for histology (for control purposes) a piece of tissue immediately adjacent to the one frozen and identify as such.

IMPRINTS (TOUCH PREPARATIONS)

(Adapted from Berard CW, Bowling MC: Technical factors in evaluation of lymph node biopsies. Tutorial on Neoplastic Hematopathology, Henry Rappaport, M.D., Director, Pasadena, California, Feb. 5-9, 1979; presented in cooperation with The City of Hope National Medical Center and The University of Chicago Center for Continuing Education.)

1 Cut a block of tissue measuring approximately 10 × 10 × 3 mm.

2 Hold the tissue gently with forceps with the freshly cut, flat surface upward.

3 With the other hand, lightly touch an alcohol-clean glass slide repeatedly in serial adjacent areas with the cut surface of the tissue. Just contact — do not compress the block. If the surface touched is excessively bloody or wet, discard the slide and repeat with another slide until the touch preparations are barely opaque. Prepare an average of four slides in this fashion.

4 As each slide is prepared, dry it rapidly by waving it in air. Do not heat or blow on the slide. It should take no more than 30-60 sec for the slide to dry; if it takes more, it means that the touches are too wet and that the resulting imprints will be unsatisfactory.

5 For standard purposes, fix (after drying) in methyl alcohol and stain two with hematoxylin-eosin and two with Wright's or Giemsa's stain.

6 After preparation of the imprints, fix and submit for histology the block used for this purpose in order to correlate its appearance with that of the imprints.

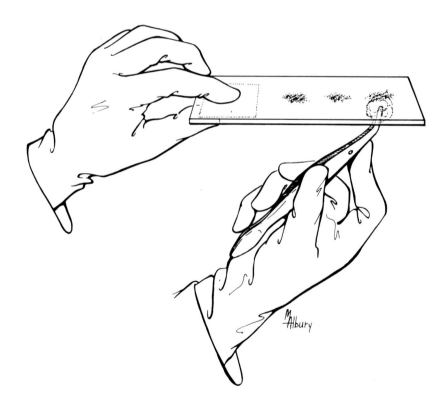

INJECTION OF SPECIMENS—GENERAL GUIDELINES

When feasible, the injection of surgical specimens may serve to illustrate more clearly the gross pathology present, as well as to ensure proper fixation. The procedure has been found most useful for lobectomies, pneumonectomies, cystectomies, colectomies, and pelvic exenterations.

1 Fill a large container partially with fixative.
2 Prepare the specimen properly (see specific instructions for the respective organs).
3 Place in container and inject with formalin.
4 Add additional fixative to the container to ensure that the entire specimen is covered by fixative.
5 Place a towel or several gauze pads over the free-floating specimen to prevent the surface from drying.
6 Cover the container with a lid.
7 Fix for twenty-four hours before dissecting.

JAW RESECTION FOR TUMOR—MANDIBULECTOMY

Procedure

1 Fix the whole specimen in formalin overnight in the refrigerator at 4° C.
2 Paint the surgical margins with India ink.
3 *For bone tumors:* Make multiple sections through bone and soft tissue with a band saw, fix further in formalin, and decalcify.
4 *For mucosal or soft tissue tumors:* Separate soft tissue from the mandible with a scalpel. The direction of the dissection should be from below to above and from the back to the anterior aspect.
5 If the specimen includes a radical neck dissection, process according to instructions for Lymph node dissection—Radical neck.

Description

1 Type of resection (partial or total) and side
2 Lesion: size, color, appearance, edges; bone invaded?
3 Nonneoplastic mucosa: leukoplakia?
4 Bone: appearance on cross sections
5 Teeth: number and appearance

Sections for histology

1 Tumor: three sections
2 Nonneoplastic mucosa
3 Mucosal surgical margins
4 Soft tissue surgical margins
5 Bone surgical margins
6 Mandibular nerve (surgical margins)
7 Bone if grossly involved or suspicious

JAW RESECTION FOR TUMOR—MAXILLECTOMY

Procedure

1 Fix the specimen in formalin overnight in the refrigerator at 4° C.

2 Paint the surgical margins with India ink.

3 Take surgical margins (anterior, posterior, external, and superior); cut the specimen with the band saw in parallel slices 0.5 cm thick. Fix them overnight. Take photographs and roentgenograms if indicated.

4 Take two Polaroid photographs and identify in one of them the site of the sections to be taken.

Description

1 Extent of resection

2 Presence of following structures: hard palate, soft palate, superior, middle, and inferior turbinates, medial and lateral pterygoid plate of sphenoid bone, air cells of ethmoid, bony floor of orbit, orbital contents, zygoma, masseter, temporalis, external and internal pterygoid muscles.

3 Tumor characteristics: location, extent, size; limited to the maxillary sinus? arise from superior, medial, lateral, anterior, posterior, or inferior part of sinus? extend into intratemporal fossa, nasal cavity, ethmoid cells, or any other of aforementioned structures? presence of tumor at surgical margins?

4 Condition of ostium of maxillary sinus and any other sinuses present; fistulae present?

Sections for histology

1 Tumor: as many sections as necessary, with minimum of three

2 Surgical margins

KIDNEY—NEEDLE BIOPSY

Procedure

The examination and sampling of this material should be carried out at the bedside or *immediately* after the specimen is received in the pathology laboratory.

1 Measure the length and diameter.

2 Try to determine by gross inspection whether the cortex is present; this can be done by identifying glomeruli with a dissecting microscope or magnifying lenses. An experienced observer can do it most of the time with the naked eye on the basis of the color.

3 If the cortex is grossly identified:

    a Take three pieces (1 mm thick each) from this area and fix in glutaraldehyde for electron microscopic examination.

    b Take one additional piece (2 mm thick) from this area and freeze in isopentane cooled with liquid nitrogen for immunofluorescence.

    c Place the remainder of the specimen in fixative for routine light microscopy. We use Zenker's fixative.

4 If the cortex cannot be identified with certainty on gross inspection, the operator may decide to perform another needle biopsy. Otherwise, the following should be done with the specimen:

    a Take two pieces (1 mm each) from *each* end and fix for electron microscopy.

    b Take two additional pieces (2 mm each) from *each* end and freeze for immunofluorescence.

    c Fix the remainder for routine histology.

5 If the amount of tissue is insufficient to divide for all these studies, electron microscopy and immunofluorescence have priority, one of the reasons being that a modified version of the light microscopic evaluation can be carried out on them.

6 If the specimen is an open wedge biopsy, the same guidelines apply, except for the fact that the cortex is always readily identifiable and therefore double sampling is not necessary.

Description

1 Number of fragments; length and diameter of each
2 Color: homogeneous or not?
3 Cortex recognizable? glomeruli: size, color, prominence

Sections for histology

1 See under Procedure
2 Needle renal biopsies routinely stained with:

    a Hematoxylin-eosin
    b Alcian blue-PAS
    c Jones' silver methenamine
    d Masson's trichrome

KIDNEY—NEPHRECTOMY
FOR NONTUMORAL CONDITION

Procedure

1 Measure and weigh the organ.
2 Two options are available depending on the type of abnormality present and the status of the organ when received in the laboratory:
   a Cut the kidney sagitally, strip the capsule, and carefully open the pelvis, calyces, and ureter.
   b Inject with formalin through the ureter and, if possible, through the renal artery, ligate the ureter (and artery), and submerge in formalin overnight. Cut sagitally the next day, strip the capsule, and open the pelvis, calyces, and ureter. This technique is especially useful in cases of hydronephrosis.
3 Take two Polaroid photographs and identify in one of them the sites of the sections to be taken.
4 If stones are present, submit for chemical analysis if indicated.

Description

1 Weight and size of kidney
2 Capsule: amount of pericapsular tissue, thickness of capsule, adherence to cortex
3 External surface: smooth? scars: number, size, shape (flat or V shaped?); cysts? (if so, number, size, location, content)
4 Cortex: color, width; glomeruli apparent? striations apparent and orderly?
5 Medulla: color, width; medullary rays apparent and orderly?
6 Pelvis: size; dilated? blunting of calyces? thickened? hemorrhage? crystalline deposits? stones; number, size, and shape; amount of peripelvic fat
7 Ureter: diameter, length, evidence of dilatation or stricture
8 Renal artery and vein; appearance

Sections for histology

1 Kidney: three sections, each including cortex and medulla
2 Pelvis: two sections
3 Ureter

Continued

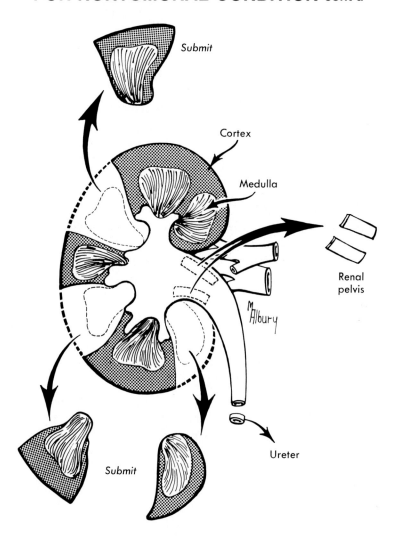

Submit

Cortex

Medulla

Renal pelvis

Ureter

Submit

KIDNEY—NEPHRECTOMY FOR TUMOR

Procedure

1 Look for and dissect any perirenal lymph nodes.
2 Look for and open the renal vein longitudinally.
3 Cut the kidney sagitally and open the pelvis, calyces, and ureter.
4 Strip the capsule and look for capsular and perirenal tumor extension.
5 If stones are present, submit for chemical analysis.
6 Take two Polaroid photographs and identify in one of them the sites of the sections to be taken.

Description

1 Weight and dimensions of specimen; length and diameter of ureter
2 Tumor characteristics: size, shape, location, extent, homogeneity, necrosis, hemorrhage; invasion of capsule, perirenal tissues, calyces, pelvis, and renal vein
3 Uninvolved kidney: external surface, cortex, medulla
4 Pelvis: dilated? blunting of calyces? stones?
5 Presence, number, size, and appearance of perirenal lymph nodes

Sections for histology

1 Tumor: three sections, including one with adjacent kidney
2 Kidney not involved by tumor: two sections
3 Pelvis: one section
4 Renal artery and vein
5 Ureter
6 Lymph nodes if present

LARGE BOWEL—COLECTOMY FOR NONTUMORAL CONDITION

Procedure

1 Dissect a few lymph nodes and remove the mesentery while the specimen is fresh.

2 Two options are available to study the bowel, depending on the type of abnormality present and the status of the specimen when received in the laboratory:

   a Open the specimen longitudinally, pin on a corkboard, and fix overnight in formalin.

   b Inject the specimen with formalin. See Injection of specimens — General guidelines. Evacuate gross fecal contents by gentle external massage of the specimen. Further cleansing may be accomplished by the use of a gentle stream of formalin or saline solution (*not* water) into the bowel lumen. One end of the specimen is tied off, the specimen is injected with formalin, and the other end is tied off. If a constricting lesion is present, be sure that adequate fixative can be easily passed through the point of constriction. If this cannot be achieved, the main mass will not be properly fixed; under these circumstances, it is better to open the specimen and fix as noted in **2 a** rather than to inject on both sides of the lesions. Injection is especially demonstrative in cases of diverticulosis.

3 Take two Polaroid photographs and identify in one of them the sites of the sections to be taken.

4 In general, take the sections *perpendicular* to the direction of the mucosal folds.

Description

1 Part of bowel removed, length of specimen, and amount of mesentery

2 Mucosa: type of lesions, extent, ulceration (linear or transverse), depth, pseudopolyps, hemorrhage, fissures

3 Wall: thickening (focal or diffuse), atrophy, fibrosis, necrosis

4 Serosa: fibrin, pus, fibrosis, adherence of mesentery

5 Diverticula: number, size, location in relation to teniae, content, evidence of inflammation, hemorrhage, or perforation

Sections for histology

1 As many as necessary to sample abnormal areas

2 Proximal and distal lines of resection in cases of colitis

3 Appendix if included in specimen

LARGE BOWEL—COLECTOMY FOR TUMOR

Procedure

1 Dissect the lymph nodes and remove the mesentery while the specimen is fresh.
2 Two options are available to study the bowel, depending on the size and location of the tumor and the status of the specimen when received in the laboratory:
   a Open the bowel longitudinally through its entire length, trying not to cut through the tumor. Pin the intestine on a corkboard and fix overnight in formalin.
   b Inject the specimen (see Injection of specimens—General guidelines and **2, b** under Procedure in the preceding section).
3 Take two Polaroid photographs and identify in one of them the sites of the sections to be taken.
4 In cases with deep penetration by tumor, dissect the veins carefully for possible tumor invasion.
5 In general, take the sections *perpendicular* to the direction of the mucosal folds.

Description

1 Part of bowel removed, length of specimen, and amount of mesentery
2 a Tumor characteristics: size (including thickness); extent around bowel; shape (fungating, flat, ulcerating); presence of necrosis or hemorrhage; extent through bowel wall; serosal involvement; satellite nodules; evidence of blood vessel invasion; invasion of adjacent organs
   b Distance of tumor to pectinate line, peritoneal reflection, each line of resection
3 Other lesions in bowel and appearance of uninvolved mucosa; if polyps absent, so state
4 Estimate of number of lymph nodes found; whether or not nodes appear involved by tumor; size of largest node

Continued

LARGE BOWEL—COLECTOMY FOR TUMOR cont'd

Sections for histology

1 Tumor: three sections

2 Representative section of subserosal connective tissue, fat, and blood vessel around tumor

3 Other lesions of bowel

4 Proximal line of resection

5 Distal line of resection

6 Bowel between tumor and distal line of resection (halfway or 5 cm, whichever suits case)

7 Appendix if included in specimen

8 Lymph nodes:

   a Around tumor

   b Distal to tumor

   c Proximal to tumor

   d At high point of resection (areas surrounding vessels ligation)

9 In abdominoperineal resections:

   a Anorectal junction

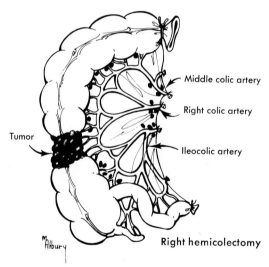

Right hemicolectomy

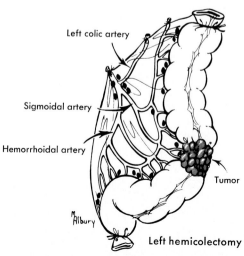

Left hemicolectomy

LARGE BOWEL—POLYPECTOMY

Procedure

1 Fix the specimen intact in formalin for several hours.
2 Measure the diameter of the head and length of the stalk.
3 For polyps with a short stalk or no stalk, identify the surgical section and cut in half longitudinally (see accompanying drawing **A**).
4 For polyps with a long stalk (1 cm or more), cut a cross section of the stalk near the surgical margin and then cut the polyp longitudinally, leaving as long a stalk as will fit in the cassette (see accompanying drawing **B**).
5 If the half of the polyp head is over 3 mm, trim to this thickness on the convex side.

Description

1 Dimensions of polyp; diameter of head and length of stalk
2 Polyp sessile or pedunculated? ulcerated? surface smooth or papillary? any cysts on cross section? stalk appear normal?

Sections for histology

1 One longitudinal section (including surgical margin in polyps with short stalk or no stalk)
2 One cross section of base of stalk (in polyps with long stalk)

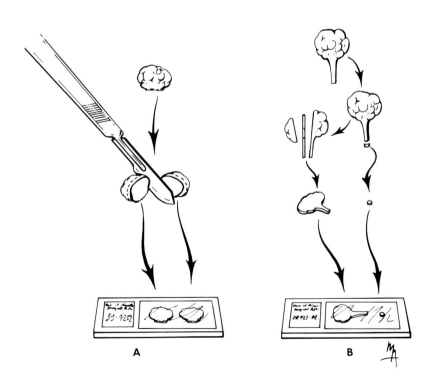

A

B

LARYNX—LARYNGECTOMY

Procedure

1 Separate the larynx from the radical neck dissection if accompanied by the latter.
2 Open the larynx along the posterior midline and keep it open with wires or by pinning to a corkboard.
3 Photograph if indicated.
4 Fix overnight in formalin.
5 Remove the hyoid bone, thyroid cartilage, and cricoid cartilage, trying to keep the soft tissue as a single piece even if the bone and cartilage need to be fragmented in the process.
6 Take two Polaroid photographs and identify in one of them the sites of the sections to be taken.
7 Paint the surgical margins (lingual, pharyngeal, and tracheal) with India Ink.
8 Section the whole specimen longitudinally in parallel slices.
9 Handle the radical neck dissection according to instructions for Lymph node dissection—Radical neck.

Description

1 Type of laryngectomy: total, hemi, supraglottic or infraglottic; presence of pharynx and/or radical neck dissection
2 Tumor characteristics: location, size, extent, ulceration, depth of invasion; glottic, supraglottic, infraglottic, or transglottic? cross midline? extralaryngeal spread? features of nonneoplastic mucosa, especially in true vocal cords

Sections for histology

1 Entire tumor (unless massive, in which case minimum of three sections)
2 Representative step sections of larynx, including epiglottis
3 Cartilage and bone if pertinent
4 Lymph nodes (see under Lymph node dissection—Radical neck)

LIP—V EXCISION

Procedure

1 Fix the specimen for several hours.
2 Paint all surgical margins with India ink.
3 Cut the specimen as shown in the accompanying drawing.

Description

1 Size of specimen
2 Tumor characteristics: size, shape (ulcerated, polypoid, etc.), location (vermilion border, skin), distance to margins

Sections for histology

1 Cross section through center (**A** in accompanying drawing)
2 Lateral margins, without trimming (**B** and **C** in accompanying drawing)

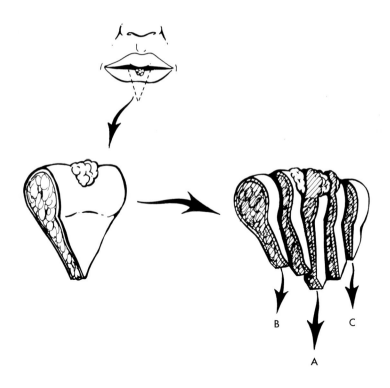

LUNG—RESECTION FOR NONTUMORAL CONDITION

Procedure

1 Obtain cultures from lesions suspected of being infectious.
2 Weigh the specimen.
3 Two options are available depending on the type of abnormality present and the status of the organ when received in the laboratory:
   a Open the bronchi longitudinally with scissors and cut the lung parenchyma (including the lesion) in slices with a sharp knife.
   b Inject with formalin through the main bronchus, tie off or clamp the bronchus, fix overnight, and section at 0.5-1 cm intervals with a sharp knife or meat cutter. The sections should be frontal, perpendicular to the hilum. The slices formed by this procedure can be kept in order by stringing them on a piece of twine.
4 For lungs with tuberculosis and other contagious diseases (proved or suspected): fix in formalin for forty-eight hours; keep the specimen in the same container while dissecting and cutting the sections; send the contaminated instruments for sterilization; carefully wrap the contaminated material in a plastic bag and place in a scrap bucket.
5 If a rib was submitted as part of the thoracotomy, examine according to instructions under Bone Marrow—Rib from thoracotomy.

Description

1 Weight of specimen and type of resection (pneumonectomy, lobectomy, wedge resection)
2 Pleura: thickness; fibrosis? fibrin? parietal pleura present? (identified by presence of subserosal fat)
3 Bronchi: mucosa, lumen (diameter and content)
4 Parenchyma: appearance; if localized lesion is present: appearance; lobe and, if possible, bronchopulmonary segment in which located; relationships to bronchi, vessels, pleura, and lymph nodes
5 Lymph nodes: number, size, and appearance

Sections for histology

1 Main lesion: three sections
2 Uninvolved lung: one section per lobe
3 Bronchus
4 Lymph nodes if present: at least one section

LUNG—RESECTION FOR TUMOR

Procedure

1 Dissect hilar lymph nodes as a single group and take out a cross section from the bronchial line of resection while the specimen is fresh.

2 Two options are available depending on the location of the tumor and the status of the organ when received in the laboratory:

   a Open all major bronchi and their branches longitudinally with scissors, and follow this by cutting parallel slices of the lung, including the tumor.

   b Inject with formalin through the main bronchus, tie off or clamp the bronchus, fix overnight, and section at 0.5-1 cm intervals with a sharp knife or meat cutter. The slices formed by this procedure can be kept in order by stringing them on a piece of twine.

3 If a rib was submitted as part of the thoracotomy, examine according to instructions under Bone marrow—Rib from thoracotomy.

Description

1 Weight of fresh specimen and type of resection (pneumonectomy, lobectomy, etc.)

2 Pleura: fibrosis, fibrin, tumor invasion; parietal pleura present? (identified by presence of fat)

3 Tumor characteristics: size, location, relation with bronchi, hemorrhage, necrosis, cavitation, blood vessel invasion, extension to pleura; distance to bronchial line of resection and pleura

4 Appearance of nonneoplastic lung

5 Number and appearance of regional lymph nodes

Sections for histology

1 Tumor: three sections, including one showing relationship to bronchus if any

2 Nonneoplastic lung, including pleura: three sections, at least one from lung distal to tumor

3 Bronchial line of resection: one cross section comprising entire circumference

4 Lymph nodes: bronchopulmonary (hilar) and mediastinal

5 If rib submitted, process according to instructions under Bone marrow—Rib from thoracotomy

LYMPH NODE—BIOPSY

Procedure

1 If the lymph node is received in the fresh state, cut in halves with a sterile blade and:

    a Take a small portion for culture if an infectious disease is suspected or needs to be ruled out.

    b Make four imprints of the cut surface on alcohol-cleaned slides, fix in methanol, and stain two with hematoxylin-eosin and two with Wright's stain. See instructions for Imprints (Touch preparations).

    c Take a representative cross section of the entire node 3 mm in thickness, place in a fixative, and send through as *biopsy* the same day.

    d Fix the rest of the specimen overnight and submit the next day as *biopsy*.

    e If adequate tissue is available, fix a slice in alternative fixative (such as Zenker's, Bouin's, or B5).

    f In cases of suspected lymphoreticular processes, and if facilities are available, place a 2 × 2 × 1 cm piece (or a piece as large as possible) of fresh tissue in a Petri dish containing a paper filter wet with saline solution and submit for evaluation of cell surface markers (see instructions for Cell surface markers — Sampling).

2 If the specimen is received already fixed in formalin, cut in 3 mm slices and submit representative sections.

Description

    1 State whether node received fresh or fixed

    2 Size of node and condition of capsule

    3 Appearance of cut surface: color, nodularity, hemorrhage, necrosis

Sections for histology

Cross section of node, including at least portion of capsule: one to three sections depending on size of node

LYMPH NODE DISSECTION—
GENERAL INSTRUCTIONS

Procedure

1 Dissect the node-containing fat from the organ in the fresh state, using forceps and sharp scissors. Make the fat dissection as close as possible to the wall of the organ (this is where most lymph nodes are located). Divide them in groups according to specific instructions.
2 Two options are available:
   a Search the fat for nodes while specimen is fresh, under a strong light, with the use of scissors, forceps, and scalpel. Avoid crushing the nodes by rough palpation. If not enough nodes are identified, contact the senior pathologist or surgeon.
   b Fix overnight in formalin or Carnoy's solution and search for nodes the next day. The latter fixative is preferred because it clears the fat somewhat.

Description

1 Number of nodes in each group
2 Size of largest and smallest nodes
3 Appearance; obvious involvement by tumor?

Sections for histology

1 *All* lymph nodes should be submitted for histology.
2 Small nodes (up to 3 mm in thickness after fat is removed) are submitted as a single piece.
3 Several small node groups may be submitted in the same cassette.
4 Larger nodes are bisected and, if necessary, further sectioned into 2-3 mm slices. A slice as large as will fit the cassette should be submitted for each one of these larger nodes.
5 Store the remainder in the formalin container, properly identified as of lymph node group.

LYMPH NODE DISSECTION—AXILLARY

See under Breast—Mastectomy.

LYMPH NODE DISSECTION—INGUINAL

1 All lymph nodes are submitted as a single group unless the surgeon has submitted the superficial and deep groups separately. A minimum of twelve lymph nodes should be found.
2 A cross section of the internal saphenous vein also should be submitted for histology.

LYMPH NODE DISSECTION—RADICAL NECK

Procedure

1 Orient the specimen and divide it into submaxillary gland, platysma, sternomastoid muscle, internal jugular veins, and node-containing fat.
2 Divide the lymph nodes into six groups depending upon whether they are on the upper or lower portion of the specimen and upon their relationship with the sternomastoid muscle (see accompanying drawing). A minimum of forty lymph nodes should be found.

Description

1 Site and type of primary neoplasm (see specific instructions)
2 Length of sternomastoid muscle
3 Jugular vein included? length? invaded by tumor?
4 Presence of tumor in lymph nodes, submaxillary gland, soft tissue, or muscle

Sections for histology

1 Superior anterior cervical lymph nodes
2 Superior jugular cervical lymph nodes
3 Superior posterior cervical lymph nodes
4 Inferior anterior cervical lymph nodes
5 Inferior jugular cervical lymph nodes
6 Inferior posterior cervical lymph nodes
7 Submaxillary gland
8 Jugular vein
9 Sternocleidomastoid muscle
10 Thyroid gland if present

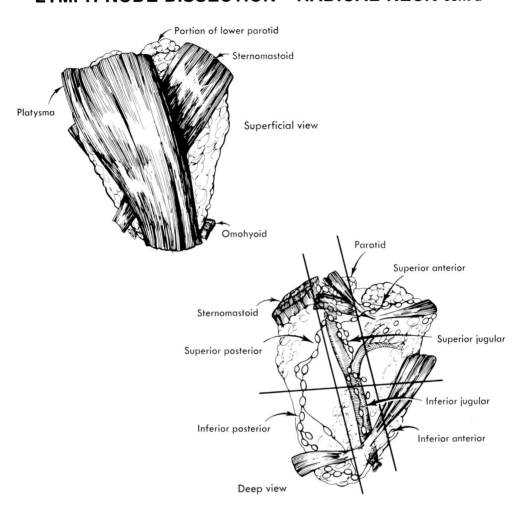

Portion of lower parotid

Sternomastoid

Platysma

Superficial view

Omohyoid

Parotid

Superior anterior

Sternomastoid

Superior jugular

Superior posterior

Inferior jugular

Inferior posterior

Inferior anterior

Deep view

LYMPH NODE DISSECTION—RETROPERITONEAL

1 For the proper evaluation of this specimen, it is essential for the surgeon to divide the lymph nodes in groups at the time he is doing the dissection and submit them to the laboratory in separate containers. In our institution, urologic surgeons divide the node groups as follows:
- Suprahilar (above level of renal artery)
- Superior interaortocaval
- Inferior interaortocaval
- Pericaval
- Periaortic
- Common iliac (usually excised only on side of tumor)

2 If the specimen is submitted as a single piece, it is necessary to identify, with the help of the surgeon, the upper and lower borders and the periaortic and pericaval regions. When this is established, the lymph nodes can be divided in the following groups:
- Superior periaortic
- Middle periaortic
- Inferior periaortic
- Superior pericaval
- Middle pericaval
- Inferior pericaval
- Common iliac (specify side)

3 If the surgeon is unavailable or unable to orient the specimen, all lymph nodes are submitted as one group. A minimum of twenty-five lymph nodes should be found.

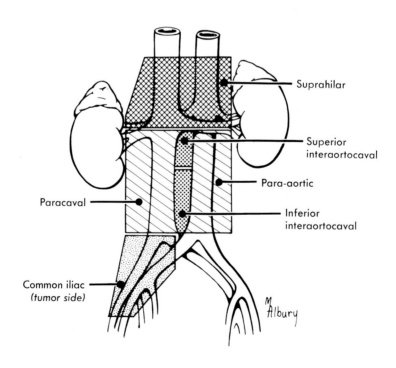

A58

NEEDLE BIOPSIES

Procedure

1 Remove the tissue from the fixative without squeezing it with a forceps; do not use toothed forceps; handle the tissue in such a manner as to keep it intact; do not cut it transversely but rather coil it inside the cassette if overly long.

2 Always search the container, including the undersurface of the lid, for tiny fragments of tissue that may be overlooked.

3 Carefully wrap the tissue in a tea bag, without squeezing.

4 If the amount of the tissue core permits (a core over 1 cm long or two tissue cores) and if it would be anticipated that a fat stain may be useful, save a 3-5 mm portion in formalin.

Description

1 Length and diameter of core; number of fragments; color

2 Homogeneity or lack of it

Sections for histology

All material received (except if fat stains desired, see under Procedure)

ORBITAL EXENTERATION

Procedure

1 Pin down the elliptical piece of orbicular skin and fix overnight at 4° C.
2 Paint the surgical margins with India ink.
3 Take surgical margins: cutaneous, soft tissue, optic nerve
4 Cut skin, soft tissue, and ocular globe.

Description

1 Skin: shape and length; appearance; if lesion present: size, shape, depth of invasion, color
2 Soft tissues
3 Ocular globe: dimensions, appearance, length of optic nerve

Sections for histology
For skin tumors

1 Tumor: three sections
2 Cutaneous surgical margins (superior, inferior, internal, and external)
3 Soft tissue surgical margins
4 Ocular globe

For ocular tumors

1 Globe with tumor
2 Orbital soft tissue adjacent to tumor
3 Surgical margin of optic nerve

ORIENTATION OF SPECIMENS WITH AGAR

1 Prepare beforehand a 3% solution of "bacteriologic" agar, divide in 1-2 ml samples, and place in small test tubes. Keep these samples at 4° C in the refrigerator until the time of use.

2 Heat the test tube on a specially prepared hot plate until the agar acquires a semiviscid consistency. The temperature should be around 60° C, and it is important to keep it as close as possible to this figure (otherwise, the agar will not melt or become too fluid). The melting of the agar should take no more than one to two minutes. It is convenient to heat as many test tubes in the morning as will be needed during the working day. However, it is advised not to keep the agar at 60° C longer than twenty-four to forty-eight hours.

3 Pick up the specimen gently with a small forceps and place it in the desired position ("on edge") on top of a glass slide (see accompanying drawing).

4 While holding the specimen in this position with one hand, use the other hand to drop a small amount of melted agar on top of the specimen with a Pasteur pipette. Do not use an excessive amount. The solidifying process can be speeded up by gently blowing in the agar. When the agar has solidified just enough for the tissue to remain in the desired position without support (it should take no more than one minute), remove the forceps and wait an additional one or two minutes.

5 Detach the tissue surrounded by the agar from the glass slide by sliding a blade beneath it (see accompanying drawing), and transfer the material to the cassette. If the size is very small, it may be necessary to wrap it in lens paper or a tea bag.

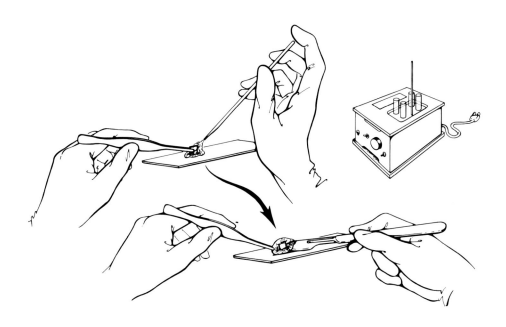

OVARY—OOPHORECTOMY

Procedure

1 Measure the organ. Weigh it if it is obviously abnormal.
2 If the specimen is received fresh:
  a Normal-sized or nearly normal–sized organ: Bivalve and fix for several hours.
  b Enlarged organ: Make several cuts and fix for several hours.

Description

1 Size and shape; weight if enlarged
2 Capsule: thickened? adhesions? hemorrhage? rupture? external surface smooth or irregular?
3 Cut section: character of cortex, medulla, and hilum; cysts (size and content); corpus luteum? calcification? hemorrhage?
4 Tumors: size; external appearance: smooth or papillary? solid or cystic? content of cystic masses; hemorrhage, necrosis, or calcification?

Sections for histology

1 For incidental oophorectomies: one sagittal section of each entire ovary labeled as to side
2 For cysts: up to three sections of cyst wall (particularly from areas with papillary appearance)
3 For tumors: three sections or one section for each centimeter of tumor, whichever is greater; also, one section of nonneoplastic ovary if identifiable

PANCREAS—PANCREATECTOMY

Procedure

1 Dissect lymph nodes while the specimen is fresh and divide them according to groups (see accompanying drawing).

2 Fill the stomach and duodenum with gauze or cotton impregnated with formalin.

3 Pin the whole specimen on a corkboard, trying to preserve the anatomic relationships.

4 Place in a large container, cover with formalin, and fix overnight at 4° C.

5 Paint with India ink the common bile duct surgical margin, as well as the pancreatic surgical margin in a Whipple's procedure.

6 Divide the specimen into anterior and posterior halves as follows: with scissors, cut the lesser curvature of the stomach and the free border of the duodenum; with scissors, cut the gastric greater curvature up to the pancreas, as well as the fourth portion of the duodenum; with a large sharp knife, cut the peripancreatic border of the duodenum and the pancreas. The orientation of the latter cut can be better controlled by introducing a catheter through the common bile duct and cutting in front of it. It may be necessary to postfix the two halves overnight before proceeding to further dissection, as indicated.

Description

1 Type of operation: Whipple's procedure,* total pancreatectomy,† regional pancreatectomy‡

2 Organs present in specimen and their dimensions

3 Tumor characteristics: involvement of ampulla, duodenal mucosa, stomach, bile duct, pancreatic duct, and pancreas; size, shape (papillary? flat? ulcerated?), color, and consistency

4 Common bile duct and main pancreatic duct: dilated? stones? tumor?

5 Location, number, and appearance of regional lymph nodes

Whipple's procedure: partial pancreatectomy, partial gastrectomy, duodenectomy.
†*Total pancreatectomy:* total pancreatectomy, partial gastrectomy, duodenectomy, splenectomy.
‡*Regional pancreatectomy:* total pancreatectomy, partial gastrectomy, cholecystectomy, duodenectomy, splenectomy, resection of portal vein, with or without transverse colectomy, mesocolon, omentum, regional lymph nodes.

Continued

PANCREAS—PANCREATECTOMY cont'd

Sections for histology

1 Tumor: up to three sections
2 Pancreas: three sections, one from distal line of resection
3 Common bile duct: two cross sections, one from surgical margin
4 Uninvolved duodenum: two sections, one from distal line of resection
5 Stomach: two sections, including proximal line of resection
6 Lymph nodes:
   • Peripancreatic (superior and inferior)
   • Pancreaticoduodenal (anterior and posterior)
   • Common bile duct and cystic duct
   • Gastric, lesser curvature
   • Gastric, greater curvature
   • Splenic
   • Other groups if present (jejunal, midcolic, omental)
7 Other organs if present (gallbladder, spleen, portal vein, colon, omentum)

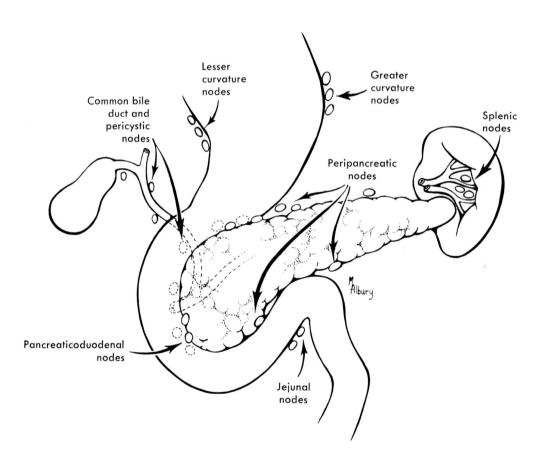

PARATHYROID GLANDS—PARATHYROIDECTOMY

Procedure

1 Accurately weigh each gland on a delicate balance after removing the surrounding fat but *before* removing any parathyroid tissue for frozen or other sections.
2 Accurately label each parathyroid gland as to site.

Description

Weight, color, consistency, and external appearance of *each* gland

Sections for histology

All parathyroid tissue (except for markedly enlarged gland, in which minimum of three sections should be taken) accurately labeled as to site

PELVIC EXENTERATION

Procedure

1 Gently express content from the rectosigmoid, wash with formalin or saline solution, and fill with cotton or gauze impregnated in formalin.
2 Fill the vagina with the same material.
3 Inject the bladder with formalin with a Foley catheter or syringe after tying the urethra.
4 Suspend the specimen in anatomic position in a large container with abundant fixative.
5 Inject formalin in the uterine cavity with a syringe through the fundus.
6 Fix for twenty-four hours.
7 Remove all cotton and gauze and cut sagitally in equal halves. The sections of large bowel, bladder, and vagina are made with scissors; that of the uterus, with a knife.
8 Take two Polaroid photographs and identify in one of them the site of the sections to be taken.
9 Remove the lymph node in the following groups: right parametrial, left parametrial, retrorectal, and mesosigmoid.
10 Paint the surgical margins with India ink.

Description

1 Type of exenteration: total, anterior, posterior; organs included; length of ureters
2 Tumor characteristics: location, invasion of other structures, size, color, consistency; fistulae? signs of radiation change?
3 Number and appearance of lymph nodes

Sections for histology

1 Tumor: three sections or one section per centimeter of tumor, whichever is greater
2 Cervix and vagina
3 Cervix and bladder
4 Cervix and rectum
5 Surgical margins (parametrial, vaginal, vesical, and rectal)
6 *In females:* vulva, vagina, cervix, endometrium, tubes, ovaries (in addition to sections from tumor)
7 *In males:* prostate
8 Lymph nodes:
   • Right parametrial
   • Left parametrial
   • Retrorectal
   • Mesosigmoid

PENIS—PENECTOMY

Procedure

1 If the specimen is accompanied by inguinal node dissections, separate them and handle according to specific instructions.
2 Introduce a catheter through the urethra.
3 Fix overnight at 4° C.
4 Paint the surgical margins (including the urethra) with India ink.
5 Cut longitudinally through the center; the section should cut the urethra in two.
6 Take two Polaroid photographs and identify in one of them the site of the sections to be taken.

Description

1 Type of operation: partial, total, with or without scrotal skin, testicles, inguinal nodes
2 Length and diameter of specimen
3 Tumor: location in relation to glans, prepuce, skin, and urethra; size, color, borders, depth of invasion
4 Glans penis: balanitis? atrophy? leukoplakia?
5 Urethra: invaded by tumor?

Sections for histology

1 Tumor: three sections
2 Glans penis and urethra
3 Surgical margin (including urethra)

PERIPHERAL NERVE—BIOPSY

Procedure

1 The examination and sampling of this material should be carried out at the bedside or *immediately* after the specimen is received in the pathology laboratory. Be careful to avoid stretching or crushing.

2 Measure the length and diameter (biopsies of the sural nerve usually measure between 1 and 3 cm).

3 Cut a portion 2-4 mm long from one end, divide in 1-2 mm³ fragments, and fix in glutaraldehyde for electron microscopy.

4 Cut a 2 mm portion from one end and a 3-4 mm portion form the other end and fix in formalin for routine light microscopy. The first is to be embedded in cross section and the second longitudinally.

5 If facilities are available for whole-mount teased preparations, fix the remaining portion of the nerve in 2% glutaraldehyde solution in 0.1M cacodylate buffer at ph 7.4 and process further according to specific instructions (Ellefson RD, Lais AC, Smith RC, Taylor WE, Van Dyke, RA: Mayo Clin Proc **45**:286-327, 1970).

Description

1 Length and diameter
2 Color
3 Irregularities

Sections for histology

1 One cross section and one longitudinal section for paraffin embedding
2 For other portions of biopsy, see under Procedure

PLACENTA—SINGLETON

Procedure/Description

1 Examine as soon as possible after delivery in the fresh state; handle the specimen with great care, avoiding lacerations.

2 Note the amount of blood and clots in the container, and search for separate pieces of membranes, cord, or placenta.

3 Examine in this order: membranes, cord, fetal surface, and maternal surface.

4 Measure the distance from the placental margin to the nearest point of rupture (zero: marginal placenta previa).

5 Examine membranes for completeness (if a portion is missing, notify the obstetrician), insertion, decidual necrosis, edema, extra-amniotic pregnancy, and retromembranous hemorrhage.

6 Take a long, 2-3 cm wide section of membranes beginning with the point of rupture and extending to and including a small portion of placental margin. Roll the specimen with the amniotic surface inward, fix for twenty-four hours, take a 3 mm section from the center (taking care not to strip the amnion off), and submit for histology.

7 Trim the remaining membranes from the placental margin.

8 Measure the length of the cord and the shortest distance from the cord insertion to the placental margin.

9 Examine the cord: insertion (nonmembranous or membranous; if latter, are vessels intact?), number of umbilical vessels (by sectioning the cord transversely at two or more points), color, true knots, torsion, stricture, hematoma, thrombosis.

10 Remove the cord from the placenta 3 cm proximal to the insertion and take a 2-4 cm segment from its midpoint; fix this segment for twenty-four hours, take a 3 mm section, and submit for histology.

11 Examine the fetal surface: color, opacity, subchorionic fibrin, cysts (number and size), amnion nodosum, squamous metaplasia, thrombosis of fetal surface vessels, chorangioma.

12 Examine the maternal surface: completeness, normal fissures, laceration (extent), depressed areas, retroplacental hemorrhage (size and distance from margin).

13 Measure the maximum diameter, thickness in the center, weight (after trimming cord and membranes), shape.

14 Hold the placenta, maternal side up, gently with one hand on a flat surface and make parallel sections with a large sharp knife at 2 cm intervals. The fetal surface will not be cut through and will hold the specimen together.

15 Remove a 2 cm piece that includes the fetal surface and intact maternal surface, about 3-4 cm from the cord insertion. Select the piece so that the fetal surface vessels are cut at right angles to their long axis; fix for twenty-four hours, trim a 3 mm section (through and through), and submit for histology.

16 Examine all cross sections for infarcts (location, size, number), intervillous thrombi (number; laminated or not?), perivillous fibrin deposition, pallor, consistency, calcification (extent), cysts, tumors.

Continued **A69**

Sections for histology

1 Placenta (as indicated previously plus abnormal areas if present)
2 Membranes
3 Cord

PLACENTA—TWIN

Procedure/Description

1 If placentas are separate (nonfused): Examine each placenta as a singleton.
2 If placentas are fused:
  a Note whether the two cords are labeled twin A and twin B. If not, label them arbitrarily and make a statement to that effect.
  b Determine the presence and type of dividing membranes:
    (1) If absent (monochorionic-monoamniotic), so state.
    (2) If present:
      (a) Remove a square of the dividing membrane, roll it, fix it for twenty-four hours, take a 3 mm section, and submit for histology.
      (b) Attempt to determine grossly whether the dividing membrane has chorion or not, according to the accompanying tables.
      (c) Record the kind and number of vascular anastomoses in monochorionic-diamniotic placentas: artery-to-artery, vein-to-vein, artery-to-vein (arteriovenous shunts). The latter can be better demonstrated by injecting the artery of one twin along the plane of fusion of the placenta with 30-50 cc of saline solution containing a dye and noting whether the fluid emerges from the vein of the other twin through one or more common villous lobules. The placenta must be intact to perform this test. Arteries always run over veins.
  c Divide the fused twin placenta along the ''vascular equator'' (rather than through the base of the dividing membrane).
  d Examine each half as a singleton placenta.

Sections for histology

1 Placenta from twin A
2 Membranes from twin A
3 Cord from twin A
4 Placenta from twin B
5 Membranes from twin B
6 Cord from twin B
7 Dividing membrane if present

PLACENTA—TWIN cont'd

Dividing membrane in twin placentas

Features	Dichorionic-diamniotic (fused)	Monochorionic-diamniotic
Appearance	Thick and opaque	Thin and transparent
Separation of membranes by stripping	Difficult	Easy
Point of attachment to fetal surface	Ridge or tearing of chorion	Smooth and continuous, without ridge
Vascular anastomoses	Very rare	Numerous

Types of twin placentas

Type	Incidence	Gross	Twin type
Dichorionic-diamniotic (separate)	35%		Monozygotic or dizygotic
Dichorionic-diamniotic (fused)	34%		Monozygotic or dizygotic
Monochorionic-diamniotic	30%		Monozygotic
Monochorionic-monoamniotic	1%		Monozygotic

PROSTATE GLAND—RADICAL PROSTATECTOMY

Procedure

1 Fix the whole specimen in formalin at 4° C overnight.
2 Paint the surgical margins with India ink.
3 Make parallel transverse slices, about 5 mm thick, and examine the cut surfaces carefully.
4 Take two Polaroid photographs of the slices to be submitted for histology and identify in one of them the site of the sections taken.

Description

1 Weight and dimensions of specimen
2 Organs present: whole prostate? urethra (length), seminal vesicles, vas, lymph nodes
3 a Prostate: tumor (location in lobes, size, color, borders, capsular and periprostatic extension)
  b Nonneoplastic prostate: nodular hyperplasia?
4 Urethra: patent? impinged by tumor?
5 Seminal vesicles: involved by tumor?

Sections for histology

1 Tumor: three sections, including capsule and urethra
2 Nonneoplastic prostate (all lobes)
3 Seminal vesicles
4 Urethral surgical margin

PROSTATE GLAND— SUPRAPUBIC PROSTATECTOMY

Procedure

1 Step section the specimen in 3 mm slices, either in the fresh state or after formalin fixation.
2 Examine *each slice* carefully for areas suspicious of carcinoma (yellow areas or foci that are harder or softer than the rest of the specimen).

Description

1 Weight of specimen
2 Shape, color, and consistency
3 Presence of hyperplastic nodules, cysts, calculi, areas suspicious of carcinoma

Sections for histology

1 Left lobe: three sections
2 Right lobe: three sections
3 Middle lobe

PROSTATE GLAND—TRANSURETHRAL RESECTION (TUR)

Procedure

1 Weigh with accurate balance.
2 Carefully examine all the fragments. Carcinoma of the prostate is often yellow and/or hard; submit for histology chips with these gross characteristics.

Description

1 Weight of specimen
2 Size, shape, and color of chips

Sections for histology

1 *If all fragments received in a single container:*
   a All of specimen until four cassettes filled
   b If an excess, one additional cassette for each additional 10 gm of tissue (each cassette holds approximately 2 gm)
2 *If fragments received are identified as to lobe from which they were taken,* submit as follows *for each* specimen (lobe) received:
   a All of specimen until four cassettes filled
   b If an excess, one additional cassette for each additional 10 gm of tissue
   c Identify in following order (not all lobes may have been biopsied in some cases):
   • Anterior lobe
   • Middle lobe
   • Posterior lobe
   • Left lateral lobe
   • Right lateral lobe

SKELETAL MUSCLE—BIOPSY

Procedure

The proper evaluation of a skeletal muscle biopsy includes routine processing and staining, enzyme histochemistry, and electron microscopic examination.

1. *Routine processing:* The specimen is usually received stretched on a special muscle biopsy clamp. It should remain on the clamp for overnight fixation. If the specimen is received fresh, pin it to a corkboard and fix overnight.
2. *Enzyme histochemistry:* Freeze a small fragment in liquid nitrogen.
3. *Electron microscopy:* See instructions under Electron microscopy—Sampling.

Description

1. Dimensions of specimen
2. Color and consistency; fibrosis? edema? necrosis?

Sections for histology

1. One longitudinal section
2. One cross section

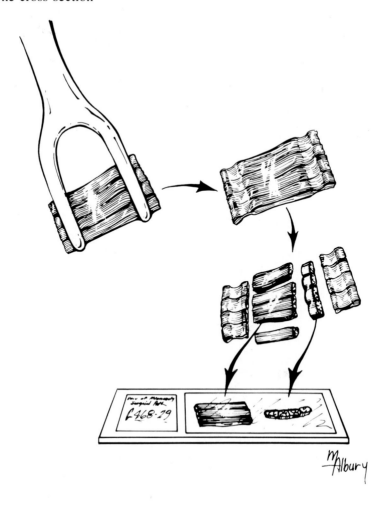

SKIN—EXCISION FOR BENIGN LESION

Procedure

1 Pigmented nevi, seborrheic keratoses, and other benign skin conditions (as well as small basal cell carcinomas) are usually removed with narrow margins, and the size of the specimen mainly depends on the size of the lesion.
2 Fix well before processing.
3 If there is any clinical or gross suggestion that the tumor may be malignant, paint margins with India ink.

Description

1 Size and shape of specimen; features of surface; lesion present? size, color, other features; margin grossly involved?
2 If specimen transected, description of appearance of cross section

Sections for histology

Note: In specimens from vesicular diseases, the vesicle should be submitted intact. Do not cut through the vesicle under any circumstances.

1 For specimens measuring 3 mm or less (see accompanying drawing **A**): Submit *in toto* without cutting.
2 For specimens measuring between 4 and 6 mm in width (see accompanying drawing **B**): Cut through the center and submit both halves.
3 For specimens with a width of 7 mm or more (see accompanying drawing **C**): Cut a 2-3 mm slice from the center for histology and save the remainder in formalin.
4 Make sure that sections will be embedded on edge.

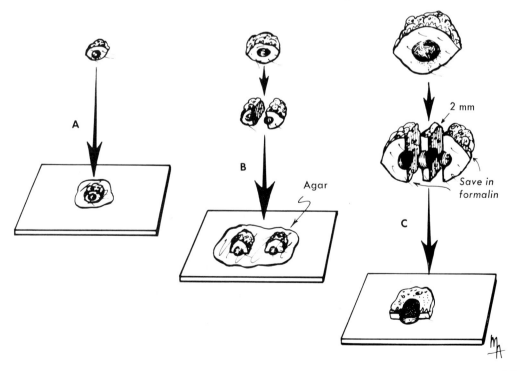

SKIN—EXCISION FOR MALIGNANT TUMOR

Procedure

1 Paint all excision margins with India ink.
2 Take two Polaroid photographs in cases of large tumors and identify in one of them the site of the sections to be taken.

Description

1 Shape and dimensions of specimen
2 Characteristics of lesion: size, shape, color or colors, configuration; elevated or depressed? ulceration? types of margins (sharp or ill-defined? flat or elevated?); distance from margins of resection; satellite nodules?

Sections for histology

1 *Small specimens* —up to 5 cm in greatest length (see accompanying drawing **I**):
   a Cross section—one piece if feasible; cut in two halves if longer than 3 cm; make sure this section made through what appears to be narrowest surgical margin (**I, A**)
   b Longitudinal sections—two pieces (**I, B** and **C**)
2 *Larger specimens* (see accompanying drawing **II**):
   a Tumor: two to four sections depending on size (**II, A, B,** and **C**)
   b Surgical margins: four or more depending on case (**II, D, E, F,** and **G**)
3 *Notes:*
   a In pigmented lesions, take parallel sections of the entire lesion, unless inordinately large.
   b An alternate method of examining the surgical margins (which we do not prefer) is shown in accompanying drawing **III**. This can be combined with the aforedescribed method, as shown in accompanying drawing **IV**. Some authors prefer these alternate methods of tangential margins for multicentric basal cell carcinoma and malignant melanoma.

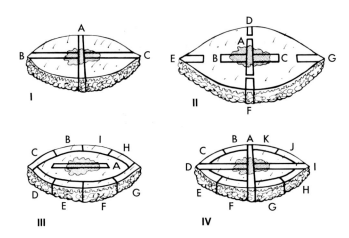

SKIN—PUNCH BIOPSY

Procedure

1 Submit *in toto* if 4 mm in diameter or smaller (see accompanying drawing **A**); cut in half longitudinally if 5 mm or larger and submit both halves for histology (see accompanying drawing **B**).
2 If the specimen is from a vesicular disease, the vesicle should be submitted *intact* for histology.

Description

1 Diameter and thickness of biopsy
2 Appearance of surface; subcutis included?

Sections for histology

1 Entire biopsy (see under Procedure)
2 Make sure section oriented on edge

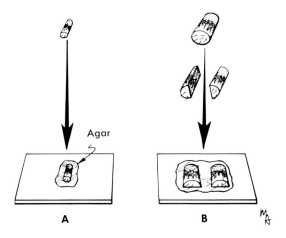

A   B

SKIN—SHAVE BIOPSY

Procedure

Shave biopsies of the skin, usually done for keratoses or basal cell carcinomas, can be quite thin, often of round or oval shape.

Description

1 Size of specimen
2 Number of fragments
3 Features of surface

Sections for histology

1 If width is 3 mm or less: Submit *in toto* without cutting.
2 If width is 4 mm or more: Cut in parallel slices, about 2-3 mm thick, and submit all for histology.
3 Make sure all sections are oriented on edge.

SMALL BOWEL—BIOPSY

Procedure

1 The specimen is usually received attached to a piece of filter paper or Gelfoam, mucosal side up; let it fix well before processing.
2 Examine with dissecting microscope and determine mucosal pattern; avoid drying of the specimen and traumatizing the mucosa during this procedure.

Description

1 Size and color of specimen
2 Mucosal pattern with dissecting microscope (see accompanying drawings)

Sections for histology

1 The entire specimen is submitted. It is essential for it to be oriented on edge.
2 It specimen comes attached to Gelfoam, the latter can be processed together with the specimen.

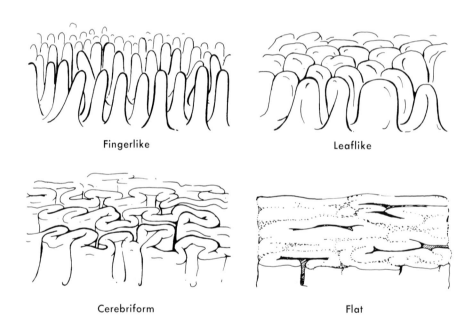

Fingerlike   Leaflike

Cerebriform   Flat

SMALL BOWEL—EXCISION

Procedure

1 Two options are available depending on the length of the bowel and the type of pathology present:

    a Cut longitudinally through the antimesenteric border, pin on corkboard, and fix overnight.

    b Wash out contents gently with formalin or saline solution (not with water), tie one end, fill the lumen with formalin, and tie the other end. Fix overnight and open longitudinally along the antimesenteric border.

Description

1 Length and diameter of specimen

2 Mucosa: appearance; edema? hemorrhage? ulcerations? tumor? (size, location, circumferential involvement? depth of invasion)

3 Wall: thickness, abnormalities

4 Serosa: fibrosis, peritonitis, adhesions

5 Lymph nodes: size and appearance

6 Mesentery; mesenteric blood vessels

Sections for histology

1 Depends on pathology present

2 In cases of infarct: several cross sections of mesenteric vessels

SPLEEN—SPLENECTOMY

Procedure

1 Measure and weigh the specimen.
2 Cut parallel slices as thin as possible with a sharp knife or meat cutter while the specimen is fresh and examine each slice carefully for focal lesions; do not wash the cut surface in tap water. Fix each slice flat in a large container.
3 Take cultures if an inflammatory condition is suspected.
4 Prepare four imprints of the cut surface in all cases in which splenic pathology is suspected; stain two with hematoxylin-eosin and two with Wright's stain.
5 If sickle cell disease is suspected, fix a block of tissue in formalin *immediately* after it has been cut from the interior of the organ.
6 Look for lymph nodes and accessory spleens in the splenic hilum.

Description

1 Weight and dimensions
2 Hilum: nature of vessels, presence of lymph nodes, presence of accessory spleens
3 Capsule: color, thickness, focal changes, adhesions, lacerations (location, length and depth)
4 Cut surface: color; consistency; bulging; malpighian corpuscles (size; color; conspicuous?); fibrous trabeculae; nodules or masses; diffuse infiltration?

Sections for histology

1 For incidental splenectomies: one section, including capsule
2 For traumatically ruptured spleen: one section through tear and one away from it
3 For diseased spleens: at least three sections, one to include hilum and two to include capsule

STAGING LAPAROTOMY FOR MALIGNANT LYMPHOMA

Procedure

1 Spleen: Handle as described under Spleen—Splenectomy except that *the entire spleen* should be sliced carefully, 3-4 mm apart, and each slice should be carefully examined. Any nodules, no matter how small, that differ from the adjacent normal malpighian corpuscles should be processed for histology. Square blocks containing these suspicious nodules, in addition to other obvious lesions, should be cut out and fixed separately for several hours or overnight in formalin.

2 Lymph nodes: These will usually include splenic hilar, para-aortic, and possibly mesenteric nodes. Dissect carefully the splenic hilum for the former.

3 Liver wedge biopsies (right and left lobes): Keep separate; trim into several slices if necessary.

4 Open iliac crest biopsy: fix, decalcify, and trim if necessary.

Description

1 Proceed as per instructions for the respective organs.

2 Presence or absence of grossly identifiable nodes in the splenic hilum must be noted.

Sections for histology

1 Spleen: all grossly abnormal or suspicious areas; if no gross abnormalities seen, four random pieces

2 Lymph nodes: all, properly identified as to site

3 Liver: all, properly identified as to lobe

4 Bone marrow: all

STOMACH—GASTRECTOMY FOR TUMOR

Procedure

1 Open the specimen along the greater curvature (unless the lesion is in this location; if it is, open the specimen along the lesser curvature).
2 Dissect the lymph node groups according to the accompanying diagram and remove the omentum.
3 If a splenectomy is included, dissect the hilar lymph nodes, measure and weigh the spleen, and cut in 1 cm longitudinal slices.
4 Pin the stomach on a corkboard and fix overnight in formalin before sectioning.
5 Take two Polaroid photographs and identify in one of them the sites of the sections to be taken.
6 Paint the surgical margins with India ink.
7 In general, take the sections *perpendicular* to the direction of the mucosal folds.
8 Another way to examine these specimens is as follows: Inject the stomach with formalin (in cases of total gastrectomy) or fill it with gauze or cotton impregnated in formalin (in partial gastrectomies). Fix overnight. Cut the side opposite the tumor with scissors and the tumor side with a long knife.

Description

1 Type of resection (total or subtotal); length of greater curvature, lesser curvature, and duodenal cuff
2 Tumor characteristics: location, size (including thickness), shape (fungating, spreading, ulcerated); depth of invasion; presence of serosal involvement; blood vessel invasion; extension into duodenum; distance from both lines of resection
3 Appearance of nonneoplastic mucosa

Sections for histology (see accompanying drawings)

1 Tumor: four sections through wall and including tumor border
2 Nonneoplastic mucosa: midstomach, two sections
3 Proximal line of resection along lesser curvature: two sections
4 Proximal line of resection along greater curvature: two sections
5 Distal line of resection (along pylorus and duodenum if present): two sections
6 Spleen if present
7 Pancreas if present
8 Lymph nodes:
  a Pyloric
  b Lesser curvature
  c Greater curvature
  d Omentum
  e Perisplenic

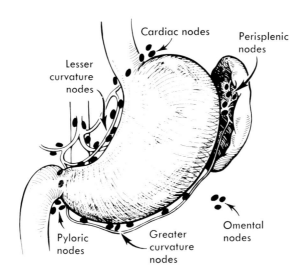

Cardiac nodes

Perisplenic nodes

Lesser curvature nodes

Pyloric nodes

Greater curvature nodes

Omental nodes

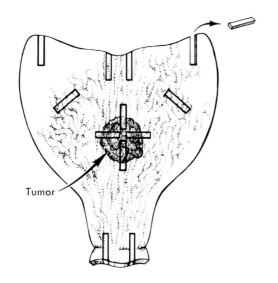

Tumor

STOMACH—GASTRECTOMY FOR ULCER

Procedure

1 Examine specimen in the fresh state.
2 Open the specimen along the greater curvature (unless the lesion is in this location; if it is, open the specimen along the lesser curvature).
3 Dissect the lymph node groups and remove the omentum.
4 Look carefully for small mucosal erosions and irregularities and for intramural or subserosal nodules.
5 Pin the stomach on a corkboard and fix overnight in formalin before sectioning.
6 Take two Polaroid photographs and identify in one of them the sites of the sections to be taken.

Description

1 Type of resection; length of greater curvature, lesser curvature, and duodenal cuff
2 Ulcer characteristics: location, size, depth of penetration, shape, and color of edges (flat or elevated? converging folds?); presence of large vessels and/or perforation at ulcer base; appearance of serosa.
   (If the clinicoroentgenographic diagnosis is peptic ulcer but no ulcer is identified in the specimen, contact the surgeon or assistant to find out whether the ulcer was not resected. Record this information as part of the gross dictation.)
3 Appearance of uninvolved mucosa: atrophy, edema, hemorrhage, etc.

Sections for histology

1 Ulcer: four sections
2 Lesser curvature: two sections cut from proximal margin of excision (Paint line of resection with India ink.)
3 Greater curvature: two sections cut from proximal margin of excision (Paint line of resection with India ink.)
4 Pylorus and duodenum: two sections, including distal line of resection
5 Other lesions if present
6 Lymph nodes: up to three sections

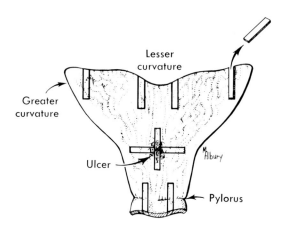

TESTICLE—ORCHIECTOMY

Procedure

1 Open the tunica vaginalis; weigh and measure the testicle.
2 Cut the testicle sagitally while it is in the fresh state and fix in formalin.
3 Take two Polaroid photographs and identify in one of them the sites of the sections to be taken.
4 Cut serial slices, about 3 mm thick, of each testicular half, perpendicular to the original section, stopping just as the level of the tunica albuginea (to keep them together) and examine each surface carefully.
5 Cut the epididymis longitudinally throughout its entire length.
6 Make several cross sections of the spermatic cord at several levels.

Description

1 Weight and dimensions of testicle
2 Length of spermatic cord
3 Features of tumor if present: size, color; consistency; homogeneity or lack of it; presence of cysts, necrosis, hemorrhage, bone, or cartilage; tumor extension to tunica albuginea, epididymis, cord, and other structures
4 Features of nonneoplastic testicle: atrophy? fibrosis? nodules?

Sections for histology

1 Tumor: at least three sections, or one section for each centimeter of tumor, whichever is greater, at least one of which should include some uninvolved testicle
(Always submit sections from hemorrhagic or necrotic areas of tumor, as well as from solid or fleshy areas.)
2 Uninvolved testicle: two sections
3 Epididymis
4 Spermatic cord and surrounding soft tissue at point about 1 cm from testicle: one cross section
5 Spermatic cord and surrounding soft tissue at line of resection: one cross section

THYMUS GLAND—THYMECTOMY

Procedure

1 Weigh the total organ. Cut parallel slices (while the specimen is fresh or after formalin fixation).
2 Look carefully for lymph nodes around the thymus.

Description

1 Weight and dimensions; both lobes identifiable?
2 Relative amount of fat and thymic parenchyma
3 Tumor characteristics: size, shape, external appearance (lobulated or smooth), cut section, color, necrosis, hemorrhage, fibrous bands, calcification, cysts (size, content)
4 Attached structures (pleura, pericardium, lung, lymph nodes)

Sections for histology

1 Tumor: three or more sections, at least two of which should include capsule
2 Uninvolved thymus: two sections
3 Other organs if present (lung, lymph nodes, etc.)

THYROID GLAND—THYROIDECTOMY

Procedure

1 Weigh and measure the specimen.
2 Orient the specimen and cut parallel longitudinal slices 5 mm each either in the fresh state or after formalin fixation.
3 Search for parathyroid glands in the surrounding fat.

Description

1 Type of specimen: lobectomy, isthmectomy, subtotal thyroidectomy, total thyroidectomy
2 Weight, shape, color, and consistency of specimen
3 Cut surface: smooth or nodular? if nodular: number, size, and appearance of nodules (cystic? calcified? hemorrhagic? necrotic?); encapsulated or invasive? distance to line of resection

Sections for histology

1 For diffuse and/or inflammatory lesions: three sections from each lobe and one from isthmus
2 For a solitary encapsulated nodule: four sections, including capsule
3 For multinodular thyroid glands: one section of each nodule (up to five nodules), including rim and adjacent normal gland; more than one section for larger nodules
4 For papillary carcinoma: block entire thyroid gland and (separately) line of resection
5 For carcinoma other than papillary: three sections of tumor, three of non-neoplastic gland, and one from line of resection
6 For all cases: submit parathyroid glands if found on gross inspection

UTERUS—CERVICAL BIOPSY

Procedure

1 Do not cut the specimen unless the individual pieces are greater than 4 mm in diameter.
2 It is essential that *all of the tissue* received be processed, no matter how small.
3 Always search the container and the underside of the lid carefully for tiny fragments of tissue.

Description

1 Number of pieces received, shape and color
2 Measurement in aggregate
3 Presence of absence of epithelium; epithelial erosions or ulcers? irregularity in epithelial thickness?
4 Any evidence of tumors or cysts?

Sections for histology

1 Submit the material in its entirety.
2 If specimens are received with a specific identification (e.g., anterior lip, posterior lip, etc.), label and submit them separately.
3 If a specimen from endocervical scraping is received, submit this as a separate specimen in its entirety (including the endocervical mucus).

UTERUS—CERVICAL CONIZATION

Procedure

1 Ideally, the specimen should be received intact, in the fresh state, and with a suture or other material identifying the 12 o'clock position.
2 Open the specimen by inserting a sharp pointed scissors into the cervical canal and cutting longitudinally along the 12 o'clock position. If the specimen has not been oriented as to position, open at any site.
3 Pin on a corkboard with the mucosal side up and fix in formalin for several hours.
4 Paint both surgical margins with India ink, taking special care that the epithelial border of the margins are well stained along their entire length.
5 Cut the entire cervix by making parallel sections, 2-3 mm apart, along the plane of the endocervical canal starting at the 12 o'clock position (or left-hand side of the specimen) and moving clockwise. Sections should be taken in such a way that the epithelium (including the squamocolumnar junction) is present in each section; some trimming of the stroma may be necessary (see accompanying drawing).

Description

1 Size (diameter and depth) and shape of cone; complete cast of cervix or fragmented?
2 Epithelium: color; presence of irregularities, erosions, healed or recent lacerations, masses (size, shape, location), cysts (size, content), previous biopsy sites

Sections for histology

1 All of the tissue must be submitted (except for trimming of the stroma).
2 If the cone has been oriented as to the 12 o'clock position, identify separately:
   a Sections from 12 to 3 o'clock (**A-1** on accompanying drawings)
   b Sections from 3 to 6 o'clock (**A-2** on accompanying drawings)
   c Sections from 6 to 9 o'clock (**A-3** on accompanying drawings)
   d Sections from 9 to 12 o'clock (**A-4** on accompanying drawings)
3 If an accurate mapping of the lesions is desired, identify sequentially each section with a letter, beginning from the 12 o'clock position.

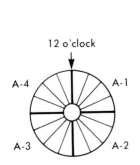
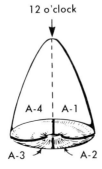
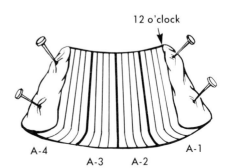

UTERUS—ENDOMETRIAL CURETTINGS OR BIOPSY

Procedure

1 Use a metal strainer or 4 × 4 inch gauze to collect the specimens.
2 Clean the forceps, other instruments, and the table carefully before handling the next case.

Description

1 Measurement in the aggregate
2 Color and consistency; blood clots present? proportion of clots in relation to whole specimen; any unusually large or firm pieces? globular tissue? evidence of necrosis? tissue suggestive of products of conception?

Sections for histology

1 For endometrial biopsy or diagnostic curettage: Submit *all* tissue. Do not fill the cassettes more than half full.
2 For endometrial curettage for incomplete abortion: Submit representative sections of tissue with the appearance of placenta, fetal parts, and decidua unless the entire specimen is small enough to fit into three cassettes. If the microscopic sections do not show products of conception, submit the rest of the material.

UTERUS—HYSTERECTOMY
(GENERAL INSTRUCTIONS)

Procedure

1 If operation was done for endometrial hyperplasia, endometrial carcinoma, or cervical (in situ or invasive) carcinoma, read specific instructions before proceeding.

2 Measure and weigh the specimen.

3 If the uterus is received fresh and intact:

  a Open it by cutting with scissors through both lateral walls, from the cervix to the uterine cornua.

  b Make a mark as to which half is anterior (e.g., by cutting a small wedge on one side) and complete the division but cutting with a sharp knife horizontally through the fundus. The uterus can be oriented by examining the level of peritoneal reflection (lower in the posterior side) and, if the tubes are attached, by the fact that their insertion is anterior to that of the round ligament.

  c Make additional cuts through any large mass in the wall.

  d Fix for several hours or overnight.

  e Make parallel transverse sections through each half, about 1 cm apart, beginning at the upper level of the endocervical canal and stopping short of completing them on one side (in order to keep them together) and examine carefully each surface.

  f Make several sections of the cervix along the endocervical canal.

  g Make at least one cross section of every myoma present and examine carefully; larger myomas need additional cuts.

  h If tubes and/or ovary accompany the specimen, follow instructions for these organs.

Description

1 Type of hysterectomy: total? radical? with salpingo-oophorectomy?

2 Shape of uterus: deformed? subserosal bulgings?

3 Serosa: fibrous adhesions?

4 Wall: thickness, abnormalities

5 Endometrium: appearance; thickness; polyps? (size, shape); cysts?

6 Cervix: appearance of exocervix, squamocolumnar junction, endocervical canal; erosions? polyps? cysts?

7 Myomas: number, location (subserosal, intramural, submucosal); size; sessile or pedunculated? hemorrhage, necrosis, or calcification? ulceration of overlying endometrium?

Continued

Sections for histology

1 Cervix: one section from anterior half and one from posterior half
2 Corpus: at least two sections taken close to fundus and including endometrium, good portion of myometrium and, if thickness permits, serosa; additional sections from any grossly abnormal areas
3 Myomas: at least one section per myoma, up to three; sections from any grossly abnormal area (e.g., soft, fleshy, necrotic, cystic, etc.)
4 Cervical or endometrial polyps: to be submitted in entirety unless extremely large

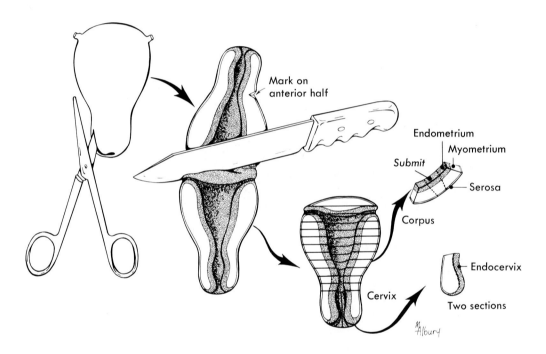

UTERUS—HYSTERECTOMY FOR CERVICAL CARCINOMA (IN SITU OR INVASIVE)

Procedure

1 If lymph nodes are included (radical hysterectomy), dissect while fresh and separate into left and right obturator, interiliac, and left and right iliac (high nodes) groups (not all of these groups will be present in every specimen).

2 Measure and weigh the specimen; orient as to anterior and posterior sides; see under Uterus—Hysterectomy (General instructions).

3 Amputate the cervix from the corpus about 2.5 cm above the external with a sharp knife.

4 Handle the uterus as described under Uterus—Hysterectomy (General instructions) and the tubes and ovary if present according to instructions for these organs.

5 Open the cervix with scissors through the endocervical canal at the 12 o'clock position and carefully pin stretched on a corkboard with the mucosal side up. Be careful to avoid tearing or rubbing the epithelial surface.

6 Fix by floating the cork for several hours or overnight with the tissue on the underside in a formalin container.

7 Paint the vaginal surgical margin with India ink.

8 Cut the entire cervix by making parallel longitudinal sections, 2-3 mm apart, along the plane of the endocervical canal starting at the 12 o'clock position and moving clockwise. Sections should be taken in such a way that the epithelium (including the squamocolumnar junction) is present in each section; some trimming of the stroma may be necessary (see accompanying drawing).

Description

1 Cervix: color of epithelium; presence of irregularities, erosions, healed or recent lacerations, masses (size, shape, location), cysts (size, content), previous biopsy, or conization sites

2 Rest of uterus: see under Uterus—Hysterectomy (General instructions).

3 Ovaries and tubes if present: see Instructions for respective organs.

4 Lymph nodes if present: approximate number; gross appearance; seem involved by tumor?

Continued

UTERUS—HYSTERECTOMY FOR CERVICAL CARCINOMA (IN SITU OR INVASIVE) cont'd

Sections for histology

1 Cervix: all tissue is submitted (except for trimming of stroma) and identified separately as follows:
   a Sections from 12 to 3 o'clock (**A-1** on accompanying drawings)
   b Sections from 3 to 6 o'clock (**A-2** on accompanying drawings)
   c Sections from 6 to 9 o'clock (**A-3** on accompanying drawings)
   d Sections from 9 to 12 o'clock (**A-4** on accompanying drawings)
   (If accurate mapping of lesions desired, identify sequentially each section with a letter, beginning from 12 o'clock position)
2 Vaginal cuff (entire line of resection)
3 Left soft tissue (for invasive cases only)
4 Right soft tissue (for invasive cases only)
5 Rest of uterus: see under Uterus—Hysterectomy (General instructions)
6 Ovaries and tubes: see Instructions for respective organs
7 Lymph nodes if present:
   • Left obturator
   • Right obturator
   • Interiliac
   • Left iliac (high nodes)
   • Right iliac (high nodes)

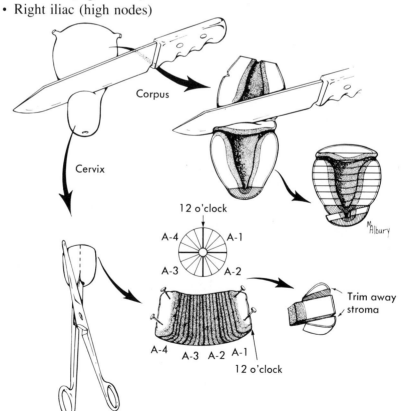

UTERUS—HYSTERECTOMY FOR ENDOMETRIAL HYPERPLASIA OR CARCINOMA

Procedure

1 If lymph nodes are included (radical hysterectomy), dissect while fresh and separate into left and right obturator, interiliac, and left and right iliac (high nodes) groups (not all of these groups will be present in every specimen).
2 Open and fix the uterus as indicated under Uterus—Hysterectomy (General instructions).
3 If ovaries and tubes are present, handle according to respective instructions.

Description

1 Type of operation: radical? total? with salpingectomy and oophorectomy?
2 Tumor: exact location; size; appearance (solid, papillary, ulcerated, necrotic, hemorrhagic); color; extent of endometrial extension; presence of myometrial, serosal, parametrial (soft tissue), venous, cervical, or tubal extension
3 Rest of uterus: see under Uterus—Hysterectomy (General instructions)
4 Ovaries and tubes: see respective instructions.
5 Lymph nodes if present: approximate number; gross appearance; seem involved by tumor?

Sections for histology

1 If obvious tumor present:
  a Three sections, one of which should be through area of deepest invasion and be complete section from surface of endometrium through serosa
    (If too thick for a cassette, divide in half and identify both halves appropriately.)
  b Two sections from nonneoplastic endometrium; do not need to be through entire wall
  c Soft tissue from left and right parametria
2 If no obvious tumor present (previous irradiation, very superficial carcinoma, endometrial hyperplasia):
  a Sample entire endometrium by making complete transverse parallel sections, 2-3 mm apart, of both uterine halves; one section should comprise entire thickness of organ, from mucosa to serosa; trim away from all others deepest two-thirds of myometrium. Label separately as anterior and posterior halves.
  b Rest of uterus: see under Uterus—Hysterectomy (General instructions)
  c Ovaries and tubes: see respective instructions
  d Lymph nodes if present:
    • Left obturator
    • Right obturator
    • Interiliac
    • Left iliac (high nodes)
    • Right iliac (high nodes)

Continued

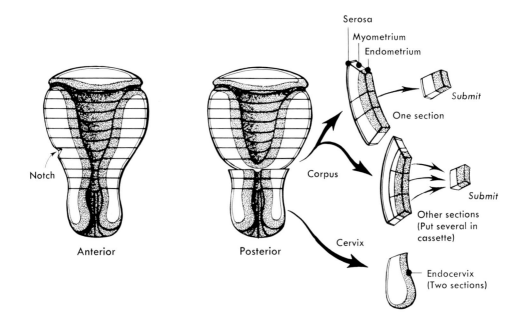

Serosa
Myometrium
Endometrium

Submit

One section

Notch

Corpus

Submit

Other sections
(Put several in cassette)

Anterior

Posterior

Cervix

Endocervix
(Two sections)

VULVA—VULVECTOMY

Procedure

1 Measure size of the specimen, including the inguinal region if present; also measure the size of the lesion.
2 In radical vulvectomy specimens, separate lymph nodes into groups and fix overnight in separate jars; Carnoy's fluid is preferable.
3 Pin on a corkboard and fix overnight; be careful to pin down the entire external borders and the vaginal margins. The latter is better preserved when it is pinned down on a cork placed in the introitus.
4 Take two Polaroid photographs and identify in one of them the sites of the sections to be taken.

Description

1 Type of vulvectomy: simple, subcutaneous, radical; lymph node groups present
2 Size of specimen
3 Lesion: size, location, extent, invasion into adjacent structures or vessels, color, surface (verrucous? ulcerated?), borders (distinct? rolled?), depth of stromal invasion
4 Appearance of nonneoplastic surface: atrophy, keratosis, ulceration
5 Lymph nodes: size of largest; appear grossly involved?

Sections for histology

1 Tumor: three sections, including edge with normal skin and deepest area of invasion
2 Nonneoplastic skin from labia majora and minora (left and right)
3 Lymph nodes (divided into groups)

Index

1